THE PITUITARY

THIRD EDITION

THE PITUITARY

THIRD EDITION

Edited by

SHLOMO MELMED

Senior Vice President, Academic Affairs
Dean of the Medical Faculty, Helene A. and Philip E. Hixon Chair in Investigative Medicine,
Cedars-Sinai Medical Center, Los Angeles, CA, USA

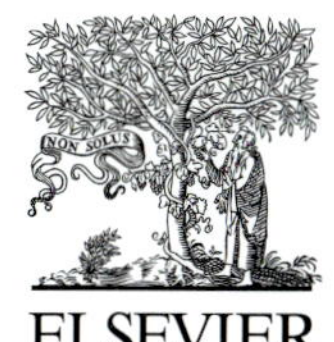

AMSTERDAM • BOSTON • HEIDELBERG • LONDON • NEW YORK • OXFORD
PARIS • SAN DIEGO • SAN FRANCISCO • SINGAPORE • SYDNEY • TOKYO

Academic Press is an imprint of Elsevier

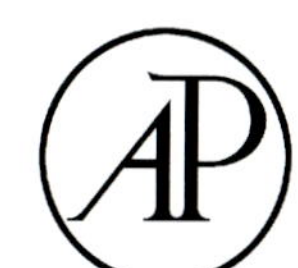

Academic Press is an imprint of Elsevier
32 Jamestown Road, London NW1 7BY, UK
30 Corporate Drive, Suite 400, Burlington, MA 01803, USA
525 B Street, Suite 1800, San Diego, CA 92101-4495, USA

First edition published by Blackwell Science, Inc. 1995
Second edition published by Blackwell Science, Inc. 2002
Third edition 2011

British Library Cataloguing-in-Publication Data
A catalogue record for this book is available from the British Library

Library of Congress Cataloging-in-Publication Data
A catalog record for this book is available from the Library of Congress

ISBN: 978-0-12-380926-1

For information on all Academic Press publications visit our website at www.elsevierdirect.com

Typeset by TNQ Books and Journals

Printed and bound in China

10 11 12 13   10 9 8 7 6 5 4 3 2 1

Dedicated to my wife Ilana, children and grandchildren,
in appreciation of their devoted support and continued inspiration.

In appreciation of the superb expertise and professionalism of
all my colleagues who contributed to this text.

Contents

Contributors

Steffen Albrecht, MD, FRCPC Department of Pathology, The Montreal's Children Hospital, McGill University Health Centre, Montréal, QC, Canada

Anat Ben-Shlomo, MD Pituitary Center, Cedars-Sinai Medical Center, Los Angeles, USA

Xavier Bertagna, MD Service des Maladies Endocriniennes et Métaboliques, Centre de Référence des Maladies Rares de la Surrénale, Hôpital Cochin, Paris, France and Département Endocrinologie-Diabète, Institut Cochin, Faculté de Médecine Paris Descartes, Paris, France

Daniel G. Bichet, MD Université de Montréal, Hôpital du Sacré-Coeur de Montréal, Montréal, QC, Canada

Juan M Bilbao, MD, FRCPC Sunnybrook Health Sciences Centre, University of Toronto, Toronto, Ontario, Canada

Glenn D. Braunstein, MD Department Of Medicine, Cedars-Sinai Medical Center, Los Angeles, CA, USA

Michael Buchfelder, MD Neurosurgical Department, University of Erlanger-Nuremberg, Germany

John D. Carmichael, MD Pituitary Center, Cedars-Sinai Medical Center, Los Angeles, CA, USA

Harold E. Carlson, MD Division of Endocrinology, Department of Medicine, Stony Brook University, Stony Brook, NY, USA

Jacques Drouin, PhD, FRSC Laboratoire de génétique moléculaire, Institut de recherches cliniques de Montréal (IRCM), Montréal, QC, Canada

Rudolf Fahlbusch, MD Endocrine Neurosurgery, International Neuroscience Institute Hannover, Germany

Mary P. Gillam, MD Endocrinologist, Chicago, IL, USA

François Girard, MD Clinique des Maladies Endocriniennes et Métaboliques, Hôpital Cochin, Paris, France

David F. Gordon, PhD Division of Endocrinology, Metabolism and Diabetes, University of Colorado Denver, Aurora, CO, USA

Yona Greenman, MD Sackler School of Medicine, Tel Aviv University, Institute of Endocrinology, Metabolism and Hypertension, Tel Aviv-Sourasky Medical Center, Tel Aviv, Israel

Laurence Guignat, MD Service des Maladies Endocriniennes et Métaboliques, Centre de Référence des Maladies Rares de la Surrénale, Hôpital Cochin, Paris, France

Brigitte Guilhaume, MD Service des Maladies Endocriniennes et Métaboliques, Hôpital Cochin, Paris, France

Vivien S. Herman-Bonert, MD Pituitary Center, Cedars Sinai Medical Center, Los Angeles, USA

Ursula B. Kaiser, MD Division of Endocrinology, Diabetes and Hypertension, Brigham and Women's Hospital, Harvard Medical School, Boston, MA, USA

Kalman Kovacs, MD, PhD, FRCPC University of Toronto, St. Michael's Hospital, Toronto, ON, Canada

Joseph A. Majzoub, MD Division of Endocrinology, Children's Hospital Boston, Harvard Medical School, Boston, MA, USA

Marcel M. Maya, Department of Imaging, Cedars-Sinai Medical Center, Los Angeles, CA, USA

Shlomo Melmed, MD Pituitary Center, Cedars-Sinai Medical Center, Los Angeles, USA

Mark E. Molitch, MD Division of Endocrinology, Metabolism and Molecular Medicine, Northwestern University Feinberg School of Medicine, Chicago, IL, USA

Olga Moshkin, MD, PhD, FRCPC Laboratory Medicine, PRHC, Peterborough, ON, Canada

Barry D. Pressman, MD, FACR Department of Imaging, Cedars-Sinai Medical Center, Los Angeles, CA, USA

Marie-Charles Raux-Demay, MD Laboratoire d'Explorations Fonctionnelles Endocriniennes Hôpital Trousseau, Paris, France

Vanessa Rouach, MD Institute of Endocrinology, Metabolism and Hypertension, Tel Aviv-Sourasky Medical Center, Tel Aviv, Israel

Mary H. Samuels, MD Division of Endocrinology, Diabetes and Clinical Nutrition, OHSU, Clinical Research Center, Oregon Health and Science University, Portland, Oregon, USA

Virginia D. Sarapura, MD Division of Endocrinology, Metabolism and Diabetes, University of Colorado Denver, Aurora, CO, USA

Peter J. Snyder, MD University of Pennsylvania, Philadelphia, PA, USA

Oulu Wang, BS Program in Neuroscience, Harvard Medical School, Division of Endocrinology, Children's Hospital Boston, Boston, MA, USA

Preface

The third edition of *The Pituitary* follows two successful prior volumes published in 1995 and 2002. This textbook continues the tradition of a cogent blend of basic science and clinical medicine which was the successful hallmark of prior editions. This comprehensive text is devoted to pathogenesis, diagnosis and treatment of pituitary disorders. The new edition is now extensively revised to reflect new knowledge derived from advances in molecular and cell biology, biochemistry, diagnostics and therapeutics as they apply to the pituitary gland. Notably, a new chapter devoted to functional development of the pituitary gland has been added to complement a comprehensive description of pituitary physiology, as well as management options for patients harboring pituitary tumors.

The wide spectrum of clinical disorders emanating from dysfunction of the "master gland" is described in detail by experts in the field. Fundamental mechanisms underlying disease pathogenesis are presented to provide the reader with an in-depth understanding of mechanisms subserving both normal and disordered pituitary hormone secretion and action.

I am especially indebted to my erudite colleagues for their scholarly contributions and dedicated efforts in compiling this extensive body of knowledge for students, trainees, physicians and scientists geared to understanding pituitary function and caring for patients with pituitary disorders. Our desire is to provide medical students, clinical and basic endocrinology trainees, endocrinologists, internists, pediatricians, gynecologists and neurosurgeons with a comprehensive yet integrated text devoted to the science and art of pituitary medicine.

Shlomo Melmed MD

Cedars-Sinai Medical Center, Los Angeles, California, USA

SECTION I

HYPOTHALAMIC–PITUITARY FUNCTION

CHAPTER

1

Pituitary Development

Jacques Drouin

Institut de recherches cliniques de Montréal (IRCM), Montréal, QC, Canada

THE PITUITARY GLAND

The pituitary gland was ascribed various roles by anatomists over the centuries, including the source of phlegm that drained from the brain to the nose or the seat of the soul. It was at the beginning of the 20th century that its endocrine functions became recognized [1] and thereafter the various hormones produced by the pituitary were characterized, isolated and their structure determined. The major role of the hypothalamus in the control of pituitary function was recognized by Harris in the mid-20th century and that marked the beginning of the new discipline of neuroendocrinology [2]. The adult pituitary is linked to the hypothalamus through the pituitary stalk that harbors a specialized portal system through which hypophysiotropic hypothalamic hormones directly reach their pituitary cell targets [3,4]. The adult pituitary is composed of three lobes, the anterior and intermediate lobes that have a common developmental origin from the ectoderm, and the posterior lobe that is an extension of the ventral diencephalon or hypothalamus. Whereas the intermediate pituitary is a relatively homogenous tissue containing only melanotroph cells that produce α-melanotropin (αMSH), the anterior lobe contains five different hormone-secreting lineages, including the corticotropes that produce adrenocorticotropin (ACTH), the gonadotropes that produce the gonadotropins luteinizing hormone (LH) and follicle-stimulating hormone (FSH), the somatotropes that produce growth hormone (GH), the lactotropes that produce prolactin (PRL) and finally, the thyrotropes that produce thyroid-stimulating hormone (TSH). In addition, these tissues contain support cells, known as pituicytes or folliculostellate cells. The neural or posterior lobe of the pituitary is largely constituted of axonal projections from the hypothalamus that secrete vasopressin (AVP) and oxytocin (OT) as well as support cells. The intermediate lobe is present in many species, in particular in rodents, mice and rats, that have been used extensively to study pituitary development and function, but it regresses in humans at about the 15th week of gestation: it is thus absent from the adult human pituitary gland. Most of our recent insight into the mechanisms of pituitary development has come from studies in mice: the review of our current knowledge presented in this chapter will therefore primarily focus on mouse development with references to other species (including humans) when significant differences are known or in cases of direct clinical relevance.

FORMATION OF RATHKE'S POUCH

The glandular or endocrine part of the pituitary gland derives from the most anterior segment of surface ectoderm. It ultimately comprises the anterior and intermediate lobes of the pituitary. This was shown using chick-quail chimeras [5,6]. It is thus the most anterior portion of the midline surface ectoderm, the anterior neural ridge, which harbors the presumptive pituitary. Interestingly, fate-mapping studies also indicated that the adjoining neural territory will form the ventral diencephalon and hypothalamus. As head development is initiated and the neuroepithelium expands to form the brain, the anterior neural ridge is displaced ventrally and eventually occupies the lower facial and oral area. It is thus the midline portion of the oral ectoderm that invaginates to become the pituitary anlage, Rathke's pouch. This invagination does not form through an active process but it rather appears to result from sustained contact between neuroepithelium and oral ectoderm at the time when derivatives of prechordal mesoderm and neural crest invade the space between neuroepithelium and surface ectoderm and thus separate these tissue layers everywhere except in the midline

The Pituitary, Third Edition, DOI: 10.1016/B978-0-12-380926-1.10001-X

at the pouch level. Rathke's pouch is thus a simple epithelium that is a few cells thick extending at the back of the oral cavity towards the developing diencephalon, with which it maintains intimate contact. This contact is essential for proper pouch and pituitary development since its rupture either physically [7–10] or through genetic manipulations [11,12] leads to aborted pituitary development. Indeed, a number of transcription factors expressed in diencephalon and infundibulum, but not in the pituitary itself such as Nkx2.1 [11,13], Sox3 [14] and Lhx2 [12], are required for proper diencephalon development and secondarily affect pituitary formation. In humans, *SOX3* mutations have been associated with hypopituitarism [14]. Collectively, these data have supported the importance of signal exchange between diencephalon and forming pituitary [15] for proper development of both tissues.

Rathke's pouch rapidly forms a closed gland through disruption of its link with the oral ectoderm. This occurs through apoptosis of the intermediate epithelial tissue [16]. The oral ectoderm and Rathke's pouch are marked by expression of transcription factors that are essential for early pouch development (Figure 1.1). The earliest factors are the pituitary homeobox (Pitx, Ptx) factors, Pitx1 and Pitx2 [17,18]. Indeed, these two related transcription factors are co-expressed throughout the oral ectoderm and their combined inactivation results in blockade of development at the early pouch stage [16]. The double mouse mutant *Pitx1*$^{-/-}$;*Pitx2*$^{-/-}$ exhibits delayed and incomplete disruption of tissues between

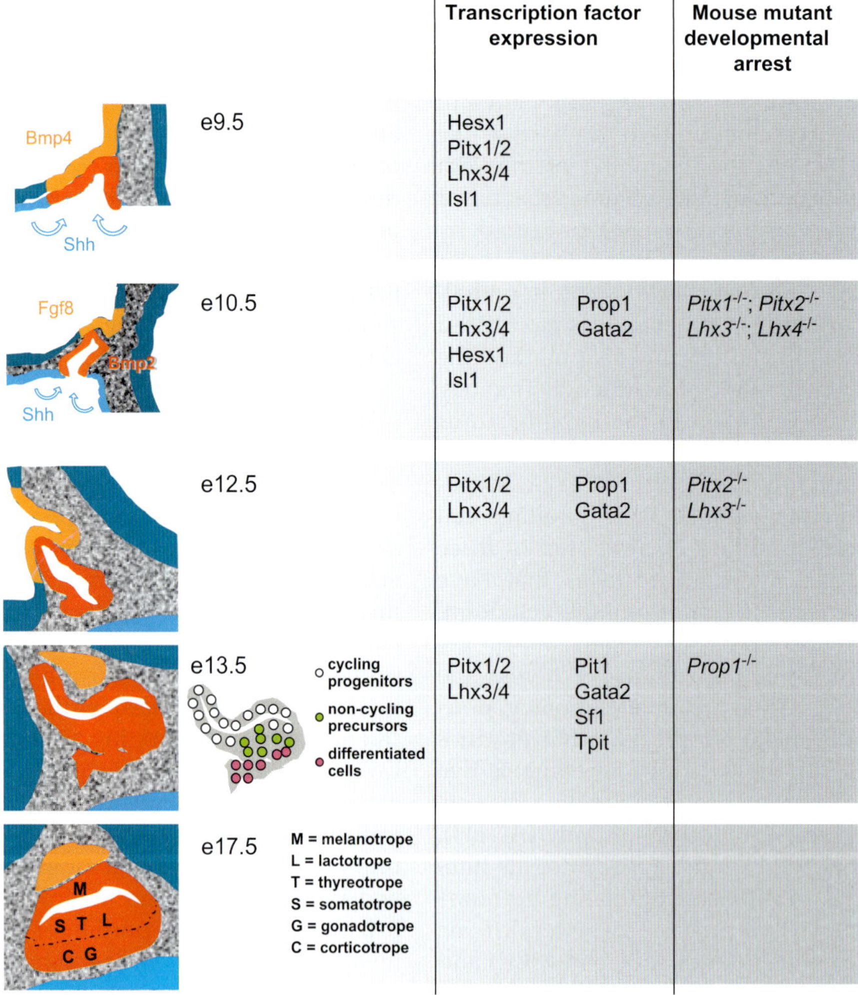

FIGURE 1.1 Development of the pituitary gland in mouse. Critical steps, signaling molecules and transcription factors for pituitary development are highlighted on drawings representing the developing pituitary or Rathke's pouch (red) from e9.5 to e17.5 of mouse embryonic development. At e9.5 and e10.5, the ventral diencephalon sequentially expresses Bmp4 and Fgf8 that are critical for Rathke's pouch development; also, sonic hedgehog (Shh) expressed throughout the oral ectoderm, but excluded from Rathke's pouch, is important for pituitary formation. The expression of critical transcription factors for either pituitary organogenesis or cell differentiation is listed in the middle column whereas the consequence of their gene inactivation is listed on the left. The position of the various mouse genotypes along the developmental time sequence indicates the stage at which pituitary development is interrupted by these mutations.

developing pituitary and oral ectoderm, and pituitary development does not appear to be able to progress beyond this stage. The single *Pitx2*$^{-/-}$ mutant is somewhat less affected, reaching the late pouch stage [19–21]. The *Pitx1*$^{-/-}$ mutant has relatively normal pituitary organogenesis, except for under-representation of the gonadotrope and thyrotrope lineages [22] that express higher levels of Pitx1 protein in the adult [23]. The two Pitx factors thus have partly redundant roles in early pituitary development with Pitx2 having predominant and unique functions in organogenesis.

Another pair of homeodomain transcription factors, the Lim-homeo factors Lhx3 and Lhx4, are also expressed in Rathke's pouch after Pitx1 and Pitx2. The expression of Lhx3 and Lhx4 is in fact dependent on Pitx factors, and thus, the Pitx pair of factors may be considered to be at the top of a regulatory cascade for pituitary development. Interestingly, the double *Lhx3*$^{-/-}$;*Lhx4*$^{-/-}$ mutant mice pituitary exhibits blocked development at the early pouch stage; it is thus a phenocopy of the double *Pitx1/2* mutant [24]. The single *Lhx3* and *Lhx4* mutants have less-pronounced phenotypes, indicating that the action of the two Lhx factors is also partly redundant with each other [25]. The phenocopy of the *Pitx1*$^{-/-}$;*Pitx2*$^{-/-}$ and *Lhx3*$^{-/-}$;*Lhx4*$^{-/-}$ pituitary phenotypes clearly suggests that many of the actions of the Pitx factors are mediated through the Lhx3/4 factors. Consistent with these mouse studies, mutations in the *LHX3* and *LHX4* genes have been associated with combined pituitary hormone deficiency (CPHD), together with neck and/or skull malformations [26–29].

Rathke's pouch is also marked by expression of the paired-like homeodomain factor Hesx1 (also known as Rpx). This factor has a complex pattern of expression in the early pre-chordal area, but its expression becomes restricted to the ventral diencephalon and Rathke's pouch by e9.5 [30,31]. It thus marks the two sides of the developing neuroendocrine hypothalamo–pituitary system [15,32]. Pituitary *Hesx1* expression is transient and is extinguished by about e12.5 following a pattern that is complementary to the appearance of Prop1 which antagonizes Hesx1 [15,33,34]. Inactivation of the mouse *Hesx1* gene results in complex brain, optic and olfactory developmental defects; pituitary development is also perturbed, ranging from complete absence to multiple invaginations and nascent glands [35]. *Hesx1* thus appears to be involved in restriction of the neuroepithelium–ectoderm contact at the midline where Rathke's pouch is normally induced. This restriction/induction may be mediated through FGF10 since its expression is extended rostrally in *Hesx1*$^{-/-}$ mutants [34].

Hesx1 is a transcriptional repressor that recruits the Groucho-related corepressor Tle1 [34]. Other Tle-related proteins are expressed during pituitary development and interestingly, inactivation of *Aes* that is transiently expressed in the pituitary results in bifurcated pouches and dysplastic pituitaries [36]. Consistent with mouse studies, mutations of human *HESX1* have been associated with septo-optic dysplasias (SOD) that cause brain and optic nerve defects, together with hypopituitarism ranging from GH deficiency to CPHD [35,37–39].

GLANDULAR OR ENDOCRINE GLAND DEVELOPMENT

The early pituitary gland is constituted of an epithelial layer that is a few cells thick and encloses a lumen that will become the pituitary cleft between intermediate and anterior lobes. The portion of this pouch that is in close contact with the infundibulum will differentiate into the intermediate lobe. The first sign of glandular development is observed at the ventro-rostral tip of the early gland where cells appear to leave the epithelial layer to take a more disorganized mesenchymal appearance. This period of transition is accompanied by intense cell proliferation and differentiated cells appear at the same time, as discussed below. This process is similar to epithelium–mesenchyme transition (EMT) and it appears to be dependent on the homeodomain transcription factor, Prophet-of-Pit (Prop1). Prop1 is transiently expressed in the e10.5–e14.5 developing pituitary [40]. The *Prop1* mutation prevents epithelium–mesenchyme transition and exhibits extensive expansion of the epithelial pituitary that becomes convoluted with an extended lumen [41,42]. At early stages, this mutant gland appears to be larger than normal but it then decreases in size through cell loss by apoptosis [42,43]. The *Prop1*$^{-/-}$ mutant is not entirely deficient in epithelium–mesenchyme transition and anterior lobe development eventually proceeds. However, Prop1 is also required for activation of the *Pit1* transcription factor gene, as indicated by its name, [40,44] which is itself required for differentiation of the somatotrope, lactotrope and thyrotrope lineages. Hence, *Prop1* mutants are deficient in these lineages [40,44,45] but the mutation does not prevent corticotrope, melanotrope or gonadotrope differentiation. The *Prop1* mutant mice are thus dwarfed because of their deficit in GH and indeed, *PROP1* mutations have been associated with dwarfism and CPHD in humans [46]. With age, patients with PROP1 mutations often develop more extensive pituitary hormone deficiencies [47,48].

SIGNALS CONTROLLING PITUITARY DEVELOPMENT

One of the early evidences for asymmetry and signaling at the onset of pituitary– hypothalamic development is the expression of BMP4 in the region of the ventral diencephalon that is overlying the area of stomodeal oral ectoderm where Rathke's pouch will develop (Figure 1.1). This expression is present at e8.5, and by around e10.5 it is replaced by Fgf8. Although inactivation of the BMP4 gene is early-lethal, analysis of a few surviving embryos at e9.5 suggested a failure of ectoderm thickening and initiation of Rathke's pouch development [13].

The early phases of pituitary development are accompanied by complex and dynamic patterns of expression for many signaling molecules involved in development and organogenesis [49,50]. The BMPs are actually a good illustration of this complex interplay. As noted above, early expression of BMP4 in the ventral diencephalon appears to be important for induction of the ectodermal pituitary anlage and experiments designed to further test this role have used transgenic overexpression of the BMP antagonist *Noggin* in the oral ectoderm, including Rathke's pouch, driven by the *Pitx1* promoter [49]. This blockade of BMP signaling led to arrested pituitary development at the pouch stage, without much cell differentiation except for a few corticotropes. This phenotype is similar to that of *Pitx2*$^{-/-}$ and *Lhx3*$^{-/-}$ mice [25]. BMP4 signaling may thus regulate *Lhx3* expression or even the upstream Pitx factors, but this experiment tested the importance of continued BMP signaling more than its initial action as assessed in *BMP4*$^{-/-}$ embryos. Inactivation of the *Noggin* gene itself supported the critical role of BMPs in pituitary induction [51]. The early expression of BMP4 in ventral diencephalon is thus on the dorsal side of the developing pouch; in parallel with its extinction, the related BMP2 is expressed on the ventral side of the developing pituitary and in the surrounding mesenchyme (around e10.5). It has been proposed that ventral BMP2 may promote differentiation of so-called "ventral" lineages such as corticotropes and this has been supported through transgenic gain-of-function experiments [49]. However, the use of organ culture systems to test the role of BMP2/4 in differentiation rather led to the conclusion that BMP signaling is repressing the corticotrope fate [50]. This latter finding is actually in agreement with a repressor effect of BMP signaling on POMC gene transcription [52].

Whereas the highly dynamic pattern of expression of these two related BMPs, BMP4 and BMP2, and the consequences of their manipulation are highly suggestive of important roles in pituitary development and cell differentiation, the same rapid changes in expression and seemingly contradictory experimental results also hint that BMPs have multiple effects depending on the timing of action and target cells. We are thus still lacking a coherent and complete picture for the multiple actions of these signaling molecules.

Another important signaling molecule for pituitary development is Sonic Hedgehog (Shh). Indeed, Shh is expressed in the ventral diencephalon and fairly widely in the oral ectoderm, but it is specifically excluded from the region of the oral ectoderm that becomes Rathke's pouch [53]. In contrast, Shh target genes such as *Patched1* are expressed in the developing pituitary, indicating that it is responsive to Shh signaling. These patterns are thus suggestive of an important role for the Shh pathway in pituitary induction. However, the *Shh*$^{-/-}$ mutant mouse was not extremely informative in precisely defining this role since Shh is critical for formation of midline structures and the bulk of these structures are affected in the *Shh* mutants [54]. Nonetheless, the importance of Shh signaling for early pituitary development is also supported by mouse mutants for the Gli zinc finger transcription factors that mediate the effects of the Shh pathway. Indeed, the double mouse mutant *Gli1*$^{-/-}$;*Gli2*$^{-/-}$ fails to develop the pituitary whereas the single *Gli2*$^{-/-}$ mutant exhibits variable defects in pituitary formation [55]. Further, over-expression of the Shh antagonist HIP blocked Rathke's pouch development [53].

As indicated above, the early expression of BMP4 in the ventral diencephalon is replaced from about e10.5 by FGF8 and FGF10 and the expression of these growth factors is maintained throughout the active phase of pituitary expansion (e11.5–e14.5). The FGFs appear to be important for survival of early pituitary cells since mutant mice for FGF10 or for its receptor FGFR2IIIb initially form Rathke's pouch and then it regresses because of widespread apoptosis [56,57]. In agreement with this, transgenic over-expression of FGF8 led to pituitary hyperplasia [49]; further, these experiments suggested that FGF8 stimulates *Lhx3* expression. This idea was also supported by analyses of the *Nkx2.1* mutant mice that fail to express FGF8 in diencephalon and pituitary Lhx3 [13]. It is thus possible that the FGF effect on proliferation and/or maintenance of early pituitary cells is mediated through induction of *Lhx3*.

The Wnt pathway also appears important for proliferation and/or survival of pituitary cells, but again the large number of Wnt molecules and their receptors expressed in and around the developing pituitary make it difficult to develop a coherent and complete picture of their role. Canonical Wnt signaling involves beta-catenin and targeted deletion of this gene using a *Pitx1-Cre* transgene resulted in a small pituitary, together with deficient *Pit1* expression and Pit1-dependent lineages [33]. It was suggested that beta-catenin is acting directly on the *Pit1* gene to regulate its expression through interaction with the upstream factor Prop1. Further, the canonical Wnt/beta-catenin pathway is acting through the transcription factors related to Lef/TCF and targeted deletion of some members of this family altered pituitary development [33,36]. The involvement of these factors, such as TCF4, in both ventral diencephalon and Rathke's pouch produces complex mutant phenotypes that result from intrinsic pituitary defects as well as from defective pituitary induction by overlying diencephalon [58]. Finally, the Notch pathway is also active in early pituitary development and recent work has suggested that its major involvement may be in pituitary progenitor cells; hence, this aspect is discussed below.

PROGENITORS AND STEM CELLS

Expansion of the early anterior pituitary between e12 and e15 of mouse development is due to the rapid proliferation of cells that do not express any marker of terminal cell differentiation, such as hormones or cell-restricted transcription factors. These cells have thus been considered to be progenitors but their level of commitment or partial differentiation cannot be evaluated because of a lack of appropriate markers. These cells contribute to significant growth of the gland during this transient period of expansion. Otherwise, it is the recent characterization of putative adult pituitary stem cells that has provided clues to the origin and early differentiation steps of pituitary lineages. Putative pituitary stem cells were first identified through a cell sphere assay and using cell markers developed in other tissues [59]. These pituisphere-forming cells appear to have the potential to differentiate into most hormone-producing lineages. It is, however, the realization that these putative adult pituitary stem cells express the embryonic marker of stem cells, Sox2, that allowed their better characterization [60]. The Sox2-positive pituitary stem cells are primarily found along the cleft of the adult gland, and they are similarly positioned but far more abundant in the developing gland. An initial step in their differentiation involves expression of the related Sox9 transcription factor and it has been suggested that cells double positive for Sox2 and Sox9 may represent committed progenitors [60]. Further, these cells also appear to express Prop1 and the Ret coreceptor GFRa2 [61]. Putative adult pituitary stem cells were also characterized using a transgenic marker dependent on a *nestin* gene promoter [62] and these putative precursors were found to undergo differentiation through Lhx3 and Lhx4 double-positive cells and then single Lhx3-positive cells. All these putative pituitary stem or progenitor cells express Pitx factors and sequential expression of the *Lhx* genes suggests that they may initiate differentiation by mimicking the fetal pattern of expression.

Undifferentiated cells of Rathke's pouch and of the early pituitary express a subset of Notch pathway genes and their expression is lost upon differentiation [63]. Further, ectopic expression of the Notch downstream effector Hes1 inhibited gonadotroph differentiation [64] as well as Pit1-dependent lineages [65], suggesting that Notch signaling may be required to maintain the progenitor state. This was indeed supported by gene inactivation of the Notch direct target transcription factor Rbp-J or its downstream target Hes1 [65–67]. In the knockout models, differentiation into corticotropes that occurs early in organogenesis is accelerated, whereas differentiation into the later Pit1-dependent lineages is impaired. The premature differentiation observed in these models is correlated with decreased progenitor proliferation and increased expression of cell cycle inhibitors of the Cip/Kip family [68] that have been implicated in progenitor cell cycle exit [69]. Collectively, these data support the idea that Notch signaling maintains the pituitary progenitor state and that during development it is essential for the sequential action of differentiation cues and the emergence of distinct lineages.

The presence of putative stem cells in the adult pituitary has suggested that cell renewal takes place in the adult gland. At this time, the relative contribution of stem-derived cell renewal or proliferation of differentiated cells in adult tissue renewal remains an open question since data supporting both have been reported. Indeed, the bulk of cells positive for proliferation markers in the adult gland do not express markers of the hormone-producing lineages and the organ ablation models, such as adrenalectomy and gonadectomy, have shown expansion of mostly hormone-negative cells before the appearance of hormone-positive cells [70]. Interestingly, the combination of these two end-organ ablation paradigms [70] has suggested expansion of a common pool of undifferentiated cells, in agreement with the existence of a common precursor for corticotropes and gonadotropes [71]. Nonetheless, this work [70] and previous studies have also documented proliferation of differentiated cells [72]. These data argue in favor of a model in which stem cells expand before differentiation for tissue adaptation to major loss of feedback regulation. In contrast, the use of lineage markers [62] or of a conditional system to kill proliferating differentiated cells [73] has rather suggested that adult tissue maintenance relies on division of differentiated cells. Although apparently contradictory, expansion of each compartment (stem and/or differentiated) may take place in different physiological or pathophysiological conditions.

CELL DIFFERENTIATION

Cell differentiation starts early during pituitary development, as assessed by expression of the hormone genes characteristic of each lineage [74]. The hormone-coding genes have also served as a starting point to identify cell-autonomous transcription factors that are involved in their own expression but also in lineage-restricted functions and differentiation. Hence, most of what we know about pituitary cell differentiation relates to the terminal stages of differentiation for each lineage and involves cell-restricted transcription factors that are responsible for terminal differentiation. The transcription factors that mark terminal differentiation are usually expressed 12–24 h before the hormone gene itself and they have so far not been useful in directly identifying or studying multivalent progenitors of the developing or adult pituitary. However, the analysis of their loss-of-function mutations has provided considerable insight into the relationships between different lineages. Investigation of the *Jackson* and *Snell* dwarf mice that carry *Pit1* mutations thus revealed the requirement for this Pou-homeo transcription factor for differentiation of three lineages, the somatotropes, lactotropes and thyrotropes [75,76]. Analyses of *Pit1* mutants in both mice and humans thus supported the model of a common precursor for these three lineages [77].

Similarly, the $Tpit^{-/-}$ mutant mice revealed an antagonistic relationship between corticotropes/melanotropes and gonadotropes, suggesting that these lineages share a common precursor [71]. Taken collectively, the data on these mutants have suggested a binary model of pituitary cell differentiation (Figure 1.2). Although consistent with current data, this model has not been ascertained more directly, for example through characterization of the putative common progenitors. Nonetheless, it provides a useful framework for ongoing investigation of the mechanisms of early commitment to each pituitary lineage. The salient features of this model and its regulatory molecules are discussed below in greater detail for each lineage.

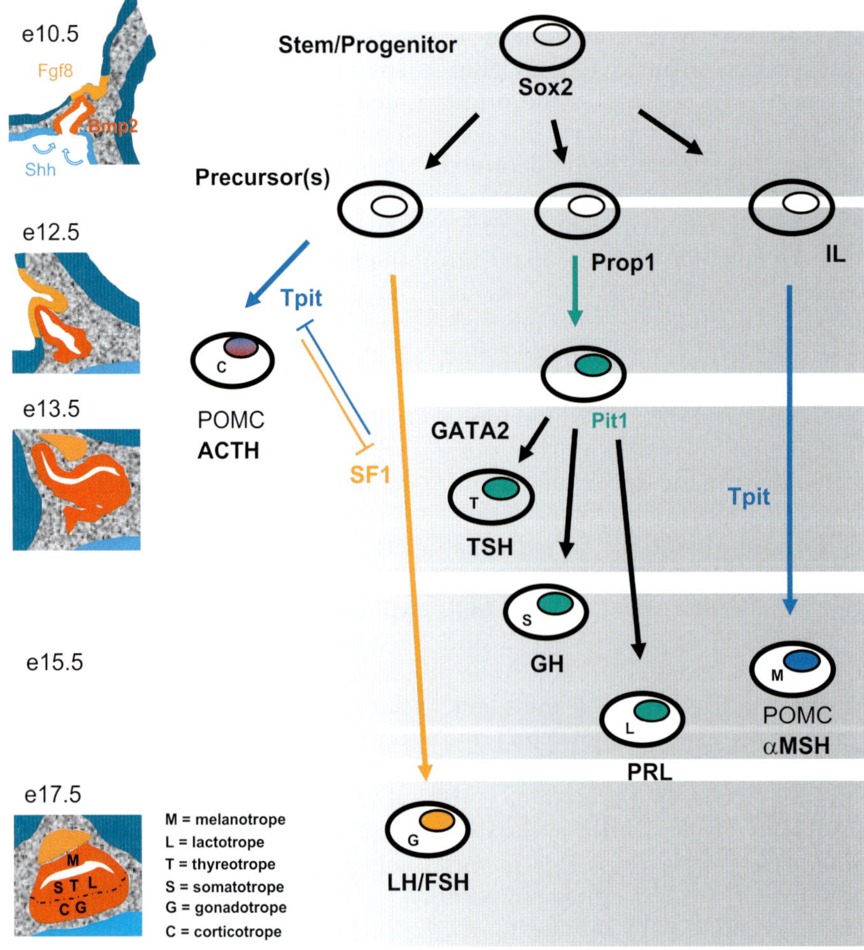

FIGURE 1.2 Differentiation of pituitary cells. A scheme for sequential differentiation of cells in the developing pituitary was derived from studies of mutants for the critical cell-restricted regulators of differentiation. Putative pituitary stem and progenitor cells are marked by expression of Sox2. While critical regulators of terminal differentiation such as Tpit, SF1 and Pit1 have been well characterized, regulators for the early commitment of putative precursors are still elusive. IL, intermediate lobe.

PITUITARY CELL CYCLE CONTROL

The expansion phase that takes place during early fetal pituitary organogenesis involves proliferation of presumed progenitors that are negative for known markers of differentiation. These proliferating progenitors do not express significant levels of cell cycle inhibitors such as the inhibitors of the Cip/Kip family, $p21^{Cip1}$, $p27^{Kip1}$ and $p57^{Kip2}$, or of the INK4 family [69]. They express detectable protein levels of the cyclins that are involved in cell cycle progression such as cyclin A and cyclins D1, D2, D3 (Figure 1.3). During this expansion phase, the proliferating progenitors are most abundant around the lumen of the developing gland where Sox2-positive cells are also found [60]. These progenitors exit the cell cycle upon expression of the cell cycle inhibitor $p57^{Kip2}$; the same cells co-express detectable levels of cyclin E [69]. These double-positive cells do not express any markers of hormone-producing cells and thus appear to be progenitors that have recently exited the cell cycle. They appear to represent a transient cell population from which differentiated cells arise: this interpretation is supported by the temporal sequence of appearance of appropriate markers and by their physical distribution going from the periluminal area of the developing anterior lobe that contains the proliferating progenitors towards the mid-gland that contains most of the non-cycling $p57^{Kip2}$ and cyclin E double-positive progenitors, and finally, more ventrally, the first differentiated cells (Figure 1.1, e13.5). The first differentiated cells appear to express Tpit and POMC and they are followed by αGSU-expressing cells. These differentiated cells switch off $p57^{Kip2}$ expression and switch on the related $p27^{Kip1}$ in its place. Expression of $p27^{Kip1}$ is maintained throughout adulthood in normal differentiated pituitary cells, whereas $p57^{Kip2}$ is undetectable in differentiated pituitary cells. Both loss-of-function mutations for $p57^{Kip2}$ and gain-of-function transgenic experiments have supported the model that $p57^{Kip2}$ is responsible for driving pituitary progenitors out of the cell cycle [68,69].

Expression of $p27^{Kip1}$ in differentiated cells is required to restrain cell cycling of these cells as supported by the presence of cycling differentiated cells in $p27^{Kip1-/-}$ pituitaries [69]. Furthermore, the loss of $p27^{Kip1}$ expression in the adult pituitary leads to the formation of pituitary tumors, particularly in the intermediate lobe [78–80] and the double mutant $p57^{Kip2-/-};p27^{Kip1-/-}$ presents fetal pituitaries in which all cells are proliferating, both progenitors and differentiated cells [69]. These

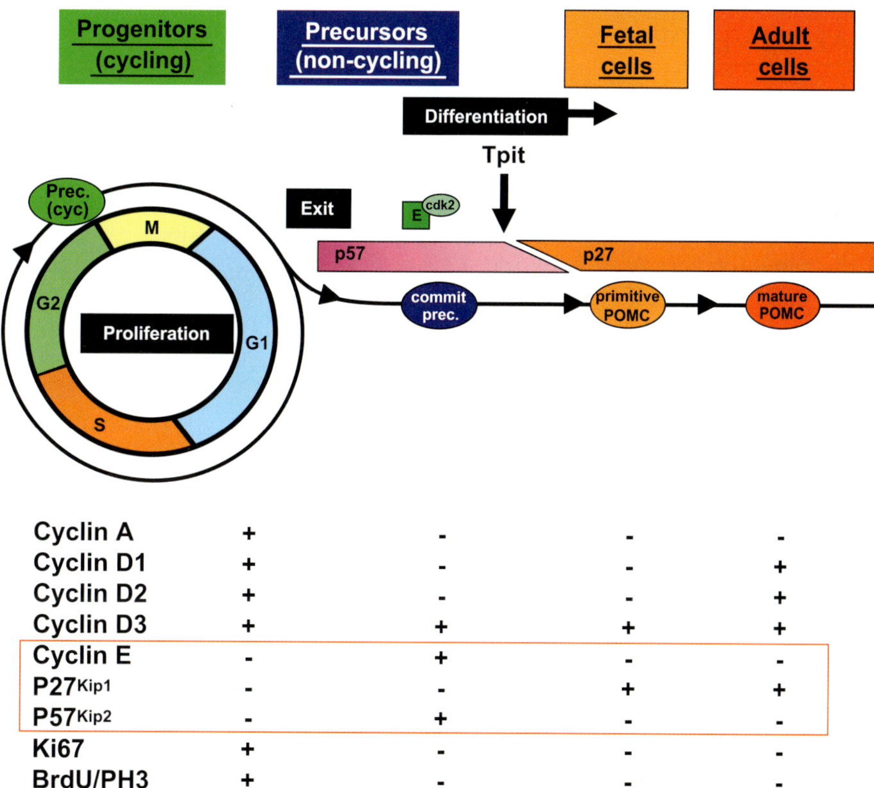

FIGURE 1.3 Cell cycle exit of pituitary progenitors. The expression of various cyclins and cell cycle inhibitors of the Cip/Kip family is shown below a diagram representing different stages of pituitary cell differentiation, starting from cycling progenitors to differentiated adult hormone-producing cells. Although the scheme of differentiation highlights the Tpit-dependent differentiation into POMC lineages, expression of the various cell cycle regulators is similar during the course of differentiation of the other pituitary lineages. *From [69].*

later observations clearly indicate that mechanisms of cell differentiation are independent of cell cycle exit. Conversely, at least one model of blocked pituitary differentiation, the *Tpit*$^{-/-}$ intermediate lobe, indicated that expression of *p27*^{Kip1} is not dependent on differentiation, although switch-off of *p57*^{Kip2} expression appears to be partly dependent on this process [69]. Collectively, the mechanisms for control of cell cycle and differentiation during pituitary development appear to be largely independent but the exact nature of the specific signals that are involved remains to be identified.

It is noteworthy that the third member of the Cip/Kip family p21^{Cip1} that is expressed at low levels in adult differentiated pituitary cells does not appear to play a major role in control of cell cycle progression or in pituitary tumorigenesis compared to p27^{Kip1} [81]. Rather, it was involved in control of cellular senescence [82]. Cellular senescence controlled by p21^{Cip1} may thus play a watchdog role by counterbalancing the effect of oncogenes associated with pituitary tumor development [83,84]. Interestingly, the impairment of progenitor state resulting from *Hes1* inactivation in developing pituitaries increased p21^{Cip1} expression and led to apoptosis [68], consistent with a purported watchdog role for abnormal pituitary cell proliferation.

POSTNATAL DEVELOPMENT

Until quite recently, the pituitary anterior lobe was considered to be a patchwork of intermingled cells of the different lineages. This idea was challenged by the discovery that all somatotropes are interconnected and form a homotypic network [85]. All cells of the gland may thus be part of the same (or very few) network(s) and the tri-dimensional (3D) organization of the GH cell network is unique compared to cell networks of other lineages or to the vasculature [86,87]. The exchange of signals between cells of homotypic networks may serve to mount a strong and coordinated secretory response to secretagogues [85] and to adjust local blood flow accordingly [86]. Thus, these 3D networks appear to increase the efficiency of hormone response and possibly to alter the patterns of response following endocrine re-setting such as occurs at sexual maturity [85]. It appears that all pituitary lineages participate in 3D homotypic cell networks and their establishment may rely on surface molecules such as cadherins [87].

CORTICOTROPES

The corticotropes are the first cells to reach terminal differentiation, and in the mouse they are first detected around e12.5 in the nascent anterior gland [74]. In fact, they appear to be the only cells to differentiate in mutant pituitaries that exhibit blocked organogenesis at the early pouch stage, such as in *Pitx1/2* or *Lhx3/4* mutants [16,24]. A highly cell-restricted transcription factor, the Tbox factor Tpit, was identified on the basis of its action on cell-specific regulatory elements of the *POMC* promoter [88]. Inactivation of the mouse *Tpit* gene showed that Tpit is critical for corticotrope differentiation; in addition, it is required for corticotrope expansion and/or maintenance [71]. In accordance with its late expression during differentiation (a half-day before POMC), Tpit deficiency does not appear to impair commitment of a subset of pituitary progenitors to the corticotrope lineage but rather blocks their terminal differentiation. Tpit is thus a positive regulator for differentiation of corticotropes (Figure 1.2).

Tpit is also a negative regulator of the gonadotrope fate, and as a result, *Tpit*$^{-/-}$ anterior pituitaries have an increased number of gonadotropes [71]. At least part of this antagonism is exerted between Tpit and the gonadotrope-specific transcription factor SF1 on their respective gene targets through a mechanism of transrepression [71]. This reciprocal mechanism results in blockade of SF1 target genes by Tpit, and vice versa; it is thus an excellent mechanism to implement a molecular switch between two cell fates. For this mechanism to be relevant, common precursors of corticotropes and gonadotropes would need to express both Tpit and SF1 and the balance between the two only needs to be tipped one way in order to ensure selection of one cell fate at the exclusion of the other. Such double-positive cells were indeed observed (albeit at very low frequency) in the fetal pituitary.

As was predicted from its highly restricted cell distribution, mutations in the human *TPIT* gene result in isolated ACTH deficiency (IAD), a condition that was barely recognized before the discovery of *Tpit* [88,89]. IAD is a recessive inherited condition caused by the deficiency of pituitary ACTH resulting in secondary adrenal glucocorticoid deficiency; it can be lethal for newborns and neonates because of abrupt and severe hypoglycemia [90]. IAD patients have no detectable pituitary ACTH and hypoplastic adrenal glands. The hormonal deficit is corrected by glucocorticoid therapy resulting in normal development. Many different *TPIT* gene mutations have been identified including premature stops, splice defects, genomic deletions and point mutations [88–90]. Many point mutations affect DNA binding and transcriptional activity and one particularly interesting mutation, Tpit M86R, is specifically deficient in protein–protein interactions but not in DNA binding per se [91]. As a highly restricted marker of corticotrope cells, Tpit is a very convenient marker of corticotroph adenoma cells, particularly since its expression is not affected by glucocorticoids in these glucocorticoid-resistant tumors [92].

NeuroD1, a basic helix-loop-helix (bHLH) transcription factor, is another factor identified on the basis of its action on cell-specific transcription of the *POMC* promoter [93–95]. During fetal pituitary development, NeuroD1 is expressed transiently at high levels in corticotropes but it is excluded from melanotropes [94]. Consistent with this pattern, inactivation of the *NeuroD1* gene results in a delay of POMC expression in anterior pituitary corticotropes [95]. However, this delay is fully recovered by e15.5, a time when normal *NeuroD1* expression has decreased in corticotropes. This is suggestive of a transient requirement on NeuroD1 but not necessarily on its target sequence, the $Ebox_{neuro}$, within the *POMC* promoter and indeed, mutagenesis of this target sequence in a transgenic mouse assay indicated sustained dependence on the $Ebox_{neuro}$ for POMC expression throughout development and adulthood [96]. It has thus been suggested that other bHLH factors take over the role of NeuroD1 at mid-development and throughout adult corticotrope function.

Corticotrope function is highly dependent on activation by hypothalamic signals and feedback repression by glucocorticoids. Activation of corticotrope function, POMC transcription and ACTH release occurs primarily through the action of corticotropin-releasing hormone (CRH) and its membrane receptor [97,98]. Expression of the CRH-R1 receptor appears upon corticotrope differentiation and corticotrope sensitivity to CRH action becomes active at mid-fetal development when the portal system between hypothalamus and pituitary becomes functional [99]. Similarly, the onset of glucocorticoid feedback repression on corticotropes and ACTH secretion occurs at the same time [99,100]. These regulatory mechanisms are maintained throughout adult life at apparently constitutive levels. However, they can be perturbed in pathological conditions. Notably, feedback repression of corticotrope POMC becomes desensitized in chronic stress and depressive states, but the mechanism of this mis-regulation is complex and not well understood [101–107].

Pituitary corticotrope adenomas that cause Cushing's disease are also characterized by relative resistance to glucocorticoid feedback. In rare cases, these adenomas express a mutant GR [108]. Recent studies have identified more frequent deficiencies in two proteins that are required for glucocorticoid feedback and that may account for hormone resistance in corticotropinomas. Indeed, about 50% of corticotropinomas are deficient in nuclear expression of either Brg1, the ATPase subunit of the chromatin remodeling Swi/snf complex, or in the histone deacetylase HDAC2 [109]. The loss of these proteins provides a molecular explanation for resistance to glucocorticoid feedback.

MELANOTROPES

All hormone-producing cells of the intermediate pituitary are melanotropes and they express the same single-copy POMC gene as anterior lobe corticotropes. However, regulation of melanotrope function is quite different compared to corticotropes [110]. During fetal development, POMC expression starts around e15.5 in melanotropes (Figure 1.2) and it is preceded by expression of Tpit [88]. Tpit is as essential for melanotrope POMC expression as it is for corticotropes and $Tpit^{-/-}$ pituitaries maintain POMC expression in only a few percent of melanotropes [69,71]. In the absence of Tpit, a significant proportion (10–15%) of intermediate lobe cells switch fate and become bona fide gonadotropes. Cells that switch fate in this model do not express markers of melanotropes and thus it appears that melanotrope and gonadotrope markers are mutually exclusive, in agreement with the observed antagonism between Tpit and SF1 [71]. Interestingly, a significant portion of $Tpit^{-/-}$ intermediate pituitary cells that do not differentiate retain expression of the fetal cell cycle inhibitor $p57^{Kip2}$. Nonetheless, these $p57^{Kip2}$-positive putative precursors as well as all cells in the mutant intermediate lobe switch on the related $p27^{Kip1}$ [69]. This model has suggested that differentiation, whether driven by Tpit, SF1 or by default, results in switching off $p57^{Kip2}$; in this context, $p57^{Kip2}$ may represent the last (temporally) marker of the precursor state.

GONADOTROPES

Gonadotropes appear to be specified relatively early during pituitary organogenesis despite the fact that their marker hormones, LH and FSH, are the last to be expressed at e16.5 of mouse development. Indeed, gonadotropes are first marked by the restricted expression of the nuclear receptor transcription factor SF1 and this expression starts at around e13.5 [111]. In addition to its expression in pituitary gonadotropes, SF1 marks every tissue of the hypothalamo–pituitary–gonadal axis as well as another steroidogenic tissue, the adrenals [112,113]. And accordingly, inactivation of the *SF1* gene results in gonadal and adrenal agenesis, hypothalamic defects and deficient LHβ, FSHβ and GnRH receptor expression in the pituitary [111,114–116]. Although these studies supported the idea that SF1 is important for function of gonadotropes and gonadotropin gene expression, expression of LHβ and FSHβ is restored in $SF1^{-/-}$ mice by treatment with GnRH [117] suggesting that SF1 is not essential for gonadotrope cell fate. Hence, it may be a relatively late regulator of differentiation.

The action of GnRH on gonadotrope function is in part mediated by the zinc finger transcription factor

Egr1 which acts in synergism with SF1 on the LHβ promoter [118–121]. The compensation of SF1 deficiency may thus be exerted through Egr1 in GnRH-treated $SF1^{-/-}$ mice. In the context of this promoter, both SF1 and Egr1 activate transcription by synergism with Pitx1 [119], thus suggesting a mechanism by which they may partially replace each other.

It thus appears that although completely gonadotrope-restricted in the pituitary, SF1 is not the earliest effector of the gonadotrope cell fate. Another factor that may contribute to gonadotrope differentiation is GATA-2 since *GATA-2* gene inactivation led to reduced gonadotropin expression [122] and GATA-2 is expressed earlier than SF1 [123]. It is possible that GATA-2 function in gonadotropes is partially redundant with the related GATA-3 [122] and hence, the true importance of GATA factors in gonadotrope differentiation remains to be defined.

Other transcription factors have been shown to be important for gonadotrope function, including Pitx1 that is expressed at higher protein levels in gonadotropes than in other lineages [23]. The level of Pitx1 protein appears to play a role in regulating the abundance of gonadotropes relative to other cells, since the *Pitx1* knockout has fewer gonadotropes [124]. Sites of direct Pitx1 action have been identified in the LHβ and FSHβ promoters [125,126]. Also, the related paired homeodomain transcription factor of bicoid specificity Otx1 is expressed in the pituitary and $Otx1^{-/-}$ mice have transient deficiencies of LH, FSH and GH, resulting in hypogonadism and dwarfism at pre-pubertal stages [127]. Further, mutations in the related OTX2 were found to cause CPHD [128]. In summary, SF1 is likely not the only gonadotrope transcription factor that contributes to differentiation of this lineage, and the relatively late action of this factor in gonadotrope differentiation suggests that other factors precede SF1 action. Similarly, other transcription factors must be involved in specific activation of LHβ versus FSHβ genes.

SOMATOTROPES

Somatotropes represent one of the three lineages, together with lactotropes and thyrotropes, that are marked by and require the Pou homeodomain transcription factor Pit1 for terminal differentiation (Figure 1.2). Expression of Pit1 starts at about e13.5 of mouse development in the medial region of the developing anterior lobe (Figure 1.1); its expression is maintained throughout adult life in somatotropes, lactotropes and thyrotropes. The consequences of Pit1 loss-of-function were first established when the *Jackson* and *Snell* dwarf mice were studied and found to carry mutations of the *Pit1* gene [75,76]. These *Pit1* mutant mice are deficient in the three Pit1-expressing lineages: this factor is thus critical for their terminal differentiation. In addition, Pit1 is required for transcription of the GH, PRL, TSHβ and GHRH receptor genes [129]; the factor was in fact first identified on the basis of this transcriptional activity [130,131]. A similar requirement on Pit1 was also shown recently in zebrafish [132] and human mutations of PIT1 are responsible for some forms of CPHD [77].

Initial expression of Pit1 requires Prop1 [40] as suggested by the name of this factor (prophet-of-Pit) but other factors, such as AtbF1, contribute to high-level *Pit1* expression [133]. Maintenance of *Pit1* expression is also dependent on a positive regulatory feedback exerted on a distal enhancer of the *Pit1* gene [134]. The importance of this autoregulatory feedback was well supported by studies of the *Snell* mutant in which initial activation of the *Pit1* gene occurs but where Pit1 expression then fails to be maintained [134]. PROP1 mutations also cause CPHD [46,77,135]. Although other transcription factors have been identified for their role in transcription of the GH gene, we still do not understand the molecular/transcriptional basis for somatotrope versus lactotrope specificity, both in terms of cell differentiation and marker hormone gene expression.

LACTOTROPE DIFFERENTIATION

Although lactotropes appear to be specified early in part through the critical action of Pit1 [76], Prl expression is mostly up-regulated postnatally. Analysis of *Prl* gene expression has led to identification of transcription factors that are required for *Prl* expression but these studies have not yet defined the basis for lactotrope-specific mechanisms of differentiation. A critical signal for lactotrope function and Prl expression is provided by estrogens, and their receptor ER was shown to act synergistically with Pit1 on a *Prl* gene enhancer [136–138]. The importance of ER and estrogen action on *Prl* expression was supported in mice inactivated for the *ERα* gene that exhibit fewer lactotropes and marked reduction of Prl expression [139]. However, specification of the lactotrope lineages is not affected in the $ER\alpha^{-/-}$ mice. Similarly, Ets transcription factors were found to be important for Prl expression [140] and the action of Ets factors is synergistic with Pit1 [141,142]. Ets factors integrate Ras-MAPK signaling through phosphorylation of Ets1 [143] and synergism with Pit1 [144]. Different Ets transcription factors have been involved in Prl expression and target sites of the Prl promoter appear to show preference for ets factors GABPα and GABPβ [145]. In addition, Prl expression depends on the Pitx factors [124,146–148] and on c/EBPα [149].

In addition to the strong activation of lactotrope function by estrogens, their function and *Prl* expression are under sustained negative action of hypothalamic dopamine. On the *Prl* promoter, dopamine repression may be exerted in part by the Ets repressor factor ERF [150]. The repressive action of dopamine is mediated through the dopamine D2 receptor (D2R) and the importance of this constitutive negative control was best exemplified in D2R mutant mice. These mice exhibit lactotrope hyperplasia and excessive prolactin production leading to formation of lactotrope adenomas in old mice [151,152]. Since de-repressed growth of lactotropes appears to predispose to lactotrope adenoma development, the balance between the inhibitory action of dopamine and the stimulatory action of estrogens on proliferation of these cells may serve in part to control the size of the lactotrope population but also to control lactotrope adenoma development.

THYROTROPES

The third Pit1-dependent lineage is thyrotropes and they are also deficient as a result of mouse and human *Pit1* mutations [75,76]. The thyrotropes are an intriguing and interesting lineage compared to the others since they share properties and regulatory transcription factors of both branches of the pituitary cell differentiation tree (Figure 1.2). Indeed, these cells are dependent on Pit1 and they are thus related to the somatotrope and lactotrope lineages. But also, they express and are dependent on GATA-2, a factor that is shared with gonadotropes [123]. The importance of GATA-2 for thyrotrope differentiation was directly assessed by conditional knockout of its gene in gonadotropes and thyrotropes using an *αGSU-cre* transgene for *GATA-2* inactivation [122]. These mutant pituitaries have fewer thyrotropes and gonadotropes in agreement with the importance of this factor for both lineages. Notwithstanding the possibility that GATA-2 function is partially compensated by GATA-3, these studies do not as yet define the basis for specificity of the thyrotrope program relative to the somato-lactotropes or to gonadotropes.

Transcription of the *TSHβ* gene was shown to depend on Lhx3 as well as GATA-2 [123,153,154]. Thyrotrope function and *TSHβ* gene transcription are stimulated by the hypothalamic hormone TRH and subject to feedback inhibition by thyroid hormones. TRH stimulation of *THSβ* transcription was recently shown to require Lhx3, activated CBP and Pit1 [154,155]. Thyroid hormone repression of *TSHβ* transcription requires the thyroid receptor β (TRβ) that appears to be acting downstream of transcription initiation within the *TSHβ* gene [156,157].

The thyrotrope lineage thus appears to represent an interesting case since its specification may respond to signals that positively control both gonadotrope and somato-lactotrope lineages as exemplified by their expression of GATA-2 and Pit1. It will be interesting to determine whether an active mechanism is responsible for maintenance of these two signals/transcription factors or whether it is the default maintenance of these factors that otherwise mark other lineages that are responsible for specification of the thyrotrope fate.

PERSPECTIVES

The last decades have been rich in teachings about regulators and mechanisms of pituitary cell differentiation with the discovery of the transcription factors Pit1, Prop1, SF1 and Tpit that control pituitary cell differentiation. Mutations in the genes encoding these factors are important causes of pituitary hormone deficiencies. Many other factors involved in development of either the pituitary itself and/or of surrounding tissues have provided candidates and culprits for various pituitary malformations that result in multiple hormone deficiencies. There is still much that we do not understand: mechanisms and regulators for many cell fate choices remain to be identified. For example, what controls the difference between somatotropes and lactotropes; and between corticotrophs and melanotrophs? What is (are) the positive regulator(s) of thyrotrope differentiation? Answers to these questions will no doubt provide tools for diagnosis of pituitary hormone deficiencies in addition to information on the underlying mechanisms of cell differentiation.

This knowledge will be of even greater importance, now that we have identified putative pituitary stem cells and that we are developing the means to manipulate stem cells. As for stem cells of any other tissue, we now realize that the greatest challenge ahead will be the control of differentiation if we are to realize the promise offered by these multipotent cells for treatment of various deficits. It is thus critical that we identify the missing regulators of pituitary cell differentiation. Further, the sequential differentiation of cells starting from progenitors towards terminally differentiated cells likely involves multiple steps and epigenetic reprogramming of precursors as cell fate is determined and differentiation choices are made. These epigenetic choices likely involve reprogramming of pituitary stem cells in order for these cells to lose their 'stemness' character and its underlying active proliferation state, towards a differentiated program and tightly controlled cell growth. It is quite likely that growth control mechanisms that shift during development and differentiation of pituitary cells are also relevant in adenoma tissues that may contain pituitary (cancer) stem cells together with hormone-producing differentiated cells. The developmental mechanisms for control of growth are thus very likely to be informative about processes that are deregulated when pituitary adenomas or tumours develop. The investigation of developmental processes is thus likely to have a major impact not only on our understanding of inherited forms of hormone deficiencies, but also on mechanisms of pituitary tumorigenesis and the hormone excesses that accompany some pituitary adenomas.

Finally, we are just realizing the nature and importance of tri-dimensional cell network organization in the pituitary: the direct contacts between cells of the same lineage and their organization within unique 3D networks are likely critical for the efficient delivery of synchronous and rapid hormone responses, and hence for appropriate function of the gland. The molecular bases for establishment of these homotypic cell networks as well as for heterotypic cell contacts remain unknown, but are likely critical for optimal function. Conversely, mis-regulation of these mechanisms may be associated with pituitary dysfunction, in particular partial or progressive loss-of-function that we may still need to appreciate at the clinical level. Establishment of these networks during fetal development but also during the post-fetal period, is likely critical to transform fetal hormone-producing pituitary cells into the hormone factories that these cells become in the adult gland. Conversely, impaired reorganization of these networks during critical phases of life such as during puberty, pregnancy or lactation, may have serious clinical implications that it is now our challenge to understand. Whereas developmental biologists have so far focused most of their interest on embryonic and fetal development, it now appears that post-natal development also includes critical events for the formation of a functional pituitary and hence our focus should in the future also include this period of development.

Acknowledgments

We are grateful to many colleagues and lab members who have contributed over the years to decipher the regulatory mechanisms responsible for pituitary development. The help of Lionel Budry for figure preparation and the secretarial assistance of Lise Laroche are gratefully acknowledged. Work in the author's laboratory has been supported by grants from the Canadian Institutes of Health Research and the Canadian Cancer Society.

References

[1] H. Cushing, The Pituitary Body and Its Disorders, JB Lippincott, Philadelphia, 1912.

[2] G.W. Harris, Neural control of pituitary gland, Physiol Rev 28 (1948) 139–179.

[3] G.W. Harris, The function of the pituitary stalk. Bull, Johns Hopkins Hosp 97 (5) (1955) 358–375.

[4] R. Guillemin, Peptides in the brain: The new endocrinology of the neuron, Science 202 (4366) (1978) 390–402.

[5] G.F. Couly, N.M. Le Douarin, Mapping of the early neural primordium in quail-chick chimeras. I. Developmental relationships between placodes, facial ectoderm, and prosencephalon, Dev Biol 110 (1985) 422–439.

[6] G.F. Couly, N.M. Le Douarin, Mapping of the early neural primordium in quail-chick chimeras. II. The prosencephalic neural plate and neural folds: Implications for the genesis of cephalic human congenital abnormalities, Dev Biol 120 (1987) 198–214.

[7] S. Daikoku, M. Chikamori, T. Adachi, Y. Maki, Effect of the basal diencephalon on the development of Rathke's pouch in rats: A study in combined organ cultures, Dev Biol 90 (1) (1982) 198–202.

[8] Y.G. Watanabe, Effects of brain and mesenchyme upon the cytogenesis of rat adenohypophysis in vitro. I. Differentiation of adrenocorticotropes, Cell Tissue Res 227 (2) (1982) 257–266.

[9] S. Kikuyama, H. Inaco, B.G. Jenks, K. Kawamura, Development of the ectopically transplanted primordium of epithelial hypophysis (anterior neural ridge) in *Bufo japonicus* embryos, J Exp Zool 266 (3) (1993) 216–220.

[10] K. Kawamura, S. Kikuyama, Induction from posterior hypothalamus is essential for the development of the pituitary proopiomelacortin (POMC) cells of the toad (*Bufo japonicus*), Cell Tissue Res 279 (2) (1995) 233–239.

[11] S. Kimura, Y. Hara, T. Pineau, P. Fernandez-Salguero, C.H. Fox, J.M. Ward, et al., The *T/ebp* null mouse: Thyroid-specific enhancer-binding protein is essential for the organogenesis of the thyroid, lung, ventral forebrain, and pituitary, Genes Dev 10 (1996) 60–69.

[12] Y. Zhao, C.M. Mailloux, E. Hermesz, M. Palkovits, H. Westphal, A role of the LIM-homeobox gene Lhx2 in the regulation of pituitary development, Dev Biol 337 (2) (2010) 313–323.

[13] N. Takuma, H.Z. Sheng, Y. Furuta, J.M. Ward, K. Sharma, B.L. Hogan, et al., Formation of Rathke's pouch requires dual induction from the diencephalon, Development 125 (23) (1998) 4835–4840.

[14] K. Rizzoti, S. Brunelli, D. Carmignac, P.Q. Thomas, I.C. Robinson, R. Lovell-Badge, SOX3 is required during the formation of the hypothalamo–pituitary axis, Nat Genet 36 (3) (2004) 247–255.

[15] E. Hermesz, L. Williams-Simons, K.A. Mahon, A novel inducible element, activated by contact with Rathke's pouch, is present in the regulatory region of the Rpx/Hesx1 homeobox gene, Dev Biol 260 (1) (2003) 68–78.

[16] M.A. Charles, H. Suh, J. Drouin, S.A. Camper, P.J. Gage, PITX genes are required for cell survival and *Lhx3* activation, Mol Endocrinol 19 (7) (2005) 1893–1903.

[17] T. Lamonerie, J.J. Tremblay, C. Lanctôt, M. Therrien, Y. Gauthier, J. Drouin, PTX1, a *bicoid*-related homeobox transcription factor involved in transcription of pro-opiomelanocortin (POMC) gene, Genes Dev 10 (10) (1996) 1284–1295.

[18] P.J. Gage, H. Suh, S.A. Camper, The bicoid-related Pitx gene family in development, Mamm Genome 10 (2) (1999) 197–200.

[19] A.K. Ryan, B. Blumberg, C. Rodriguez-Esteban, S. Yonei-Tamura, I. Tamura, T. Tsukui, et al., Pitx2 determines left-right asymmetry of internal organs in vertebrates, Nature 394 (6693) (1998) 545–551.

[20] P.J. Gage, H.Y. Suh, S.A. Camper, Dosage requirement of Pitx2 for development of multiple organs, Development 126 (20) (1999) 4643–4651.

[21] H. Suh, P.J. Gage, J. Drouin, S.A. Camper, *Pitx2* is required at multiple stages of pituitary organogenesis: Pituitary primordium formation and cell specification, Development 129 (2002) 329–337.

[22] D.P. Szeto, C. Rodriguez-Esteban, A.K. Ryan, S.M. O'Connell, F. Liu, C. Kioussi, et al., Role of the Bicoid-related homeodomain factor Pitx1 in specifying hindlimb morphogenesis and pituitary development, Genes Dev 13 (4) (1999) 484–494.

[23] C. Lanctôt, Y. Gauthier, J. Drouin, Pituitary homeobox 1 (Ptx1) is differentially expressed during pituitary development, Endocrinology 140 (3) (1999) 1416–1422.

[24] H.Z. Sheng, K. Moriyama, T. Yamashita, H. Li, S.S. Potter, K.A. Mahon, et al., Multistep control of pituitary organogenesis, Science 278 (5344) (1997) 1809–1812.

[25] H.Z. Sheng, A.B. Zhadanov, B. Mosinger, T. Fujii, S. Bertuzzi, A. Grinberg, et al., Specification of pituitary cell lineages by the LIM homeobox gene Lhx3, Science 272 (5264) (1996) 1004–1007.

[26] I. Netchine, M.L. Sobrier, H. Krude, D. Schnabel, M. Maghnie, E. Marcos, et al., Mutations in LHX3 result in a new syndrome revealed by combined pituitary hormone deficiency, Nat Genet 25 (2) (2000) 182–186.

[27] K. Machinis, J. Pantel, I. Netchine, J. Leger, O.J. Camand, M.L. Sobrier, et al., Syndromic short stature in patients with a germline mutation in the LIM homeobox LHX4, Am J Hum Genet 69 (5) (2001) 961–968.

[28] M.L. Sobrier, T. Attie-Bitach, I. Netchine, F. Encha-Razavi, M. Vekemans, S. Amselem, Pathophysiology of syndromic combined pituitary hormone deficiency due to a LHX3 defect in light of LHX3 and LHX4 expression during early human development, Gene Expr Patterns 5 (2) (2004) 279–284.

[29] A.P. Bhangoo, C.S. Hunter, J.J. Savage, H. Anhalt, S. Pavlakis, E.C. Walvoord, et al., A novel LHX3 mutation presenting as combined pituitary hormonal deficiency, J Clin Endocrinol Metab 91 (2006) 747–753.

[30] P.Q. Thomas, B.V. Johnson, J. Rathjen, P.D. Rathjen, Sequence, genomic organization, and expression of the novel homeobox gene hesx1, J Biol Chem 270 (8) (1995) 3869–3875.

[31] E. Hermesz, S. Mackem, K.A. Mahon, Rpx: A novel anterior-restricted homeobox gene progressively activated in the prechordal plate, anterior neural plate and Rathke's pouch of the mouse embryo, Development 122 (1) (1996) 41–52.

[32] K. Kawamura, S. Kikuyama, Evidence that hypophysis and hypothalamus constitute a single entity from the primary stage of histogenesis, Development 115 (1992) 1–9.

[33] L.E. Olson, J. Tollkuhn, C. Scafoglio, A. Krones, J. Zhang, K.A. Ohgi, et al., Homeodomain-mediated beta-catenin-dependent switching events dictate cell-lineage determination, Cell 125 (3) (2006) 593–605.

[34] J.S. Dasen, J.P. Barbera, T.S. Herman, S.O. Connell, L. Olson, B. Ju, et al., Temporal regulation of a paired-like homeodomain repressor/TLE corepressor complex and a related activator is required for pituitary organogenesis, Genes Dev 15 (23) (2001) 3193–3207.

[35] M.T. Dattani, J.P. Martinez-Barbera, P.Q. Thomas, J.M. Brickman, R. Gupta, I.L. Martensson, et al., Mutations in the homeobox gene HESX1/Hesx1 associated with septo-optic dysplasia in human and mouse, Nat Genet 19 (2) (1998) 125–133.

[36] M.L. Brinkmeier, M.A. Potok, K.B. Cha, T. Gridley, S. Stifani, J. Meeldijk, et al., TCF and Groucho-related genes influence pituitary growth and development, Mol Endocrinol 17 (11) (2003) 2152–2161.

[37] J.M. Brickman, M. Clements, R. Tyrell, D. McNay, K. Woods, J. Warner, et al., Molecular effects of novel mutations in Hesx1/HESX1 associated with human pituitary disorders, Development 128 (24) (2001) 5189–5199.

[38] M.T. Dattani, I.C. Robinson, The molecular basis for developmental disorders of the pituitary gland in man, Clin Genet 57 (5) (2000) 337–346.

[39] M.T. Dattani, Novel insights into the aetiology and pathogenesis of hypopituitarism, Horm Res 62 (Suppl 3) (2004) 1–13.

[40] M.W. Sornson, W. Wu, J.S. Dasen, S.E. Flynn, D.J. Norman, S.M. O'Connell, et al., Pituitary lineage determination by the Prophet-of-Pit-1 homeodomain factor defective in Ames dwarfism, Nature 384 (6607) (1996) 327–333.

[41] L.T. Raetzman, R. Ward, S.A. Camper, Lhx4 and Prop1 are required for cell survival and expansion of the pituitary primordia, Development 129 (18) (2002) 4229–4239.

[42] R.D. Ward, L.T. Raetzman, H. Suh, B.M. Stone, I.O. Nasonkin, S.A. Camper, Role of PROP1 in pituitary gland growth, Mol Endocrinol 19 (3) (2005) 698–710.

[43] R.D. Ward, B.M. Stone, L.T. Raetzman, S.A. Camper, Cell proliferation and vascularization in mouse models of pituitary hormone deficiency, Mol Endocrinol 20 (6) (2006) 1378–1390.

[44] P.J. Gage, M.L. Brinkmeier, L.M. Scarlett, L.T. Knapp, S.A. Camper, K.A. Mahon, The ames dwarf gene, df, is required early in pituitary ontogeny for the extinction of rpx transcription and initiation of lineage-specific cell proliferation, Mol Endocrinol 10 (12) (1996) 1570–1581.

[45] I.O. Nasonkin, R.D. Ward, L.T. Raetzman, A.F. Seasholtz, T.L. Saunders, P.J. Gillespie, et al., Pituitary hypoplasia and respiratory distress syndrome in Prop1 knockout mice, Hum Mol Genet 13 (22) (2004) 2727–2735.

[46] W. Wu, J.D. Cogan, R.W. Pfaffle, J.S. Dasen, H. Frisch, S.M. O'Connell, et al., Mutations in PROP1 cause familial combined pituitary hormone deficiency, Nat Genet 18 (2) (1998) 147–149.

[47] S. Vallette-Kasic, A. Barlier, C. Teinturier, A. Diaz, M. Manavela, F. Berthezene, et al., PROP1 gene screening in patients with multiple pituitary hormone deficiency reveals two sites of hypermutability and a high incidence of corticotroph deficiency, J Clin Endocrinol Metab 86 (9) (2001) 4529–4535.

[48] A. Bottner, E. Keller, J. Kratzsch, H. Stobbe, J.F. Weigel, A. Keller, et al., PROP1 mutations cause progressive deterioration of anterior pituitary function including adrenal insufficiency: A longitudinal analysis, J Clin Endocrinol Metab 89 (10) (2004) 5256–5265.

[49] M. Treier, A.S. Gleiberman, S.M. O'Connell, D.P. Szeto, J.A. McMahon, A.P. McMahon, et al., Multistep signaling requirements for pituitary organogenesis in vivo, Genes Dev 12 (11) (1998) 1691–1704.

[50] J. Ericson, S. Norlin, T.M. Jessell, T. Edlund, Integrated FGF and BMP signaling controls the progression of progenitor cell differentiation and the emergence of pattern in the embryonic anterior pituitary, Development 125 (6) (1998) 1005–1015.

[51] S.W. Davis, S.A. Camper, Noggin regulates Bmp4 activity during pituitary induction, Dev Biol 305 (1) (2007) 145–160.

[52] M. Nudi, J.F. Ouimette, J. Drouin, Bone morphogenic protein (Smad)-mediated repression of proopiomelanocortin transcription by interference with Pitx/Tpit activity, Mol Endocrinol 19 (5) (2005) 1329–1342.

[53] M. Treier, S. O'Connell, A. Gleiberman, J. Price, D.P. Szeto, R. Burgess, et al., Hedgehog signaling is required for pituitary gland development, Development 128 (3) (2001) 377–386.

[54] C. Chiang, Y. Litingtung, E. Lee, K.E. Young, J.L. Corden, H. Westphal, et al., Cyclopia and defective axial patterning in mice lacking Sonic hedgehog gene function, Nature 383 (6599) (1996) 407–413.

[55] H.L. Park, C. Bai, K.A. Platt, M.P. Matise, A. Beeghly, C.C. Hui, et al., Mouse Gli1 mutants are viable but have defects in SHH signaling in combination with a Gli2 mutation, Development 127 (8) (2000) 1593–1605.
[56] H. Ohuchi, Y. Hori, M. Yamasaki, H. Harada, K. Sekine, S. Kato, et al., FGF10 acts as a major ligand for FGF receptor 2 IIIb in mouse multi-organ development, Biochem Biophys Res Commun 277 (3) (2000) 643–649.
[57] L. De Moerlooze, B. Spencer-Dene, J. Revest, M. Hajihosseini, I. Rosewell, C. Dickson, An important role for the IIIb isoform of fibroblast growth factor receptor 2 (FGFR2) in mesenchymal-epithelial signalling during mouse organogenesis, Development 127 (3) (2000) 483–492.
[58] M.L. Brinkmeier, M.A. Potok, S.W. Davis, S.A. Camper, TCF4 deficiency expands ventral diencephalon signaling and increases induction of pituitary progenitors, Dev Biol 311 (2) (2007) 396–407.
[59] J. Chen, N. Hersmus, D.V. Van, P. Caesens, C. Denef, H. Vankelecom, The adult pituitary contains a cell population displaying stem/progenitor cell and early embryonic characteristics, Endocrinology 146 (9) (2005) 3985–3998.
[60] T. Fauquier, K. Rizzoti, M. Dattani, R. Lovell-Badge, I.C. Robinson, SOX2-expressing progenitor cells generate all of the major cell types in the adult mouse pituitary gland, Proc Natl Acad Sci USA 105 (8) (2008) 2907–2912.
[61] M. Garcia-Lavandeira, V. Quereda, I. Flores, C. Saez, E. Diaz-Rodriguez, M.A. Japon, et al., A GRFa2/Prop1/stem (GPS) cell niche in the pituitary, PLoS ONE 4 (3) (2009) e4815.
[62] A.S. Gleiberman, T. Michurina, J.M. Encinas, J.L. Roig, P. Krasnov, F. Balordi, et al., Genetic approaches identify adult pituitary stem cells, Proc Nat Acad Sci USA 105 (17) (2008) 6332–6337.
[63] L.T. Raetzman, S.A. Ross, S. Cook, S.L. Dunwoodie, S.A. Camper, P.Q. Thomas, Developmental regulation of Notch signaling genes in the embryonic pituitary: Prop1 deficiency affects Notch2 expression, Dev Biol 265 (2) (2004) 329–340.
[64] L.T. Raetzman, B.S. Wheeler, S.A. Ross, P.Q. Thomas, S.A. Camper, Persistent expression of Notch2 delays gonadotrope differentiation, Mol Endocrinol 20 (11) (2006) 2898–2908.
[65] X. Zhu, J. Zhang, J. Tollkuhn, R. Ohsawa, E.H. Bresnick, F. Guillemot, et al., Sustained Notch signaling in progenitors is required for sequential emergence of distinct cell lineages during organogenesis, Genes Dev 20 (19) (2006) 2739–2753.
[66] L.T. Raetzman, J.X. Cai, S.A. Camper, Hes1 is required for pituitary growth and melanotrope specification, Dev Biol 304 (2) (2007) 455–466.
[67] A. Kita, I. Imayoshi, M. Hojo, M. Kitagawa, H. Kokubu, R. Ohsawa, et al., Hes1 and Hes5 control the progenitor pool, intermediate lobe specification, and posterior lobe formation in the pituitary development, Mol Endocrinol 21 (6) (2007) 1458–1466.
[68] P. Monahan, S. Rybak, L.T. Raetzman, The notch target gene HES1 regulates cell cycle inhibitor expression in the developing pituitary, Endocrinology 150 (9) (2009) 4386–4394.
[69] S. Bilodeau, A. Roussel-Gervais, J. Drouin, Distinct developmental roles of cell cycle inhibitors p57Kip2 and p27Kip1 distinguish pituitary progenitor cell cycle exit from cell cycle re-entry of differentiated cells, Mol Cell Biol 29 (7) (2009) 1895–1908.
[70] L.A. Nolan, A. Levy, A population of non-luteinising hormone/non-adrenocorticotrophic hormone-positive cells in the male rat anterior pituitary responds mitotically to both gonadectomy and adrenalectomy, J Neuroendocrinol 18 (9) (2006) 655–661.
[71] A.M. Pulichino, S. Vallette-Kasic, J.P.Y. Tsai, C. Couture, Y. Gauthier, J. Drouin, Tpit determines alternate fates during pituitary cell differentiation, Genes Dev 17 (6) (2003) 738–747.
[72] M. Gulyas, L. Pusztai, G. Rappay, G.B. Makara, Pituitary corticotrophs proliferate temporarily after adrenalectomy, Histochemistry 96 (2) (1991) 185–189.
[73] D. Gregoire, M. Kmita, Recombination between inverted loxP sites is cytotoxic for proliferating cells and provides a simple tool for conditional cell ablation, Proc Nat Acad Sci USA 105 (38) (2008) 14492–14496.
[74] M.A. Japon, M. Rubinstein, M.J. Low, In situ hybridization analysis of anterior pituitary hormone gene expression during fetal mouse development, J Histochem Cytochem 42 (1994) 1117–1125.
[75] S.A. Camper, T.L. Saunders, R.W. Katz, R.H. Reeves, The Pit-1 transcription factor gene is a candidate for the murine snell dwarf mutation, Genomics 8 (3) (1990) 586–590.
[76] S. Li, E.B.I. Crenshaw, E.J. Rawson, D.M. Simmons, L.W. Swanson, M.G. Rosenfeld, Dwarf locus mutants lacking three pituitary cell types result from mutations in the POU-domain gene pit-1, Nature 347 (1990) 528–533.
[77] L.E. Cohen, S. Radovick, Molecular basis of combined pituitary hormone deficiencies, Endocr Rev 23 (4) (2002) 431–442.
[78] M.L. Fero, M. Rivkin, M. Tasch, P. Porter, C.E. Carow, E. Firpo, et al., A syndrome of multiorgan hyperplasia with features of gigantism, tumorigenesis, and female sterility in p27(Kip1)-deficient mice, Cell 85 (5) (1996) 733–744.
[79] H. Kiyokawa, R.D. Kineman, K.O. Manova-Todorova, V.C. Soares, E.S. Hoffman, M. Ono, et al., Enhanced growth of mice lacking the cyclin-dependent kinase inhibitor function of p27(Kip1), Cell 85 (5) (1996) 721–732.
[80] K. Nakayama, N. Ishida, M. Shirane, A. Inomata, T. Inoue, N. Shishido, et al., Mice lacking p27(Kip1) display increased body size, multiple organ hyperplasia, retinal dysplasia, and pituitary tumors, Cell 85 (5) (1996) 707–720.
[81] S. Jirawatnotai, D.S. Moons, C.O. Stocco, R. Franks, D.B. Hales, G. Gibori, et al., The cyclin-dependent kinase inhibitors p27Kip1 and p21Cip1 cooperate to restrict proliferative life span in differentiating ovarian cells, J Biol Chem 278 (19) (2003) 17021–17027.
[82] V. Chesnokova, S. Zonis, K. Kovacs, A. Ben Shlomo, K. Wawrowsky, S. Bannykh, et al., p21(Cip1) restrains pituitary tumor growth, Proc Nat Acad Sci USA 105 (45) (2008) 17498–17503.
[83] V. Chesnokova, S. Zonis, T. Rubinek, R. Yu, A. Ben Shlomo, K. Kovacs, et al., Senescence mediates pituitary hypoplasia and restrains pituitary tumor growth, Cancer Res 67 (21) (2007) 10564–10572.
[84] V. Chesnokova, S. Melmed, Pituitary tumour-transforming gene (PTTG) and pituitary senescence, Horm Res 71 (Suppl 2) (2009) 82–87.
[85] X. Bonnefont, A. Lacampagne, A. Sanchez-Hormigo, E. Fino, A. Creff, M.N. Mathieu, et al., Revealing the large-scale network organization of growth hormone-secreting cells, Proc Nat Acad Sci USA 102 (46) (2005) 16880–16885.
[86] C. Lafont, M.G. Desarmenien, M. Cassou, F. Molino, J. Lecoq, D. Hodson, et al., Cellular in vivo imaging reveals coordinated regulation of pituitary microcirculation and GH cell network function, Proc Nat Acad Sci USA 107 (9) (2010) 4465–4470.
[87] N. Chauvet, T. El Yandouzi, M.N. Mathieu, A. Schlernitzauer, E. Galibert, C. Lafont, et al., Characterization of adherens junction protein expression and localization in pituitary cell networks, J Endocrinol 202 (3) (2009) 375–387.

[88] B. Lamolet, A.M. Pulichino, T. Lamonerie, Y. Gauthier, T. Brue, A. Enjalbert, et al., A pituitary cell-restricted T-box factor, Tpit, activates POMC transcription in cooperation with Pitx homeoproteins, Cell 104 (6) (2001) 849–859.

[89] A.M. Pulichino, S. Vallette-Kasic, C. Couture, Y. Gauthier, T. Brue, M. David, et al., Human and mouse Tpit gene mutations cause early onset pituitary ACTH deficiency, Genes Dev 17 (6) (2003) 711–716.

[90] S. Vallette-Kasic, T. Brue, A.M. Pulichino, M. Gueydan, A. Barlier, M. David, et al., Congenital isolated adrenocorticotropin deficiency: An underestimated cause of neonatal death, explained by TPIT gene mutations, J Clin Endocrinol Metab 90 (3) (2005) 1323–1331.

[91] S. Vallette-Kasic, C. Couture, A. Balsalobre, Y. Gauthier, L.A. Metherell, M. Dattani, et al., The TPIT gene mutation M86R associated with isolated ACTH deficiency interferes in protein:protein interactions, J Clin Endocrinol Metab. 92 (10) (2007) 3991–3999.

[92] S. Vallette-Kasic, D. Figarella-Branger, M. Grino, A.M. Pulichino, H. Dufour, F. Grisoli, et al., Differential regulation of proopiomelanocortin and pituitary-restricted transcription factor (TPIT), a new marker of normal and adenomatous human corticotrophs, J Clin Endocrinol Metab 88 (7) (2003) 3050–3056.

[93] M. Therrien, J. Drouin, Cell-specific helix-loop-helix factor required for pituitary expression of the pro-opiomelanocortin gene, Mol Cell Biol 13 (1993) 2342–2353.

[94] G. Poulin, B. Turgeon, J. Drouin, NeuroD1/BETA2 contributes to cell-specific transcription of the POMC gene, Mol Cell Biol 17 (11) (1997) 6673–6682.

[95] G. Poulin, M. Lebel, M. Chamberland, F.W. Paradis, J. Drouin, Specific protein:protein interaction between basic Helix-Loop-Helix transcription factors and homeoproteins of the Pitx family, Mol Cell Biol 20 (2000) 4826–4837.

[96] P.L. Lavoie, L. Budry, A. Balsalobre, J. Drouin, Developmental Dependence on NurRE and EboxNeuro for Expression of Pituitary POMC, Mol Endocrinol 22 (7) (2008) 1647–1657.

[97] G.W. Smith, J.M. Aubry, F. Dellu, A. Contarino, L.M. Bilezikjian, L.H. Gold, et al., Corticotropin releasing factor receptor 1-deficient mice display decreased anxiety, impaired stress response, and aberrant neuroendocrine development, Neuron 20 (6) (1998) 1093–1102.

[98] T.L. Bale, R. Picetti, A. Contarino, G.F. Koob, W.W. Vale, K.F. Lee, Mice deficient for both corticotropin-releasing factor receptor 1 (CRFR1) and CRFR2 have an impaired stress response and display sexually dichotomous anxiety-like behavior, J Neurosci 22 (1) (2002) 193–199.

[99] D.I. Lugo, J.E. Pintar, Ontogeny of basal and regulated secretion from POMC cells of the developing anterior lobe of the rat pituitary gland, Dev Biol 173 (1) (1996) 95–109.

[100] D.I. Lugo, J.E. Pintar, Ontogeny of basal and regulated pro-opiomelanocortin-derived peptide secretion from fetal and neonatal pituitary intermediate lobe cells: Melanotrophs exhibit transient glucocorticoid responses during development, Dev Biol 173 (1) (1996) 110–118.

[101] I. Heuser, Anna-Monika-Prize paper. The hypothalamic-pituitary-adrenal system in depression, Pharmacopsychiatry 31 (1) (1998) 10–13.

[102] F. Holsboer, N. Barden, Antidepressants and hypothalamic-pituitary-adrenocortical regulation, Endocr Rev 17 (2) (1996) 187–205.

[103] F. Holsboer, R. Liebl, E. Hofschuster, Repeated dexamethasone suppression test during depressive illness. Normalisation of test result compared with clinical improvement, J Affect Disord 4 (2) (1982) 93–101.

[104] C.B. Nemeroff, E. Widerlov, G. Bissette, H. Walleus, I. Karlsson, K. Eklund, et al., Elevated concentrations of CSF corticotropin-releasing factor-like immunoreactivity in depressed patients, Science 226 (4680) (1984) 1342–1344.

[105] T.W. Pace, F. Hu, A.H. Miller, Cytokine-effects on glucocorticoid receptor function: Relevance to glucocorticoid resistance and the pathophysiology and treatment of major depression, Brain Behav Immun 21 (1) (2007) 9–19.

[106] S. Watson, P. Gallagher, I.N. Ferrier, A.H. Young, Post-dexamethasone arginine vasopressin levels in patients with severe mood disorders, J Psychiatr Res 40 (4) (2006) 353–359.

[107] C. Schule, T.C. Baghai, D. Eser, R. Rupprecht, Hypothalamic-pituitary-adrenocortical system dysregulation and new treatment strategies in depression, Expert Rev Neurother 9 (7) (2009) 1005–1019.

[108] S.W.J. Lamberts, Glucocorticoid receptors and Cushing's disease, Mol Cell Endocrinol 197 (1–2) (2002) 69–72.

[109] S. Bilodeau, S. Vallette-Kasic, Y. Gauthier, D. Figarella-Branger, T. Brue, F. Berthelet, et al., Role of Brg1 and HDAC2 in GR *trans*-repression of pituitary POMC gene and misexpression in Cushing disease, Genes Dev 20 (20) (2006) 2871–2886.

[110] L. Proulx-Ferland, H. Meunier, J. Côté, D. Dumont, B. Gagné, F. Labrie, Multiple factors involved in the control of ACTH and a-MSH secretion, J Steroid Biochem 19 (1983) 439–445.

[111] H.A. Ingraham, D.S. Lala, Y. Ikeda, X. Luo, W.H. Shen, M.W. Nachtigal, et al., The nuclear receptor steroidogenic factor 1 acts at multiple levels of the reproductive axis, Genes Dev 8 (1994) 2302–2312.

[112] Y. Ikeda, D.S. Lala, X. Luo, E. Kim, M.P. Moisan, K.L. Parker, Characterization of the mouse FTZ-F1 gene, which encodes a key regulator of steroid hydroxylase gene expression, Mol Endocrinol 7 (7) (1993) 852–860.

[113] Y. Ikeda, W.H. Shen, H.A. Ingraham, K.L. Parker, Developmental expression of mouse steroidogenic factor-1, an essential regulator of the steroid hydroxylases, Mol Endocrinol 8 (5) (1994) 654–662.

[114] X. Luo, Y. Ikeda, K.L. Parker, A cell-specific nuclear receptor is essential for adrenal and gonadal development and sexual differentiation, Cell 77 (4) (1994) 481–490.

[115] K. Shinoda, H. Lei, H. Yoshii, M. Nomura, M. Nagano, H. Shiba, et al., Developmental defects of the ventromedial hypothalamic nucleus and pituitary gonadotroph in the Ftz-F1 disrupted mice, Dev Dyn 204 (1) (1995) 22–29.

[116] L. Zhao, M. Bakke, Y. Krimkevich, L.J. Cushman, A.F. Parlow, S.A. Camper, et al., Steroidogenic factor 1 (SF1) is essential for pituitary gonadotrope function, Development 128 (2) (2001) 147–154.

[117] Y. Ikeda, X. Luo, R. Abbud, J.H. Nilson, K.L. Parker, The nuclear receptor steroidogenic factor 1 is essential for the formation of the ventromedial hypothalamic nucleus, Mol Endocrinol 9 (4) (1995) 478–486.

[118] P. Topilko, S. Schneider-Maunoury, G. Levi, A. Trembleau, D. Gourdji, M.A. Driancourt, et al., Multiple pituitary and ovarian defects in Krox-24 (NGFI-A, Egr-1)-targeted mice, Mol Endocrinol 12 (1) (1998) 107–122.

[119] J.J. Tremblay, J. Drouin, Egr-1 is a downstream effector of GnRH and synergizes by direct interaction with Ptx1 and SF-1 to enhance luteinizing hormone b gene transcription, Mol Cell Biol 19 (4) (1999) 2567–2576.

[120] C. Dorn, Q. Ou, J. Svaren, P.A. Crawford, Y. Sadovsky, Activation of luteinizing hormone beta gene by gonadotropin-releasing hormone requires the synergy of early growth response-1 and steroidogenic factor-1, J Biol Chem 274 (20) (1999) 13870–13876.

[121] M.W. Wolfe, G.B. Call, Early growth response protein 1 binds to the luteinizing hormone-beta promoter and mediates gonadotropin-releasing hormone-stimulated gene expression, Mol Endocrinol 13 (5) (1999) 752–763.

[122] M.A. Charles, T.L. Saunders, W.M. Wood, K. Owens, A.F. Parlow, S.A. Camper, et al., Pituitary-specific Gata2 knockout: Effects on gonadotrope and thyrotrope function, Mol Endocrinol 20 (6) (2006) 1366–1377.

[123] J.S. Dasen, S.M. O'Connell, S.E. Flynn, M. Treier, A.S. Gleiberman, et al., Reciprocal interactions of Pit1 and GATA2 mediate signaling gradient-induced determination of pituitary cell types, Cell 97 (5) (1999) 587–598.

[124] D.P. Szeto, A.K. Ryan, S.M. O'Connell, M.G. Rosenfeld, P-OTX: A PIT-1-interacting homeodomain factor expressed during anterior pituitary gland development, Proc Nat Acad Sci USA 93 (15) (1996) 7706–7710.

[125] C.C. Quirk, K.L. Lozada, R.A. Keri, J.H. Nilson, A single Pitx1 binding site is essential for activity of the LHbeta promoter in transgenic mice, Mol Endocrinol 15 (5) (2001) 734–746.

[126] M.M. Zakaria, K.H. Jeong, C. Lacza, U.B. Kaiser, Pituitary homeobox 1 activates the rat FSHbeta (rFSHbeta) gene through both direct and indirect interactions with the rFSHbeta gene promoter, Mol Endocrinol 16 (8) (2002) 1840–1852.

[127] D. Acampora, S. Mazan, F. Tuorto, V. Avantaggiato, J.J. Tremblay, D. Lazzaro, et al., Transient dwarfism and hypogonadism in mice lacking *Otx1* reveal prepubescent stage-specific control of pituitary levels of GH, FSH and LH. Development 125 (7) (1998) 1229–1239.

[128] T. Tajima, A. Ohtake, M. Hoshino, S. Amemiya, N. Sasaki, K. Ishizu, et al., OTX2 loss of function mutation causes anophthalmia and combined pituitary hormone deficiency with a small anterior and ectopic posterior pituitary, J Clin Endocrinol Metab 94 (1) (2009) 314–319.

[129] B. Andersen, M.G. Rosenfeld, POU domain factors in the neuroendocrine system: Lessons from developmental biology provide insights into human disease, Endocr Rev 22 (1) (2001) 2–35.

[130] M. Bodner, J.L. Castrillo, L.E. Theill, T. Deerinck, M. Ellisman, M. Karin, The pituitary-specific transcription factor GHF-1 is a homeobox-containing protein, Cell 55 (3) (1988) 505–518.

[131] H.A. Ingraham, R. Chen, H.J. Mangalam, H.P. Elsholtz, S.E. Flynn, C.R. Lin, et al., A tissue-specific transcription factor containing a homeodomain specifies a pituitary phenotype, Cell 55 (3) (1988) 519–529.

[132] G. Nica, W. Herzog, C. Sonntag, M. Hammerschmidt, Zebrafish pit1 mutants lack three pituitary cell types and develop severe dwarfism, Mol Endocrinol 18 (5) (2004) 1196–1209.

[133] Y. Qi, J.A. Ranish, X. Zhu, A. Krones, J. Zhang, R. Aebersold, et al., Atbf1 is required for the Pit1 gene early activation, Proc Nat Acad Sci USA 105 (7) (2008) 2481–2486.

[134] S.J. Rhodes, R. Chen, G.E. DiMattia, K.M. Scully, K.A. Kalla, S.C. Lin, et al., A tissue-specific enhancer confers Pit-1-dependent morphogen inducibility and autoregulation on the pit-1 gene, Genes Dev 7 (1993) 913–932.

[135] P.E. Mullis, Genetic control of growth, Eur J Endocrinol 152 (1) (2005) 11–31.

[136] R.N. Day, S. Koike, M. Sakai, M. Muramatsu, R.A. Maurer, Both pit-1 and the estrogen receptor are required for estrogen responsiveness of the rat prolactin gene, Mol Endocrinol 4 (12) (1990) 1964–1971.

[137] E.B. Crenshaw III, K. Kalla, D.M. Simmons, L.W. Swanson, M.G. Rosenfeld, Cell-specific expression of the prolactin gene in transgenic mice is controlled by synergistic interactions between promoter and enhancer elements, Genes Dev 3 (1989) 959–972.

[138] B.E. Nowakowski, R.A. Maurer, Multiple Pit-1-binding sites facilitate estrogen responsiveness of the prolactin gene, Mol Endocrinol 8 (12) (1994) 1742–1749.

[139] K.M. Scully, A.S. Gleiberman, J. Lindzey, D.B. Lubahn, K.S. Korach, M.G. Rosenfeld, Role of estrogen receptor-alpha in the anterior pituitary gland, Mol Endocrinol 11 (6) (1997) 674–681.

[140] A. Gutierrez-Hartmann, D.L. Duval, A.P. Bradford, ETS transcription factors in endocrine systems, Trends Endocrinol Metab 18 (4) (2007) 150–158.

[141] A.P. Bradford, C. Wasylyk, B. Wasylyk, A. Gutierrez-Hartmann, Interaction of Ets-1 and the POU-homeodomain protein GHF-1/Pit-1 reconstitutes pituitary-specific gene expression, Mol Cell Biol 17 (3) (1997) 1065–1074.

[142] A.P. Bradford, K.E. Conrad, C. Wasylyk, B. Wasylyk, A. Gutierrez-Hartmann, Functional interaction of c-Ets-1 and GHF-1/Pit-1 mediates Ras activation of pituitary-specific gene expression: Mapping of the essential c-Ets-1 domain, Mol Cell Biol 15 (5) (1995) 2849–2857.

[143] B. Wasylyk, J. Hagman, A. Gutierrez-Hartmann, Ets transcription factors: Nuclear effectors of the Ras-MAP-kinase signaling pathway, Trends Biochem Sci 23 (6) (1998) 213–216.

[144] A.P. Bradford, K.E. Conrad, P.H. Tran, M.C. Ostrowski, A. Gutierrez-Hartmann, GHF-1/Pit-1 functions as a cell-specific integrator of Ras signaling by targeting the Ras pathway to a composite Ets-1/GHF-1 response element, J Biol Chem 271 (40) (1996) 24639–24648.

[145] R.E. Schweppe, A.A. Melton, K.S. Brodsky, L.D. Aveline, K.A. Resing, N.G. Ahn, et al., Purification and mass spectrometric identification of GA-binding protein (GABP) as the functional pituitary Ets factor binding to the basal transcription element of the prolactin promoter, J Biol Chem 278 (19) (2003) 16863–16872.

[146] J.J. Tremblay, C. Lanctôt, J. Drouin, The pan-pituitary activator of transcription, Ptx-1 (pituitary homeobox1), acts in synergy with SF-1 and Pit1 and is an upstream regulator of the Lim-homeodomain gene Lim3/Lhx3, Mol Endocrinol 12 (3) (1998) 428–441.

[147] J.J. Tremblay, C.G. Goodyer, J. Drouin, Transcriptional properties of Ptx1 and Ptx2 isoforms, Neuroendocrinol 71 (2000) 277–286.

[148] M.H. Quentien, I. Manfroid, D. Moncet, G. Gunz, M. Muller, M. Grino, et al., Pitx factors are involved in basal and hormone-regulated activity of the human prolactin promoter, J Biol Chem 277 (46) (2002) 44408–44416.

[149] K.K. Jacob, F.M. Stanley, CCAAT/enhancer-binding protein alpha is a physiological regulator of prolactin gene expression, Endocrinology 140 (10) (1999) 4542–4550.

[150] J.C. Liu, R.E. Baker, C. Sun, V.C. Sundmark, H.P. Elsholtz, Activation of Go-coupled dopamine D2 receptors inhibits ERK1/ERK2 in pituitary cells. A key step in the transcriptional suppression of the prolactin gene, J Biol Chem 277 (39) (2002) 35819–35825.

[151] A. Saiardi, Y. Bozzi, J.H. Baik, E. Borrelli, Antiproliferative role of dopamine: Loss of D2 receptors causes hormonal dysfunction and pituitary hyperplasia, Neuron 19 (1) (1997) 115–126.

[152] S.L. Asa, M.A. Kelly, D.K. Grandy, M.J. Low, Pituitary lactotroph adenomas develop after prolonged lactotroph hyperplasia in dopamine D2 receptor-deficient mice, Endocrinology 140 (11) (1999) 5348–5355.

[153] D.F. Gordon, S.R. Lewis, B.R. Haugen, R.A. James, M.T. Mcdermott, W.M. Wood, et al., Pit-1 and GATA-2 interact and functionally cooperate to activate the thyrotropin beta-subunit promoter, J Biol Chem 272 (39) (1997) 24339–24347.

[154] K. Hashimoto, M. Yamada, T. Monden, T. Satoh, F.E. Wondisford, M. Mori, Thyrotropin-releasing hormone (TRH) specific interaction between amino terminus of P-Lim and CREB binding protein (CBP), Mol Cell Endocrinol 229 (1–2) (2005) 11–20.

[155] K. Hashimoto, K. Zanger, A.N. Hollenberg, L.E. Cohen, S. Radovick, F.E. Wondisford, cAMP response element-binding protein-binding protein mediates thyrotropin-releasing hormone signaling on thyrotropin subunit genes, J Biol Chem 275 (43) (2000) 33365–33372.

[156] S. Sasaki, L.A. Lesoon-Wood, A. Dey, T. Kuwata, B.D. Weintraub, G. Humphrey, et al., Ligand-induced recruitment of a histone deacetylase in the negative-feedback regulation of the thyrotropin beta gene, EMBO J 18 (19) (1999) 5389–5398.

[157] E.D. Abel, E.G. Moura, R.S. Ahima, A. Campos-Barros, C.C. Pazos-Moura, M.E. Boers, et al., Dominant inhibition of thyroid hormone action selectively in the pituitary of thyroid hormone receptor-beta null mice abolishes the regulation of thyrotropin by thyroid hormone, Mol Endocrinol 17 (9) (2003) 1767–1776.

CHAPTER

2

Hypothalamic Regulation of Anterior Pituitary Function

Anat Ben-Shlomo, Shlomo Melmed

Pituitary Center, Cedars-Sinai Medical Center, Los Angeles, USA

Establishing the concept that the pituitary is centrally regulated by the hypothalamus required participation from several disciplines, including neuroanatomy, biochemistry and physiology [1], and discoveries that critically contributed to this idea ultimately produced three Nobel prizes.

Hormones were recognized as chemical messengers in the 1920s, and in the ensuing decade, the pituitary gland emerged as the "conductor of the endocrine orchestra" and the existence of neuromediators was finally established. Morphological and functional relationships between the nervous and endocrine systems [2] formed the background for the notion, first suggested in 1928 by Ernst Scharrer, that the pituitary is regulated by the hypothalamus [2]. Scharrer proposed that hypothalamic neurons secreted hormones and speculated that these neurons control the pituitary [2].

Santiago Ramón y Cajal identified the hypothalamic–neurohypophyseal (posterior pituitary) connection and also showed unmyelinated nerve fibers crossing from the murine hypothalamus to the neurohypophysis, later localized by I.L. Pines to the supraoptic and paraventricular hypothalamic nuclei [3]. The functional significance of this neuroanatomic support for the concept of hypothalamic regulation of the pituitary was developed in the 1930s by Fisher and colleagues, who demonstrated that bilateral interruption of the feline supraoptico–hypophyseal tract dramatically increased urine output and caused atrophy of the neurohypophysis, sparing the anterior pituitary. These observations were abolished by injection of posterior pituitary extracts, but in contrast, extracts of the atrophic posterior pituitary had no pressor, oxytocic, or antidiuretic effects. Ranson later showed that transection of the monkey median eminence but not the infundibular stem, resulted in severe polyuria. Thus, across species, the posterior pituitary was later shown to be directly regulated by hypothalamic antidiuretic hormone and oxytocin produced by hormone-secreting neurons in the supraoptic nucleus, traveling through axons in the pituitary stalk, was stored and secreted by the posterior pituitary gland [3,4].

A physical connection between the hypothalamus and the anterior pituitary had been established, and loose physical communication via connective tissue between the hypothalamus and the anterior pituitary was described at the end of the 19th century by Berkeley [5]. Blood flow communication via complex hypophysio-portal vessels was subsequently observed by Popa and Fielding [6]. The idea that the hypothalamus could neuroregulate the anterior pituitary was formulated by Berta and Ernst Scharrer in the 1930s, and supported by the work of Geoffrey Harris, who used conscious female rabbits to show that direct and highly selective hypothalamic but not pituitary electrical stimulation induced ovulation, even though it was known that the intact pituitary gland was required for ovulation. This finding argued against neural pathways passing from the hypothalamus to the anterior pituitary, and supported a humoral mechanism whereby hormones pass from the hypothalamus, through the hypothalamic–pituitary portal vein system to the anterior pituitary [7].

The concept that hypothalamic factors regulate anterior pituitary functions through the portal vessels was crystallized in Harris' milestone textbook of physiology published in 1955, *Neural Control of the Pituitary Gland*, and marked the beginning of a new era in neuroendocrinology – the search for hypothalamic neurohormones that regulate the pituitary [2].

The Pituitary, Third Edition, DOI: 10.1016/B978-0-12-380926-1.10002-1

Between the 1930s and 1950s several pituitary hormones were discovered. Ovine luteinizing hormone (oLH) was isolated by Evans et al. in Berkeley in 1940, and this was followed by isolation of oACTH in 1943, growth hormone (GH) in 1945 and follicle-stimulating hormone (FSH) in 1949. Evans' student Cho Hao Li isolated a non-hydrolyzed (α) oACTH and determined its amino acid sequence in 1955. The discovery of pituitary hormones had a significant impact on medicine, and was followed by the discovery of hypothalamic regulators of their respective synthesis and release. Accordingly, three investigators received the Nobel Prize for this work, Du Vigneaud characterized and synthesized oxytocin and ADH (vasopressin), Guillemin discovered thyrotropin-releasing hormone (TRF, TRH), gonadotropin-releasing hormone (GnRH, LHF, LHRH), and somatostatin [8], and Schally discovered gonadotropin-releasing hormone (GnRH) [9].

During the last 30 years our understanding of the hypothalamic–pituitary unit has continued to expand. Key milestones have included cloning and recombinant production of all known pituitary and hypothalamic hormones, cloning and characterization of their receptors, mostly seven transmembrane domain G-protein-coupled receptors, discovery of other hypothalamic peptides regulating the pituitary, achieving an in-depth understanding of hypothalamic–pituitary physiology and pathophysiology, and development of a pharmacotherapeutic armamentarium to treat hypothalamic–pituitary disorders.

ANATOMY AND HISTOLOGY OF THE HYPOTHALAMIC–PITUITARY UNIT

The Hypothalamus

The hypothalamus constitutes less than 1% of brain volume and weighs approximately 5 g [10,11]. The hypothalamic sulcus defines the upper border and extends from the interventricular foramen to the cerebral aqueduct, above which lies the thalamus. The anterior delineation is roughly defined as a line through the anterior commissure, lamina terminalis and optic chiasm. The posterior border is adjacent to the midbrain tegmentum superiorly and the mammillary bodies inferiorly. The lateral borders are defined by the substantia innominata, the internal capsule, the subthalamic nucleus, and the cerebral peduncle.

Hypothalamic neuronal bodies that produce factors controlling the pituitary are clustered in different nuclei, and any given hypothalamic hormone is often produced in more than one nucleus, and often a single nucleus may express several hormones. Nuclei predominantly involved in pituitary regulation are mostly located in the medial hypothalamus.

The median eminence is the major functional link between the hypothalamus and the pituitary, and lies outside the blood–brain barrier, receiving blood supply separately from the rest of the hypothalamus, and largely shared with the pituitary [12–14]. The median eminence is composed of ependymal, internal and external zones [15]. The innermost ependymal layer in the floor of the third ventricle contains tight junctions to prevent exchange of large molecules between the cerebrospinal fluid (CSF) and extracellular median eminence spaces. Other cells in this zone termed tanycytes send processes to other median eminence zones [16]. Tight junctions and tanycytes likely prevent back-trafficking of releasing factors into the hypothalamus. The internal zone consists of axons arising from the supraoptic and paraventricular nuclei to the posterior pituitary, and axons from the hypophyseotropic neurons to the external zone of the median eminence. The external zone of the median eminence contains axons from periventricular hypophyseotropic neurons, including the periventricular hypothalamic nucleus, paraventricular and arcuate nucleus. Axons from peptidergic neurons release peptides including TRH, GnRH, corticotropin-releasing hormone (CRH), growth-hormone-releasing hormone (GHRH) and somatostatin. Axons from monoamine-secreting neurons release dopamine and serotonin. Releasing factors are transferred into the hypophyseal–portal circulation in the external zone of the median eminence, and from there, they eventually reach anterior pituitary trophic hormone-secreting cells [15]. There is an intimate anatomic connection between the axon termini and the fenestrated capillary endothelium of the hypothalamic–pituitary circulation in both the anterior and posterior pituitary.

However, many releasing factors do not reach the hypophyseal–portal circulation, but are released locally to regulate secretion by other nerve terminals in the zone [17]. The hypophyseal–portal circulation originates from the superior hypophyseal artery, a branch of the internal carotid artery, forming a capillary loop network that penetrates and surrounds the internal and external median eminence zones. Arterial blood in this network receives releasing factors secreted upon depolarization of hypothalamic neurons, and transports these peptides to a large network of sinusoids surrounding the pituitary stalk and supplying the entire anterior pituitary [15,18]. The large surface area of this fenestrated vascular network [19,20] facilitates diffusion of hypothalamic releasing factors to pituitary cells. Recently, staining with plasmalemmal vesicle-associated protein 1 (PV1), which constitutes individual radial fibrils in the fenestrated diaphragm, demonstrated the hypothalamic–pituitary vascular unit to be fenestrated, especially at the median eminence, arcuate nucleus and proximal to the pituitary stalk [21]. Moreover, PV1 in this area was not glycosylated, suggesting greater permeability to vascular fenestrations which are estrous-cycle dependent. During the pre-ovulatory LH surge, PV1 expression increased, coinciding with increased fenestrations, suggesting anticipation of the mediobasal hypothalamus to feedback regulators from the pituitary/periphery [21]. Hypophyseal–portal circulation blood likely flows predominantly, if not exclusively, from the hypothalamus to the pituitary [18], however humoral feedback regulation on hypothalamic neurons controlling the pituitary likely also occurs. Potential routes for peripheral humoral factors regulating the hypothalamus include transcytosis through glial and endothelial cells in the blood–brain barrier, permeable capillaries that allow access of peripheral factors to the CSF and the presence of bidirectional fenestrated capillaries.

Non-neuroendocrine supporting cell types including pituicytes and tanycytes also contribute to hypothalamic–pituitary regulation. Pituicytes engulf axon terminals of vasopressin neurons when the hormone is not required, but retract when vasopressin secretion is increased, for example during dehydration [22]. Tanycytes, activated by growth factors and adhesion molecules, operate similarly on axon terminals of GnRH neurons [16,23].

Pituitary Anatomy

The human pituitary gland (hypophysis) is subdivided into the anterior pituitary (adenohypophysis) and the posterior pituitary (neurohypophysis) (Figure 2.1). The adult human pituitary weighs about 0.6 g and its dimensions are about 13 mm (longest transverse dimension) by 6–9 mm (vertical dimension) by 9 mm (anteroposterior dimension). The pituitary is lined

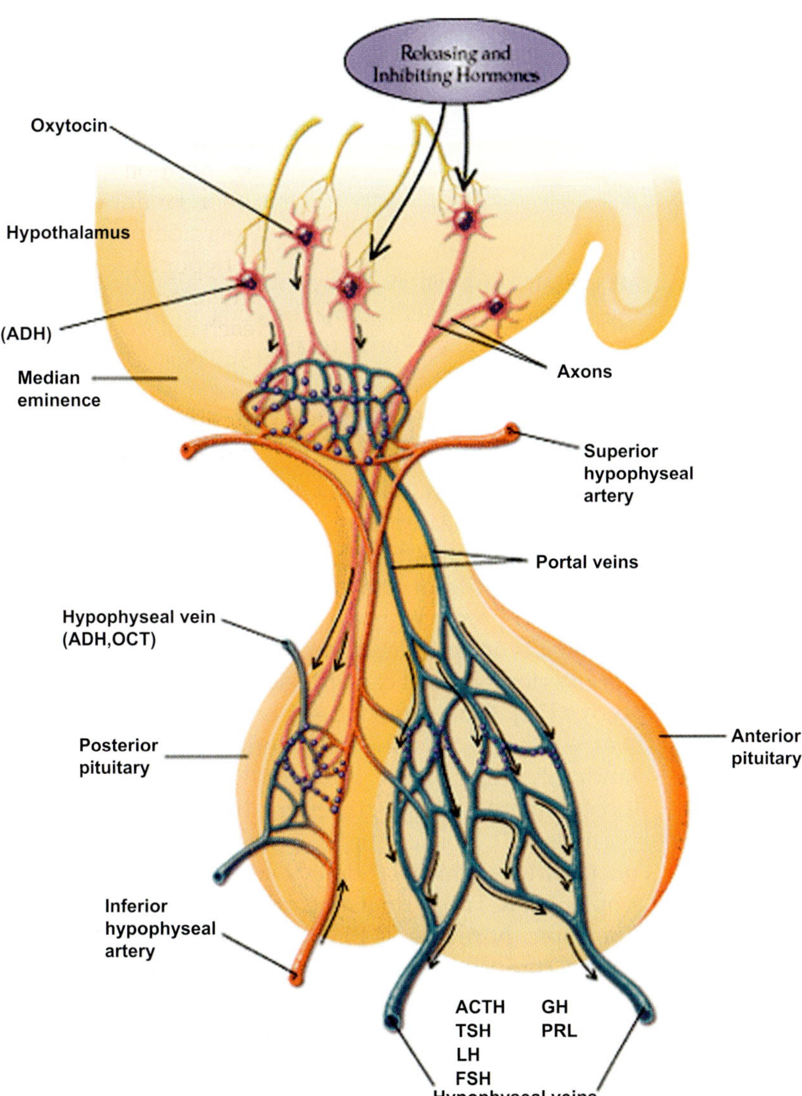

FIGURE 2.1 Structural–functional humoral, endocrine and neuroendocrine relationships within the hypothalamic–pituitary unit emphasize the unique and intimate interdependence of neural structures and hormone secretion with the circulation. Oxytocin (OCT) and vasopressin (ADH) neuron bodies located in the hypothalamus send axons through the pituitary stalk that terminate in the posterior pituitary, where they release OCT and ADH into blood vessels within the posterior pituitary. Hypothalamic neurons that produce growth-hormone-releasing hormone (GHRH), corticotropin-releasing hormone (CRH), thyrotropin-releasing hormone (TRH) and gonadotropin-releasing hormone (GnRH) send their axons through the median eminence to terminate and release their hormones into the hypophyseal–portal circulation. This network of blood vessels is located at the median eminence, which surrounds the pituitary stalk and penetrates into the anterior lobe of the pituitary. These hypothalamic neurohormones stimulate responsive anterior pituitary cells to secrete growth hormone (GH), adrenocorticotropin hormone (ACTH), thyroxin-stimulating hormone (TSH), lutenizing hormone (LH) and follicular-stimulating hormone (FSH), respectively. Dopamine neurons reaching the median eminence are responsible for tonic inhibition of prolactin secretion from the anterior pituitary, while somatostatin released from somatostatinergic neurons inhibits GH and TRH release. *Adapted from Melmed S. in Pituitary, David C. Dale and Daniel D. Federman (Eds.) In ACP Medicine Vol. 1 (2006) pp 571–586.*

by dura mater and lies in the hypophyseal fossa (sella turcica), a bony convection in the upper surface of the sphenoid bone. Within the sella turcica, the pituitary is separated from the sphenoid sinus by a thin bony plate. The sella turcica protects the lower, anterior and posterior pituitary margins. The tuberculum sella is a bony ridge located anterior to the pituitary, while the middle and anterior clinoid processes are anterolateral bony protrusions in the sphenoid bone. The posterior edge of the sella turcica is marked by the dorsum sella and the posterior clinoid processes on two sides. On its upper end, the pituitary is protected from CSF pressure by the diaphragma sella, which is an extension of the dura mater with a small central opening traversed by the pituitary stalk. The optic chiasm is located just anterior to the pituitary stalk. On its two lateral ends the pituitary is adjacent to the cavernous sinuses, large networks of thin-walled veins bordered by the temporal bone, the sphenoid bone and the dura lateral to the sella turcica (Figure 2.2). Cranial nerves III (oculomotor), IV (trochlear), V_1 (the ophthalmic nerve, a branch of the trigeminal nerve), V_2 (the maxillary nerve, a branch of the trigeminal nerve) and VI (abducens) pass through this space arranged from superior to inferior within the lateral wall of the cavernous sinus. Cranial nerve VI (abducens) runs medially to the other nerves and the internal carotid artery medial to the abducens nerve. The internal carotid artery ascends from the neck, enters the cavernous sinus, then traverses the roof of the cavernous sinus medial to the anterior clinoid process, to enter the supra-cavernous portion. This vascular path constitutes the carotid siphon.

The posterior pituitary lobe is visually distinguished from the anterior lobe by T_1-weighted magnetic resonance imaging (MRI) as a bright small area in the posterior part of the gland. It comprises the pars nervosa, which is the neural posterior pituitary, the infundibular stalk, the hypothalamic median eminence and a part of the base of the hypothalamus called tuber cinereum. Histologically, the posterior pituitary is a collection of axon terminals originating from the magnocellular secretory neuron bodies located in the hypothalamic paraventricular and supraoptic nuclei. These axons traverse the infundibular stalk, terminating at the posterior pituitary, and store and secrete vasopressin and oxytocin into the systemic circulation. Glial-like cells called pituicytes are scattered between axon terminals.

The anterior lobe of the pituitary can be divided into the pars distalis (pars glandularis) that constitutes ~80% of the gland, the pars intermedia, and the pars tuberalis. The pars intermedia (the intermediate lobe) lies between the pars distalis and the pars tuberalis, and is rudimentary in the human, although in other species it is more developed. The pars tuberalis (pars infundibularis) is

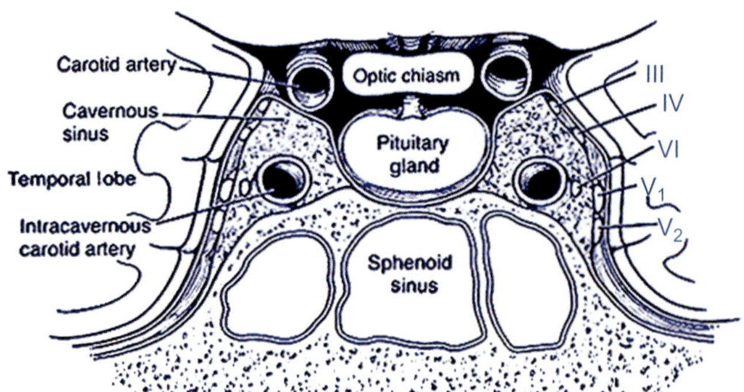

FIGURE 2.2 Coronal view of the pituitary gland within the human skull. The borders of the pituitary are composed of the sella turcica below, the optic chiasm above, and the cavernous sinuses on both sides. The sella turcica is situated immediately above the sphenoid sinus. The cavernous sinuses constitute a thin-walled venous network that receive blood from the superior and inferior ophthalmic veins, the sphenoparietal sinus, and the superficial middle cerebral veins. Blood from the cavernous sinuses drains into the superior and inferior petrosal sinuses, the emissary veins and the pterygoid plexus. Structures crossing the cavernous sinuses lateral to the pituitary gland include the carotid artery, cranial nerve III (oculomotor), cranial nerve IV (trochlear), cranial nerve VI (abducens) nerve), two branches of cranial nerve V (trigeminal nerve), the ophthalmic branch V1 and the maxillary branch V2. *Adapted from Stiver SI, Sharpe JA. Neuro-ophthalomologic evaluation of pituitary tumors. In Thapar K, Kovacs K, Scheithauer BW, Lloyd RV (eds). Diagnosis and management of pituitary tumors. Totowa, NJ, Humana Press, 2001, pp 173–200.*

an upward extension of the anterior lobe that engulfs the infundibular stalk that descends from the median eminence to the posterior lobe.

Cellular Composition of the Anterior Pituitary

The anterior pituitary is derived from oral ectoderm and has an appearance typical of an endocrine gland, with cells grouped in cords and follicles. Approximately 50% of the cells of the anterior pituitary are somatotrophs that produce growth hormone (GH) (Figure 2.3). These cells are primarily located in the lateral wings of the anterior lobe, but can also be scattered in the median wedge [24]. Prolactin (PRL)-secreting lactotrophs represent ~15% of cells in the anterior pituitary and are randomly distributed throughout the lobe, but are most numerous in the posteromedial and posterolateral portions [24]. Corticotrophs express proopiomelanocortin (POMC), which is the precursor of adrenocorticotropin (ACTH), melanocortin hormone (MSH), lipotropic hormone (LPH) and endorphins. Corticotrophs comprise about 15% of anterior pituitary cells. They mostly cluster in the central mucoid wedge, but are also scattered in the lateral wings, and are the predominant cell type in the poorly developed human intermediate lobe. Gonadotroph cells produce

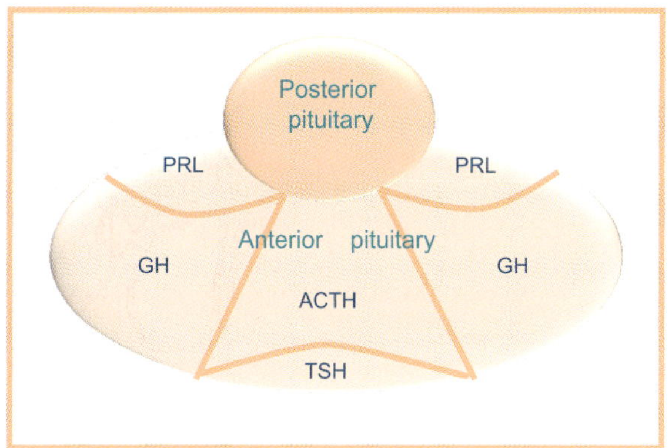

FIGURE 2.3 Distribution and percentage of anterior pituitary cell subtypes, horizontal view. Gonadotroph cells are scattered throughout the anterior pituitary and consistute ~10% of cells. PRL, prolactin-secreting cells (15%); GH, growth-hormone-secreting cells (50%); ACTH, adrenocorticotropin-secreting cells (15%); TSH, thyrotropin-secreting cells (5%). *Adapted from Scheithauer BW, Horvath E, Lloyd RV, Kovacs K. Pathology of pituitary adenoma and pituitary hyperplasia. In Thapar K, Kovacs K, Scheithauer BW, Lloyd RV (eds). Diagnosis and management of pituitary tumors. Totowa, NJ, Humana Press, 2001, pp 91–154.*

luteinizing hormone (LH) and follicle-stimulating hormone (FSH), and represent up to 10% of the human anterior pituitary cell population. In the rat, gonadotroph cell number varies with age, sex and hormonal status [25]. Gonadotrophs are scattered throughout the pars distalis and are the major constituent of the pars tuberalis [26]. Thyrotrophs are the least abundant cell type in the anterior pituitary, comprising ~5% of the total cell population, and are mostly found in the anteromedial portion of the gland [24], but are also located in the pars tuberalis [26].

Many supporting and/or non-neuroendocrine cells are scattered throughout the anterior pituitary. These include follicular cells surrounding follicles [24,27], agranular folliculostellate cells with long branched cytoplasmic processes [28,29], incompletely differentiated null cells that do not secrete specific hormones [30] and mitochondria rich oncocytes [24].

HYPOTHALAMIC FACTORS REGULATING PITUITARY FUNCTION

The hypothalamic–pituitary unit is a neuro-endocrine transducer that mediates input trafficking between the brain and the peripheral hormone-secreting target glands. Positive and negative feedback regulators are critical mediators in the fine-tuning of brain control biological processes that maintain life in health and illness. In response to specific circadian, pulsatile or acute brain stimuli, relevant hypothalamic neurons (Table 2.1) secrete hypothalamic releasing or inhibiting neurohormones locally and/or into the hypophyseal–portal circulation to impinge upon pituitary cells and regulate trophic hormone synthesis and release. Pituitary peptidic hormones are secreted to the systemic circulation to reach their distal target organs and regulate peripheral hormone release by specific endocrine glands (Figure 2.4). Negative feedback regulation of hormone secretion exists at all levels of control, but is mostly by target gland hormones suppressing the pituitary and hypothalamus. At all levels of the hypothalamic–pituitary unit, other local factors lincluding cytokines, growth factors, nutrients, neuropeptides and neurotransmitters add further paracrine/autocrine complexity and can alter the delicate hormonal balance along each respective axis.

Thus, the hypothalamic pituitary unit is the major brain–endocrine connection transducing neuronal messages into humoral signals that effectively and extensively reach all target organs. Accordingly, pituitary hormonal secretion is regulated at three tiers (Figure 2.5). The first tier comprises hypothalamic releasing and inhibiting hormones impinging upon the pituitary. The second tier involves paracrine and autocrine intrapituitary hormone, cytokine and growth factors signals. The third tier involves feedback regulation enabled by specific hormones secreted by target glands and organs which regulate their respective pituitary or hypothalamic control.

This chapter describes the major hypothalamic neuropeptides responsible for regulation of pituitary thyrotrophs, lactotrophs, somatotrophs, corticotrophs and gonadotrophs (Table 2.2).

Thyrotropin-releasing Hormone

Thyrotropin-releasing hormone (TRH) is the major endogenous stimulator of the hypothalamic–pituitary–thyroid axis (Figure 2.6). TRH is a phylogenetically ancient tripeptide, synthesized and released from TRH-neurons with cell bodies in the paraventricular nucleus [31]. High concentrations of TRH-positive terminals are found in the median eminence. The human TRH prepro-hormone gene encodes six copies of TRH [32]. Translation produces a peptide precursor that is subsequently cleaved by several prohormone convertases (PC1/3, PC2, carboxipeptidase E), which is then further processed to the active hormone pyroGlu-His-Pro-NH_2 [33].

Two subtypes of mammalian TRH receptor have been reported, TRH-R1 and TRH-R2, but only TRH-R1 exists in humans [34]. TRH-R1 is highly expressed in the anterior pituitary, neuroendocrine brain regions, the autonomic nervous system and the brainstem. In rodents, TRH-R2 is highly expressed in brain regions responsible for somatosensory signals and advanced CNS functions. TRH receptors are seven transmembrane domain G-protein-coupled receptors (GPCR) that are members

TABLE 2.1 Neuropeptides, Neurotransmitters and Receptors in Hypothalamic-Pituitary Neuroendocrine Regulation

Group and Ligand	Receptor Family	Receptor Protein*	Receptor Gene*	Dominant Mode of Action#
Classic Neurotransmitters				
• Catecholamines (NE,E)	α1-Adrenoreceptors	ADA1A (α1A)	ADRA1A	7-TM, $G_{q/11}$
		ADA1B (α1B)	ADRA1B	7-TM, $G_{q/11}$
		ADA1D (α1D)	ADRA1D	7-TM, $G_{q/11}$
	α2-Adrenoreceptors	ADA2A (α2A)	ADRA2A	7-TM, $G_{i/o}$
		ADA2B (α2B)	ADRA2B	7-TM, $G_{i/o}$
		ADA2C (α2C)	ADRA2C	7-TM, $G_{i/o}$
	β-Adrenoreceptors	ADRB1 (β1)	ADRB1	7-TM, G_s
		ADRB3 (β2)	ADRB2	7-TM, G_s
		ADRB3 (β3)	ADRB3	7-TM, G_s
• Serotonin (5-OH-tryptamine)	5-HT1 receptors	5HT1A (5HT1A-α)	HTR1A	7-TM, $G_{i/o}$
		5HT1B (5HT1D-β)	HTR1B	7-TM, $G_{i/o}$
		5HT1D (5HT1D-α)	HTR1D	7-TM, $G_{i/o}$
		5HT1E	HTR1E	7-TM, $G_{i/o}$
	5-HT2 receptors	5HT2A	HTR2A	7-TM, $G_{q/11}$
		5HT2B	HTR2B	7-TM, $G_{q/11}$
		5HT2C (5HT1C)	HTR2C	7-TM, $G_{q/11}$
	5-HT3 receptors	5HT3	Pentamer	Cation flux
		Subunit genes:	HTR3A, HTR3B	
	5-HT4 receptors	5HT4R	HTR4	7-TM, G_S
• Dopamine	Dopamine receptors	DRD1 (D1-R, D1A)	DRD1	7-TM, G_S
		DRD2 (D2-R)	DRD2	7-TM, $G_{i/o}$
		DRD3 (D3-R)	DRD3	7-TM, $G_{i/o}$
		DRD4 (D4-R, D2C)	DRD4	7-TM, $G_{i/o}$
		DRD5 (D5-R, D1B)	DRD5	7-TM, G_S
• Histamine	Histamine receptors	HRH1 (H1-R)	HRH1	7-TM, $G_{q/11}$
		HRH2 (H2-R)	HRH2	7-TM, G_s
		HRH3 (H3-R)	HRH3	7-TM, $G_{i/o}$
• Melatonin	Melatonin receptors	MT1RA (Mel1AR, MT1)	MTNR1A	7-TM, $G_{i/o}$ PLC-β
		MT1RB (Mel1BR, MT2)	MTNR1B	7-TM, $G_{i/o}$ $G_{q/11}$
		MT3 (quinone reductase 2)	NQO2	Cystosolic enzyme
• Trace amines	Trace amine receptor	TAAR1 (TaR-1)	TAAR1	7-TM,
• Acetylcholine	Muscarinic receptors	ACM 1 (M1)	CHRM1	7-TM, $G_{q/11}$
		ACM 2 (M2)	CHRM2	7-TM, $G_{q/11}$
		ACM 3 (M3)	CHRM3	7-TM, $G_{q/11}$
		ACM 4 (M4)	CHRM4	7-TM, $G_{i/o}$
		ACM 5 (M5)	CHRM5	7-TM, $G_{q/11}$
	Nicotinic receptors	ACHA-P, ACH1-7	Pentamer	Cation flux
		Subunit genes	CHRNA, CHRNB	
• Glutamate	Ionotropic receptors	NMDA (NR1, NR2A-D)	Oligomer	Cation flux
		NMZ1 subunit gene:	GRIN1 (NMDAR1)	Cation flux
		AMPA (GluR1-4)	Oligomer	Cation flux
		GRIA1 subunit gene	GRIA1 (GLUR1)	
		Kainate (GluR5-7, KA-1/2)	Oligomer	
		LK1 subunit gene:	GRIK1 (GLUR5)	
	Metabotropic receptors	MGR1 (mGluR1)	GRM1	7-TM, $G_{q/11}$
		MGR2 (mGluR2)	GRM2	7-TM, $G_{i/o}$
		MGR3 (mGluR3)	GRM3	7-TM, $G_{i/o}$
		MGR4 (mGluR4)	GRM4	7-TM, $G_{i/o}$
		MGR5 (mGluR5)	GRM5	7-TM, $G_{q/11}$
		MGR6 (mGluR6)	GRM6	7-TM, $G_{i/o}$
		MGR7 (mGluR7)	GRM7	7-TM, $G_{i/o}$
• γ-aminobutyric acid (GABA)	Ionotropic	GAA-E (GABA-A-R)	Pentamer	[Cl] ion flux
		GAA1 (α1) subunit gene	GABRA1	
	Heterodimeric	GABR1 (GABA-B-R1)	GABBR1	7-TM, $G_{i/o}$
		GABR2 (GABA-B-R2)	GABBR2	7-TM, $G_{i/o}$

TABLE 2.1 Neuropeptides, Neurotransmitters and Receptors in Hypothalamic-Pituitary Neuroendocrine Regulation—cont'd

Group and Ligand	Receptor Family	Receptor Protein*	Receptor Gene*	Dominant Mode of Action#
Neuropeptides				
Neurohypophyseal hormones				
• Vasopressin	Vasopressin receptors	V1AR (V1a) V1BR (V1b,V3) V2R (ADH-R)	AVPR1A AVPR1B AVPR2	7-TM, $G_{q/11}$ 7-TM, $G_{q/11}$ 7-TM, G_S
• Oxytocin	Oxytocin receptor	OXYR (OT-R)	OXTR	7-TM, $G_{q/11}$
Hypophyseotropic hormones				
• TRH	TRH receptor	TRFR (TRH-R)	TRHR	7-TM, $G_{q/11}$
• GHRH	GHRH receptor	GHRHR (GRFR)	GHRHR	7-TM, G_s
• GHRP/Ghrelin	GHS receptor	GHSR (GHRP-R)	GHSR	7-TM, $G_{q/11}$
• GnRH	GnRH receptor	GNRHR (GnRH-R)	GNRHR	7-TM, $G_{q/11}$
• CRH/Urocortin	CRH receptor	CRFR1 (CRH-R1) CRFR2 (CRH-R2)	CRHR1 CRHR2	7-TM, G_s 7-TM, G_s
• Somatostatin/ Cortistatin	Somatostatin receptors	SSTR1 (SS1R, SRIF-2) SSTR2 (SS2R, SRIF-1) SSTR3 (SS3R, SSR-28) SSTR4 (SS4R) SSTR5 (SS5R)	SSTR1 SSTR2 SSTR3 SSTR4 SSTR5	7-TM, $G_{i/o}$ 7-TM, $G_{i/o}$ 7-TM, $G_{i/o}$ 7-TM, $G_{i/o}$ 7-TM, $G_{i/o}$
Endogenous opioid peptides				
• β-endorphin	Mu opioid receptor	OPRM (μ, MOR-1)	OPRM1	7-TM, $G_{i/o}$
• Enkephalin	Delta opioid receptor	OPRD (δ, DOR-1) OPRK (κ, KOR-1) OPRX (KOR-3)	OPRD1 OPRK1 OPRL1	7-TM, $G_{i/o}$ 7-TM, $G_{i/o}$ 7-TM, $G_{i/o}$
Melanocortin peptides				
• MSH	MSH receptor	MSHR (MC1-R)	MC1R	7-TM, G_S
• ACTH	ACTH receptor	ACTHR (MC2-R)	MC2R	7-TM, G_S
• γMSH, MSH	Melanocortin receptor 3	MC3R (MC3-R)	MC3R	7-TM, G_S
• MSH, βMSH	Melanocortin receptor 4	MC4R (MC4-R)	MC4R	7-TM, G_S
• MSH	Melanocortin receptor 5	MC5R (MC5-R)	MC5R	7-TM, G_S
Tachykinins (neurokinins)				
• Substance P	Neurokinin receptors	NK1R (SPR)	TACR1	7-TM, $G_{i/o}$
• Substance K		NK2R (SKR)	TACR2	7-TM, $G_{i/o}$
• Neurokinin B		NKR3 (NKR)	TACR3	7-TM, $G_{i/o}$
Vasoactive peptides				
• Angiotensin II	Angiotensin receptors	AGTR1 (AT1) AGTTR2 (AT2)	AGTR1 AGTR2	7-TM, $G_{q/11}$ 7-TM, $G_{i/o}$
• Atrial natriuretic peptide	ANP receptors	ANPRA (NPR-A) ANPRB (NPR-B)	NPR1 NPR2	cGMP, 1-TM cGMP, 1-TM
• Endothelin	Endothelin receptors	ENDRA (ETA-R) ENDRB (ETB-R)	EDNRA EDNRB	7-TM, $G_{q/11}$ 7-TM, $G_{q/11}$

(Continued)

TABLE 2.1 Neuropeptides, Neurotransmitters and Receptors in Hypothalamic-Pituitary Neuroendocrine Regulation—cont'd

Group and Ligand	Receptor Family	Receptor Protein*	Receptor Gene*	Dominant Mode of Action#
Miscellaneous neuropeptides				
• CART	No receptor identified			7-TM, $G_{i/o}$
• Orexin/hypocretin	Orexin receptors	OX1R (HCRTR-1) OX2R (HCRTR-2)	HCRTR1 HCRTR2	7-TM, many 7-TM, many
• Melanin-concentrating hormone	MCH receptor	MCHR1 (GPCR24)	MCHR1	7-TM, $G_{i/q}$
• Prolactin-releasing peptide	PRP receptor	PRLHR (GPCR10)	PRLHR	7-TM, $G_{i/o/q}$
• Kisspeptins/Metastin	Kisspeptin receptor	KISSR (GPCR54)	KISS1R	7-TM, $G_{q/11}$
• Gonadotropin inhibitory peptide or RF-amide related peptides (RFRP)	GnIH (or RFRP) receptor	GnIH1 (NPFF-1, GPR147)	GnIH1	7-TM, unknown
• Neuromedin U	Neuromedin receptors	NMUR1 (GPCR66) NUMR2	NMUR1 NMUR2	7-TM, $G_{q/11}$ 7-TM, $G_{q/11}$
• Neurotensin	Neurotensin receptor	NTR1 (NTRH)	NTSR1	7-TM, $G_{q/11}$
• PACAP	PACAP receptor	PACR (PACAP-R-1)	ADCYAR1R1	7-TM, G_s
• Vasoactive intestinal peptide	VIP receptors	VIPR1 (PACAP-R-2) VIPR2 (PACAP-R-3)	VIPR1 VIPR3	7-TM, G_s 7-TM, G_s
• Galanin/GALP	Galanin receptors	GALR1 (GAL1-R) GALR2 (GAL2-R) GALR3 (GAL3-R)	GALR1 GALR2 GALR3	7-TM, $G_{i/o}$ 7-TM, $G_{i/o}$ 7-TM, $G_{i/o}$
• Glucagon-like peptide	GLP receptor	GLP1R	GLP1R	7-TM, G_s
• CCK/Gastrin	CCK receptor	CCKAR (CCK1-R) GASR (CCK2-R)	CCKAR CCKBR	7-TM, $G_{q/11}$ 7-TM, $G_{q/11}$
• Neuropeptide Y	NPY/PYY/PP receptors	NPY1R (NPY-Y1)	NPY1R	7-TM, $G_{i/o}$
• PYY (3-32)		NPY2R (NPY-Y2)	NPY2R	7-TM, $G_{i/o}$
• Pancreatic polypeptide		NPY4R (PP1)	PPYR1	7-TM, $G_{i/o}$
• Neuropeptide Y		NPY5R (NPY-Y5)	NPY5R	7-TM, $G_{i/o}$
Other				
• Cannabinoids	Cannabinoid receptor	CNR1 (CB1)	CNR1	7-TM, $G_{i/o}$

* *Swiss-Prot identifiers (alternative names) were obtained from GPCRDB information system at www.gpcr.org/7tm/ as described in: Horn F, Bettler E, Oliveira L, Campagne F, Cohen FE, Vriend G (2003) GPCRDB information system for G protein-coupled receptors. Nucleic Acid Res. 31: 294–297.*

#*Describes the most dominant Gα subunit activated by the receptor, however, many of the neuropeptides and neurotransmitters can activate more than one Gα subunit subtype.*

AMPA , α-amino-3-hydroxy-5-methyl-4-isoxazdepropionic acid; CART, cocain and amphetamine responsive transcript; CCK, cholecystokinine; CRH, corticotropin-releasing hormone; E, epinephrine; GALP, galanin-like peptide; GHRH, growth hormone releasing factor; GnRH, gonadotropin releasing factor; NE, norepinephrine; NMDA, N-methyl-D-aspartate; NPFF, neuropeptide FF; OFQ, orphanin FQ; PACAP, pituitary adenylyl cyclase activating peptide; PYY, peptide YY; TRH, thyrotropin-releasing hormone.

Adapted from: Low, MJ, Neuroendocrinology, in Williams Textbook of Endocrinology, Eds: Kronenberg HM, Melmed S, Polonsky, KS & Larsen, PR, 11th edition, Saunders Elsevier, 2008.

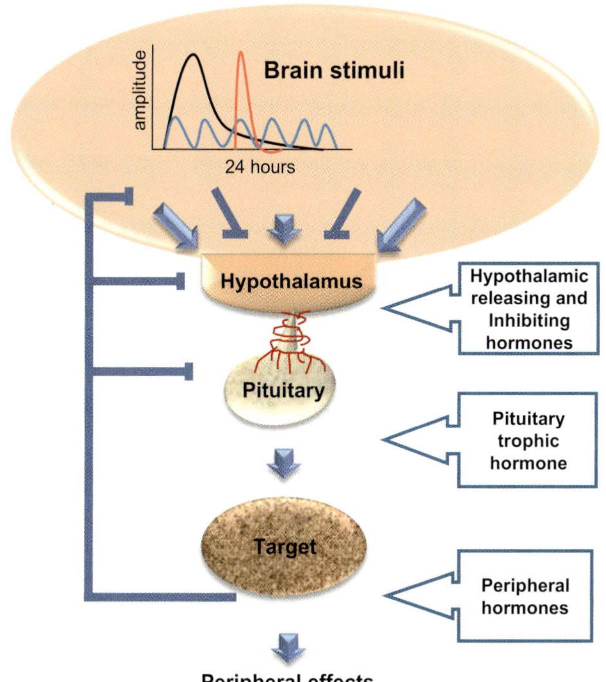

FIGURE 2.4 The three control levels of hypothalamic–pituitary–target organ regulation. The first level is composed of hypothalamic neurons that secrete releasing and inhibiting hormones into the hypophyseal–portal circulation that allow communication between the hypothalamus and the pituitary. The second control level involves the release of pituitary hormones to the circulation, reaching target glands and organs. The third control level constitutes the distal target organs secreting hormones that elicit the required effect on peripheral tissues. Secreted hormones negatively regulate respective stimulating hormone release in each axis.

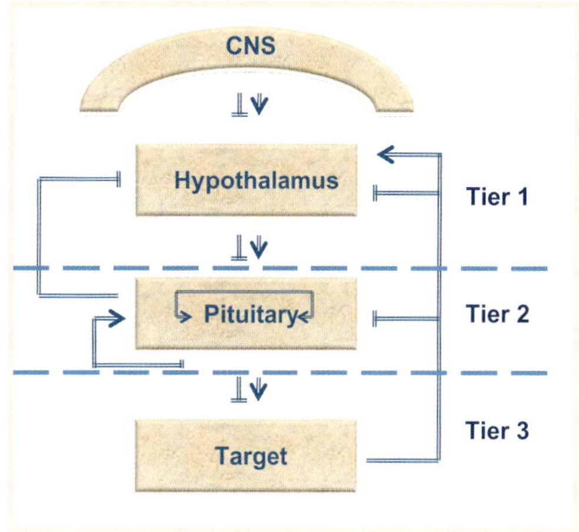

FIGURE 2.5 Three tiers regulating pituitary function. → stimulation; ⊣ inhibition. *Reproduced from Ray D. & Melmed S. Pituitary cytokine and growth factor expression and action. Endocrin Rev 18 (1997) 206-228.*

of group A7 of the rhodopsin-like receptor family (class 1). TRH-R1 signaling is mediated primarily by $G_{q/11}$ proteins. Upon TRH binding, activation of phosphoinositide stimulates phospholipase C, which in turn induces hydrolysis of phosphatidylinositol 4,5,-P_2 (PIP_2) to form inositol 1,4,5-triphosphate ($InsP_3$) and 1,2-diacylglycerol. This leads to increased intracellular Ca^{2+} concentrations $[Ca^{2+}]_i$ and phosphokinase C (PKC) activation. TRH-R1 also increases $[Ca^{2+}]_i$ by coupling to G_{i2} or G_{i3} [34]. TRH also activates calcium/calmodulin-dependent protein kinase and mitogen-activated protein kinase (MAPK) [34]. Pituitary TRH-R1 expression is regulated by thyroid hormone but not by TRH [35].

TRH injection in humans elicits up to a 22-fold increase in pituitary thyroid-stimulating hormone (TSH, thyrotropin) levels within about 30 minutes [36]. TRH induces both TSH secretion and synthesis. A sustained infusion of TRH over 4 hours results in a biphasic TSH increase. The first peak represents the early release of preformed TSH, and the second peak represents release of newly synthesized TSH [37]. TRH also affects TSH bioactivity by altering its glycosylation pattern [38]. TSH secretion increases thyroid T_4 secretion, which is converted to the more active form, triiodothyronine (T_3) [39].

TRH also stimulates pituitary prolactin secretion [40] and may cause hyperprolactinemia in some hypothyroid patients. TRH-null mice have PRL levels that are 60% of those seen in WT, and although TRH is not essential for pregnancy and lactation, it is required for full lactotroph function, particularly during murine lactation [41]. TRH may stimulate GH release in acromegaly, renal or liver failure, anorexia nervosa, psychotic depression and in some hypothyroid children [40].

Multiple factors, either directly or indirectly, regulate TRH neuron activity (Figure 2.7). Thyroid hormones are the most potent negative regulators of TRH. T_4, efficiently taken up by epithelial cells of the choroid system in the lateral ventricle, binds to transthyretin (T_4-binding prealbumin) and is secreted across the blood–brain barrier into the CSF. In the paraventricular nucleus, type II deiodinase converts T_4 to T_3, which interacts with thyroid hormone receptors on TRH neurons to reduce TRH synthesis and secretion. Almost 80% of T_3 at the paraventricular nucleus originates from peripheral T_4. Only 20% of hypothalamic T_3 crosses the blood–brain barrier directly from the periphery [42,43]. Type II deiodinase, mainly expressed in third ventricle tanycytes, is an important regulator of TRH neuron activity and plays a major role in T_3 availability in the paraventricular nucleus. Fasting and infection upregulate tanycyte type II deiodinase expression, resulting in local increases of hypothalamic T_3 which may partially explain the reactive decrease in peripheral TSH observed during fasting or inflammatory diseases [43]. T_3 inhibits TRH gene transcription [31,44] and TSH synthesis and release in vitro [45] and in thyrotroph

TABLE 2.2 Hypothalamic—Pituitary- Target Overview

		Stimulatory				***Inhibitory***	
Hypothalamus	*Neuron*	**TRH**	**CRH**	**GHRH**	**GnRH**	**Somatostatin**	**Dopamine**
	Hypothalamic nucleus	Paraventricular	Paraventricular	arcuate ventromedial	medio-basal, infundibular, periventricular regions	Periventricular paraventricular arcuate ventromedial	Arcuate periventricular
	Gene	*TRH*	*CRH*	*GHRH*	*GNRH-1*	*SST*	
	Precursor	Prepro-TRH	Prepro-CRH	Prepro-GHRH	Prepro-GnRH	Prepro-somatostatin	Tyrosine L-DOPA
	Human chromosome	3q13.3-q21	8q13	20q11.2	8p21-p11.2	3q28	
	Amino acid sequence	pGlu-His-Pro-NH_2	Ser-Glu-Glu-Pro-Pro-Ile-Ser-Leu-Asp-Leu-Thr-Phe-His-Leu-Leu-Arg-Glu-Val-Leu-Glu-Met-Ala-Arg-Ala-Glu-Gln-Leu-Ala-Gln-Gln-Ala-His-Ser-Asn-Arg-Lys-Leu-Met-Glu-Ile-Ile-NH_2	Tyr-Ala-Asp-Ala-Ile-Phe-Thr-Asn-Ser-Tyr-Arg-Lys-Val-Leu-Gly-Gln-Leu-Ser-Ala-Arg-Lys-Leu-Leu-Gln-Asp-Ile-Met-Ser-Arg-Gln-Gln-Gly-Glu-Ser-Asn-Gln-Glu-Arg-Gly-Ala ***or*** [-Arg-Ala-Arg-Leu-NH_2]	pGlu-His-Trp-Ser-Tyr-Gly-Leu-Arg-Pro-Gly-NH_2	Ala-Gly-*Cys-Lys-Asn-Phe-Phe-Trp-Lys-Thr-Phe-Thr-Ser-Cys*	
	Neuro-hormone	TRH	CRH	GHRH(1-40) GHRH(1-44)	GnRH	somatostatin	dopamine
Pituitary	*Dominant GPCR*	TRH-R1	CRH-R1 CRH-R2	GHRHR	GnRHR	SSTR1, SSTR2, SSTR3, SSTR5	D2R
	G_α protein subunits	$G_{\alpha q/11}$($G_{\alpha i2}$, $G_{\alpha i3}$)	$G_{\alpha s}$ ($G_{\alpha q}$, $G_{\alpha i}$)	$G_{\alpha s}$	$G_{\alpha q/11}$ ($G_{\alpha s}$, $G_{\alpha i/o}$)	$G_{\alpha i/o}$	$G_{\alpha i/o}$
	Signaling pathways Shown to be involved in signaling	-PLC -Calcium -MAPK	-Adenylate cyclase-cAMP-PKA -MAPK -PLC -PKC -Calcium	-Adenylate cyclase-cAMP-PKA-MAPK -PLC-Calcium	-PLC -Calcium -MAPK	-Adenylate cyclase-cAMP-PKA -MAPK -Calcium -PTP	-Adenylate cyclase-cAMP-PKA -PLC -Calcium -PTP
	Pituitary cell	Thyrotroph lactotroph	Corticotroph	Somatotroph	Gonadotroph	Somatotroph Thyrotroph Corticotroph	Lactotroph Thyrotroph Melanotroph
	Pituitary hormone affected	TSH PRL	ACTH	GH	LH, FSH	GH, TSH, ACTH	PRL, TSH, MSH
	Pituitary hormone GPCR	TSHR PRLR	Mc2R	GHR	LHR, FSHR		
Target	*Target gland*	thyroid	Adrenal cortex	liver	Gonads		
	Peripheral hormone	T4, T3	Cortisol Androgens	IGF-1	Estrogen, Testosterone Progesterone		
	Receptors	$TR_{\alpha 1}$, $TR_{\beta 2}$	GCR type I, type II	IGF-1R	ERα, ERβ, AR, PR		
Effects		Metabolic Homeostasis	Metabolic Homeostasis Stress response	Tissue growth	Sexual development fertility		

TRH, thyrotropin releasing hormone; CRH, corticotrophin releasing hormone; GHRH, growth hormone releasing hormone; GnRH, gonadotropin releasing hormone; L-DOPA, 3,4-*d*ihydr*o*xy*p*henyl*a*lanine; PKA, phosphokinase A; PKC, phosphokinase C; PLC, phospholipase C; MAPK, mitogen activating phosphokinase; PTP, phosphotyrosine kinase; TSH, thyroxin stimulating hormone; ACTH, adrenocorticotropin hormone; GH, growth hormone; LH, lutenizing hormone; FSH, follicular stimulating hormone; PRL, prolactin; TSHR, TSH receptor; PRLR, prolactin receptor; Mc2R, melanocortin receptor type 2; GHR, GH receptor; LHR, LH receptor; FSHR, FSH receptor; T4, thyroxine; T3, triiodothyroxine; GCR, glucocorticoid receptor; IGF-1, insulin-like growth factor type 1; IGF-1R, IGF-1 receptor; ER, estrogen receptor; AR, androgen receptor; PR, progesterone receptor.

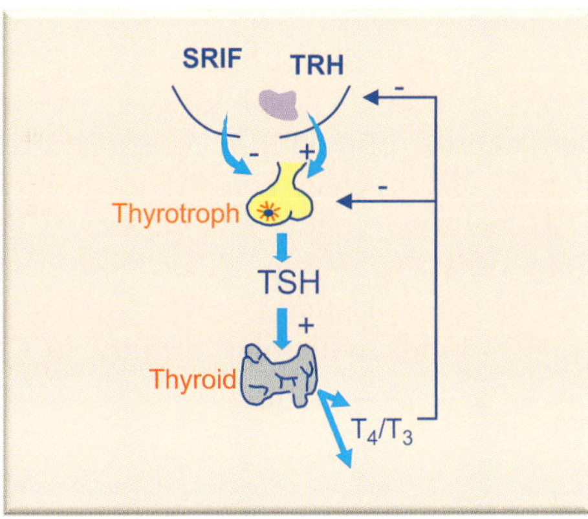

FIGURE 2.6 Specific hypothalamic neurons release thyrotropin-releasing hormone (TRH), which stimulates pituitary thyrotrophs to release thyroxine-stimulating hormone (TSH). TSH then induces the thyroid to produce and release thyroxine (T4 and T3). T4 and T3 negatively regulate further release of both TSH and TRH, thus constituting a negative feedback loop. Somatostatin (SRIF) inhibits both TRH and TSH release. *Reproduced from Melmed, S. Mechanisms for Tumorigenesis: The Plastic Pituitary, J Clin Invest 112 (2003) 1603–1618.*

xenografts [46]. T_3 also influences processing of proTRH by altering paraventricular nucleus prohormone convertase (PC) levels [38]. T_4 also reduces TRH levels measured in the hypophyseal portal circulation [47].

Other factors regulate pituitary TSH response to TRH, but it has been difficult to distinguish between direct hypothalamic vs. pituitary effects. Somatostatin (SRIF) inhibits TRH-induced pituitary TSH and PRL release in cultured rat anterior pituitary cells and TRH-induced TSH in hypothyroid rats [48]. Injection of somatostatin antibodies into rat cerebral ventricles increases both TSH and GH levels, suggesting that TRH increases when somatostatin release is inhibited [49]. Dopamine inhibits TRH stimulation of TSH in normal and hyperprolactinemic females, while the dopamine synthesis inhibitor alpha-methyl-p-tyrosine (AMPT) enhanced the TSH response to TRH [50].

The medulla oblongata mediates temperature regulation of TRH neurons. Cold exposure mediates adrenergic input from the medulla and stimulates TRH release, mainly through $\alpha 1$ adrenoreceptors, and reverses T_3 suppression of TRH transcription [38]. Cocaine- and amphetamine-regulated transcript (CART) stimulates TRH release and potentiates epinephrine action on TRH neurons, and neuropeptide Y (NPY) inhibits TRH transcription [38], both are released by adrenergic medullary neurons.

TRH appears to play a role in appetite control. The arcuate nucleus contains leptin neurons that regulate appetite and leptin upregulates TRH expression. However, leptin also indirectly modulates TRH through POMC and NPY-agouti-related peptide (AgRP) neurons in the arcuate nucleus [51]. Leptin reduction during fasting is associated with reduced preproTRH transcription, and hypothyroidism in leptin null mice can be corrected with exogenous leptin [52]. TRH neurons express glucocorticoid receptors, the TRH gene contains glucocorticoid response elements and glucocorticoids inhibit the TRH–TSH–T_4 axis either directly or indirectly.

Corticotropin-releasing Hormone

Corticotropin-releasing hormone (CRH) is the dominant stimulator of the hypothalamic–pituitary–adrenal (HPA) axis [53] (Figure 2.8). CRH is highly conserved among human, mouse and rat species, but the ovine peptide differs by seven amino acids, increasing ovine CRH potency. The earliest members of the CRH family appeared during the Precambrian eon (>540 million years ago) and include mammalian CRH, urocortin I, II (stresscopin-related peptide) and III (stresscopin) all have a role in the coordination of the stress response

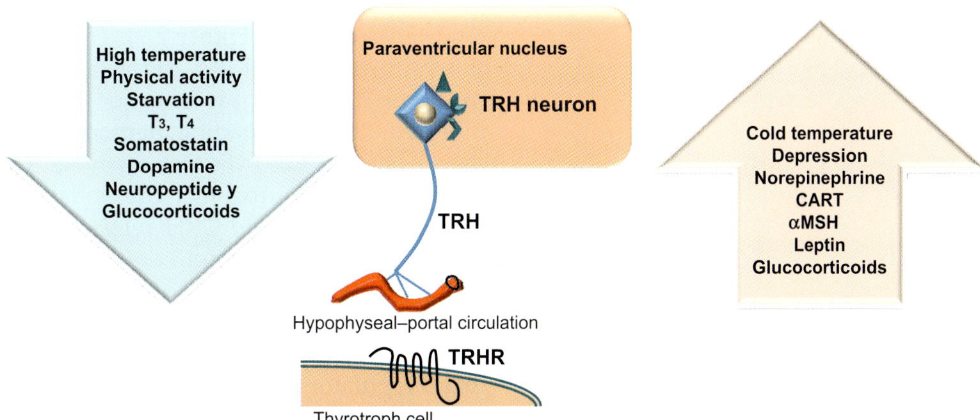

FIGURE 2.7 Stimulators (up arrow) and inhibitors (down arrow) of the thyrotropin-releasing hormone (TRH) neuron in the hypothalamic paraventricular nucleus. ▲ thyroid hormone receptor; ❯ glucocorticoid receptor; leptin receptor. CART, cocaine and amphetamine responsive transcript; αMSH, α melanocortin-stimulating hormone.

[53,54]. CRH pre-prohormone precursor is produced in the parvocellular neurons of the hypothalamic paraventricular nucleus along with vasopressin, enkephalin and neurotensin [54,55]. The amidated 41-amino-acid CRF peptide is cleaved from its carboxyl terminus by PC1,3 and PC2 [56].

CRHR1 is the predominant receptor subtype in pituitary corticotrophs [54], and is also highly expressed in the adrenal medulla and to a lesser extent in the adrenal cortex, specifically in the zona fasiculata and reticularis [57]. CRHR2 has several splice variants. CRHR2α mRNA is localized to the hypothalamus, hippocampus and lateral brain septum, while CRHR2β is expressed in the brainstem, vasculature, heart, lung, skeletal muscle and gastrointestinal tract. CRHR2 variants are also expressed in human adrenals, with greater expression in the cortex compared to the medulla [57]. Stress results in significant upregulation of CRHR1 in the paraventricular nucleus in rodents, specifically in CRH neurons after somatosensory stress [54], suggesting the existence of a CRH autocrine feedback. The CRH peptide family and their respective receptors have also been identified in the adrenals indicating an intra-adrenal CRH-dependent circuit distinct from the hypothalamic–pituitary CRH unit [57].

CRH and urocortin I bind both CRHR1 and CRHR2, while urocortin II and III bind only CRHR2 [58]. Both receptors are GPCRs coupled to the $G_{\alpha s}$ unit and stimulate adenylyl cyclase to increase cAMP levels and activate phophokinase-A (PKA). $G_{\alpha q}$, $G_{\alpha i}$ and also $G_{\alpha s}$ mediate increased calcium levels in vitro [59], an effect mediated through stimulation of phospholipase-C (PLC)-β, and PLC-ε. CRHR1 is rapidly phosphorylated, desensitized and internalized upon stimulation with either CRH or urocortin [54]. PKC rather than PKA mediates CRHR1 phosphorylation and desensitization [54].

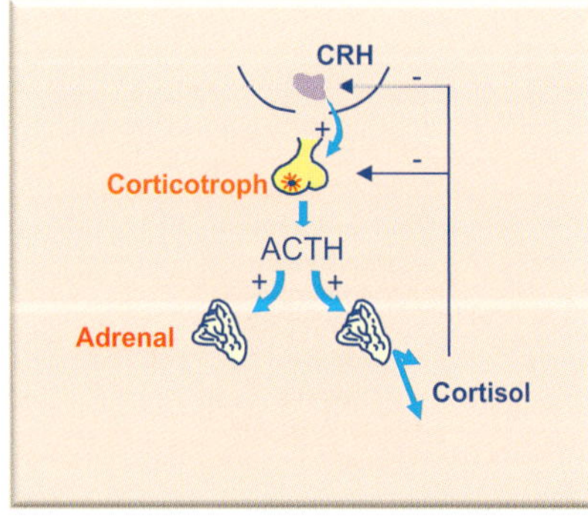

FIGURE 2.8 Hypothalamic corticotropin-releasing hormone (CRH) stimulates the corticotroph to release adrenocorticotropin hormone (ACTH) which in turn stimulates the adrenal glands to produce and release cortisol and androgens. Cortisol inhibits further release of both CRH and ACTH. *Reproduced from Melmed, S. Mechanisms for Tumorigenesis: The Plastic Pituitary, J Clin Invest 112 (2003) 1603–1618.*

CRH action on the pituitary is modified by CRH-binding protein (CRH-BP), a highly conserved 37-kDa glycoprotein abundantly expressed in the pituitary and hypothalamus, but with very low expression in the paraventricular nucleus and the median eminence where CRH neurons reside. Cytoplasmic CRH-BP is localized in cells expressing CRH receptors, and is also found in the plasma [54,57]. CRH-BP rapidly but transiently binds with high affinity to CRH and urocortins, and hence competitively inhibits ligand action [57].

CRH administration is followed by a rapid release of ACTH (peaks at 30 minutes) followed by cortisol (peaks at 60 minutes) [60] and androgen release. Urocortin 1 injection also increases ACTH (peak at 60 minutes) and cortisol (peak at 90 minutes) [61]. CRH and urocortin have other extra-pituitary functions that are beyond the scope of this chapter, for example increased sympathetic activity, behavioral changes such as arousal, locomotion, reward and feeding, and immune, cardiac, gastrointestinal and reproductive functions.

ACTH and cortisol follow a 24-h circadian rhythm that is believed to be driven by CRH [62]. ACTH diurnal variation is essential for maintaining normal adrenal function [63]. Human ACTH and cortisol begin rising between 1 and 4 am, peak during the early morning, a lower peak occurs in the early afternoon, then fall during the rest of the day to reach a nadir at around midnight. CRH null mice have atrophic adrenals without overt ACTH deficiency, and do not exhibit a normal circadian ACTH–corticosterone rhythm [64]. Continuous CRH infusion to these mice produced marked diurnal changes in corticosterone levels, indicating that CRH is necessary for maintaining a normal ACTH circadian rhythm [64].

CRH neurons are tightly regulated by a wide array of stimulators and inhibitors that arrive from the periphery, and also by an extensive network of afferent neurons from the hypothalamus, the limbic forebrain and the brainstem (Figure 2.9). These influences enable finely tuned control of CRH action at baseline and in response to stress. Systemic or physiologic stressors like cytokines, salt loading, hemorrhage, adrenalectomy, hypoglycemia and fasting activate CRH release in rodents [65]. Neurogenic, emotional, or psychological stressors can activate CRH release, but since the paraventricular nucleus is not known to receive direct input from the cerebral cortex or the thalamus, these CRH responses are likely indirect [65,66].

Glucocorticoids (GC), the dominant negative feedback regulators of CRH, freely cross the blood–brain barrier, and bind GC type I and II receptors. GC inhibit CRH gene expression, peptide levels and rate of secretion of CRH. However, severe stress and increased CRH levels can override GC inhibition [55]. GC receptors are widely distributed in the brain and pituitary, inhibit CRH in the parvocellular neurons of the paraventricular nucleus, but either stimulate or have no effect on CRH transcription in CRH-secreting neurons not involved in pituitary regulation [55]. GC may regulate CRH expression through direct action on the CRH neuron, although the *CRH* gene does not contain a glucocorticoid response element [55]. Indirect action may occur through afferents that make synaptic contact with CRH neurons in the arcuate nucleus and catecholaminergic neurons, and via afferents that regulate neuronal input from other brain areas. This extensive network allows a wide range of control of neural influences on CRH function [55].

Other potent regulators of CRH include inflammatory cytokines and neurotransmitters. During inflammation, cytokines like IL-1, TNFα and IL-6 secreted from white blood cells increase CRH release and mediate CNS responses [67–69] to stimulate ACTH and adrenal secretion. Increased GC levels limit inflammation by inhibiting lymphocyte proliferation and production of immunoglobulins and cytokines, all important anti-inflammatory factors. Glutamatergic and GABAergic neurotransmission have been implicated as critical regulators of the stress response. Glutamate stimulates while GABA inhibits CRH release and both neurotransmitters also influence each other [70,71]. Leptin stimulates CRH release from CRH neurons. As leptin receptor mRNA has not been detected in the paraventricular nucleus, but is mostly concentrated in the arcuate nucleus, the effect of leptin is likely indirect [72,73]. Somatostatin neurons are in close proximity to CRH neurons in the paraventricular nucleus [74] and somatostatin inhibits hypothalamic CRH release [75,76]. Catecholamines including dopamine increase CRH expression directly and indirectly [77,78]. Ghrelin may also stimulate CRH directly via efferents terminating on CRH neurons, but mostly indirectly, through GABAergic NPY/Agouti-related protein neurons [79].

Growth-hormone-releasing Hormone (GHRH)

The existence of a putative hypothalamic factor that controls pituitary growth hormone secretion was predicted from animal studies involving hypothalamic lesions [80] and pituitary cell treatment with hypothalamic extracts [81]. This hypothesis was also supported by the observed GH depletion after stalk resection [82], the circadian nature of GH release [83], and acute GH response to stress [84] and somatostatin (the GH-inhibiting factor) [85]. The predicted growth-hormone-releasing hormone (GHRH) was discovered in 1982 from two patients with ectopic GHRH secreted from a pancreatic adenoma [86,87].

GHRH neurons are located in the arcuate nucleus and around the ventromedial nucleus that project into the median eminence, terminate on the capillaries of the hypophyseal–portal circulation, and release GHRH [88]. GHRH is detected in the human hypothalamus between 18 and 29 weeks gestation, and coincides with the appearance of fetal pituitary somatotrophs. In vitro, fetal pituitary cells respond to GHRH and somatostatin in mid-gestation. During mid-puberty, GHRH levels increase significantly, in girls more than boys, but then decline with age, in part accounting for age-related somatopause [89]. Sex steroids activate both somatostatin and GHRH neurons, accounting at least in part for the sexual dimorphism of GH secretion patterns [90]. These effects depend on neonatal and pubertal estrogen and testosterone exposure. Adult males have higher somatostatin and GHRH mRNA expression in their respective neurons, corresponding to higher peaks and lower troughs in GH secretion. Somatostatin levels in male rats are mediated by the androgen receptor,

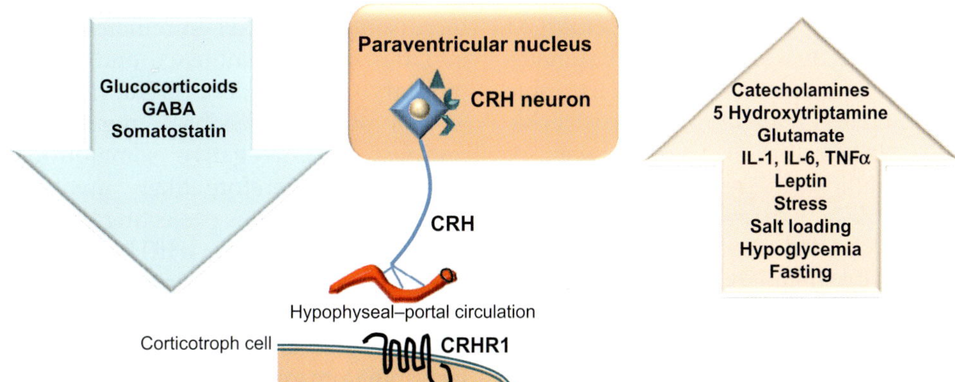

FIGURE 2.9 Stimulators (up arrow) and inhibitors (down arrow) of the corticotropin-releasing hormone (CRH) neuron in the hypothalamic paraventricular nucleus. ▲ cytokine receptors; ❯ glucocorticoid receptor; leptin receptor; GABA; γ aminobutiric acid; CRHR1, CRH receptor subtype 1; IL, interleukin; TNF, tumor necrosis factor.

while expression is dependent on signaling by estrogen receptors. Moreover, males have more GHRH neurons than females but there is no gender difference in somatostatin neuron numbers. The synaptic organization in the arcuate nucleus also differs between genders: females exhibit more synapses, and synapse number varies with the estrous cycle [90].

The *GHRH* gene includes five exons and is located on chromosome 20 in humans, but on chromosome 2 in mice. The precursor GHRH preprotein contains 108 amino acids, and is subsequently processed into GHRH (1-40)-OH and GHRH(1-44)-NH_2, which comprise 40 and 44 amino acids, respectively. While the NH_2-terminal is essential for GHRH bioactivity, the COOH-terminal is not, and fragments as short as GHRH(1-29)-NH_2 are active [91]. The circulating enzyme dipeptidylpeptidase type IV inactivates GHRH to a stable metabolite, GHRH (3-44)-NH_2, which is the most abundant GHRH plasma metabolite [91]. The COOH-terminal of GHRH accounts for the most interspecies sequence diversity [92].

GHRH receptor (GHRHR), mostly expressed on pituitary somatotroph cells, is a GPCR coupled to the $G_{\alpha s}$ subunit. Activation of GHRHR increases intracellular calcium levels and stimulates adenylyl cyclase, which then increases intracellular cAMP concentrations [93]. GHRHR also activates pituitary phosphatidyl inositol and MAPK pathways [94].

Pituitary GHRH action includes effects on GH synthesis and release and somatotroph cell proliferation (Figure 2.10). A single intravenous GHRH bolus dose-dependently increases serum GH levels, peaking at 15–45 minutes, and returning to baseline within 90–120 minutes [95]. Repeated or constant administration of GHRH maintains elevated GH and IGF-1 levels without axis down-regulation [96]. GHRH stimulation of GH is enhanced by estrogens, glucocorticoids and starvation, and is inhibited by somatostatin, obesity and aging. GHRH also directly induces somatotroph proliferation, hyperplasia and even neoplastic transformation [97]. Transgenic mice over-expressing GHRH exhibit somatotroph hyperplasia in enlarged pituitaries and ultimately develop multifocal somatotroph adenomas. Clinical examples for GHRH trophic effect include ectopic GHRH release by neuroendocrine tumors, increased GHRH action as a consequence of activating somatic mutations in the $G_{\alpha s}$ subunit gene observed in up to 40% of patients with acromegaly and loss-of-function *PRKAR1A* gene mutations, which encode type 1A regulatory subunit of PKA in some families with Carney complex. These clinical conditions result in somatotroph hyperplasia and adenomatous transformation [97].

Negative feedback control of GHRH release is achieved mainly by direct GH and probably IGF-1 stimulatory effects on somatostatin neurons, but also

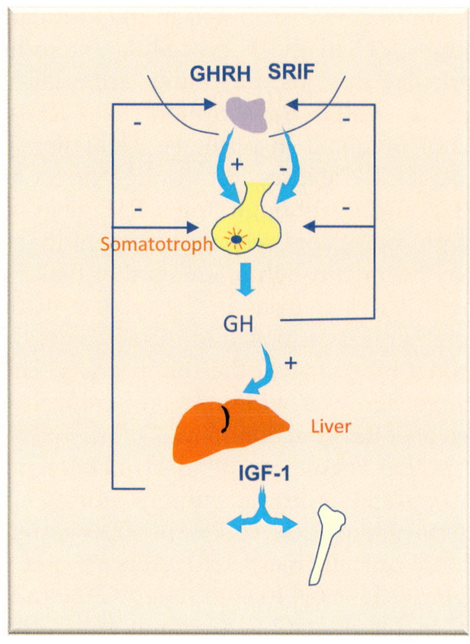

FIGURE 2.10 Hypothalamic growth-hormone-releasing hormone (GHRH) stimulates the somatotroph to release growth hormone (GH), which in turn stimulates the liver to produce and release insulin-like growth factor 1 (IGF-1). Both GH and IGF-1 negatively regulate further release of both GHRH and GH. Somatostatin (SRIF) inhibits both GHRH and GH release. *Reproduced from Melmed, S. Mechanisms for Tumorigenesis: The Plastic Pituitary, J Clin Invest 112 (2003) 1603–1618.*

by an indirect effect on GHRH neurons (Figure 2.11). Neuroanatomic and neurofunctional bidirectional interactions have been demonstrated between somatostatinergic neurons in the periventricular and paraventricular nuclei and GHRH neurons in the arcuate nucleus [98,99]. GHRH neurons express Somatostatin receptor subtype 2 (SSTR2) but not GHR, while somatostatin neurons express both GHR and GHRHR. GH injection into rat cerebral ventricles reduces GHRH-induced GH release; this effect was abolished by treatment with either cysteamine (which depletes somatostatin), or pretreatment with anti-SRIF serum [100]. Increased serum GH stimulates somatostatin release into the median eminence and subsequently inhibits pituitary GH secretion. SSTR2 null mice are refractory to GH negative feedback regulation in the arcuate nucleus [101]. Negative somatotroph regulation by somatostatin therefore likely involves GH-stimulated somatostatin neurons projecting into the arcuate nucleus that directly inhibit GHRH release, in addition to releasing somatostatin into the hypophyseal–portal circulation to directly inhibit pituitary GH secretion.

IGF-1 inhibits GH secretion by direct action on pituitary somatotrophs [102] and also indirect action on the hypothalamus, especially at the arcuate nucleus and median eminence [98]. Both the pituitary and the hypothalamus abundantly express IGF-1 receptors

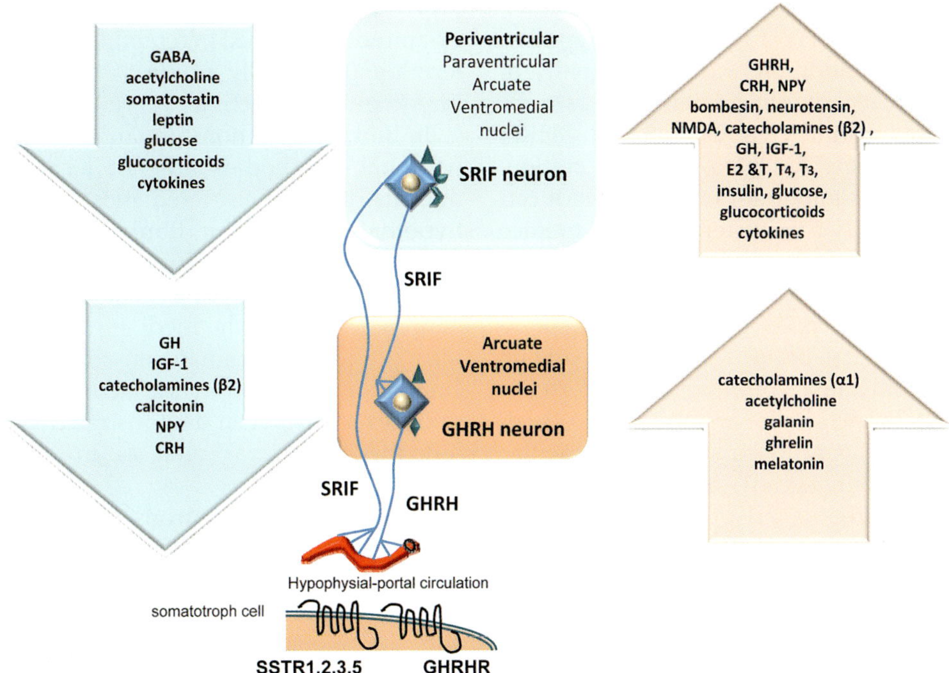

FIGURE 2.11 Stimulators (up arrow) and inhibitors (down arrow) of the growth-hormone-releasing hormone (GHRH) neuron and somatostatin (SRIF) neuron in the hypothalamic nulei. ▲ SRIF receptors; GH receptor; ❯ GHRH receptor; ♦ GH secretagogue receptor. GABA, γ-aminobutiric acid; SRIF, somatostatin; GHRH, growth-hormone releasing hormone; CRH, corticotropin-releasing hormone; NPY,Neuropeptide Y; NMDA, N-methyl-D-aspartate; GH, growth hormone; IGF-1, insulin-like growth factor 1; E2, estradiol; T, testosterone.

[103–105]. IGF-1 also reaches the hypothalamus from the periphery, as the median eminence and parts of the arcuate nucleus are outside the blood–brain barrier. Up-regulation of endogenous hypothalamic IGF-1 may also block pituitary GH secretion by inhibiting GHRH and stimulating somatostatin release [106].

Several other hormones and neurotransmitters regulate pituitary GH secretion. However, in some cases, it is difficult to distinguish between direct pituitary effects and indirect effects on GHRH or somatostatin neurons. Both GHRH and somatostatin neurons express receptors for several neurotransmitters and peptides, and multiple extrahypothalamic brain regions project to GHRH and somatostatin neurons. Some neurotransmitters regulate hypothalamic control of GH secretion. For example, activation of β_2 adrenoreceptor inhibits GH secretion through stimulation of somatostatin neurons while activation of α_2 adrenoreceptor stimulates GH secretion, in part by a dual effect that involves stimulation of GHRH and inhibition of somatostatin. Acetylcholine also enhances GHRH-induced GH secretion, mostly by activation of muscarinic receptor subtype 1 (M1) on somatostatin neurons, which inhibits somatostatin release. In addition, acetylcholine was recently discovered to activate M3 on hypothalamic GHRH neurons. M3 null mice exhibit pronounced anterior pituitary gland hypoplasia and a marked decrease in pituitary and serum growth hormone and prolactin. These deficits can be corrected by exogenous GHRH treatment [107].

Neuropeptides that regulate rodent GH secretion include galanin, ghrelin and melatonin which stimulate GH secretion, and calcitonin, neuropeptide Y (NPY) and CRH, which inhibit GH secretion. Galanin is a 29-amino-acid peptide expressed in the paraventricular and arcuate nuclei, and is co-expressed with GHRH. Both central and peripheral galanin administration induce GH secretion and potentiate GHRH-stimulated GH secretion [108]. In humans, galanin caused a significant increase in plasma GH through both direct GHRH stimulation [109] and somatostatin inhibition [108]. Interestingly, galanin mRNA expression in GHRH neurons is also considerably higher in males than females [108], suggesting that sexually dimorphic GH pulsatility may be related to galanin expression.

Ghrelin is a gut-derived 28-amino acid GH secretagogue that acts on the ghrelin receptor (GHS-R) to increase intracellular calcium concentration via inositol phosphate and stimulate GH release. GHS-R mRNA is expressed in arcuate and ventromedial hypothalamic nuclei and in the pituitary. Ghrelin dose dependently stimulates GH release from pituitary somatotrophs both in vitro and in vivo. Intravenous ghrelin injection stimulates GH release in both rats and humans [110]. Direct ghrelin action on hypothalamic GHRH to stimulate GH secretion is likely, since ghrelin does not stimulate GH release in patients with hypothalamic lesions, but does increase GHRH release from hypothalamic tissue in vitro. In addition, in rats, the ability of ghrelin to induce GH in primary pituitary cell cultures is significantly lower than in vivo. Ghrelin and GHRH co-treatment have a synergistic effect on GH secretion, suggesting that GHRH is important for ghrelin-induced GH release [110]. Centrally administered ghrelin to mice initiates a GH pulse, by both stimulating GHRH and inhibiting somatostatin release.

Neuropeptide Y (NPY) is a 36-amino-acid peptide widely distributed in the brain and in sympathetic neurons. In the hypothalamic–pituitary unit, NPY-containing neurons are located in the arcuate nucleus and, to a lesser extent, in paraventricular and periventricular nuclei. In the rat, intracerebral NPY injection or chronic infusion inhibit GH secretion, most likely through activation of somatostatin [111–113].

Gonadotropin-releasing Hormone (GnRH)

Gonadotropin-releasing hormone (GnRH) is a hypothalamic neuropeptide that regulates release of follicular-stimulating hormone (FSH) and luteinizing hormone (LH) by pituitary gonadotroph cells (Figure 2.12). Mammals express two GnRH genes. GnRH-I is located on chromosome 8, and GnRH-II is on chromosome 20 [114]. GnRH-I is the predominant peptide in the brain and hypothalamus and is the regulator of gonadotroph function. GnRH-II is expressed mostly outside the brain. The *GnRH-I* gene encodes a precursor protein of 92 amino acids that is further processed by prohormone convertase to create the 10-amino acid GnRH, retaining a pyroGlu at the N-terminus and a Gly-amide at the C-terminus that are important for bioactivity [114].

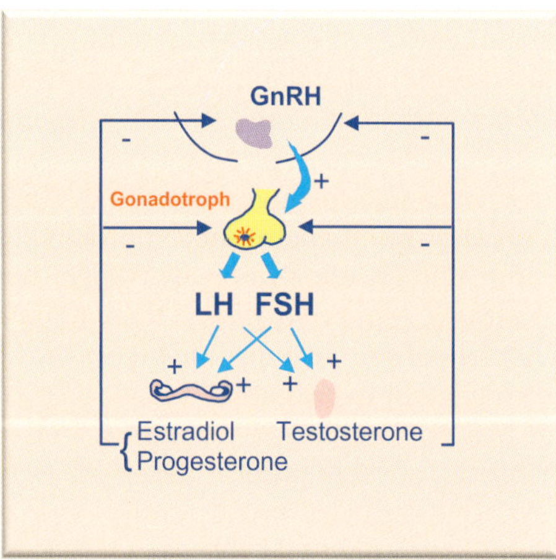

FIGURE 2.12 Hypothalamic gonadotropin-releasing hormone (GnRH) stimulates the gonadotroph to release follicular-stimulating hormone (FSH) and luteinizing hormone (LH). These two hormones in turn stimulate gonads to produce and release estradiol and testosterone and regulate germ cell function. Both estradiol and testosterone negatively regulate further release of GnRH, FSH and LH. *Reproduced from Melmed, S. Mechanisms for Tumorigenesis: The Plastic Pituitary, J Clin Invest 112 (2003) 1603–1618.*

In humans and non-human primates, small GnRH-I neuronal cell bodies are not localized to a specific nucleus, but are scattered mostly in the medio-basal hypothalamus, infundibular and periventricular regions, and form a diffuse neural network that coordinates the GnRH pulse generator [115,116]. GnRH-I neurons project to the median eminence and infundibular stalk and terminate on the hypophyseal–portal circulation and also in the neurohypophysis. GnRH-I mRNA has also been demonstrated in both the normal human pituitary as well as in pituitary adenomas [117].

Unlike the other neurons discussed in this chapter, GnRH neurons originate from outside the CNS and migrate to the hypothalamus depending upon a scaffold of neurons and glial cells, as well as chemotactic and adhesion molecules. GnRH neurons were believed to arise from the olfactory placode, supported by observations that GnRH deficiency in humans is accompanied by loss of the sense of smell (Kallmann syndrome) and by studies showing that ablation of the olfactory placode in animals causes loss of GnRH cells. However, GnRH-I neurons have also been proposed to arise from the region giving rise to the anterior pituitary placode, as demonstrated in chick and fish. Zebrafish mutants lacking a pituitary but with normal olfactory organs also lose hypothalamic GnRH-I neurons [118].

The GnRH receptor (GnRHR) is a small G-protein-coupled receptor that lacks a typical intracellular C-terminal cytoplasmic domain [117]. It mostly binds $G_{\alpha q/11}$ but may also bind $G_{\alpha s}$ and $G_{\alpha i}$. Dose-dependent coupling transition from one G_{α} subunit to another is likely important for an autocrine mechanism that maintains pulsatile GnRH-I secretion crucial for maintenance of normal gonadotropin release profiles. Upon binding, phospholipase C is activated and stimulates the diacylglycerol–PKC and inositol-3-phosphate pathways to increase intracellular calcium levels and stimulate FSH secretion [117,119]. These signaling pathways also activate MAPK cascades [117,119]. In the normal anterior pituitary, GnRHR immunopositivity colocalizes with α-subunit-, FSHβ-, LHβ-, TSHβ- and GH-producing cells, suggesting GnRHR expression in gonadotrophs, thyrotrophs and somatotrophs. GnRH levels regulate gonadotroph GnRHR expression levels [117]. When GnRH levels are low (e.g., during lactation and malnutrition), GnRHR expression declines substantially. Exposure of gonadotrophs to GnRH up-regulates GnRHR in the cell membrane. Long-term deprivation of GnRH necessitates longer periods of pituitary priming with repeated (but not continuous) pulses of

GnRH until optimal sensitivity to GnRH is achieved. Continuous exposure to GnRH down-regulates GnRH receptors by enhancing receptor internalization and degradation, rendering the gonadotroph insensitive to GnRH [120–122].

GnRH neurons exhibit a pulsatile pattern of coordinated, repetitive GnRH release into the hypophyseal–portal circulation. This GnRH pulse generator is controlled by both intrinsic [123] and external regulators [116]. Pulse frequency determines the rate of pulsatile FSH/LH release from gonadotrophs, the ratio between FSH and LH, and the degree to which FSH and LH are glycosylated, which determines their stability and potency. Although GnRH pulses match LH surges, FSH is not always pulsatile and is only partially concordant with LH surges. Therefore, LH, and not FSH, is used as an indicator for GnRH pulsatility. Higher GnRH frequencies increase LH and decrease FSH, thus increasing the LH/FSH ratio, while lower frequencies decrease the LH/FSH ratio [124]. Glycosylation of FSH and LH, especially the addition of terminal sialic acid, is important for physiological action, protecting from liver degradation, thereby prolonging their half life, however potency is decreased. Slow GnRH frequencies increase FSH glycosylation during the ovarian follicular phase and support follicle development, however, increased GnRH frequencies prior to ovulation generate more potent FSH with a shorter half life [125].

Multiple factors regulate GnRH neurons (Figure 2.13). GnRH regulates GnRH hypothalamic neurons that express GnRHR via an autocrine and/or paracrine effect. In addition, pituitary gonadotroph GnRH communicates with the hypothalamic GnRH system through hypothalamo–pituitary portal vessels and retrograde neurohypophyseal flow. Theoretically, linking two autocrine-controlled GnRH systems provides an additional regulatory mechanism, a short-loop feedback, that controls LH and GnRH secretion [116].

Kisspeptin (metastin) and its GPCR 54 (GPR54) are expressed in GnRH neurons and regulate their function [116,126,127]. Kisspeptin-1 enhances GnRH pulse amplitude and duration while GnRH inhibits kisspeptin-1 secretion. Moreover, GnRHR and GPR54 can heterodimerize, and this receptor complex may preferentially couple $G_{\alpha i}$ and thereby inhibit GnRH release. Galanin-like peptide (GALP) has a direct stimulatory action on GnRH secretion and is dependent on estradiol presence [128,129]. Both GALP and kisspeptin neurons express leptin receptors and are stimulated by leptin, linking GnRH neuron function, and thus the reproductive system, to nutrition and energy reserves [130].

Sex steroid hormones have a dramatic effect on GnRH release pattern. Estrogen receptors α and β (ERα and ERβ) [131], progesterone (PR) [132] and androgen receptors (AR) [133] exhibit considerable overlap, and are found in hypothalamic areas involved with reproduction and sexual behavior. GnRH neurons are regulated indirectly by sex steroids, as they are surrounded by cells, and receive terminals from other neurons that express sex steroid receptors [116]. Whether or not GnRH neurons express estrogen receptors and are directly regulated by estrogen is unclear [116,134]. In

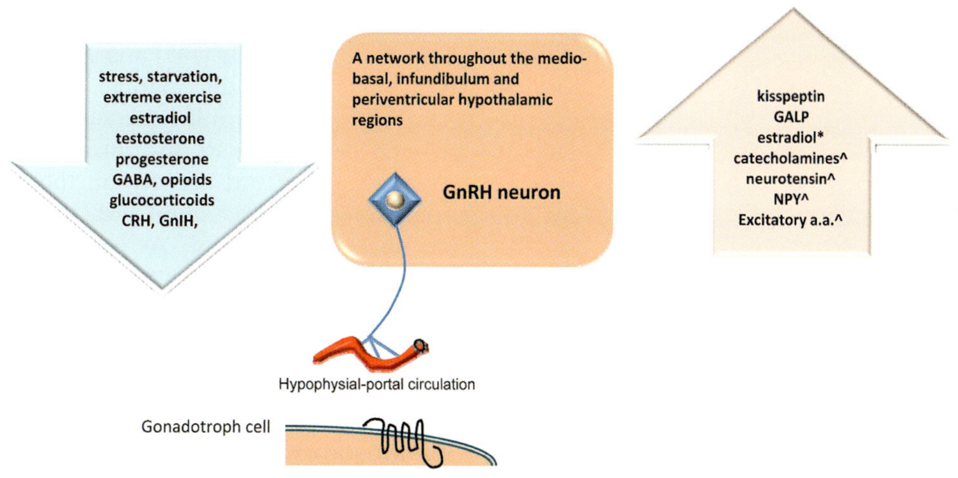

FIGURE 2.13 Stimulators (up arrow) and inhibitors (down arrow) of the gonadotropin-releasing hormone (GnRH) neuron in the hypothalamic medio-basal, infundibulum and periventricular hypothalamic regions. * Under certain physiological conditions including mid-cycle LH-surge, estradiol stimulates GnRH release. ^ hypothalamic factors enhancing estradiol-induced GnRH release. GnRH, gonadotropin-releasing factor; GALP, galanin-like peptide; NPY, neuropeptide Y; GABA, γ-aminobutiric acid; CRH, corticotropin-releasing hormone; GnIH, gonadotropin-inhibiting hormone; LH, luteinizing hormone; FSH, follicular-stimulating hormone; GnRHR1, gonadotropin-releasing hormone receptor subtype 1; a.a., amino acids.

general, estradiol, progesterone and testosterone reduce GnRH pulse frequency and GnRH release to the hypophyseal–portal circulation [135]. As sex steroids regulate pituitary LH and FSH in a species-specific manner, it is challenging to discriminate between the extent of inhibition in the hypothalamus and that of the pituitary in different species. In humans, estradiol inhibition of LH/FSH is dominant at the pituitary level, while progesterone and testosterone inhibition is mostly hypothalamic [135]. Estradiol also stimulates GnRH release and action during the pre-ovulatory LH surge in mid-estrous cycle depending on plasma concentration and duration of elevated estradiol. Estradiol-positive feedback increases GnRH release from GnRH neurons and synthesis and expression of GnRHR on gonadotroph membranes, increasing their sensitivity to GnRH. Mechanisms mediating the dual inhibitory/stimulatory effect of estradiol on GnRH neurons and the switch between the two forms are unclear, but are likely due to afferents from other estradiol-responsive neurons that directly regulate GnRH neurons.

Neural enhancers of the estradiol stimulatory effect on GnRH include excitatory amino acids, catecholamines, NPY and neurotensin [136]. Glutamate and aspartate, directly or indirectly, lead to GnRH stimulation and increased LH release [137]. Aspartate- and glutamate-induced GnRH release are strongly affected by sex steroids, and are important in regulating the GnRH pulse generator and synchronizing the estrous cycle.

Noradrenergic and adrenergic neurons stimulate both pulsatile and pre-ovulatory release of GnRH, mostly through the α1-adrenergic receptor. Some NPY neurons in the arcuate nucleus express ERα, and NPY expression is regulated by estrogen. NPY neurons also send efferents that terminate on GnRH neurons. NPY levels are increased before the LH surge, and inhibition of NPY synthesis prevents the LH surge. Neurotensin expressed by neurons in the preoptic area mediates estrogen-induced release of GnRH, mostly through the NT1 receptor subtype. Neurotensin neurons express ER, and neurotensin synthesis is induced by estrogen. Inhibition of NPY synthesis attenuates the LH surge.

Neural inhibitors of the stimulatory effect of estradiol on GnRH include GABA and opioids, and a significant decrease in their tone prior to the LH surge is critical for surge generation [136]. GABA inhibits the LH surge. GABA neurons express ERα and are sensitive to estradiol action. GABA likely acts on GnRH neurons directly, as GABAergic neuron synapses terminate on GnRH neurons that express functional $GABA_A$. Endogenous opioids contribute to inhibition of the stimulatory estradiol effect on GnRH neurons through indirect neural circuits, since GnRH neurons do not express opioid receptors.

Recently, gonadotropin inhibitory hormone (GnIH) was discovered in birds [138]. Orthologous peptides were then discovered in mammals belonging to the RF-amide peptide superfamily (RFRP). In mammals including humans, RFRP 1, 2 and 3 are similar in function to the avian GnIH, and should therfore similarly be called GnIH 1, 2 and 3. GnIH neurons localize to hypothalamic nuclei and project to GnRH neurons in the median eminence, where expression of the cognate GnIH receptor (GnIH-R) can be found. GnIH neurons also project to orexin and melanin-concentrating hormone (MCH) neurons, pro-opiomelanocortin (POMC) and NPY cells. GnIH receptors, previously named neuropeptide FF receptor subtype 1 (NPFF1), are GPCR highly expressed in the hypothalamus. GnIH reduce the firing rate of GnRH neurons and GnRH release. GnIH is also involved in appetite and energy balance, and increases food intake when administered centrally [138].

GnRH release decreases during the postnatal period and begins to increase again in late childhood. Increased GnRH during puberty results from a combination of increased stimulatory tone and a simultaneous decrease in inhibitory tone [139]. Hypothalamic GABAergic tone is reduced in monkeys in early puberty, and premature activation of GnRH neurons followed inhibition of GABAergic tone in pre-puberty [139]. During the same time, increased hypothalamic glutaminergic effect, increased NPY, norepinephrine, kisspeptin and GALP stimulate GnRH neurons at puberty.

Multiple physical and psychological stressors suppress GnRH neuron activity, including starvation, intense exercise, extreme temperature, pain, trauma and infection [140]. CRH, increased glucocorticoid levels [141], GABA, opioids [142] and leptin are also involved in a stress-type-specific manner. Activins and inhibins, members of transforming growth factor β (TGF-β), are secreted by the gonads and indirectly affect the GnRH pulse generator and activity on the pituitary through regulation of FSH secretion and GnRH receptor expression on the gonadotroph. Activin, produced by both the gonads and the pituitary, stimulates FSH release and increases GnRHR expression mostly in an autocrine/paracrine way, while inhibin suppresses FSH secretion in an endocrine fashion [143].

Somatostatin

Somatotropin release-inhibiting hormone (SRIF) or somatostatin 14 was inadvertently discovered in 1973 during the search for a hypothalamic growth-hormone-releasing factor [76]. SRIF28, a 28-amino acid somatostatin peptide that is a longer form of SRIF14, was discovered immediately thereafter [76]. The somatostatin gene is located on the long arm of chromosome 3 and comprises two exons and one intron. The two exons encode prepro-somatostatin however, only exon 2 encodes SRIF14 and SRIF28. Both peptides are derived from post-translational cleavage of pro-somatostatin by PC1 and PC2 and carboxypeptidase E [76]. Somatostatins are cyclic peptides with a single covalent bond between two Cys residues and a bioactive core composed of a Phe-Trp-Lys-Thr amino acid sequence. SRIF14 is the predominant peptide in the brain, while SRIF28 is the predominant peptide in the GI tract [76]. The name somatostatin was given as this peptide was primarily discovered to inhibit pituitary GH release, however, this peptide also inhibits TSH, ACTH and other central and peripheral hormones [144]. Moreover, in some tissues SRIF14 exhibits both stimulatory and inhibitory acute actions [144].

Members of the SRIF family of peptides are derived from a common primordial gene that divided at about the time of the advent of chordates to create two parallel genes, preprosomatostatin and preprocortistatin, that were later independently mutated. Preprosomatostatin was further duplicated into preprosomatostatin I and preprosomatostatin II ~400 million years ago [76]. While fish and amphibians both have preprosomatostatin I and II, mammals have a single preprosomatostatin similar to preprosomatostatin I that gives rise to SRIF14 and SRIF28. Preprosomatostatin II gives rise to other SRIF products, for example angelfish SRIF28 or catfish SRIF 22. SRIF14 is identical in all vertebrates and exhibits a high degree of homology to SRIF14 in invertebrates and protozoa [76]. SRIF14 is the main form in the brain including the hypothalamus, while cortistatin is mostly expressed in the hippocampus and cortex [76].

Somatostatin is expressed widely throughout the brain, however hypothalamic SRIF14 is the major regulator of pituitary function. Hypothalamic somatostatin is produced predominantly in the anterior periventricular nucleus, as well as in the paraventricular, arcuate and ventromedial hypothalamic nuclei. These neurons project into the median eminence, and their fibers terminate on the hypophyseal–portal circulation, where they release somatostatin into the blood reaching anterior pituitary cells [76]. Some axons terminate in the posterior pituitary [145]. Additional minor routes for somatostatin to reach the pituitary include CSF leakage from the third ventricle to the portal system, peripheral somatostatin and short portal blood vessels crossing from the posterior to the anterior pituitary [145]. Thus somatostatin acts as an endocrine hormone on the anterior pituitary.

The primary function of somatostatin is to inhibit pituitary hormone secretion and, to a lesser extent, pituitary cell growth. These are accomplished by inhibition of hypothalamic peptides responsible for pituitary hormone synthesis and secretion and by direct effects on pituitary cells themselves. In the hypothalamus, somatostatin inhibits release of several hypothalamic hormones and neurotransmitters, including CRH, TRH, dopamine, norepinephrine [76] and GHRH [101,146]. Somatostatin also inhibits its own secretion from the periventricular nucleus [76]. In the pituitary, somatostatin inhibits secretion of GH, TSH and ACTH in the presence of low glucocorticoid levels, and estrogen-induced PRL [147].

Somatostatin signals through five somatostatin receptor subtypes, SSTR1, 2, 3, 4 and 5. These are G-PCR encoded by specific genes on different chromosomes. SSTR2 is alternatively spliced to SSTR2a and SSTR2b in rodents but not in humans; however, only the SSTR2a isoform is expressed in the pituitary [147]. Somatostatin 14 exhibits high binding affinities to all the receptor subtypes, but has greatest affinity to SSTR2, which is the subtype largely responsible for inhibiting pituitary hormone secretion. Most studies on somatostatin receptor action in pituitary cells have involved SSTR2 and SSTR5. Upon ligand binding, the receptors bind the $G_{\alpha i/o}$ subunit, which in turn inhibits adenylyl cyclase and thus reduces cytoplasmic cAMP levels. Receptor activation also initiates opening of potassium channels and closure of calcium channels. These mechanisms result in suppression of hormone secretion [147].

Multiple factors regulate hypothalamic somatostatin secretion, including ions and nutrients, neuropeptides, neurotransmitters, classical hormones, growth factors and cytokines (Figure 2.11). Intracellular stimulators of somatostatin include stimuli that induce membrane depolarization, calcium, cAMP, cGMP and nitric oxide. Stimulators of hypothalamic somatostatin include GHRH, CRH, bombesin, neurotensin, NMDA, GH, IGF-I, estrogen, testosterone, thyroxin, insulin and glucagon, and cytokines such as IL-1, IL-6, IL-10, INFγ and TNFα. Inhibitors of somatostatin release include opiates, GABA, leptin, glucose and TGFβ. Glucocorticoids have a dual effect on somatostatin release from the hypothalamus: at low doses, glucocorticoids stimulate stomatastatin secretion, but high doses inhibit somatostatin release [76].

Somatostatin receptor expression is also regulated by multiple factors. For example, pituitary SSTR2 is up-regulated by prolonged exposure to somatostatin, GHRH, testosterone and by short exposure to glucocorticoids and TGFβ. In contrast, somatastatin receptor expression is down-regulated by ghrelin and chronic glucocorticoid exposure. SSTR5 is up-regulated by sustained exposure to somatostatin and thyroxine, and down-regulated by GHRH, ghrelin and estrogen [147].

Prolactin-inhibitory Factors (PIF)

Pituitary prolactin secretion is under tonic inhibition by hypothalamic dopamine (Figure 2.14). In the absence of this inhibition (such as when the pituitary stalk is damaged, or when the gland is ectopically transplanted), a marked increase in lactotroph production and secretion of prolactin ensues [148]. Studies in rats demonstrated that hypothalamic dopamine is released from neurons located in the arcuate and anterior periventricular nuclei. Tuberoinfundibular dopaminergic (TIDA) neurons project into the external zone of the median eminence, and are considered the major source of dopamine to the anterior pituitary. Tuberohypophyseal dopamine (THDA) neurons also project into the posterior and intermediate pituitary, while periventricular hypophyseal dopaminergic (PHDA) neurons project to the intermediate pituitary lobe. The anterior pituitary also receives inhibitory dopaminergic input from the posterior and intermediate pituitary through interconnecting short portal veins [149]. Dopamine also inhibits MSH release from melanotrophs located in the intermediate lobe, which is rudimentary in humans. Increased dopamine release from rat THDA and PHDA is associated with decreased melanotroph POMC gene expression, proliferation [150] and serum MSH levels [151].

Dopamine is a catecholamine with a catechol nucleus (benzene ring with two adjacent hydroxyl groups) and one amine group. Catecholamine neurotransmitters share a common synthetic pathway: the amino acid tyrosine is metabolized to dihydroxyphenylalanine (DOPA) by thyrosine hydroxylase; DOPA is then decarboxylated to dopamine by aromatic L-amino acid decarboxylase. In dopaminergic neurons, further metabolism of dopamine does not occur, but in noradrenergic neurons, dopamine is subsequently hydroxylated to norepinephrine by dopamine β hydroxylase, and then to epinephrine by phenylethanolamine N-methyl transferase (PNMT).

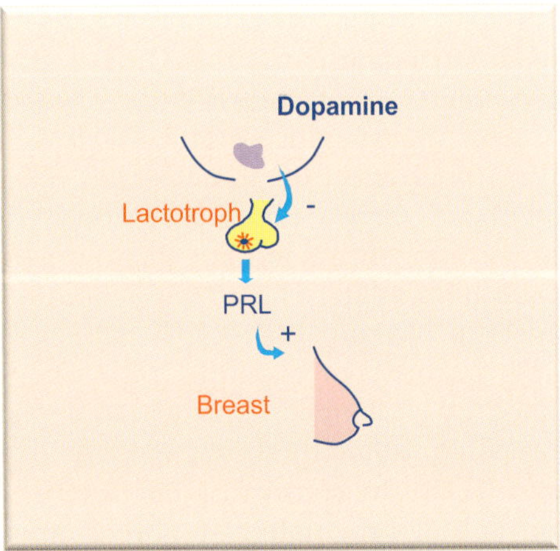

FIGURE 2.14 Hypothalamic dopamine neurons release dopamine that exerts tonic pituitary lactotroph inhibition, reducing prolactin (PRL) synthesis and secretion. *Reproduced from Melmed, S. Mechanisms for Tumorigenesis: The Plastic Pituitary, J Clin Invest 112 (2003) 1603–1618.*

Dopamine binds dopamine receptor subtype 2 (D2R) on pituitary lactotrophs, to inhibit prolactin synthesis and release, and lactotroph proliferation. D2R null mice develop lactotroph hyperplasia, hyperprolactinemia and lactotroph adenomas, which indicates that at least in mice, D2R is the predominant dopamine receptor mediating the dopamine effect on prolactin [152]. D2R is a GPCR that couples the $G_{\alpha i/o}$ subunit to decrease adenylyl cyclase and intracellular cAMP levels, increase potassium influx, inhibit inositol phosphate production and decrease intracellular calcium concentration. These signaling pathways acutely inhibit prolactin secretion [153], and to a lesser extent secretion of TSH. Multiple downstream signaling pathways involved in lactotroph proliferation inhibition include adenylyl cyclase-PKA, MAPK [154] and phosphotyrosine phosphatase [155]; however, the exact mechanisms are unclear.

Although dopamine is considered the main prolactin-inhibitory factor, there are frequent inconsistencies between dopamine levels in the hypophyseal–portal circulation and rat serum prolactin levels. For instance, even though serum prolactin levels are similar in males and females, dopamine levels in the hypophyseal–portal circulation are five to seven times lower in males. The apparent inconsistency between dopaminergic activity and prolactin secretion has been attributed to other hypothalamic factors that can alter prolactin release in vitro and in vivo, including γ-aminobutyric acid (GABA), somatostatin that inhibit and calcitonin that stimulate prolactin [148].

Prolactin-releasing Factors (PRF)

Reduced dopamine availability to lactotroph cells causes increased prolactin synthesis and release. However, a number of hypothalamic factors inconsistently stimulate prolactin secretion. These include TRH, oxytocin, vasopressin, VIP, angiotensin II, NPY, galanin, substance P, bombesin-like peptides (gastrin-releasing peptide, neuromedin B and C) and neurotensin [148]. TRH, oxytocin, vasopressin and VIP concentrations in the hypophyseal–portal circulation are higher than in the periphery, and are sufficient to stimulate prolactin release in vitro. Blocking these peptide activities decreases prolactin release.

Neurons in the paraventricular nucleus that project into the median eminence secrete TRH into the hypophyseal–portal circulation. TRH stimulates pituitary prolactin secretion in vitro and in vivo in estrogen-primed male rats [156]. Interestingly, transient dopamine antagonism or withdrawal enhances the stimulatory effect of TRH on prolactin secretion [148].

Oxytocin and vasopressin reach anterior pituitary lactotrophs through both the long and short hypophyseal–portal circulation. Oxytocin inconsistently functions as a PRF. Oxytocin increases male rat prolactin levels while inhibition of oxytocin reduces prolactin surges induced by suckling or by estrogen, and blocks endogenous stimulatory rhythms controlling prolactin secretion in female rats. In contrast, low-dose oxytocin injections reduced basal and stress-induced prolactin secretion in male rats. In addition, blocking vasopressin activity with antiserum attenuates suckling-induced rise of plasma prolactin [148].

VIP, peptide histidine-isoleucine (PHI), or its human homologue PHM, influence pituitary prolactin secretion, are synthesized from the same prohormone precursor, and are released simultaneously with CRH from neurons located in the paraventricular nucleus. Both stimulate prolactin release in rats and in vitro. PACAP, a VIP-like hypothalamic peptide, dose-dependently stimulates pituitary prolactin in both male and non-suckled lactating female rats [148].

At very low (pM) concentrations, dopamine may actually stimulate prolactin secretion, but the physiological relevance of these studies in humans is unclear [157–159].

Prolactin receptors are expressed on all dopaminergic neurons that supply the pituitary, enabling a short negative feedback loop of prolactin on dopamine synthesis. Increasing prolactin levels increases thyrosine hydroxylase expression that in turn increases dopamine expression and leads to decreased prolactin levels [160,161]. Factors that increase prolactin secretion eventually increase dopamine synthesis and release; examples include estrogen [162] and placental lactogens [148]. Estrogen increases prolactin mainly by reducing expression of lactotroph dopamine receptors. Long-term estrogen treatment also reduces levels of tyrosine hydroxylase and dopamine content in TIDA neurons. Placental lactogens also inhibit tyrosine hydroxylase and dopamine content [163].

Multiple neural systems regulate dopaminergic neurons and PIF and PRF neurons, and subsequently regulate prolactin secretion. TIDA neurons are stimulated by acetylcholine, glutamate and opioids, and inhibited by stress, high levels of glucocorticoids and histamine. PRF neurons in the paraventricular nucleus are stimulated by serotonin. TIDA neurons are also controlled by light, constituting the major neuroendocrine mechanism underlying the prolactin circadian rhythm. Since both the pituitary and the hypothalamus express dopamine receptors, most neuroleptics that inhibit dopamine secretion also increase prolactin levels [164].

SUMMARY

There has been considerable progress in our knowledge of the anatomical, physiological and pathophysiological aspects of the hypothalamic pituitary unit since their intimate interaction was recognized almost a century ago. Discovery of pituitary hormones was followed by isolation of hypothalamic neuropeptides that regulate their synthesis, their cognate receptors and multiple signaling pathways which they activate. Extensive feedback mechanisms, essential for neuroendocrine fine-tuning and complex brain networking widely regulate hypothalamic neuropeptides to alter pituitary and target gland responses. Though the need to unravel hypothalamic–pituitary interaction is crucial for understanding health and disease, inaccessibility of the human hypothalamus and pituitary tissue for research and the complexity of scientific techniques required for these studies will continue to challenge progress in this field.

References

[1] C.T. Sawin, Berta and Ernst Scharrer and the concept of neurosecretion, The Endocrinologist 13 (2003) 73–75.

[2] M.M. Klavdieva, The history of neuropeptides 1, Front Neuroendocrinol 16 (1995) 293–321.

[3] G.W. Harris, Neural control of the pituitary gland. I. The neurohypophysis, Br Med J 2 (1951) 559–564.

[4] E. Scharrer, Neurosecretion. X. A relationship between the paraphysis and the paraventricular nucleus in the garter snake (Thamnophis sp.), Biological bulletin 101 (1951) 106–113.

[5] H.J. Berkeley, The finer anatomy of the infundibular region of the cerebrum including the pituitary gland, Brain 17 (1894) 515–547.

[6] G.T. Popa, U. Fielding, Hypophysio-portal vessels and their colloid accompaniment, J Anat 67 (1933) 221, 227–232.

[7] G.W. Harris, Electrical stimulation of the hypothalamus and the mechanism of neural control of the adenohypophysis, J Physiol 107 (1948) 418–429.

[8] R. Guillemin, 2008 Somatostatin: The beginnings, Mol Cell Endocrinol 286 (1972) 3–4.

[9] A.V. Schally, M. Saffran, B. Zimmermann, A corticotrophin-releasing factor: Partial purification and amino acid composition, Biochem J 70 (1958) 97–103.

[10] H.L. Sheehan, K. Kovacs, Neurohypophysis and hypothalamus, in: J.M.B Bloodworth Jr. (Ed.), Endocrine Pathology, General and Surgical, Williams & Wilkins, Baltimore, 1982, pp. 45–99.

[11] B.W. Scheithauer, The hypothalamus and neurohypophysis, in: K. Kovacs, S.L. Asa (Eds.), Functional Endocrine Pathology, second ed)., Blackwell Science, Boston, 1991, pp. 171–296.

[12] G. Ambach, M. Palkovits, J. Szentagothai, Blood supply of the rat hypothalamus. IV. Retrochiasmatic area, median eminence, arcuate nucleus, Acta Morphol Acad Sci Hung 24 (1976) 93–119.

[13] R.D. Broadwell, B.J. Balin, M. Salcman, R.S. Kaplan, Brain–blood barrier? Yes and no, Proc Nat Acad Sci USA 80 (1983) 7352–7356.

[14] R.B. Page, The anatomy of the hypothalamo–hypophyseal complex, in: E. Knobil, J. Neill, L.L. Ewing, G.S. Greenwald, C.L. Markert, D.W. Pfaff (Eds.), The Physiology of Reproduction, Raven Press, New York, 1988, pp. 1161–1233.
[15] K.M. Knigge, D.E. Scott, Structure and function of the median eminence, Am J Anat 129 (1970) 223–243.
[16] E.M. Rodriguez, J.L. Blazquez, F.E. Pastor, B. Pelaez, P. Pena, B. Peruzzo, et al., Hypothalamic tanycytes: A key component of brain-endocrine interaction, Int Rev Cytol 247 (2005) 89–164.
[17] I. Clarke, D. Jessop, R. Millar, M. Morris, S. Bloom, S. Lightman, et al., Many peptides that are present in the external zone of the median eminence are not secreted into the hypophysial portal blood of sheep, Neuroendocrinology 57 (1993) 765–775.
[18] R.B. Page, Pituitary blood flow, Am J Physiol 243 (1982) E427–442.
[19] D.J. Begley, M.W. Brightman, Structural and functional aspects of the blood–brain barrier, Prog Drug Res 61 (2003) 39–78.
[20] S.W. Shaver, J.J. Pang, D.S. Wainman, K.M. Wall, P.M. Gross, Morphology and function of capillary networks in subregions of the rat tuber cinereum, Cell Tissue Res 267 (1992) 437–448.
[21] P. Ciofi, M. Garret, O. Lapirot, P. Lafon, A. Loyens, V. Prevot, et al., Brain–endocrine interactions: A microvascular route in the mediobasal hypothalamus, Endocrinology 150 (2009) 5509–5519.
[22] G.I. Hatton, L.S. Perlmutter, A.K. Salm, C.D. Tweedle, Dynamic neuronal-glial interactions in hypothalamus and pituitary: Implications for control of hormone synthesis and release, Peptides 5 (Suppl 1) (1984) 121–138.
[23] S.R. Ojeda, A. Lomniczi, U.S. Sandau, Glial-gonadotrophin hormone (GnRH) neurone interactions in the median eminence and the control of GnRH secretion, J Neuroendocrinol 20 (2008) 732–742.
[24] S.L. Asa, Tumors of the pituitary gland. Atlas of tumor pathology, Fascicle 22, Third series, Armed Forces Institute of Pathology, Washington DC, 1998.
[25] E. Horvath, K. Kovacs, Fine structural cytology of the adenohypophysis in rat and man, J Electron Microsc Tech 8 (1988) 401–432.
[26] P.J. Morgan, L.M. Williams, The pars tuberalis of the pituitary: A gateway for neuroendocrine output, Rev Reprod 1 (1996) 153–161.
[27] E. Horvath, K. Kovacs, G. Penz, C. Ezrin, Origin, possible function and fate of "follicular cells" in the anterior lobe of the human pituitary, Am J Pathol 77 (1974) 199–212.
[28] C. Girod, J. Trouillas, M.P. Dubois, Immunocytochemical localization of S-100 protein in stellate cells (folliculo-stellate cells) of the anterior lobe of the normal human pituitary, Cell Tissue Res 241 (1985) 505–511.
[29] H. Hofler, G.F. Walter, H. Denk, Immunohistochemistry of folliculo-stellate cells in normal human adenohypophyses and in pituitary adenomas, Acta Neuropathol 65 (1984) 35–40.
[30] K. Kovacs, E. Horvath, N. Ryan, C. Ezrin, Null cell adenoma of the human pituitary, Virchows Arch A Pathol Anat Histol 387 (1980) 165–174.
[31] E.M. Dyess, T.P. Segerson, Z. Liposits, W.K. Paull, M.M. Kaplan, P. Wu, et al., Triiodothyronine exerts direct cell-specific regulation of thyrotropin-releasing hormone gene expression in the hypothalamic paraventricular nucleus, Endocrinology 123 (1988) 2291–2297.
[32] M. Yamada, S. Radovick, F.E. Wondisford, Y. Nakayama, B.D. Weintraub, J.F. Wilber, Cloning and structure of human genomic DNA and hypothalamic cDNA encoding human prepro-thyrotropin-releasing hormone, Mol Endocrinol 4 (1990) 551–556.
[33] M. Perello, E.A. Nillni, The biosynthesis and processing of neuropeptides: Lessons from prothyrotropin releasing hormone (proTRH), Front Biosci 12 (2007) 3554–3565.
[34] Y. Sun, X. Lu, M.C. Gershengorn, Thyrotropin-releasing hormone receptors – similarities and differences, J Mol Endocrinol 30 (2003) 87–97.
[35] M. Mori, M. Yamada, S. Kobayashi, Role of the hypothalamic TRH in the regulation of its own receptors in rat anterior pituitaries, Neuroendocrinology 48 (1988) 153–159.
[36] G. Faglia, The clinical impact of the thyrotropin-releasing hormone test, Thyroid 8 (1998) 903–908.
[37] J.M. Hartnell, A.E. Pekary, J.M. Hershman, Comparison of the effects of pulsatile and continuous TRH infusion on TSH release in men, Metabolism 36 (1987) 878–882.
[38] M.I. Chiamolera, F.E. Wondisford, Minireview: Thyrotropin-releasing hormone and the thyroid hormone feedback mechanism, Endocrinology 150 (2009) 1091–1096.
[39] J. Weeke, The response of thyrotropin and triiodothyronine to various doses of thyrotropin releasing hormone in normal man, Eur J Clin Invest 5 (1975) 447–453.
[40] I.M. Jackson, Thyrotropin-releasing hormone, N Engl J Med 306 (1982) 145–155.
[41] M. Yamada, N. Shibusawa, S. Ishii, K. Horiguchi, R. Umezawa, K. Hashimoto, et al., Prolactin secretion in mice with thyrotropin-releasing hormone deficiency, Endocrinology 147 (2006) 2591–2596.
[42] R.M. Lechan, C. Fekete, Role of thyroid hormone deiodination in the hypothalamus, Thyroid 15 (2005) 883–897.
[43] C. Fekete, R.M. Lechan, Negative feedback regulation of hypophysiotropic thyrotropin-releasing hormone (TRH) synthesizing neurons: Role of neuronal afferents and type 2 deiodinase, Front Neuroendocrinol 28 (2007) 97–114.
[44] A.N. Hollenberg, T. Monden, T.R. Flynn, M.E. Boers, O. Cohen, F.E. Wondisford, The human thyrotropin-releasing hormone gene is regulated by thyroid hormone through two distinct classes of negative thyroid hormone response elements, Mol Endocrinol 9 (1995) 540–550.
[45] M.A. Shupnik, W.W. Chin, J.F. Habener, E.C. Ridgway, Transcriptional regulation of the thyrotropin subunit genes by thyroid hormone, J Biol Chem 260 (1985) 2900–2903.
[46] M.A. Shupnik, E.C. Ridgway, Triiodothyronine rapidly decreases transcription of the thyrotropin subunit genes in thyrotropic tumor explants, Endocrinology 117 (1985) 1940–1946.
[47] G.E. Dahl, N.P. Evans, L.A. Thrun, F.J. Karsch, A central negative feedback action of thyroid hormones on thyrotropin-releasing hormone secretion, Endocrinology 135 (1994) 2392–2397.
[48] J. Drouin, A. De Lean, D. Rainville, R. Lachance, F. Labric, Characteristics of the interaction between thyrotropin-releasing hormone and somatostatin for thyrotropin and prolactin release, Endocrinology 98 (1976) 514–521.
[49] F. Rodriguez, T. Jolin, The role of somatostatin and/or dopamine in basal and TRH-stimulated TSH release in food-restricted rats, Acta Endocrinol (Copenh) 125 (1991) 186–191.
[50] I. Nicoletti, P. Filipponi, L. Fedeli, F. Ambrosi, C. Giammartino, F. Spinozzi, et al., Catecholamines and pituitary function. IV. Effects of low-dose dopamine infusion and long-term bromocriptine treatment on the abnormal thyrotroph (TSH) dynamics in patients with pathological hyperprolactinaemia, Acta Endocrinol (Copenh) 111 (1986) 154–161.
[51] R.M. Lechan, C. Fekete, Feedback regulation of thyrotropin-releasing hormone (TRH): Mechanisms for the non-thyroidal illness syndrome, J Endocrinol Invest 27 (2004) 105–119.

[52] R.S. Ahima, D. Prabakaran, C. Mantzoros, D. Qu, B. Lowell, E. Maratos-Flier, et al., Role of leptin in the neuroendocrine response to fasting, Nature 382 (1996) 250–252.

[53] D.A. Lovejoy, Structural evolution of urotensin-I: Reflections of life before corticotropin releasing factor, Gen Comp Endocrinol 164 (2009) 15–19.

[54] G. Aguilera, M. Nikodemova, P.C. Wynn, K.J. Catt, Corticotropin releasing hormone receptors: Two decades later, Peptides 25 (2004) 319–329.

[55] A.G. Watts, Glucocorticoid regulation of peptide genes in neuroendocrine CRH neurons: A complexity beyond negative feedback, Front Neuroendocrinol 26 (2005) 109–130.

[56] S. Shibahara, Y. Morimoto, Y. Furutani, M. Notake, H. Takahashi, S. Shimizu, et al., Isolation and sequence analysis of the human corticotropin-releasing factor precursor gene, EMBO J 2 (1983) 775–779.

[57] C. Tsatsanis, E. Dermitzaki, M. Venihaki, E. Chatzaki, V. Minas, A. Gravanis, et al., The corticotropin-releasing factor (CRF) family of peptides as local modulators of adrenal function, Cell Mol Life Sci 64 (2007) 1638–1655.

[58] K. Gysling, M.I. Forray, P. Haeger, C. Daza, R. Rojas, Corticotropin-releasing hormone and urocortin: Redundant or distinctive functions? Brain Res Brain Res Rev 47 (2004) 116–125.

[59] E. Gutknecht, I. Van der Linden, K. Van Kolen, K.F. Verhoeven, G. Vauquelin, F.M. Dautzenberg, Molecular mechanisms of corticotropin-releasing factor receptor-induced calcium signaling, Mol Pharmacol 75 (2009) 648–657.

[60] P.W. Gold, D.L. Loriaux, A. Roy, M.A. Kling, J.R. Calabrese, C.H. Kellner, et al., Responses to corticotropin-releasing hormone in the hypercortisolism of depression and Cushing's disease. Pathophysiologic and diagnostic implications, N Engl J Med 314 (1986) 1329–1335.

[61] M.E. Davis, C.J. Pemberton, T.G. Yandle, J.G. Lainchbury, M.T. Rademaker, M.G. Nicholls, et al., Urocortin-1 infusion in normal humans, J Clin Endocrinol Metab 89 (2004) 1402–1409.

[62] M.A. Kling, M.D. DeBellis, D.K. O'Rourke, S.J. Listwak, T.D. Geracioti Jr., I.E. McCutcheon, et al., Diurnal variation of cerebrospinal fluid immunoreactive corticotropin-releasing hormone levels in healthy volunteers, J Clin Endocrinol Metab 79 (1994) 233–239.

[63] L.J. Muglia, L. Jacobson, S.C. Weninger, C.E. Luedke, D.S. Bae, K.H. Jeong, et al., Impaired diurnal adrenal rhythmicity restored by constant infusion of corticotropin-releasing hormone in corticotropin-releasing hormone-deficient mice, J Clin Invest 99 (1997) 2923–2929.

[64] L. Muglia, L. Jacobson, P. Dikkes, J.A. Majzoub, Corticotropin-releasing hormone deficiency reveals major fetal but not adult glucocorticoid need, Nature 373 (1995) 427–432.

[65] P.E. Sawchenko, H.Y. Li, A. Ericsson, Circuits and mechanisms governing hypothalamic responses to stress: A tale of two paradigms, Prog Brain Res 122 (2000) 61–78.

[66] J.P. Herman, H. Figueiredo, N.K. Mueller, Y. Ulrich-Lai, M.M. Ostrander, D.C. Choi, et al., Central mechanisms of stress integration: Hierarchical circuitry controlling hypothalamo–pituitary–adrenocortical responsiveness, Front Neuroendocrinol 24 (2003) 151–180.

[67] S. Reichlin, Neuroendocrinology of infection and the innate immune system, Recent Prog Horm Res 54 (1999) 133–181 discussion 181–183.

[68] H. Besedovsky, A. del Rey, E. Sorkin, C.A. Dinarello, Immunoregulatory feedback between interleukin-1 and glucocorticoid hormones, Science 233 (1986) 652–654.

[69] I. Berczi, A. Quintanar-Stephano, K. Kovacs, Neuroimmune regulation in immunocompetence, acute illness, and healing, Ann NY Acad Sci 1153 (2009) 220–239.

[70] D. Durand, M. Pampillo, C. Caruso, M. Lasaga, Role of metabotropic glutamate receptors in the control of neuroendocrine function, Neuropharmacology 55 (2008) 577–583.

[71] K.J. Kovacs, I.H. Miklos, B. Bali, GABAergic mechanisms constraining the activity of the hypothalamo–pituitary–adrenocortical axis, Ann NY Acad Sci 1018 (2004) 466–476.

[72] M.W. Schwartz, R.J. Seeley, L.A. Campfield, P. Burn, D.G. Baskin, Identification of targets of leptin action in rat hypothalamus, J Clin Invest 98 (1996) 1101–1106.

[73] M. Jang, A. Mistry, A.G. Swick, D.R. Romsos, Leptin rapidly inhibits hypothalamic neuropeptide Y secretion and stimulates corticotropin-releasing hormone secretion in adrenalectomized mice, J Nutr 130 (2000) 2813–2820.

[74] N. Liao, H. Vaudry, G. Pelletier, Neuroanatomical connections between corticotropin-releasing factor (CRF) and somatostatin (SRIF) nerve endings and thyrotropin-releasing hormone (TRH) neurons in the paraventricular nucleus of rat hypothalamus, Peptides 13 (1992) 677–680.

[75] X.M. Wang, J.J. Tresham, J.P. Coghlan, B.A. Scoggins, Intracerebroventricular infusion of a cyclic hexapeptide analogue of somatostatin inhibits hemorrhage-induced ACTH release, Neuroendocrinology 45 (1987) 325–327.

[76] Y.C. Patel, Somatostatin and its receptor family, Front Neuroendocrinol 20 (1999) 157–198.

[77] A. Szafarczyk, V. Guillaume, B. Conte-Devolx, G. Alonso, F. Malaval, N. Pares-Herbute, et al., Central catecholaminergic system stimulates secretion of CRH at different sites, Am J Physiol 255 (1988) E463–468.

[78] M.J. Eaton, S. Cheung, K.E. Moore, K.J. Lookingland, Dopamine receptor-mediated regulation of corticotropin-releasing hormone neurons in the hypothalamic paraventricular nucleus, Brain Res 738 (1996) 60–66.

[79] M.A. Cowley, R.G. Smith, S. Diano, M. Tschop, N. Pronchuk, K.L. Grove, et al., The distribution and mechanism of action of ghrelin in the CNS demonstrates a novel hypothalamic circuit regulating energy homeostasis, Neuron 37 (2003) 649–661.

[80] S. Reichlin, Thyroid function, body temperature regulation and growth in rats with hypothalamic lesions, Endocrinology 66 (1960) 340–354.

[81] R.R. Deuben, J. Meites, Stimulation of pituitary growth hormone release by a hypothalamic extract in vitro, Endocrinology 74 (1964) 408–414.

[82] G.J. Antony, J.J. Van Wyk, F.S. French, R.P. Weaver, G.S. Dugger, R.L. Timmons, et al., Influence of pituitary stalk section on growth hormone, insulin and TSH secretion in women with metastatic breast cancer, J Clin Endocrinol Metab 29 (1969) 1238–1250.

[83] W.M. Hunter, J.A. Friend, J.A. Strong, The diurnal pattern of plasma growth hormone concentration in adults, J Endocrinol 34 (1966) 139–146.

[84] F.C. Greenwood, J. Landon, Growth hormone secretion in response to stress in man, Nature 210 (1966) 540–541.

[85] P. Brazeau, W. Vale, R. Burgus, N. Ling, M. Butcher, J. Rivier, et al., Hypothalamic polypeptide that inhibits the secretion of immunoreactive pituitary growth hormone, Science 179 (1973) 77–79.

[86] J. Rivier, J. Spiess, M. Thorner, W. Vale, Characterization of a growth hormone-releasing factor from a human pancreatic islet tumour, Nature 300 (1982) 276–278.

[87] K.E. Mayo, W. Vale, J. Rivier, M.G. Rosenfeld, R.M. Evans, Expression-cloning and sequence of a cDNA encoding human growth hormone-releasing factor, Nature 306 (1983) 86–88.

[88] B. Bloch, R.C. Gaillard, P. Brazeau, H.D. Lin, N. Ling, Topographical and ontogenetic study of the neurons producing growth hormone-releasing factor in human hypothalamus, Regul Pept 8 (1984) 21–31.

[89] K. Lin-Su, M.P. Wajnrajch, Growth hormone releasing hormone (GHRH) and the GHRH receptor, Rev Endocr Metab Disord 3 (2002) 313–323.
[90] J.A. Chowen, L.M. Frago, J. Argente, The regulation of GH secretion by sex steroids, Eur J Endocrinol 151 (Suppl 3) (2004) U95–100.
[91] L.A. Frohman, T.R. Downs, E.P. Heimer, A.M. Felix, Dipeptidylpeptidase IV and trypsin-like enzymatic degradation of human growth hormone-releasing hormone in plasma, J Clin Invest 83 (1989) 1533–1540.
[92] L.A. Frohman, T.R. Downs, P. Chomczynski, M.A. Frohman, Growth hormone-releasing hormone: Structure, gene expression and molecular heterogeneity, Acta Paediatr Scand Suppl 367 (1990) 81–86.
[93] K.E. Mayo, P.A. Godfrey, S.T. Suhr, D.J. Kulik, J.O. Rahal, Growth hormone-releasing hormone: Synthesis and signaling, Recent Prog Horm Res 50 (1995) 35–73.
[94] C.M. Pombo, J. Zalvide, B.D. Gaylinn, C. Dieguez, Growth hormone-releasing hormone stimulates mitogen-activated protein kinase, Endocrinology 141 (2000) 2113–2119.
[95] A. Giustina, J.D. Veldhuis, Pathophysiology of the neuroregulation of growth hormone secretion in experimental animals and the human, Endocr Rev 19 (1998) 717–797.
[96] M.L. Vance, D.L. Kaiser, J. Rivier, W. Vale, M.O. Thorner, Dual effects of growth hormone (GH)-releasing hormone infusion in normal men: Somatotroph desensitization and increase in releasable GH, J Clin Endocrinol Metab 62 (1986) 591–594.
[97] L.A. Frohman, R.D. Kineman, Growth hormone-releasing hormone and pituitary development, hyperplasia and tumorigenesis, Trends Endocrinol Metab 13 (2002) 299–303.
[98] E.E. Muller, V. Locatelli, D. Cocchi, Neuroendocrine control of growth hormone secretion, Physiol Rev 79 (1999) 511–607.
[99] M. Fodor, C. Kordon, J. Epelbaum, Anatomy of the hypophysiotropic somatostatinergic and growth hormone-releasing hormone system minireview, Neurochem Res 31 (2006) 137–143.
[100] A. Torsello, G. Panzeri, P. Cermenati, M.C. Caroleo, E. Ghigo, F. Camanni, et al., Involvement of the somatostatin and cholinergic systems in the mechanism of growth hormone autofeedback regulation in the rat, J Endocrinol 117 (1988) 273–281.
[101] H. Zheng, A. Bailey, M.H. Jiang, K. Honda, H.Y. Chen, M.E. Trumbauer, et al., Somatostatin receptor subtype 2 knockout mice are refractory to growth hormone-negative feedback on arcuate neurons, Mol Endocrinol 11 (1997) 1709–1717.
[102] S. Yamashita, M. Weiss, S. Melmed, Insulin-like growth factor I regulates growth hormone secretion and messenger ribonucleic acid levels in human pituitary tumor cells, J Clin Endocrinol Metab 63 (1986) 730–735.
[103] F. Aguado, J. Rodrigo, L. Cacicedo, B. Mellstrom, Distribution of insulin-like growth factor-I receptor mRNA in rat brain. Regulation in the hypothalamo–neurohypophysial system, J Mol Endocrinol 11 (1993) 231–239.
[104] L.M. Garcia-Segura, J.R. Rodriguez, I. Torres-Aleman, Localization of the insulin-like growth factor I receptor in the cerebellum and hypothalamus of adult rats: An electron microscopic study, J Neurocytol 26 (1997) 479–490.
[105] S. Melmed, Insulin-like growth factor I – a prototypic peripheral-paracrine hormone? Endocrinology 140 (1999) 3879–3880.
[106] K. Becker, S. Stegenga, S. Conway, Role of insulin-like growth factor I in regulating growth hormone release and feedback in the male rat, Neuroendocrinology 61 (1995) 573–583.
[107] D. Gautam, J. Jeon, M.F. Starost, S.J. Han, F.F. Hamdan, Y. Cui, et al., Neuronal M3 muscarinic acetylcholine receptors are essential for somatotroph proliferation and normal somatic growth, Proc Nat Acad Sci USA 106 (2009) 6398–6403.
[108] I. Mechenthaler, Galanin and the neuroendocrine axes, Cell Mol Life Sci 65 (2008) 1826–1835.
[109] A.L. Hulting, B. Meister, L. Carlsson, A. Hilding, O. Isaksson, On the role of the peptide galanin in regulation of growth hormone secretion, Acta Endocrinol (Copenh) 125 (1991) 518–525.
[110] M. Kojima, K. Kangawa, Ghrelin: Structure and function, Physiol Rev 85 (2005) 495–522.
[111] J.M. Danger, M.C. Tonon, B.G. Jenks, S. Saint-Pierre, J.C. Martel, A. Fasolo, et al., Neuropeptide Y: Localization in the central nervous system and neuroendocrine functions, Fundam Clin Pharmacol 4 (1990) 307–340.
[112] M.T. Bluet-Pajot, J. Epelbaum, D. Gourdji, C. Hammond, C. Kordon, Hypothalamic and hypophyseal regulation of growth hormone secretion, Cell Mol Neurobiol 18 (1998) 101–123.
[113] C. Wagner, S.R. Caplan, G.S. Tannenbaum, Interactions of ghrelin signaling pathways with the GH neuroendocrine axis: A new and experimentally tested model, J Mol Endocrinol 43 (2009) 105–119.
[114] V.H. Lee, L.T. Lee, B.K. Chow, Gonadotropin-releasing hormone: Regulation of the GnRH gene, FEBS J 275 (2008) 5458–5478.
[115] P.M. Conn, W.F. Crowley Jr., Gonadotropin-releasing hormone and its analogues, N Engl J Med 324 (1991) 93–103.
[116] L.Z. Krsmanovic, L. Hu, P.K. Leung, H. Feng, K.J. Catt, The hypothalamic GnRH pulse generator: Multiple regulatory mechanisms, Trends Endocrinol Metab 20 (2009) 402–408.
[117] C.K. Cheng, P.C. Leung, Molecular biology of gonadotropin-releasing hormone (GnRH)-I, GnRH-II, and their receptors in humans, Endocr Rev 26 (2005) 283–306.
[118] K.E. Whitlock, Origin and development of GnRH neurons, Trends Endocrinol Metab 16 (2005) 145–151.
[119] Z. Naor, Signaling by G-protein-coupled receptor (GPCR): Studies on the GnRH receptor, Front Neuroendocrinol 30 (2009) 10–29.
[120] R.N. Clayton, Mechanism of GnRH action in gonadotrophs, Hum Reprod 3 (1988) 479–483.
[121] P.M. Conn, W.F. Crowley Jr., Gonadotropin-releasing hormone and its analogs, Annu Rev Med 45 (1994) 391–405.
[122] L.A. Rispoli, T.M. Nett, Pituitary gonadotropin-releasing hormone (GnRH) receptor: Structure, distribution and regulation of expression, Anim Reprod Sci 88 (2005) 57–74.
[123] G. Martinez de la Escalera, A.L. Choi, R.I. Weiner, Generation and synchronization of gonadotropin-releasing hormone (GnRH) pulses: Intrinsic properties of the GT1-1 GnRH neuronal cell line, Proc Nat Acad Sci USA 89 (1992) 1852–1855.
[124] L. Wildt, A. Hausler, G. Marshall, J.S. Hutchison, T.M. Plant, P.E. Belchetz, et al., Frequency and amplitude of gonadotropin-releasing hormone stimulation and gonadotropin secretion in the rhesus monkey, Endocrinology 109 (1981) 376–385.
[125] S.C. Chappel, A. Ulloa-Aguirre, C. Coutifaris, Biosynthesis and secretion of follicle-stimulating hormone, Endocr Rev 4 (1983) 179–211.
[126] S.B. Seminara, Metastin and its G protein-coupled receptor, GPR54: Critical pathway modulating GnRH secretion, Front Neuroendocrinol 26 (2005) 131–138.
[127] H.M. Dungan, D.K. Clifton, R.A. Steiner, Minireview: Kisspeptin neurons as central processors in the regulation of gonadotropin-releasing hormone secretion, Endocrinology 147 (2006) 1154–1158.
[128] Y. Uenoyama, H. Tsukamura, M. Kinoshita, S. Yamada, K. Iwata, V. Pheng, et al., Oestrogen-dependent stimulation of luteinising hormone release by galanin-like peptide in female rats, J Neuroendocrinol 20 (2008) 626–631.
[129] A.L. Gundlach, Galanin/GALP and galanin receptors: Role in central control of feeding, body weight/obesity and reproduction? Eur J Pharmacol 440 (2002) 255–268.

[130] A. Crown, D.K. Clifton, R.A. Steiner, Neuropeptide signaling in the integration of metabolism and reproduction, Neuroendocrinology 86 (2007) 175–182.
[131] P. Shughrue, P. Scrimo, M. Lane, R. Askew, I. Merchenthaler, The distribution of estrogen receptor-beta mRNA in forebrain regions of the estrogen receptor-alpha knockout mouse, Endocrinology 138 (1997) 5649–5652.
[132] C.L. Bethea, N.A. Brown, S.G. Kohama, Steroid regulation of estrogen and progestin receptor messenger ribonucleic acid in monkey hypothalamus and pituitary, Endocrinology 137 (1996) 4372–4383.
[133] R.B. Simerly, C. Chang, M. Muramatsu, L.W. Swanson, Distribution of androgen and estrogen receptor mRNA-containing cells in the rat brain: An in situ hybridization study, J Comp Neurol 294 (1990) 76–95.
[134] L. Hu, R.L. Gustofson, H. Feng, P.K. Leung, N. Mores, L.Z. Krsmanovic, et al., Converse regulatory functions of estrogen receptor-alpha and -beta subtypes expressed in hypothalamic gonadotropin-releasing hormone neurons, Mol Endocrinol 22 (2008) 2250–2259.
[135] T.M. Plant, Gonadal regulation of hypothalamic gonadotropin-releasing hormone release in primates, Endocr Rev 7 (1986) 75–88.
[136] M.J. Smith, L. Jennes, Neural signals that regulate GnRH neurones directly during the oestrous cycle, Reproduction 122 (2001) 1–10.
[137] D.W. Brann, V.B. Mahesh, Excitatory amino acids: Function and significance in reproduction and neuroendocrine regulation, Front Neuroendocrinol 15 (1994) 3–49.
[138] J.T. Smith, I.J. Clarke, Gonadotropin inhibitory hormone function in mammals, Trends Endocrinol Metab (2010).
[139] T.M. Plant, Neurobiological bases underlying the control of the onset of puberty in the rhesus monkey: A representative higher primate, Front Neuroendocrinol 22 (2001) 107–139.
[140] J.L. Cameron, Stress and behaviorally induced reproductive dysfunction in primates, Semin Reprod Endocrinol 15 (1997) 37–45.
[141] K.M. Breen, F.J. Karsch, New insights regarding glucocorticoids, stress and gonadotropin suppression, Front Neuroendocrinol 27 (2006) 233–245.
[142] H. Dobson, S. Ghuman, S. Prabhakar, R. Smith, A conceptual model of the influence of stress on female reproduction, Reproduction 125 (2003) 151–163.
[143] L.M. Bilezikjian, A.L. Blount, C.J. Donaldson, W.W. Vale, Pituitary actions of ligands of the TGF-beta family: Activins and inhibins, Reproduction 132 (2006) 207–215.
[144] A. Ben-Shlomo, S. Melmed, Pituitary somatostatin receptor signaling, Trends Endocrinol Metab 21 (2010) 123–133.
[145] Y.C. Patel, C.B. Srikant, Somatostatin mediation of adenohypophysial secretion, Annu Rev Physiol 48 (1986) 551–567.
[146] R.J. Ross, S. Tsagarakis, A. Grossman, L. Nhagafoong, R.J. Touzel, L.H. Rees, et al., GH feedback occurs through modulation of hypothalamic somatostatin under cholinergic control: Studies with pyridostigmine and GHRH, Clin Endocrinol (Oxf) 27 (1987) 727–733.
[147] A. Ben-Shlomo, S. Melmed, Pituitary somatostatin receptor signaling, Trends Endocrinol Metab (2010) 123–133.
[148] M.E. Freeman, B. Kanyicska, A. Lerant, G. Nagy, Prolactin: Structure, function, and regulation of secretion, Physiol Rev 80 (2000) 1523–1631.
[149] A. Lerant, M.E. Herman, M.E. Freeman, Dopaminergic neurons of periventricular and arcuate nuclei of pseudopregnant rats: Semicircadian rhythm in Fos-related antigens immunoreactivities and in dopamine concentration, Endocrinology 137 (1996) 3621–3628.
[150] B.M. Chronwall, W.R. Millington, W.S. Griffin, J.R. Unnerstall, T.L. O'Donohue, Histological evaluation of the dopaminergic regulation of proopiomelanocortin gene expression in the intermediate lobe of the rat pituitary, involving in situ hybridization and [3H]thymidine uptake measurement, Endocrinology 120 (1987) 1201–1211.
[151] S.E. Lindley, J.W. Gunnet, K.J. Lookingland, K.E. Moore, Effects of alterations in the activity of tuberohypophysial dopaminergic neurons on the secretion of alpha-melanocyte stimulating hormone, Proc Soc Exp Biol Med 188 (1988) 282–286.
[152] S.L. Asa, M.A. Kelly, D.K. Grandy, M.J. Low, Pituitary lactotroph adenomas develop after prolonged lactotroph hyperplasia in dopamine D2 receptor-deficient mice, Endocrinology 140 (1999) 5348–5355.
[153] L. Vallar, J. Meldolesi, Mechanisms of signal transduction at the dopamine D2 receptor, Trends Pharmacol Sci 10 (1989) 74–77.
[154] S. Suzuki, I. Yamamoto, J. Arita, Mitogen-activated protein kinase-dependent stimulation of proliferation of rat lactotrophs in culture by 3′,5′-cyclic adenosine monophosphate, Endocrinology 140 (1999) 2850–2858.
[155] T. Florio, M.G. Pan, B. Newman, R.E. Hershberger, O. Civelli, P.J. Stork, Dopaminergic inhibition of DNA synthesis in pituitary tumor cells is associated with phosphotyrosine phosphatase activity, J Biol Chem 267 (1992) 24169–24172.
[156] M. Piercy, S.H. Shin, Comparative studies of prolactin secretion in estradiol-primed and normal male rats induced by ether stress, pimozide and TRH, Neuroendocrinology 31 (1980) 270–275.
[157] C. Denef, D. Manet, R. Dewals, Dopaminergic stimulation of prolactin release, Nature 285 (1980) 243–246.
[158] J.B. Hill, G.M. Nagy, L.S. Frawley, Suckling unmasks the stimulatory effect of dopamine on prolactin release: Possible role for alpha-melanocyte-stimulating hormone as a mammotrope responsiveness factor, Endocrinology 129 (1991) 843–847.
[159] B.J. Arey, T.P. Burris, P. Basco, M.E. Freeman, Infusion of dopamine at low concentrations stimulates the release of prolactin from alpha-methyl-p-tyrosine-treated rats, Proc Soc Exp Biol Med 203 (1993) 60–63.
[160] L. Milenkovic, A.F. Parlow, S.M. McCann, Physiological significance of the negative short-loop feedback of prolactin, Neuroendocrinology 52 (1990) 389–392.
[161] L.A. Arbogast, J.L. Voogt, Prolactin (PRL) receptors are colocalized in dopaminergic neurons in fetal hypothalamic cell cultures: Effect of PRL on tyrosine hydroxylase activity, Endocrinology 138 (1997) 3016–3023.
[162] T.W. Toney, D.E. Pawsat, A.E. Fleckenstein, K.J. Lookingland, K.E. Moore, Evidence that prolactin mediates the stimulatory effects of estrogen on tuberoinfundibular dopamine neurons in female rats, Neuroendocrinology 55 (1992) 282–289.
[163] K.T. Demarest, N.J. Duda, G.D. Riegle, K.E. Moore, Placental lactogen mimics prolactin in activating tuberoinfundibular dopaminergic neurons, Brain Res 272 (1983) 175–178.
[164] M.E. Molitch, Drugs and prolactin, Pituitary 11 (2008) 209–218.

CHAPTER

3

Adrenocorticotropin

Oulu Wang, Joseph A. Majzoub

Division of Endocrinology, Children's Hospital Boston, Harvard Medical School, Boston, MA, USA

CELLS OF ORIGIN

Fetal Anatomy

The anterior pituitary forms via invagination of the pharyngeal stomodeum in the region of contact with the diencephalon. By week 5 of human gestation, this invagination, termed Rathke's diverticulum, has formed, but the downward migration of the diencephalic diverticulum, destined to be the neurohypophysis, has not yet commenced. It is at this time that adrenocorticotropin (ACTH) is first detectable by immunocytochemistry in the collection of cells within Rathke's diverticulum which are furthest from contact with the diencephalon [1]. By 8 weeks of gestation, ACTH is detectable by radioimmunoassay of both fetal pituitary tissue and fetal blood [1]. The hypophyseal–portal vascular system forms between 8 and 14 weeks gestation, dating the earliest time after which hypothalamic corticotropin-releasing factors may function to regulate fetal pituitary ACTH [1]. By 14 weeks gestation, release of ACTH from human fetal corticotrophs is highly responsive to exposure to corticotropin-releasing hormone (CRH) in vitro [2]. The intensity of immunohistochemical ACTH staining in the anterior pituitary increases progressively from the mid-first through to the end of the second trimester. In contrast, it is only after 21 weeks gestation that ACTH-positive cells begin to appear in the pars intermedia of the human fetal pituitary, defined as that region between Rathke's cleft anteriorly and the neurohypophysis posteriorly. The ACTH-containing cells in this region are epithelial-like, in contrast to the large, angular, ovoid appearance of corticotrophs in the anterior pituitary [1].

Adult Anatomy

Corticotrophs were initially identified by their basophilic staining. This has been subsequently found to be due to the presence of complex sugars in corticotrophs, principally those containing α-L-fucose and complex N-glyosyl-protein, as well as terminal ß-galactose. Corticotrophs constitute between 10 and 20% of the cell population of the anterior pituitary [3]. They occur either singly or in clumps. They are most numerous in the midsagittal region of the pituitary (median wedge) but also occur in the lateral wings of the gland. Although the adult human pituitary does not contain an intermediate lobe, the junctional zone between the anterior and posterior lobes is known as the zona intermedia. This region, derived from the portion of Rathke's diverticulum posterior to Rathke's cleft, contains scattered cells immunopositive for ACTH. Some of these ACTH-containing cells appear to extend into the posterior pituitary, a feature known as basophilic invasion [3]. These areas of apparent migration of corticotrophs from the zona intermedia into the posterior pituitary occur focally along the border between these two regions.

In humans, in addition to the sellar pituitary, there is a pharyngeal pituitary which is located in either the sphenoid sinus or within the sphenoid bone. It consists of pituitary-like tissue approximately 2–5 mm by 0.2 mm in size. It is connected to the sellar gland by trans-sphenoidal vessels [4]. Only 1–2% of the cells in the pharyngeal pituitary contain immunoreactive ACTH, in contrast to approximately 14% of the cells in the sellar pituitary [4]. The pharyngeal pituitary is thought to arise as a rest of tissue resulting from the normal migration of cells from Rathke's pouch to the sella turcica. There have been several reports of Cushing's disease, a disorder

The Pituitary, Third Edition, DOI: 10.1016/B978-0-12-380926-1.10003-3

characterized by elevated ACTH and cortisol, due to corticotroph adenomas arising in the pharyngeal pituitary [4].

MOLECULAR EMBRYOLOGY

Tremendous progress has been made in recent years concerning the molecular mechanisms controlling pituitary organogenesis and pituitary cell-lineage specification in animal models. A complex network of transcriptional events mediated by extrinsic and intrinsic signals has been implicated in the determination and a stereotypical spatio-temporal differentiation of the five trophic cell types of the mature anterior pituitary gland.

Intrinsic Signals

Rpx (Rathke's pouch homeobox), also known as Hesx1 (homeobox gene expression in embryonic stem cells) is the earliest known marker for the pituitary primordium [5]. Hesx1/Rpx is a member of the *paired-like* class of homeobox genes. Early Hesx1/Rpx expression occurs in the anterior midline endoderm and prechordal plate precursor followed by expression in the cephalic neural plate [5]. Expression becomes progressively restricted anteriorly in the cephalic neural plate in a distribution consistent with tissue known by fate-mapping studies to form the primordium of the anterior pituitary [1]. Hesx1/Rpx expression ultimately becomes restricted to Rathke's pouch, and down-regulation of Hesx1/Rpx in the pouch coincides with the differentiation of pituitary-specific cell types [5]. Embryonic mice lacking Rpx demonstrate variable abnormalities of hypothalamic and pituitary morphogenesis, reduced prosencephalon, anophthalmia or microophthalmia, and defective olfactory development. Neonatal mice have abnormalities in the corpus callosum, the anterior and hippocampal commissures, and the septum pellucidum [1,6]. These abnormalities are reminiscent of defects seen in a heterogeneous group of human disorders known as septo-optic dysplasia (SOD). Deficits in SOD include optic nerve hypoplasia, abnormalities of the midline brain structures and abnormalities of the hypothalamic–pituitary axis. Patients commonly present with endocrinopathies including hypoglycemia and adrenal crisis, which may signal growth hormone, ACTH, or thyroid-stimulating hormone deficiency [1]. Dattani and colleagues have identified two siblings with SOD who are homozygous for missense mutations within the *HESX1* homeodomain which prevents it from binding target DNA [6]. The siblings identified with *HESX1* mutations presented with hypoglycemia hours after birth and demonstrated panhypopituitarism, substantiating a role for *HESX1* in human pituitary development [6].

The corticotroph lineage appears to diverge relatively early from the other cell types of the anterior pituitary. Lhx3, a LIM-type homeodomain protein, is essential for the growth of Rathke's pouch and determination of pituitary cell lineages [7]. In Lhx3-deficient mice, proopiomelanocortin (POMC), an ACTH precursor, was detected in a small cohort of cells at the ventral base of the pouch remnant, which roughly corresponds to the position of the first presumptive corticotroph cells to differentiate in the wild-type pouch [7]. Although some pouch cells were able to differentiate and express POMC, these cells failed to proliferate. An insufficient or non-functional corticotroph cell mass may have caused the hypoplastic adrenal cortices noted in these animals [7].

Ptx1 is a *bicoid*-related homeobox transcription factor identified based upon its ability to activate transcription of POMC in the corticotroph derived AtT-20 cell line and its ability to interact with the transactivation domain of Pit-1 [1,8]. It is expressed in the primordial Rathke's pouch, oral epithelium, first branchial arch, the duodenum and hindlimb [8]. Ptx1 is expressed in all mature pituitary cells, but is differentially expressed during pituitary development in different cell types [9]. In the mature pituitary, the highest levels of expression are found within corticotrophs. In addition to activating transcription of POMC, Ptx1 is required for sustained expression of Lhx3 [10], directly activates transcription of the common α-glycoprotein subunit (α-GSU) [8], synergizes with Pit-1 on the growth hormone and prolactin promoter [10], and synergizes with SF-1 on the promoter of the lutenizing hormone β (LH-β) gene [10]. Ptx2, also known as RIEG, is an additional *bicoid*-related homeobox gene 97% identical to Ptx1 [11]. Ptx2 is also differentially expressed in the pituitary and is excluded from corticotrophs, suggesting that some of the functions ascribed to Ptx1 may be performed by Ptx2. Expression of Pit-1, a POU domain transcription factor, is restricted to the anterior pituitary and is required for the development of thyrotrophs, lactotrophs and somatotrophs [12]. Consistent with this, patients with mutations in Pit-1 have normal hypothalamic–pituitary–adrenal (HPA) axis function. Prophet of Pit-1 (Prop-1) is required for Pit-1 expression, and mutation of its gene is also associated with deficiencies in the development of thyrotophs, lactotrophs and somatotrophs in the Ames dwarf mouse and in humans. In a small number of patients with mutations in *PROP1*, modest impairment of ACTH secretion has been reported [1].

Developmentally essential, cell-line-restricted factors have been identified for a number of different pituitary cell types. SF-1, an orphan nuclear receptor, is necessary for the development of gonadotrophs [1]. However, no essential corticotroph-specific factor has yet been clearly identified. NeuroD, also known as Beta2, is a cell-restricted basic helix-loop-helix (bHLH) transcription factor implicated in late neuronal differentiation [13] which has also been isolated as a cell-specific transcription factor of the insulin gene [14]. NeuroD is expressed in a number of tissues including pancreatic endocrine cells, the intestine and brain, including the mouse corticotroph AtT-20 cell line, but not the rat somatotroph pituitary cell line (GH3) [14]. Drouin and colleagues have demonstrated that NeuroD expression does appear to be restricted to corticotrophs in the mouse pituitary, and that NeuroD, in association with ubiquitous bHLH dimerization partners, specifically recognizes and activates transcription from the POMC promoter E box that confers transcriptional specificity of POMC to corticotrophs [15]. However, the necessity of this transcription factor for corticotroph specification or differentiation is still undetermined. A corticotroph-restricted transcription factor, Tpit (also known as Tbx19), has been identified, which interacts with Ptx1 and is required for *POMC* transcription, as discussed subsequently. However, it is not required for corticotroph lineage commitment, as *Tpit* knockout mice develop Acth-deficient corticotrophs [1]. Moreover, neither POMC nor its various cleavage products are themselves required for differentiation or maintenance of corticotrophs, because these cells are present in Pomc knockout mice [16]. Because no intrinsic factor has yet been identified that is absolutely required for the development of corticotrophs in situ, it is possible that they arise elsewhere during fetal life and migrate into the anterior pituitary. One possible source could be neural crest, as this is the origin of POMC-producing melanocytes which migrate to the skin [17]. This is consistent with the finding that zebrafish Pomc is first expressed in the early embryo asymmetrically as two bilateral groups of cells anterior to the neural ridge midline before migrating to the anterior pituitary [18].

Extrinsic Signals

The oral ectoderm, from which Rathke's pouch forms, and the neural ectoderm of the ventral diencephalon, from which the hypothalamus arises, are in direct contact at the time of the formation of Rathke's pouch [1]. Classical explant experiments have indicated that inductive signals arising from mesenchyme and neural ectoderm adjacent to Rathke's pouch are required for pituitary organogenesis and cell line specification. The necessity for extrinsic signals for development of corticotrophs is supported by the demonstration that the expression of POMC in ectoderm explants requires coculture with mesoderm [1]. Direct evidence confirming the necessity of the ventral diencephalon for proper pituitary organogenesis has been obtained from examination of mice bearing null mutations in the Nkx2.1 homeobox gene, also known as T/ebp or Ttf1 [19]. This gene is not expressed in the oral ectoderm or in the developing pituitary at any time during embryogenesis, but Nkx2.1 null mice demonstrate severe defects in the development of the diencephalon and also fail to develop a pituitary gland [19].

The nature of the extrinsic signals that promote pituitary organogenesis and cause cell line specification is an area of active investigation. A number of secreted factors have been implicated in pituitary development and cell line specification including bone morphogenic proteins (BMP4, BMP2), fibroblast growth factor 8 (FGF8), Sonic hedgehog (Shh) and Wnt5a [1]. A model of coordinate control of anterior pituitary progenitor cell identity, proliferation and differentiation imposed by FGF8 secreted from the dorsally located infundibulum and BMP2 from ventrally located mesenchyme has been proposed. It has been suggested that corticotroph progenitors progress to a definitive corticotroph state only after escaping both FGF8 and BMP2 signaling. While the precise signals and interactions required for pituitary organogenesis and corticotroph specification are incompletely understood, it is clear that signals from the mature hypothalamus like CRH and AVP are not required for corticotroph specification. The anterior pituitary appears to develop normally in a CRH null mouse [20]. Furthermore, deletion of the class III POU transcription Brn-2 results in failed maturation of AVP, CRH and oxytocin producing neurons of the hypothalamus, and failed maturation of the posterior pituitary with no apparent defect in the maturation of any anterior pituitary cell type [21].

LOCALIZATION OF NON-ACTH PEPTIDES WITHIN CORTICOTROPHS

Many other neuropeptides have been found to be colocalized with ACTH within corticotrophs, although in most cases it is not clear whether this is due to synthesis or binding of the peptide within the cell. Neurophysin (but not vasopressin) colocalizes with ACTH in both normal and adenomatous corticotrophs. Neurophysin immunocytochemical staining is especially prominent in corticotrophs in the zona intermedia, which appear to project into the posterior pituitary. Chromogranin A has been described in the majority of corticotroph adenomas, although only a fraction of these patients have elevations of circulating plasma chromogranin A levels. Galanin is present in all normal corticotrophs as well as in the majority of corticotroph adenomas that have been examined [22]. Galanin has also been found in those corticotrophs in the zona intermedia which appear to be migrating into the posterior pituitary. It has also been described in corticotrophs which have undergone Crooke's hyalinization. Calpastatin, an inhibitor of the calcium-dependent cysteine proteases, calpain I and calpain II, has been found in all ACTH-containing cells of the anterior pituitary, including those in the median wedge as well as those extending into the posterior pituitary [23]. Vasoactive intestinal peptide has been found in corticotroph adenomas, but only rarely in normal corticotrophs [22].

Normal corticotrophs contain small amounts of cytokeratin, whereas corticotrophs which have undergone Crooke's hyalinization are markedly positive for this protein [24]. Corticotrophs appear to have few structural characteristics associated with neuronal cell types, for they are negative for neurofilament, vimentin, glial fibrillary acidic protein and desmon [24]. Likewise, corticotrophs in the zona intermedia, unlike those in the pars intermedia of rodents, appear not to be innervated by neurons, since they do not stain with any of these neuron-specific markers. Similarly, synaptophysin, a 38 kDa integral membrane glycoprotein found in presynaptic vesicles of neurons, stains only weakly in corticotrophs [23]. These findings, together with a lack in humans of an anatomically discrete intermediate lobe with large numbers of α-MSH-containing cells, has led most investigators to conclude that there is no functional counterpart of the rodent pituitary intermediate lobe in humans.

EXTRAPITUITARY LOCALIZATION OF ACTH AND RELATED PEPTIDES

Although the vast majority of ACTH is synthesized in anterior pituitary corticotrophs, it is also expressed in several nonpituitary human tissues, both within and outside of the central nervous system. Within the central nervous system, ACTH and its related peptides are expressed to the greatest degree in cell bodies of the infundibular nucleus of the basal hypothalamus (analogous to the rodent arcuate nucleus) [25]. The cell bodies of these hypothalamic ACTH neurons are located at the base of the third ventricle, adjacent to the median eminence and pituitary stalk. These neurons project to limbic, diencephalic, mesencephalic and amygdaloid sites. Lesser amounts of ACTH and related peptides are found in substantia nigra, periventricular gray matter and hippocampus [26]. Interestingly, POMC expression in the hypothalamus occurs in areas also known to express the orexigenic neuropeptides NPY and AGRP and projects to many of the same hypothalamic targets [27]. The rodent arcuate nucleus prominently expresses the leptin receptor, implicating POMC products in the regulation of appetite and energy homeostasis (see melanocortin receptors) [28]. The brain areas containing ACTH also coincide with areas mediating stimulation analgesia, suggesting that expression of ACTH, or another product of the POMC gene (such as ß-endorphin), in these sites may regulate pain perception.

Outside of the central nervous system, ACTH and other POMC gene products, including α-MSH and ß-endorphin, are synthesized in a large number of human tissues, including in descending order of abundance, adrenal, testis, peripheral mononuclear cells, spleen, kidney, ovary, lung, thyroid, liver, colon and duodenum [29]. In most of these tissues, POMC peptides are translated from truncated messenger RNAs lacking signal peptide sequences, suggesting that they cannot be secreted extracellularly [30], raising the question of their functional significance. However, adrenal and testis in addition express full-length POMC mRNA, suggesting that these tissues may also secrete POMC-related peptides [29]. Recently, several additional cell types have been shown to produce POMC peptides including monocytes, astrocytes, gastrin-producing cells of the gastrointestinal tract, keratinocytes, skin melanocytes and atrial myocytes.

GENE STRUCTURE

ACTH is derived from a 266-amino acid precursor, proopiomelanocortin (POMC), so named because it encodes opioid, melanotropic and corticotropic activities [31]. The human *POMC* gene is a single copy gene located on chromosome 2p23. It and the genes encoding the highly homologous opioid peptides, preproenkephalin A and preproenkephalin B (dynorphin), are all located on different chromosomes.

The human *POMC* gene is 8 kilobases (kb) long (Figure 3.1). It consists of a promoter of at least 400 basepairs (bp) at the 5′ end of the gene, followed by three exons, 86 (exon 1), 152 (exon 2) and 833 (exon 3) bp long, and two introns, 3708 (intron 1) and 2886 (intron 2) bp in length. Exon 1 is not translated. Perhaps because of this, exon 1 of the human and other mammalian POMC genes are less than 50% identical. The initiator methionine is located 20 bp into exon 2, and is followed by a 26-amino acid hydrophobic signal peptide. Except for the signal peptide and 18 amino acids of the amino-terminal glycopeptide, the majority of the POMC precursor is encoded by exon 3 [31]. Exon 2 is close to 90% identical between the *POMC* genes of humans and other mammals. Within exon 3 of *POMC* are located all known peptide products of the *POMC* gene, including N-terminal glycopeptide, γ-MSH, joining peptide, ACTH, α-MSH, corticotropin-like intermediate lobe peptide (CLIP), ß-lipotropin (ß-LPH), ß-MSH

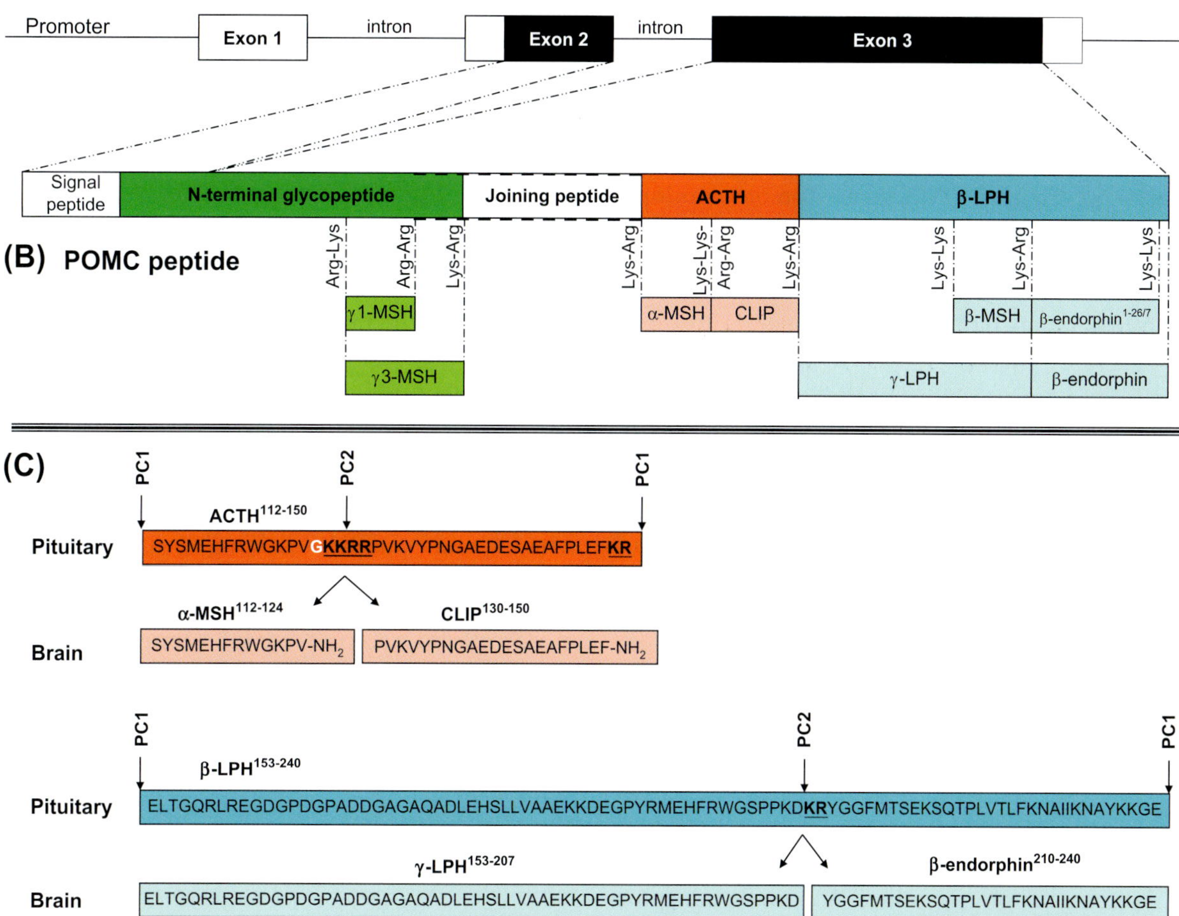

FIGURE 3.1 Organization of the proopiomelanocortin gene and peptide. Structure of proopiomelanocortin (POMC) gene and peptide products. (A) Schematic diagram of the *POMC* gene, consisting of 3 exons (rectangles) separated by two introns (thin lines). Translated regions are shown in black with the corresponding peptide regions indicated by dotted lines. (B) The 240-amino acid precursor is formed after removal of the 26-amino acid N-terminal signal peptide. The POMC precursor can be divided into three domains: (1) N-terminal glycopeptide and joining peptide; (2) adrenocorticotropic hormone (ACTH); and (3) β-lipotropin (β-LPH). These are further cleaved by prohormone convertase enzymes, PC1 and PC2, at arginine-arginine, arginine-lysine, or lysine-lysine residues, to produce site-specific expression. The *POMC* gene is highly conserved except in the joining peptide and latter portion of γ3-MSH, denoted by dashed lines. (C) Pituitary- and brain-specific peptides are cleaved from the POMC precursor. Amino acids at proteolytic cleavage sites are indicated in bold, underlined letters (lysine **K**, arginine **R**). The glycine (G) residue in white indicates a C-terminal amidation site. MSH, melanocyte stimulating hormone; CLIP, corticotropin-like intermediate lobe peptide; α-MSH, α-melanocyte stimulating hormone.

and ß-endorphin. Within exon 3, the regions encoding the N-terminal glycopeptide, α-MSH, ACTH and ß-endorphin, are greater than 95% identical between the human and other mammals. In contrast, joining peptide, the region between the N-terminal glycopeptide and ACTH, is very poorly conserved among mammals, which has suggested to some workers that it does not encode a biologically important function [31].

POMC Gene Promoter Structure

The promoter of the human POMC gene contains typical TATA and CAAT boxes 28 and 62 bp, respectively, upstream from the transcription start site. Using in vitro transcription and transfection of the human POMC gene into heterologous cells [32], the POMC gene promoter has been shown to contain DNA elements which mediate increased transcription by cyclic AMP and decreased transcription by glucocorticoids. Although these DNA elements have not been precisely localized in the human POMC gene promoter, they are present within the 700 bp 5′ to the transcription start site [32]. The rat POMC gene promoter has been studied more extensively. Drouin and coworkers, using DNA-mediated gene transfer into transgenic mice and tissue culture cells, found that the DNA sequences needed for corticotroph-specific expression and negative transcriptional regulation by glucocorticoid are contained within 543 bp of the transcription start site. These workers have reported the presence of a DNA sequence which mediates negative regulation by glucocorticoids (nGRE), located in the region of the CAAT box, which also binds nuclear proteins of the chicken ovalbumin upstream promoter (COUP) family. Using DNAase footprint and gel retardation analysis of the rat POMC gene promoter, multiple synergistic DNA elements have been reported to be necessary for correct pituitary-specific expression of the gene. These workers have identified NeuroD, Ptx1 and Tpit as transcription factors which cooperate to cause corticotroph-specific expression of *POMC* [15].

POMC mRNA Transcription, Splicing and Polyadenylation

In addition to the major transcriptional initiation site present in corticotrophs, at least six other start sites have been found in several non-pituitary tissues, including adrenal, thymus and testes of the human [30]. These sites are all between 41 and 162 nucleotides downstream from the 5′ end of exon 3. The mRNAs transcribed from these sites thus would be intronless, and the only truncated molecules that might be translated would be devoid of a signal peptide and therefore could not be secreted. Tissues containing these shorter forms of POMC mRNA, including adrenal, testis, spleen, kidney, ovary, lung, thyroid and gastrointestinal tract, express ACTH, N-terminal glycopeptide$^{1-61}$ and ß-endorphin [29]. These truncated mRNAs are capable of being translated both in cell-free translation systems and in heterologous cells transfected with the appropriate fragment of the human POMC gene, although the peptide products are not secreted. The significance of the expression of these truncated forms of POMC mRNA and their translated peptide products in human non-pituitary tissue is not clear.

A canonical polyadenylation signal is present in human POMC mRNA 23 bases upstream from the poly (A) addition site. The length of the polyadenylate tail, attached to the 3′ end of POMC mRNA and believed to play a role in translational efficiency of mRNA stability, is much longer in hypothalamic compared with pituitary cells in the rat, although this has not been studied in the human.

GENE REGULATION

In human anterior pituitary corticotrophs, POMC mRNA levels are increased by CRH and inhibited by glucocorticoids [32]. Similar results are seen in normal and adenomatous corticotrophs, although the glucocorticoid inhibition of POMC mRNA expression is less in the latter cells. The same results are seen in rat anterior pituitary corticotrophs, where the opposing effects of CRH and glucocorticoids are due to their opposite influence on the transcription rate of the POMC gene [33]. Of interest, glucocorticoids have no effect on the POMC mRNA content of rat intermediate pituitary lobe corticotrophs [33].

CRH, acting via the type 1 CRH receptor, increases cAMP content in anterior pituitary corticotrophs [34]. CRH, vasopressin and glucocorticoids all inhibit expression of CRH receptor 1 mRNA, which may limit the effect of these agents during the stress response, as discussed subsequently. The CRH-induced rise in cAMP is responsible for both the increase in *POMC* transcription and peptide synthesis as well as for the rise in intracellular calcium which results in ACTH secretion [32]. CRH mediates its stimulation of *POMC* transcription via the POMC CRH responsive element (PCRH-RE), which binds PCRH-RE binding protein [32]. The negative effect of glucocorticoids upon POMC gene transcription is thought to be mediated by a glucocorticoid–glucocorticoid receptor complex binding to *cis*-acting DNA sequences within the POMC promoter, although definitive evidence for this is lacking. The possibility exists that the glucocorticoid receptor complex does not bind directly to the POMC gene, but instead binds to another protein such as a positive transcription factor, and in this way mediates its negative effect on POMC gene expression. Glucocorticoid stimulates, rather than inhibits, POMC gene expression in the arcuate nucleus of the hypothalamus, the site of α-MSH production. The significance of this is not clear, but could be involved in the inhibition of appetite by glucocorticoids in the post-absorptive state, when glucocorticoid levels are high.

Insights into the development and regulation of the HPA axis have come from the discovery that leukemia-inhibitory factor (LIF) has an important role in these events [32]. LIF is a cytokine expressed in corticotrophs and folliculostellate cells beginning as early as 14 weeks gestation. LIF stimulates transcription of *POMC* and expression of ACTH [32]. In many tissues, including pituitary, LIF expression is up-regulated by inflammatory stimuli. The LIF receptor is a member of the class I cytokine receptor superfamily which heterodimerizes with gp130. In common with other family members, the LIF receptor signals through the Jak-STAT pathway, particularly utilizing Jak1 and STAT-3 [32]. As with other receptors coupled via these mediators, SOCS-3 inhibits POMC expression following its simulation by LIF [35]. Mice which over-express a LIF transgene develop Cushing's syndrome [36]. Their pituitary glands have corticotroph hyperplasia and multiple Rathke-like cysts lined by ciliated cells. Mice with targeted deletion of *Lif* have secondary adrenal insufficiency. LIF may interact with CRH and CREB to regulate POMC transcription [32]. All of these data point towards LIF playing an important role in the regulation of ACTH secretion, perhaps most importantly by immune and inflammatory stimuli. In addition, the data suggest that LIF might be involved in the pathogenesis of Rathke-cleft tumors. Finally, AMP kinase may play a role in the activation of the *POMC* promoter [37], and FoxO1 may inhibit leptin regulation of *POMC* promoter activity by blocking STAT-3 [38].

Vasopressin potentiates the action of CRH on ACTH secretion, both in vitro and in vivo [39]. Vasopressin's effect is mediated by the vasopressin V1b (or V3) protein kinase C. Despite this positive effect on ACTH secretion, vasopressin has been reported to decrease both basal and CRH-stimulated POMC mRNA levels in anterior pituitary cells. ß-adrenergic catecholamines, like CRH, also increase POMC mRNA levels in corticotrophs via a cAMP mechanism. Insulin-induced hypoglycemia also causes an increase in POMC mRNA content in rat anterior pituitary corticotrophs [40], but whether this is secondary to an increase in hypothalamic CRH, vasopressin, or catecholamines is not known. The inhibitory neurotransmitter GABA causes a decrease in POMC mRNA levels in intermediate, but not anterior, pituitary corticotrophs [22].

POMC BIOSYNTHESIS AND PROCESSING

The human POMC precursor has the potential to encode several overlapping peptides of biological importance (Figure 3.1). Within the precursor, these peptides are separated from one another by two or more basic amino acids which serve as recognition sites for prohormone cleavage enzymes. In addition, POMC-derived peptides contain potential signals for amidation, glycosylation, acetylation and phosphorylation. Because the nomenclature of the various proteolytic products of POMC has been derived from both peptide-mapping studies as well as molecular biological studies in which putative peptides had been predicted from inspection of nucleotide sequences [31], the terminology can be confusing. To avoid confusion, amino acid (aa) positions in this chapter are numbered as superscripts with reference to the 240-aa-long human POMC precursor, formed after removal of the 26-aa-long signal peptide.

The 240 aa POMC precursor can be considered to be composed of three domains (Figure 3.1). Domain I (aa 1–111), the N-terminal domain, encodes the 76-aa-long N-terminal glycopeptide$^{1-76}$ within its first 78 aa, and the 30-aa-long C-terminal joining, or hinge, peptide (JP$^{79-108}$) within its last 33 aa. The middle Domain II (aa 112–152), 41-aa-long, encodes the 39-aa ACTH$^{112-150}$ peptide, which may be further processed to α-melanocyte-stimulating hormone (MSH)$^{112-124}$. The C-terminal Domain III, termed ß-LPH$^{153-240}$, is 88 aa long. It contains within it the 31-aa-long ß-endorphin$^{210-240}$. Beside these peptides, several other products have been identified, although evidence for their existence and/or biological importance in man is not clear [31]. These include gamma$_1$-MSH$^{51-61}$, gamma$_2$-MSH$^{51-62}$, and gamma$_3$-MSH$^{51-76}$ in Domain I, corticotropin-like intermediate lobe peptide (CLIP)$^{130-150}$ in Domain II, and gamma-LPH$^{153-206}$ and ß-MSH$^{191-206}$ in Domain III (Figure 3.1).

Glycosylation of POMC

Within the ER, POMC undergoes initial glycosylation. Human POMC is glycosylated solely at two sites in the N-terminal glycopeptide$^{1-76}$ of Domain I. Carbohydrate is added via an O-linked glycosylation to Thr^{45} and via an N-linked glycosylation to Asn^{65}.

C-terminal Amidation of POMC

Three human POMC products undergo C-terminal amidation [31]. These include N-terminal glycopeptide$^{1-61}$, JP$^{79-108}$ and α-MSH$^{112-124}$. In addition, these three products are also present in their Gly-extended forms, which may be incompletely processed intermediates. C-terminal amidation is common among neuropeptides and is usually essential for bioactivity. This reaction is mediated by a bifunctional enzyme consisting of peptidylglycine-α-amidating monooxygenase (PAM) and peptidyl-α-hydroxyglycine α-amidating lyase (PAL) activities, which transfer the amino group of a C-terminal Gly to the carboxyl group of the adjacent amino acid. Human PAM/PAL exists in both a membrane-bound and free cytoplasmic form.

N-terminal Acetylation of POMC

Two human POMC products undergo N-terminal acetylation. These are α-MSH and ß-endorphin. In humans α-MSH exists predominantly in the nonacetylated form [31]. N-terminal acetylation of ACTH$^{1-13}$-amide to form α-MSH results in increased melanotrophic activity and decreased corticotrophic activity.

Proteolytic Processing of POMC

POMC gives rise to several smaller, biologically active peptide products. These are generated by post-translational cleavage of POMC by trypsin-like prohormone convertase endopeptidase enzymes which cleave the precursor on the C-terminal side of regions of two or more basic amino acid residues [31]. These basic amino acids are subsequently removed by carboxypeptidase activity. Some POMC proteolytic products subsequently undergo amidation at their C-terminus or acetylation at their N-terminus, as described above. The post-translational processing of POMC exhibits a remarkable degree of tissue-specificity, which recently has been postulated to be due to the differential distribution of processing enzymes in the various tissues which synthesize POMC (see below).

Proteolytic Processing Enzymes

All proteolytic processing of human POMC occurs at either lys-arg or arg-arg residues (Figure 3.1). Every lys-arg and arg-arg site within the human precursor is capable of being cleaved in vivo, whereas in the mouse and rat, additional arg-lys and lys-lys sequences at the N-termini of gamma$_1$-MSH and ß-MSH, respectively, appear to be utilized [31]. It is likely that the proteolytic digestion of human POMC at all sites is mediated by either of two structurally related endopeptidases, prohormone convertase 1 (PC1) or prohormone convertase 2 (PC2). These enzymes, best studied in rodents thus far, are part of a seven-member family of subtilisin/kexin-like mammalian proteinases, and are distributed specifically within endocrine cells and neurons. Both enzymes are capable of cleaving neuropeptide precursors, including POMC, proinsulin and proglucagon, at dibasic sites, and each appears to manifest distinct preferences for different sites within the same precursor prohormone, with PC2 able to cleave at a wider selection of available dibasic sites than PC1 [31].

The tissue distributions of PC1 and PC2 mRNAs are distinctly different. PC1 is abundant in ~20% of anterior pituitary cells (presumably including corticotrophs), in all intermediate lobe pituitary cells (of the rodent) and in the supraoptic nucleus of the hypothalamus [41]. In contrast, PC2 is absent from the anterior pituitary, but is highly expressed in rodent pituitary intermediate lobe, multiple sites within the central nervous system, including cerebral cortex, hippocampus and thalamus, and in pancreatic islet cells [41]. The differential tissue-specific distribution of these enzymes matches nicely with the known tissue-specific differences in POMC proteolytic processing (see below), suggesting that PC1 is responsible for the POMC cleavage products found in anterior pituitary corticotrophs, whereas PC2 cleaves POMC in the pituitary intermediate lobe (of lower mammals) and in the brain. This suggestion is supported by studies of the differential processing of POMC by PC1 and PC2 [41].

A patient with severe childhood obesity and hyperproinsulinemia with postprandial hypoglycemia has been identified with compound heterozygous mutations in the PC1 gene [42]. The patient presented with multiple endocrine abnormalities including impaired glucose tolerance and post prandial hypoglycemia which has been attributed to the secretion of large amounts of proinsulin given its partial insulin-like action and long biological half life. She also suffered from hypogonadotropic hypogonadism with primary amenorrhea, but normal development of secondary sexual characteristics. Ovulation was induced with exogenous gonadotropins, and the patient delivered healthy quadruplets. The pregnancy was complicated by gestational diabetes requiring insulin treatment. She also suffered from mild adrenal cortical insufficiency with complaints of fatigue and excessive daytime somnolence reversed by glucocorticoid administration. The adrenal cortical insufficiency was attributed to defective POMC processing with elevated levels of serum ACTH precursors confirming a role for PC1 in human POMC processing [42].

Following the generation of peptide products by prohormone convertase enzymes, the C-terminal basic amino acids are removed by carboxypeptidase activity. Carboxypeptidase E (Cpe) is required for the excision of paired dibasic residues of various peptide prohormone intermediates, including those derived from proinsulin and POMC [43]. The mutation in a strain of hyperproinsulinemic, late-onset obese mouse, the fat/fat mouse, has recently been mapped to the carboxypeptidase E gene [43]. A missense mutation has been identified in the Cpe^{fat} allele and these mice demonstrated a 20-fold decrease in CPE enzymatic activity in pituitaries and isolated islets.

The sorting of POMC into secretory granules is probably mediated by a signal patch, located within the tertiary structure of the molecule, which directs it to the granules. The presence of all POMC processed products in equimolar amounts within secretory granules suggests that this sorting precedes proteolytic cleavage of POMC. This suggestion is supported by data which demonstrate that initiation of proteolytic processing of POMC begins in the trans-Golgi system and continues in secretory vesicles and is also consistent with data demonstrating localization of PC1 and PC2 within the TGN and/or dense core secretory granules [44]. Since POMC as well as PC1 and PC2 all contain signal peptides and are presumably colocalized throughout the endoplasmic reticulum, prohormone convertase activity must be inhibited in the endoplasmic reticulum and cis-Golgi regions. PC activity may be regulated by the local intracellular environment of these compartments and/or by control of catalytic activation of prohormone convertase.

7B2 is a small, hydrophobic acidic protein originally isolated from porcine and human anterior pituitary glands that is widely distributed in neuroendocrine tissues and found to associate specifically with PC2 [45]. The 27-kDa 7B2 precursor protein is cleaved to a 21-kDa protein and a small carboxy-terminal peptide (CT peptide). Interaction of 7B2, particularly the 21-kDa fragment, with proPC2 appears necessary for the generation of mature and active PC2 in the *trans*-Golgi region. The 7B2 CT peptide is a nanomolar inhibitor of PC2 in vitro, but its role in vivo has not been defined. The role of 7B2 in activating proPC2 has been confirmed in vivo in 7B2 null mice [46]. 7B2 null mice are devoid of PC2 activity and deficiently process islet hormones and proopiomelanocortin. The mice are hypoglycemic and demonstrate hyperproinsulinemia and hypoglucagonemia. These mice also demonstrate profound intermediate lobe ACTH hypersecretion with minimal conversion of this peptide to α-MSH resulting in a severe Cushing's syndrome that causes death by 9 weeks of age [46]. Curiously, PC2 null mice demonstrate similar islet cell dysfunction resulting in hypoglycemia, but do not abnormally produce a Cushingoid syndrome [47]. This discrepancy suggests additional functional roles for 7B2 which are further suggested by the localization of 7B2 in regions of the brain lacking PC2.

Recently, the suggestion that 7B2 may represent one member of a family of related convertase inhibitor proteins has been proposed with the identification of the protein proSAAS [48]. ProSAAS is a 26-kDa granin-like neuroendocrine peptide precursor isolated from rodents and humans with structural similarity to 7B2 including a proline-rich sequence in the first half of the molecule and a C-terminal peptide (SAAS CT peptide) following a dibasic cleavage sequence [48]. Overexpression of proSAAS in AtT-20 cells reduces the rate of POMC processing and the SAAS CT peptide is a nanomolar competitive inhibitor of PC1, but not PC2 [48].

Tissue Specificity of POMC Processing

In human corticotrophs, POMC is processed predominantly into N-terminal glycopeptide$^{1-76}$, joining peptide (JP)$^{79-108}$, ACTH$^{112-150}$ and ß-LPH$^{153-240}$ (Figure 3.1) [31]. Much smaller amounts of α-MSH$^{112-124}$, CLIP$^{130-150}$, ß-endorphin$^{210-240}$ and a truncated form of N-terminal glycopeptide$^{1-61}$, also known as "big" gamma-MSH, are also present [31]. There is no evidence for cleavage after arg^{50}, and therefore no evidence for the presence of gamma$_1$-MSH$^{51-61}$ in the human pituitary. JP$^{79-108}$ exists as both a monomer and homodimer, most likely joined via disulfide bonding between the single Cys^{87} of two molecules. A function for N-terminal glycopeptide has also not been assigned, although one intriguing study reported that it is capable of stimulating aldosterone release from adrenal cells.

Whereas the production of distinct POMC peptide derivatives is clearly segregated between the anterior and intermediate lobes of the rodent, in the human, small, acetylated POMC peptide derivatives colocalize with larger desacetylated POMC peptides in corticotrophs of the anterior pituitary suggesting that the strict dichotomy between corticotrope and melanotrope POMC processing observed in rodents and other species does not extend to human pituitaries [31].

Levels of desacetyl-α-MSH are elevated in pituitary corticotrophs and plasma of patients with Addison's disease, Cushing's disease and Nelson's syndrome [31]. Desacetyl-α-MSH has approximately 75% of the melanotrophic activity of α-MSH, whereas ACTH is only 5% as potent as α-MSH in this regard. Because the serum levels of ACTH are 50- to 100-fold higher than levels of desacetyl-α-MSH in patients with Cushing's disease, Addison's disease and Nelson's syndrome, it is likely that the hyperpigmentation associated with these disorders is largely due to the melanotrophic effect of ACTH, and not MSH.

Thus, in human anterior pituitary corticotrophs, the POMC precursor is predominantly cleaved at limited Lys-Arg sites into two peptides in Domain I (N-terminal glycopeptide$^{1-76}$ and JP$^{79-108}$), one peptide in Domain II (ACTH$^{112-150}$) and one peptide in Domain III (ß-LPH$^{153-240}$) (see Figure 3.1). As discussed above, human POMC is also expressed in several brain sites outside of the anterior pituitary, predominantly in the arcuate nucleus of the anterior hypothalamus. In these extrapituitary locations, POMC is processed to a greater extent than in anterior pituitary. In brain, ACTH$^{112-150}$ is cleaved to α-MSH$^{112-124}$ and CLIP$^{130-150}$, such that the amount of α-MSH relative to ACTH is 300-fold higher in hypothalamus, telencephalon and mesencephalon than it is in anterior pituitary [31]. As in anterior pituitary, α-MSH is almost exclusively present in the desacetyl form.

Adding additional levels of complexity to the issue of tissue specificity of POMC processing are results from a dopamine D2 receptor (D2R) deficient mouse. Similar to dopaminergic tonic inhibitory control of prolactin expression in lactotrophs, POMC expression in the rodent intermediate lobe is under inhibitory dopaminergic control mediated via D2 receptors. D2R-deficient mice demonstrate mild intermediate lobe hyperplasia accompanied by up-regulation of both PC1 and PC2 [49]. These mice present with unexpectedly high levels of ACTH with corresponding adrenal hypertrophy and increases in corticosteroid secretion [49]. The altered prohormone convertase levels in these mice suggest the possibility of dynamic regulation of prohormone processing within specific tissues.

HORMONE MEASUREMENT

ACTH was one of the first substances to be measured by radioimmunoassay (RIA) [50]. In pioneering work using polyclonal antisera, Yalow described the measurement of ACTH and related peptides in normal persons and those with ectopic ACTH production by lung cancer. These studies provided among the first data that ACTH was synthesized from larger precursors, which were termed 'big' and 'big-big' ACTH. The ACTH RIA can be performed on unextracted plasma, but suffers from a limit of sensitivity of ~25 pg/ml, and is therefore often unable to detect levels of plasma ACTH in the normal basal range.

Radioimmunoassay remained the standard method for the measurement of plasma ACTH until the development of the immunoradiometric assay (IRMA). ACTH IRMAs employ two antibodies, one or both monoclonal, against ACTH. The solution-phase antibody is radiolabeled, and the solid-phase antibody is linked to a bead or other solid support. In general, the ACTH IRMA on unextracted plasma compares very favorably with RIA, being more sensitive, more reproducible and more rapid [51]. Most IRMAs have lower limits of detection of 3–5 pg/ml and coefficients of variation of less than 10% up to 5000 pg/ml. Depending on the antigenic specificity of the chosen antibodies, the ACTH IRMA may detect only intact ACTH, both ACTH and POMC precursor peptides, or only POMC precursors. It is essential to know the sequence specificity of any IRMA in clinical use, for some, unlike most polyclonal RIAs, are incapable of detecting ACTH precursors which may be secreted by lung carcinomas. Despite the wide availability of the ACTH IRMA, results from different laboratories are difficult to compare because of lack of agreement on a suitable ACTH reference standard. An immunofluorometric assay (IFMA) for ACTH has also been developed [52]. Its sensitivity and accuracy are similar to those of the IRMA. Its principal advantage is its speed and the use of nonradioactive label which is stable for over 1 year. A direct comparison of IRMA and RIA tests for ACTH found them to be comparable [51]. Furthermore, a nonradioactive electrochemiluminescent adrenocorticotropic hormone (ACTH) immunoassay was found to be precise and reliable in combination with reduced turnaround time [53]. Recently, an assay for Synacthen (1–24 ACTH) in urine by tandem mass spectrometry has been developed to detect illegal doping activity in athletes [54].

Plasma assay of POMC products other than ACTH, including ß-endorphin and N-terminal glycopeptide, has been suggested as an adjunct in the evaluation of the hypothalamic–pituitary–adrenal (HPA) axis. In general, the levels of these hormones parallel that of ACTH in various HPA axis abnormalities. However, except for use as a screening test for lung carcinoma associated with preferential secretion of N-terminal glycopeptide$^{1-61}$ or pro-ACTH$^{1-150}$, such tests are much less helpful than the ACTH IRMA because of the low concentration of other POMC peptide fragments compared with ACTH in most physiologic and pathologic settings.

Secretion of ACTH: Biochemistry and Pharmacology

Secretion of ACTH from the corticotrophs of the anterior pituitary is mediated by several factors (Figure 3.2). CRH and vasopressin are the primary secretagogues for ACTH, although a number of other agents may also affect its release, and glucocorticoids are the major negative regulators of ACTH secretion. Once a ligand has bound to its receptor, release of ACTH from the corticotroph is mediated by second messengers through one of four signal transduction pathways, involving either protein kinase A, protein kinase C, glucocorticoids, or the Janus kinase/STAT system. (This last pathyway, regulated by LIF, was described in a previous section.) These pathways result in changes in the phosphorylation pattern of specific cellular proteins, and/or in intracellular calcium levels, impacting on ACTH synthesis and release. Circulating ACTH then binds to receptors, primarily in the adrenal gland, leading to steroid biosynthesis.

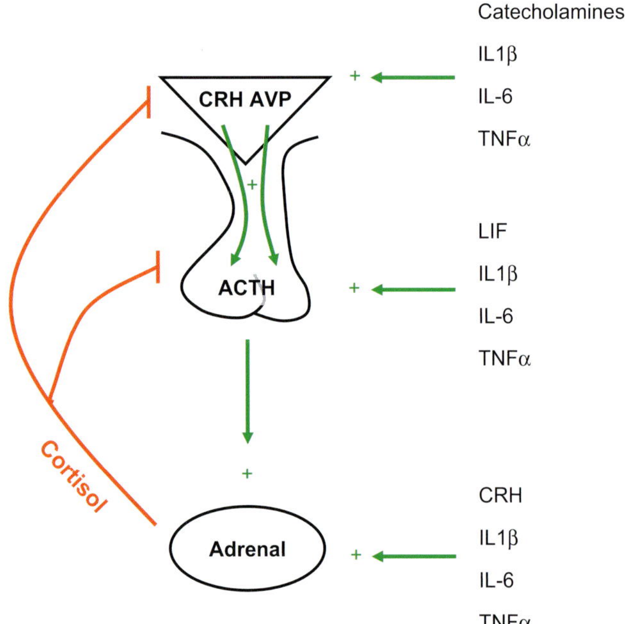

FIGURE 3.2 Regulation of ACTH secretion.

CRH

CRH Stimulation of ACTH Secretion

CRH is the most important physiologic ACTH secretagogue. Stressors, endogenous circadian rhythms and glucocorticoids influence CRH release. In the rat, afferent inputs to the PVN may mediate the action of stressors by controlling the release of CRH [55]. Sources of neuronal afferents to the hypothalamus include the amygdala and hippocampus of the limbic system, and brainstem regions involved in autonomic functions [55]. In rats, acetylcholine, norephinephrine, angiotensin II and possibly CRH itself, increase CRH concentrations in the hypophyseal portal plasma. On the other hand, ß-endorphin and GABA inhibit the ACTH response to stress [56].

Perfused human fetal pituitaries and cultured human fetal pituitary cells in culture secrete ACTH in response to CRH [2]. Rats have been used extensively in the study of ACTH secretion, as it is difficult to culture human corticotroph cells in vitro. In dispersed rat anterior pituitary cells, CRH stimulates a 9-fold increase in ACTH release that is sustained for as long as the cells are exposed to CRH. Even with maximal CRH stimulation, only 6% of cultured pituitary cells release ACTH.

Most of the CRH released into the hypophyseal blood is derived from the PVN. Concentrations of CRH that are similar to the concentrations of CRH found in rat portal plasma have been shown to increase secretion of ACTH in human fetal hemipituitaries in vitro [57]. The CRH content in the hypophyseal portal blood of anesthetized male rats is about 100 pM, which exceeds the in vitro threshold of 10–20 pM CRH to stimulate ACTH release [58]. In addition to stimulating ACTH expression and release, CRH can also directly stimulate secretion of glucocorticoids from the adrenal gland [59].

CRH stimulates ACTH synthesis as well as release. In humans, the biphasic response may reflect secretion of a ready pool of ACTH, followed by later release of newly synthesized protein [60]. Exposing cells to CRH for a long period of time results in an increase in ACTH in the cell and in the medium. Thus, the sustained phase of ACTH secretion may represent later release of newly synthesized ACTH peptide.

Modulators of CRH Release

Interleukin-1 beta stimulates ACTH release in conscious rats by acting on the hypothalamus to induce secretion of CRH [56]. Interleukin-1 does not cross the blood–brain barrier, but activates noradrenergic neurons in the brainstem and hypothalamus, which may stimulate CRH secretion, especially in the median eminence. Prostaglandins may be involved in the response to interleukin-1, since ibuprofen, which blocks the formation of prostaglandins, blocks endotoxin-induced ACTH release in humans [61].

In humans and other mammals, the impact of angiotensin II on basal or CRH-stimulated ACTH release is unclear. In humans, infusion of angiotensin II alone does not increase ACTH release [62]. However, in dispersed rat anterior pituitary cells, angiotensin II does stimulate release of ACTH [63]. Angiotensin II has a synergistic effect with CRH in stimulating ACTH release in humans in vivo [62]. Angiotensin II potentiates CRH-stimulated ACTH release from cultured anterior pituitary cells [64], although it is less effective than AVP, and potentiates the CRH-stimulated increase in cAMP. Angiotensin II and AVP do not potentiate each other's effect on ACTH release, suggesting that they act via the same mechanism.

CRH Receptors

In human pituitaries, CRH has been shown to bind to sites in the anterior lobe. The distribution of binding sites in human pituitary correlates with the distribution of corticotrophs. CRH receptors in the anterior pituitary gland are low-capacity, high-affinity receptors, with a K_d for CRH binding of about 1 nM. To date, two CRH receptor genes have been identified in humans and other mammals, with a third additional one being described in the catfish [34]. The type 1 receptor is expressed predominantly in anterior pituitary corticotroph cells, whereas the type 2 receptor is more widely distributed in the brain and periphery, particularly in cardiovascular tissue [34]. The type 1 receptor binds and is activated by CRH as well as the CRH-like peptide, urocortin [34]. This receptor mediates the actions of CRH at the corticoctroph. In addition, the type 1 receptor mediates fear and anxiety behaviors following stressors, even in CRH-deficient mice [65]. Mice with deletion of the CRH type 1 receptor gene show reduced fear and anxiety [34]. These data suggest that a CRH-related peptide, possibly urocortin or another unknown member of the CRH family, mediates fear responses via the CRH type 1 receptor. The CRH type 2 receptor binds urocortin with over 20-fold higher affinity compared to CRH. Its distribution, along with the hypotensive cardiovascular response to infused urocortin which is abolished in CRH type 2 receptor-deficient mice [34], suggests that the receptor may be involved in blood pressure control. This may underlie the hypotension observed during the CRH stimulation test. Several peptide antagonists to CRH receptors were synthesized, with hopes of treating conditions from anxiety to depression, but these were unable to pass through the blood–brain barrier. In 1996, a CRH type 1 receptor-specific antagonist, called antalarmin, was developed [66]. Antalarmin is non-peptide and orally active. It features a central ring core with a basic nitrogen group that modulates the confirmation of an agonist-binding site [66]. Male rhesus macaques were treated orally with antalarmin and challenged with an intense social stressor, two unfamiliar males separated by a transparent screen [66]. Treatment with antalarmin significantly decreased ACTH and cortisol responses. Additionally, behaviors typically associated with social stress, such as body tremors, grimacing, teeth gnashing, urination and defecation, were decreased. Exploratory and sexual behaviors that are typically suppressed during stress were increased in antalarmin-treated primates.

AVP

AVP Stimulation of ACTH Secretion

AVP is synthesized in the same parvocellular hypothalamic paraventricular nuclear neurons which express CRH [56], and appears to be co-released with CRH at the median eminence into the portal hypophyseal system. However, a substantial amount of AVP in the portal blood is released from projections from the supraoptic nuclei in the median eminence [56]. AVP from the posterior pituitary may also reach the anterior pituitary through portal vessels that connect the two. This raises the possibility that increased vasopressin secretion from the posterior pituitary, in response to hyperosmolality, may also stimulate ACTH secretion.

In rat anterior pituitary cells, AVP causes an increase in ACTH release [56]. AVP elicits an initial rapid release of ACTH, observable within 5 seconds, reaching a maximum in less than 1–2 minutes, and lasting less than 3–6 minutes. This is followed by a second phase lasting for several hours. In humans, AVP infusion by itself has only a small effect on ACTH release.

In rodents, central catecholamines stimulate ACTH release, and the effects of catecholamines on ACTH secretion appear to be mediated via secretion of CRH, and possibly AVP, into the hypophyseal portal circulation [67]. However, in humans, catecholamines have little direct effect on ACTH secretion from the pituitary. Peripheral catecholamines, increased by a variety of stresses, do not cross the blood–brain barrier to reach the hypothalamus, but do reach the pituitary, yet do not increase basal or CRH-stimulated plasma ACTH levels. This suggests that the increased peripheral levels of epinephrine and norepinephrine generated during stress are probably not responsible for the increase in ACTH, and that catecholamines do not act directly on the pituitary to stimulate ACTH release.

Modulators of AVP Release

Tumor necrosis factor is a potent secretagogue for ACTH, and when administered to human subjects, leads to an increase in ACTH, cortisol and AVP, but inhibits CRH-, AVP- and angiotensin-II-stimulated ACTH secretion. Tumor necrosis factor may stimulate ACTH secretion by stimulating CRH release from the hypothalamus [68]. However, there is evidence that the site of action of tumor necrosis factor is peripheral to the pituitary and hypothalamus [68]. Bacterial endotoxin, when administered to human subjects, increases ACTH, cortisol and AVP release [61]. Tumor necrosis factor may mediate the hormonal responses to endotoxin, since tumor necrosis factor levels increase after endotoxin administration [69]. Endotoxin does not increase ACTH release from cultured rat adenohypophyseal cells.

In rats and humans, interleukin-6 leads to ACTH secretion via CRH-dependent [70] and CRH-independent pathways, most likely via a prostaglandin-dependent pathway [71]. GABA inhibits the secretion of ACTH by inhibiting the release of CRH and possibly AVP. GABAergic inputs into the PVN of the hypothalamus have been characterized in animals, including inputs from the hippocampus [72]. Opiates and opiate agonists decrease ACTH secretion, and may tonically inhibit ACTH secretion [73], although some studies demonstrate no effect of naloxone, an opiate antagonist, on the basal levels of cortisol [74]. Opiates inhibit CRH- and AVP-stimulated ACTH release, and different opiate agonists differentially affect CRH- versus AVP-stimulated release [75]. In humans, morphine blunts CRH-stimulated ACTH release without decreasing AVP or catecholamine levels [75]. Modulation of CRH-stimulated ACTH secretion by opiates most likely occurs at a level above the corticotroph [75]. Met-enkephalin analogues inhibit ACTH secretion, and controversy exists as to whether inhibition occurs at the hypothalamus or pituitary. In humans CRH-induced ACTH release is almost completely abolished with pre-treatment with a met-enkephalin analogue [76].

AVP Receptors

A single population of specific AVP receptors has been identified in rat anterior pituitaries, which are distinct from CRH receptors. Most corticotrophs have AVP receptors, since 80% of the ACTH-secreting cells in the pituitary bind AVP. The anterior pituitary AVP receptors are distinct from the V2 renal receptors and the V1 hepatic/pressor receptors. This has led to the classification of hepatic/pressor receptors as V1a receptors and anterior pituitary receptors as V1b [150], or V3, receptors. V1a, V1b and V2 receptors can be distinguished by their patterns of recognition of AVP analogues [77]. V1a binding sites in the rat anterior pituitary have a K_d of about 1 nM, and the minimal effective dose of AVP is 0.1 nM [78]. DdAVP (desmopressin), an AVP analogue with V2 receptor affinity, has an insignificant effect on plasma ACTH levels, though it does increase, but is not additive to, CRH-stimulated ACTH release [62].

The genes for all three vasopressin receptors (V1, V2 and V1b) have been identified. They are highly related members of the seven-transmembrane, G-protein-coupled receptor family. V1b receptor mRNA is highly expressed in anterior pituitary corticotrophs, and is coupled to stimulation of POMC gene expression and ACTH secretion via the protein kinase C pathway [79].

Second Messenger Regulation of ACTH Secretion

Protein Kinase A Pathway

CRH stimulates ACTH release via the cAMP-protein kinase A pathway. CRH stimulates adenylate cyclase activity, which then increases cAMP [32]. Forskolin, a direct stimulator of adenylate cyclase activity, and 8-bromo-cAMP, a cAMP analogue, both markedly stimulate ACTH release and increase CRH-stimulated ACTH release, but do not potentiate ACTH release from cells maximally stimulated by CRH. The CRH-stimulated increase in cAMP activates cAMP-dependent protein kinase A.

Protein Kinase C Pathway

AVP V1 and V2 receptors are coupled to different second messenger systems. V1 receptors in the pituitary mobilize calcium through activation of phospholipase C, whereas V2 receptors activate adenylate cyclase, increasing cAMP. AVP-stimulated ACTH release is mediated via the protein kinase C pathway. Evidence that AVP acts through the protein kinase C pathway in the anterior pituitary includes the finding that AVP stimulates accumulation of inositol phosphates in rat anterior pituitary cells. Phorbol esters, which activate protein kinase C directly by substituting for diacylglycerol and binding to protein kinase, induce ACTH release in rat pituitary cell cultures. Activation of protein kinase C appears more important in the sustained phase of AVP-stimulated ACTH release, not in the initial phase.

Synergism Between CRH and AVP

Alone, AVP is a less important physiologic ACTH secretagogue than CRH. AVP potentiates CRH-stimulated release of ACTH from cultivated rat anterior pituitary cells by two-fold. When cells are first exposed to CRH, reaching the sustained phase of CRH-stimulated ACTH release, and AVP is then added, the usual initial spike of AVP-stimulated ACTH secretion is superimposed on top of the CRH-induced plateau of secretion. Despite continued exposure to AVP, ACTH secretion decreases down to the level of the plateau phase of CRH-stimulated secretion [80]. In cells exposed to AVP before CRH, CRH does not potentiate AVP-stimulated ACTH secretion [80]. This, together with the presence of AVP and CRH in the same parvocellular neurons of the PVN, suggests that the two neuropeptides cooperate to regulate ACTH release. However, this remains to be proven in humans, as there are no examples of persons with defects in AVP synthesis or release who have impaired ACTH secretion.

Oxytocin

In humans, low-dose oxytocin perfusion decreases plasma ACTH and cortisol levels, and infusion of oxytocin completely inhibits CRH-stimulated ACTH release [81]. Oxytocin acts via a similar mechanism as AVP. Oxytocin binds competitively to AVP receptors in the anterior pituitary, but is much weaker than AVP at stimulating ACTH release. Like AVP, oxytocin stimulates ACTH secretion through the protein kinase C pathway.

Glucocorticoids

Glucocorticoids are the primary negative regulators of ACTH secretion. Glucocorticoids act on corticotrophs to inhibit the secretion of ACTH induced by AVP and CRH, the synergism between CRH and AVP, and substances that provoke production of inositol phosphates and cAMP. Glucocorticoids' negative impact on ACTH regulation is also due to their inhibition of the principal stimulators of ACTH, CRH and AVP.

In the rat, glucocorticoid receptors are widely distributed in the brain, including the PVN. The PVN is a site for glucocorticoid negative feedback, since dexamethasone decreases the amount of basal CRH in the hypothalami explant and in the PVN, and the CRH response to secretagogues like serotonin and to stress. Glucocorticoids inhibit CRH release and decrease intracellular CRH in the PVN, and dexamethasone has a local effect on the hypothalamus, decreasing CRH mRNA expression, and preventing the rise in intracellular CRH and AVP usually seen after adrenalectomy.

Glucocorticoids increase, and adrenalectomy decreases, the amount of GABA in the hypothalamus and the hippocampus [82]. Glucocorticoids appear to feedback to increase the GABA activity of the hippocampus and hypothalamus, and thus inhibit CRH release [82]. In the anterior pituitary, glucocorticoid inhibition of ACTH secretion in vitro is mediated via glucocorticoid receptors, and lack of glucocorticoid effect in the intermediate lobe of the pituitary is most likely because functional receptors are not present in these cells. The negative effect of glucocorticoids on CRH-, AVP-, angiotensin II- and norepinephrine-stimulated ACTH release is biphasic, which may reflect an initial inhibition of ACTH release, followed by an inhibition of POMC biosynthesis. Glucocorticoids inhibit POMC secretion, gene transcription and mRNA levels in the anterior pituitary.

Mediation of the Effects of POMC-derived Peptides

The melanocortin receptors are a family of seven-transmembrane spanning, G-protein-coupled receptors that are activated by melanocortin derivatives of POMC including α-MSH and ACTH. Activation of all five receptors results in adenylate cyclase activity and cAMP production. Cloning of the melanocyte MSH receptor (melanocortin 1 receptor – MC1R) [83] and the adrenal ACTH receptor (melanocortin 2 receptor – MC2R) [83] was quickly followed by the cloning of three additional family members. The five known melanocortin receptors show distinct tissue distributions throughout the nervous system and periphery and distinct selectivities for the various melanocortin peptides. Prior to the cloning of this receptor family, the actions of melanocortins were primarily known through the effects of MSH on pigmentation and the effects of ACTH on glucocorticoid secretion from the adrenals. However, many additional roles including cognitive and behavioral effects, effects on the immune system and effects on the cardiovascular system have also been attributed to the melanocortins. With the cloning of this family of receptors, the physiologic roles of ACTH, MSH and other melanocortin derivatives are beginning to be elucidated.

Ligand Specificity

The pharmacology of melanocortin receptor activation with a large number of natural and synthetic melanocortin peptides is the subject of extensive investigation. All five melanocortin receptors are activated by ACTH. However, MC2R binds only ACTH and is not activated by other melanocortin peptides [84]. The synthetic agonist 4-norleucine,7-D-phenylalanine-α-MSH (NDP-MSH) is the most potent agonist of MC1R, MC3R, MC4R and MC5R [85]. The endogenous non-ACTH melanocortin peptides generally bind the melanocortin receptors with an order of potency MC1R > MC3R > MC4R > MC5R when expressed in COS cells and measurements are obtained in competition with NDP-MSH [85]. γ-MSH is relatively selective for MC3R over MC4R and MC5R [85]. Whether the differences in melanocortin receptor specificity for different melanocortin ligands are physiologically relevant is unknown. Interestingly, Org 2766 and BIM 22015, two ACTH4-10 analogues, have no activity at any of the cloned MCRs, but have potent effects on central and peripheral nervous systems, suggesting the possibility of undiscovered melanocortin receptors [86].

Melanocortin 1 Receptor

The MC1R was initially cloned from primary melanoma tumors [87]. MC1R gene expression has also been confirmed in primary human melanocytes by northern blotting [87]. Other cutaneous cells including keratinocytes and dermal fibroblasts have also been reported to express MC1R, although the presence of MC1R in keratinocytes could not be confirmed in other studies [88]. Recent evidence demonstrates that the MC1R is expressed in keratinocytes and that its expression is induced by calcium and UV light treatments [89]. Corresponding to its expression in the skin, its function is perhaps most fully understood with respect to its role in cutaneous pigmentation. Activation of melanocyte MC1R, via activation of adenylate cyclase, stimulates tyrosinase activity, the rate-limiting enzyme in melanogenesis [88]. The activation of tyrosinase results in an increased proportion of eumelanin (brown-black pigment) formation over pheomelanin (red-yellow pigment) formation resulting in increased pigmentation.

Mutations and variant alleles in the MC1R gene have been linked to variation in mammalian pigmentation. The extension locus has long been known to regulate pigmentation in mammalian species. The extension locus has been shown to encode the mouse MC1R [90]. The recessive yellow allele (e) at this locus results from a frameshift that produces a prematurely terminated, nonfunctioning receptor [90]. The sombre (E^{so} and E^{so-3j}) alleles and tobacco darkening (E^{tob}) alleles, which have dominant melanizing effects, result from point mutations that produce constitutively active or hyperactive receptors [90].

The human MC1R is highly polymorphic, and mutant alleles have been associated with fair skin and blond or red hair [91]. Analysis of five naturally occurring common variants of MC1R associated with fair skin and red hair have revealed decreased stimulation of cAMP synthesis with no changes in or only slightly reduced α-MSH binding. In addition, MC1R variants have recently been shown to determine sun-sensitivity in humans with dark hair [92]. Melanocytes, which express POMC and several of its processed peptides, are derived from the neural crest [17]. It is likely that α-MSH produced via POMC expression in melanocytes is responsible for the pigmenting effects of ultraviolet light, and together with variations in MC1R discussed above, for the different degrees of skin pigmentation observed among ethic groups.

MC1R has been detected in Leydig cells of the testis, luteal cells of the corpus luteum and in the placenta. In the central nervous system, detection of MC1R mRNA and protein has been confined to a few scattered neurons of the periaqueductal gray in rat and human brains.

With the cloning of the melanocortin receptors, the role of melanocortins as anti-inflammatory agents has gained renewed interest [93]. Systemic administration of α-MSH has been shown to be beneficial in animal models of arthritis, adult respiratory distress syndrome and septic shock. Consistent with this role, MC1R expression has been documented on macrophages and monocytes [94]. Treatment of activated macrophages with α-MSH resulted in decreased nitric oxide production by inhibiting the induction of nitric oxide synthase II [94]. LPS and interferon treatments of neutrophils induced increases in neutrophil MC1R mRNA and treatment with α-MSH inhibited neutrophil chemotaxis by a cAMP-dependent process [95]. Constitutive expression of MC1R has also been found on dermal microvascular endothelial cells where its expression can be increased by stimulation with IL-1β or α-MSH itself [96]. A potential role for melanocortins to regulate local inflammation in the brain has been proposed based on the evidence that TNF-alpha secretion by an anaplastic astrocytoma cell line (A-172) is decreased by α-MSH and that these cells express MC1R.

Melanocortin 2 Receptor: The ACTH Receptor

Early in the study of receptor biology, Haynes demonstrated the action of ACTH in generating cyclic adenosine monophosphate (cAMP) in adrenal cells. The ACTH receptor was the first receptor that was shown to bind its ligand with high affinity and specificity. In human adrenal glands, the ACTH receptor has a K_d of 1.6 nmol/l and about 3500 sites/cell. The ED50 of ACTH for cAMP production is 0.11 nmol/l, 20-fold less than the K_d for binding. The ED50 of ACTH for cortisol production is 2 pmol/l, 720-fold less than the K_d for ACTH binding, and 35-fold less than the concentration of ACTH needed to obtain a half-maximal increase in cAMP production. Only a small percentage of ACTH receptors need to be occupied to achieve a maximal effect on steroidogenesis, which occurs at an ACTH concentration of 0.01 nmol/L. Because the adrenal gland may express more than one of the five melanocortin receptors it is not possible to assign the biochemical characterizations to a specific melanocortin receptor.

The human ACTH receptor (MC2R) was cloned based on its homology to MC1R. In situ hybridization with the adrenal gland of the rhesus monkey demonstrated the presence of message in the zona glomerulosa and fasciculata cells, and a weaker signal in the zona reticularis. Initial attempts at characterizing the ligand specificity and cAMP signal generation in response to ACTH and other melanocortins was confounded by either poor levels of expression or the presence of endogenous melanocortin receptors in transfected cells. Recently, human MC2R has been stably transfected into the Y6 cell line, a mutant derived from the mouse Y1 adrenocortical cell line, that fails to express any endogenous MC2R [97]. Y6 cells alone demonstrated no cAMP response to micromolar ACTH, and MC2R transfected cells displayed an EC50 of 6.8 nmol/l [97].

MRAP and MRAP2

Genome-wide array studies of patients with familial glucocorticoid deficiency (FGD) but without MC2R mutations revealed a new protein linked to the disease. The melanocortin 2 receptor accessory protein, MRAP, is required to traffic MC2R to the plasma membrane [98], where it binds ACTH (Figure 3.3). MRAP is a 19-kDa single-transmembrane domain protein and maps to chromosome 21q22.1 in humans [98]. The *MRAP* gene consists of six exons, and the last two exons may be alternatively spliced to encode MRAP-α or MRAP-β isoforms.

Co-immunoprecipitation studies showed that MC2R physically associated with MRAP. Heterologous cells only responded to ACTH when MRAP and MC2R were transfected together, not when MC2R was transfected alone [98]. Mouse Y1 cells, one cell line known to endogenously respond to ACTH, was shown to express MRAP. When MRAP was knocked down by RNAi, these cells lost ACTH responsiveness [99]. MC2R was localized to the endoplasmic reticulum and plasma membrane. In transfected CHO cells, markers for both the N- and C-termini of the MRAP protein were localized externally [100]. Endogenous MRAP also presented both N- and C-termini externally in adrenal cells. Half of MRAP was glycosylated at a single endogenous N-terminal glycosylation site, and mutant MRAP with potential glycosylation sites on both sides of the membrane were glycosylated only at one domain. MRAP forms an antiparallel homodimer that stably complexes with MC2R. MRAP was the first antiparallel homodimeric membrane protein identified in eukaryotic cells. MRAP was initially thought to be highly specific for MC2R and did not increase cell surface expression of other melanocortin receptors, β2-adrenergic receptors, or TSH-releasing hormone receptors [100]. More recently, however, it was shown that MRAP co-precipitated with MC5R and blocked MC5R dimerization and cell surface localization [101].

Human genome analysis has identified a single MRAP paralogue, which was named *MRAP2*, because it also interacts with MC2R. Though *MRAP2* bears only 27% sequence homology to *MRAPα*, there is greater interspecies conservation of *MRAP2* than *MRAP*, and it

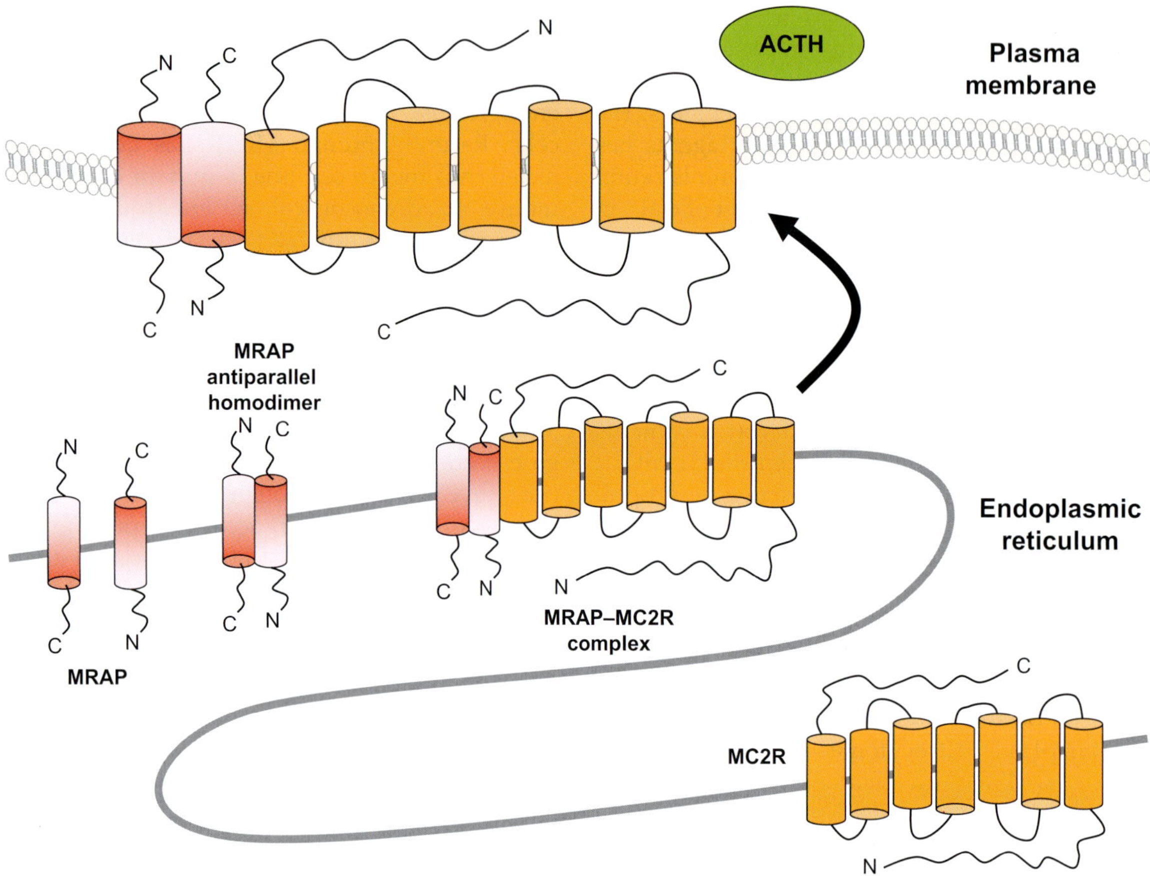

FIGURE 3.3 Interaction between MRAP and MC2R. The melanocortin 2 receptor accessory protein, MRAP, is required to traffic MC2R to the plasma membrane, where it interacts with ACTH. MRAP was localized to the endoplasmic reticulum and plasma membrane, and both C- and N-termini of MRAP were found to face externally in the membranes. MRAP is the first eukaryotic protein known to function as an antiparallel homodimer. In this conformation, MRAP stably binds MC2R, and the complex is trafficked to the plasma membrane. In the plasma membrane, MC2R interacts with and responds to ACTH. Knock down of MRAP confers the inability of MC2R to respond to ACTH. In human patients, MRAP mutations are responsible for approximately 25% of cases of familial glucocorticoid deficiency (FGD).

is believed that *MRAP2* most closely resembles the ancestral protein. There is 87% sequence homology between human and mouse *MRAP2* [102]. MRAP2 is a 205-amino acid single-transmembrane domain protein that is primarily expressed in the human adult adrenal gland and ventromedial hypothalamus in the brain, a site of MC3R and MC4R expression.

Adrenal Actions of ACTH

The critical role of ACTH in regulating the synthesis and secretion of steroids from the adrenal gland has long been recognized. In adrenocortical cells, ACTH regulates lipoprotein uptake by receptor-mediated endocytosis from the plasma to lipid droplets by stimulation of lipoprotein receptors. Within the lipid droplets, ACTH regulates hydrolysis of cholesterol esters by activation of cholesterol esterases or suppression of cholesterol acyltransferase, through cAMP-dependent protein kinase. ACTH stimulates the transport of cholesterol to the mitochondria, principally via stimulation of steroidogenic acute regulatory protein (StAR) [103]. The rate-limiting step in steroidogenesis is the side-chain cleavage of cholesterol to pregnenolone, and is catalyzed by cytochrome P450 side-chain cleavage enzyme in the inner membrane of mitochondria of the adrenal, probably on the matrix side. ACTH stimulation results in long-term and short-term effects on steroid hormone biosynthesis in the mitochondria. The long-term effect of ACTH leads to an increase in the amounts of steroid hormone enzymes by increasing transcription of these genes. StAR is the key protein which regulates cholesterol transport into the mitochondrion [103]. Mutations in this protein result in defects in adrenal and gonadal steroidogenesis, which had been previously attributed to defects in side-chain cleavage enzyme activity [103]. Beginning several hours after ACTH administration, ACTH increases the levels of steroidogenic enzyme mRNAs in primary cultures of human adrenals by several-fold, including cholesterol side-chain cleavage enzyme, 17-α-hydroxylase/17,20-lyase, 11-ß-hydroxylase/18-hydroxylase/18-methyloxidase and 21-hydroxylase cytochrome P450 enzyme. ACTH has a positive regulatory effect on its own receptors, and on the cAMP response to binding of ACTH to the receptor. With sustained stimulation, down-regulation does occur, but physiologically this effect is minor since ACTH causes proliferation as well as steroid secretion.

In addition to its prominent role in regulating adrenal steroidogenesis, ACTH exerts profound trophic effects upon the adrenal. Hypophysectomy results in adrenal atrophy and ACTH replacement restores adrenal gland weight in a dose-dependent manner. While the role of ACTH in adrenal hypertrophy is well established, its role in adrenocortical mitogenesis and hyperplasia is incompletely understood. The absence of ACTH induces apoptotic cell death in the adrenal cortex. Prolonged ACTH administration not only blocks apoptosis, but also increases the adrenal DNA content in the rat and ACTH increases mRNA levels for c-fos and ß-actin, proteins involved in cellular proliferation. However, ACTH paradoxically inhibits mitosis of adrenocortical cells in culture. ACTH-antiserum administered to intact rats caused a highly significant decrease in corticosterone levels, but had no effect on adrenal weight. Furthermore, ACTH inhibits the rapid compensatory proliferation of the remaining adrenal that normally occurs after unilateral adrenalectomy. Another anterior pituitary-derived candidate for the stimulation of adrenal proliferation is the 28-amino acid N-terminal proopiomelanocortin peptide (N-POMC). This peptide is mitogenic in vitro and in vivo for the adrenal cortex, and N-POMC antiserum significantly diminishes adrenal mitotic activity after enucleation [104]. The compensatory adrenal growth that occurs after unilateral adrenalectomy may be mediated by a neural reflex that includes afferent neurons originating from the disrupted adrenal gland, the ventromedial nuclei of the hypothalamus and efferent neurons innervating the remaining gland.

In 1947, Albright coined the term adrenarche to denote the developmental increase in adrenal androgens that occurs several years before the onset of gonadal maturation [105]. Adrenal androgen secretion may be sufficient for the development of some secondary sexual changes including the development of pubic and axillary hair and the maturation of sebaceous glands. A condition in which axillary and pubic hair develop prematurely as a result of early adrenal androgen secretion has been termed premature adrenarche. The mechanisms controlling adrenarche have remained obscure. Many hypotheses have been advanced, and many factors including ACTH, estrogens, prolactin, gonadotropins, growth hormone, glucocorticoids, androgens and other POMC-derived products have been suggested as modulators of adrenal androgen secretion. ACTH is widely accepted as a modulator of adrenal androgen secretion although, after administration of corticotropin, increases in DHEA and DHEAS tend to be small. Furthermore, the increase in adrenal androgens that occurs in adrenarche is not accompanied by an increase in serum cortisol levels, leading to the suggestion that factors other than ACTH are responsible for adrenarche. However, cortisol production rates do increase at the same time as the increase in adrenal androgen secretion, suggesting a possible common link that could be due to ACTH stimulation of both steroid pathways [106]. Dissection of the physiology of adrenarche has proven difficult as the only animal showing an adrenarche similar to that of humans is the chimpanzee. Recent data from patients with genetic defects in MC2R provide definitive evidence for the participation of this receptor in the process of adrenarche, as discussed subsequently.

Nonadrenal Actions of ACTH

ACTH binds with high affinity to rat adipocytes and has potent lipolytic effects. High levels of MC2R mRNA expression have been demonstrated in all murine adipose tissues examined, but MC5R mRNA expression was also found in a subset of these tissues [107]. Both MC2R and MC5R mRNA were identified in the 3T3-L1 cell line after these cells were induced to differentiate into adipocytes. The physiologic importance of the actions of melanocortins on adipose tissue is unclear. Primate adipose tissues have been reported to be insensitive to the lipolytic actions of ACTH [108]. MC2R mRNA expression was not detected in human adipose tissue.

In order to examine whether the MC2R might play roles in the hypothalamic–pituitary–adrenal axis in sites other than the adrenal gland, MC2R expression has been examined in the hypothalamus and the pituitary. MC2R mRNA could not be detected in the hypothalamus or the pituitary. The expression of an ACTH receptor on human mononuclear leukocytes was suggested after a finding that high-affinity ACTH binding did not occur in a patient with FGD [109]. However, this finding is puzzling in retrospect as MC2R mRNA expression has not been demonstrated in leukocytes.

Human skin cells express MC2R along with mRNA for three obligatory enzymes of steroid synthesis, the cytochromes P450scc (CYP11A1), P450c17 (CYP17) and P450c21 (CYP21A2). Slominski et al. have hypothesized that an equivalent of the HPA axis composed of locally produced CRH, CRH-receptor, POMC and cortisol operate in mammalian skin as a local response to stress [110]. Recently, it was demonstrated that ACTH can induce

DNA synthesis and cell proliferation in an oral keratinocyte cell line [111].

Melanocortin 3 Receptor

Expression of the third cloned melanocortin receptor, MC3R, has been identified in the brain, placenta, gut and heart. Detailed mapping of the MC3R in the central nervous system by in situ hybridization localized the highest densities of MC3R mRNA to the hypothalamus and limbic system [90]. MC3R mRNA was found in the arcuate nucleus [90], the site of POMC expression within the hypothalamus.

An autoradiographic approach using the non-selective [^{125}I]NDP-MSH in competition with the relatively MC3R-selective γ-MSH or an MC4R-selective synthetic agent HS014 has been used to visualize the MC3R and MC4R distributions within the central nervous system [112]. In the nucleus accumbens shell, the medial preoptic area and the ventromedial nucleus of the hypothalamus, the MC3R dominates. In the lateral septum and the olfactory tubercle, both MC3R and MC4R seem to be present. The lack of overlap between the autoradiographic data and the data concerning MC3R mRNA expression may indicate the presence of MC3R on nerve terminals projecting from the arcuate nucleus. A physiologic role for MC3R has not yet been identified.

In a murine model of experimental gout, systemic treatment of mice with $ACTH_{4-10}$ inhibited neutrophil accumulation [113]. This effect was blocked by the melanocortin receptor type 3/4 antagonist SHU9119. MC3R, but not MC4R, mRNA was detected in murine macrophages suggesting that MC3R may play a role in modulating inflammation. A mouse with targeted deletion of the MC3R gene has been created [114]. Although this mouse has a normal body weight, it has an increased fat-to-lean weight ratio, which seems to be due to an increased efficiency of converting ingested food into stored fuel. Thus, a function of melanocortins acting via MC3R may be to promote the conversion of energy in food into either lean body mass or forms of energy other than fat. This raises the possibility that in humans, mutations in MC3R may contribute to the "thrifty" genotype, as is found in Pima Indians [115].

Melanocortin 4 Receptor

The MC4R is localized to the brain and, in contrast to the MC3R, its expression has been documented throughout the central nervous system including the cortex, thalamus, hypothalamus, brainstem and spinal cord [116]. In humans, the MC4R has not been detected in any peripheral tissue, although this distribution does not hold true for all animals as the MC4R is expressed in many peripheral tissues of the chicken. The MC4R has garnered considerable attention as this melanocortin receptor subtype appears to play a central role in weight regulation. Mice homozygous for an Mc4r-null allele demonstrate autosomal dominant, maturity-onset obesity, hyperphagia, hyperinsulinemia and hyperglycemia [111]. Heterozygotes have an intermediate phenotype. The MC4R-null mouse also demonstrates increased linear growth [111], a feature unique to the agouti yellow mice (discussed subsequently) and the MC4R-null mouse among rodent obesity models.

The role of MC4R in weight regulation in humans has been confirmed with the identification of individuals with dominantly inherited obesity segregating with mutations in the MC4R gene that result in frameshift errors [117]. Recent studies suggest that haploinsufficiency of MC4R may be a frequent, but incompletely penetrant, cause of human obesity [118,119]. The incomplete penetrance is highlighted by the absence of obesity in individuals with large deletions of chromosome 18q, a region that spans the MC4R gene [120]. A dominant-negative effect of mutant MC4R has been proposed, but cotransfection studies of mutant and wild-type MC4R in vitro showed that mutants affected neither signaling nor cell surface expression of wild-type MC4R [121]. More recently, single-nucleotide polymorphisms near MC4R have been identified in association with obesity and insulin resistance in several genome-wide association studies [122].

Leptin Signaling

MC4R impacts energy metabolism through its role in second-order leptin-responsive neurons. Though leptin signaling has attracted attention for its potential as a weight loss agent in the current obesity pandemic, its evolutionary role is more likely derived from starvation. Animals faced food scarcity and starvation far more often than overabundance and obesity. For these animals, depleted fat stores and consequently decreased leptin signaling elicited feeding and overfeeding responses at the next availability of food. The leptin-deficient *ob/ob* mouse is severely hyperphagic and consumes nearly twice as much food as its wild-type counterpart, and is significantly obese as a result.

Leptin is a hormone secreted by adipose tissues in proportion to metabolic energy stores in fat [123]. Leptin binds the long isoform of the leptin receptor (LepR), called Ob-Rb, and activates tyrosine kinases JAK (Janus kinase)/STAT (signal transducer and activator of transcription). Leptin crosses the blood–brain barrier from the periphery, and for many years, LepR in the arcuate nucleus of the hypothalamus was believed to be the main site of action for energy metabolism. Receptors are also expressed peripherally and in many other sites in the central nervous system, including other nuclei of the hypothalamus. In the arcuate nucleus, LepRs are expressed in two disparate populations: proopiomelanocortin/cocaine-and-amphetamine-regulated transcript (POMC/CART) and neuropeptide Y/agouti-related peptide (NPY/AGRP) neurons.

POMC/CART neurons produce α-MSH (a proteolytic product of POMC; Figure 3.1), which activates downstream MC4R-expressing neurons to decrease food intake. In NPY/AGRP neurons, NPY inhibits POMC neurons, and AGRP binds MC4R as an inverse agonist to inhibit MC4R neuron activity. Together, these serve to increase food intake and decrease energy expenditure. Thus POMC/CART neurons are considered anorexigenic and NPY/AGRP orexigenic. One important MC4R-expressing target for these POMC/CART and NPY/AGRP neurons is the paraventricular nucleus (PVN) of the hypothalamus. Administration of melanocortin receptor agonist, MTII, into the PVN inhibited feeding and increased energy expenditure [124]. Antagonist administration into the PVN elicited opposite effects [125].

Recently, Cre/loxP technology has facilitated the manipulation of genes in very specific subsets of cells. Using this method, LepR was deleted specifically from POMC neurons. Unlike global leptin- or leptin-receptor-deficient mice, POMC-specific LepR knockout mice were only mildly obese [123]. Mice lacking LepR in both POMC and AGRP neurons were also mildly obese [123]. Leptin receptors are also expressed in other hypothalamic sites, including the ventromedial hypothalamus (VMH). Conditional LepR removal from VMH neurons resulted in mildly obese mice that are especially sensitive to diet-induced obesity [126]. Together these data indicate that sites of LepR expression beyond the arcuate nucleus contribute to energy metabolism and merit further study.

Using Cre/loxP technology, MC4R was specifically reactivated in the PVN of global MC4R-deficient mice [123]. MC4R-deficient animals were obese, and mice with PVN-specific MC4R-reactivation had only ~60% amelioration of obesity. Hyperphagia, but not energy expenditure, was rescued. MC4R signaling in the PVN was previously believed to be the predominant effector of energy metabolism. It is now believed that food intake and energy expenditure are mediated by divergent pathways, and MC4R in the PVN is responsible primarily for food intake. Other poorly understood sites of MC4R may be responsible for energy expenditure.

Leptin Resistance

In leptin-deficient *ob/ob* mice, leptin administration reduced food intake and rescued body weight [127]. Leptin was initially considered a breakthrough in treatment of obesity. However, obesity caused by a high-fat diet was not sensitive to leptin in humans or animal models, and a high-fat diet itself caused significant elevation of circulating leptin levels. Most forms of obesity are unresponsive to these high levels of leptin, which has been termed "leptin resistance." The mechanism by which leptin resistance develops is unclear. One purported mechanism is that leptin is no longer able to cross the blood–brain barrier. Peripheral leptin levels in obese patients were over three-fold higher than in lean controls, but leptin levels centrally, as measured by cerebrospinal fluid (CSF), were only 30% higher in obese subjects [128].

Another well-studied mechanism is that leptin resistance is mediated through endoplasmic reticulum (ER) stress. The endoplasmic reticulum is responsible for protein folding, and stress impairs ER function, causing accumulation of misfolded proteins. This accumulation activates the unfolded protein response (UPR), which alleviates ER stress by increasing folding capacity, increasing degradation of misfolded proteins, or decreasing general translation. Prolonged exposure to ER stress causes cells to undergo apoptosis via activation of the apoptotic transcription factor, CHOP (CCAAT/enhancer-binding protein-homologous protein). Three ER proteins, inositol-requiring protein 1 (IRE1), double-stranded-RNA-dependent protein kinase-like ER kinase (PERK) and activating transcription factor 6 (ATF6), are sensors of ER stress, and when activated, these activate an ER chaperone protein, GRP78, that uses ATP to promote folding and prevent accumulation. Activated IRE1 induces translation of XBP1, which is a transcription factor for GRP78. Activated PERK decreases eIF2 (eukaryotic initiation factor 2) activity and represses translation. ER stress is known to inhibit leptin-induced phosphorylation of STAT3, and ER stress-inducing agents cause leptin resistance in vitro and in vivo [129]. High-fat diet-induced obesity caused ER stress in the hypothalamus, as measured by PERK phosphorylation [130]. Obesity caused ER stress and lead to insulin resistance and type 2 diabetes [131]. Reversal of ER stress by several different methods results in a reduction in leptin resistance and reversal of obesity [132]. *Xbp1*-deficient mice developed insulin resistance. *Eif2ak3* (PERK)-deficient mice have diabetes and abnormal pancreas function. Human *EIF2AK3* mutations were found in patients with Wolcott-Rallison syndrome, a disorder characterized by insulin-dependent diabetes at a young age [133]. The diabetic Akita mouse had hyperglycemia, apoptosis of pancreatic β-cells and CHOP expression; disruption of CHOP delayed the onset of diabetes [134].

Melanocortin 5 Receptor

Expression of the fifth melanocortin receptor has been recognized in the brain and at low levels in many tissues including the adrenal glands, skin, adipocytes, skeletal muscle, kidneys, lung, stomach, liver, spleen, thymus, lymph nodes, mammary glands, ovary, pituitary, testis and uterus. In situ hybridization studies showed that within the adrenal, MC5R is predominantly expressed in the aldosterone-producing zona glomerulosa cells. High levels of MC5R mRNA expression have been documented in the secretory epithelia of a number of exocrine and endocrine glands including Harderian, preputial, lacrimal, sebaceous and prostate glands and pancreas [135]. Melanocortins have been reported to affect a number of exocrine glands. Removal of the neurointermediate lobe of the pituitary reduces sebaceous lipid production, and this reduction is restored by administration of α-MSH. Exogenous ACTH and MSH increase secretion from the lacrimal gland. Deletion of the murine MC5R resulted in the loss of detectable binding of [^{125}I]NDP-MSH to Harderian, lacrimal and preputial glands and skeletal muscle, indicating that MC5R is the predominant melanocortin receptor in these tissues [135]. Development of the MC5R-null mouse confirmed a physiologic role for the melanocortins in regulating exocrine gland function; the mice demonstrate severe deficits in water repulsion and thermoregulation as a result of decreased sebaceous lipid production [135]. MC5R also appears to be essential for hormonally regulated release of porphyrins from the Harderian gland [135]. The preputial gland is a specialized sebaceous gland implicated in pheromone production. Exogenous α-MSH stimulates the release of a preputial odorant into the urine of male mice which stimulates aggressive attacks. Chen and colleagues have hypothesized the existence of a hypothalamic–pituitary–exocrine axis which might provide a mechanism by which stress could alter behavior via the regulation of olfactory cues [135].

Diseases Caused by Melanocortin Receptor Ligands

POMC Deficiency

Several unrelated individuals have been identified with genetic defects in the *POMC* gene [136,137]. The first patient was a compound heterozygote for two mutations in exon 3 which interfere with appropriate synthesis of ACTH and α-MSH (Figure 3.1). The second patient was homozygous for a mutation in exon 2 which abolishes POMC translation. Both patients presented with adrenal insufficiency, early-onset obesity, fair skin and red hair pigmentation. Additional patients have had nonsense or frameshift mutations. One proteolytic cleavage product of POMC in the pituitary is ACTH, which binds MC2R in the adrenal gland to stimulate cortisol production. In the absence of ACTH due to these *POMC* gene mutations, adrenal glands are hypotrophied and patients present with adrenal insufficiency. In the brain, *POMC*-expressing neurons are activated by leptin binding. Unlike in the pituitary, neuronal ACTH is further cleaved into α-MSH, which binds MC4R to decrease food intake and increase energy expenditure. α-MSH also activates MC1R, which contributes to skin and hair pigmentation. In the absence of α-MSH due to these *POMC* gene mutations, patients are hyperphagic, obese, and have fair skin with red hair pigmentation. Humans with polymorphic variants in MC1R have also been found to have fair skin and red hair pigmentation [138]. No symptoms related to β-endorphin deficiencies have been noted. The brother of patient one had died at the age of 7 months of hepatic failure following severe cholestasis and was found to have bilateral adrenal hypoplasia in the postmortem examination. All other anterior pituitary-derived hormones were normal. The heterozygous parents were normal in both families.

Isolated ACTH deficiency of the pituitary due to other causes is also rare. It most commonly appears to be acquired in later life, and is more common in men [139]. Most cases have been reported in Japan, and are often associated with other autoimmune endocrinopathies, including Hashimoto's thyroiditis and type 1 diabetes mellitus. It is likely that only pituitary ACTH, and not hypothalamic α-MSH, is affected in these patients, as they are not obese and do not have red hair, unlike patients with POMC gene mutations [136]. *Tpit* has been identified as a transcription factor specific to pituitary corticotrophs and melanotrophs, and absent in hypothalamic neurons which also express *POMC*. It interacts with the *POMC*-specific transcription factor, Ptx1, to regulate *POMC* transcription. Twelve recessive mutations in *TPIT* have been described [15]. Consistent with its sites of expression, these patients have congenital, secondary adrenal insufficiency, but not obesity or red hair.

A POMC-deficient mouse was produced whose phenotype was similar to the human POMC-deficient syndrome and confirmed the known functions of melanocortins [140]. The phenotype includes obesity, increased body length, yellow pigmentation, deficits in sebaceous gland function and thermoregulation, and adrenal hypoplasia and glucocorticoid deficiency. Adrenal glands could not be identified. In addition to undetectable corticosterone levels, aldosterone levels were also undetectable. The mutant mice lost 40% of their excess weight after 2 weeks of treatment with a stable α-MSH agonist. Although some of this weight loss was clearly attributable to decreased food intake, these same authors have clearly shown that α-MSH administration has additional lipolytic effects and results in increased energy expenditure [141]. Consistent with the lack of dependence of aldosterone activity upon ACTH, these mice have normal aldosterone function [142].

Agouti and Agouti-related Protein

The agouti gene locus was identified over half a century ago as a genetic locus that controls the amount and distribution of eumelanin (brown/black) and pheomelanin (yellow/red) pigmentation in the mammalian coat [143]. However, analyses of mutations at the agouti gene locus have occupied investigators for nearly a century. The lethal yellow mutation at the agouti locus was the first murine embryonic lethal mutation and the first murine obesity syndrome to be characterized [144].

Agouti is a small 131-amino acid protein that is secreted by dermal papillae cells and acts to block melanocortin action on follicular melanocytes at MC1R in the mouse [145,146]. The recombinant murine agouti protein is a potent nanomolar competitive antagonist for melanocortin receptors at MC1R and MC4R, relatively weaker at MC3R, and only a micromolar inhibitor of MC5R [145] which represents the first known endogenous antagonist for a G-protein-coupled receptor. In wild-type rodents, agouti expression is restricted to the hair follicle [146]. The human agouti gene which is 85% identical to the mouse gene is expressed much more widely including in adipose tissue, testis, ovary and heart, and at lower levels in liver, kidney and foreskin. The human agouti protein the agouti-signaling protein (ASIP), displays a similar pharmacologic profile for antagonism of melanocortin receptors as compared to the murine agouti protein, except that ASIP may display both competitive and non-competitive antagonism at MC4R and also appears to act as a non-competitive antagonist of MC2R.

The heterozygous lethal yellow agouti mouse is characterized by a yellow coat color, late-onset obesity associated with hyperphagia, hyperinsulinemia and hyperglycemia, increased linear growth, and susceptibility to a wide variety of epithelial and mesenchymal tumors. This phenotype is the result of a 170-kb deletion which removes all but the promoter and noncoding first exon of the Raly gene 5′ to the exons of the agouti gene and results in ubiquitous overexpression of agouti in all tissues examined to date [146]. The lethal yellow phenotype is presumably the result of agouti antagonism of the widely distributed melanocortin receptors and is consistent with the known actions of melanocortin receptors described above.

The agouti-related protein (AGRP) gene was identified based on its homology to agouti and is expressed in the hypothalamus, adrenal medulla, and at low levels in the testis, lung and kidney [147]. In contrast to the divergent expression patterns of murine and human agouti, the expression pattern of murine and human AGRP appears identical. Within the hypothalamus, AGRP expression is confined to the arcuate nucleus and AGRP-immunoreactive terminals paralleled POMC-immunoreactive terminals projecting from the arcuate nucleus [27]. AGRP is a selective, nanomolar competitive antagonist of MC3R and MC4R clearly implicating it as the endogenous melanocortin antagonist involved in energy homeostasis [148]. Whereas germline deletion of Agrp has only a mild impact to retard weight gain in older mice, ablation of the gene in adult mice is associated with a profound decrease in feeding and death [149]. This puzzling observation suggests that early loss of Agrp causes some sort of adaptative response.

Corticostatins are a family of related low-molecular-weight members of the defensin family of peptides that are competitive inhibitors of ACTH-induced steroidogenesis in the adrenal cortex, which act by blocking the ACTH receptor. In rats, corticostatins block the corticosterone response to stress. Corticostatins and the agouti peptides are the two known endogenous competitive inhibitors of melanocortin receptors, but do not appear to be structurally related.

Additional Potential Melanocortin Actions

Additional physiologic roles for melanocortins have been proposed that do not clearly correlate with the known functions of specific melanocortin receptors as surmised from human or mouse mutants. A multitude of behavioral and psychological effects have been attributed to melanocortins. Intracerebroventricular administration of ACTH or α-MSH elicits excessive grooming behavior, yawning, stretching and penile erection. The grooming, stretching and yawning behavior, but not erectile function, may be mediated by MC4R as deduced through the use of MC4R-selective antagonists [150]. In a double-blind, placebo-controlled crossover study, a cyclic α-MSH analogue initiated erections in men with psychogenic erectile dysfunction [151]. Roles for the actions of melanocortins in neuromuscular development, promotion of the regeneration of crushed nerves, and CNS protection from injury have also been postulated [86]. Melanocortins have a potential role in fetal growth and brain development. Data indicating a role for melanocortins as modulators of inflammation have been discussed previously. Centrally administered MSH is a potent antipyretic agent and, in an endogenous pyrogen-induced fever model in rabbits, is approximately 25,000-fold more potent than acetaminophen [152]. Physiologic roles for melanocortins in maintenance of cardiovascular homeostasis have also been proposed. Peripheral or central administration of γMSH causes tachycardia and pressor effects [153]. Central administration of α-MSH results in bradycardia and depressor effects [153]. Melanocortins may further influence cardiovascular homeostasis through their effects on electrolyte regulation. α-MSH and γ-MSH are potent natriuretics.

SECRETION OF ACTH: PHYSIOLOGY

Physiologically a number of factors interact to determine the final pattern of ACTH release, including circadian rhythms, stress and negative feedback by glucocorticoids. These factors impact on each other in an integrated fashion to control ACTH release. The stage of development, from fetal life through puberty, and pregnancy and parturition, also impact on ACTH secretion. Finally, the immune system interacts with the HPA axis, adding another facet to the complexity of ACTH release.

Secretion Dynamics of ACTH in Vivo

ACTH secretion is characterized by pulsatile release of ACTH from the corticotroph in a burst-like pattern, with no interpulse secretion [154]. Fifteen-minute sampling reveals approximately 12 ACTH and cortisol pulses over a 24-hour period, whereas more frequent 10-minute sampling reveals 40 ACTH pulses in 24 hours [154]. Blood ACTH rises by an average of 24 pg/ml per pulse [154]. ß-endorphin secretion parallels the pulsatile release of ACTH.

Spontaneous ACTH and cortisol pulses correlate highly. There is a strong relationship between the magnitude of concomitant ACTH and cortisol pulses, particularly if a 15-minute phase delay in cortisol secretion is allowed for [154,155]. Not all spontaneous ACTH and cortisol pulses are concomitant: approximately 50–75% of spontaneous ACTH pulses are followed by a cortisol pulse, whereas approximately 60–90% of spontaneous cortisol pulses are preceded by an ACTH pulse.

The 24-hour pattern of ACTH pulses, but not the cortisol pattern, differs between males and females. Males have more pulses, greater mean peak ACTH amplitude, greater 24-hour ACTH secretion and higher mean ACTH levels. The sensitivity of the adrenal cortex, or the availability of ACTH to the adrenal cortex, may be greater in females. Alternatively, males and females may have different set points for cortisol feedback. CRH may also be secreted in a pulsatile fashion, accounting for pulsatile ACTH secretion. When exogenous CRH is given continuously, there is a progressive desensitization of the ACTH response to CRH. However, when CRH is given in a prolonged pulsatile manner, it does not desensitize the corticotroph CRH receptor, and the releasable ACTH pool is not depleted. Recently, ACTH pulsatile secretion has been shown to increase with increasing body mass index [154], consistent with the known relationship between cortisol production rate and body size.

Negative Regulation of ACTH Secretion

Negative feedback can be defined as long, short, or ultrashort depending on the location and nature of the hormone mediating the feedback.

Long Feedback by Glucocorticoids

Long feedback refers to the effects of adrenal glucocorticoids on ACTH secretion at the pituitary and in the hypothalamus. Glucocorticoid-mediated negative feedback can be subdivided into fast and delayed, which can be further subdivided into intermediate and slow feedback. In animals, the initial fast negative effect of glucocorticoids occurs within seconds to minutes, involves inhibition of stimulated ACTH and CRH release, not synthesis, and occurs during the period when plasma glucocorticoid levels are increasing. Cortisol given to patients at the start of surgery attenuates the surgery-induced ACTH rise, and may be an example of fast feedback.

Delayed feedback has two components, intermediate and slow [156]. Intermediate feedback is the component of delayed feedback that is due to inhibition of ACTH release, but not synthesis, and may be important after short durations of glucocorticoid exposure, or after noncontinuous, repeated exposures [156]. Intermediate delayed feedback develops after 45–120 minutes, and maximal inhibition occurs 2–4 hours after administration of one dose of glucocorticoid. Unlike ACTH, CRH synthesis as well as release may be affected by intermediate feedback [156].

The slow component of delayed feedback is most important after long exposures to a moderately high dose of glucocorticoid, and is a function of the total dose of glucocorticoids, the glucocorticoid level achieved, and the amount of time since the steroid was given [156]. Slow feedback occurs after more than 24 hours of exposure to glucocorticoids and can persist for days. POMC biosynthesis is inhibited, leading to inhibition of basal and stimulated ACTH secretion [156], and intracellular ACTH decreases implying decreased synthesis.

In humans, negative feedback by glucocorticoids takes 30–60 minutes to be manifest. When endogenous cortisol is suppressed with metyrapone, the effects of exogenous glucocorticoids on the morning ACTH rise, or on CRH-stimulated ACTH release, are not seen initially but appear 30 minutes after glucocorticoid administration. In addition, glucocorticoids have little effect on the initial CRH-induced increase in ACTH release, but decrease CRH-induced ACTH release after 60 minutes. Cortisol given to patients at the start of surgery attenuates the surgery-induced ACTH rise.

Cortisol modulates the responsiveness of the pituitary. The corticotroph is dependent on CRH stimulation to maintain ACTH secretion, and glucocorticoids suppress CRH-induced ACTH secretion in vivo and in vitro. On the other hand, when endogenous cortisol levels are suppressed by metyrapone, basal ACTH and CRH-induced ACTH release are increased. Glucocorticoid inhibition of ACTH secretion from the corticotroph may recover more quickly than CRH secretion from the hypothalamus. Secondary adrenal insufficiency due to long-term glucocorticoid therapy may in part be due to continued suppression of hypothalamic CRH secretion. Adrenalectomized patients on exogenous glucocorticoid therapy have a blunted ACTH response to CRH that normalizes after several CRH boluses, suggesting that lack of stimulation of the corticotroph by CRH suppresses the ACTH response. On the other hand, corticotrophs of patients recovering from trans-sphenoidal surgery for Cushing's disease are profoundly unresponsive to CRH, which cannot be attributed solely to deficient CRH priming.

Glucocorticoids inhibit AVP secretion. In most studies, patients with hypopituitarism or primary adrenal insufficiency are unable to maximally dilute their urine in response to a water load, and this is corrected by glucocorticoid administration [157]. However, it is unclear if elevated AVP levels or lack of glucocorticoids is responsible for the inability to maximally dilute the urine in the hypocortisolemic state. Glucocorticoids inhibit nitric oxide synthase, and nitric oxide is capable of stimulating the insertion of the water channel, aquaporin 2, in the luminal membrane of the renal collecting cell [158]. This may provide an explanation for why glucocorticoid deficiency is associated with decreased free water clearance.

Short Feedback

Short feedback refers to the effect of pituitary ACTH to inhibit CRH release. In normal subjects, the administration of ACTH does not affect CRH levels, most likely because of the negative effects of cortisol present prior to ACTH administration. However, in patients with elevated CRH levels due to Addison's disease or hypopituitarism, ACTH decreases CRH and ß-endorphin levels, suggesting that ACTH inhibits CRH secretion. ACTH may act in the median eminence or in the hypothalamus to inhibit CRH release.

Circadian Regulation of ACTH Secretion

There is an endogenous circadian rhythm to the pulsatile pattern of ACTH secretion which leads to a circadian rhythm of glucocorticoid release. The function of this circadian rhythm in cortisol secretion is not known, although one hypothesis suggests that the early morning rise in cortisol causes a delayed-phase rise in insulin resistance, which may play a role in altered glucose metabolism [159]. For instance, since the brain does not require insulin for glucose uptake, peripheral insulin resistance might cause a rise in glucose levels, leading to greater uptake in the brain. The circadian rhythm is generated in the suprachiasmatic nucleus (SCN), and the signals travel via efferent inputs to the PVN to modulate CRH release. This circadian rhythm is due to variation in ACTH pulse amplitude, not frequency [155]. The amount of ACTH secreted per pulse varies by 3.8-fold over a 24-hour period [155]. Basal ACTH and cortisol levels parallel each other and are the highest upon awakening in the morning between 06:00 h and 09:00 h, decline through the day to intermediate levels at 16:00 h, and are lowest between 23:00 h and 03:00 h [155]. From 23:00 h to 02:00 h, there is a quiescent period of minimal secretory activity, corresponding to the nadir of ACTH and cortisol levels. Secretion of ACTH and cortisol abruptly increases in the early morning. The diurnal secretory pattern is similar for free and total cortisol, although the relative increase in free cortisol is about 1.5 times greater than the relative increase in total cortisol.

Alterations in feeding and sleep impact on cortisol secretion. Cortisol briefly increases postprandially, especially after the midday meal. Exercise or administration of ACTH at 10:00 h leads to a rise in cortisol and blunts the midday cortisol surge, and at 14:00 h leads to a rise in cortisol. Overall, the major features of the diurnal cortisol pattern persist under conditions of complete fasting, continuous feeding, or total sleep deprivation. However, the circadian rhythm of cortisol secretion fully adapts to permanent changes in environmental time and the sleep–wake pattern. This adaptation takes about 3 weeks, the limiting factor being the time it takes for the quiescent period of secretion to fully adapt. The acrophase adapts much more quickly and is partially synchronized after one day and totally synchronized after 10 days.

There is circadian regulation of the sensitivity of the response of the adrenal cortex to ACTH. Injection of ACTH at 07:00 h, just at the time of the endogenous cortisol peak, causes a significant increase in cortisol. The absolute increment in cortisol secretion in response to an ACTH stimulation test is greater when the test is performed at circadian nadir compared to the peak, although in one study this was true in males only. The incremental increase in cortisol secretion in response to a CRH stimulation test is also greatest at night when basal levels are lowest, although the total amount of cortisol released is greatest in the morning when the basal cortisol levels are highest. The basal cortisol level, not the time of day, seems to be the important factor determining the cortisol response to oCRH, and the higher the basal cortisol level, the lower the peak cortisol response to oCRH. On the other hand, the maximum

ACTH blood level in response to oCRH occurs at 07:00 h, the time of the minimum cortisol increment to oCRH.

The factors governing the circadian rhythm in ACTH release in humans are not clear. On the one hand, it may be regulated by a diurnal rhythm in CRH secretion. The highest CRH levels occur at 06:00 h (7.0 pg/ml) and the lowest at 18:00 h and 22:00 h (about 1.8 pg/ml), which parallels the pattern of ACTH and cortisol secretion. Serotoninergic and cholinergic pathways may play a role in the CRH circadian rhythm, and display circadian periodicity in their hypothalamic concentrations. On the other hand, when the pituitary is exposed to constant levels of CRH 30-fold higher than those found in portal hypophyseal blood, such as during CRH infusion and in pregnancy [160], the circadian rhythms in ACTH and cortisol persist. CRH clearly plays a role in the ACTH rhythm, as CRH-deficient mice have an absent or markedly attenuated diurnal rise in ACTH [161]. However, in these mice, constant infusion of CRH restores the ACTH rhythm. This indicates that changes in CRH amplitude are not necessary to drive the ACTH rhythm, but that a tonic level of CRH is required to maintain ACTH responsiveness [162] to circadian cues. Many peripheral cells express circadian clocks. Recently, glucocorticoids have been shown to be required for clock function in several, but not all, peripheral tissues [163].

Physical Stress Regulation of ACTH Secretion

Glucocorticoid release mediated by ACTH plays a major role in the response to stress. An interaction exists between stress-mediated ACTH release, which leads to glucocorticoid secretion, and glucocorticoid-mediated negative feedback, which inhibits further ACTH and glucocorticoid release. A number of stressful stimuli lead to ACTH secretion. Most physical stressors activate the HPA axis. The magnitude of the rise in ACTH and cortisol is dependent upon many factors, including the nature of the stress, its magnitude including the rapidity of its appearance and the time of day it is experienced. In general, stressors have a larger impact on ACTH release when they develop rapidly, are of high magnitude and occur during the circadian nadir in ACTH release.

Hypoglycemia

In humans, insulin-induced hypoglycemia is associated with a 5–6-fold increase in plasma ACTH levels [164], from a basal level of about 40 pg/ml to a peak of 250 pg/ml at 45 minutes [164]. Cortisol levels increase over 2-fold, from a basal level of about 11 μg/dl to a peak of about 25 μg/dl at 60–90 minutes [164]. Insulin-induced hypoglycemia causes a 4–5-fold greater increase in ACTH secretion than oCRH alone, and a 1.3-fold greater increase than AVP plus CRH.

CRH may play a permissive rather than a dynamic role in the ACTH response to hypoglycemia, whereas AVP may play a more direct role. AVP levels have been shown to increase 2.5–7-fold at 30–45 minutes after insulin. When AVP levels are raised endogenously by saline infusion or lowered to undetectable levels by waterloading, the hypoglycemia-induced AVP increase is greater after saline, even though saline blunts the hypoglycemic response to insulin. Catecholamines increase in response to hypoglycemia, and may act at the hypothalamus to mediate ACTH release. Epinephrine appears to play more of a role than norepinephrine, increasing at least 13-fold at 30 minutes after insulin, whereas norepinephrine increases 2.4-fold at 60 minutes.

Exercise

Exercise increases ACTH and ß-endorphin levels, and the response is dependent on the intensity of exercise and the level of training. Exercising to exhaustion, or exercise of short duration and high intensity, increases ACTH, ß-endorphin and cortisol levels. Hypercortisolism is seen in highly trained athletes, who need a higher level of oxygen consumption to stimulate ACTH release, and have elevated basal ACTH levels [165]. Physical exercise and stress both lead to analgesia in man [166]. Naloxone reverses exercise-induced analgesia from certain types of pain, suggesting a role for endorphins. Dexamethasone reverses exercise-induced analgesia from other types of pain, like dental pain, that are not reversed by naloxone, suggesting a role for ACTH, although dexamethasone also suppresses ß-endorphin release.

Starvation

Essential bodily functions, such as reproduction, growth and immune responses, require adequate energy from food. The ability to survive famine through various adaptive changes, from increased food seeking to decreased metabolic function, is evolutionarily advantageous. The HPA axis is activated during starvation. In humans and animal models, all hormones in the HPA axis (CRH, ACTH and cortisol) are increased following acute food deprivation [167]. Cortisol is known to induce glucose release via stimulation of glycogenolysis, gluconeogenesis and lipolysis, which provides interim energy during fasting. Cortisol also stimulates hypothalamic AGRP, which stimulates appetite and likely causes "rebound hyperphagia" once food becomes available after a period of starvation [168]. The circadian peak of cortisol coincides with morning awakening and mobilizes glucose reserves for activity after overnight fasting. Nocturnal animals have circadian rhythmicity in which the corticosterone peak corresponds to night-time awakening and activity. High levels of cortisol also correlate with increased food-seeking behaviors in both food-deprived animal models and human dieters. Following prolonged food deprivation, however, levels of CRH and ACTH are decreased. This is likely because sustained elevation of cortisol or corticosterone provides negative feedback to inhibit CRH and ACTH [167]. Activation of the HPA axis correlates with inhibited reproductive function and decreased bone and muscle density, suggesting a role in stress-induced inhibition of nonessential functions.

Lower Body Negative Pressure and Acute Hemorrhage

Lower body negative pressure in humans simulates acute hemorrhage. Lower body negative pressure increases ACTH secretion to peak values of 60–250 pg/ml at 2–10 minutes after cessation of the stimulus, and the increase in ACTH is reversed by dexamethasone [169]. Hypovolemia may be the physiologically important stress. In animals, hemorrhage stimulates ACTH secretion primarily mediated by CRH and, to some degree, by AVP. Hypovolemia increases portal blood CRH, AVP, epinephrine and oxytocin, whereas hypotension, also a component of hemorrhage, induced by nitroprusside, increases portal blood CRH only.

Surgical Stress

Surgery induces a large increase in plasma ACTH levels. Patients undergoing surgery may have increased sensitivity of the adrenal cortex to ACTH [170]. Fentanyl, an opiate agonist, attenuates the ACTH response to surgery. Evidence in adrenalectomized primates suggests that supraphysiological doses of glucocorticoids are not necessary for the animal to withstand surgical stress, but that a minimal level is necessary.

Psychological and Emotional Stress

Psychological and emotional stress play a role in the hormonal stress response. ACTH levels are high in patients awaiting an insulin-tolerance test. During physical exercise, psychological and physical stress may act synergistically to increase ß-endorphin and ACTH levels. With increasing experience in performing a set level of exhaustive physical exercise, plasma ACTH and cortisol levels declined [171].

Fetal and Postnatal Regulation of ACTH Secretion

In utero, maternal cortisol influences alterations of fetal heart rate, movement and behavioral states [172]. By 35 weeks of gestation, there is a circadian rhythm in fetal behavioral states that is altered if the maternal diurnal variation in ACTH and cortisol secretion are abolished by maternal administration of triamcinolone [172]. Neonates, even when born prematurely, have an endogenous cortisol rhythm. Minimally and severely stressed neonates in the neonatal intensive care unit, born between 23 and 38 weeks of gestation, have a significant diurnal rhythm in cortisol and endorphin secretion, although ACTH levels do not vary significantly. Others have suggested that diurnal rhythmicity is a function of maturation, and is not present before 6 months of age [173].

Regulation of ACTH Secretion During Puberty

Normal children between the ages of 1 year and 16 years do not differ from adults in ACTH, ß-endorphin and cortisol responses to CRH, and the responses of boys do not differ from girls. Some of the other adrenal steroids and adrenal androgens demonstrate basal and stimulated variation with age. The CRH-stimulated androstenedione to 17-hydroxyprogesterone ratio increases with sexual maturation, suggesting that the 17,20-desmolase activity increases with puberty. The dehydroepiandrosterone response to CRH increases as children progress from stage 1 to stage 5 of puberty, and by stage 5 of puberty, dehydroepiandrosterone levels do not differ from those of adults.

Regulation of Reproduction by Stress

Stress responses to acute stressors are designed to improve the chances of immediate survival at the expense of immediate reproductive fitness. Thus, stress responses consist of fight-or-flight physiology, including enhancement of cognition, physical strength and fuel production, as well as inhibition of nonessential activities such as reproductive function, growth, feeding and fuel storage. Reproduction is especially energetically expensive for vertebrates, and under unfavorable conditions, reproductive behaviors and hormones are actively suppressed. Though stress is a potent inhibitor of the hypothalamic–pituitary–gonadal (HPG) reproductive axis, the mechanisms by which stressors target this axis are unknown. Most studies have focused on the downstream consequences of reproductive inhibition. A robust phenomenon known for several decades is that anorexic female patients can become amenorrheic and infertile [174]. Anorexic females also had high levels of cortisol. In rats, hamsters and zebrafish, food deprivation triggered reproductive inhibition [167]. Food deprivation in rodent models correlated with high levels of corticosterone [175]. Disparate stressors also elicit reproductive inhibition, as measured by decreased levels of pituitary luteinizing hormone, follicle-stimulating hormone and gonadal estradiol or testosterone. These include immobilization stress, cold exposure, insulin-induced hypoglycemia, endotoxin administration, tissue injury and foot shock [175,176]. Though all these stressors inhibited the HPG axis, only some stimulated the HPA axis. Increased CRH, ACTH and glucocorticoids cannot wholly explain stress-induced reproductive inhibition. The CRH knockout mouse, which is deficient in Crh and Acth, and has low corticosterone, is able to suppress luteinizing hormone and testosterone after food deprivation and immobilization stressors [175].

HPA-AXIS–IMMUNE INTERACTIONS

The immune system and the neuroendocrine system communicate with each other, and share a common set of structurally identical hormones and receptors [177]. Cells of the immune system synthesize biologically active neuroendocrine peptide hormones, immune cells contain receptors for neuroendocrine hormones, neuroendocrine hormones modulate immune function, and lymphokines modulate neuroendocrine function. The neuroendocrine system and the immune system work together in the regulation of both the stress and the immune response, and the components include lymphoid cells, cholinergic and adrenergic neurons, cytokines and lymphokines, hormones and neuropeptides released by the endocrine glands and the CNS, receptors, and higher CNS activity which modulates these responses.

Effect of Immune System on HPA Axis

Immune cells, particularly monocytes, macrophages and lymphocytes, produce cytokines involved in the immune response, and these cytokines activate the HPA axis. Bacterial-derived endotoxin and lipopolysaccharide stimulate the release of interleukin-1, interleukin-6 and tumor necrosis factor-α, which are regulated by glucocorticoid feedback. The effects of cytokines on the HPA axis at the level of the brain, pituitary and adrenal gland, are the best examples of immune modulation of a neuroendocrine system. Interleukin-1 is produced by stimulated macrophages and monocytes, and stimulates CRH release. Interleukin-1 also directly stimulates the adrenal cortex. Tumor necrosis factor is produced primarily by activated monocytes, and has many of the same biological activities and responds to many of the same immune challenges as interleukin-1. Tumor necrosis factor stimulates ACTH release, most likely at an extrapituitary site. Interleukin-6 has actions similar to interleukin-1 and TNF, and stimulates the HPA axis [70]. Interleukin-2 is synthesized by T cells after an antigenic challenge, and increases ACTH and cortisol levels in humans, although this may be indirect and due to the stress response generated by fever and chills. Gamma-interferon causes an increase in steroid production by adrenal cells. As discussed above, leukemia-inhibitory factor (LIF) may be a major activator of POMC gene transcription and ACTH release following immune or inflammatory stimulation.

Effect of HPA Axis on Immune System

Stress suppresses immune function. Following an infection or most immunization procedures, and the presence of bacterial endotoxin, a stress-like response of the pituitary occurs leading to the release of ACTH and cortisol which tends to suppress the immune system. However, in humans, there is no clear evidence that the rise in cortisol following an immune or inflammatory stimulus plays a significant role in modulating the subsequent immune response. In fact, prior to the treatment of patients with primary adrenal insufficiency, there were no substantive reports that these patients suffered from overactivity of their immune systems. Receptors for CRH, ACTH and glucocorticoids most likely mediate the effect of these hormones on the immune system. ACTH receptors on human peripheral monocytes have been characterized, and glucocorticoid receptors are present on human lymphocytes.

Glucocorticoids inhibit many aspects of immune function, establishing a negative feedback loop between the immune and neuroendocrine systems. Glucocorticoids block lymphocyte activation, block the production and action of interleukin-2, interleukin-1, gamma-interferon, tumor necrosis factor and prostaglandins, and interfere with the interaction of certain effector molecules with target cells.

HPA Axis Within Immune System

Cells of the immune system produce CRH, ACTH and endorphins. Human peripheral mononuclear leukocytes synthesize three molecular forms of immunoreactive ACTH, and lymphocytes produce ß-endorphins. Mouse spleen macrophages and virally infected mouse splenocytes contain ß-endorphin and POMC mRNA. CRH mRNA and peptide are found in monocytes in acute inflammatory reactions [178] and in T-cell lymphocytes [179].

Releasing hormones and cytokines interact to stimulate ACTH production from immune cells. CRH and AVP stimulate a dramatic increase in biologically active ACTH and ß-endorphin from human peripheral leukocytes in some studies. Unstimulated leukocytes produce little ACTH. In humans, only B lymphocytes secrete ß-endorphin in response to CRH and AVP, and monocyte-secreted interleukin-1 mediates the effect. A feedback loop exists between the immune and neuroendocrine systems [180]. Cytokines released by immune cells stimulate secretion of ACTH and glucocorticoids which are active in the fight against infection. Subsequently, these hormones suppress the further synthesis of cytokines.

Secretion of ACTH: Pathophysiology

Abnormal secretion of ACTH occurs in ACTH-secreting pituitary adenomas responsible for Cushing's disease or Nelson's syndrome; in Cushing's syndrome due to an ectopic pituitary adenoma or an ectopic ACTH-secreting tumor.

Familial Glucocorticoid Deficiency Syndrome

The familial glucocorticoid deficiency (FGD) syndrome is a rare autosomal recessive syndrome originally described by Shepard et al. in 1959 [181]. Patients typically present in early childhood with symptoms resulting from their glucocorticoid insufficiency including hyperpigmentation, hypoglycemia, lethargy and weakness [181]. The clinical course may be complicated by frequent infections [181]. Patients with FGD typically have low or undetectable plasma cortisol and high ACTH levels (often >1000 pg/mL) in conjunction with normal aldosterone and plasma renin levels. Occasionally FGD patients have low normal cortisol values, which respond subnormally to exogenous corticotropin. Patients with FGD do not present with symptoms related to salt wasting, dehydration, or electrolyte disturbances, as the renin–aldosterone axis is preserved. The preservation of the renin–aldosterone axis clearly distinguishes this syndrome from childhood Addison's disease. FGD also shares symptoms with Allgrove, also called triple-A, syndrome, but Allgrove can be distinguished by its presentation of alacrima, achalasia and neurological defects in addition to adrenal insufficiency. A feature of FGD is that many of the patients are reported to be unusually tall [181]. The mechanism is unclear, but excessive growth is reduced upon glucocorticoid replacement, suggesting that glucocorticoid deficiency or ACTH excess may be the cause. Melanocortin receptors are present in bone and the growth plate, and one hypothesis is that excess ACTH stimulates growth via these receptors. The adrenal glands are atrophic, and only occasional cortical cells remained in the zona glomerulosa with no remnants of the zona fasciculata or reticularis, but the adrenal medulla appears normal [181]. This adrenal atrophy substantiates the physiologic relevance of ACTH's trophic action on the adrenal gland. Recently, an examination of 11 patients with FGD revealed a discrepancy between partial glucocorticoid deficiency and significantly diminished DHEAS secretion, confirming a significant contribution for ACTH (or at least for MC2R) in the onset of adrenarche [182].

For many years, there were no animal models of FGD. The *Mc2r* knockout mouse was first generated and characterized in 2007 [183]. Like human patients with FGD, these mice had high levels of ACTH and undetectable levels of corticosterone. Adrenal histology in these animals showed atrophied zona fasciculata but intact zona glomerulosa. *Mc2r* knockout mice also presented with neonatal hypoglycemia, which frequently led to death. However, they did not present with excessive longitudinal growth. These mice also differed from humans in that they were deficient in aldosterone and aldosterone synthase. ACTH is thought to regulate zona glomerulosa development in rodents more so than in humans [84].

A number of different homozygous or compound heterozygous missense and nonsense mutations in MC2R have been reported in patients with FGD, and in all cases these mutations cosegregate with disease in the affected families [184]. Transient expression of the S741 mutant MC2R ($ser^{74} \rightarrow$ ile) in COS-7 cells resulted in an EC50 for cAMP production of 67 nmol/l, approximately 12-fold higher than the normal EC50 MC2R of 5.5 nmol/l. Expression of a Asp107 $\rightarrow$ Asn mutation in Cloudman S91 melanoma cells resulted in a 6–9-fold increase in the EC50 for cAMP generation. These results were confounded by endogenous melanocortin receptors, making it difficult to determine whether the mutant receptor, demonstrated defective ligand binding or defective coupling to adenylate cyclase [84]. FGD caused by receptor mutations are classified as FGD type 1, and mutations in *MC2R* account for approximately 25% of FGD.

ACTH-MC2R signaling in adrenal cells requires the presence of the MC2R accessory protein, MRAP. MRAP traffics MC2R from the endoplasmic reticulum to the plasma membrane, where MC2R interacts ACTH. In the absence of MRAP, MC2R remains sequestered in the endoplasmic reticulum [100], and cells are unable to bind and respond to ACTH. Mutations in *MC2R* account for roughly 25% of FGD. FGD without *MC2R* mutations is called FGD type 2. In 2005, whole-genome SNP analyses of families with FGD but no *MC2R* mutations demonstrated that mutations in *MRAP* were linked to familial glucocorticoid deficiency type 2 [98]. Sequence analysis revealed a slice site mutation that led to a defective protein [98], and further sequencing of FGD type 2 families revealed similar mutations. Mutations in *MC2R* and *MRAP* account for approximately half of all cases of the disease.

ACTH-independent Activation of ACTH Receptor Pathways

Several rare causes of ACTH-independent Cushing's syndrome are due to ACTH-independent pathological activation of ACTH receptor pathways. In the McCune-Albright syndrome, a mutation in the GTPase region of the stimulatory alpha subunit G-protein, $G_s\alpha$, can result in constitutive activation of protein kinase A in the adrenal cortex, leading to hypersecretion of cortisol and adrenal adenoma formation [185]. Ectopic expression of other seven-transmembrane G-protein-coupled receptors, including those which bind gastric inhibitory polypeptide, luteinizing hormone, vasopressin and catecholamines, in the adrenal cortex, may occur [186]. In this situation, Cushing's syndrome results from the cognate hormone binding to the ectopically expressed receptor, leading to stimulation of adenylate cylase, activation of cyclic AMP and cortisol hypersecretion [186]. Finally, patients with mutations in the regulatory subunit of protein kinase A, R1α, may develop Cushing's syndrome secondary to micronodular adrenocortical hyperplasia [187]. This disorder, termed Carney complex, may be associated with myxomas of the cardiac atria and other tissues, and freckling of the skin [186].

Pituitary Adenomas

ACTH immunoreactivity in an abnormal pituitary is usually due to a single functional adenoma, but can be associated with nodular hyperplasia or a silent corticotrophic adenoma. Diffuse or nodular corticotroph hyperplasia, which could result from an ectopic or hypothalmic CRH-producing tumor, or to Addison's disease, is a rare cause of a pituitary adenoma or ACTH hyperfunction. Pituitary adenomas constitute about 15% of intracranial tumors [3]. Approximately 56% of pituitary adenomas are active, and about one-third of active pituitary adenomas produce ACTH; 10–15% of pituitary adenomas are pleurihormonal, some of which secrete ACTH. When discovered, ACTH-producing adenomas are often functional, small, highly vascular and prone to hemorrhage [188]. Corticotroph adenomas tend to be located in the central portion of the adenohypophysis, in the "mucoid wedge," and form micronodular aggregates [188]. Invasive adenomas are more frequently found among undifferentiated, extremely laterally localized, or large adenomas, and recur more frequently than non-invasive tumors. There is no correlation between the size of an adenoma and the cortisol level or rate of recurrence. The majority of adenomas responsible for Cushing's disease or Nelson's syndrome are microadenomas. ACTH-producing adenomas are usually monoclonal, but may be polyclonal. Pleurihormonal adenomas are usually polyclonal.

The biochemical structure and ultrastructure of ACTH-secreting pituitary adenoma cells differ from nonadenomatous pituitary cells. The cells may look normal, but be increased in number [188]. Cells are oval to polygonal in shape, with eccentric spherical nuclei and well-developed rough endoplasmic reticulim. Crooke's hyaline is characteristic of ACTH-producing tumors, is associated with either endogenous or exogenous hypercortisolism and is due to massive accumulation of intermediate cytoplasmic filaments that are normally present in small numbers [3]. Clinically, an increased number of Crooke's cells is correlated with a requirement for a longer postoperative replacement dose of cortisol.

Pituitary adenomas may produce products in addition to ACTH. Some ACTH-producing corticotroph adenomas contain a form of gastrin that is smaller than gastrin found in normal adenohypophysis. 7B2 is a secretory granule-associated protein, which may be involved in proconvertase activtion [189], is sometimes secreted by ACTH-producing tumors; it is secreted in the highest levels from nonfunctional pituitary tumor.

A variant of Cushing's disease is due to ACTH-producing pituitary adenomas occurring ectopically, which have been described to arise in the mucosa of the sphenoid sinus, within a benign cystic ovarian teratoma and intrahemispherically in a 6-year-old male [190]. Rarely, both Cushing's disease and Nelson's syndrome have been preceded by generalized glucocorticoid resistance due to a mutation in the glucocorticoid receptor. In these cases, the high rate of ACTH secretion, stimulated by the generalized glucocorticoid resistance, in some way led to adenoma formation, perhaps following a second oncogenic transformation.

Pituitary carcinomas are malignant pituitary tumors associated with extracranial metastases, including liver and lung. Pituitary carcinomas cannot be histologically differentiated from adenomas [3]. A large number of pituitary carcinomas produce Cushing's disease [3]. In patients with Cushing's disease due to a pituitary carcinoma, the primary tumor and metastases stain immunochemically for ACTH, ß-LPH, ß-endorphin and α-MSH, and production of both CRH and ACTH from a pituitary carcinoma has been described.

Ectopic ACTH-secreting Tumors

Several neuroendocrine neoplasms occur in the bronchopulmonary tract, including small-cell neuroendocrine carcinomas, carcinoids, well-differentiated neuroendocrine carcinomas and intermediate-cell neuroendocrine carcinomas. These neoplasms express neuroendocrine markers including chromogranins and synaptophysin; 34% of small-cell carcinomas of the lung show immunoreactivity to one or more peptide hormones, and patients with peptide-positive small-cell lung carcinomas have a shorter mean survival than patients with nonreactive tumors. ACTH is by far the most common hormone present, and is seen in 24% of small-cell carcinomas. However, 56% of small-cell lung cancer cell lines secrete significant concentrations of ACTH precursors, with little, if any, processing to ACTH. Oat-cell lung carcinomas may also produce ACTH, leading to Cushing's syndrome.

Carcinoid tumors often produce more than one hormone, and can be responsible for the ectopic ACTH syndrome. Bronchial carcinoids occasionally contain ACTH and related opioid peptides, which does not alter the overall favorable prognosis of these tumors. Cushing's syndrome caused by ACTH secretion by pulmonary tumorlets has been described [191]. Upon radiologic imaging, such tumorlets, which may be over 100 in number, present a very unusual appearance.

Most nonpituitary POMC-secreting tumors do not produce CRH. However, some patients with ectopic ACTH syndrome due to lung cancer have tumors that produce ACTH and CRH, and secrete ACTH in response to CRH. Bronchial carcinoid tumors may contain CRH and ACTH, and be associated with high plasma ACTH and CRH levels and Cushing's syndrome, or with normal plasma CRH levels. Cushing's syndrome has been associated with ectopic ACTH secretion from a unilateral adrenal pheochromocytoma, and from bilateral pheochromocytomas in a case of multiple endocrine neoplasia type 2A [192].

A number of other ectopic tumors have been described that secrete ACTH, including an adenoid cystic carcinoma of the lung, a renal cell carcinoma, a neuroendocrine tumor of the nasal roof and an ACTH-producing tumor metastatic to the liver. In general, POMC mRNA from nonpituitary tumors responsible for the ectopic ACTH syndrome is identical to normal and to POMC mRNA from pituitary tumors. However, some tumors contain a larger POMC mRNA species that is increased in amount from 0.3% of the overall POMC mRNA in normal pituitaries, to up to 35–40% in the tumor, and is transcribed from an alternative upstream promoter. Pancreatic islet cell tumors responsible for Cushing's syndrome have been demonstrated to contain ACTH, ß-endorphin and POMC mRNA [193].

References

[1] D. Kelberman, K. Rizzoti, R. Lovell-Badge, I.C. Robinson, M.T. Dattani, Genetic regulation of pituitary gland development in human and mouse, Endocr Rev 30 (7) (2009) 790–829.

[2] Z. Blumenfeld, R.B. Jaffe, Hypophysiotropic and neuromodulatory regulation of adrenocorticotropin in the human fetal pituitary gland, J Clin Invest 78 (1) (1986) 288–294.

[3] I. Doniach, Histopathology of the pituitary, Clin Endocrinol Metab 14 (4) (1985) 765–789.

[4] L.A. Puy, D.R. Ciocca, Human pharyngeal and sellar pituitary glands: Differences and similarities revealed by an immunocytochemical study, J Endocrinol 108 (2) (1986) 231–238.

[5] E. Hermesz, S. Mackem, K.A. Mahon, Rpx: A novel anterior-restricted homeobox gene progressively activated in the prechordal plate, anterior neural plate and Rathke's pouch of the mouse embryo, Development 122 (1996) 41–52.

[6] M.T. Dattani, J.P. Martinez-Barbera, P.Q. Thomas, J.M. Brickman, R. Gupta, I.L. Martensson, et al., Mutations in the homeobox gene HESX1/Hesx1 associated with septo-optic dysplasia in human and mouse, Nat Genet 19 (1998) 125–133.

[7] H.Z. Sheng, A.B. Zhadanov, B.J. Mosinger, T. Fujii, S. Bertuzzi, A. Grinberg, et al., Specification of pituitary cell lineages by the LIM homeobox gene Lhx3, Science 272 (1996) 1004–1007.

[8] D.P. Szeto, A.K. Ryan, S.M. O'Connell, M.G. Rosenfeld, P-OTX: A PIT-1-interacting homeodomain factor expressed during anterior pituitary gland development, Proc Nat Acad Sci USA 93 (1996) 7706–7710.

[9] C. Lanctot, Y. Gauthier, J. Drouin, Pituitary homeobox 1 (Ptx1) is differentially expressed during pituitary development, Endocrinology 140 (1999) 1416–1422.

[10] J.J. Tremblay, C. Lanctot, J. Drouin, The pan-pituitary activator of transcription, Ptx1 (pituitary homeobox 1), acts in synergy with SF-1 and Pit1 and is an upstream regulator of the Lim-homeodomain gene Lim3/Lhx3, Mol Endocrinol 12 (1998) 428–441.

[11] E.V. Semina, R. Reiter, N.J. Leysens, W.L. Alward, K.W. Small, N.A. Datson, et al., Cloning and characterization of a novel bicoid-related homeobox transcription factor gene, RIEG, involved in Rieger syndrome, Nat Genet 14 (1996) 392–399.

[12] S. Li, E.B. Crenshaw 3rd, E.J. Rawson, D.M. Simmons, L.W. Swanson, M.G. Rosenfeld, Dwarf locus mutants lacking three pituitary cell types result from mutations in the POU-domain gene pit-1, Nature 347 (1990) 528–533.

[13] J.E. Lee, S.M. Hollenberg, L. Snider, D.L. Turner, N. Lipnick, H. Weintraub, Conversion of *Xenopus* ectoderm into neurons by NeuroD, a basic helix-loop-helix protein, Science 268 (1995) 836–844.

[14] F.J. Naya, C.M. Stellrecht, M.J. Tsai, Tissue-specific regulation of the insulin gene by a novel basic helix-loop-helix transcription factor, Genes Dev 9 (1995) 1009–1019.

[15] J. Drouin, S. Bilodeau, S. Vallette, Of old and new diseases: Genetics of pituitary ACTH excess (Cushing) and deficiency, Clin Genet 72 (3) (2007) 175–182.

[16] J. Karpac, D. Ostwald, G.Y. Li, S. Bui, P. Hunnewell, M.B. Brennan, et al., Proopiomelanocortin heterozygous and homozygous null mutant mice develop pituitary adenomas, Cell Mol Biol (Noisy-le-grand) 52 (2) (2006) 47–52.

[17] K.J. Dunn, B.O. Williams, Y. Li, W.J. Pavan, Neural crest-directed gene transfer demonstrates Wnt1 role in melanocyte expansion and differentiation during mouse development, Proc Nat Acad Sci USA 97 (18) (2000) 10050–10055.

[18] N.A. Liu, H. Huang, Z. Yang, W. Herzog, M. Hammerschmidt, S. Lin, et al., Pituitary corticotroph ontogeny and regulation in transgenic zebrafish, Mol Endocrinol 17 (5) (2003) 959–966.

[19] S. Kimura, Y. Hara, T. Pineau, P. Fernandez-Salguero, C.H. Fox, J.M. Ward, et al., The T/ebp null mouse: Thyroid-specific enhancer-binding protein is essential for the organogenesis of the thyroid, lung, ventral forebrain, and pituitary, Genes Dev 10 (1996) 60–69.

[20] L. Muglia, L. Jacobson, P. Dikkes, J.A. Majzoub, Corticotropin-releasing hormone deficiency reveals major fetal but not adult glucocorticoid need, Nature 373 (1995) 427–432.

[21] M.D. Schonemann, A.K. Ryan, R.J. McEvilly, S.M. O'Connell, C.A. Arias, K.A. Kalla, et al., Development and survival of the endocrine hypothalamus and posterior pituitary gland requires the neuronal POU domain factor Brn-2, Genes Dev 9 (1995) 3122–3135.

[22] C. Denef, Paracrinicity: The story of 30 years of cellular pituitary crosstalk, J Neuroendocrinol 20 (1) (2008) 1–70.

[23] A. Kitahara, E. Takano, H. Ohtsuki, Y. Kirihata, Y. Yamagata, R. Kannagi, et al., Reversed distribution of calpains and calpastatin in human pituitary gland and selective localization of calpastatin in adrenocorticotropin-producing cells as demonstrated by immunohistochemistry, J Clin Endocrinol Metab 63 (2) (1986) 343–348.

[24] Y. Uei, Immunohistological study of Crooke's cells, Pathol Res Pract 183 (5) (1988) 636–637.

[25] L. Desy, G. Pelletier, Immunohistochemical localization of alpha-melanocyte stimulating hormone (alpha-MSH) in the human hypothalamus, Brain Res 154 (2) (1978) 377–381.

[26] P.C. Emson, R. Corder, S.J. Ratter, S. Tomlin, P.J. Lowry, L.H. Ress, et al., Regional distribution of pro-opiomelanocortin-derived peptides in the human brain, Neuroendocrinology 38 (1) (1984) 45–50.

[27] C. Broberger, J. Johansen, C. Johansson, M. Schalling, T. Hokfelt, The neuropeptide Y/agouti gene-related protein (AGRP) brain circuitry in normal, anorectic, and monosodium glutamate-treated mice, Proc Nat Acad Sci USA 95 (1998) 15043–15048.

[28] C.C. Cheung, D.K. Clifton, R.A. Steiner, Proopiomelanocortin neurons are direct targets for leptin in the hypothalamus, Endocrinology 138 (1997) 4489–4492.

[29] C.R. DeBold, J.K. Menefee, W.E. Nicholson, D.N. Orth, Pro-opiomelanocortin gene is expressed in many normal human tissues and in tumors not associated with ectopic adrenocorticotropin syndrome, Mol Endocrinol 2 (9) (1988) 862–870.

[30] T. Lacaze-Masmonteil, Y. de Keyzer, J.P. Luton, A. Kahn, X. Bertagna, Characterization of proopiomelanocortin transcripts in human nonpituitary tissues, Proc Nat Acad Sci USA 84 (1987) 7261–7265.

[31] A.B. Bicknell, The tissue-specific processing of pro-opiomelanocortin, J Neuroendocrinol 20 (6) (2008) 692–699.

[32] B.G. Jenks, Regulation of proopiomelanocortin gene expression: An overview of the signaling cascades, transcription factors, and responsive elements involved, Ann NY Acad Sci 1163 (2009) 17–30.

[33] R.T.J. Fremeau, J.R. Lundblad, D.B. Pritchett, J.N. Wilcox, J.L. Roberts, Regulation of pro-opiomelanocortin gene transcription in individual cell nuclei, Science 234 (1986) 1265–1269.

[34] G. Aguilera, M. Nikodemova, P.C. Wynn, K.J. Catt, Corticotropin releasing hormone receptors: Two decades later, Peptides 25 (3) (2004) 319–329.

[35] C. Bousquet, C. Susini, S. Melmed, Inhibitory roles for SHP-1 and SOCS-3 following pituitary proopiomelanocortin induction by leukemia inhibitory factor, J Clin Invest 104 (9) (1999) 1277–1285.

[36] H. Yano, C. Readhead, M. Nakashima, S.G. Ren, S. Melmed, Pituitary-directed leukemia inhibitory factor transgene causes Cushing's syndrome: Neuro-immune-endocrine modulation of pituitary development, Mol Endocrinol 12 (11) (1998) 1708–1720.

[37] Y. Iwasaki, M. Nishiyama, T. Taguchi, M. Kambayashi, M. Asai, M. Yoshida, et al., Activation of AMP-activated protein kinase stimulates proopiomelanocortin gene transcription in AtT20 corticotroph cells, Am J Physiol Endocrinol Metab 292 (6) (2007) E1899–E1905.

[38] G. Yang, C.Y. Lim, C. Li, X. Xiao, G.K. Radda, X. Cao, et al., FoxO1 inhibits leptin regulation of pro-opiomelanocortin promoter activity by blocking STAT3 interaction with specificity protein 1, J Biol Chem 284 (6) (2009) 3719–3727.

[39] K. Kageyama, T. Suda, Regulatory mechanisms underlying corticotropin-releasing factor gene expression in the hypothalamus, Endocr J 56 (3) (2009) 335–344.

[40] B.G. Robinson, K. Mealy, D.W. Wilmore, J.A. Majzoub, The effect of insulin-induced hypoglycemia on gene expression in the hypothalamic–pituitary–adrenal axis of the rat, Endocrinology 130 (2) (1992) 920–925.

[41] J. Korner, J. Chun, D. Harter, R. Axel, Isolation and functional expression of a mammalian prohormone processing enzyme, murine prohormone convertase 1, Proc Nat Acad Sci USA 88 (15) (1991) 6834–6838.

[42] R.S. Jackson, J.W. Creemers, S. Ohagi, M.L. Raffin-Sanson, L. Sanders, C.T. Montague, et al., Obesity and impaired prohormone processing associated with mutations in the human prohormone convertase 1 gene [see comments], Nat Genet 16 (1997) 303–306.

[43] J.K. Naggert, L.D. Fricker, O. Varlamov, P.M. Nishina, Y. Rouille, D.F. Steiner, et al., Hyperproinsulinaemia in obese fat/fat mice associated with a carboxypeptidase E mutation which reduces enzyme activity, Nat Genet 10 (1995) 135–142.

[44] D. Malide, N.G. Seidah, M. Chretien, M. Bendayan, Electron microscopic immunocytochemical evidence for the involvement of the convertases PC1 and PC2 in the processing of proinsulin in pancreatic beta-cells, J Histochem Cytochem 43 (1995) 11–19.

[45] J.A. Braks, G.J. Martens, 7B2 is a neuroendocrine chaperone that transiently interacts with prohormone convertase PC2 in the secretory pathway, Cell 78 (1994) 263–273.

[46] C.H. Westphal, L. Muller, A. Zhou, X. Zhu, S. Bonner-Weir, M. Schambelan, et al., The neuroendocrine protein 7B2 is required for peptide hormone processing in vivo and provides a novel mechanism for pituitary Cushing's disease, Cell 96 (1999) 689–700.

[47] M. Furuta, H. Yano, A. Zhou, Y. Rouille, J.J. Holst, R. Carroll, et al., Defective prohormone processing and altered pancreatic islet morphology in mice lacking active SPC2, Proc Nat Acad Sci USA 94 (1997) 6646–6651.

[48] L.D. Fricker, A.A. McKinzie, J. Sun, E. Curran, Y. Qian, L. Yan, et al., Identification and characterization of proSAAS, a granin-like neuroendocrine peptide precursor that inhibits prohormone processing, J Neurosci 20 (2000) 639–648.

[49] A. Saiardi, E. Borrelli, Absence of dopaminergic control on melanotrophs leads to Cushing's-like syndrome in mice, Mol Endocrinol 12 (1998) 1133–1139.

[50] R.S. Yalow, Radioimmunoassay: A probe for the fine structure of biologic systems, Science 200 (4347) (1978) 1236–1245.

[51] J.R. Lindsay, V.K. Shanmugam, E.H. Oldfield, A.T. Remaley, L.K. Nieman, A comparison of immunometric and radioimmunoassay measurement of ACTH for the differential diagnosis of Cushing's syndrome, J Endocrinol Invest 29 (11) (2006) 983–988.

[52] S. Dobson, A. White, M. Hoadley, T. Lovgren, J. Ratcliffe, Measurement of corticotropin in unextracted plasma: Comparison of a time-resolved immunofluorometric assay and an immunoradiometric assay, with use of the same monoclonal antibodies, Clin Chem 33 (10) (1987) 1747–1751.

[53] I. Verschraegen, E. Anckaert, J. Schiettecatte, M. Mees, A. Garrido, D. Hermsen, et al., Multicenter evaluation of a rapid electrochemiluminescent adrenocorticotropic hormone (ACTH) immunoassay, Clin Chim Acta 380 (1–2) (2007) 75–80.

[54] A. Thomas, M. Kohler, W. Schanzer, M. Kamber, P. Delahaut, M. Thevis, Determination of Synacthen in urine for sports drug testing by means of nano-ultra-performance liquid chromatography/tandem mass spectrometry, Rapid Commun Mass Spectrom 23 (17) (2009) 2669–2674.
[55] G. Aguilera, C. Rabadan-Diehl, M. Nikodemova, Regulation of pituitary corticotropin releasing hormone receptors, Peptides 22 (5) (2001) 769–774.
[56] D.S. Jessop, Review: Central non-glucocorticoid inhibitors of the hypothalamo–pituitary–adrenal axis, J Endocrinol 160 (2) (1999) 169–180.
[57] D.M. Gibbs, R.D. Stewart, W. Vale, J. Rivier, S.S. Yen, Synthetic corticotropin-releasing factor stimulates secretion of immunoreactive beta-endorphin/beta-lipotropin and ACTH by human fetal pituitaries in vitro, Life Sci 32 (5) (1983) 547–550.
[58] C.R. DeBold, W.R. Sheldon Jr., G.S. DeCherney, R.V. Jackson, W.E. Nicholson, D.P. Island, et al., Effect of subcutaneous and intranasal administration of ovine corticotropin-releasing hormone in man: Comparison with intravenous administration, J Clin Endocrinol Metab 60 (5) (1985) 836–840.
[59] R. Smith, S. Mesiano, E.C. Chan, S. Brown, R.B. Jaffe, Corticotropin-releasing hormone directly and preferentially stimulates dehydroepiandrosterone sulfate secretion by human fetal adrenal cortical cells, J Clin Endocrinol Metab 83 (8) (1998) 2916–2920.
[60] C.R. DeBold, G.S. DeCherney, R.V. Jackson, W.R. Sheldon, A.N. Alexander, D.P. Island, et al., Effect of synthetic ovine corticotropin-releasing factor: Prolonged duration of action and biphasic response of plasma adrenocorticotropin and cortisol, J Clin Endocrinol Metab 57 (2) (1983) 294–298.
[61] H.R. Michie, J.A. Majzoub, S.T. O'Dwyer, A. Revhaug, D.W. Wilmore, Both cyclooxygenase-dependent and cyclooxygenase-independent pathways mediate the neuroendocrine response in humans, Surgery 108 (2) (1990) 254–259, discussion 9–61.
[62] R.C. Gaillard, A.M. Riondel, N. Ling, A.F. Muller, Corticotropin releasing factor activity of CRF 41 in normal man is potentiated by angiotensin II and vasopressin but not by desmopressin, Life Sci 43 (23) (1988) 1935–1944.
[63] T. Watanabe, Y. Oki, D.N. Orth, Kinetic actions and interactions of arginine vasopressin, angiotensin-II, and oxytocin on adrenocorticotropin secretion by rat anterior pituitary cells in the microperifusion system, Endocrinology 125 (4) (1989) 1921–1931.
[64] P. Schoenenberg, R.C. Gaillard, P. Kehrer, A.F. Muller, cAMP-dependent ACTH secretagogues facilitate corticotropin releasing activity of angiotensin II on rat anterior pituitary cells in vitro, Acta Endocrinol (Copenh) 114 (1) (1987) 118–123.
[65] S.C. Weninger, A.J. Dunn, L.J. Muglia, P. Dikkes, K.A. Miczek, A.H. Swiergiel, et al., Stress-induced behaviors require the corticotropin-releasing hormone (CRH) receptor, but not CRH, Proc Nat Acad Sci USA 96 (14) (1999) 8283–8288.
[66] E. Zoumakis, K.C. Rice, P.W. Gold, G.P. Chrousos, Potential uses of corticotropin-releasing hormone antagonists, Ann NY Acad Sci 1083 (2006) 239–251.
[67] C. Rivier, W. Vale, Effects of corticotropin-releasing factor, neurohypophyseal peptides, and catecholamines on pituitary function, Fed Proc 44 (1 Pt 2) (1985) 189–195.
[68] B.M. Sharp, S.G. Matta, P.K. Peterson, R. Newton, C. Chao, K. McAllen, Tumor necrosis factor-alpha is a potent ACTH secretagogue: Comparison to interleukin-1 beta, Endocrinology 124 (6) (1989) 3131–3133.
[69] H.R. Michie, K.R. Manogue, D.R. Spriggs, A. Revhaug, S. O'Dwyer, C.A. Dinarello, et al., Detection of circulating tumor necrosis factor after endotoxin administration, N Engl J Med 318 (23) (1988) 1481–1486.
[70] Y. Naitoh, J. Fukata, T. Tominaga, Y. Nakai, S. Tamai, K. Mori, et al., Interleukin-6 stimulates the secretion of adrenocorticotropic hormone in conscious, freely-moving rats, Biochem Biophys Res Commun 155 (3) (1988) 1459–1463.
[71] P. Navarra, S. Tsagarakis, M.S. Faria, L.H. Rees, G.M. Besser, A.B. Grossman, Interleukins-1 and -6 stimulate the release of corticotropin-releasing hormone-41 from rat hypothalamus in vitro via the eicosanoid cyclooxygenase pathway, Endocrinology 128 (1) (1991) 37–44.
[72] J.I. Koenig, Pituitary gland: Neuropeptides, neurotransmitters and growth factors, Toxicol Pathol 17 (2) (1989) 256–265.
[73] J. Volavka, D. Cho, A. Mallya, J. Bauman, Naloxone increases ACTH and cortisol levels in man, N Engl J Med 300 (18) (1979) 1056–1057.
[74] I. Wakabayashi, R. Demura, N. Miki, E. Ohmura, H. Miyoshi, K. Shizume, Failure of naloxone to influence plasma growth hormone, prolactin, and cortisol secretions induced by insulin hypoglycemia, J Clin Endocrinol Metab 50 (3) (1980) 597–599.
[75] R.S. Rittmaster, G.B. Cutler Jr., D.O. Sobel, D.S. Goldstein, M.C. Koppelman, D.L. Loriaux, et al., Morphine inhibits the pituitary–adrenal response to ovine corticotropin-releasing hormone in normal subjects, J Clin Endocrinol Metab 60 (5) (1985) 891–895.
[76] B. Allolio, U. Deuss, D. Kaulen, U. Leonhardt, D. Kallabis, E. Hamel, et al., FK 33-824, a met-enkephalin analog, blocks corticotropin-releasing hormone-induced adrenocorticotropin secretion in normal subjects but not in patients with Cushing's disease, J Clin Endocrinol Metab 63 (6) (1986) 1427–1431.
[77] A. Schmidt, S. Audigier, C. Barberis, S. Jard, M. Manning, A.S. Kolodziejczyk, et al., A radioiodinated linear vasopressin antagonist: A ligand with high affinity and specificity for V1a receptors, FEBS Lett 282 (1) (1991) 77–81.
[78] E. Spinedi, A. Negro-Vilar, Arginine vasopressin and adrenocorticotropin release: Correlation between binding characteristics and biological activity in anterior pituitary dispersed cells, Endocrinology 114 (6) (1984) 2247–2251.
[79] G. Aguilera, S. Volpi, C. Rabadan-Diehl, Transcriptional and post-transcriptional mechanisms regulating the rat pituitary vasopressin V1b receptor gene, J Mol Endocrinol 30 (2) (2003) 99–108.
[80] T. Watanabe, D.N. Orth, Detailed kinetic analysis of adrenocorticotropin secretion by dispersed rat anterior pituitary cells in a microperifusion system: Effects of ovine corticotropin-releasing factor and arginine vasopressin, Endocrinology 121 (3) (1987) 1133–1145.
[81] S.R. Page, V.T. Ang, R. Jackson, S.S. Nussey, The effect of oxytocin on the plasma glucagon response to insulin-induced hypoglycaemia in man, Diabetes Metab 16 (3) (1990) 248–251.
[82] T.M. Mishunina, V.Y. Kononenko, Specific GABA binding in the adrenals and blood corticosteroid levels in stress in intact rats and rats with changes in the functional activity of the hypothalamo–pituitary–adrenal system, Neurosci Behav Physiol 32 (2) (2002) 109–112.
[83] K.G. Mountjoy, L.S. Robbins, M.T. Mortrud, R.D. Cone, The cloning of a family of genes that encode the melanocortin receptors, Science 257 (1992) 1248–1251.
[84] A.J. Clark, L.F. Chan, T.T. Chung, L.A. Metherell, The genetics of familial glucocorticoid deficiency, Best Pract Res Clin Endocrinol Metab 23 (2) (2009 Apr) 159–165.
[85] H.B. Schioth, R. Muceniece, J.E. Wikberg, Characterisation of the melanocortin 4 receptor by radioligand binding, Pharmacol Toxicol 79 (1996) 161–165.

[86] F.L. Strand, C. Saint-Come, T.S. Lee, S.J. Lee, J. Kume, L.A. Zuccarelli, ACTH/MSH(4-10) analog BIM 22015 aids regeneration via neurotrophic and myotrophic attributes, Peptides 14 (1993) 287–296.
[87] R.D. Cone, K.G. Mountjoy, L.S. Robbins, J.H. Nadeau, K.R. Johnson, L. Roselli-Rehfuss, et al., Cloning and functional characterization of a family of receptors for the melanotropic peptides, Ann NY Acad Sci 680 (1993) 342–363.
[88] I. Suzuki, R.D. Cone, S. Im, J. Nordlund, Z.A. Abdel-Malek, Binding of melanotropic hormones to the melanocortin receptor MC1R on human melanocytes stimulates proliferation and melanogenesis, Endocrinology 137 (1996) 1627–1633.
[89] A.K. Chakraborty, Y. Funasaka, J.M. Pawelek, M. Nagahama, A. Ito, M. Ichihashi, Enhanced expression of melanocortin-1 receptor (MC1-R) in normal human keratinocytes during differentiation: Evidence for increased expression of POMC peptides near suprabasal layer of epidermis, J Invest Dermatol 112 (1999) 853–860.
[90] L.S. Robbins, J.H. Nadeau, K.R. Johnson, M.A. Kelly, L. Roselli-Rehfuss, E. Baack, et al., Pigmentation phenotypes of variant extension locus alleles result from point mutations that alter MSH receptor function, Cell 72 (1993) 827–834.
[91] P. Valverde, E. Healy, I. Jackson, J.L. Rees, A.J. Thody, Variants of the melanocyte-stimulating hormone receptor gene are associated with red hair and fair skin in humans [see comments], Nat Genet 11 (1995) 328–330.
[92] E. Healy, N. Flannagan, A. Ray, C. Todd, I.J. Jackson, J.N. Matthews, et al., Melanocortin-1-receptor gene and sun sensitivity in individuals without red hair [letter], Lancet 355 (2000) 1072–1073.
[93] T.A. Luger, T. Scholzen, T. Brzoska, E. Becher, A. Slominski, R. Paus, Cutaneous immunomodulation and coordination of skin stress responses by alpha-melanocyte-stimulating hormone, Ann NY Acad Sci 840 (1998) 381–394.
[94] R.A. Star, N. Rajora, J. Huang, R.C. Stock, A. Catania, J.M. Lipton, Evidence of autocrine modulation of macrophage nitric oxide synthase by alpha-melanocyte-stimulating hormone, Proc Nat Acad Sci USA 92 (1995) 8016–8020.
[95] A. Catania, N. Rajora, F. Capsoni, F. Minonzio, R.A. Star, J.M. Lipton, The neuropeptide alpha-MSH has specific receptors on neutrophils and reduces chemotaxis in vitro, Peptides 17 (1996) 675–679.
[96] M. Hartmeyer, T. Scholzen, E. Becher, R.S. Bhardwaj, T. Schwarz, T.A. Luger, Human dermal microvascular endothelial cells express the melanocortin receptor type 1 and produce increased levels of IL-8 upon stimulation with alpha-melanocyte-stimulating hormone, J Immunol 159 (1997) 1930–1937.
[97] L.L. Elias, A. Huebner, G.D. Pullinger, A. Mirtella, A.J. Clark, Functional characterization of naturally occurring mutations of the human adrenocorticotropin receptor: Poor correlation of phenotype and genotype, J Clin Endocrinol Metab 84 (1999) 2766–2770.
[98] L.A. Metherell, J.P. Chapple, S. Cooray, A. David, C. Becker, F. Ruschendorf, et al., Mutations in MRAP, encoding a new interacting partner of the ACTH receptor, cause familial glucocorticoid deficiency type 2, Nat Genet 37 (2) (2005) 166–170.
[99] S.N. Cooray, L. Chan, L. Metherell, H. Storr, A.J. Clark, Adrenocorticotropin resistance syndromes, Endocr Dev 13 (2008) 99–116.
[100] J.A. Sebag, P.M. Hinkle, Melanocortin-2 receptor accessory protein MRAP forms antiparallel homodimers, Proc Nat Acad Sci USA 104 (51) (2007) 20244–20249.
[101] J.A. Sebag, P.M. Hinkle, Regions of melanocortin 2 (MC2) receptor accessory protein necessary for dual topology and MC2 receptor trafficking and signaling, J Biol Chem 284 (1) (2009) 610–618.
[102] T.R. Webb, A.J. Clark, Minireview: The melanocortin 2 receptor accessory proteins, Mol Endocrinol 24 (3) (2009) 475–484.
[103] W.L. Miller, J.F. Strauss 3rd, Molecular pathology and mechanism of action of the steroidogenic acute regulatory protein, StAR, J Steroid Biochem Mol Biol 69 (1–6) (1999) 131–141.
[104] F.E. Estivariz, F. Iturriza, C. McLean, J. Hope, P.J. Lowry, Stimulation of adrenal mitogenesis by N-terminal proopiocortin peptides, Nature 297 (1982) 419–422.
[105] F. Albright, Osteoporosis, Annals of Internal Medicine 27 (1947) 861–882.
[106] B.L. Linder, N.V. Esteban, A.L. Yergey, J.C. Winterer, D.L. Loriaux, F. Cassorla, Cortisol production rate in childhood and adolescence, J Pediatr 117 (6) (1990) 892–896.
[107] B.A. Boston, R.D. Cone, Characterization of melanocortin receptor subtype expression in murine adipose tissues and in the 3T3-L1 cell line, Endocrinology 137 (1996) 2043–2050.
[108] A. Bousquet-Melou, J. Galitzky, M. Lafontan, M. Berlan, Control of lipolysis in intra-abdominal fat cells of nonhuman primates: Comparison with humans, J Lipid Res 36 (1995) 451–461.
[109] E.M. Smith, P. Brosnan, W.J. Meyer, J.E. Blalock, An ACTH receptor on human mononuclear leukocytes. Relation to adrenal ACTH-receptor activity, N Engl J Med 317 (1987) 1266–1269.
[110] A. Slominski, G. Ermak, J. Hwang, J. Mazurkiewicz, D. Corliss, A. Eastman, The expression of proopiomelanocortin (POMC) and of corticotropin releasing hormone receptor (CRH-R) genes in mouse skin, Biochim Biophys Acta 1289 (1996) 247–251.
[111] S. Kapas, F.M. Cammas, J.P. Hinson, A.J. Clark, Agonist and receptor binding properties of adrenocorticotropin peptides using the cloned mouse adrenocorticotropin receptor expressed in a stably transfected HeLa cell line, Endocrinology 137 (1996) 3291–3294.
[112] J. Lindblom, H.B. Schioth, A. Larsson, J.E. Wikberg, L. Bergstrom, Autoradiographic discrimination of melanocortin receptors indicates that the MC3 subtype dominates in the medial rat brain, Brain Res 810 (1998) 161–171.
[113] S.J. Getting, R.J. Flower, M. Perretti, Agonism at melanocortin receptor type 3 on macrophages inhibits neutrophil influx, Inflamm Res 48 (1999) S140–S141.
[114] A.S. Chen, D.J. Marsh, M.E. Trumbauer, E.G. Frazier, X.M. Guan, H. Yu, et al., Inactivation of the mouse melanocortin-3 receptor results in increased fat mass and reduced lean body mass, Nat Genet 26 (1) (2000) 97–102.
[115] D.E. Cummings, M.W. Schwartz, Melanocortins and body weight: A tale of two receptors, Nat Genet 26 (1) (2000) 8–9.
[116] K.G. Mountjoy, M.T. Mortrud, M.J. Low, R.B. Simerly, R.D. Cone, Localization of the melanocortin-4 receptor (MC4-R) in neuroendocrine and autonomic control circuits in the brain, Mol Endocrinol 8 (1994) 1298–1308.
[117] C. Vaisse, K. Clement, E. Durand, S. Hercberg, B. Guy-Grand, P. Froguel, Melanocortin-4 receptor mutations are a frequent and heterogeneous cause of morbid obesity [see comments], J Clin Invest 106 (2000) 253–262.
[118] C. Vaisse, K. Clement, B. Guy-Grand, P. Froguel, A frameshift mutation in human MC4R is associated with a dominant form of obesity [letter], Nat Genet 20 (1998) 113–114.
[119] I.S. Farooqi, G.S. Yeo, J.M. Keogh, S. Aminian, S.A. Jebb, G. Butler, et al., Dominant and recessive inheritance of morbid obesity associated with melanocortin 4 receptor deficiency [see comments], J Clin Invest 106 (2000) 271–279.

[120] J.D. Cody, X.T. Reveles, D.E. Hale, D. Lehman, H. Coon, R.J. Leach, Haplosufficiency of the melancortin-4 receptor gene in individuals with deletions of 18q, Hum Genet 105 (1999) 424–427.

[121] G. Ho, R.G. MacKenzie, Functional characterization of mutations in melanocortin-4 receptor associated with human obesity, J Biol Chem 274 (1999) 35816–35822.

[122] J.C. Chambers, P. Elliott, D. Zabaneh, W. Zhang, Y. Li, P. Froguel, et al., Common genetic variation near MC4R is associated with waist circumference and insulin resistance, Nat Genet 40 (6) (2008) 716–718.

[123] N. Balthasar, Genetic dissection of neuronal pathways controlling energy homeostasis, Obesity (Silver Spring) 14 (Suppl 5) (2006) 222S–227S.

[124] M.A. Cowley, N. Pronchuk, W. Fan, D.M. Dinulescu, W.F. Colmers, R.D. Cone, Integration of NPY, AGRP, and melanocortin signals in the hypothalamic paraventricular nucleus: evidence of a cellular basis for the adipostat, Neuron 24 (1999) 155–163.

[125] A. Kask, H.B. Schioth, Tonic inhibition of food intake during inactive phase is reversed by the injection of the melanocortin receptor antagonist into the paraventricular nucleus of the hypothalamus and central amygdala of the rat, Brain Res 887 (2) (2000) 460–464.

[126] H. Dhillon, J.M. Zigman, C. Ye, C.E. Lee, R.A. McGovern, V. Tang, et al., Leptin directly activates SF1 neurons in the VMH, and this action by leptin is required for normal body-weight homeostasis, Neuron 49 (2) (2006) 191–203.

[127] J.M. Friedman, Obesity: Causes and control of excess body fat, Nature 459 (7245) (2009) 340–342.

[128] J.F. Caro, J.W. Kolaczynski, M.R. Nyce, J.P. Ohannesian, I. Opentanova, W.H. Goldman, et al., Decreased cerebrospinal-fluid/serum leptin ratio in obesity: A possible mechanism for leptin resistance, Lancet 348 (9021) (1996) 159–161.

[129] T. Hosoi, M. Sasaki, T. Miyahara, C. Hashimoto, S. Matsuo, M. Yoshii, et al., Endoplasmic reticulum stress induces leptin resistance, Mol Pharmacol 74 (6) (2008) 1610–1619.

[130] X. Zhang, G. Zhang, H. Zhang, M. Karin, H. Bai, D. Cai, Hypothalamic IKKbeta/NF-kappaB and ER stress link overnutrition to energy imbalance and obesity, Cell 135 (1) (2008) 61–73.

[131] U. Ozcan, Q. Cao, E. Yilmaz, A.H. Lee, N.N. Iwakoshi, E. Ozdelen, et al., Endoplasmic reticulum stress links obesity, insulin action, and type 2 diabetes, Science 306 (5695) (2004) 457–461.

[132] L. Ozcan, A.S. Ergin, A. Lu, J. Chung, S. Sarkar, D. Nie, et al., Endoplasmic reticulum stress plays a central role in development of leptin resistance, Cell Metab 9 (1) (2009) 35–51.

[133] M. Delepine, M. Nicolino, T. Barrett, M. Golamaully, G.M. Lathrop, C. Julier, EIF2AK3, encoding translation initiation factor 2-alpha kinase 3, is mutated in patients with Wolcott-Rallison syndrome, Nat Genet 25 (4) (2000) 406–409.

[134] S. Oyadomari, A. Koizumi, K. Takeda, T. Gotoh, S. Akira, E. Araki, et al., Targeted disruption of the Chop gene delays endoplasmic reticulum stress-mediated diabetes, J Clin Invest 109 (4) (2002) 525–532.

[135] W. Chen, M.A. Kelly, X. Opitz-Araya, R.E. Thomas, M.J. Low, R.D. Cone, Exocrine gland dysfunction in MC5-R-deficient mice: Evidence for coordinated regulation of exocrine gland function by melanocortin peptides, Cell 91 (1997) 789–798.

[136] H. Krude, H. Biebermann, W. Luck, R. Horn, G. Brabant, A. Gruters, Severe early-onset obesity, adrenal insufficiency and red hair pigmentation caused by POMC mutations in humans, Nat Genet 19 (1998) 155–157.

[137] H. Krude, H. Biebermann, D. Schnabel, M.Z. Tansek, P. Theunissen, P.E. Mullis, et al., Obesity due to proopiomelanocortin deficiency: Three new cases and treatment trials with thyroid hormone and ACTH4-10, J Clin Endocrinol Metab 88 (10) (2003) 4633–4640.

[138] N. Flanagan, E. Healy, A. Ray, S. Philips, C. Todd, I.J. Jackson, et al., Pleiotropic effects of the melanocortin 1 receptor (MC1R) gene on human pigmentation, Hum Mol Genet 9 (17) (2000) 2531–2537.

[139] T. Kikuchi, S. Yabe, T. Kanda, I. Kobayashi, Antipituitary antibodies as pathogenetic factors in patients with pituitary disorders, Endocr J 47 (4) (2000) 407–416.

[140] L. Yaswen, N. Diehl, M.B. Brennan, U. Hochgeschwender, Obesity in the mouse model of pro-opiomelanocortin deficiency responds to peripheral melanocortin [see comments], Nat Med 5 (1999) 1066–1070.

[141] S. Forbes, S. Bui, B.R. Robinson, U. Hochgeschwender, M.B. Brennan, Integrated control of appetite and fat metabolism by the leptin-proopiomelanocortin pathway, Proc Nat Acad Sci USA 98 (7) (2001) 4233–4237.

[142] K.B. Linhart, J.A. Majzoub, Pomc knockout mice have secondary hyperaldosteronism despite an absence of adrenocorticotropin, Endocrinology 149 (2) (2008) 681–686.

[143] W.K. Silvers, E.S. Russell, An experimental approach to action of genes at the agouti locus in the mouse, J Exp Zool 130 (1955) 199–220.

[144] L. Cuneot, Les races pures et leurs combinaisons chez les souris, Arch Xool Exp Gen 3 (1905) 123–132.

[145] D. Lu, D. Willard, I.R. Patel, S. Kadwell, L. Overton, T. Kost, et al., Agouti protein is an antagonist of the melanocyte-stimulating-hormone receptor, Nature 371 (1994) 799–802.

[146] S.J. Bultman, E.J. Michaud, R.P. Woychik, Molecular characterization of the mouse agouti locus, Cell 71 (1992) 1195–1204.

[147] M.M. Ollmann, B.D. Wilson, Y.K. Yang, J.A. Kerns, Y. Chen, I. Gantz, et al., Antagonism of central melanocortin receptors in vitro and in vivo by agouti-related protein [published erratum appears in Science (1998) 281 (5383) 1615], Science 278 (1997) 135–138.

[148] Y.K. Yang, D.A. Thompson, C.J. Dickinson, J. Wilken, G.S. Barsh, S.B. Kent, et al., Characterization of Agouti-related protein binding to melanocortin receptors, Mol Endocrinol 13 (1999) 148–155.

[149] S. Luquet, F.A. Perez, T.S. Hnasko, R.D. Palmiter, NPY/AgRP neurons are essential for feeding in adult mice but can be ablated in neonates, Science 310 (5748) (2005) 683–685.

[150] A. Argiolas, M.R. Melis, S. Murgia, H.B. Schioth, ACTH- and alpha-MSH-induced grooming, stretching, yawning and penile erection in male rats: Site of action in the brain and role of melanocortin receptors [In Process Citation], Brain Res Bull 51 (2000) 425–431.

[151] H. Wessells, K. Fuciarelli, J. Hansen, M.E. Hadley, V.J. Hruby, R. Dorr, et al., Synthetic melanotropic peptide initiates erections in men with psychogenic erectile dysfunction: Double-blind, placebo controlled crossover study, J Urol 160 (1998) 389–393.

[152] M.T. Murphy, D.B. Richards, J.M. Lipton, Antipyretic potency of centrally administered alpha-melanocyte stimulating hormone, Science 221 (1983) 192–193.

[153] S.J. Li, K. Varga, P. Archer, V.J. Hruby, S.D. Sharma, R.A. Kesterson, et al., Melanocortin antagonists define two distinct pathways of cardiovascular control by alpha- and gamma-melanocyte-stimulating hormones, J Neurosci 16 (1996) 5182–5188.

[154] J.D. Veldhuis, F. Roelfsema, A. Iranmanesh, B.J. Carroll, D.M. Keenan, S.M. Pincus, Basal, pulsatile, entropic

(patterned), and spiky (staccato-like) properties of ACTH secretion: Impact of age, gender, and body mass index, J Clin Endocrinol Metab 94 (10) (2009) 4045–4052.

[155] J.D. Veldhuis, S.M. Anderson, N. Shah, M. Bray, T. Vick, A. Gentili, et al., Neurophysiological regulation and target-tissue impact of the pulsatile mode of growth hormone secretion in the human, Growth Horm IGF Res 11 (Suppl A) (2001) S25–S37.

[156] M.F. Dallman, Fast glucocorticoid actions on brain: Back to the future, Front Neuroendocrinol 26 (3–4) (2005) 103–108.

[157] W. Oelkers, Hyponatremia and inappropriate secretion of vasopressin (antidiuretic hormone) in patients with hypopituitarism, N Engl J Med 321 (8) (1989) 492–496.

[158] R. Bouley, S. Breton, T. Sun, M. McLaughlin, N.N. Nsumu, H.Y. Lin, et al., Nitric oxide and atrial natriuretic factor stimulate cGMP-dependent membrane insertion of aquaporin 2 in renal epithelial cells, J Clin Invest 106 (9) (2000) 1115–1126.

[159] E. Van Cauter, Putative roles of melatonin in glucose regulation, Therapie 53 (5) (1998) 467–472.

[160] A. Sasaki, O. Shinkawa, K. Yoshinaga, Placental corticotropin-releasing hormone may be a stimulator of maternal pituitary adrenocorticotropic hormone secretion in humans, J Clin Invest 84 (6) (1989) 1997–2001.

[161] L.J. Muglia, L. Jacobson, S.C. Weninger, C.E. Luedke, D.S. Bae, K.H. Jeong, et al., Impaired diurnal adrenal rhythmicity restored by constant infusion of corticotropin-releasing hormone in corticotropin-releasing hormone-deficient mice, J Clin Invest 99 (12) (1997) 2923–2929.

[162] L.J. Muglia, L. Jacobson, C. Luedke, S.K. Vogt, M.L. Schaefer, P. Dikkes, et al., Corticotropin-releasing hormone links pituitary adrenocorticotropin gene expression and release during adrenal insufficiency, J Clin Invest 105 (9) (2000) 1269–1277.

[163] A.Y. So, T.U. Bernal, M.L. Pillsbury, K.R. Yamamoto, B.J. Feldman, Glucocorticoid regulation of the circadian clock modulates glucose homeostasis, Proc Nat Acad Sci USA 106 (41) (2009) 17582–17587.

[164] M.J. Ellis, R.S. Schmidli, R.A. Donald, J.H. Livesey, E.A. Espiner, Plasma corticotrophin-releasing factor and vasopressin responses to hypoglycaemia in normal man, Clin Endocrinol (Oxf) 32 (1) (1990) 93–100.

[165] P.A. Deuster, G.P. Chrousos, A. Luger, J.E. DeBolt, L.L. Bernier, U.H. Trostmann, et al., Hormonal and metabolic responses of untrained, moderately trained, and highly trained men to three exercise intensities, Metabolism 38 (2) (1989) 141–148.

[166] M.N. Janal, E.W. Colt, W.C. Clark, M. Glusman, Pain sensitivity, mood and plasma endocrine levels in man following long-distance running: Effects of naloxone, Pain 19 (1) (1984) 13–25.

[167] T. Wang, C.C. Hung, D.J. Randall, The comparative physiology of food deprivation: From feast to famine, Annu Rev Physiol 68 (2006) 223–251.

[168] D.L. Drazen, M.D. Wortman, M.W. Schwartz, D.J. Clegg, G. van Dijk, S.C. Woods, et al., Adrenalectomy alters the sensitivity of the central nervous system melanocortin system, Diabetes 52 (12) (2003) 2928–2934.

[169] A.F. Pitts, M.A. Preston 2nd, R.S. Jaeckle, W. Meller, R.G. Kathol, Simulated acute hemorrhage through lower body negative pressure as an activator of the hypothalamic–pituitary–adrenal axis, Horm Metab Res 22 (8) (1990) 436–443.

[170] R. Udelsman, J.A. Norton, S.E. Jelenich, D.S. Goldstein, W.M. Linehan, D.L. Loriaux, et al., Responses of the hypothalamic–pituitary–adrenal and renin–angiotensin axes and the sympathetic system during controlled surgical and anesthetic stress, J Clin Endocrinol Metab 64 (5) (1987) 986–994.

[171] K. Voigt, M. Ziegler, M. Grunert-Fuchs, U. Bickel, G. Fehm-Wolfsdorf, Hormonal responses to exhausting physical exercise: The role of predictability and controllability of the situation, Psychoneuroendocrinology 15 (3) (1990) 173–184.

[172] D. Arduini, G. Rizzo, E. Parlati, C. Giorlandino, H. Valensise, S. Dell'Acqua, et al., Modifications of ultradian and circadian rhythms of fetal heart rate after fetal–maternal adrenal gland suppression: A double blind study, Prenat Diagn 6 (6) (1986) 409–417.

[173] S. Onishi, G. Miyazawa, Y. Nishimura, S. Sugiyama, T. Yamakawa, H. Inagaki, et al., Postnatal development of circadian rhythm in serum cortisol levels in children, Pediatrics 72 (3) (1983) 399–404.

[174] A. Keys, The residues of malnutrition and starvation, Science 112 (2909) (1950) 371–373.

[175] K.H. Jeong, L. Jacobson, E.P. Widmaier, J.A. Majzoub, Normal suppression of the reproductive axis following stress in corticotropin-releasing hormone-deficient mice, Endocrinology 140 (4) (1999) 1702–1708.

[176] C. Rivier, Inhibitory effect of neurogenic and immune stressors on testosterone secretion in rats, Neuroimmunomodulation 10 (1) (2002) 17–29.

[177] B.S. McEwen, The neurobiology of stress: From serendipity to clinical relevance, Brain Res 886 (1–2) (2000) 172–189.

[178] K. Karalis, H. Sano, J. Redwine, S. Listwak, R.L. Wilder, G.P. Chrousos, Autocrine or paracrine inflammatory actions of corticotropin-releasing hormone in vivo, Science 254 (5030) (1991 Oct 18) 421–423.

[179] L.J. Muglia, N.A. Jenkins, D.J. Gilbert, N.G. Copeland, J.A. Majzoub, Expression of the mouse corticotropin-releasing hormone gene in vivo and targeted inactivation in embryonic stem cells, J Clin Invest 93 (5) (1994) 2066–2072.

[180] S. Reichlin, Neuroendocrinology, Williams Textbook of Endocrinology, W.B. Saunders Company, Philadelphia, 1998, pp. 165–248.

[181] T.H. Shepard, B.H. Landing, D.G. Mason, Familial Addison's disease. Case reports of two sisters with corticoid deficiency unassociated with hypoaldosteronism, Am J Dis Child 97 (1959) 154–162.

[182] A. Weber, A.J. Clark, L.A. Perry, J.W. Honour, M.O. Savage, Diminished adrenal androgen secretion in familial glucocorticoid deficiency implicates a significant role for ACTH in the induction of adrenarche, Clin Endocrinol (Oxf) 46 (1997) 431–437.

[183] D. Chida, S. Nakagawa, S. Nagai, H. Sagara, H. Katsumata, T. Imaki, et al., Melanocortin 2 receptor is required for adrenal gland development, steroidogenesis, and neonatal gluconeogenesis, Proc Nat Acad Sci USA 104 (46) (2007) 18205–18210.

[184] A.J. Clark, L. McLoughlin, A. Grossman, Familial glucocorticoid deficiency associated with point mutation in the adrenocorticotropin receptor, Lancet 341 (1993) 461–462.

[185] C.A. Stratakis, Cushing syndrome caused by adrenocortical tumors and hyperplasias (corticotropin-independent Cushing syndrome), Endocr Dev 13 (2008) 117–132.

[186] I. Bourdeau, A. Lampron, M.H. Costa, M. Tadjine, A. Lacroix, Adrenocorticotropic hormone-independent Cushing's syndrome, Curr Opin Endocrinol Diabetes Obes 14 (3) (2007) 219–225.

[187] L.S. Kirschner, J.A. Carney, S.D. Pack, S.E. Taymans, C. Giatzakis, Y.S. Cho, et al., Mutations of the gene encoding the protein kinase A type I-alpha regulatory subunit in patients with the Carney complex, Nat Genet 26 (1) (2000) 89–92.

[188] B.W. Scheithauer, Surgical pathology of the pituitary: The adenomas, Part II. Pathol Annu 19 (Pt 2) (1984) 269–329.

[189] E.V. Apletalina, L. Muller, I. Lindberg, Mutations in the catalytic domain of prohormone convertase 2 result in decreased binding to 7B2 and loss of inhibition with 7B2 C-terminal peptide, J Biol Chem 275 (2000) 14667–14677.
[190] K. Neilson, J.P. de Chadarevian, Ectopic anterior pituitary corticotropic tumour in a six-year-old boy. Histological, ultrastructural and immunocytochemical study, Virchows Arch A Pathol Anat Histopathol 411 (3) (1987) 267–273.
[191] E. Arioglu, J. Doppman, M. Gomes, D. Kleiner, D. Mauro, C. Barlow, et al., Cushing's syndrome caused by corticotropin secretion by pulmonary tumorlets, N Engl J Med 339 (13) (1998) 883–886.
[192] B.B. Mendonca, I.J. Arnhold, W. Nicolau, V.A. Avancini, W. Boise, Cushing's syndrome due to ectopic ACTH secretion by bilateral pheochromocytomas in multiple endocrine neoplasia type 2A, N Engl J Med 319 (24) (1988) 1610–1611.
[193] S. Melmed, S. Yamashita, K. Kovacs, J. Ong, S. Rosenblatt, G. Braunstein, Cushing's syndrome due to ectopic proopiomelanocortin gene expression by islet cell carcinoma of the pancreas, Cancer 59 (4) (1987) 772–778.

CHAPTER

4

Growth Hormone

Vivien S. Herman-Bonert, Shlomo Melmed

Pituitary Center, Cedars-Sinai Medical Center, Los Angeles, USA

GROWTH HORMONE (GH) GENE STRUCTURE

The human GH genomic locus spans approximately 66 kb and contains a cluster of five highly conserved genes located on the long arm of human chromosome 17 at bands q22–24. The 5′ to 3′ arrangement of these genes is hGH-N, hCS-L, hCS-A, hGH-V and hCS-B [1], all of which have the same basic structure consisting of five exons separated by four introns [1]. The hGH-N gene is transcribed only in somatotrophs of the anterior pituitary while the hCS-A and hCS-B genes are expressed in placental trophoblasts [2]. hGH-N codes for a 22-kDa protein consisting of 191 amino acids. Approximately 10% of pituitary GH circulates as a 20-kDa variant lacking amino acid residues 32–46 [3], and probably arising as a result of an alternate splicing mechanism. hGH-V is expressed by the syncytiotrophoblast of the placenta during the second and third trimesters of gestation [4], hGH-V messenger RNA (mRNA) encodes a 22-kDa protein secreted form which can be detected in the maternal circulation from midpregnancy [5] and a minor form hGH-V2 which is predicted to be a 26-kDa protein product [6]. The role of hGH-V is unknown, however, the rise in hGH-V concentrations in maternal serum correlates with a fall in hGH-N concentrations, suggesting the possibility of a feedback loop on the maternal hypothalamic–pituitary axis [7]. Postpartum, GH-V levels drop rapidly and are undetectable in the circulation after 1 hour [8]. hGH-V has a greater binding affinity than hGH-N for somatogen vs. lactogen receptors [9]. hGH-V and hGH-N also differ in their ratio of somatogen to lactogen bioactivities, with hGH-V having the greater ratio [8]. In addition, hGH-V has been shown to influence carbohydrate and fat metabolism in rat adipose tissues in a manner similar to that of hGH-N. The hCS-L gene is not known to yield a product [9].

Somatotroph Development and Differentiation

GH is specifically expressed in the somatotroph cell of the anterior pituitary which develops in a time- and space-dependent manner. Expression of the α-subunit transcript in the hypophyseal placode within ectoderm of the pharynx prior to the formation of Rathke's pouch defines the onset of pituitary organogenesis [10,11]. The mammalian anterior pituitary develops from Rathke's pouch during the early stages of embryonic development [12], and a process of cytodifferentiation gives rise to the different hormone-producing cells. Acidophil cells are the progenitors for both GH-producing somatotrophs and prolactin-producing lactotrophs (PRL).

The transcription factors PROPI and POUIFI determine somatotroph and lactotroph growth, differentiation and commitment to expressing the GH or PRL gene product [10] (Figure 4.1). The *Pit*-I gene transcript and POUIFI protein are expressed in somatotrophs, lactotrophs and thyrotrophs [10]. Actions of Pit-1 are complemented by other factors required to achieve physiologic patterns of cell-specific gene activation [10]. Inherited syndromes of GH deficiency or GH action may be attributed to mutations of transcription factors, the GH-1 gene, the GHRH receptor, the GH receptor, or rarely IGF-related molecules.

Experimental evidence obtained from transgenic mice studies suggests that most PRL-expressing cells arise from GH-producing cells [13]. Ablation of somatotrophs by expression of GH-diphtheria toxin and GH-thymidine kinase fusion genes inserted into the germline of transgenic mice results in the elimination of the majority of lactotrophs; however a small percentage of lactotrophs escape destruction [13,14]. This suggests that the majority of PRL-producing cells arise from postmitotic somatotrophs.

The Pituitary, Third Edition, DOI: 10.1016/B978-0-12-380926-1.10004-5

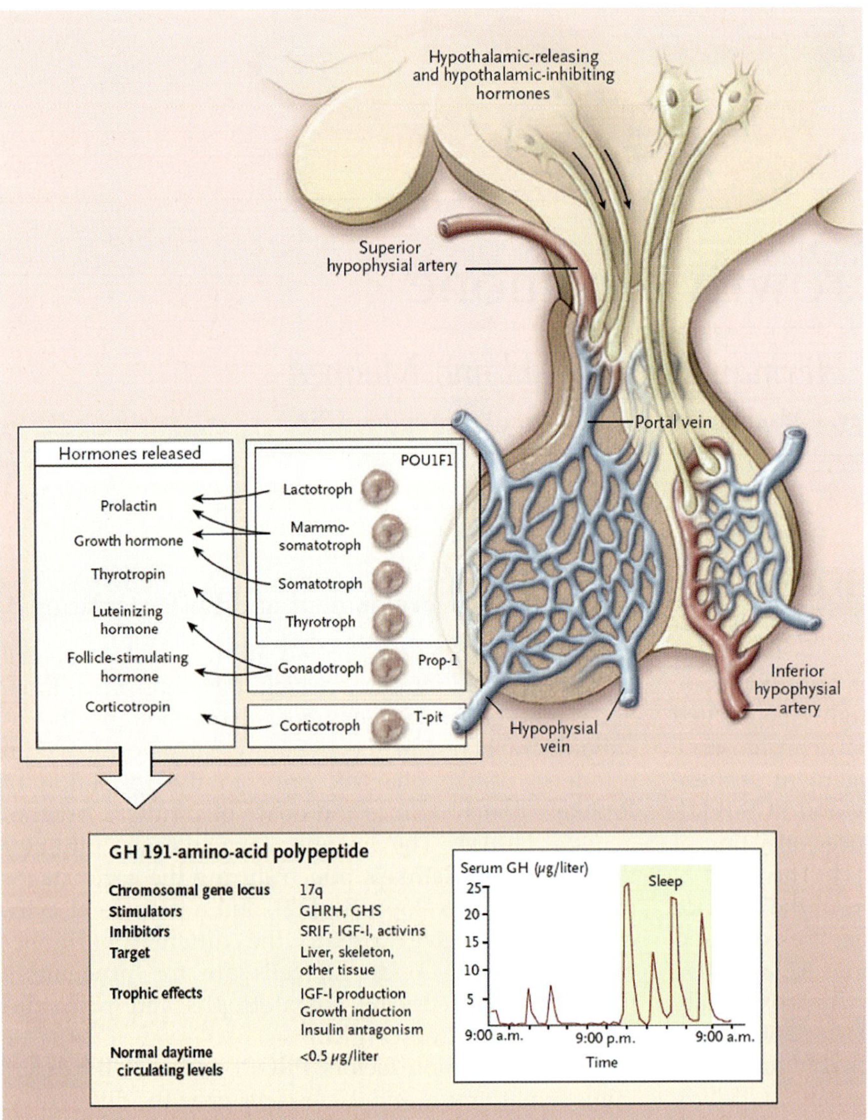

FIGURE 4.1 Hypothalamic–pituitary control of growth hormone (GH) secretion. Control of the secretion of GH is achieved by hypothalamic GH-releasing hormone (GHRH) and somatostatin, which traverse the portal vein, somatotroph-specific transcription factors, and negative feedback control of insulin-like growth factor I (IGF-I). Accurate measurement of pulsatile secretion of GH requires ultrasensitive assays. POU1F1 denotes POU domain, class 1, transcription factor 1; Prop-1 Prophet of Pit-1; GHS growth hormone secretagogues (e.g., ghrelin and GHRH, growth-hormone-releasing hormone); and SRIF somatostatin. *Reproduced with permission from [272].*

Promoter Structure

PROP-1, a paired homeobox protein, is required for initial commitment of Pit-1 cell lineages [15]. PROP-1 represses Rpx expression, and missense and spliced mutations of PROP-1 leading to loss of DNA binding or transactivation leads to pituitary failure with short stature and varying degrees of thyroid failure, hypogonadism and ACTH deficiency [16]. Footprinting analysis revealed SPI binding to the distal Pit-1 site [17,18]. Pit-1 binds to its distal site with a lower affinity [19,20] and, in addition, Pit-1 and Sp1 bind in a mutually exclusive manner to the GH promoter [17,18]. In vivo, both sites contribute to rat GH promoter activation [18]. Abrogation of Sp1 binding results in a 50% reduction of promoter activity, suggesting that GH activation by Pit-1 and Sp1 may occur through a multistage mechanism. Sequences −266/−252 of the hGH promoter contain an 8-bp recognition site for the adenoviral major late transcription factor (MLTF), also termed upstream stimulating factor (USF) [21], and a USF-like protein also binds the upstream hGH promoter [17,21,22].

POUIFI [23] mutations may also lead to pituitary failure. Patients with combined pituitary hormone deficiency have predominantly GH and PRL deficiency, with variable degrees of hypothyroidism [23].

Numerous factors bind to the GH promoter in response to diverse hormones. In the absence of Pit-1 the promoter region is inactive, and binding of Pit-1 to the transcriptional machinery facilitates the interaction between this factor and other ubiquitous activators already bound to the promoter or subsequently activated to enhance GH transcription. This model of cooperative interaction likely underlies tissue-specific expression of the hGH gene by a single-cell type-specific activator.

CONTROL OF GH SECRETION

Somatotrophs, comprising up to 45% of pituitary cells, are located predominantly in the lateral wings of the anterior pituitary gland which contains a total of 5–15 mg of GH. The GH molecule, a single-chain polypeptide hormone consisting of 191 amino acids (Figure 4.2), is synthesized, stored and secreted by somatotroph cells. The crystal structure of human GH reveals four alpha helixes and several structural features confer functional characteristics which determine GH signaling. These include the third α-helix with amphiphilic domains and a large helical loop [24,25]. Circulating GH molecules comprise at least three monomeric forms and several oligomers. The monomeric moieties include a 22- and 20-kDa form, acetylated 22K, and two desamido GHs. The 22-kDa peptide is the major physiologic GH component. The 20-kDa GH has a slower metabolic clearance than the 22-kDa form, which accounts for the plasma 20:22 ratio being higher than in the pituitary gland. The 22-kDa and 20-kDa peptides have similar growth-promoting activity. Monomeric GH forms found in the plasma of acromegaly patients are qualitatively similar to those found in normal plasma [26].

Circulating GH is first detectable in fetal serum at the end of the first trimester, peaks at a concentration of 100–150 ng/ml at 20 weeks of gestation, and subsequently falls to 30 ng/ml at birth. GH levels continue to

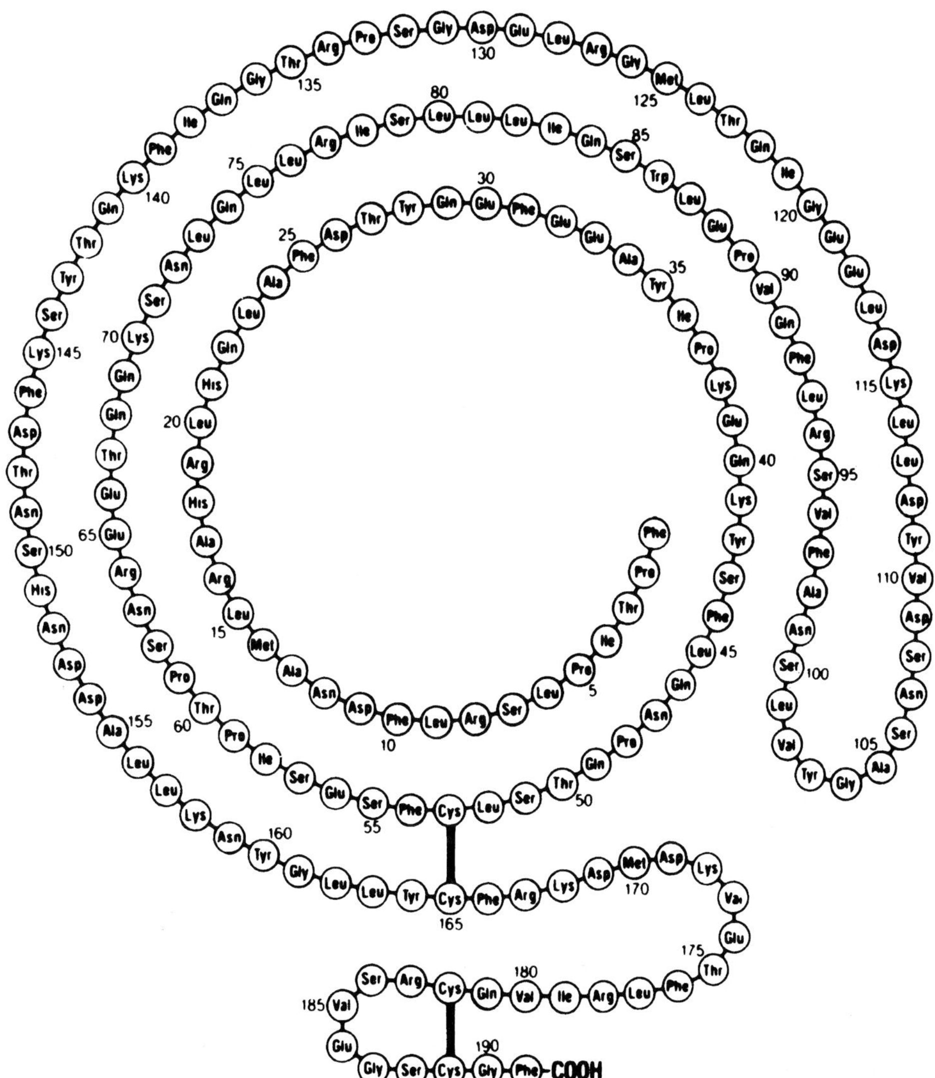

FIGURE 4.2 Amino acid structure of human growth hormone (GH). GH is a 191-amino acid single-chain 21.5-kDa polypeptide with two intramolecular disulfide bonds. Fifteen percent of GH is deleted from amino acid (32–46) and is secreted as a 20-kDa protein.

fall during infancy. During childhood, levels are similar to those in adulthood until puberty, when circulating levels are elevated. GH levels decline after adolescent growth and remain stable until mid-adulthood, when they decline progressively through old age [27].

Physiologic Factors Affecting GH Secretion

GH secretion is pulsatile, the anterior pituitary gland secreting bursts of GH, with almost undetectable basal levels occurring between these peaks [28]. The number of GH pulses detected depends on the frequency of blood sampling. Integrated GH levels are higher in women than in men, and are also enhanced in postmenopausal women following estrogen replacement [28].

Effects of Sleep

A major GH secretory pulse occurs shortly after the onset of sleep, associated with the first episode of slow-wave sleep.

Sleep stimulates GH secretion and 60–70% of daily GH secretion occurs during early sleep, in association with slow-wave sleep [29]. Rapid eye movement (REM) sleep is reduced by approximately 50% after age 50 years with significant sleep fragmentation. Endogenous GHRH may mediate the nocturnal GH surge; however, the mechanism is uncertain [30]. Although increased PRL and ACTH concentrations occur later during sleep, their secretion is not as tightly linked to sleep patterns as is GH secretion. "Jet lag" transiently increases the height of GH peaks during the day and night, resulting in a transient increase of 24-hour GH secretion. Jet lag also shifts the major GH secretory spike from early to late sleep [31].

Exercise

Exercise is one of the most potent stimulants of GH secretion and increases GH secretion, probably mediated by a cholinergic mechanism [32].

Stress

GH release is stimulated by physical stress, including trauma with hypovolemic shock and sepsis. However, chronic debilitating diseases, including cancer, are not associated with increased GH levels. Increased GHRH release, mediated by adrenergic pathways, is thought to mediate stress-induced GH secretion. Emotional deprivation is associated with suppressed GH secretion, and subnormal GH responses to provocative stimuli have been described in endogenous depression.

Nutritional and Metabolic Effects

Nutritional and metabolic factors profoundly influence GH secretion. Chronic malnutrition and voluntary 5-day fasting [33] are associated with elevated GH levels, most likely as a result of direct somatotroph stimulation by decreasing IGF-I levels [34]. Both pulse frequency and amplitude of GH secretory peaks increase with fasting. Obesity decreases basal and stimulated GH secretion. The degree of GH attenuation correlates with the amount of total and visceral body fat [35]. Obese subjects demonstrate decreased somatotroph response to GHRH and GHS [36] suggesting increased SRIF activity or a direct pituitary suppressive effect of free fatty acids. Insulin-induced hypoglycemia stimulates GH release 30–45 minutes after the glucose trough, whereas acute hyperglycemia inhibits GH secretion for 1–3 hours [37], followed by a GH increase 3–5 hours after oral glucose administration. Insulin-induced hypoglycemia forms the basis of the insulin tolerance test, which is a gold-standard GH provocative test. Diabetic patients with chronic hyperglycemia, however, do not have suppressed GH levels and in fact many poorly controlled diabetic patients have increased basal and exercise-induced GH levels. Central nervous system glucoreceptors appear to sense fluctuations, rather than absolute glucose levels. However, glucose homeostasis is not the major determinant of GH secretion, this being overridden by effects of sleep, exercise, stress and by random GH bursts.

A high-protein meal, and single amino acids (including arginine and leucine) administered intravenously stimulate GH secretion. Arginine may suppress endogenous somatostatin secretion and thereby stimulate GH secretion [38]. Decreased serum free fatty acid (FFA) levels cause acute GH release and increased serum FFA blunt the effects of various stimuli, including arginine infusion, sleep, L-dopa and exercise on GHRH-stimulated GH release [39].

In acromegaly patients, dexamethasone suppresses GH secretion [40], and supraphysiologic serum glucocorticoid concentrations retard growth. Cushing's disease is associated with growth retardation, decreased serum GH [41] and decreased pituitary GH content in tissue surrounding the adenoma [42]. A single dose of dexamethasone administered to normal subjects suppresses GHRH-induced GH release. Glucocorticoids administered to normal subjects produce a dose-dependent inhibition of GHRH-stimulated GH secretion, identical to that seen in Cushing's syndrome. In contrast, acute glucocorticoid administration induces GH levels [43]. Thus glucocorticoids exhibit short-term stimulatory effects on GH secretion and delayed inhibitory effects.

Neuroendocrine Control of GH Secretion

The central neurogenic control of GH is complex. Neuropeptides, neurotransmitters and opiates impinge on the hypothalamus and modulate GHRH and somatostatin (SRIF) release. The net effect of these complex influences determines the final secretory pattern of GH.

Leptin, a 167-amino acid cytokine, is the product of the *ob* gene and plays a key role in the regulation of body fat mass [44], regulating food intake and energy expenditure. As GH secretion is markedly impaired in obese subjects, leptin may act as a metabolic signal to regulate GH secretion. In the fasted state, leptin levels decrease rapidly, prior to and out of proportion to changes in fat mass [45], which triggers a neuroendocrine adaptive response to acute energy deprivation including decreased reproductive and thyroid hormone levels that slow metabolic rate, increased GH levels that mobilize energy and reduced IGF-I levels, which may slow growth-related processes [46]. Interactions between leptin and the growth hormone and adrenal axes may be less important in humans than in animal models, as patients with congenital leptin deficiency have normal linear growth and adrenal function [46].

Dopamine (DA) is a precursor of epinephrine and norepinephrine. Apomorphine, a central dopamine receptor agonist, stimulates GH secretion. GH-deficient children have been shown to increase their growth velocity after 6 months of levodopa treatment. Sixty to 90 minutes after oral L-dopa administration, adults increase their serum GH levels from 0 to 5–20 ng/ml.

Norepinephrine increases GH secretion via α-adrenergic pathways and inhibits GH release via β-adrenergic pathways. Insulin-induced hypoglycemia increases GH secretion via an α_2-adrenergic pathway, whereas clonidine acts on α_1-adrenergic receptors to increase GH secretion. Arginine administration, exercise, L-dopa and antidiuretic hormone (ADH) facilitate GH secretion by α-adrenergic effects [47]. β-adrenergic blockade increases GHRH-induced GH release, possibly due to a β-adrenergic effect at the pituitary level or via decreased hypothalamic somatostatin release. β-blockade also enhances GH release elicited by insulin-induced hypoglycemia, ADH, glucagon and L-dopa [47]. Epinephrine may regulate GH release by decreasing somatostatin release.

Cholinergic and serotoninergic neurons have been implicated in the etiology of sleep-induced GH secretion.

The lateral hypothalamus expresses Orexin-A (Hypocretin-1) and Orexin-B (Hypocretin-2), derived from a common precursor [48]. Orexins primarily regulate food intake and modulate the sleep–wake cycle and arousal, and also play a role in control of several endocrine axes. Orexin-A is expressed mostly in lactotrophs and to a lesser extent in thyrotrophs, somatotrophs and gonadotrophs, but not in corticotroph cells. Orexin-B is expressed in almost all pituitary corticotroph cells [49]. Orexin A markedly reduces spontaneous GH secretion and GH pulsatility as well as GH response to ghrelin in rats [50] in vivo. This hypothalamic inhibitory role on in vivo GH secretion is mediated via somatostatinergic neurons [51]. Furthermore, loss of orexin function in knock-out mice results in narcolepsy [52], implicating orexins in the regulation of arousal and the sleep–wake cycle. GH secretion is linked to the sleep–wake cycle and feeding state in humans. Thus, pituitary-derived orexins may play a role in coordinating sleep and energery homeostasis.

Several gastrointestinal neuropeptides stimulate GH secretion in animal models, including substance P, neurotensin, vasoactive intestinal polypeptide, peptide histidine isoleucine amide (PHI), motilin, galanin, cholecystokinin and glucagon [53].

HYPOTHALAMIC HORMONES

Thyrotropin-releasing hormone (TRH) does not stimulate GH secretion in normal subjects, but induces GH secretion in about 70% of patients with acromegaly, and in patients with liver disease, renal disease, ectopic GHRH-releasing carcinoid tumors [54], anorexia nervosa [55] and depression. A novel group of reproductive kisspeptin neuropeptides, encoded by the KISS-1 gene, stimulate hypothalamic GnRH neurons, and also induce GH release in peripubertal rats [56]. The physiological relevance in humans has not been elucidated.

Growth-hormone-releasing Hormone

Hypothalamic growth-hormone-releasing hormone (GHRH) was characterized from ectopic pancreatic GHRH-secreting tumors causing acromegaly [54,57]. Analysis of one tumor revealed a 44-amino acid GHRH residue; the other contained 37-, 40-, and 44-amino acid forms [58]. GHRH (1–40) and GHRH (1–44) are both found in extracts derived from the human hypothalamus. GHRH is secreted from neurons in the hypothalamic arcuate nucleus and premammillary area, with axons that project to the median eminence. The *hGHRH* gene encodes a 108-amino acid prepro-hormone for GHRH-44 [59,60], which has a free amino terminal and amidated carboxy terminal residue. The amino terminal appears to bestow biological activity on the GHRH molecule.

There is considerable structural homology between GHRH and several gut peptides. The highest is between GHRH and PHI, which have 12 amino acids in common in equivalent positions [61]. Varying degrees of homology exist between GHRH and VIP, glucagon, secretin and GIP. All of these peptides stimulate GH secretion in various physiologic systems, but with lower potency than GHRH.

GHRH binds to a specific receptor on the somatotroph membrane, resulting in increased intracellular 3′,

5′cAMP levels [62]. The GHRH receptor encodes a 47-kDa protein of 423 amino acids [63]. GHRH has a selective action on GH synthesis as well as secretion, and stimulates GH gene transcription. GHRH stimulates GH release from both stored and newly synthesized intracellular GH pools [64]. Somatostatin suppresses both basal and GHRH-stimulated GH release, but does not affect GH biosynthesis [65]. GHRH administered to normal adults elicits a prompt increase in serum GH levels, with higher levels occurring in female subjects [66]. Furthermore, GHRH facilitates GH responses to several pharmacological stimuli including levodopa, arginine, clonidine, insulin hypoglycemia, pyridostigmine and GHRP-6 [67]. GHRH is the principal regulator of pulsatile GH secretion, and age-related decline in GH secretion (somatopause) is likely GHRH-mediated [68]. Age-associated decrease in GH output is due to decreased GH pulse amplitude, with no demonstrated changes in GH pulse frequency or nadir levels, implicating reduced GHRH pulse amplitude in the somatopause [69]. Sexual dimorphism of GH secretion may also be attributed to GHRH. In males, GH is secreted at night, with low daytime baseline secretion, whereas females exhibit more daytime GH secretory pulses with higher basal GH levels [70], mirroring increased nocturnal GHRH secretion in males, with elevated daytime GHRH levels in females [70].

Somatostatin

Somatostatin (SRIF), a cyclic peptide, includes quantitatively predominant, but less bioactive SRIF-14, and more bioactive SRIF-28 [71]. The SRIF precursor is a 116-amino acid pro-hormone consisting of a 24-amino acid signal peptide, a 64-amino acid connecting region, followed by SRIF-28 [72] which incorporates SRIF-14. Prosomatostatin is synthesized in the anterior hypothalamic periventricular nuclei and transported by axonal flow to nerve terminals ending near the hypophyseal portal vessels. SRIF has also been isolated from pancreatic islets, gastrointestinal, neural and epithelial cells, and extrahypothalamic central nervous system neurons. SRIF has a short plasma half life of 2–3 minutes [71] and inhibits GH, ACTH and TSH release, TRH stimulation of TSH but not PRL [73], and pancreatic secretion of insulin and glucagon [74].

SRIF-28 binds to pituitary receptors with a three-fold greater affinity than SRIF-14 [75]. Both SRIF-14 and SRIF-28 block GHRH effects on GH, SRIF also blocks GH secretory responses to insulin-induced hypoglycemia, exercise, arginine, morphine, levodopa and sleep-related GH release.

Somatostatin exerts its biologic effects through specific membrane-bound high-affinity receptors. Five somatostatin receptor (SSTR) subtypes, termed SSTRs 1–5 have been cloned [76]. Somatostatin receptors are coupled to guanine nucleotide protein (G), and comprise seven transmembrane domains. There is 42–60% amino acid homology among the five somatostatin receptor subtypes. Somatostatin receptors mediate their responses via several cellular effectors including adenylyl cyclase, protein phosphatases, Na^+-H^+ exchanger, cyclic GMP-dependent protein kinases, phospholipase C, potassium and calcium channels [76]. The human pituitary gland expresses predominantly SSTR1, 2 and 5 [77], whereas human pituitary adenomas contain SSTR1, 2, 3 and 5 [77–79]. Somatostatin analogues, used to control GH hypersecretion in acromegaly, bind with high affinity to SSTR2 and less efficiently to SSTR5 [80]. SRIF receptors may also signal constitutively in the absence of ligand, to regulate basal pituitary hormone release [76].

GHRH and SRIF Interaction in Regulating GH Secretion

SRIF and GHRH secreted in independent waves from the hypothalamus interact to generate pulsatile GH release. SRIF inhibits GH secretion, while GHRH stimulates GH synthesis and secretion. GH secretion is further regulated by its target growth factor, IGF-I, which participates in a hypothalamic–pituitary–peripheral regulatory feedback system [81,82]. GH stimulates the liver and other peripheral tissues to produce IGF-I, which exerts a feedback effect on the hypothalamus and pituitary. IGF-I also induces hypothalamic SRIF release [74]. Specific antibodies directed against GHRH or SRIF have been used to dissect the respective contributions of these two peptides in the generation of GH pulsatility in rats. Anti-SRIF administration results in elevated baseline GH levels, with intact intervening GH pulses [83]. These studies imply that hypothalamic SRIF secretion generates GH troughs. Anti-GHRH antibodies eliminate spontaneous GH surges and GH pulsatility persists when GHRH is tonically elevated due to ectopic GHRH production by a tumor or during GHRH infusion [84], suggesting that hypothalamine SRIF is mainly responsible for GH pulsatility. The rat hypothalamus releases GHRH and SRIF 180° out of phase every 3–4 hours, resulting in pulsatile GH levels [83]. GHRH and SRIF also act synergistically, in that pre-exposure to SRIF enhances subsequent somatotroph sensitivity to GHRH stimulation [85]. Hence, during a normal GH trough period, high SRIF levels likely prime the somatotroph to respond maximally to subsequent GHRH pulses, thus optimizing GH release. In addition, SRIF exerts a central inhibitory effect on GHRH release via direct synaptic connections between SRIF-containing axons and GHRH-containing perikarya in the arcuate nucleus [86].

GH Autoregulation

Chronic GHRH stimulation results in decreased GH release in humans [87] due to somatotroph desensitization. Loss of GH sensitivity to administered GHRH does not occur in acromegaly [88] or in somatotroph adenomas in vitro [89], possibly reflecting larger intracellular pools of GH or abnormal signaling. GHRH pretreatment in vitro also leads to a 50% decrease in somatotroph GHRH binding sites [90].

Feedback loops exist between GH and IGF-I and the release of SRIF and GHRH (Figure 4.3). GH stimulates hypothalamic SRIF release in vitro [91], and in vivo, GH administration decreases GH responses to GHRH [92], most likely by increasing hypothalamic SRIF release [93]. GHRH and SRIF also autoregulate their own secretion. GHRH inhibits its own secretion but stimulates SRIF secretion in vitro, while SRIF inhibits its own secretion in vitro [94].

Growth Hormone Secretagogues (GHS) and Ghrelin

Small synthetic molecules termed growth hormone secretagogues (GHS) [95] stimulate and amplify pulsatile pituitary GH release, via a separate pathway distinct from GHRH/SRIF. GH secretagogues (GHS), administered alone or in combination with GHRH, are potent and reproducible GH releasers and are useful tools for the diagnosis of GH deficiency [96].

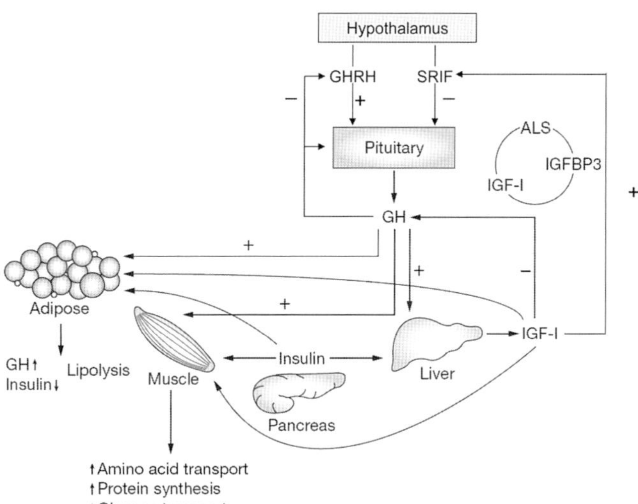

FIGURE 4.3 Schematic diagram of insulin, growth hormone, and insulin-like growth factor 1 regulation. In the liver, insulin enables increased insulin-like growth factor 1 synthesis in response to growth hormone. Free insulin-like growth factor 1 exerts negative feedback on growth-hormone production in the pituitary. In muscle, insulin and growth hormone increase protein synthesis, and transport of amino acids; insulin also increases transport of glucose. +, variables that stimulate growth hormone secretion; −, variables that inhibit growth hormone secretion; ALS, acid-labile subunit; GH, growth hormone; IGF-I, insulin-like growth factor 1; IGFBP3, IGF-binding protein 3. *Adapted from [271].*

The GHS receptor, a heterotrimeric GTP-binding protein (G-protein)-coupled protein [97] comprises seven alpha helical membrane-spanning domains and three intracellular and extracellular loops. The GHS receptor is expressed in pituitary somatotroph cells and in both hypothalamic and nonhypothalamic brain regions. The ligand of the GHS receptor is a 28-amino acid peptide, ghrelin, isolated from the gastrointestinal tract, and is n-octanoylated at the serine 3 residue [98]. Ghrelin releases GH both in vivo and in vitro and n-octanoylation is essential for GH-releasing activity. Ghrelin is expressed in the arcuate nucleus of the hypothalamus, and also in the pituitary gland [98,99]. Ghrelin modulates GH secretion at both a hypothalamic and pituitary level [100] and stimulates GHS receptors to induce GH release [98]. In vitro, GHRH and GHS or ghrelin have additive effects on GH release, whereas in vivo administration of GHRH with GHS/ghrelin is synergistic [101]. This implies that ghrelin acts predominantly at the hypothalamic level, and that GH secretagogues and GHRH act via different mechanisms [101]. Furthermore, GHRP-6 which activates GHS receptors does not elicit GH release following hypothalamic–pituitary disconnection [102].

There is still uncertainty as to whether circulating ghrelin directly influences pituitary GH secretion, as well as how the hypothalamic peptide modulates GH. Transgenic mice with decreased GHS receptor mRNA expression demonstrate reduced GH and IGF-I levels [103], and GHS-receptor knockout mice have lower IGF-I levels and decreased body weight [104]. However, ghrelin-null mice do not exhibit dwarfism [105]. Recently identified missence mutations in the GHS receptor, with markedly attenuated ghrelin binding, result in partial isolated GH deficiency [102,106]. Furthermore, healthy volunteers demonstrated synchronicity between ghrelin and GH pusatility suggesting stimulation of GH by ghrelin or possibly co-regulation of both by other neuroendocrine factors [107].

Ghrelin amplifies the GH secretory pattern [108] and enhances GH responsiveness to GHRH [101,109–111]. These observations may be explained by findings that GHRH acts as an allosteric co-agonist for the ghrelin (GHS) receptor [112]. Ghrelin thus appears to act coordinately with GHRH to regulate GH secretion and energy balance [113].

Functional GHS receptors are detected in the human pituitary by the fifth week of gestation [114]. GH secretogogue-mediated GH-release is demonstratable at birth, continues through infancy, increases at puberty and then decreases thereafter. Estrogen and testosterone increase GH secretogogue-mediated GH release in childhood.

As GH secretogogues elicit a synergy with GHRH on GH release, which is minimally altered by age, sex, or adiposity and is devoid of potential side effects (unlike insulin-induced hypogylcemia), this combined test is a useful diagnostic tool in the diagnosis of adult GHD, and no serious side effects have been reported. Although highly specific for GH release, slight increases in prolactin and ACTH/cortisol have been reported with some GH secretogogues [115] leading to the development of new more selective GHSs with no ACTH- or PRL-releasing effects.

GH-binding Proteins (GHBP)

Circulating GH is attached to specific binding proteins (BP). Two circulating GHBPs have been identified, one of high affinity and one of low affinity. The 60-kDa high-affinity BP corresponds to the extracellular domain of the hepatic GH receptor, produced by proteolytic cleavage with receptor ectodomain shedding. Under basal conditions, half of the circulating 22-kDa GH is bound to the high-affinity BP when GH levels are up to 10–15 ng/ml [116], while 20-kDa GH binds preferentially to the low-affinity BP [117]. Binding to plasma GHBP prolongs GH plasma half life by decreasing GH metabolic clearance rate [117]. The high-affinity BP also inhibits GH binding to surface receptors by competing for the ligand [118]. Thus GHBP dampens acute oscillations in serum GH levels caused by pulsatile pituitary GH secretion. High-affinity BP levels are low in the fetus and neonate, rise most rapidly in the first 1–2 years after birth [119], and stay constant throughout adult life, with similar levels found in males and females.

GH resistance, demonstrated in Laron dwarfism [120] and in African Pygmies, is characterized by decreased plasma levels of high-affinity BP. Other syndromes of growth retardation with low GHBP levels include the Pygmies of Zaire and Little Women of Loja. GHBP measurement has no diagnostic value in adulthood, but in childhood-onset GHD, GHBP levels are low, and increase during the first 6–12 months of GH replacement therapy, after which GHBP levels plateau.

In the adult GH deficiency syndrome associated with changes in body composition and increased fat mass, GHBP levels are either normal or increased. GH replacement in adult GHD patients is not associated with changes in GHBP levels. In acromegaly, measuring GHBP levels offers no diagnostic utility.

Circulating GHBP levels correlate with fat mass, as well as with circulating leptin levels [121]. GHBP levels increase gradually during pregnancy and peak in the second trimester, declining to normal levels before term. Placental GH levels are inversely correlated with serum GHBP levels [122].

Peripheral GH Action

GH Receptor

GH binds to its peripheral receptor and induces intracellular signaling by a phosphorylation cascade involving the JAK/STAT pathway [24]. GH also acts indirectly by inducing synthesis of IGF-I, the potent growth and differentiation factor. The GH receptor (GHR) is a 70-kDa protein member of the class I cytokine/hematopoietin receptor superfamily [123,124]. GHR consists of an extracellular ligand-binding domain, a single membrane-spanning domain, and a cytoplasmic signaling component. The GH ligand complexes with a preformed dimer of two GHR components leading to receptor internal rotation. This ligand–receptor interaction is critical for subsequent GH signaling. GHR rotation is followed by rapid activation of JAK2 tyrosine kinase, leading to phosphorylation of cytoplasmic signaling molecules, including the GHR itself, and signal transducing activators of transcription proteins (STAT), critical signaling components for GH action [24]. Phosphorylated cytoplasmic proteins are translocated to the cell nucleus where they elicit GH-specific target gene expression by binding to nuclear DNA [24]. STAT1 and STAT5 may also interact directly with the GH receptor molecule [125]. Other target actions induced by GH include c-fos induction, IRS-1 phosphorylation, and insulin synthesis, cell proliferation and cytoskeletal changes. As a differentiating and growth factor, IGF-I is a critical protein induced by GH, and is likely responsible for most of the growth-promoting activities of GH [126]. GH-activated STAT5b directly induces GH transcription [127]. IGF-I itself may also directly regulate GH [126] and GH receptor function [128]. The liver contains abundant GH receptors and several peripheral tissues also express modest amounts of receptor, including muscle and fat. GH-mediated postnatal growth, adipocyte functions and sexual dimorphism of GH hepatic actions all require STAT5b [24]. Transgenic mice with deleted STAT5b exhibit impaired growth, with low IGF-1 levels, and are insensitive to injected GH [129].

Mutations of the GH receptor are associated with partial or complete GH insensitivity and growth failure. These syndromes are associated with normal or high circulating GH levels, decreased circulating GHBP levels and low levels of circulating IGF-I. Multiple homozygous or heterozygous exonic and intronic GHR mutations have been described, most of which occur in the extracellular ligand-binding domain of the receptor.

Tissue responses to GH signaling may be determined by the pattern of GH secretion, rather than the absolute amount of circulating hormone. Thus, linear growth patterns, liver enzyme induction and STAT5b activity may be phenotypically distinct for male animals due to their higher rates of GH pulse frequency [130]. STAT5b is sensitive to repeated pulses of injected GH [131], unlike other GH-induced patterns which are desensitized by repeated GH pulsing. Mice harboring a disrupted STAT5b transgene exhibit impaired male

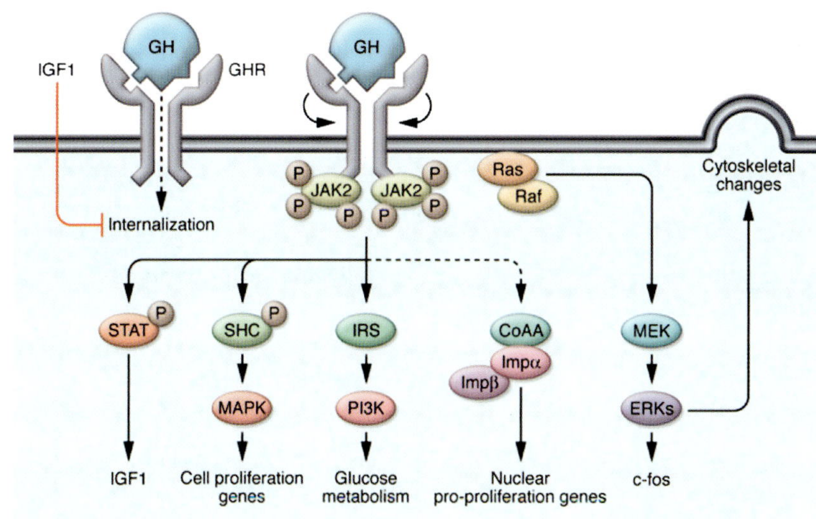

FIGURE 4.4 GH action. GH binds to the GHR dimer, which undergoes internal rotation, resulting in JAK2 phosphorylation (P) and subsequent signal transduction. GH signaling is mediated by JAK2 phosphorylation of depicted signaling molecules or by JAK2-independent signaling including Src/ERK pathways (S42). Ligand binding to a preformed GHR dimer results in internal rotation and subsequent phosphorylation cascades. GH targets include IGF-I, c-fos, cell proliferation genes, glucose metabolism and cystoskeletal proteins. GHR internalization and translocation (dotted lines) induce nuclear pro-proliferation genes via importin α/β (Impα/Impβ) coactivator (CoAA) signaling. IGF-I may also block GHR internalization, acting in a feedback loop. The GHR antagonist, pegvisomant, blocks GHR signaling; SRLs also attenuate GH binding and signaling (not shown). *Reproduced with permission from [113].*

pattern body growth [129] with IGF-I and testosterone levels normally seen in female mice. Thus, the sexual dimorphic pattern of GH secretion and GH tissue targeting appear to be determined by STAT5b. The requirement for appropriate GH pulsatility to determine body growth also appears to be mediated by STAT5b [132]. In contrast, STAT5 does not appear to be critical for metabolic effects of GH on carbohydrate metabolism. In humans, STAT mutations result in short stature and relative GH insensitivity [133]. Intracellular GH signaling is also abrogated by SOCS proteins, which disrupt the JAK/STAT pathway and thus exert a further level of control over the action of GH [134] (Figure 4.4).

IGF-I and IGF-II Structure and Synthesis

IGF-I and IGF-II are single-chain polypeptide molecules with three intrachain sulfide bridges (Figure 4.5). IGF-I, composed of 70 amino acids, and IGF-II, consisting of 67 amino acids, have a sequence homology of 62%.

The IGFs consist of B and A peptide domains (structurally homologous with the insulin B and A chains), a C domain analogous to the connecting (C) peptide of proinsulin and a D domain. IGF-I and IGF-II are single distinct gene loci, localized on chromosome 12 (12q22-q24.1) and chromosome 11 (11p15), respectively. The IGF-I gene primary transcript can be alternately spliced to different products resulting in IGF-Ia (exons 1, 2, 3, 5) or IGF-Ib (exons 1, 2, 3, 4). Several IGF-I mRNA species have been isolated from adult and fetal tissues. The liver is the main source of circulating IGF-I levels.

The IGF-I gene is expressed in human fetal connective tissues and cells of mesenchymal origin [135]. This ubiquitous localization of IGFs favors a paracrine/autocrine

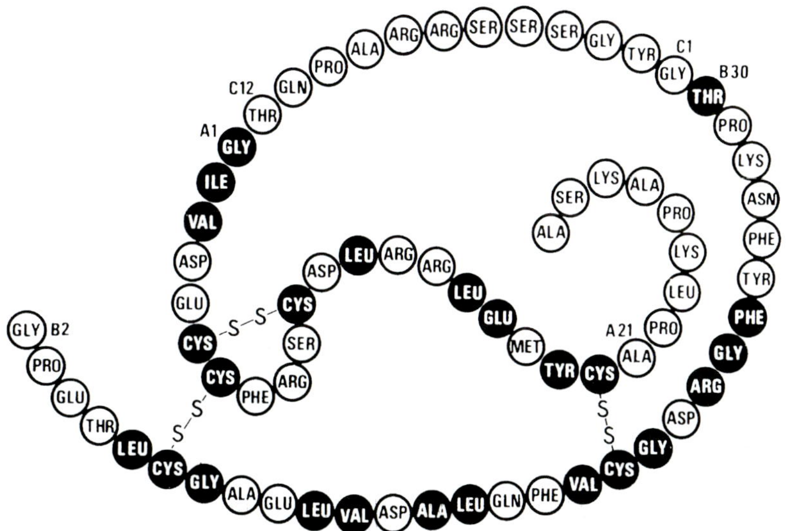

FIGURE 4.5 Amino acid sequence of human insulin-like growth factor I (IGF-I). The black amino acids are identical to those in human insulin. The numbering corresponds to the numbering of residues in the proinsulin molecule. IGF-I consists of a 70-amino acid single-peptide chain with A, B, C and D domains. A and B domains are structurally homologous to the A and B chains in the insulin molecule, and the C domain is equivalent to the connecting (C) peptide in proinsulin. *From Humbel [273].*

function as well as an endocrine function of IGF-I. GH is the major regulator of IGF-I gene expression in adult liver, heart, lung and pancreas [136], and acts at the level of IGF-I transcription. Fetal IGF-I production is GH-independent [137], and platelet-derived growth factor (PDGF) and fibroblast growth factor (FGF) also stimulate IGF-I production from human fibroblasts in vitro [138]. ACTH, TSH, LH and FSH stimulate paracrine production of IGF-I in their respective target tissues. Nutritional status is also an important regulator of IGF-I production at all ages [139].

IGF-I and IGF-II are bound to carrier proteins in the serum. IGFs are found in lymph, breast milk, saliva and amniotic fluid. IGF-I levels are low before birth, rise during childhood to high levels during puberty, and decline with age [140].

IGFs play an important role in regulating somatic growth and ensure that development proceeds appropriately to nutritional supply. Multiple cellular actions of IGF-I are mediated via the IGF-I receptor, a transmembrane tyrosine kinase cell surface receptor with high homology to the insulin receptor. IGFs are expressed widely throughout most tissues in the body, are not stored in cellular secretory granules and are secreted associated with high-affinity circulating binding proteins, the IGF binding proteins (IGFBPs).

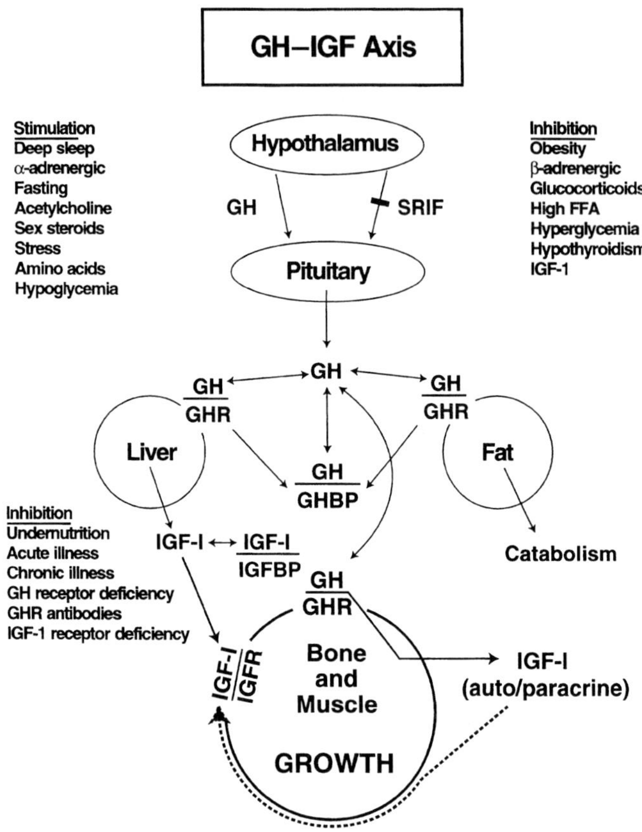

FIGURE 4.6 Simplified diagram of GH–IGF-I axis involving hypophysiotropic hormones controlling pituitary GH release, circulating GH-binding protein and its GH receptor source, IGF-I and its largely GH-dependent binding proteins, and cellular responsiveness to GH and IGF-I interacting with their specific receptors. IGFR, IGF-I receptor; FFA, free fatty acids. *From Rosenbloom [274].*

IGF-binding Proteins (IGFBPs)

IGF-I and IGF-II are complexed to six specific binding proteins in biological fluids [141] (Figure 4.6 and Table 4.1). IGFBPs are cysteine-rich proteins, with similar amino acid sequences. They have a unique ability to bind IGFs with high affinity. The major form of binding protein present in the human circulation is IGFBP-III, a glycoprotein associated with an IGF molecule and an 80-kDa acid-labile subunit (ALS) to form a 150–200-kDa complex [141].

Actions of the IGFBPs include modulation of IGF actions, storage of IGFs in extracellular matrices and the carrier protein function of IGFBPs. Most IGF circulates as a 150 000 dalton complex that consists of IGF-I or IGF-II plus IGFBP-III and a non-IGF binding component, the acid labile subunit (ALS). Binding of IGF-I or -II to IGFBP-III in the presence of ALS results in the formation of an IGF–IGFBP–ALS ternary complex, which is stabilized by IGF binding [142]; 75% of circulating IGF-I and IGF-II is carried in this ternary 150-kDa complex. When associated with the 150-kDa complex, the IGFs do not readily leave the vascular compartment and have prolonged half lives [143] compared to the half life of free IGF-I which is less than 10 minutes [144]. A circulating protease acting specifically on IGFBP-III, results in limited cleavage of IGFBP-III, with subsequent decreased binding affinity of IGF-I. There is little detectable IGFBP-III protease activity in normal serum, due to the presence of inhibitors which protect IGFBP-III from proteolysis. A pregnancy-associated plasma protein A system cleaves IGFBP-IV [145].

Plasma concentrations of IGFBPs are hormonally regulated. Serum IGFBP-III levels correlate with IGF-I and -II levels, increase in patients with acromegaly, and are reduced in hypopituitarism [146]. Malnutrition, insulin-dependent diabetes mellitus and cirrhosis are associated with decreased IGF-I levels, as well as suppressed IGFBP-III levels [147]. IGFBP-I levels are high at birth and decline until puberty [148]. There is a diurnal variation with a nocturnal peak in serum IGFBP-I levels [149]. However, IGFBP-I levels are elevated in hypopituitarism [150] and decreased in acromegaly. IGFBP-I levels are regulated by insulin, increased IGFBP-I levels associated with insulin-dependent diabetes mellitus [141] are normalized by insulin, and insulinoma is associated with suppressed IGFBP-I levels. Octreotide increases IGFBP-I levels in acromegaly patients [151]. When normal subjects ingest glucose, the fall in IGFBP-I levels correlates inversely with the rise in insulin levels [152]. Hypophysectomy is associated

TABLE 4.1 General Characteristics of Human IGF Binding Proteins

	No. of Amino Acids	Core Molecular Mass (kDa)	Chromosomal Localization	IGF Affinity	Modulation of IGF Action	Source in Biological Fluids
IGFBP-I	234	25.3	7	I = II	Inhibition and/or potentiation	Amniotic fluid, serum, placenta, endometrium, milk, urine, synovial fluid, interstial fluid and seminal fluid
IGFBP-II	289	31.4	2	II > I	Inhibition	CSF, serum, milk, urine, synovial fluid, interstitial fluid, lymph follicular fluid, seminal fluid and amniotic fluid
IGFBP-III	264	28.7	7	I = II	Inhibition and/or potentiation	Serum, follicular fluid, milk, urine, CSF, amniotic fluid, synvovial fluid, interestitial fluid and seminal fluid
IGFBP-IV	237	25.9	17	I = II	Inhibition	Serum follicular fluid, seminal fluid, interstitital fluid and synovial fluid
IGFBP-V	252	28.5	5	II > I	Potention	Serum and CSF
IGFBP-VI	216	22.8	12	II > I	Inhibition	CSF, serum and amniotic fluid

Modified from Rajaram S et al. [276].

with elevated IGFBP-II levels in rats, which fall with GH administration [147], while insulin increases IGFBP-II levels [147].

Paracrine GH Action

GH and GH-releasing factors are also produced in tissues outside the hypothalamic–pituitary axis. Extrapituitary actions of GH are likely autocrine/paracrine and complement the classic endocrine action between the GH-releasing factors, GH and target tissues. GH gene expression is not restricted to the pituitary gland. GH immunoreactivity and GH mRNA have been localized to several extrapituitary tissues including placenta, mammary gland, muscle, spleen lymphocyte, suggesting an extrapituitary paracrine/autocrine action for GH. Paracrine mammary cell GH has been implicated in control of miotic activity and regulating pro-proliferative genes [153].

Role of GH/IGF-I in Growth and Development Throughout the Lifespan

Longitudinal bone growth is initiated in the epiphyseal growth plate of long bones. When growth occurs, chondrocytes in the resting zone of long bone epiphyseal growth plates proliferate and replicate rapidly with subsequent differentiation into hypertrophic chondrocytes. Extracellular matrix is secreted, resulting in new cartilage formation (chondrogenesis). GH and IGF-I affect chondrogenesis in that chondrocytes in the skeletal growth plate express GH receptors which are down-regulated by local and systemic IGF-I and up-regulated when IGF-I binds to IGFBPs [154]. GH affects the fate of mesenchymal precursors favoring chondrogenesis and osteoblastogenesis over adipogenesis [155]. IGF-I regulates chondrocyte differentiation, as evidenced by impaired chondrocyte maturation and shortened femoral length in IGF-I null mutants [156].

Blood vessels and bone cell precursors then invade newly formed cartilage, facilitating calcification into bone trabeculae [157] (endochondral ossification). Genetic, hormonal and nutritional factors influence endochondral ossification [157]. In addition to longitudinal bone growth, bone tissue also undergoes remodeling and modeling. Bone modeling occurs mostly during growth; whereas bone remodeling removes potentially damaged bone and is also necessary for calcium homeostasis. Bone remodeling is thus a process of coordinated bone resorption and formation occurring in multicellular units throughout the lifespan [158]. During the remodeling process, multinucleated osteoclasts are attracted to specific sites to resorb bone, and osteoblasts are attracted to fill the cavity with newly synthesized matrix. Osteoblast and osteoclast activity are thus coupled. GH stimulates proliferation of osteoblast cells, whereas IGF-I is required for selected anabolic effects of GH in osteoblasts [159]. GH also stimulates expression

TABLE 4.2 Effects of GH on Bone

Functions	Effects
GROWTH PLATE	
Chondrocyte replication	↑ ↑
Endochondral bone formation	↑ ↑
BONE REMODELING UNIT	
Osteoblastogenesis	↑
Osteoblast proliferation	↑
Function of mature osteoblasts	↔ ↑
Osteoprotegerin production	↑
RANK-L production	↔
Phosphate retention	↑

Effects of GH on bone. ↔ no effect; ↑ minor stimulating effect; ↑ ↑ major stimulating effect [164].

of bone morphogenetic proteins, important for osteoblast differentiation and for bone formation [160]. In addition to effects on osteoblast lineage, GH stimulates, either directly or indirectly through IGF-I, functions of the mature osteoblast, and also stimulates carboxylation of osteocalcin, a marker of osteoblastic function [161] (Table 4.2; Figure 4.7).

Low serum IGF-I levels in GH-receptor-mutated mice manifest small growth plates, osteopenia and reduced cortical bone with normal trabecular bone [162], suggesting a more pronounced effect of systemic IGF-I on cortical than on trabecular bone; whereas mice with osteoblast-specific knockout of the IGF receptor gene exhibit decreased osteoblast number and function, causing reduced bone formation and trabecular volume [163] indicating a more significant role for skeletal IGF-I in the maintenance of trabecular bone.

GH and IGF-I influence bone metabolism throughout the lifespan [164]. During embryonic development, IGF-I and IGF-II are key determinants of bone growth, acting independently of GH. GH deficiency, or insensitivity (caused by GH receptor mutations or defects in GH signaling pathways) markedly impairs postnatal, but not prenatal growth [165]. Postnatally and through puberty, both GH and IGF-I are critical in determining longitudinal skeletal growth [166], as well as skeletal maturation and acquisition of bone mass in the prepubertal period. Children with GH deficiency manifest short stature, while GH excess in childhood causes gigantism. In contrast, an IGF-I gene mutation causing IGF-I deficiency [167] and IGF-I resistance due to IGF receptor gene mutations [168] is associated with both pre- and postnatal growth deficits.

Late adolescence and adulthood are critical periods for achievement of peak bone mass [164]. Anabolic effects of GH and IGF-I (systemic and local skeletal) are important in the acquisition of bone mass and maintenance of skeletal architecture.

Bone Metabolism in Adult Growth Hormone Deficiency (Adult GHD)

Adults with GHD manifest low bone turnover osteoporosis and increased fracture risk, with decreased osteoid and mineralizing surfaces and reduced bone formation rate. Decreased osteocalcin and bone resorption markers reflect low bone turnover. Cortical bone loss is greater than trabecular bone loss [169], and bone loss is proportional to age of onset of GHD and duration and severity of the disease. Childhood-onset

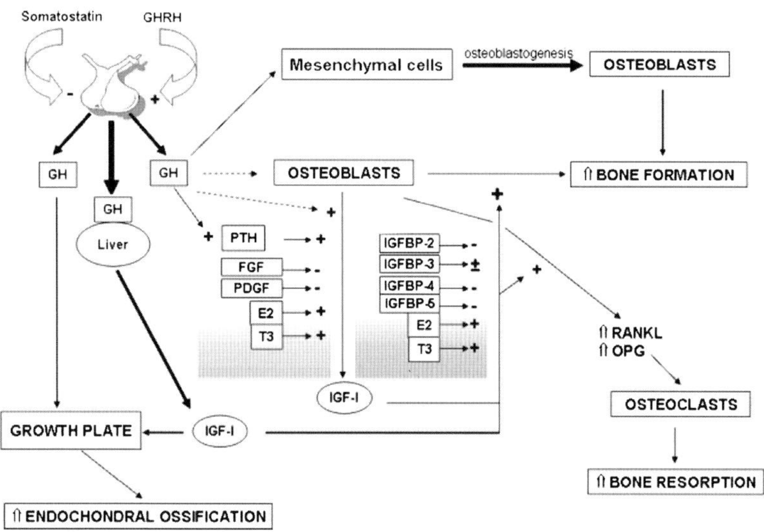

FIGURE 4.7 Effects of GH and IGF-I on bone. The skeletal effects of GH and IGF-I are modulated by complex interactions between circulating IGF-I and IGFBPs and locally produced IGF-I and IGFBPs. IGF-I and IGF-II are the most abundant growth factors in skeletal tissue and their synthesis and activity are regulated by systemic hormones, such as GH and PTH. GH may have direct effects on skeletal cells and also induce IGF-I action in bone. FGF, Fibroblast growth factor; E2, estradiol; OPG, osteoprotegerin. RANKL induces osteoclast formation. —>_ not consistently demonstrated effect; —> minor stimulating effect; —> major stimulating effect. *From [164].*

GHD is associated with more severely reduced vertebral bone mineral density than adult-onset patients, possibly due to failure to attain peak bone mass [170]. Nonvertebral fracture risk is increased three-fold in untreated GHD patients with fractures frequently localized to the radius [171].

GH AND METABOLISM

In childhood, multiple GH actions contribute to linear growth. However, GH continues to be secreted in adulthood after growth cessation, implying important metabolic functions in adult life. Metabolic actions of GH are either acute insulin-like or are chronically antagonistic to insulin action, and may be directly, or indirectly mediated by IGF-I.

GH predominantly stimulates adipocyte lipolysis, with increased circulating free fatty acids (FFAs), and increased muscle and liver lipoprotein lipase expression with enhanced triglyceride uptake. GH effects on carbohydrate metabolism are dominantly anti-insulin with a net anabolic effect on protein metabolism (Table 4.3).

GH Effect on Adipose Tissue

GH-deficient children are mildly obese, with a decreased total number of fat cells that are larger in size, with increased lipid content. GH replacement therapy leads to decreased body fat and, eventually, decreased size and lipid content of subcutaneous adipocytes. GH-deficient adults have altered body composition, with increased fat mass and decreased lean body mass. Initial acute effects of GH on lipid metabolism are antilipolytic (insulin-like) and subsequently, GH exerts a chronic lipolytic (anti-insulin) effect.

Lipolysis

GH increases fat lipolysis largely in visceral adipose tissue, and somewhat in subcutaneous adipose tissue, with release of circulatory FFAs [172]. GH activates hormone-sensitive lipase [173] via enhanced agonist-induced stimulation of β-adrenergic receptors [174], resulting in increased hydrolysis of triglycerides to free fatty acids and glycerol (lipolysis). GH also facilitates differentiation of small pre-adipocytes into large, mature adipocytes, with increased capacity to store triglycerides and a higher lipolytic potential. Activation of STAT5 and possibly subsequent association with PPAR-γ may be associated with GH-induced adipogenesis [175].

TABLE 4.3 Metabolic Effects of Growth Hormone

EFFECTS ON CARBOHYDRATE METABOLISM
Antagonism of insulin action
EFFECTS ON LIPID METBOLISM
Adipose tissue: increased lipolysis → increased free fatty acids
Muscle/liver: increased lipoprotein lipase expression → increased triglyceride uptake
EFFECTS ON PROTEIN METABOLISM
Increased protein synthesis

In the liver, however, GH has the opposite effect to that observed in adipose tissue, and induces triglyceride uptake by increasing LPL and/or hepatic lipase expression. GH treatment increases hepatic triglyceride storage. In skeletal muscle, GH promotes lipid utilization by increasing LPL expression which stimulates triglyceride uptake, with subsequent storage as intramyocellular triglyceride, or stimulates lipid oxidation with energy release.

GH-deficient adults have elevated total cholesterol, low-density-lipoprotein cholesterol (LDL) and apolipoprotein B (ApoB) [176], with decreased high-density lipoprotein (HDL) and high triglyceride levels. This lipid profile is associated with premature atherosclerosis and cardiovascular disease. GH replacement decreases total cholesterol [177], LDL cholesterol and ApoB, and increases HDL levels. Long-term surveillance is required to determine whether long-term GH replacement therapy reverses premature atheroclerosis and reduces cardiovascular morbidity and mortality in GH-deficient adults. Furthermore, low-dose GH replacement decreased total and visceral adipose tissue and reduced the elevated levels of inflammatory markers, including highly sensitive C-reactive protein (hsCRP) and interleukin-6 (IL-6) in hypopituitary women, with a relatively modest increase in IGF-I levels and without worsening insulin resistance [178].

GH Effects on Body Composition

Anabolic, lipolytic and antinatriuretic GH actions impact body composition affecting fat mass, lean body mass and fluid volume in GH-deficient adults. Lean body mass (LBM) is reduced, and fat mass is increased in GH-deficient adults compared to predicted values for age-, sex- and height-matched normal controls. With GH deficiency, excess fat accumulates mostly in the visceral compartment in a central, mainly abdominal, distribution and total body water is reduced.

GH replacement therapy reverses these effects on body composition by increasing LBM. GH replacement also reduces fat mass by 4–6 kg in GH-deficient adults with the most significant reduction in visceral fat. GH therapy increases total body water, especially extracellular water, within 3–5 days. Total blood volume increases after 3 months of treatment. GH and IGF-I stimulate sodium reabsorption via epithelial sodium channels (ENaC) in the rat distal nephron [179], contributing to the antinatriuretic action of GH.

Effects on Carbohydrate Metabolism

GH decreases glucose uptake in adipose tissue, and regulates the glucose transporter-I (GLUT-I) in adipose-tissue-derived cell lines [180]. GH may antagonize adipocyte insulin, lower serum leptin levels, while effects on adiponectin are unclear. In the liver, GH increases glycogenolysis, thereby increasing hepatic glucose production, possibly as a result of insulin antagonism.

GH-deficient children have decreased fasting glucose levels [181], decreased insulin secretion [181], contradictory impairment of glucose tolerance [182], and increased insulin sensitivity due to increased glucose utilization and blunted hepatic glucose release. GH replacement increases fasting glucose levels [182], insulin levels [182] and hepatic glucose production. Endogenous GH secretion antagonizes insulin action. Normally, GH secretion increases 3–5 hours after oral glucose ingestion, resulting in decreased disposal of a second oral glucose challenge, associated with hyperinsulinemia occurring 2 hours after GH levels peak. Both intravenous and oral glucose tolerance tests are impaired if performed during periods of increased GH secretion, such as sleep onset.

GH-deficient adults have elevated fasting insulin levels and a positive correlation between fasting plasma insulin and both fat mass and waist girth, suggesting the presence of insulin resistance. GH replacement initially further increases insulin resistance, in the first 1–6 weeks of therapy, but subsequently, long-term studies suggest unchanged insulin sensitivity [183].

Effects on Protein Metabolism

Somatic growth is under the primary control of GH and, as such, GH is an anabolic hormone. GH causes urinary nitrogen retention and decreases plasma urea levels in normal and GH-deficient children. Both insulin and IGF-I have been implicated in the anabolic effects of GH on protein metabolism, especially as insulin is a protein anabolic hormone and GH induces circulating insulin levels.

GH Effects on Muscle Strength and Exercise Performance

GH deficiency is associated with reduced muscle strength, due to altered body composition. Reduction in muscle cross-sectional area, as well as lack of conditioning and training, may contribute to weakness. Prolonged GH replacement therapy is required to significantly increase muscle mass, which may not result in improved strength.

GH Effects on Cardiovascular Function

GH and IGF-I influence both cardiac structure and function. Increased cardiovascular morbidity and mortality are associated with both GH deficiency and GH excess [184]. Epidemiological studies suggest that lower-normal range IGF-I levels in the general population may increase the risk of ischemic heart disease [185] and of cardiac failure [186]. Cultured rat cardiac myocytes express GH and IGF-I receptors and IGF-I induces cultured rat myocytes and delays apoptosis. IGF-I sensitizes cultured rat myofilaments to calcium, thereby enhancing myocardial contractility. Moreover, locally produced IGF-I promotes arterial cell growth and paracrine IGF-I effects contribute to inflammatory angiogenesis during atherosclerosis [187].

GHD adults manifest increased abdominal adiposity, insulin resistance, hypercoagulability, high total and LDL cholesterol and low HDL cholesterol, decreased exercise performance and pulmonary capacity, all of which are cardiovascular risk factors for coronary artery disease [188]. Furthermore, GHD adults manifest less aortic distensibility and endothelial dysfunction with higher fibrinogen, tissue plasminogen activator antigen and plasminogen activator inhibitor activity, and increased blood vessel intima-medial thickness. Left ventricular posterior wall and interventricular septal thickness is reduced resulting in decreased LV mass index, and decreased LV internal diameter in children and adolescents with childhood-onset GHD. GH replacement improves peak exercise cardiac performance, and reduces carotid artery intima-medial thickness. GH replacement also has beneficial effects on lean body and fat mass, total and LDL cholesterol levels, and diastolic blood pressure [177]. GH replacement therapy may reduce the risk of premature cardiovascular mortality [176,189].

TESTS OF GH SECRETION

Because of the pulsatile nature of pituitary GH secretion, a single random blood sample for GH measurement is not helpful in the diagnosis of GH hypersecretory or deficiency states, or GH neurosecretory disorders. Nonphysiologic provocative or suppression tests, or measurement of spontaneous GH secretion by 24-hour integrated serum GH concentration (IC-GH), are therefore employed to assess GH secretion.

Measurement of Spontaneous GH Secretion

Integrated 24-hour GH Concentrations

Pituitary GH secretion occurs episodically during waking hours, as well as during sleep, necessitating measurement over 24 hours [53] to accurately assess integrated GH secretion. Constant blood collection over a 24-hour period allows determination of a true mean or IC-GH, requiring a nonthrombogenic continuous withdrawal pump or patent indwelling catheter from subjects whose food intake and physical activity are not limited. Sampling intervals of 20 minutes are most widely used, but 5-minute and 30-second sampling frequencies detect significantly more pulses per hour. Samples from collection periods may be pooled, producing a combined aliquot in which the IC-GH concentration is measured. The 24-hour IC-GH reflects the average GH concentration over a 24-hour period, eliminating peak or trough levels that might otherwise be obtained by single random sampling of GH when the latter is released in a pulsatile manner. The discriminating power of continuous GH measurement in the diagnosis of GH deficiency has been disputed, and is also very costly. Measuring spontaneous GH secretion in prepubertal short children was found to be an insensitive test, with no clear diagnostic advantage over GH stimulation tests and considerable overlap between values obtained in normal, short children and children with GHD. As young normal control subjects have IC-GH levels which overlap those of organic hypopituitary patients [190], measurement of spontaneous GH secretion has limitations in the diagnosis of organic GH deficiency in adults.

However, others have found 24-hour IC-GH measurements to be consistently more reproducible and sensitive than repeated pharmacologic stimulation tests [190]. These conflicting findings may be attributable to differences in control groups in the discrepant studies.

Evaluation of GH Hypersecretion

Increased serum IGF-I levels are a consistent finding in acromegaly [191]. Integrated 24-hour serum GH levels are elevated and show a log (dose) response correlation with serum IGF-I levels [192]. The currently accepted diagnostic test of GH hypersecretion is failure of GH levels to be suppressed to less than 1 ng/ml within 2 hours following a 75-g oral glucose load using an IRMA (two site immunoradiometric assay) or chemiluminescent assay [193]. In normal subjects receiving oral glucose loading, serum GH levels initially fall and then subsequently increase as plasma glucose declines. However, in acromegaly, oral glucose fails to suppress GH to the normal range. GH levels may paradoxically increase in response to an oral glucose load in up to 30% of acromegaly patients, remain unchanged (in approximately 36%), or fall (in approximately 36% of patients). In acromegaly, basal GH secretion is tonically elevated with minor bursts. A random GH value of less than 0.4 ng/ml excludes the diagnosis of acromegaly [193].

Evaluation of GH Deficiency

Random GH and 1GF-I Measurements

Random GH measurements are not helpful for diagnosis of GH deficiency, as GH secretion is pulsatile and daytime levels are often low in normal subjects. Low IGF-I levels are suggestive of GH deficiency, but are also encountered in malnutrition, acute illness, celiac disease, poorly controlled diabetes mellitus, liver disease and estrogen ingestion. Fifteen percent of children diagnosed as GH deficient by stimulation tests may have normal IGF-I levels [194]. IGF-I levels are normally very low before 3 years of age and are highest in adolescence. Normal and GH-deficient children may have IGF-I levels which overlap those observed in infancy [195]. Furthermore, both normal and low IGF-I levels are present in children with growth delay and genetic short stature [196]. IGF-I levels do not always correlate with GH levels after provocative GH stimulation and low IGFBP-III levels are encountered in children with GH deficiency.

The diagnosis of adult GHD is more reliably established by provocative testing of GH secretion, as a single age-adjusted IGF-I level has limitations. Whereas in acromegaly there is an excellent correlation between IC-GH and IGF-I [192], in adult GH deficiency, age-adjusted IGF-I should not be regarded as a simple screening test, because of the limitations outlined above.

Provocative Tests

Dynamic testing of GH reserve involves stimulation of somatotrophs to secrete GH in response to a pharmacological stimulus. Several GH stimulatory agents have been utilized, including insulin, clonidine, arginine, L-dopa, GHRH, propranolol and glucagon.

Insulin-induced Hypoglycemia (Insulin Tolerance Test, ITT)

This reliable stimulus for GH secretion is the historical gold standard provocative test [197]. Regular insulin 0.1 IU/kg is administered intravenously to decrease basal glucose levels by 50% to a value below 40 mg/dI. Maximal GH secretion peaks at 30–60 minutes. Patients may experience symptoms of hypoglycemia, including light-headedness, anxiety, tremulousness, sweating, tachycardia seizures and rarely, unconsciousness. Insulin-induced hypoglycemia is contraindicated in patients with a history of seizure disorder, coronary artery disease, or over the age of 55 years. The test should be performed under close supervision, and intravenous glucose (50%) should be readily at hand for rapid administration. The risk of inducing profound hypoglycemia is greater in GH-deficient patients because of increased insulin sensitivity.

Clonidine

This alpha-adrenergic agonist stimulates GH release via a central action. Clonidine (0.15 mg/m^2) is administered orally, with a maximum GH secretory peak occurring after 60–90 minutes. Patients may experience some drowsiness, with a decrease in systolic blood pressure in sodium-depleted GH-deficient adults at doses required to release GH (0.25–0.30 mg orally). Clonidine, frequently used as a stimulus for GH release in children, is not reliable to assess GHD in adults.

L-dopa/Propranolol

L-dopa, the immediate metabolic precursor of dopamine, stimulates GH release by stimulating hypothalamic dopaminergic receptors. Adrenergic blockade (propranolol) enhances the GH response to L-dopa. L-dopa is administered orally according to the patient's weight (125 mg if weighing <30 kg); 250 mg if 10–30 kg; 500 mg if >30 kg) together with propranolol 0.75 mg/kg (maximum dose 40 mg) after an overnight fast. Maximum GH secretion occurs after 60–90 minutes.

Arginine/GHRH

Arginine potentiates maximal somatotroph responsiveness to GHRH [198]. GHRH directly elicits GH secretion from pituitary somatotroph cells, potentiated by arginine. After an overnight fast, GHRH (1 μg/kg) is administered as an intravenous bolus at 0 minutes with arginine (30 g) in 100 ml infused from 0–30 minutes, with subsequent blood sampling for GH performed every 15 minutes for 90 minutes. Combined arginine/GHRH responses are age-independent and this is a highly reproducible GH provocative test [198], at least as sensitive as insulin-induced hypoglycemia [199].

GHRH/GHRP-6

GHRH (1 μg/kg) plus GHRP-6 (1 μg/kg) is given intravenously at 0 minutes and blood drawn for GH sampling at 0 and 120 minutes [200]. GH releasing peptide-6 (GHRP-6) is an artificial hexapeptide [96] that activates the ghrelin receptor [98]. Combined administration of GHRP-6 and GHRH is the most potent stimulus to GH release, with excellent reproducibility and no serious side effects [96]. GHRH/GHRP-6 is a viable alternative to the ITT in patients with organic pituitary disease, however there is overlap between GH levels attained in the control group and severely GH-deficient patients. Since GHRH and GHRP act directly on the pituitary, it is possible that their administration restores GH secretion in patients with a deficiency of these secretagogues because of hypothalamic disease [201].

Glucagon

The mechanism of glucagon-induced GH release is not fully understood. After fasting for at least 8 hours, 1 mg glucagon (1.5 mg if patient's weight >90 kg) is administered intramuscularly, with serum GH and capillary blood glucose levels measured every 30 minutes for 4 hours. Glucagon stimulation is contraindicated in malnourished patients or in patients who are not fasting for 48 hours. Side effects include nausea and late hypoglycemia. A normal response is defined as a GH peak above 3 μg/L. In adults with GHD, GH levels do not rise above 3 μg/L.

GH Provocative Testing

Multiple sampling of GH levels most accurately reflects GH secretion, but is not practical in clinical practice. Provocative tests of GH secretion are employed when patients suspected of having GHD require confirmation of the diagnosis [197].

Serum IGF-I levels below the age-adjusted normal range, in the absence of liver dysfunction and catabolic disorders usually indicate GH deficiency [202]. However, the finding of normal IGF-I levels does not exclude the diagnosis of GHD [199] and GH provocative testing is required for diagnosis in the appropriate clinical setting [197]. One GH stimulation test is sufficient to confirm the diagnosis of adult GHD in patients who require provocative testing [202]. Provocative GH testing is not required for hypopituitary patients, those with serum IGF-I levels below the reference range, as well as those exhibiting three or more other pituitary hormone deficits, as these patients have a >97% chance of being GHD [203].

Historically, the insulin tolerance test (ITT) has been the "gold standard" GH provocative test, but is contraindicated in patients with seizure disorders or cardiovascular disease and requires intensive monitoring. Combined arginine-GHRH testing is considered a reliable alternative with 95% sensitivity and 91% specificity at a GH cutoff of 4.1 ng/ml, compared to 96% sensitivity and 92% specificity for the ITT with an optimal GH cutoff of 5.1 ng/ml [199]. A caveat for the arginine-GHRH test is the falsely normal GH response in patients with GHD due to hypothalamic disease, in whom GHRH directly stimulates the pituitary gland [204]. The relative performance of ITT and arginine-GHRH stimulation is comparable; however arginine alone, clonidine, levodopa and the combination of arginine plus levodopa are less robust tests for the diagnosis of adult GHD [199]. The GH cut-off for diagnosis of GHD varies with the test used. A peak GH response of <3 ng/ml during ITT and glucagon test confirms the diagnosis of GHD. Relative adiposity in the abdominal region blunts GH responses to stimulation [205], and thus cutoffs for arginine-GHRH testing have been validated by body mass index (BMI): for patients with BMI <25 kg/m^2 a peak GH <11 ng/ml, for BMI 25–30 kg/m^2 a peak GH <8 ng/ml, for BMI >30 kg/m^2 a peak GH <4 ng/ml define validated GH cutoff levels [206].

In addition to the stimulus used for provocative GH testing, lack of age- and gender-adjusted normative data, and assay variability influence definition of GH cut off diagnostic criteria. GH levels between 3 and 5 ng/ml were previously defined using polyclonal RIAs [207]. Cutoff values for newer, more sensitive, two-site assays have not been rigorously defined [202]. However, GH values of 5.1 ng/ml and 4.1 ng/ml have been proposed using ITT and arginine-GHRH respectively, using immunochemiluminescent two-site assays in one study [199].

Pediatric patients with idiopathic GHD (either isolated or with one additional hormone deficit) should be retested for GHD after completion of puberty [208] and after discontinuing GH treatment for at least a month [197]. Patients with a high likelihood of permanent GHD, who do not require re-testing after puberty, include those with radiologically confirmed sellar/suprasellar abnormality, those with a transcription factor mutation, those with acquired hypothalamic–pituitary disease, patients who have had hypothalamic–pituitary surgery, and those who have had hypothalamic–pituitary radiation.

Lack of international assay standardization further hinders the definition of GH cutoff values. Analytic methods used in individual assays influence GH results and ideally assay-specific cutoff values should be defined for each provocative test [202]. The calibrant used in the assay, GH isoform detected, as well as the presence or absence of GH-binding protein all influence GH assay results. Adoption of a universal GH calibration standard would be valuable in the international harmonization and standardization of GH provocative test results.

IGF-I measurements are also challenged by lack of a universal calibrator and lack of large age- and gender-matched normative databases.

Variability of GH Assays

The comparison of results of various GH assays obtained in different laboratories is difficult because of differences between several aspects of the immunoassays. Older radioimmunoassay methods employed polyclonal competitive techniques and were relatively insensitive. Newer sensitive non-competitive sandwich-type GH immunoassays employ two antibodies directed against different epitopes on the surface of the GH molecule. One antibody captures the GH molecules, whereas the second labeled antibody generates a signal proportional to the amount of GH in the sample. Older radioimmunoassays used radiolabelled GH, whereas newer non-radioactive sandwich-type assays employ various labels including enzyme-linked, fluorescence and chemiluminescence (most common).

Different circulating forms of GH are not all recognized in GH assays. Because monomeric 22k is the only GH form available as a standard in sufficient purity and quantity, and because monomeric 22k is also the most abundant circulating form, it is used as the basis for GH measurement. Other GH forms are recognized to varying and largely unknown degrees. Thus different antibodies or assay designs yield different results. Polyclonal antibodies were used in the early RIAs inducing higher estimates of GH, because they recognized several molecular forms of GH compared to newer immunometric assays employing highly specific monoclonal antibodies.

GH standards also affect comparison of GH values in different laboratories. In 1994, the first international standard for somatotropin, IRP 88/624, was prepared by the WHO, using recombinant technology in contrast to the previous standards prepared from pituitary extracts. Use of an international standard enables uniformity of calibration between different GH kits. The recent recombinant International Standard (IS) preparation, WHOIS 98/574, is a recombinant 22-kDa growth hormone of >95% purity which provides an opportunity for international use of a single calibrant for GH assays. As different antibodies employed in immunoassays bind to a different spectrum of GH isoforms, GH concentrations measured by immunoassay likely depend on the particular antibody used. Furthermore, as distribution of GH isoforms varies between individuals, results from different GH immunoassays should be compared. GH-binding proteins (GHBPs) may influence GH estimates by interfering in some GH assays. Approximately 50% of circulating GH is complexed to GHBP. As low-affinity GHBP has a greater affinity for the 20-kDa GH molecule, it presumably does not interfere in GH estimates in the new GH assays, specific for the 22-kDa GH molecule. GHBP present in high concentrations in serum samples can block epitope accessibility of respective antibodies used in GH assays, and lead to underestimation of GH concentrations in the sample. GHBP steric hindrance is less of a problem when older assays using polyclonal antisera with longer incubation times are used, compared to the more specific newer monoclonal antibody assays with defined epitopes and shorter incubation times [209].

GH immunoassay heterogeneity thus poses a major challenge in the definition of standards for the diagnosis of GHD. Different conversion factors are used to report GH assay results in mass units, which is a further cause for assay result variability. A borderline GH value,

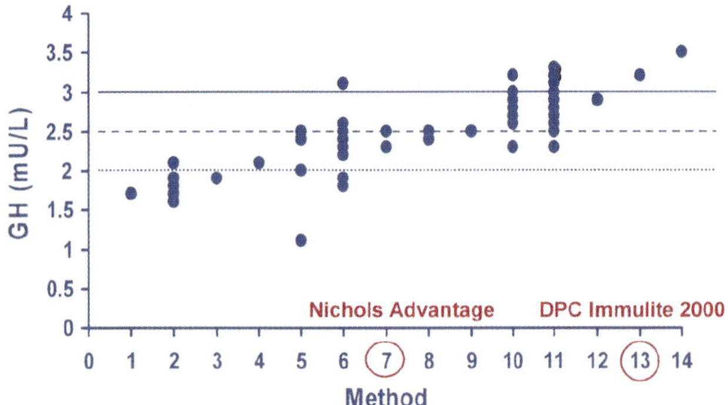

FIGURE 4.8 The impact of conversion factors (CFs) on GH results. 1, Immunotech IRMA; 2, Wallac DELFIA; 3, NETRIA IRMA; 4, Nichols Allegro IRMA; 5, Tosoh AIA; 6, Nichols Advantage; 7, Nichols ICMA; 8, Beckman Access; 9, DSL ELISA; 10, DPC Immulite; 11, DPC Immulite 2000; 12, in-house ELISA; 13, DiaSorin IRMA; 14, in-house IRMA. The lines present the Cortina Consensus cut-off value transformed into mU/L using various CFs: solid line, CF 3, 11% of results consistent with active acromegaly; wide dashed line, CF 2·6, 55% acromegaly; narrow dashed line, CF 2, 86% active acromegaly. *Reproduced with permission from [210].*

obtained from a patient with suspected acromegaly, was sent to 104 laboratories for analysis [210] (Figure 4.8). The median GH was 2.6 mU/L (range 1.04–3.5 mU/L). When a conversion factor of 3.0 (1 μg/L = 3 mU/L) was used, 11% of result values were consistent with acromegaly; with a conversion factor of 2.6, 55% were diagnosed with acromegaly, whereas using a conversion factor of 2.0, 86% of patients had acromegaly. Reliable and harmonious GH assays with robust reference standards still need to be developed.

Variability of IGF Assays

Serum IGF-I levels are regulated by GH, as well as nutrient intake, estrogen, thyroid, coritsol levels and IGF-binding proteins. Testosterone, age, gender, ethnicity and BMI also influence IGF-1 levels [211]. IGF-I levels increase until puberty and then decline (Figure 4.9), necessitating adequate age-adjusted ranges with large numbers of healthy male and female control subjects within each age range [212]. IGFBPs interfere with IGF-I antibody recognition, and thus reliable removal of binding proteins is important. Commonly used methods include acid-ethanol extraction, size-exclusion gel chromatography and addition of excess IGF-II.

Commonly used commercial IGF-I assays, although calibrated against a standard preparation, (WHO 87/518), have similar sensitivities and coefficients of variation; however they exhibit marked nonlinear differences in comparative studies [213]. The reason for these discrepancies is not clear; however awareness of these differences is important when comparing data from different assays. Reliable immunoassays require validation of recovery of exogenous IGF-I, cross-reactivity with IGF-II and assay reproducibility, as well as comparison of sample types, in order to ensure accurate data. Validation of reported results should be published in the kit inserts of commercial assays [214].

CLINICAL USE OF GH (TABLE 4.4)

GH Therapy in Childhood

Recombinant hGH is administered to promote linear growth in short children. The FDA has approved GH treatment for the following conditions: GH deficiency, idiopathic short stature, chronic kidney disease, Turner syndrome, Prader-Willi syndrome, SHOX gene haploinsufficiency, Noonan syndrome and small-for-gestational-age (SGA) infants. Higher GH doses are recommended in children with non-GHD growth disorders. The efficacy of GH treatment in children with non-GHD growth disorders is well-established. However,

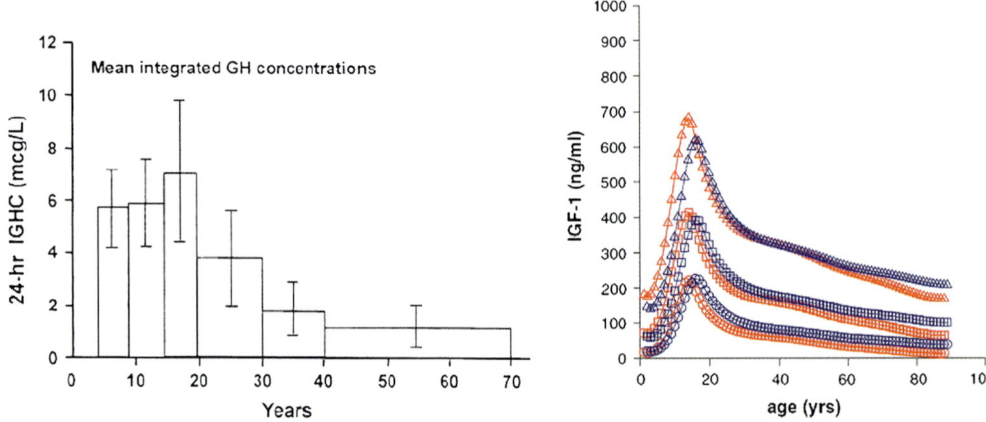

FIGURE 4.9 (Left panel) Twenty-four hour integrated GH levels in 173 non-obese subjects, aged 7–65 years, stratified by age decades. *Reproduced with permission from [275].* (Right panel) Age- and gender-specific IGF-I levels in 3900 healthy subjects. Serum IGF-I levels measured by Nichols Advantage Assay. *Reproduced with permission from [140].*

TABLE 4.4 Indications for GH Therapy

APPROVED USE
GH deficiency
AIDS-associated muscle wasting
Idiopathic short stature
Turner's syndrome
Children born small-for-gestational-age (SGA)
Chronic renal insufficiency
SHOX gene deficiency
INVESTIGATIONAL USE
Frailty of aging
Osteoporosis
Catabolic states
Cachexia
Burns
Postoperative recovery
Wound healing
Parenteral nutrition
Ovulation induction
Immune deficiency

individual responses are variable, and prediction of adult height is guarded. Long-term follow-up studies do not confirm a higher incidence of neoplasia in children or adults who received GH therapy in childhood. However, in light of high GH doses employed, careful monitoring of IGF-I and IGFBP-III is recommended [215].

Classic GH Deficiency

Childhood GH deficiency ranges from complete absence of GH associated with severe growth retardation to partial GH deficiency resulting in short stature. Diagnosis is based on decreased height (more than 2.5 standard deviations [SD] below the mean for age-matched normal children), poor growth velocity (less than the twenty-fifth percentile), delayed bone age, and a predicted adult height below mean parental height [216].

GH deficiency (GHD) is usually confirmed by inadequate pituitary GH responses to standard provocative stimuli. Combined clinical evaluation and provocative testing are used in assessment of childhood GH deficiency. Concomitant endocrine deficiencies, especially hypothyroidism, should be corrected to maximize the growth-promoting benefits of hGH.

GH replacement should be started as early as possible before height drops below the third percentile, as total height gain is inversely proportional to the pretreatment chronological and bone age, as well as severity of GH deficiency. The most pronounced acceleration in linear growth rate occurs during the first 2 years of treatment. Dose and frequency of administration of hGH both influence height velocity.

Idiopathic Short Stature

Idiopathic short stature describes otherwise normal children who are at or below the fifth percentile for height, with normal growth hormone responses to provocative stimuli. Children with ISS are normal size at birth, but grow slowly during early childhood so that the average height falls below −2.0 SD by school-age, maintaining a height velocity within the lower normal range, growing below but parallel to the normal centile channels. Untreated adult height is below the normal range and below mid-parental height by about 1 SD. Historical evidence has suggested that children with ISS have disorganized GH secretion. Recently, genetic defects in several of the genes associated with GH/IGF-I secretion/growth, resulting in short stature, and dismissed as ISS, have been described [217]. GH administered to children with ISS induced an adult height gain of between 3 and 7 cm, depending on the duration of treatment [218]. Rates of adverse events associated with GH therapy in children with ISS are lower compared to side effect profiles observed in other GH-treated disorders, as these children are generally healthy.

Turner's Syndrome

Patients with Turner's syndrome manifest dysmorphic body features, ovarian failure and reduced growth rate, starting during intrauterine life and continuing through childhood and puberty, resulting in reduced final adult height. GH therapy in girls with Turner's syndrome has been shown to significantly increase predicted height, with a greater increase in height in girls treated with GH early and in whom estrogen replacement was postponed until at least age 14 years. In a randomized controlled study, mean adult height was 7 cm greater than the untreated group after 6 years [219]. However, GH-treated Turner's syndrome patients manifest increased incidence of type 2 diabetes mellitus [220].

Children Born Small-for-gestational-age (SGA)

Children with a birth length at least 2 SD below the mean are defined as SGA. Poor fetal growth may be idiopathic due to maternal toxins or associated with defined syndromes. Almost 90% of SGA infants experience catch-up growth within the first or second year of life; the remaining 10–15% increase adult height by approximately 1.0–1.4 SD with long-term GH treatment [221].

Chronic Renal Insufficiency

Chronic renal insufficiency is frequently associated with growth failure, which may be due to protein-calorie malnutrition, acid–base disturbances, hyperparathyroidism, or GH insensitivity manifest by reduced IGF-I:IGFBP ratios with decreased free IGF-I concentrations. The indication for GH treatment in chronic renal insufficiency is growth failure (subnormal height velocity) rather than short stature. GH treatment elicits a doubling of pretreatment height velocity in the first year of treatment [222]. Children with chronic renal insufficiency on GH treatment must be carefully monitored for impaired glucose tolerance, as they have relative glucose intolerance, even in the absence of GH treatment.

SHOX *Gene Deficiency*

The *SHOX* gene, at the distal ends of the X and Y chromosomes, encodes a homeodomain transcription factor responsible for a significant proportion of long bone growth. The *SHOX* gene plays a role in the short stature of Turner's syndrome, Leri-Weill syndrome and some cases of ISS. Patients may not manifest dysmorphic signs or alternatively may have disproportionate shortening of the middle segments of the upper and lower limbs. GH treatment significantly increases first and second year height velocity.

GH Therapy in Adults

GH is administered to promote physiological and psychological well-being and altered body composition in adults with GH deficiency, muscle wasting due to HIV/AIDS and short bowel syndrome [214].

Adult GHD Syndrome

ETIOLOGY

The diagnosis of adult GHD should be suspected in patients with hypothalamic or pituitary disease, or with a history of having received cranial irradiation or pituitary adenoma treatment, or prior traumatic brain injury or subarachonid hemorrhage. Adult GHD may be isolated or can occur in association with several other pituitary hormone deficiencies (panhypopituitarism).

Childhood-onset GHD is most commonly idiopathic, but may be genetic, or associated with congenital anatomical malformations in the brain or sella turcica region (Table 4.5). Idiopathic GHD is the commonest cause of GHD in childhood. Adult GHD may follow childhood-onset GHD, which persists into adulthood or can be acquired in adulthood secondary to structural sella and parasellar lesions or may be secondary to head trauma. The commonest cause of adult GHD is a pituitary macroadenoma (30–60% of which are associated with single or multiple pituitary hormone deficiencies),

TABLE 4.5 Causes of Adult Growth Hormone (GH) Deficiency

PRESENTING IN CHILDHOOD
Congenital
Idiopathic
Genetic
Transcription factor defect
GHRH receptor defect
GH gene defect
GH receptor/post receptor defect
Embryologic defects (structural)
Agenesis of corpus callosum
Hydrocephalus
Septo-optic dysplasia
Arachnoid cyst
Empty sella syndrome
GH resistance
Laron dwarfism
Pygmy
Neurosecretory defects
Radiation for brain tumors, leukemia
Head trauma
Perinatal birth injury
Child abuse
Accidental
Inflammatory diseases
Viral encephalitis
Meningitis, bacterial, fungal, tuberculosis
ACQUIRED IN ADULTHOOD
Pituitary/hypothalamic/tumors
Pituitary adenoma
Craniopharyngioma
Rathke's cleft cyst
Metastasis
Parasellar tumors
Germinoma
Astrocytoma
Postpituitary surgery
Head trauma
Hemochromatosis
Sickle cell disease
Thalassemia
Autoimmunity
Lymphocytic hypophysitis
Cranial irradiation
Infiltrative/granulomatous infectious disease
Histiocytosis
Sarcoidosis
Idiopathic
Infection
Tuberculosis
Syphilis
Vascular

or pituitary adenoma treatment (surgery or radiotherapy). Twenty-five percent of patients who sustain traumatic brain injury subsequently develop GHD with varying degrees of concomitant hypopituitarism. GHD is usually the first hormone deficiency to develop when pituitary damage occurs; thus in patients diagnosed with multiple pituitary hormone deficits, the likelihood of GHD is very high. The incidence of hypopituitarism associated with pituitary irradiation increases over time, with 50% of patients diagnosed with varying degrees of hypopituitarism 10 years after having received conventional radiotherapy.

DIAGNOSIS

GHD adults have altered body composition with increased fat mass, decreased lean body mass and decreased muscle volume and strength, decreased bone mineral density, altered glucose and lipid metabolism, lower psychosocial achievement, and possibly increased mortality due to cardiovascular disease (Table 4.6).

IGF-I is a robust screening test in lean, younger patients (<40 years) suspected of having GHD. However, at any age, in hypopituitary adults screening IGF-I levels may be normal in the presence of severe GHD. Other causes of low IGF-I levels include liver disease and malnutrition. In well-nourished subjects without liver disease, low serum IGF-I levels strongly predict severe GHD.

The diagnosis of GHD is confirmed by provocative testing of GH secretion. Other hormonal deficits should be adequately replaced prior to GH provocative testing. A single stimulation test is adequate for the diagnosis of AGHD. Not all patients suspected of having GHD, however, require a GH stimulation test for diagnosis. Adult patients with three or four pituitary hormone deficits and a low IGF-I level do not require GH stimulation testing to establish the diagnosis [203].

The insulin-tolerance test (ITT) remains the test of reference despite concerns about reproducibility, safety and specificity. There are tests that are as reliable as ITT. ITT is contraindicated in adults with ischemic heart disease and seizure disorders, and is a potential risk in elderly patients as occult vascular disease increases with age. ITT requires close monitoring by trained medical personnel to attain adequate hypoglycemia, with reversal of severe insulin-induced hypoglycemia to avoid neuroglycopenia.

TABLE 4.6 Physical Findings in the Adult Growth Hormone Deficiency Syndrome.

Truncal adiposity
Increased waist/hip ratio
Thin, dry, cool skin
Reduced exercise performance
Reduced muscle strength
Reduced bone mineral density
Depressed mood
Psychosocial impairment

Adapted from Carroll et al. [277].

Sensitive and reliable alternative GH stimulants have been evaluated. The GHRH-arginine test, with 95% sensitivity and 91% specificity, at a GH cutoff of 4.1 μg/L compares very favorably to the ITT, with a GH cutoff of 5.1 μg/L (96% sensitivity and 92% specificity) [199]. Arginine alone, clonidine, levo-dopa and arginine plus levo-dopa are not reliable alternatives to the ITT.

GHRH-ARG is well-tolerated and requires less monitoring than the ITT. However, two caveats should be considered when interpreting results of GHRH-ARG stimulation testing – the impact of increased BMI on GH secretion and whether the GHD is due to hypothalamic or pituitary damage.

Obese subjects have reduced spontaneous and stimulated GH secretion negatively associated with body mass index [205]. Diagnostic GH cutoff values have been evaluated for lean (BMI <25 kg/m^2), overweight (BMI >25 but <30 kg/m^2) and obese (BMI >30 kg/m^2) subjects, with high sensitivity and specificity for GH deficiency. In lean subjects, a peak GH cutoff point of 11.5 μg/L had the highest sensitivity and specificity using ROC analysis; in the overweight and obese population lower cutoff points were determined, at 8–4.2 μg/L [206]. To avoid false-positive responses in overweight and obese subjects, and false-negative results in lean subjects, BMI must be considered in the interpretation of GH responses to GHRH-ARG provocative stimulation, and approximate GH cutoff points must be considered.

GHRH stimulates the pituitary directly, and thus falsely "normal" responses can be elicited in patients with hypothalamic GHD, because exogenously administered GHRH directly stimulates pituitary somatotroph cells. Therefore, in patients with suspected hypothalamic damage (e.g., after cranial irradiation), the peak GH response to GHRH and arginine may be normal, whereas the ITT may reveal an abnormal response [204].

GHRH-arginine is now widely recognized as a reliable alternative to the ITT [197,202]; however, since October 2008 GHRH has not been available in the USA. Glucagon stimulation testing is a well-tolerated alternative GH provocative test to GHRH-arginine [223]. Glucagon is relatively inexpensive and widely available for treating hypoglycemia in patients with diabetes mellitus. Glucagon is contraindicated in patients who have fasted for more than 48 hours. Glucagon is well-tolerated. Side effects may include nausea and late hypoglycemia, which can be prevented by eating small frequent meals after completing the test. Glucagon is administered intramuscularly and GH is measured half-hourly for 4 hours. In adults with GHD, GH levels do not rise above 3 μg/L. A GH cutoff value of 3 μg/L provides the best sensitivity (100 and 97% respectively) and specificity (100 and 88% respectively), using ROC analysis [223]. Unlike the GHRH-arginine test, there is no inverse correlation between BMI and peak GH response to glucagon.

GH REPLACEMENT THERAPY

Prior to the advent of recombinant hGH, the scarcity of GH limited GH replacement therapy to GH-deficient children. The primary therapeutic goal was to increase linear growth and in the past, treatment was terminated after epiphyseal fusion, when a certain height had been achieved. However, GH secretion normally continues into adulthood, and GH influences many metabolic systems other than growth (Tables 4.7 and 4.8). The goal of GH replacement therapy in adulthood is to correct the metabolic, functional and psychological deficiencies associated with AGHD. The numerous beneficial effects of GH replacement in adulthood are described in Table 4.7. GH replacement in GH-deficient adults is associated with increased energy levels, improved mood, vitality and emotional reactions and less feeling of social isolation. GH replacement therapy is associated with significantly improved Nottingham Health Profile (NHP) energy scores.

GH doses in adulthood are adjusted to individual needs (Table 4.8). As more GH is secreted in younger, lean individuals and in females, elderly, male, or obese individuals require lower GH replacement doses. The use of oral estrogen replacement affects the GH replacement dose. Premenopausal women or postmenopausal women using transdermal estrogen replacement require lower GH doses than postmenopausal women receiving oral estrogen replacement [224]. Oral, but not transdermal, estrogens antagonize GH actions and reduce IGF-I levels (Figure 4.10). Historically, GH treatment regimens were weight-based, resulting in a higher incidence of side effects as well as higher maintenance doses than in currently used individualized dose-titration GH replacement regimens. Current dosing recommendations suggest a starting GH dose of 0.2 mg/day in young men,

TABLE 4.7 Beneficial Effects of GH Replacement in Adults

Body composition	Increased lean body mass
	Decreased fat mass
	Increased bone mass
Physical performance	Increased max O_2 uptake
	Increased max power
Metabolic	Increased IGF-I levels
	Increased BMR
	Decreased LDL with probable increased HDL
	Transient hyperglycemia
	Increased T_3 levels
	Salt and water retention
Cardiovascular	Increased stroke volume
	Increased diastolic volume
	Increased LV wall mass
	Atherosclerosis impact
Psychological	Mood and energy uplift
	Enhanced vitality
	Improved physical mobility
	Social isolation decreased
Adipose tissue	Decreased adipocyte size
	Increased lipolysis
	Decreased lipogenesis

TABLE 4.8 Factors Determining Side Effects of GH Replacement

Patient age, gender
Enhanced IGF-I response
Greater body weight and body mass index
Adult onset vs. childhood onset of GH deficiency

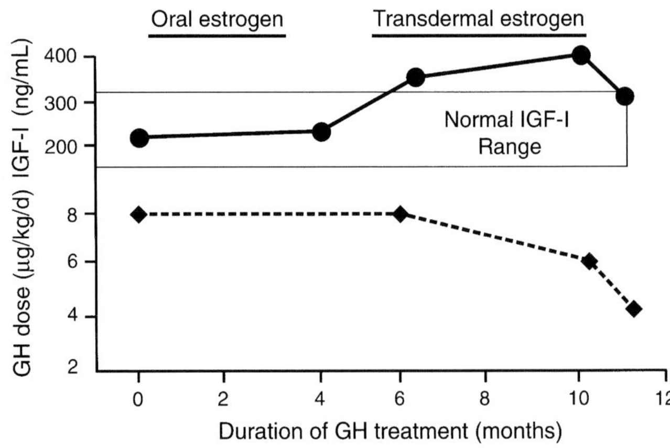

FIGURE 4.10 Time course of GH dose and serum IGF-I concentration in a representative patient (38-year-old woman) who was switched from oral to transdermal estrogen therapy during the course of GH replacement. *Reproduced with permission from Cook et al. [224].*

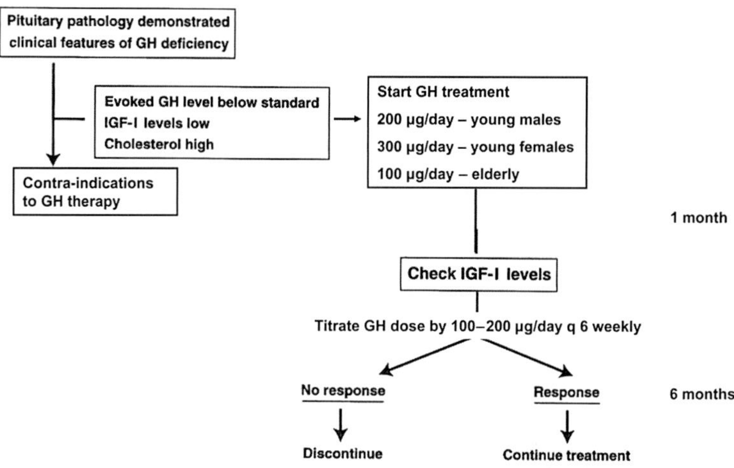

FIGURE 4.11 Algorithm for the management of adult GH deficiency.

0.3 mg/day in young women and 0.1 mg/day in the elderly [223]. GH is self-administered as a single subcutaneous evening injection, to mimic normal physiological nocturnal GH secrtion.

Daily doses are titrated by 100–200 μg/day every 6 weeks according to clinical responses, side effects and IGF-I levels [197,223]. After maintenance doses have been established, patients can be monitored at 6–12-monthly intervals, for clinical evaluation, side effects and serum IGF-I levels. GH doses are adjusted until IGF-I levels reach mid-normal range for age and sex (Figure 4.11). Lipid profile and fasting blood glucose levels should be evaluated annually [197]. If the pretreatment bone DEXA scan is abnormal, follow-up DEXA scan is evaluated at 1–2-year intervals. Hypopituitary patients may require evaluation of thyroid and adrenal axes, after initiation of GH therapy.

Duration of GH therapy depends on benefits of treatment. Discontinuing GH therapy may be appropriate, if objective benefits are not apparent after at least 1 year of treatment; however, if objective clinical benefits are obtained from GH replacement, GH treatment is continued.

Side effects of GH replacement are usually transient and include arthralgias, edema and carpal tunnel syndrome due to fluid retention. However, dose reduction may be required. As GH may reduce insulin sensitivity, glycemic control should be monitored. In a placebo-controlled study, GH therapy induced impaired glucose tolerance in 13% of patients and diabetes mellitus in 4%, with a significant number of patients developing worsening of glucose tolerance in the GH-treated group [225]. GH replacement therapy is contraindicated in patients with active malignancy, benign intracranial hypertension and proliferative diabetic retinopathy (Table 4.9).

The growth-promoting and mitogenic effects of GH and IGF-I could potentially increase cancer risk and promote tumor regrowth. However, increases in the occurrence of either intracranial or extracranial tumors have not been reported in adult GHD patients on long-term GH replacement therapy [226]. Increased rates of tumor regrowth have not been reported following GH replacement either in patients with previous craniopharyngiomas [227] or other childhood brain tumors [228] or adult pituitary macroadenomas [229]. GH therapy does not impose a need for more frequent pituitary MRIs than would be performed for the regular clinical follow-up of residual pituitary tumor.

Serum IGF-I levels in the upper-normal range may be of predictive value for risk of developing prostate cancer [230], breast cancer in healthy premenopausal females [231] and colorectal cancer in healthy men [232]. Furthermore, cancer risk was inversely correlated with serum IGFBP-3 levels. These studies, which have not been uniformly reproduced, provide a clear rationale for maintaining IGF-I in the mid-normal age-adjusted range, in AGHD or patients on GH replacement therapy.

TABLE 4.9 Contraindications to GH Therapy in Adults

ABSOLUTE
Active neoplasm
Intracranial hypertension
Proliferative diabetic retinopathy
RELATIVE
Uncontrolled diabetes
Untreated thyroid dysfunction
Cost benefit
Need for injections

EFFECTS OF GH REPLACEMENT THERAPY ON HYPOPITUITARISM

Complex hormonal interactions occur between GH and other pituitary hormones which impact diagnosis as well as optimal hormone replacement therapy. Thyroid, adrenal and sex steroid replacement must be optimized for at least 3 months prior to testing for GHD. In addition, GH replacement may unmask incipient adrenal and thyroid insufficiency, necessistating monitoring of these hormonal interactions in order to achieve optimal hormone replacement.

THYROID HORMONE

TSH levels are not helpful in the diagnosis of central hypothyroidism in hypopituitary patients, as the pituitary secretes abnormally glycosylated TSH, with reduced bioactivity. Decreased serum T_4 is therefore the best marker for diagnosis of central hypothyroidism.

GH replacement increases conversion of T_4 to T_3 and decreases conversion of T_4 to reverse T_3 [233]. Initiation of GH replacement therapy may therefore be associated with a fall in serum T_4 levels, unmasking pre-existing central hypothyroidism [233]. Careful monitoring of thyroid function is important in patients taking thyroid replacement who are initiated on GH replacement therapy, as thyroid hormone dose adjustments may be required.

GONADAL STEROIDS

Female patients taking oral estrogens require at least two-fold greater doses of GH [224], as estrogen administered orally impairs GH action. Therefore, to reduce GH requirements, a nonoral route (such as a transdermal patch) for estrogen replacement in hypopituitary women should be considered.

Recommendations for sex steroid replacement in hypopituitary patients after menopause should follow guidelines for the general population. If adjustments are made in the dose of oral estrogens in hypopituitary female patients, the GH replacement dose should be re-evaluated, as it may need to be changed. Changes in dose or route of androgen replacement therapy do not require re-evaluation of GH dosage.

GLUCOCORTICOIDS

GH or IGF-I decrease 11 β-hydroxysteroid dehydrogenase type I activity, resulting in reduced conversion of inactive cortisone to active cortisol [234], and thus may unmask secondary hypoadrenalism. The hypothalamic–pituitary–adrenal axis should therefore be re-evaluated during initiation of GH therapy as increased glucocorticoid replacement therapy or initiation of steroid replacement therapy may be required.

GH in the Healthy Elderly

Serum GH and IGF-I levels decline progressively with age, a phenomenon referred to as "somatopause" (Figure 4.9). Increased adiposity and decreased lean body mass observed in the adult GHD syndrome also occur with aging. The purported rationale for GH use as an antiaging therapy is the potential for improvement in body composition, bone density and cholesterol levels observed in GH-deficient adults treated with GH replacement therapy. GH is not approved for use as an antiaging hormone by the US Food and Drug Administration, but abuse of GH for this purpose continues to escalate [235].

Randomized controlled studies evaluating safety and efficacy of GH in the healthy elderly are limited [235]. The scant data suggest small but clinically nonsignificant improvements in body composition with adverse events including impaired fasting glucose, onset of diabetes mellitus, carpal tunnel syndrome, edema, arthralgias and no beneficial effect on strength or physical function. Thus, available evidence does not validate physiological benefits from augmenting the declining GH levels in the normal aging process.

In animal models mutations resulting in suppression of the GH/IGF-I axis with reduced GH/IGF-I signaling increase lifespan [236]. Snell and Ames dwarf mice with defects in anterior pituitary function due to Pit-1 and PROP-1 mutations respectively, exhibit severely reduced insulin, IGF-I, glucose and thyroid hormone levels, female infertility and increased longevity [237]. Lit/Lit drwarf mice with mutations in the extracellular domain of the GHRH receptor had reduced serum IGF-I levels, increased adiposity and ~25% increased longevity. Herterozygous IGF-I-receptor-gene-disrupted mice have a 50% reduction in receptor levels, and a 33% increased lifespan in females, who are not dwarf [238]. In contrast, mice expressing a transgene for a GH antagonist, with reduced GH-induced intracellular signaling, and decreased IGF-I levels are dwarf, but do not exhibit increased longevity [239]. Mice with a disrupted hepatic IGF-I receptor gene exhibit reduced IGF-I and elevated GH levels, four-fold increase in serum insulin with normal glucose levels, with normal longevity [240].

Caloric restriction, another mechanism of decreasing circulating IGF-I levels, also prolongs lifespan in several species [241].

Sarcopenia (loss of muscle mass) increases with age and contributes to frailty. The mechanism of loss of muscle mass is unclear, and may be due to intrinsic muscle factors or other factors, nutrition, exercise, or hormones. Clinical trials using GH in the healthy elderly have not proven to enhance muscle strength or quality of life. Ghrelin may be beneficial in catabolic states, and increases appetite and lean body mass in healthy older men [242].

Although associated with some positive effects on body composition, GH has not proven beneficial as an antiaging agent. A recent study evaluating the contribution of physiological supplementation with GH and testosterone for 16 weeks in elderly community-dwelling males showed improved lean body mass, muscle strength and performance, with reduced total body and truncal fat [243].

GH Abuse in Sport

Use of GH by Athletes

Exercise is a potent stimulus of GH secretion and GH levels increase within 10–20 minutes of the onset of exercise, and are sustained for up to 2 hours following exercise. Furthermore, healthy subjects who exercise regularly demonstrate increased 24-hour GH secretion rates. Short- and long-term effects of GH are thus potentially important in the physiological demands of exercise and training. Age, gender, BMI, physical fitness, duration and intensity of exercise influence the magnitude of the GH response to exercise [244].

Beneficial effects of GH replacement therapy on exercise capacity in truly GHD adults have encouraged unapproved use of GH by athletes. GH-deficient adults demonstrate reduced VO_2 max (maximum capcity to take in and use oxygen) with impaired exercise capacity. A recent meta-analysis of 268 GHD patients treated with 3.3–15.7 mg/week GH for 6–18 months in 11 randomized placebo-controlled studies, demonstrated significant improvement in exercise capacity evaluated by maximally increased work rate and VO_2 max [245]. Lipolytic effects of GH increase availability of circulating free fatty acids to exercising muscle during prolonged exercise [246], with potential conservation of glycogen stores. GH-enhanced increase in the cardiac LV ejection fraction potentially improves oxygen delivery to exercising muscle [247,248].

GHD adults manifest reduced skeletal muscle mass, with reduced isometric muscle strength and possibly reduced isokinetic strength. GH and IGF-I exert anabolic effects on skeletal muscle [249], with increased protein synthesis and reduced protein oxidation, an effect which is enhanced with concurrent administration of testosterone [250]. GH replacement in GHD adults increases isometric and isokinetic strength into the normal range, especially in those patients with the most compromised baseline muscle strength; an effect which is sustained for 5 years [251]. GH replacement also improves body composition and enhances thermoregulation with increased sweat secretion rates during heat exposure and exercise in GHD adults.

Supraphysiological doses of GH to pituitary-replete athletes increase free fatty acid availability, with no effect however on fat oxidation, during or following exercise [252]. Furthermore, oxidative protein loss at rest, during and following exercise is reduced [253], as well as increasing lean body mass in young healthy subjects and trained athletes. Beneficial effects of GH replacement in GHD adults as well as all those of supraphysiological GH doses to healthy subjects, have not been documented to enhance performance. Despite lack of proven efficacy, inappropriate use of rhGH by athletes increased from 6% in 2001 to 24% in 2006 [254].

Safety and Efficacy of GH to Enhance Athletic Performance

Administration of hGH to athletes is termed "doping." Evidence based on rigorous clinical studies is not available to support enhanced athletic performance associated with GH use in young adults. There are also no supportive data of enhanced athletic performance using rhGH in combination with anabolic steroids, in young athletes. A recent systematic review [255] of 56 articles reported 303 young recreational athletes, average age 27 years who had received GH for an average of 20 days, many of whom received only one hGH injection. The average GH dose was 36 μg/kg/day (approximately 5–10-fold the replacement dose used in GH-deficient adults). Lean body mass (LBM) increased in the treatment group, compared to those not treated, with a statistically insignificant decrease in fat mass. There was no improvement in muscle strength after 24 and 84 days of GH administration in two studies. This analysis revealed little beneficial effect of GH in recreational athletes and failed to document improved performance. However, the studies were of short duration and likely do not reflect either the GH dose or duration of administration of GH to competitive athletes. In a single study of a highly select group of abstinent dependent users of anabolic androgenic steroids, hGH (19 μg/kg/day) for 1 week improved strength, peak power output and IGF-I levels [256].

Testing for GH Doping in Athletes

GH is not FDA approved for enhancement of athletic performance, and the International Olympic Committee (IOC) has prohibited GH doping. Development of reliable routine tests to detect GH doping was delayed until the GH-2000 project because of lack of scientific research to develop appropriate tests, as well as the requirement for blood rather than urine for testing. The GH-2000 project comprised endocrinologists from four European countries, who proposed a test based on the measurement of two GH-sensitive markers, IGF-I and type III pro-collagen [257].

The GH isoform test based on the measurement of GH isoforms was used at the Olympic Games in Athens in 2004, in Turin in 2006 and in Beijing in 2008. Pituitary GH contains several different GH isoforms, while recombinant human GH comprises only the 22kD isoform [258]. Administration of rhGH suppresses endogenous GH secretion, with increased 22kD GH to total GH ratios. To detect the 22kD GH isoform, the test must be performed within 24 hours of GH administration, thus discontinuation of GH the day before the test will result in a false-negative result. No positive isoform tests were reported during 2004, 2006, or 2008 Olympics testing. The GH-2004 project demonstrated minor ethnic differences in IGF-I and procollagen III peptide levels in athletes, which did not affect test performance [259]. However, a recent large cross-sectional study in over 1000 athletes from 12 countries, representing four major ethnic groups and ten major sport types showed that age and gender are major determinants of variability in IGF-I and collagen markers. Age, gender, BMI, ethnicity and sport type contributed to 56% of the variability of IGF-I axis markers (IGF-I, IGFBP-3 and ALS) and collagen markers (type I procollagen, c-terminal telopeptide of type I collagen and N-terminal propeptide of type III procollagen) [260]. Thus, demographic factors, especially age and gender must be taken into account in interpretation of tests using IGF-I and collagen markers to detect GH doping.

Recently gene expression analysis of peripheral blood leukocytes was attempted as a method to detect GH doping. The rationale is that GH induces subtle alterations in gene expression in peripheral blood lymphocytes which could potentially be effective in detecting GH doping. However, this approach was not found to be clinically valuable for widespread screening [261].

Complications of GH Treatment

Complications of GH treatment have been described in GH-deficient patients inappropriately treated with GH (Table 4.10). Non-GH-deficient patients receiving GH can be likened to acromegaly patients, with increased GH levels. Adverse reactions, including glucose intolerance, arthralgias, myalgias, backache, parasthesias, peripheral edema, carpel tunnel syndrome, headache, hypertension and rhinitis are frequent, often transient or disappear with lowering of the GH dose and are more common in adult-onset than childhood-onset GH deficiency.

TABLE 4.10 Side Effects of GH Replacement Therapy

METABOLIC	
Glucose homeostasis	
Salt and fluid retention; peripheral edema	
Unmasking of thyroid dysfunction	
JOINT	
Adults	Athralgias and myalgias
	Carpal tunnel syndrome
Children	Slipped capital femoral epiphysis
	Hydrocephalus

Elevated (but still within normal range) endogenous IGF-I concentrations have been epidemiologically correlated with prostate, breast, colon [262] and lung cancer risk [263].

Decreased IGF-I Levels

Protein-Calorie Malnutrition, Starvation, Anorexia Nervosa

Short-term fasting in normal healthy subjects results in moderately elevated basal GH levels [231]. However, protein-calorie malnutrition is associated with low IGF-I levels and markedly elevated GH levels [264]. This may reflect an uncoupling of the IGF-I feedback regulation of GH secretion. In patients with anorexia nervosa, basal GH levels are also elevated [265]. GH abnormalities in anorexia nervosa are due to weight loss and to the concomitant psychiatric disturbance, which may influence hypothalamic–pituitary function.

Diabetes Mellitus

Poorly controlled diabetes mellitus (both insulin-dependent and noninsulin-dependent) is associated with elevated basal GH levels and increased GH response to exercise. Elevated GH levels return to normal with improved diabetic control after insulin administration.

IGF-I levels are low in children with poorly controlled insulin-dependent diabetes, including those entering puberty, suggesting insulin resistance. Anti-insulin actions of increased GH may exacerbate the insulin resistance.

Laron Syndrome

Laron syndrome, an autosomal recessive disorder, is a condition of peripheral unresponsiveness to GH. Serum GH levels are normal or elevated, circulating IGF-I is absent, and there is no IGF-I response to exogenously administered GH [120]. Inactivating mutations of the GH receptor [266] cause insensitivity to exogenous GH. IGF-I therapy increases height velocity, with improved body composition as evidenced by loss of fat mass [267].

Decreased GH Clearance

Chronic Renal Failure

Approximately one-third of children with chronic renal insufficiency (CRI), have heights below the third centile [268]. The growth pattern in children with CRI varies depending on age of onset of renal insufficiency. Many factors contribute to the abnormal linear growth in childhood CRI including etiology of renal disease, protein-calorie malnutrition, acid–base disturbance and abnormalities of the GH/IGF-I axis. There is apparent insensitivity to endogenous GH, with high basal GH levels in patients with chronic renal failure [269], primarily due to reduced renal GH clearance. GH rises paradoxically in response to a glucose load in these patients [269]. GH is degraded by the kidney. GH insensitivity is manifest by reduced IGF-I:IGFBP ratios, resulting in decreased free IGF-I levels.

Despite high GH levels, children with renal failure are short. Following renal transplantation, return to normal growth is variable. The indication for GH treatment in chronic renal failure is not short stature, but rather growth failure (subnormal height velocity). A meta-analysis of randomized controlled trials of GH treatment to children with chronic renal insufficiency, concluded that catch-up growth occurred in the first year of treatment and continued GH treatment likely prevents progressive growth failure [270].

References

[1] W.L. Miller, N.L. Eberhardt, Structure and evolution of the growth hormone gene family, Endocr Rev 4 (2) (1983) 97–130.

[2] E.Y. Chen, Y.C. Liao, D.H. Smith, H.A. Barrera-Saldana, R.E. Gelinas, P.H. Seeburg, The human growth hormone locus: Nucleotide sequence, biology, and evolution, Genomics 4 (4) (1989) 479–497.

[3] U.J. Lewis, L.F. Bonewald, L.J. Lewis, The 20,000-dalton variant of human growth hormone: Location of the amino acid deletions, Biochem Biophys Res Commun 92 (2) (1980) 511–516.

[4] F. Frankenne, F. Rentier-Delrue, M.L. Scippo, J. Martial, G. Hennen, Expression of the growth hormone variant gene in human placenta, J Clin Endocrinol Metab 64 (3) (1987) 635–637.

[5] F. Frankenne, J. Closset, F. Gomez, M.L. Scippo, J. Smal, G. Hennen, The physiology of growth hormones (GHs) in pregnant women and partial characterization of the placental GH variant, J Clin Endocrinol Metab 66 (6) (1988) 1171–1180.

[6] C.L. Boguszewski, P.A. Svensson, T. Jansson, R. Clark, L.M. Carlsson, B. Carlsson, Cloning of two novel growth hormone transcripts expressed in human placenta, J Clin Endocrinol Metab 83 (8) (1998) 2878–2885.

[7] J. Ray, H. Okamura, P.A. Kelly, N.E. Cooke, S.A. Liebhaber, Human growth hormone-variant demonstrates a receptor binding profile distinct from that of normal pituitary growth hormone, J Biol Chem 265 (14) (1990) 7939–7944.

[8] J.N. MacLeod, I. Worsley, J. Ray, H.G. Friesen, S.A. Liebhaber, N.E. Cooke, Human growth hormone-variant is a biologically active somatogen and lactogen, Endocrinology 128 (3) (1991) 1298–1302.

[9] H. Hirt, J. Kimelman, M.J. Birnbaum, E.Y. Chen, P.H. Seeburg, N.L. Eberhardt, et al., The human growth hormone gene locus: Structure, evolution, and allelic variations, DNA 6 (1) (1987) 59–70.

[10] X. Zhu, C.R. Lin, G.G. Prefontaine, J. Tollkuhn, M.G. Rosenfeld, Genetic control of pituitary development and hypopituitarism, Curr Opin Genet Dev 15 (3) (2005) 332–340.

[11] A.M. Pulichino, S. Vallette-Kasic, C. Couture, T. Brue, J. Drouin, [Tpit mutations reveal a new model of pituitary differentiation and account for isolated ACTH deficiency], Med Sci (Paris) 20 (11) (2004) 1009–1013.

[12] Y.G. Watanabe, S. Daikoku, An immunohistochemical study on the cytogenesis of adenohypophysial cells in fetal rats, Dev Biol 68 (2) (1979) 557–567.

[13] R.R. Behringer, L.S. Mathews, R.D. Palmiter, R.L. Brinster, Dwarf mice produced by genetic ablation of growth hormone-expressing cells, Genes Dev 2 (4) (1988) 453–461.

[14] E. Borrelli, R.A. Heyman, C. Arias, P.E. Sawchenko, R.M. Evans, Transgenic mice with inducible dwarfism, Nature 339 (6225) (1989) 538–541.

[15] M.W. Sornson, W. Wu, J.S. Dasen, S.E. Flynn, D.J. Norman, S.M. O'Connell, et al., Pituitary lineage determination by the Prophet of Pit-1 homeodomain factor defective in Ames dwarfism, Nature 384 (6607) (1996) 327–333.

[16] W. Wu, J.D. Cogan, R.W. Pfaffle, J.S. Dasen, H. Frisch, S.M. O'Connell, et al., Mutations in PROP1 cause familial combined pituitary hormone deficiency, Nat Genet 18 (2) (1998) 147–149.

[17] F.P. Lemaigre, S.J. Courtois, D.A. Lafontaine, G.G. Rousseau, Evidence that the upstream stimulatory factor and the Sp1 transcription factor bind in vitro to the promoter of the human-growth-hormone gene, Eur J Biochem 181 (3) (1989) 555–561.

[18] F. Schaufele, B.L. West, T.L. Reudelhuber, Overlapping Pit-1 and Sp1 binding sites are both essential to full rat growth hormone gene promoter activity despite mutually exclusive Pit-1 and Sp1 binding, J Biol Chem 265 (28) (1990) 17189–17196.

[19] H.A. Ingraham, R.P. Chen, H.J. Mangalam, H.P. Elsholtz, S.E. Flynn, C.R. Lin, et al., A tissue-specific transcription factor containing a homeodomain specifies a pituitary phenotype, Cell 55 (3) (1988) 519–529.

[20] M. Bodner, J.L. Castrillo, L.E. Theill, T. Deerinck, M. Ellisman, M. Karin, The pituitary-specific transcription factor GHF-1 is a homeobox-containing protein, Cell 55 (3) (1988) 505–518.

[21] L.N. Peritz, E.J. Fodor, D.W. Silversides, P.A. Cattini, J.D. Baxter, N.L. Eberhardt, The human growth hormone gene contains both positive and negative control elements, J Biol Chem 263 (11) (1988) 5005–5007.

[22] D. Prager, S. Gebremedhin, S. Melmed, An insulin-induced DNA-binding protein for the human growth hormone gene, J Clin Invest 85 (5) (1990) 1680–1685.

[23] C. Romero, S. Nesi-França, S. Radovick, The molecular basis of hypopituitarism, Trends Endocrinol Metab 20 (2009) 506–516.

[24] N.J. Lanning, C. Carter-Su, Recent advances in growth hormone signaling, Rev Endocr Metab Disord 7 (4) (2006) 225–235.

[25] X.Z. Chen, A.W. Shafer, J.S. Yun, Y.S. Li, T.E. Wagner, J.J. Kopchick, Conversion of bovine growth hormone cysteine residues to serine affects secretion by cultured cells and growth rates in transgenic mice, Mol Endocrinol 6 (4) (1992) 598–606.

[26] G. Baumann, J.G. MacCart, K. Amburn, The molecular nature of circulating growth hormone in normal and acromegalic man: Evidence for a principal and minor monomeric forms, J Clin Endocrinol Metab 56 (5) (1983) 946–952.

[27] D. Rudman, M.H. Kutner, C.M. Rogers, M.F. Lubin, G.A. Fleming, R.P. Bain, Impaired growth hormone secretion in the adult population: Relation to age and adiposity, J Clin Invest 67 (5) (1981) 1361–1369.

[28] N. Goldenberg, A. Barkan, Factors regulating growth hormone secretion in humans, Endocrinol Metab Clin North Am 36 (1) (2007) 37–55.

[29] E. Van Cauter, R. Leproult, L. Plat, Age-related changes in slow wave sleep and REM sleep and relationship with growth hormone and cortisol levels in healthy men, JAMA 284 (7) (2000 Aug 16) 861–868.

[30] C.A. Jaffe, D.K. Turgeon, R.D. Friberg, P.B. Watkins, A.L. Barkan, Nocturnal augmentation of growth hormone (GH) secretion is preserved during repetitive bolus administration of GH-releasing hormone: Potential involvement of endogenous somatostatin – a clinical research center study, J Clin Endocrinol Metab 80 (11) (1995) 3321–3326.

[31] J. Golstein, E. Van Cauter, D. Desir, P. Noel, J.P. Spire, S. Refetoff, et al., Effects of "jet lag" on hormonal patterns. IV. Time shifts increase growth hormone release, J Clin Endocrinol Metab 56 (3) (1983) 433–440.

[32] F.F. Casanueva, L. Villanueva, J.A. Cabranes, J. Cabezas-Cerrato, A. Fernandez-Cruz, Cholinergic mediation of growth hormone secretion elicited by arginine, clonidine, and physical exercise in man, J Clin Endocrinol Metab 59 (3) (1984) 526–530.

[33] N. Moller, J.O. Jorgensen, Effects of growth hormone on glucose, lipid, and protein metabolism in human subjects, Endocr Rev 30 (2) (2009) 152–177.

[34] L.E. Katz, D.D. DeLeon, H. Zhao, A.F. Jawad, Free and total insulin-like growth factor (IGF)-I levels decline during fasting: Relationships with insulin and IGF-binding protein-1, J Clin Endocrinol Metab 87 (6) (2002) 2978–2983.

[35] J.L. Clasey, A. Weltman, J. Patrie, J.Y. Weltman, S. Pezzoli, C. Bouchard, et al., Abdominal visceral fat and fasting insulin are important predictors of 24-hour GH release independent of age, gender, and other physiological factors, J Clin Endocrinol Metab 86 (8) (2001) 3845–3852.

[36] P. Alvarez-Castro, M.L. Isidro, J. Garcia-Buela, A. Leal-Cerro, F. Broglio, F. Tassone, et al., Marked GH secretion after ghrelin alone or combined with GH-releasing hormone (GHRH) in obese patients, Clin Endocrinol (Oxf) 61 (2) (2004) 250–255.

[37] J. Roth, S.M. Glick, R.S. Yalow, Bersonsa. Hypoglycemia: A potent stimulus to secretion of growth hormone, Science 140 (1963) 987–988.

[38] J. Alba-Roth, O.A. Muller, J. Schopohl, K. von Werder, Arginine stimulates growth hormone secretion by suppressing endogenous somatostatin secretion, J Clin Endocrinol Metab 67 (6) (1988) 1186–1189.

[39] F.F. Casanueva, L. Villanueva, C. Dieguez, Y. Diaz, J.A. Cabranes, B. Szoke, et al., Free fatty acids block growth hormone (GH) releasing hormone-stimulated GH secretion in man directly at the pituitary. J Clin Endocrinol Metab 65 (4) (1987) 634–642.

[40] K. Nakagawa, K. Akikawa, M. Matsubara, M. Kubo, Effect of dexamethasone on growth hormone (GH) response to growth hormone releasing hormone in acromegaly, J Clin Endocrinol Metab 60 (2) (1985) 306–310.

[41] J.B. Tyrrell, J. Wiener-Kronish, M. Lorenzi, R.M. Brooks, P.H. Forsham, Cushing's disease: Growth hormone response to hypoglycemia after correction of hypercortisolism, J Clin Endocrinol Metab 44 (1) (1977) 218–221.

[42] T. Suda, H. Demura, R. Demura, K. Jibiki, F. Tozawa, K. Shizume, Anterior pituitary hormones in plasma and pituitaries from patients with Cushing's disease, J Clin Endocrinol Metab 51 (5) (1980) 1048–1053.

[43] F.F. Casanueva, B. Burguera, C. Muruais, C. Dieguez, Acute administration of corticoids: A new and peculiar stimulus of growth hormone secretion in man, J Clin Endocrinol Metab 70 (1) (1990) 234–237.

[44] T. Kelesidis, I. Kelesidis, S. Chou, C.S. Mantzoros, Narrative review: The role of leptin in human physiology. Emerging clinical applications, Ann Intern Med 152 (2) (2010) 93–100.

[45] J.L. Chan, K. Heist, A.M. DePaoli, J.D. Veldhuis, C.S. Mantzoros, The role of falling leptin levels in the neuroendocrine and metabolic adaptation to short-term starvation in healthy men, J Clin Invest 111 (9) (2003) 1409–1421.

[46] J.L. Chan, C.J. Williams, P. Raciti, J. Blakeman, T. Kelesidis, I. Kelesidis, et al., Leptin does not mediate short-term fasting-induced changes in growth hormone pulsatility but increases IGF-I in leptin deficiency states, J Clin Endocrinol Metab 93 (7) (2008) 2819–2827.

[47] J.B. Martin, Neural regulation of growth hormone secretion, N Engl J Med 288 (26) (1973) 1384–1393.

[48] L. de Lecea, T.S. Kilduff, C. Peyron, X. Gao, P.E. Foye, P.E. Danielson, et al., The hypocretins: Hypothalamus-specific peptides with neuroexcitatory activity, Proc Nat Acad Sci USA 95 (1) (1998) 322–327.

[49] M. Blanco, R. Gallego, T. Garcia-Caballero, C. Dieguez, A. Beiras, Cellular localization of orexins in human anterior pituitary, Histochem Cell Biol 120 (4) (2003) 259–264.

[50] J.J. Hagan, R.A. Leslie, S. Patel, M.L. Evans, T.A. Wattam, S. Holmes, et al., Orexin A activates locus coeruleus cell firing and increases arousal in the rat, Proc Nat Acad Sci USA 96 (19) (1999) 10911–10916.

[51] M. Kojima, K. Kangawa, Ghrelin: Structure and function, Physiol Rev 85 (2) (2005) 495–522.

[52] R.M. Chemelli, J.T. Willie, C.M. Sinton, J.K. Elmquist, T. Scammell, C. Lee, et al., Narcolepsy in orexin knockout mice: Molecular genetics of sleep regulation, Cell 98 (4) (1999) 437–451.

[53] A. Giustina, J.D. Veldhuis, Pathophysiology of the neuroregulation of growth hormone secretion in experimental animals and the human, Endocr Rev 19 (6) (1998) 717–797.

[54] M.O. Thorner, R.L. Perryman, M.J. Cronin, A.D. Rogol, M. Draznin, A. Johanson, et al., Somatotroph hyperplasia. Successful treatment of acromegaly by removal of a pancreatic islet tumor secreting a growth hormone-releasing factor, J Clin Invest 70 (5) (1982) 965–977.

[55] K. Maeda, Y. Kato, N. Yamaguchi, K. Chihara, S. Ohgo, Growth hormone release following thyrotrophin-releasing hormone injection into patients with anorexia nervosa, Acta Endocrinol (Copenh) 81 (1) (1976) 1–8.

[56] E. Gutierrez-Pascual, A.J. Martinez-Fuentes, L. Pinilla, M. Tena-Sempere, M.M. Malagon, J.P. Castano, Direct pituitary effects of kisspeptin: Activation of gonadotrophs and somatotrophs and stimulation of luteinising hormone and growth hormone secretion, J Neuroendocrinol 19 (7) (2007) 521–530.

[57] R. Guillemin, P. Brazeau, P. Bohlen, F. Esch, N. Ling, W.B. Wehrenberg, Growth hormone-releasing factor from a human pancreatic tumor that caused acromegaly, Science 218 (4572) (1982) 585–587.

[58] J. Rivier, J. Spiess, M. Thorner, W. Vale, Characterization of a growth hormone-releasing factor from a human pancreatic islet tumour, Nature 300 (5889) (1982) 276–278.

[59] U. Gubler, J.J. Monahan, P.T. Lomedico, R.S. Bhatt, K.J. Collier, B.J. Hoffman, et al., Cloning and sequence analysis of cDNA for the precursor of human growth hormone-releasing factor, somatocrinin, Proc Nat Acad Sci USA 80 (14) (1983) 4311–4314.

[60] K.E. Mayo, W. Vale, J. Rivier, M.G. Rosenfeld, R.M. Evans, Expression-cloning and sequence of a cDNA encoding human growth hormone-releasing factor, Nature 306 (5938) (1983) 86–88.

[61] K. Tatemoto, V. Mutt, Isolation and characterization of the intestinal peptide porcine PHI (PHI-27), a new member of the glucagon–secretin family, Proc Nat Acad Sci USA 78 (11) (1981) 6603–6607.

[62] L.M. Bilezikjian, W.W. Vale, Stimulation of adenosine 3′,5′-monophosphate production by growth hormone-releasing factor and its inhibition by somatostatin in anterior pituitary cells in vitro, Endocrinology 113 (5) (1983) 1726–1731.

[63] K.E. Mayo, Molecular cloning and expression of a pituitary-specific receptor for growth hormone-releasing hormone, Mol Endocrinol 6 (10) (1992) 1734–1744.

[64] J. Fukata, D.J. Diamond, J.B. Martin, Effects of rat growth hormone (rGH)-releasing factor and somatostatin on the release and synthesis of rGH in dispersed pituitary cells, Endocrinology 117 (2) (1985) 457–467.

[65] M. Barinaga, L.M. Bilezikjian, W.W. Vale, M.G. Rosenfeld, R.M. Evans, Independent effects of growth hormone releasing factor on growth hormone release and gene transcription, Nature 314 (6008) (1985) 279–281.

[66] M.C. Gelato, O. Pescovitz, F. Cassorla, D.L. Loriaux, G.R. Merriam, Effects of a growth hormone releasing factor in man, J Clin Endocrinol Metab 57 (3) (1983) 674–676.

[67] N. Pandya, R. DeMott-Friberg, C.Y. Bowers, A.L. Barkan, C.A. Jaffe, Growth hormone (GH)-releasing peptide-6 requires endogenous hypothalamic GH-releasing hormone for maximal GH stimulation, J Clin Endocrinol Metab 83 (4) (1998) 1186–1189.

[68] M. Russell-Aulet, C.A. Jaffe, R. Demott-Friberg, A.L. Barkan, In vivo semiquantification of hypothalamic growth hormone-releasing hormone (GHRH) output in humans: Evidence for relative GHRH deficiency in aging, J Clin Endocrinol Metab 84 (10) (1999) 3490–3497.

[69] M. Russell-Aulet, E.V. Dimaraki, C.A. Jaffe, R. DeMott-Friberg, A.L. Barkan, Aging-related growth hormone (GH) decrease is a selective hypothalamic GH-releasing hormone pulse amplitude mediated phenomenon, J Gerontol A Biol Sci Med Sci 56 (2) (2001) M124–M129.

[70] S.K. Jessup, E.V. Dimaraki, K.V. Symons, A.L. Barkan, Sexual dimorphism of growth hormone (GH) regulation in humans: Endogenous GH-releasing hormone maintains basal GH in women but not in men, J Clin Endocrinol Metab 88 (10) (2003) 4776–4780.

[71] S. Reichlin, Somatostatin, N Engl J Med 309 (24) (1983) 1495–1501.

[72] L.P. Shen, R.L. Pictet, W.J. Rutter, Human somatostatin I: Sequence of the cDNA, Proc Nat Acad Sci USA 79 (15) (1982) 4575–4579.

[73] T.M. Siler, S.C. Yen, W. Vale, R. Guillemin, Inhibition by somatostatin on the release of TSH induced in man by thyrotropin-releasing factor, J Clin Endocrinol Metab 38 (5) (1974) 742–745.

[74] D.J. Koerker, W. Ruch, E. Chideckel, J. Palmer, C.J. Goodner, J. Ensinck, et al., Somatostatin: Hypothalamic inhibitor of the endocrine pancreas, Science 184 (135) (1974) 482–484.

[75] C.B. Srikant, Y.C. Patel, Receptor binding of somatostatin-28 is tissue specific, Nature 294 (5838) (1981) 259–260.

[76] A. Ben-Shlomo, S. Melmed, Pituitary somatostatin receptor signaling, Trends Endocrinol Metab 21 (3) (2010) 123–133.

[77] G.M. Miller, J.M. Alexander, H.A. Bikkal, L. Katznelson, N.T. Zervas, A. Klibanski, Somatostatin receptor subtype gene expression in pituitary adenomas, J Clin Endocrinol Metab 80 (4) (1995) 1386–1392.

[78] Y. Greenman, S. Melmed, Heterogeneous expression of two somatostatin receptor subtypes in pituitary tumors, J Clin Endocrinol Metab 78 (2) (1994) 398–403.

[79] Y. Greenman, S. Melmed, Expression of three somatostatin receptor subtypes in pituitary adenomas: Evidence for preferential SSTR5 expression in the mammosomatotroph lineage, J Clin Endocrinol Metab 79 (3) (1994) 724–729.

[80] I. Shimon, X. Yan, J.E. Taylor, M.H. Weiss, M.D. Culler, S. Melmed, Somatostatin receptor (SSTR) subtype-selective analogues differentially suppress in vitro growth hormone and prolactin in human pituitary adenomas. Novel potential therapy for functional pituitary tumors, J Clin Invest 100 (9) (1997) 2386–2392.

[81] M. Berelowitz, M. Szabo, L.A. Frohman, S. Firestone, L. Chu, R.L. Hintz, Somatomedin-C mediates growth hormone negative feedback by effects on both the hypothalamus and the pituitary, Science 212 (4500) (1981) 1279–1281.

[82] S. Yamashita, S. Melmed, Insulin-like growth factor I action on rat anterior pituitary cells: Suppression of growth hormone secretion and messenger ribonucleic acid levels, Endocrinology 118 (1) (1986) 176–182.

[83] G.S. Tannenbaum, N. Ling, The interrelationship of growth hormone (GH)-releasing factor and somatostatin in generation of the ultradian rhythm of GH secretion, Endocrinology 115 (5) (1984) 1952–1957.

[84] M.L. Vance, D.L. Kaiser, P.M. Martha Jr., R. Furlanetto, J. Rivier, W. Vale, et al., Lack of in vivo somatotroph desensitization or depletion after 14 days of continuous growth hormone (GH)-releasing hormone administration in normal men and a GH-deficient boy, J Clin Endocrinol Metab 68 (1) (1989) 22–28.

[85] G.S. Tannenbaum, J.C. Painson, A.M. Lengyel, P. Brazeau, Paradoxical enhancement of pituitary growth hormone (GH) responsiveness to GH-releasing factor in the face of high somatostatin tone, Endocrinology 124 (3) (1989) 1380–1388.

[86] S. Horvath, M. Palkovits, T. Gorcs, A. Arimura, Electron microscopic immunocytochemical evidence for the existence of bidirectional synaptic connections between growth hormone-releasing hormone and somatostatin-containing neurons in the hypothalamus of the rat, Brain Res 481 (1) (1989) 8–15.

[87] J.R. Davis, M.C. Sheppard, R.A. Shakespear, S.S. Lynch, R.N. Clayton, Does growth hormone releasing factor desensitize the somatotroph? Interpretation of responses of growth hormone during and after 10-hour infusion of GRF 1-29 amide in man, Clin Endocrinol (Oxf) 24 (2) (1986) 135–140.

[88] M. Losa, P.G. Chiodini, A. Liuzzi, A. Konig, O.A. Muller, J. Schopohl, et al., Growth hormone-releasing hormone infusion in patients with active acromegaly, J Clin Endocrinol Metab 63 (1) (1986) 88–93.

[89] A. Spada, F.R. Elahi, M. Arosio, A. Sartorio, L. Guglielmino, L. Vallar, et al., Lack of desensitization of adenomatous somatotrophs to growth-hormone releasing hormone in acromegaly, J Clin Endocrinol Metab 64 (3) (1987) 585–591.

[90] L.M. Bilezikjian, H. Seifert, W. Vale, Desensitization to growth hormone-releasing factor (GRF) is associated with down-regulation of GRF-binding sites, Endocrinology 118 (5) (1986) 2045–2052.

[91] M.C. Sheppard, S. Kronheim, B.L. Pimstone, Stimulation by growth hormone of somatostatin release from the rat hypothalamus in vitro, Clin Endocrinol (Oxf) 9 (6) (1978) 583–586.

[92] S.M. Rosenthal, J.A. Hulse, S.L. Kaplan, M.M. Grumbach, Exogenous growth hormone inhibits growth hormone-releasing factor-induced growth hormone secretion in normal men, J Clin Invest 77 (1) (1986) 176–180.

[93] R.J. Ross, F. Borges, A. Grossman, R. Smith, L. Ngahfoong, L.H. Rees, et al., Growth hormone pretreatment in man blocks the response to growth hormone-releasing hormone; evidence for a direct effect of growth hormone, Clin Endocrinol (Oxf) 26 (1) (1987) 117–123.

[94] R.A. Peterfreund, W.W. Vale, Somatostatin analogs inhibit somatostatin secretion from cultured hypothalamus cells, Neuroendocrinology 39 (5) (1984) 397–402.

[95] R.G. Smith, L.H. Van der Ploeg, A.D. Howard, S.D. Feighner, K. Cheng, G.J. Hickey, et al., Peptidomimetic regulation of growth hormone secretion, Endocr Rev 18 (5) (1997) 621–645.

[96] F.F. Casanueva, C. Dieguez, Growth hormone secretagogues: Physiological role and clinical utility, Trends Endocrinol Metab 10 (1) (1999) 30–38.

[97] A.D. Howard, S.D. Feighner, D.F. Cully, J.P. Arena, P.A. Liberator, C.I. Rosenblum, et al., A receptor in pituitary and hypothalamus that functions in growth hormone release, Science 273 (5277) (1996) 974–977.

[98] M. Kojima, H. Hosoda, Y. Date, M. Nakazato, H. Matsuo, K. Kangawa, Ghrelin is a growth-hormone-releasing acylated peptide from stomach, Nature 402 (6762) (1999) 656–660.

[99] S. Gnanapavan, B. Kola, S.A. Bustin, D.G. Morris, P. McGee, P. Fairclough, et al., The tissue distribution of the mRNA of ghrelin and subtypes of its receptor, GHS-R, in humans, J Clin Endocrinol Metab 87 (6) (2002) 2988.

[100] A.J. van der Lely, M. Tschop, M.L. Heiman, E. Ghigo, Biological, physiological, pathophysiological, and pharmacological aspects of ghrelin, Endocr Rev 25 (3) (2004) 426–457.

[101] Y. Hataya, T. Akamizu, K. Takaya, N. Kanamoto, H. Ariyasu, M. Saijo, et al., A low dose of ghrelin stimulates growth hormone (GH) release synergistically with GH-releasing hormone in humans, J Clin Endocrinol Metab 86 (9) (2001) 4552.

[102] V. Popovic, D. Miljic, D. Micic, S. Damjanovic, E. Arvat, E. Ghigo, et al., Ghrelin main action on the regulation of growth hormone release is exerted at hypothalamic level, J Clin Endocrinol Metab 88 (7) (2003) 3450–3453.

[103] Y. Shuto, T. Shibasaki, A. Otagiri, H. Kuriyama, H. Ohata, H. Tamura, et al., Hypothalamic growth hormone secretagogue receptor regulates growth hormone secretion, feeding, and adiposity, J Clin Invest 109 (11) (2002) 1429–1436.

[104] Y. Sun, P. Wang, H. Zheng, R.G. Smith, Ghrelin stimulation of growth hormone release and appetite is mediated through the growth hormone secretagogue receptor, Proc Nat Acad Sci USA 101 (13) (2004) 4679–4684.

[105] Y. Sun, S. Ahmed, R.G. Smith, Deletion of ghrelin impairs neither growth nor appetite, Mol Cell Biol 23 (22) (2003) 7973–7981.

[106] J. Pantel, M. Legendre, S. Cabrol, L. Hilal, Y. Hajaji, S. Morisset, et al., Loss of constitutive activity of the growth hormone secretagogue receptor in familial short stature, J Clin Invest 116 (3) (2006) 760–768.

[107] P. Koutkia, B. Canavan, J. Breu, M.L. Johnson, S.K. Grinspoon, Nocturnal ghrelin pulsatility and response to growth hormone secretagogues in healthy men, Am J Physiol Endocrinol Metab 287 (3) (2004) E506–E512.

[108] P. Zizzari, H. Halem, J. Taylor, J.Z. Dong, R. Datta, M.D. Culler, et al., Endogenous ghrelin regulates episodic growth hormone (GH) secretion by amplifying GH pulse amplitude: Evidence from antagonism of the GH secretagogue-R1a receptor, Endocrinology 146 (9) (2005) 3836–3842.

[109] G.S. Tannenbaum, J. Epelbaum, C.Y. Bowers, Interrelationship between the novel peptide ghrelin and somatostatin/growth hormone-releasing hormone in regulation of pulsatile growth hormone secretion, Endocrinology 144 (3) (2003) 967–974.

[110] J. Kamegai, H. Tamura, T. Shimizu, S. Ishii, A. Tatsuguchi, H. Sugihara, et al., The role of pituitary ghrelin in growth hormone (GH) secretion: GH-releasing hormone-dependent regulation of pituitary ghrelin gene expression and peptide content, Endocrinology 145 (8) (2004) 3731–3738.

[111] E. Arvat, M. Maccario, L. Di Vito, F. Broglio, A. Benso, C. Gottero, et al., Endocrine activities of ghrelin, a natural growth hormone secretagogue (GHS), in humans: Comparison and interactions with hexarelin, a nonnatural peptidyl GHS, and GH-releasing hormone, J Clin Endocrinol Metab 86 (3) (2001) 1169–1174.

[112] F.F. Casanueva, J.P. Camina, M.C. Carreira, Y. Pazos, J.L. Varga, A.V. Schally, Growth hormone-releasing hormone as an agonist of the ghrelin receptor GHS-R1a, Proc Nat Acad Sci USA 105 (51) (2008) 20452–20457.

[113] S. Melmed, Acromegaly pathogenesis and treatment, J Clin Invest 119 (11) (2009) 3189–3202.

[114] I. Shimon, X. Yan, S. Melmed, Human fetal pituitary expresses functional growth hormone-releasing peptide receptors, J Clin Endocrinol Metab 83 (1) (1998) 174–178.

[115] A.F. Massoud, P.C. Hindmarsh, C.G. Brook, Hexarelin-induced growth hormone, cortisol, and prolactin release: A dose-response study, J Clin Endocrinol Metab 81 (12) (1996) 4338–4341.

[116] C.P. Barsano, G. Baumann, Simple algebraic and graphic methods for the apportionment of hormone (and receptor) into bound and free fractions in binding equilibria; or how to calculate bound and free hormone? Endocrinology 124 (3) (1989) 1101–1106.

[117] G. Baumann, M.A. Shaw, Plasma transport of the 20,000-dalton variant of human growth hormone (20K): Evidence for a 20K-specific binding site, J Clin Endocrinol Metab 71 (5) (1990) 1339–1343.

[118] G. Baumann, K.D. Amburn, T.A. Buchanan, The effect of circulating growth hormone-binding protein on metabolic clearance, distribution, and degradation of human growth hormone, J Clin Endocrinol Metab 64 (4) (1987) 657–660.

[119] W.H. Daughaday, B. Trivedi, B.A. Andrews, The ontogeny of serum GH binding protein in man: A possible indicator of hepatic GH receptor development, J Clin Endocrinol Metab 65 (5) (1987) 1072–1074.

[120] Z. Laron, Laron syndrome (primary growth hormone resistance or insensitivity): The personal experience 1958–2003, J Clin Endocrinol Metab 89 (3) (2004) 1031–1044.

[121] B. Bulow, B. Ahren, S. Fisker, O. Dehlin, B. Hagberg, E. Jensen, et al., The gender differences in growth hormone-binding protein and leptin persist in 80-year-old men and women and is not caused by sex hormones, Clin Endocrinol (Oxf) 59 (4) (2003) 482–486.

[122] H.D. McIntyre, R. Serek, D.I. Crane, T. Veveris-Lowe, A. Parry, S. Johnson, et al., Placental growth hormone (GH), GH-binding protein, and insulin-like growth factor axis in normal, growth-retarded, and diabetic pregnancies: Correlations with fetal growth, J Clin Endocrinol Metab 85 (3) (2000) 1143–1150.

[123] A.J. Brooks, J.W. Wooh, K.A. Tunny, M.J. Waters, Growth hormone receptor; mechanism of action, Int J Biochem Cell Biol 40 (10) (2008) 1984–1989.

[124] R.J. Brown, J.J. Adams, R.A. Pelekanos, Y. Wan, W.J. McKinstry, K. Palethorpe, et al., Model for growth hormone receptor activation based on subunit rotation within a receptor dimer, Nat Struct Mol Biol 12 (9) (2005) 814–821.

[125] B.C. Xu, X. Wang, C.J. Darus, J.J. Kopchick, Growth hormone promotes the association of transcription factor STAT5 with the growth hormone receptor, J Biol Chem 271 (33) (1996) 19768–19773.

[126] S. Melmed, S. Yamashita, H. Yamasaki, J. Fagin, H. Namba, H. Yamamoto, et al., IGF-I receptor signalling: Lessons from the somatotroph, Recent Prog Horm Res 51 (1996) 189–215, discussion 216.

[127] J. Woelfle, D.J. Chia, P. Rotwein, Mechanisms of growth hormone (GH) action. Identification of conserved Stat5 binding sites that mediate GH-induced insulin-like growth factor-I gene activation, J Biol Chem 278 (51) (2003) 51261–51266.
[128] K.C. Leung, M.J. Waters, I. Markus, W.R. Baumbach, K.K. Ho, Insulin and insulin-like growth factor-I acutely inhibit surface translocation of growth hormone receptors in osteoblasts: A novel mechanism of growth hormone receptor regulation, Proc Nat Acad Sci USA 94 (21) (1997) 11381–11386.
[129] D.J. Chia, M. Ono, J. Woelfle, M. Schlesinger-Massart, H. Jiang, P. Rotwein, Characterization of distinct Stat5b binding sites that mediate growth hormone-stimulated IGF-I gene transcription, J Biol Chem 281 (6) (2006) 3190–3197.
[130] G.B. Udy, R.P. Towers, R.G. Snell, R.J. Wilkins, S.H. Park, P.A. Ram, et al., Requirement of STAT5b for sexual dimorphism of body growth rates and liver gene expression, Proc Nat Acad Sci USA 94 (14) (1997) 7239–7244.
[131] P.A. Ram, S.H. Park, H.K. Choi, D.J. Waxman, Growth hormone activation of Stat 1, Stat 3, and Stat 5 in rat liver. Differential kinetics of hormone desensitization and growth hormone stimulation of both tyrosine phosphorylation and serine/threonine phosphorylation, J Biol Chem 271 (10) (1996) 5929–5940.
[132] H.W. Davey, S.H. Park, D.R. Grattan, M.J. McLachlan, D.J. Waxman, STAT5b-deficient mice are growth hormone pulse-resistant. Role of STAT5b in sex-specific liver p450 expression, J Biol Chem 274 (50) (1999) 35331–35336.
[133] E.M. Kofoed, V. Hwa, B. Little, K.A. Woods, C.K. Buckway, J. Tsubaki, et al., Growth hormone insensitivity associated with a STAT5b mutation, N Engl J Med 349 (12) (2003) 1139–1147.
[134] C.J. Greenhalgh, E. Rico-Bautista, M. Lorentzon, A.L. Thaus, P.O. Morgan, T.A. Willson, et al., SOCS2 negatively regulates growth hormone action in vitro and in vivo, J Clin Invest 115 (2) (2005) 397–406.
[135] V.K. Han, A.J. D'Ercole, P.K. Lund, Cellular localization of somatomedin (insulin-like growth factor) messenger RNA in the human fetus, Science 236 (4798) (1987) 193–197.
[136] L.S. Mathews, G. Norstedt, R.D. Palmiter, Regulation of insulin-like growth factor I gene expression by growth hormone, Proc Nat Acad Sci USA 83 (24) (1986) 9343–9347.
[137] J.A. Romanus, A. Rabinovitch, M.M. Rechler, Neonatal rat islet cell cultures synthesize insulin-like growth factor I, Diabetes 34 (7) (1985) 696–702.
[138] D.R. Clemmons, D.S. Shaw, Variables controlling somatomedin production by cultured human fibroblasts, J Cell Physiol 115 (2) (1983) 137–142.
[139] J.P. Thissen, J.M. Ketelslegers, L.E. Underwood, Nutritional regulation of the insulin-like growth factors, Endocr Rev 15 (1) (1994) 80–101.
[140] G. Brabant, M.A. von zur, C. Wuster, M.B. Ranke, J. Kratzsch, W. Kiess, et al., Serum insulin-like growth factor I reference values for an automated chemiluminescence immunoassay system: Results from a multicenter study, Horm Res 60 (2) (2003) 53–60.
[141] D.R. Clemmons, Value of insulin-like growth factor system markers in the assessment of growth hormone status, Endocrinol Metab Clin North Am 36 (1) (2007) 109–129.
[142] R.C. Baxter, J.L. Martin, Structure of the Mr 140,000 growth hormone-dependent insulin-like growth factor binding protein complex: Determination by reconstitution and affinity-labeling, Proc Nat Acad Sci USA 86 (18) (1989) 6898–6902.
[143] H.P. Guler, J. Zapf, C. Schmid, E.R. Froesch, Insulin-like growth factors I and II in healthy man. Estimations of half-lives and production rates, Acta Endocrinol (Copenh) 121 (6) (1989) 753–758.
[144] S.C. Hodgkinson, S.R. Davis, L.G. Moore, H.V. Henderson, P.D. Gluckman, Metabolic clearance of insulin-like growth factor-II in sheep, J Endocrinol 123 (3) (1989) 461–468.
[145] J. Holly, C. Perks, The role of insulin-like growth factor binding proteins, Neuroendocrinology 83 (3-4) (2006) 154–160.
[146] R.C. Baxter, J.L. Martin, Radioimmunoassay of growth hormone-dependent insulin-like growth factor binding protein in human plasma, J Clin Invest 78 (6) (1986) 1504–1512.
[147] J. Zapf, C. Hauri, M. Waldvogel, E. Futo, H. Hasler, K. Binz, et al., Recombinant human insulin-like growth factor I induces its own specific carrier protein in hypophysectomized and diabetic rats, Proc Nat Acad Sci USA 86 (10) (1989) 3813–3817.
[148] S.L. Drop, D.J. Kortleve, H.J. Guyda, B.I. Posner, Immunoassay of a somatomedin-binding protein from human amniotic fluid: Levels in fetal, neonatal, and adult sera, J Clin Endocrinol Metab 59 (5) (1984) 908–915.
[149] M. Degerblad, G. Povoa, M. Thoren, I.L. Wivall, K. Hall, Lack of diurnal rhythm of low molecular weight insulin-like growth factor binding protein in patients with Cushing's disease, Acta Endocrinol (Copenh) 120 (2) (1989) 195–200.
[150] W.H. Busby, D.K. Snyder, D.R. Clemmons, Radioimmunoassay of a 26,000-dalton plasma insulin-like growth factor-binding protein: Control by nutritional variables, J Clin Endocrinol Metab 67 (6) (1988) 1225–1230.
[151] S. Ezzat, S.G. Ren, G.D. Braunstein, S. Melmed, Octreotide stimulates insulin-like growth factor binding protein-1 (IGFBP-1) levels in acromegaly, J Clin Endocrinol Metab 73 (2) (1991) 441–443.
[152] J.M. Holly, R.A. Biddlecombe, D.B. Dunger, J.A. Edge, S.A. Amiel, R. Howell, et al., Circadian variation of GH-independent IGF-binding protein in diabetes mellitus and its relationship to insulin. A new role for insulin? Clin Endocrinol (Oxf) 29 (6) (1988) 667–675.
[153] M.J. Waters, J.L. Barclay, Does growth hormone drive breast and other cancers? Endocrinology 148 (10) (2007) 4533–4535.
[154] M.C. Slootweg, C. Ohlsson, J.P. Salles, C.P. de Vries, J.C. Netelenbos, Insulin-like growth factor binding proteins-2 and -3 stimulate growth hormone receptor binding and mitogenesis in rat osteosarcoma cells, Endocrinology 136 (10) (1995) 4210–4217.
[155] E.F. Gevers, N. Loveridge, I.C. Robinson, Bone marrow adipocytes: A neglected target tissue for growth hormone, Endocrinology 143 (10) (2002) 4065–4073.
[156] J. Wang, J. Zhou, C.A. Bondy, Igf1 promotes longitudinal bone growth by insulin-like actions augmenting chondrocyte hypertrophy, FASEB J 13 (14) (1999) 1985–1990.
[157] O. Nilsson, R. Marino, F. De Luca, M. Phillip, J. Baron, Endocrine regulation of the growth plate, Horm Res 64 (4) (2005) 157–165.
[158] E. Canalis, The fate of circulating osteoblasts, N Engl J Med 352 (19) (2005) 2014–2016.
[159] D.J. DiGirolamo, A. Mukherjee, K. Fulzele, Y. Gan, X. Cao, S.J. Frank, et al., Mode of growth hormone action in osteoblasts, J Biol Chem 282 (43) (2007) 31666–31674.
[160] E. Canalis, A.N. Economides, E. Gazzerro, Bone morphogenetic proteins, their antagonists, and the skeleton, Endocr Rev 24 (2) (2003) 218–235.
[161] E. Hubina, P. Lakatos, L. Kovacs, I. Szabolcs, K. Racz, M. Toth, et al., Effects of 24 months of growth hormone (GH) treatment on serum carboxylated and undercarboxylated osteocalcin levels in GH-deficient adults, Calcif Tissue Int 74 (1) (2004) 55–59.

[162] N.A. Sims, P. Clement-Lacroix, F. Da Ponte, Y. Bouali, N. Binart, R. Moriggl, et al., Bone homeostasis in growth hormone receptor-null mice is restored by IGF-I but independent of Stat5, J Clin Invest 106 (9) (2000) 1095–1103.

[163] M. Zhang, S. Xuan, M.L. Bouxsein, D. von Stechow, N. Akeno, M.C. Faugere, et al., Osteoblast-specific knockout of the insulin-like growth factor (IGF) receptor gene reveals an essential role of IGF signaling in bone matrix mineralization, J Biol Chem 277 (46) (2002) 44005–44012.

[164] A. Giustina, G. Mazziotti, E. Canalis, Growth hormone, insulin-like growth factors, and the skeleton, Endocr Rev 29 (5) (2008) 535–559.

[165] R.G. Rosenfeld, A.L. Rosenbloom, J. Guevara-Aguirre, Growth hormone (GH) insensitivity due to primary GH receptor deficiency, Endocr Rev 15 (3) (1994) 369–390.

[166] B.C. van der Eerden, M. Karperien, J.M. Wit, Systemic and local regulation of the growth plate, Endocr Rev 24 (6) (2003) 782–801.

[167] K.A. Woods, C. Camacho-Hubner, M.O. Savage, A.J. Clark, Intrauterine growth retardation and postnatal growth failure associated with deletion of the insulin-like growth factor I gene, N Engl J Med 335 (18) (1996) 1363–1367.

[168] M.J. Abuzzahab, A. Schneider, A. Goddard, F. Grigorescu, C. Lautier, E. Keller, et al., IGF-I receptor mutations resulting in intrauterine and postnatal growth retardation, N Engl J Med 349 (23) (2003) 2211–2222.

[169] R.D. Murray, J.E. Adams, S.M. Shalet, A densitometric and morphometric analysis of the skeleton in adults with varying degrees of growth hormone deficiency, J Clin Endocrinol Metab 91 (2) (2006) 432–438.

[170] A.F. Attanasio, S.W. Lamberts, A.M. Matranga, M.A. Birkett, P.C. Bates, N.K. Valk, et al., Adult growth hormone (GH)-deficient patients demonstrate heterogeneity between childhood onset and adult onset before and during human GH treatment. Adult Growth Hormone Deficiency Study Group, J Clin Endocrinol Metab 82 (1) (1997) 82–88.

[171] R. Bouillon, E. Koledova, O. Bezlepkina, J. Nijs, E. Shavrikhova, E. Nagaeva, et al., Bone status and fracture prevalence in Russian adults with childhood-onset growth hormone deficiency, J Clin Endocrinol Metab 89 (10) (2004) 4993–4998.

[172] M. Pasarica, J.J. Zachwieja, L. Dejonge, S. Redman, S.R. Smith, Effect of growth hormone on body composition and visceral adiposity in middle-aged men with visceral obesity, J Clin Endocrinol Metab 92 (11) (2007) 4265–4270.

[173] R.S. Birnbaum, H.M. Goodman, Studies on the mechanism of the antilipolytic effects of growth hormone, Endocrinology 99 (5) (1976) 1336–1345.

[174] S. Yang, H. Mulder, C. Holm, S. Eden, Effects of growth hormone on the function of beta-adrenoceptor subtypes in rat adipocytes, Obes Res 12 (2) (2004) 330–339.

[175] M. Kawai, N. Namba, S. Mushiake, Y. Etani, R. Nishimura, M. Makishima, et al., Growth hormone stimulates adipogenesis of 3T3-L1 cells through activation of the Stat5A/5B-PPARgamma pathway, J Mol Endocrinol 38 (1–2) (2007) 19–34.

[176] M. Gola, S. Bonadonna, M. Doga, A. Giustina, Clinical review: Growth hormone and cardiovascular risk factors, J Clin Endocrinol Metab 90 (3) (2005) 1864–1870.

[177] P. Maison, S. Griffin, M. Nicoue-Beglah, N. Haddad, B. Balkau, P. Chanson, Impact of growth hormone (GH) treatment on cardiovascular risk factors in GH-deficient adults: A metaanalysis of blinded, randomized, placebo-controlled trials, J Clin Endocrinol Metab 89 (5) (2004) 2192–2199.

[178] C. Beauregard, A.L. Utz, A.E. Schaub, L. Nachtigall, B.M. Biller, K.K. Miller, et al., Growth hormone decreases visceral fat and improves cardiovascular risk markers in women with hypopituitarism: A randomized, placebo-controlled study, J Clin Endocrinol Metab 93 (6) (2008) 2063–2071.

[179] P. Kamenicky, S. Viengchareun, A. Blanchard, G. Meduri, P. Zizzari, M. Imbert-Teboul, et al., Epithelial sodium channel is a key mediator of growth hormone-induced sodium retention in acromegaly, Endocrinology 149 (7) (2008) 3294–3305.

[180] P.K. Tai, J.F. Liao, E.H. Chen, J. Dietz, J. Schwartz, C. Carter-Su, Differential regulation of two glucose transporters by chronic growth hormone treatment of cultured 3T3-F442A adipose cells, J Biol Chem 265 (35) (1990) 21828–21834.

[181] J. Bell, K.L. Parker, R.D. Swinford, A.R. Hoffman, T. Maneatis, B. Lippe, Long-term safety of recombinant human growth hormone in children, J Clin Endocrinol Metab 95 (1) (2010) 167–177.

[182] T.J. Merimee, P. Felig, E. Marliss, S.E. Fineberg, G.G. Cahill Jr., Glucose and lipid homeostasis in the absence of human growth hormone, J Clin Invest 50 (3) (1971) 574–582.

[183] J. Svensson, J. Fowelin, K. Landin, B.A. Bengtsson, J.O. Johansson, Effects of seven years of GH-replacement therapy on insulin sensitivity in GH-deficient adults, J Clin Endocrinol Metab 87 (5) (2002) 2121–2127.

[184] A. Colao, P. Marzullo, C. Di Somma, G. Lombardi, Growth hormone and the heart, Clin Endocrinol (Oxf) 54 (2) (2001) 137–154.

[185] G.A. Laughlin, E. Barrett-Connor, M.H. Criqui, D. Kritz-Silverstein, The prospective association of serum insulin-like growth factor I (IGF-I) and IGF-binding protein-1 levels with all cause and cardiovascular disease mortality in older adults: The Rancho Bernardo Study, J Clin Endocrinol Metab 89 (1) (2004) 114–120.

[186] R.S. Vasan, L.M. Sullivan, R.B. D'Agostino, R. Roubenoff, T. Harris, D.B. Sawyer, et al., Serum insulin-like growth factor I and risk for heart failure in elderly individuals without a previous myocardial infarction: The Framingham Heart Study, Ann Intern Med 139 (8) (2003) 642–648.

[187] A. Bayes-Genis, C.A. Conover, R.S. Schwartz, The insulin-like growth factor axis: A review of atherosclerosis and restenosis, Circ Res 86 (2) (2000) 125–130.

[188] A. Colao, C. Di Somma, M. Savanelli, M. De Leo, G. Lombardi, Beginning to end: Cardiovascular implications of growth hormone (GH) deficiency and GH therapy, Growth Horm IGF Res 16 (Suppl A) (2006) S41–S48.

[189] R. Abs, U. Feldt-Rasmussen, A.F. Mattsson, J.P. Monson, B.A. Bengtsson, M.I. Goth, et al., Determinants of cardiovascular risk in 2589 hypopituitary GH-deficient adults – a KIMS database analysis, Eur J Endocrinol 155 (1) (2006) 79–90.

[190] D.M. Hoffman, A.J. O'Sullivan, R.C. Baxter, K.K. Ho, Diagnosis of growth-hormone deficiency in adults, Lancet 343 (8905) (1994) 1064–1068.

[191] D.R. Clemmons, J.J. Van Wyk, E.C. Ridgway, B. Kliman, R.N. Kjellberg, L.E. Underwood, Evaluation of acromegaly by radioimmunoassay of somatomedin-C, N Engl J Med 301 (21) (1979) 1138–1142.

[192] A.L. Barkan, I.Z. Beitins, R.P. Kelch, Plasma insulin-like growth factor-I/somatomedin-C in acromegaly: Correlation with the degree of growth hormone hypersecretion, J Clin Endocrinol Metab 67 (1) (1988) 69–73.

[193] S. Melmed, A. Colao, A. Barkan, M. Molitch, A.B. Grossman, D. Kleinberg, et al., Guidelines for acromegaly management: An update, J Clin Endocrinol Metab 94 (5) (2009) 1509–1517.

[194] H.J. Dean, J.G. Kellett, R.M. Bala, H.J. Guyda, B. Bhaumick, B.I. Posner, et al., The effect of growth hormone treatment on somatomedin levels in growth hormone-deficient children, J Clin Endocrinol Metab 55 (6) (1982) 1167–1173.
[195] R.M. Bala, J. Lopatka, A. Leung, E. McCoy, R.G. McArthur, Serum immunoreactive somatomedin levels in normal adults, pregnant women at term, children at various ages, and children with constitutionally delayed growth, J Clin Endocrinol Metab 52 (3) (1981) 508–512.
[196] K.R. Rubin, J.M. Lichtenfels, S.K. Ratzan, M. Ozonoff, D.W. Rowe, D.E. Carey, Relationship of somatomedin-C concentration to bone age in boys with constitutional delay of growth, Am J Dis Child 140 (6) (1986) 555–558.
[197] M.E. Molitch, D.R. Clemmons, S. Malozowski, G.R. Merriam, S.M. Shalet, M.L. Vance, et al., Evaluation and treatment of adult growth hormone deficiency: An Endocrine Society Clinical Practice Guideline, J Clin Endocrinol Metab 91 (5) (2006) 1621–1634.
[198] E. Ghigo, J. Bellone, E. Mazza, E. Imperiale, M. Procopio, F. Valente, et al., Arginine potentiates the GHRH- but not the pyridostigmine-induced GH secretion in normal short children. Further evidence for a somatostatin suppressing effect of arginine, Clin Endocrinol (Oxf) 32 (6) (1990) 763–767.
[199] B.M. Biller, M.H. Samuels, A. Zagar, D.M. Cook, B.M. Arafah, V. Bonert, et al., Sensitivity and specificity of six tests for the diagnosis of adult GH deficiency, J Clin Endocrinol Metab 87 (5) (2002) 2067–2079.
[200] V. Popovic, A. Leal, D. Micic, H.P. Koppeschaar, E. Torres, C. Paramo, et al., GH-releasing hormone and GH-releasing peptide-6 for diagnostic testing in GH-deficient adults, Lancet 356 (9236) (2000) 1137–1142.
[201] K.K. Ho, Diagnosis of adult GH deficiency, Lancet 356 (9236) (2000) 1125–1126.
[202] K.K. Ho, Consensus guidelines for the diagnosis and treatment of adults with GH deficiency II: A statement of the GH Research Society in association with the European Society for Pediatric Endocrinology, Lawson Wilkins Society, European Society of Endocrinology, Japan Endocrine Society, and Endocrine Society of Australia, Eur J Endocrinol 157 (6) (2007) 695–700.
[203] M.L. Hartman, B.J. Crowe, B.M. Biller, K.K. Ho, D.R. Clemmons, J.J. Chipman, Which patients do not require a GH stimulation test for the diagnosis of adult GH deficiency? J Clin Endocrinol Metab 87 (2) (2002) 477–485.
[204] K.H. Darzy, G. Aimaretti, G. Wieringa, H.R. Gattamaneni, E. Ghigo, S.M. Shalet, The usefulness of the combined growth hormone (GH)-releasing hormone and arginine stimulation test in the diagnosis of radiation-induced GH deficiency is dependent on the post-irradiation time interval, J Clin Endocrinol Metab 88 (1) (2003) 95–102.
[205] V.S. Bonert, J.D. Elashoff, P. Barnett, S. Melmed, Body mass index determines evoked growth hormone (GH) responsiveness in normal healthy male subjects: Diagnostic caveat for adult GH deficiency, J Clin Endocrinol Metab 89 (7) (2004) 3397–3401.
[206] G. Corneli, C. Di Somma, R. Baldelli, S. Rovere, V. Gasco, C.G. Croce, et al., The cut-off limits of the GH response to GH-releasing hormone-arginine test related to body mass index, Eur J Endocrinol 153 (2) (2005) 257–264.
[207] Consensus guidelines for the diagnosis and treatment of adults with growth hormone deficiency, summary statement of the Growth Hormone Research Society Workshop on Adult Growth Hormone Deficiency, J Clin Endocrinol Metab 83 (2) (1998) 379–381.
[208] M. Tauber, P. Moulin, C. Pienkowski, B. Jouret, P. Rochiccioli, Growth hormone (GH) retesting and auxological data in 131 GH-deficient patients after completion of treatment, J Clin Endocrinol Metab 82 (2) (1997) 352–356.
[209] M. Bidlingmaier, P.U. Freda, Measurement of human growth hormone by immunoassays: Current status, unsolved problems and clinical consequences, Growth Horm IGF Res 20 (1) (2010) 19–25.
[210] A. Pokrajac, G. Wark, A.R. Ellis, J. Wear, G.E. Wieringa, P.J. Trainer, Variation in GH and IGF-I assays limits the applicability of international consensus criteria to local practice, Clin Endocrinol (Oxf) 67 (1) (2007) 65–70.
[211] D.R. Clemmons, IGF-I assays: Current assay methodologies and their limitations, Pituitary 10 (2) (2007) 121–128.
[212] C. Massart, J.Y. Poirier, Serum insulin-like growth factor-I measurement in the follow-up of treated acromegaly: Comparison of four immunoassays, Clin Chim Acta 373 (1–2) (2006) 176–179.
[213] A. Krebs, H. Wallaschofski, E. Spilcke-Liss, T. Kohlmann, G. Brabant, H. Volzke, et al., Five commercially available insulin-like growth factor I (IGF-I) assays in comparison to the former Nichols Advantage IGF-I in a growth hormone treated population, Clin Chem Lab Med 46 (12) (2008) 1776–1783.
[214] J. Frystyk, P. Freda, D.R. Clemmons, The current status of IGF-I assays – a 2009 update, Growth Horm IGF Res 20 (1) (2010) 8–18.
[215] M.A. Sperling, P.H. Saenger, H. Ray, W. Tom, S.R. Rose, Growth hormone treatment and neoplasia – coincidence or consequence? J Clin Endocrinol Metab 87 (12) (2002) 5351–5352.
[216] M.L. Vance, N. Mauras, Growth hormone therapy in adults and children, N Engl J Med 341 (16) (1999) 1206–1216.
[217] C.A. Quigley, Growth hormone treatment of non-growth hormone-deficient growth disorders, Endocrinol Metab Clin North Am 36 (1) (2007) 131–186.
[218] J. Bryant, L. Baxter, C.B. Cave, R. Milne, Recombinant growth hormone for idiopathic short stature in children and adolescents, Cochrane Database Syst Rev (3) (2007) CD004440.
[219] D.K. Stephure, Impact of growth hormone supplementation on adult height in Turner syndrome: Results of the Canadian randomized controlled trial, J Clin Endocrinol Metab 90 (6) (2005) 3360–3366.
[220] W.S. Cutfield, P. Wilton, H. Bennmarker, K. Albertsson-Wikland, P. Chatelain, M.B. Ranke, et al., Incidence of diabetes mellitus and impaired glucose tolerance in children and adolescents receiving growth-hormone treatment, Lancet 355 (9204) (2000) 610–613.
[221] F. de Zegher, A. Hokken-Koelega, Growth hormone therapy for children born small for gestational age: Height gain is less dose dependent over the long term than over the short term, Pediatrics 115 (4) (2005) e458–e462.
[222] D. Vimalachandra, J.C. Craig, C. Cowell, J.F. Knight, Growth hormone for children with chronic renal failure, Cochrane Database Syst Rev (4) (2001) CD003264.
[223] K. Yuen, B. Biller, M. Molitch, D. Cook, Clinical review: Is lack of recombinant growth hormone (GH)-releasing hormone in the United States a setback or time to consider glucagon testing for adult GH deficiency? J Clin Endocrinol Metab 94 (8) (2009) 2702–2707.
[224] D.M. Cook, W.H. Ludlam, M.B. Cook, Route of estrogen administration helps to determine growth hormone (GH) replacement dose in GH-deficient adults, J Clin Endocrinol Metab 84 (11) (1999) 3956–3960.
[225] A.R. Hoffman, J.E. Kuntze, J. Baptista, H.B. Baum, G.P. Baumann, B.M. Biller, et al., Growth hormone (GH) replacement therapy in adult-onset GH deficiency: Effects on body composition in men and women in a double-blind, randomized, placebo-controlled trial, J Clin Endocrinol Metab 89 (5) (2004) 2048–2056.

[226] G. Frajese, W.M. Drake, R.A. Loureiro, J. Evanson, D. Coyte, D.F. Wood, et al., Hypothalamo–pituitary surveillance imaging in hypopituitary patients receiving long-term GH replacement therapy, J Clin Endocrinol Metab 86 (11) (2001) 5172–5175.

[227] N. Karavitaki, J.T. Warner, A. Marland, B. Shine, F. Ryan, J. Arnold, et al., GH replacement does not increase the risk of recurrence in patients with craniopharyngioma, Clin Endocrinol (Oxf) 64 (5) (2006) 556–560.

[228] A. Jostel, A. Mukherjee, P.A. Hulse, S.M. Shalet, Adult growth hormone replacement therapy and neuroimaging surveillance in brain tumour survivors, Clin Endocrinol (Oxf) 62 (6) (2005) 698–705.

[229] E.M. Erfurth, B. Bulow, C.H. Nordstrom, Z. Mikoczy, L. Hagmar, U. Stromberg, Doubled mortality rate in irradiated patients reoperated for regrowth of a macroadenoma of the pituitary gland, Eur J Endocrinol 150 (4) (2004) 497–502.

[230] J.M. Chan, M.J. Stampfer, E. Giovannucci, P.H. Gann, J. Ma, P. Wilkinson, et al., Plasma insulin-like growth factor-I and prostate cancer risk: A prospective study, Science 279 (5350) (1998) 563–566.

[231] S.E. Hankinson, W.C. Willett, G.A. Colditz, D.J. Hunter, D.S. Michaud, B. Deroo, et al., Circulating concentrations of insulin-like growth factor-I and risk of breast cancer, Lancet 351 (9113) (1998) 1393–1396.

[232] J. Ma, M.N. Pollak, E. Giovannucci, J.M. Chan, Y. Tao, C.H. Hennekens, et al., Prospective study of colorectal cancer risk in men and plasma levels of insulin-like growth factor (IGF)-I and IGF-binding protein-3, J Natl Cancer Inst 91 (7) (1999) 620–625.

[233] M. Losa, M. Scavini, E. Gatti, A. Rossini, S. Madaschi, I. Formenti, et al., Long-term effects of growth hormone replacement therapy on thyroid function in adults with growth hormone deficiency, Thyroid 18 (12) (2008) 1249–1254.

[234] C. Giavoli, R. Libe, S. Corbetta, E. Ferrante, A. Lania, M. Arosio, et al., Effect of recombinant human growth hormone (GH) replacement on the hypothalamic–pituitary–adrenal axis in adult GH-deficient patients, J Clin Endocrinol Metab 89 (11) (2004) 5397–5401.

[235] H. Liu, D.M. Bravata, I. Olkin, S. Nayak, B. Roberts, A.M. Garber, et al., Systematic review: The safety and efficacy of growth hormone in the healthy elderly, Ann Intern Med 146 (2) (2007) 104–115.

[236] D.E. Berryman, J.S. Christiansen, G. Johannsson, M.O. Thorner, J.J. Kopchick, Role of the GH/IGF-1 axis in lifespan and healthspan: Lessons from animal models, Growth Horm IGF Res 18 (6) (2008) 455–471.

[237] A. Bartke, J.C. Wright, J.A. Mattison, D.K. Ingram, R.A. Miller, G.S. Roth, Extending the lifespan of long-lived mice, Nature 414 (6862) (2001) 412.

[238] K. Flurkey, J. Papaconstantinou, R.A. Miller, D.E. Harrison, Lifespan extension and delayed immune and collagen aging in mutant mice with defects in growth hormone production, Proc Nat Acad Sci USA 98 (12) (2001) 6736–6741.

[239] W.Y. Chen, M.E. White, T.E. Wagner, J.J. Kopchick, Functional antagonism between endogenous mouse growth hormone (GH) and a GH analog results in dwarf transgenic mice, Endocrinology 129 (3) (1991) 1402–1408.

[240] S. Yakar, J.L. Liu, B. Stannard, A. Butler, D. Accili, B. Sauer, et al., Normal growth and development in the absence of hepatic insulin-like growth factor I, Proc Nat Acad Sci USA 96 (13) (1999) 7324–7329.

[241] N. Barzilai, A. Bartke, Biological approaches to mechanistically understand the healthy life span extension achieved by calorie restriction and modulation of hormones, J Gerontol A Biol Sci Med Sci 64 (2) (2009) 187–191.

[242] R. Nass, S.S. Pezzoli, M.C. Oliveri, J.T. Patrie, F.E. Harrell Jr., J.L. Clasey, et al., Effects of an oral ghrelin mimetic on body composition and clinical outcomes in healthy older adults: A randomized trial, Ann Intern Med 149 (9) (2008) 601–611.

[243] F.R. Sattler, C. Castaneda-Sceppa, E.F. Binder, E.T. Schroeder, Y. Wang, S. Bhasin, et al., Testosterone and growth hormone improve body composition and muscle performance in older men, J Clin Endocrinol Metab 94 (6) (2009) 1991–2001.

[244] R.I. Holt, E. Webb, C. Pentecost, P.H. Sonksen, Aging and physical fitness are more important than obesity in determining exercise-induced generation of GH, J Clin Endocrinol Metab 86 (12) (2001) 5715–5720.

[245] W.M. Widdowson, J. Gibney, The effect of growth hormone replacement on exercise capacity in patients with GH deficiency: A metaanalysis, J Clin Endocrinol Metab 93 (11) (2008) 4413–4417.

[246] J. Gibney, M.L. Healy, M. Stolinski, S.B. Bowes, C. Pentecost, L. Breen, et al., Effect of growth hormone (GH) on glycerol and free fatty acid metabolism during exhaustive exercise in GH-deficient adults, J Clin Endocrinol Metab 88 (4) (2003) 1792–1797.

[247] A. Colao, C. di Somma, A. Cuocolo, L. Spinelli, N. Tedesco, R. Pivonello, et al., Improved cardiovascular risk factors and cardiac performance after 12 months of growth hormone (GH) replacement in young adult patients with GH deficiency, J Clin Endocrinol Metab 86 (5) (2001) 1874–1881.

[248] A. Colao, C. Di Somma, A. Cuocolo, M. Filippella, F. Rota, W. Acampa, et al., The severity of growth hormone deficiency correlates with the severity of cardiac impairment in 100 adult patients with hypopituitarism: An observational, case-control study, J Clin Endocrinol Metab 89 (12) (2004) 5998–6004.

[249] L.J. Woodhouse, A. Mukherjee, S.M. Shalet, S. Ezzat, The influence of growth hormone status on physical impairments, functional limitations, and health-related quality of life in adults, Endocr Rev 27 (3) (2006) 287–317.

[250] J. Gibney, T. Wolthers, G. Johannsson, A.M. Umpleby, K.K. Ho, Growth hormone and testosterone interact positively to enhance protein and energy metabolism in hypopituitary men, Am J Physiol Endocrinol Metab 289 (2) (2005) E266–E271.

[251] J. Svensson, K.S. Sunnerhagen, G. Johannsson, Five years of growth hormone replacement therapy in adults: Age- and gender-related changes in isometric and isokinetic muscle strength, J Clin Endocrinol Metab 88 (5) (2003) 2061–2069.

[252] B.A. Irving, J.T. Patrie, S.M. Anderson, D.D. Watson-Winfield, K.I. Frick, W.S. Evans, et al., The effects of time following acute growth hormone administration on metabolic and power output measures during acute exercise, J Clin Endocrinol Metab 89 (9) (2004) 4298–4305.

[253] M.L. Healy, J. Gibney, D.L. Russell-Jones, C. Pentecost, P. Croos, P.H. Sonksen, et al., High dose growth hormone exerts an anabolic effect at rest and during exercise in endurance-trained athletes, J Clin Endocrinol Metab 88 (11) (2003) 5221–5226.

[254] J.S. Baker, M.R. Graham, B. Davies, Steroid and prescription medicine abuse in the health and fitness community: A regional study, Eur J Intern Med 17 (7) (2006) 479–484.

[255] H. Liu, D.M. Bravata, I. Olkin, A. Friedlander, V. Liu, B. Roberts, et al., Systematic review: The effects of growth hormone on athletic performance, Ann Intern Med 148 (10) (2008) 747–758.

[256] M.R. Graham, J.S. Baker, P. Evans, A. Kicman, D. Cowan, D. Hullin, et al., Physical effects of short-term recombinant human growth hormone administration in abstinent steroid dependency, Horm Res 69 (6) (2008) 343–354.

[257] J.K. Powrie, E.E. Bassett, T. Rosen, J.O. Jorgensen, R. Napoli, L. Sacca, et al., Detection of growth hormone abuse in sport, Growth Horm IGF Res 17 (3) (2007) 220–226.

[258] J.D. Wallace, R.C. Cuneo, M. Bidlingmaier, P.A. Lundberg, L. Carlsson, C.L. Boguszewski, et al., Changes in non-22-kilodalton (kDa) isoforms of growth hormone (GH) after administration of 22-kDa recombinant human GH in trained adult males, J Clin Endocrinol Metab 86 (4) (2001) 1731–1737.

[259] I. Erotokritou-Mulligan, E.E. Bassett, D.A. Cowan, C. Bartlett, C. McHugh, P.H. Sonksen, et al., Influence of ethnicity on IGF-I and procollagen III peptide (P-III-P) in elite athletes and its effect on the ability to detect GH abuse, Clin Endocrinol (Oxf) 70 (1) (2009) 161–168.

[260] A.E. Nelson, C.J. Howe, T.V. Nguyen, K.C. Leung, G.J. Trout, M.J. Seibel, et al., Influence of demographic factors and sport type on growth hormone-responsive markers in elite athletes, J Clin Endocrinol Metab 91 (11) (2006) 4424–4432.

[261] C.J. Mitchell, A.E. Nelson, M.J. Cowley, W. Kaplan, G. Stone, S.K. Sutton, et al., Detection of growth hormone doping by gene expression profiling of peripheral blood, J Clin Endocrinol Metab 94 (12) (2009) 4703–4709.

[262] J. Ma, M. Pollak, E. Giovannucci, J.M. Chan, Y. Tao, C. Hennekens, et al., A prospective study of plasma levels of insulin-like growth factor I (IGF-I) and IGF-binding protein-3, and colorectal cancer risk among men, Growth Horm IGF Res 10 (Suppl A) (2000) S28–S29.

[263] A. Lukanova, P. Toniolo, A. Akhmedkhanov, C. Biessy, N.J. Haley, R.E. Shore, et al., A prospective study of insulin-like growth factor-I, IGF-binding proteins-1, -2 and -3 and lung cancer risk in women, Int J Cancer 92 (6) (2001) 888–892.

[264] G.F. Cahill Jr., M.G. Herrera, A.P. Morgan, J.S. Soeldner, J. Steinke, P.L. Levy, et al., Hormone–fuel interrelationships during fasting, J Clin Invest 45 (11) (1966) 1751–1769.

[265] W.L. Isley, L.E. Underwood, D.R. Clemmons, Dietary components that regulate serum somatomedin-C concentrations in humans, J Clin Invest 71 (2) (1983) 175–182.

[266] P.F. Backeljauw, L.E. Underwood, Therapy for 6.5–7.5 years with recombinant insulin-like growth factor I in children with growth hormone insensitivity syndrome: A clinical research center study, J Clin Endocrinol Metab 86 (4) (2001) 1504–1510.

[267] Z. Laron, B. Klinger, Comparison of the growth-promoting effects of insulin-like growth factor I and growth hormone in the early years of life, Acta Paediatr 89 (1) (2000) 38–41.

[268] S.L. Furth, Growth and nutrition in children with chronic kidney disease, Adv Chronic Kidney Dis 12 (4) (2005) 366–371.

[269] Z. Laron, S. Anin, Y. Klipper-Aurbach, B. Klinger, Effects of insulin-like growth factor on linear growth, head circumference, and body fat in patients with Laron-type dwarfism, Lancet 339 (8804) (1992) 1258–1261.

[270] D. Vimalachandra, E.M. Hodson, N.S. Willis, J.C. Craig, C. Cowell, J.F. Knight, Growth hormone for children with chronic kidney disease, Cochrane Database Syst Rev (3) (2006) CD003264.

[271] D.R. Clemmons, Clinical utility of measurements of insulin-like growth factor 1, Nat Clin Pract Endocrinol Metab 2 (8) (2006) 436–446.

[272] S. Melmed, Medical progress: Acromegaly, N Engl J Med 355 (24) (2006) 2558–2573.

[273] R.E. Humbel, Insulin-like growth factors I and II, Eur J Biochem 190 (3) (1990) 445–462.

[274] A.L. Rosenbloom, Growth hormone insensitivity: Physiologic and genetic basis, phenotype, and treatment, J Pediatr 135 (3) (1999) 280–289.

[275] Z. Zadik, S.A. Chalew, R.J. McCarter Jr., M. Meistas, A.A. Kowarski, The influence of age on the 24-hour integrated concentration of growth hormone in normal individuals, J Clin Endocrinol Metab 60 (3) (1985) 513–516.

[276] S. Rajaram, D.J. Baylink, S. Mohan, Insulin-like growth factor-binding proteins in serum and other biological fluids: Regulation and functions, Endocr Rev 18 (6) (1997) 801–831.

[277] P.V. Carroll, E.R. Christ, B.A. Bengtsson, L. Carlsson, J.S. Christiansen, D. Clemmons, et al., Growth hormone deficiency in adulthood and the effects of growth hormone replacement: A review. Growth Hormone Research Society Scientific Committee, J Clin Endocrinol Metab 83 (2) (1998) 382–395.

CHAPTER

5

Prolactin

Mary P. Gillam [1], *Mark E. Molitch* [2]

[1] Endocrinologist, Chicago, IL, USA,

[2] Northwestern University Feinberg School of Medicine, Chicago, IL, USA

HISTORICAL OVERVIEW

In the late 1920s and early 1930s, it was found that pituitary extracts could induce milk secretion [1–3]. Riddle and coworkers found that this substance, which they named prolactin (PRL), could be differentiated from the known growth- and gonad-stimulating substances [1–3]. In these experiments, they showed that PRL stimulated milk production by guinea pig mammary glands and a milk-like substance from the crop sacs of pigeons and doves, giving rise to the pigeon crop sac bioassay for PRL [1–3].

Over the ensuing years, PRL was characterized, sequenced and specific radioimmunoassays (RIAs) developed for PRL from a number of species. Because of the high lactogenic activity of even very highly purified preparations of human growth hormone (GH), however, it was impossible to separate human PRL from GH using the relatively crude pigeon crop assay. However, several human disease states provided strong evidence that these two hormones were separate. For example, it was observed that most patients with pituitary tumors in whom galactorrhea and amenorrhea were the cardinal clinical features did not have acromegalic features and patients who were known to have isolated, congenital GH deficiency were able to undergo postpartum lactation. Finally, in 1970, Frantz and Kleinberg developed a sensitive in vitro bioassay which involved staining milk produced by cultured, lactating mouse mammary tissue in response to PRL that was capable of measuring PRL levels as low as 5 ng/ml. In this assay they added excess antibody to GH to neutralize any potential lactogenic effects it had and, for the first time, were able to demonstrate measurable PRL levels in women with puerperal and nonpuerperal galactorrhea, but not in most normal men and women [4]. Shortly thereafter, an RIA for human PRL was developed which could finally measure PRL levels in the sera of normal individuals, permitting the eventual sequencing of human PRL [5] and determination of its cDNA sequence [6].

CELL OF ORIGIN

PRL is made by the pituitary lactotrophs (also known as mammotrophs). In the normal human pituitary, the lactotrophs comprise about 15–25% of the total number of cells, are similar in number in both sexes, and do not change significantly with age [7]. During pregnancy and subsequent lactation, however, substantial lactotroph hyperplasia may be observed [8], presumably as a result of lactotroph proliferation, the transdifferentiation of somatotrophs and/or expansion from a stem cell population [8–10]. The hyperplastic process involutes within several months after delivery, although breast-feeding retards this process [8]. This stimulatory effect of pregnancy on the lactotrophs also holds true for prolactinomas, which may be subject to significant pregnancy-induced tumor enlargement (see Chapter 15). Details regarding the morphology of normal and tumorous lactotrophs can be found in Chapter 22.

Lactotroph Ontogeny

Continuous hypothalamic–pituitary interaction takes place during embryological development. During the formation of Rathke's pouch, the primordium of the anterior pituitary, the ectodermal primordial cells of the anterior and intermediate lobes of the pituitary make contact with the neuroectoderm of the floor of the diencephalon; experimental studies have shown inductive interactions between these tissues that are necessary for their subsequent interdependent development. Elegant studies using a series of targeted mutations have shown that there are a number of

The Pituitary, Third Edition, DOI: 10.1016/B978-0-12-380926-1.10005-7

transcription factors (Six-3, Hesx1, Lhx3, Lhx4, Sox2, Sox 3, Pitx2, Otx2, Bmp2, Bmp4 and Gli2) that are sequentially expressed in the developing hypothalamus and pituitary that lead to the final determination of the five mature pituitary cell types and the functional integration of the hypothalamic–pituitary system [11]. Mutations in most of the genes for these factors have been shown in humans to result in disordered development of hypothalamic, pituitary and other brain structures, with varying degrees of hypopituitarism.

The POU homeodomain transcription factor Pou1f1 (also called Pit-1) gene (see below) becomes activated relatively late in development and is necessary for the activation of the PRL, GH, GHRH receptor and TSHβ genes, as well as being necessary for the differentiation and proliferation of these cell lineages. A point mutation in the POU homeodomain of Pou1f1 has been found to be the cause of the GH, PRL and TSH deficiencies found in the Snell dwarf mouse, with absence of somatotroph, lactotroph and thyrotroph cells [12]. Similar mutations in Pou1f1 have now been found to cause a similar deficiency of GH, PRL and TSH in humans [11]. A second paired-like homeodomain factor, known as Prophet of Pit-1 (Prop-1) has also been found to be necessary for the expression of Pit-1. Mutations of the Prop-1 gene cause the dwarfism in mice known as the Ames mouse (defects of somatotrophs, lactotrophs and thyrotrophs) and similar mutations in humans cause variable deficiencies of GH, PRL, TSH, LH and FSH [11].

Many lactotrophs arise from cells that at least at some point expressed the GH gene [13]. However, at least in mice, it appears that many, if not most, lactotrophs may derive from an earlier precursor [14]. Subsequent lactotroph proliferation occurs once estrogen receptors appear [13]. Estrogen stimulates PRL gene transcription (see below) only if Pou1f1 is bound to the PRL promoter [15]. Stimulation by Prop-1 is necessary for the subsequent development of all noncorticotroph cells. Pou1f1 is then necessary for the development and proliferation of thyrotrophs and somatomammotrophs, but the separation of these two cell lines occurs before the appearance of the ability to synthesize α-subunits. The final differentiation of somatomammotrophs occurs at least in part in relationship to estrogen stimulation.

PROLACTIN GENE

Prolactin belongs to the somatotropin/prolactin family, a large family of proteins that includes growth hormone (GH), placental lactogens (PL), prolactin-like and prolactin-related proteins, proliferins and proliferin-related proteins. The human prolactin gene is located on chromosome 6p22.2-p21.3 and consists of five coding exons, one noncoding exon and four introns [16]. It is believed that PRL, GH and PL arose from duplication of a common ancestral gene ~400 million years ago [6]. The entire PRL locus in both humans and rats spans a region of ~10 kb. The human PRL cDNA is 914 nucleotides long and contains a 681-nucleotide open reading frame encoding mRNA for a prohormone (pre-prolactin) of 227 amino acids. During PRL processing, the 28-amino acid signal peptide is proteolytically cleaved [5], resulting in a mature 199-amino acid PRL polypeptide with a molecular weight of 23 kDa. Genes for the related hormones GH and PL (or chorionic somatomamotropin, CS) are clustered on chromosome 17 [17].

Much of the knowledge regarding regulation of PRL gene expression has been derived from studies utilizing the rat pituitary PRL promoter. Less information is available on regulation of hPRL and mouse PRL. Although attempts have been made to investigate hPRL regulation by transfecting the hPRL promoter into rat GH3 cells, it is uncertain how reliably this type of experimental system recapitulates hPRL promoter activity, since transformed rat and human lactotrophs may not share the same repertoire of endogenous transcriptional and/or epigenetic regulators. The rPRL gene is controlled by a proximal promoter and a distal enhancer, located −433/−20 bp and 1800/−1500 bp respectively, relative to the pituitary transcriptional start site. In rats, 3 kb of 5′-flanking region is sufficient to direct lactotroph-specific transgene expression and a synergistic interaction between the distal enhancer and proximal promoter region is required for high levels of expression [18]. Sequences flanking the enhancer restrict PRL expression to pituitary lactotrophs.

Organization of the hPRL gene is more complex, and its transcription is regulated by two main independent promoter regions (Figure 5.1). The proximal 5800 bp region directs pituitary-specific expression [19], while a more upstream promoter region, designated the "superdistal PRL promoter," is responsible for directing extrapituitary expression [20]. Although most of circulating PRL in serum is produced by pituitary lactotrophs, PRL is also expressed in several extrapituitary tissues, including uterine decidualized endometrium, breast, brain, prostate, lymphocytes, skin and adipose tissue. PRL expression at these sites is cell-type-specific and Pit-1 independent [21]. In human extrapituitary tissues, PRL mRNA transcription is driven by the alternative "superdistal PRL promoter" located 5.8 kb upstream of the pituitary transcription start site, resulting in transcription of an extra exon, designated exon 1a. This alternative exon 1a of hPRL gene is noncoding, and transcription from either promoter produces mRNAs with differing 5′ untranslated regions (UTR) but identical protein-coding sequences. Although the

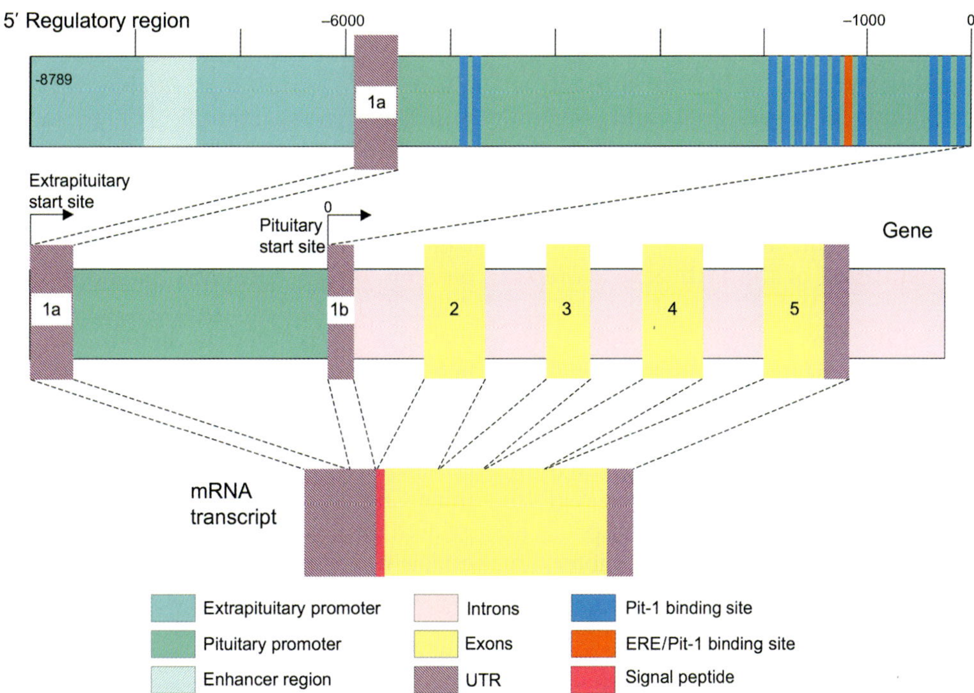

FIGURE 5.1 Schematic diagram of the human prolactin (PRL) 5′ gene regulatory region, gene and mRNA transcript. The PRL gene consists of five exons, designated by the numbers [1−5]. The region from −5800 base pairs (bp) to 0 indicates the region known to regulate pituitary PRL synthesis whereas the region from −8789 to −5800 is referred to as the "superdistal" or "extrapituitary" promoter region. Thirteen Pit1-binding sites are present in the regulatory region. A single degenerate estrogen response element (ERE) has been identified at −1189 bp. The extrapituitary PRL mRNA is ~150 bp longer than the pituitary transcript, and has a different 5′ UTR, but transcription from either promoter produces identical protein coding sequences.

purpose of the alternative promoter is not known for certain, it appears to confer tissue-specific expression, and it is likely that the variant 5′ UTRs may influence the stability or translational efficiency of the disparate PRL transcripts [22−24].

Characterization and analysis of the far upstream elements dictating extrapituitary hPRL expression are incomplete but evolving. In silico analysis of the extrapituitary hPRL promoter has revealed that the 5′ proximal region of the extrapituitary hPRL promoter, as well as exon 1a and a portion of intronic sequence, occur within a long terminal repeat-like [25] transposable element (TE) of the medium frequency reiterated repeat (MER) family. The LTR sequence, named MER39, appears to have been inserted ~30 million years ago before the divergence of monkeys from higher apes. In addition, an older TE, MER20, provides an additional 198 bp of the 5′ flanking region of exon 1a. TE-derived sequences typically regulate nearby human genes and, in most cases, the LTR acts as an alternative promoter, but does not alter the coding sequence [26,27]. Some of the transcription-factor-binding sites that mediate extrapituitary PRL expression are located within these TE sites. For example, responsiveness to cAMP is mediated by a degenerate cAMP-responsive element (CRE) located within the MER39 LTR [28]. Thus, the evolutionary acquisition of these two TEs may underlie the ability of mammals to express PRL in extrapituitary tissues.

Pit-1

Transcriptional regulators that control development of anterior pituitary lactotrophs also control PRL synthesis during adult life. Prominent among these is the Pit-1 protein, a POU-homeodomain transcription factor that dictates the terminal differentiation of pituitary somatotrophs, lactotrophs and thyrotrophs, and regulates expression of their respective protein hormone genes, GH, PRL and TSHβ. Multiple signaling pathways ultimately converge upon Pit-1, and as such Pit-1 serves as the main transcriptional regulator of PRL gene expression. Pit-1 integrates information from a wide range of signaling pathways (triiodothyronine, estradiol, glucocorticoids, protein kinase A, protein kinase C and Ras) in a cell-specific manner by functionally interacting with numerous nuclear hormone receptors and coregulators (including itself, ER, TR, GR, cJun, Oct1, GATA2, P-Lim, Ptx-1, Ets), and recruiting them to Pit-1-regulated promoters [29−37].

Through its interactions with specific DNA elements in target gene promoters, Pit-1 recruits coregulatory proteins that alter histone acetylation and modify the chromatin structure, providing either a permissive or repressive environment for transcription [38–42]. Precise homeostatic control is achieved through a network of interactions between Pit-1 and several different classes of transcription factors, including the nuclear receptors [34], other homeodomain proteins [43], Ets family proteins [32] and basic region-leucine zipper (B-Zip) transcription factors [44].

Transcriptional activation of the PRL gene requires the assembly of specific coactivator complexes at Pit-1 composite DNA-binding sites. There are eight Pit-1-binding sites (four within the proximal promoter, four within the enhancer) in the regulatory region of the rat PRL gene, whereas there are 13 known Pit-1-binding sites (three within the proximal promoter, eight within the distal enhancer, two within the superdistal region) in the human PRL promoter [45,46]. CBP/p300 is required for Pit-1 activation of PRL promoter in response to PKA activation [42].

Pit-1 contains two well-defined functional motifs that affect its activity: the transcriptional activation domain [47] and DNA-binding domain (DBD). The amino terminal TAD contains a regulatory domain and a basal and Ras-responsive region. This latter region contains a basal activation region and an overlapping, dual-function, Ras-responsive and inhibitory segment. Distinct coactivators mediate basal and Ras-activated Pit-1 TAD activity, with CBP/p300 being a key effector of Pit-1's basal TAD, and steroid receptor coactivator-1 (SRC-1) a mediator of Ras responsiveness [48–50]. DNA binding of Pit-1 is achieved through a carboxy-terminal DBD composed of two motifs, referred to as the POU-specific (POU_S) and POU-homeo (POU_{HD}) domains [51], both of which are necessary for high-affinity DNA binding. The combination of this bipartite DBD and specific DNA-binding sites generates a complex "code" which enables various subdomains within Pit-1 to adopt specific configurations; these subsequently control the recruitment of various coregulators to fine-tune PRL gene transcription [52].

A Pit-1 splice isoform known as Pit-1β contains a 26-amino acid motif inserted at amino acid 48, in the middle of the Pit-1 transcription activation domain [47], resulting from an alternative splicing event that uses an in-frame acceptor 78 nucleotides upstream of exon 2 [53]. In contrast to the activation of anterior pituitary hormone promoters by Pit-1, Pit-1β represses GH, PRL and TSHβ promoters in a pituitary cell-specific manner [54]. The Pit-1β repression is potent as it is capable of inhibiting the oncogenic Ras response of the rPRL promoter [52]. Mechanistically, this Pit-1β motif-dependent transcriptional repression results from the active recruitment of corepressors as well as interference with efficient recruitment of CBP [38,55–57].

Studies investigating Pit-1 regulation of PRL and pituitary gene expression have determined that several mechanisms exist that enable Pit-1 to respond to multiple diverse stimuli. For example, Pit-1 largely binds to DNA elements as a dimer, but under the influence of certain signaling events will bind as a monomer. Crystal structure analysis reveals that Pit-1 homodimerizes in a head-to-tail fashion to achieve optimal DNA binding on an idealized palindromic sequence [58]. The activity of Pit-1 homodimers on dimeric sites in the rPRL promoter is determined by the balance between corepressor (NCoR/SMRT, mSin3A/B) and coactivator (histone acetylases, CBP, P300/CBP) complexes at the transcriptional start site. In fact, homodimerization of Pit-1 appears to be important to maximize CBP recruitment in response to insulin and other growth factor stimulation [50,59]. In contrast, Ras or estrogen receptor alpha activation of the rPRL promoter at a monomeric Pit-1/Ets composite binding site is independent of CBP and instead relies upon a p160 SRC coactivator complex [52,60]. The recruitment of these specific transcriptional complexes is dependent upon structural features that are revealed when Pit-1 binds to DNA sites as a monomer or as a dimer. In addition, differences in the spacing between DNA contact points for the POU_S and POU_{HD} domains alter the structure of the linker region, such that the 4 bp spacing on a Pit-1 site in the PRL promoter results in an activating Pit-1 conformation, whereas a 6 bp spacing in the GH promoter coverts Pit-1 to a repressor in pituitary lactotrophs [39]. Finally, phosphorylation of Pit-1 by protein kinase A, protein kinase C and cyclin-dependent kinases modifies its conformation on DNA recognition elements and thus alters its DNA-binding affinity [61,62]. Phosphorylation specifically inhibits binding of Pit-1 to monomeric DNA sites (i.e., those used by Ras and estradiol) and consequently decreases its transcriptional activity in response to these signaling events, whereas phosphorylation has no effect on basal, dimeric Pit-1 binding [63]. Thus, a plethora of mechanisms, including monomeric versus dimeric Pit-1 binding, relative spacing of the Pit-1 POU_S and POU_{HD} binding sites, and the phosphorylation status of Pit-1 all together generate a unique structural interface for the binding of distinct coactivator/corepressor complexes to regulate the expression of the PRL gene in pituitary lactotrophs.

Estrogen

Estrogen is an important physiological activator of both PRL gene synthesis and lactotroph proliferation. At present, three identified estrogen receptors (ER) are expressed in the adenohypophysis: two classical nuclear ERs, ER alpha (α) and ER beta (β), which function as ligand-activated nuclear transcription factors; and G-protein-coupled estrogen receptor 1 (GPR30, GPER1), a seven-transmembrane GPCR that binds with high affinity to estradiol and mediates rapid signaling events. Both ERα and ERβ are expressed in human and rat lactotrophs [64,65]. The mouse pituitary expresses ERα, but not ERβ [66,67]. GPR30 expression in rodent adenohypophysis has been confirmed by in situ hybridization and immunohistochemistry, but detailed information regarding specific cell type localization of this receptor, or possible functional roles in mediating or contributing to estradiol effects in lactotrophs, are not known [68,69]. The in vivo function of ERα in regulating PRL expression has been demonstrated in mice with targeted deletion of the ERα gene (ERαKO). Although the specification of the lactotroph lineage occurs normally in these animals, there is a 10–20-fold reduction in PRL mRNA levels and a decrease in number of lactotrophs [70]. Curiously, plasma PRL levels are only slightly reduced, probably as a result of compensatory mechanisms, such as heightened sensitivity to PRL secretagogues. Pituitaries from ERβ knockout mice exhibit normal PRL expression, but the lack of ERβ expression in wild-type mouse pituitary precludes the ability to draw conclusions about the role of ERβ in human PRL expression and/or lactotroph function on the basis of this genetic mouse model [71].

The ER selectively binds to a single estrogen response element (ERE) located within the distal rPRL enhancer adjacent to the monomeric Pit-1d site at approximately 1.5 kb upstream from the transcription initiation site. This ERE has been shown to mediate a dramatic synergistic interaction between Pit-1 and ER that results in a 60-fold induction of rPRL transcription in response to estrogen [34,72]. Binding of Pit-1 to this distal enhancer site as a monomer dictates the use of a specific amino terminal transactivation domain that is necessary to synergize with ERα in a cell-specific manner [15,60]. Interestingly, this Pit-1 synergy domain is not required for synergistic events on the growth hormone promoter. Estrogen-induced PRL expression also requires an intact mitogen-activated protein kinase (MAPK) signaling transduction pathway, as interfering with MAPK activation ablates the ability of estrogen to induce PRL expression [73].

A degenerate yet functional ERE sequence also exists in the hPRL promoter at −1189 bp relative to the transcription start site. This hPRL ERE differs significantly from the rPrl ERE, although it is located within the corresponding sequence [74,75]. ERα and Pit-1 exert synergistic transcriptional effects on both the rat and human PRL promoters, suggesting that Pit-1 and ER are involved in the formation of a multiprotein complex at this site. The hPRL ERE has a relatively low binding affinity for ERα, and when stimulated by estradiol alone, exhibits modest transcriptional activity (~two-fold). However, a marked synergistic transcriptional effect is observed in the presence of estradiol and TNFα, and it appears that this particular ERE sequence is essential for the TNFα-induced, NFκB-mediated activation of the hPRL promoter [76]. Thus, the ERE sequence in the hPRL gene promoter appears to be a target for at least two signaling pathways and as such, may represent an important converging point for integrating multiple physiological endocrine signals in vivo.

Ets

Members of the Ets family of transcription factors are key regulators controlling PRL gene expression. Analyses of the rPRL promoter in somatolactotroph cell lines have identified two critical Ets binding sites (EBS): a composite Ets-1/Pit-1 binding site located at −212 and a more proximal EBS located at −96. The composite Ets-1/Pit-1 binding site confers synergy between the two proteins and mediates stimulation by the Ras/MAPK signaling transduction pathway, including those initiated by fibroblast growth factor (FGF) and thyrotropin-releasing hormone (TRH) [30–32,77–79]. Although Pit-1 and Ets interact directly, the synergistic activation of PRL gene expression does not necessitate this physical interaction, but does require the assembly of distinct Pit-1 transcriptional activation domains, as well as the specific sequence of the composite site [48,80]. The synergy between Pit-1 and Ets-1 can be prevented by an Ets-2 repressor factor apparently by preventing Pit-1 from binding to the composite site [80]. The proximal EBS centered at −96, the target of several growth factor signaling pathways, is recognized and activated by Ets factors GABPα and GABPβ [81].

Other Transcription Factors

Several additional transcription-regulating proteins identified in the pituitary have been implicated as key elements in regulation of the PRL promoter. These include Pitx factors, thyroid hormone receptor (via activating protein-1 (AP-1) transcription factor), CCAAT/enhancer-binding protein (C/EBPα), SMAD4 and Ikaros. The Pitx family is a class of bicoid homeodomain proteins required for development of several organs. Among the three members of this family, Pitx1 and Pitx2 are expressed in the anterior pituitary and in several pituitary cell lines. Both Pitx1 and Pitx2 can interact and synergize with Pit-1 in activating pituitary-specific promoters [82–85]. The synergy between Pitx2 and Pit-1 is achieved by Pit-1 binding to the carboxy-terminal tail of Pitx2, which relieves the autorepression imposed by this region, thereby increasing

DNA binding of Pitx2 to a canonical bicoid site [82]. Two bicoid sites, B1 and B2, located at −27 and −110, respectively, have been identified in the human PRL proximal promoter; the B2 site and two Pit-1 binding sites are necessary for the synergistic interaction of Pitx2 and Pit-1 [83]. Although an intact B2 Pitx binding site is necessary for full responsiveness to several signaling pathways regulating the hPRL promoter, Pitx factors play a secondary role to factors such as Pit-1 and Ets in the regulation of hPRL gene expression, since mutation of the B1 and B2 sites has only modest inhibitory impact on promoter activity [83].

Triiodothyronine (T3) down-regulates transcription of hPRL gene [36]. The hPRL promoter contains two T3 responsive regions. The first, located in the proximal promoter, mediates a strong negative effect, while the second, located in the distal promoter, mediates a weak positive effect. The overall effect of the two combined regions is negative. T3 exerts its inhibitory effect by binding to thyroid hormone receptor (TR) and interfering with the AP-1 transactivation mediated by an AP-1-binding site located in the proximal hPRL promoter. The T3/TR complex has different effects on PRL expression in the rat, where it mediates an overall activation of the rPRL promoter [86].

C/EBPα, a member of the bZip family of transcription factors, also synergizes with Pit-1 to stimulate the rPRL promoter and the rGH promoter [87]. The importance of C/EBPα interactions with Pit-1 is underscored by the observation that mutations in Pit-1 that disrupt physical binding between Pit-1 and C/EBPα lead to combined pituitary hormone deficiency (CPHD) in humans [59,88]. The DNA binding site utilized by the Pit-1-C/EBPα complex in the PRL promoter overlaps with the proximal Ets binding site, which is recognized by GABPα/GABPβ [87].

Bone morphogenetic protein-4 (BMP-4), one of the members of the TGF-β superfamily, plays a role in pituitary development from the initial induction of Rathke's pouch to cell specification in the anterior lobe and differentiation of the lactotroph lineage [89]. BMP-4, which is also overexpressed in different rodent prolactinoma models, exerts proliferative effects on postnatal lactotrophs through a complex mechanism involving cross talk among intracellular signaling pathways of BMP-4, Smad-4 and estradiol [90]. In addition to effects on lactotroph proliferation, BMP-4 and estradiol synergistically activate transcription of the rPRL promoter independently of EREs, but in a manner dependent upon an SMAD binding element located between −2000 and −1500 bp relative to the pituitary transcriptional start site [91].

Ikaros is a zinc finger transcription factor that is expressed in the pituitary, where it has been shown to regulate fibroblast growth factor receptor 4 (FGFR4) expression through its effects on histone acetylation [92]. In mammosomatotroph cells that express both GH and PRL, Ikaros suppresses GH but activates PRL gene expression [93]. The mechanism for this differential effect on hormone expression appears to rely on the state of chromatin accessibility for Pit-1, as mediated in part by Ikaros. Access of Pit-1 is modulated in a gene-specific manner such that Ikaros selectively deacetylates histone 3 residues on the GH promoter, and therefore restricts the access of Pit-1 [94]. In contrast, Ikaros acetylates histone 3 on the proximal PRL promoter and thereby facilitates Pit-1 binding to this region in the same cells [94]. Thus, Ikaros-mediated histone acetylation and chromatin remodeling provides one potential mechanism for the selective regulation of pituitary GH and PRL hormone gene expression in cells that are capable of elaborating both.

Signaling Pathways that Converge upon PRL Promoter

PRL expression is dynamically regulated by neurotransmitters, hormones and growth factors through activation or inhibition of G-protein-coupled receptors (GPCRs) and receptor tyrosine kinases that feed into several signal transduction pathways (Figure 5.2). These positive and negative signals ultimately converge upon the regulatory promoter region. The intracellular signal transduction pathway linking dopamine (DA) to the PRL gene involves inhibition of adenylate cyclase and the cAMP/protein kinase a (PKA) pathway [95−99]. PKA-dependent cAMP signals typically activate the transcription factor cAMP response element (CRE)-binding protein (CREB), leading to its homodimerization on DNA complexes. However, the human and rat PRL promoters lack functional cAMP DNA response elements (CRE), and although one-half CRE is located in the rPRL promoter, CREB does not bind to this sequence with high affinity. Therefore alternative undefined molecular mechanisms are involved in cAMP-dependent PRL gene regulation [100−103]. Growth factors and hormones, such as insulin, epidermal growth factor (EGF) and thyrotropin-releasing hormone (TRH), utilize protein kinase C (PKC)-dependent pathways to directly phosphorylate the coactivator CBP, which stimulates its subsequent recruitment to Pit-1, to regulate transcription of the PRL gene [41,42,50]. Other signaling pathways involving phosphoinositide 3-kinase (PI3K)-Akt phosphorylation of CREB have also been proposed to mediate induction of the PRL promoter by insulin and prolactin-releasing peptide [104]. In this latter pathway, CREB probably regulates PRL promoter activity through interaction with an Ets family member [105]. Extracellular signal-regulated kinase-1/2 (Erk-1/2)

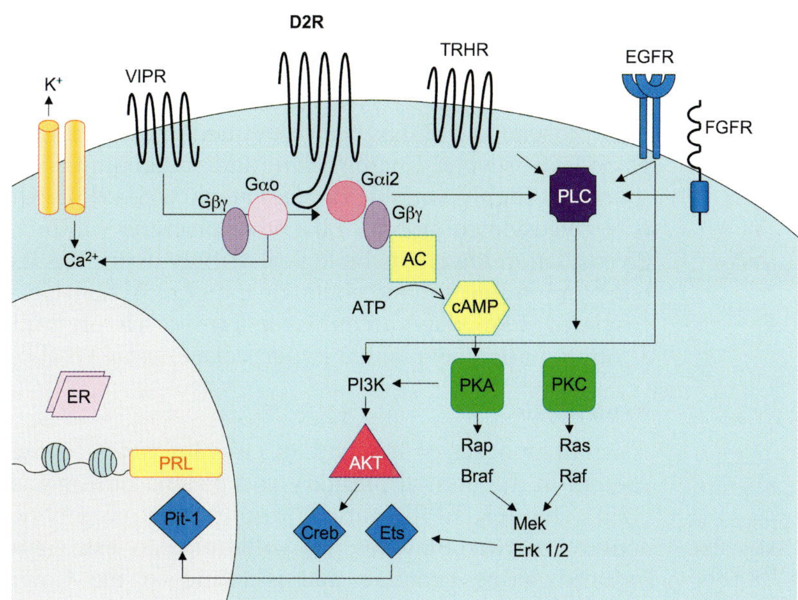

FIGURE 5.2 Schematic diagram of the membrane receptors and corresponding signal transduction pathways in pituitary lactotrophs that are involved in prolactin (PRL) gene regulation. The dopamine D_2 receptor (D2R) exerts the main, inhibitory influence upon PRL synthesis. TRHR, thyrotropin releasing hormone receptor; VIPR, vasoactive inhibitory peptide receptor; EGFR, epidermal growth factor receptor; FGFR, fibroblast growth factor receptor; PLC, phospholipase C; AC, adenylate cyclase; cAMP, cyclic adenosine monophosphate; PI3K, phosphoinositide 3-kinase; PKA, protein kinase A; PKC, protein kinase C; AKT, protein kinase B; Creb, cAMP response element binding protein; ER, estrogen receptor.

activation serves as a point of convergence for PRL gene regulation by numerous stimuli, including vasoactive intestinal peptide (VIP), insulin-like growth factor 1 (IGF-1), pituitary adenylyl cyclase activating polypeptide (PACAP) and fibroblast growth factor 2 (FGF2). These stimuli initially signal through pathways characterized by differential utilization of monomeric G proteins. Thus, vasoactive intestinal peptide (VIP) and insulin-like growth factor 1 (IGF-1) stimulate PRL gene expression through a Ras/Raf/Erk/Ets cascade [30,31,106], whereas PACAP signals through Rap1/Braf/Erk, and FGF2 signals through Rac-1/phospholipase C (PLC)/protein kinase C (PKC)/Erk to control PRL gene expression [107,108].

Some of the intra- and extracellular factors that participate in lactotroph proliferation and PRL gene expression appear to participate in complex cross-talk signaling pathways when studied in vitro. For example, BMP4 and estradiol exert a synergistic effect on PRL gene expression in a manner dependent upon SMAD1, but independent of EREs [91]. TGF-β, however, inhibits PRL transcription in a manner that overrides both BMP4 and estradiol stimulatory actions [91]. Similarly, EGFR and ERα participate in overlapping signaling pathways that modulate PRL expression and release [109–111]. The cytokine TNF-α activates the hPRL promoter through NF-κB signaling in a manner that is also dependent upon ERα [74,76]. Since most of these observations are based upon data derived from transformed rodent cell lines that lack normal dopaminergic control, the relevance of these cross-talk patterns for human PRL expression and lactotroph function remains to be confirmed.

HORMONE BIOSYNTHESIS

Prolactin Protein

Structural Characteristics and Post-translational Modifications

The mature human prolactin protein is composed of 199 amino acids [112]. A comparison of the sequence homology at the amino acid level from different species shows that the degree of conservation is highly variable among mammalian and nonmamalian species, reflecting their phylogenetic relationships. Primate PRL has 97% homology to hPRL, whereas rodent PRL has only 61–64% homology. Moreover, rat PRL is capable of activating the human prolactin receptor, whereas mouse PRL cannot [113]. The prolactin polypeptide is arranged in a single chain of amino acids with three highly conserved intramolecular disulfide bonds between six cysteine residues (Figure 5.3). According to nuclear magnetic resonance (NMR) spectroscopy, prolactin folds into four antiparallel alpha helices, similar to the tertiary structure of GH and other close relatives [114].

Post-translational modifications of the PRL polypeptide, such as glycosylation, phosphorylation, proteolytic cleavage and polymerization influence its stability, receptor binding, measurement and biological activity. Phosphorylated forms of PRL have been identified in most species, although it is not known whether these forms appear in the plasma in vivo. Mass spectrometry of standard human pituitary extracts indicates that ~19% of human PRL exists in a mono-phosphorylated form, another 19% in a di-phosphorylated form, and ~62% is unphosphorylated [115]. In the human pituitary,

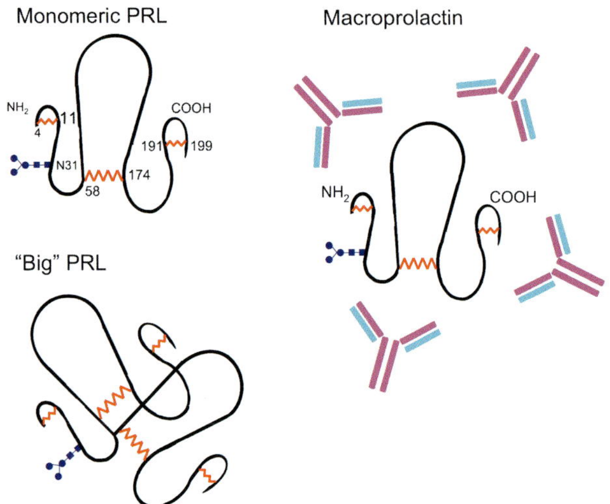

FIGURE 5.3 Schematic illustration of prolactin (PRL) proteins as they exist in the serum as three forms: monomeric 23-kDa PRL (>95%), "big PRL," consisting of PRL aggregates, and "big, big PRL," or macroprolactin, consisting of PRL bound to IgG. The native PRL protein is composed of 199 amino acids. Red hatching indicates the relative locations of the three disulfide bonds. A single N-glycosylation site has been identified on human PRL at codon 31. Two putative phosphorylation sites (not depicted) have been proposed at serines 163 and 194.

PRL is phosphorylated at serine (ser) 194 and ser 163; in sera, ser 163 is primarily dephosphorylated [116]. The major primary phosphorylation sites have been identified in bovine (ser 90) and rat (ser 177) PRL [117,118]. In the pituitary, ser 179 is the equivalent residue in human PRL (hPRL). The physiologic role of phosphorylated PRL may be inferred from investigations using a recombinant artificial mutant of PRL that has been developed as a PRLR antagonist. S179D is a mimic of mono-phosphorylated hPRL in which the putative serine phosphorylation site is replaced by an aspartate residue [119]. Phosphorylated PRL has reduced potency in standard bioassays, and it antagonizes the pro-proliferative action of the predominant unphosphorylated form [118]. As compared to unmodified PRL, S179D PRL inhibits cell proliferation, promotes differentiation, is pro-apoptotic and anti-angiogenic [119]. These biological properties may result from differential use of post-receptor signaling pathways. Although both the phosphomimetic S179D and unmodified PRL interact with the same PRLR, unmodified PRL preferentially activates the JAK-Stat signaling cascade, whereas S179D predominantly activates Erk 1/2 [120].

In the rat pituitary, the relative ratio of phosphorylated to nonphosphorylated PRL isoforms is altered during different phases of male reproductive development, and various stages of the estrous cycle, suggesting that this post-translational modification may have functional significance [121,122]. Whether phosphorylation modifications have biological relevance and the extent to which endogenous phosphorylated forms of hPRL participate in biologically significant PRLR signaling has not been conclusively determined.

Glycosylated PRL has been identified in the pituitary glands of several mammalian and nonmammalian species at highly variable degrees (1–60%) [112]. hPRL is N-glycosylated on N31. Like other prolactin variants, glycosylation lowers its biological activity as well as its receptor binding and metabolic clearance rate [123]. Glycosylated PRL may account for rare cases of mild asymptomatic unexplained hyperprolactinemia [124].

Proteolysis

Small amounts of 16K and 8K cleavage products are present in the normal pituitary and plasma of humans [125]. The 16K hPRL variant results from enzymatic activity of two enzymes: [1] kallikrein, an estrogen-induced serine protease that is found in the Golgi cisternae and secretory granules of lactotrophs [126]; and [2] bone morphogenetic protein 1, a metalloproteinase that activates latent complexes of the TGFβ superfamily members [127]. Although this 16K product has been reported to have anti-angiogenic properties in vitro, the existence and/or significance of this cleavage product in humans is indeterminate [109,128,129].

Macroprolactin

Normally, over 90% of PRL is present in serum as the 23-kDa monomer and less than 10% has alternative compositions and sizes. These other forms consist of aggregates of monomeric PRL with varying degrees of glycosylation, and they exhibit covalent and noncovalent bonding. Aside from monomeric PRL, the two other major species identified by gel filtration chromatography include "big PRL" which has a molecular weight of 48–56 kDa and "big, big PRL," referred to as macroprolactin, which has a molecular weight of >100 kDa (Figure 5.3). Macroprolactin is most often comprised of monomeric PRL bound to immunoglobulin (IgG), but sometimes it is in the form of oligomers [130,131]. The presence of macroprolactin in the sera of patients can lead to clinical dilemmas due to the potential for misinterpretations of biochemical testing (see clinical testing below).

Placental and Decidual, and Lymphoblastoid Forms

A variety of PRL-like proteins produced by the placenta have been identified in rodents, in addition to placental lactogen [132,133]. These PRL-like proteins are secreted at different times during gestation by the placenta and thus may have different functions, including alterations in blood vessel formation, hematopoiesis and lymphocyte function [132,133]. No such proteins have been identified in the human, and human placental lactogen (hPL) is much closer in structure to GH than it is to PRL [109].

PRL levels in maternal blood rise throughout gestation and are of pituitary origin [134,135]. However, PRL concentrations in amniotic fluid are 10–100-fold higher than either maternal or fetal blood levels [135]. Utilizing the "extrapituitary" or "decidual" PRL promoter (as detailed above), human chorion-decidual tissues synthesize and release a PRL species that is identical to pituitary PRL [136,137]. The two PRL mRNAs are indistinguishable except for four silent nucleotide differences [138].

The regulation of decidual PRL secretion differs from that of pituitary PRL (detailed below). Dopamine, bromocriptine and TRH have no effects on the decidual production of PRL in vitro [136]. Decidual PRL production is increased by progesterone and progesterone plus estrogen, but not by estrogen alone [139,140]. Insulin, through the insulin receptor, insulin-like growth factor I (IGF-I), through the IGF-I receptor and relaxin, a third peptide related to insulin and IGF-I have all been reported to stimulate synthesis and release of PRL [139,141].

The function of decidual PRL in the human remains obscure, although there is some evidence in animal studies that it may contribute to the osmoregulation of the amniotic fluid, fetal lung maturation and uterine contractility [142]. Human myometrial tissue also synthesizes PRL but its functional significance is unknown [143].

A human clonal lymphoblast cell line, IM-9-P3, has been established which produces a PRL that is identical to pituitary PRL in all aspects, including the sequence of their mRNAs [144]. There are differences from pituitary but not decidual PRL, however, in the 5′ untranslated region of the gene, suggesting that regulatory mechanisms may be different [144]. Indeed, studies have shown that PRL production by this cell line can be decreased by dexamethasone, but other substances known to affect pituitary PRL secretion, such as estradiol, thyroxine, TRH and VIP, have no effect [145].

HORMONE SECRETION: BIOCHEMISTRY

Studies in the early 1970s demonstrated the existence of two pools of PRL within the rat lactotroph cell, one turning over rapidly and the other turning over slowly [146]. Newly synthesized PRL is preferentially released compared to older, stored PRL in response to some stimuli and constitutes the rapidly turning over pool [146]. However, other stimuli, such as TRH, result in a preferential release of older, stored PRL [147]. These two types of secretion, rapid and slow, occur not so much due to differences in the type of stimulation for a given cell but due to functional heterogeneity of the cells so that some cells synthesize and secrete PRL rapidly while others secrete more slowly [147].

Much of the storage pool of PRL in the pituitary appears to exist in a high-molecular-weight, disulfide-bonded, poorly immunoreactive polymeric form that is converted to a releasable, immunoreactive monomeric form within the secretory granule when processed for release [148]. This conversion involves a thio-disulfide interchange mechanism and can be stimulated by reduced glutathione and decreased by aminothiols such as cysteamine [148].

Measurement of Prolactin

Assays and Bioassays

Prolactin levels in sera are measured by two-site immunoradiometric assays (IRMA) and chemiluminometric assays (ICMA) utilizing the sandwich principle, whereby the PRL molecule reacts with an immobilized capture antibody and a labeled detector antibody at two distinct sites. Following removal of unused reagents with a wash step, the signal generated is proportional to the concentration of PRL in the sample. Most immunoassays are calibrated against the WHO third international standard for prolactin, IS 84/500, consisting of human 23-kDa monomeric PRL.

The standard reference bioassay for PRL and other lactogens is the Nb2 cell proliferation assay. In this assay, cultured rat lymphoma cells that are completely dependent on lactogenic hormones for growth are incubated with a biologic sample, and the rate of cell division is quantified to provide a measurement for the amount of lactogens present. This assay is highly sensitive (10 pg/ml) but has the potential theoretical disadvantage of inaccuracy due to species differences in PRLR responsiveness. Newer bioassays for human lactogens have been developed to address this issue, as well as to analyze structure–function studies of human lactogen analogues, and to assess for the presence of macroprolactin (see below). These bioassays utilize cell lines that stably express the human PRLR [1] alone, as part of a proliferation assay, or [2] in the presence of a luciferase reporter to measure transcriptional activity [149,150]. Experience with these assays is limited and testing to determine accuracy, validity and reproducibility in a larger series of patients is awaited.

Clinical Testing

PRL is secreted episodically and some PRL levels obtained during the day may rise above the upper limit of normal established for a given laboratory. Thus the finding of minimally elevated levels in blood requires confirmation in several samples. Several nonhypothalamic–pituitary conditions can cause moderate PRL elevations, generally to levels <250 ng/ml. A careful history and physical examination, screening blood chemistries, thyroid function tests and a pregnancy test will identify virtually all causes except for hypothalamic–pituitary disease. When there is no obvious cause of the hyperprolactinemia from routine screening, radiological evaluation of the hypothalamic–pituitary area is mandatory to exclude a mass lesion. This includes patients with even mild PRL elevations. Magnetic resonance imaging [23] with gadolinium enhancement is the preferred study for pituitary imaging (see Chapter 20). It must be emphasized that it is essential to distinguish between a large nonfunctioning tumor causing modest PRL elevations (usually <250 ng/ml, see above) from a PRL-secreting macroadenoma (PRL levels usually >>250 ng/ml), as the management approaches to these two entities are different. Most PRL-secreting macroadenomas generally respond readily to DA agonist therapy with size reduction (see Chapter 15) whereas only about 10% of nonsecreting pituitary tumors respond in this manner. It is also important to be aware of potential artifacts in PRL measurement that may lead to misdiagnoses (see below). Stimulation and suppression tests using TRH, hypoglycemia, chlorpromazine, domperidone and other medications yield nonspecific results and reveal no more information than simple measurement of basal PRL levels. Thus, consensus has developed that such stimulation and suppression tests are not recommended in the differential diagnosis of hyperprolactinemia [151].

Artifacts

HOOK EFFECT

Although current PRL immunoassays are highly sensitive and specific, artifacts due to saturation of the antibodies at excessively high PRL concentrations, which prevent antibody–PRL–antibody sandwich formation may nevertheless occur (Figure 5.4). This phenomenon, referred to as the "hook effect," grossly underestimates the true PRL concentration, leading the laboratory to report a falsely low value. St. Jean et al. noted this high-end "hook effect" in 5.6% of 69 patients who were thought to have clinically nonfunctioning adenomas [152]. Interference from the "hook effect" generally becomes problematic when PRL levels exceed 100,000 mU/l [153], but the threshold for this effect varies among immunoassay platforms. Therefore, in patients with large macroadenomas if there is suspicion regarding the susceptibility of an assay to this phenomenon, PRL assessments should be performed in both undiluted and 1:100 diluted serum to exclude the "hook effect."

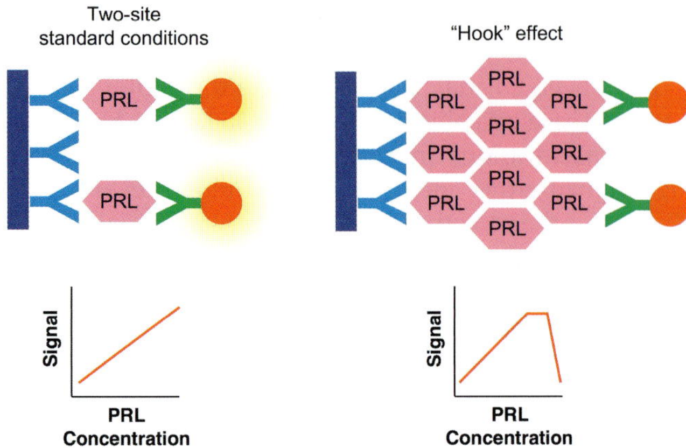

FIGURE 5.4 Schematic diagram illustrating the measurement artifact referred to as the "hook effect." Under usual circumstances (left side), PRL is detected in immunoassays by a solid-phase capture antibody and a labeled detection antibody. When PRL levels are grossly elevated (right side), the PRL protein saturates both antibodies, preventing sandwich formation and quantitative detection.

MACROPROLACTIN

A major diagnostic conundrum facing laboratories and clinicians is the differentiation of patients with true hyperprolactinemia from those with macroprolactinemia. Based on several clinical series, the estimated incidence of macroprolactin accounting for a significant proportion of hyperprolactinemic sera is approximately 10–20% [153,154]. The gold standard method to assess for macroprolactinemia is gel-filtration chromatography [153]. However, this method is laborious and expensive, and an alternative acceptable method is to perform polyethylene glycol (PEG) precipitation. With this pretreatment step, the larger-molecular-weight forms of PRL are removed by precipitation, leaving the residual monomeric forms in the supernatant [153]. Clinicians should be aware that due to methodological issues, PEG precipitation is not technically feasible on all commercial immunoassays.

Normative ranges have been published for sera treated with PEG for several of the most widely used assay systems [25]. Nevertheless, disagreement persists regarding the threshold concentration of residual monomeric PRL at which a hyperprolactinemic sample should be designated as being attributable to macroprolactin. Some investigators assert that in a patient with hyperprolactinemia, if the recovery of monomeric PRL left following PEG precipitation is less than 40% or 50% of the initial total value, then the hyperprolactinemia is due to macroprolactin [154]. Others suggest that since some macroprolactin is present in normal serum and/or some monomer is precipitated with PEG, the "normal" reference range should be recalculated from normal samples after PEG treatment; therefore, hyperprolactinemia is attributable to macroprolactin only when the level of nonprecipitated PRL is within the normal range [155]. It is clear that in many cases, especially when sera contain high concentrations of PRL, even when the amount of nonprecipitated PRL is less than 40% of the total, the residual PRL level still exceeds the normal range.

An additional issue that remains unresolved is a reliable estimation of the bioactivity of macroprolactin, as it is presumed that its presence in serum does not confer biological significance since it is unable to pass through the capillary endothelial barrier. The bioactivity of macroprolactin as measured by the classic rat Nb2 cell proliferation assay is comparable to the bioactivity of monomeric PRL [131]. However, when bioactivity is measured using human PRLR constructs, as tested in Ba/F-3 or human embryonic kidney-derived 293 (HEK-293) cell lines, the bioactivity of macroprolactin is reduced [149,150]. Technical pitfalls could potentially account for the findings in either of these cell-based systems. For example, under the bioassay conditions employed in the Nb2 cell bioassay, dissociation of macroprolactin into its constituents may free monomeric PRL to react, yielding a result suggestive of hormonal activity [156]. On the other hand, transfection conditions used to express exogenous human PRLR plasmids could alter the structure or function of the PRL added from the sample. In most clinical series investigating suspected or possible macroprolactinemia, symptoms are fewer and less severe in patients whose hyperprolactinemia is attributable to macroprolactin than in those patients who are determined to have true hyperprolactinemia [153,157]. In studies in which patients with suspected macroprolactinemia (often in retrospect) are treated with DA agonists, galactorrhea, when present, generally disappears, but oligo/amenorrhea is variably responsive [157]. Long-term follow-up studies of patients diagnosed with macroprolactinemia indicate that PRL levels show considerable instability (up to five-fold) [157].

In clinical practice, if a patient has typical symptoms, such as galactorrhea, amenorrhea, or impotence and is found to have mild hyperprolactinemia, the usual conditions should be excluded (medications, hypothyroidism, elevated creatinine, pregnancy) to be followed by pituitary MRI, primarily to exclude a large lesion such as a craniopharyngioma or clinically nonfunctioning adenoma. In patients with mild hyperprolactinemia who have equivocal symptoms (such as headaches or decreased libido) but normal menses and no galactorrhea, assessment for macroprolactin using PEG precipitation is reasonable. A decision that hyperprolactinemia is due to macroprolactin then would depend on demonstrating an abnormal amount of PRL precipitated by PEG, and a residual PRL monomer level that falls within the normal range. Under these circumstances, pituitary imaging may not be indicated, but would warrant continued clinical and biochemical assessment of such patients on a periodic basis.

Physiology

Metabolic Clearance and Production Rates of Prolactin

Using a labeled PRL method, the metabolic clearance rate has been found to be 46 ± 4 and 40 ± 6 ml/min/m^2 and the calculated production rates using the labeled PRL method were 200 ± 63 and 536 ± 218 μg/day/m^2 in two studies [158,159]. Studies in patients with chronic renal failure have shown the MCR to be reduced by 33% [159]; increased uptake by the liver has been found in nephrectomized rabbits [160].

Hormone Secretion Patterns

PRL is secreted episodically (Figure 5.5). There is an innate pulsatility to pituitary PRL secretion with an interpulse interval of about 8 minutes, as determined by studies of media obtained from primate pituitaries cultured in vitro [161]. When plasma is sampled from normal individuals in whom hypothalamic function is superimposed upon this innate pulsatility, it becomes apparent that there are 4–14 secretory episodes per day. Using cluster analysis, 13–14 peaks per day in young subjects were found with a peak duration of 67–76 min, a mean peak amplitude of 3–4 ng/ml and an interpulse interval of 93–95 min [162]. Disinhibition caused by hypothalamic tumors causes an increase in basal PRL levels due to an increase in pulse amplitude and not pulse frequency [163].

There is an increase in the amplitude of the PRL secretory pulses that begins about 60–90 minutes after the onset of sleep; the secretory pulses increase with non-REM sleep and fall prior to the next period of REM sleep [164]. Lowest PRL concentrations are found during REM sleep and highest concentrations are found during non-REM sleep [164]. When subjects are kept awake to reverse the sleep–waking cycle, PRL levels do not rise until sleep begins [165]. Thus, the diurnal variation of

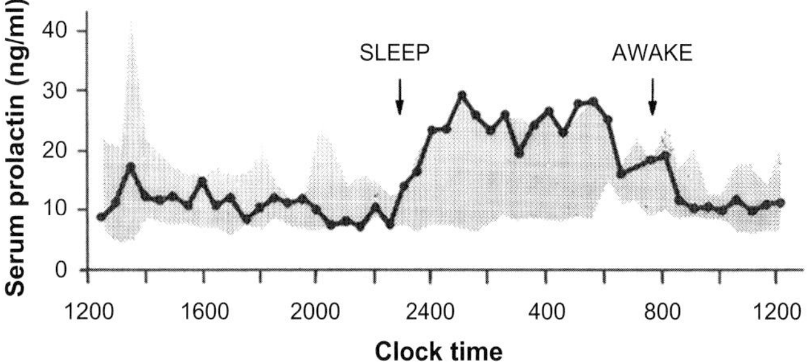

FIGURE 5.5 Prolactin levels throughout the day in a single individual superimposed upon the range from five normal individuals. Note the episodic nature of secretion and the nocturnal rise.

PRL secretion is not an inherent rhythm but depends on the occurrence of sleep. Interestingly, the diurnal variation of PRL with the sleep-induced rise persists despite other powerful physiologic influences such as breast-feeding [166].

There is an increase in circulating PRL levels of 50–100% within 30 minutes of meals that is due to the amino acids generated from the protein component of the meals, phenylalanine, tyrosine and glutamic acid being the most potent in this regard [167]. Carlson et al. have provided evidence that this stimulatory action of these amino acids is centrally mediated by showing that large neutral amino acids such as valine inhibit the transport of phenylalanine across the blood–brain barrier and blunt the stimulatory action of this amino acid [167].

Changes in Prolactin with Age

PRL levels are elevated almost ten-fold in infants following delivery but then gradually decrease so that levels of normal by 3 months of age [168]. These high levels of PRL at birth are probably related to the stimulatory effect of high maternal estrogen levels. PRL levels are lowest between the ages of 3 months and 9 years and then rise modestly during puberty to adult levels [168]. In some studies there is a gradual fall of basal PRL levels with age but in other studies no changes with age have been found [168–172]. PRL levels have been shown to fall with menopause [169], but estrogen replacement therapy has been shown to have variable effects on this fall [169,170]. In hyperprolactinemic women, estrogen replacement therapy causes no change in PRL levels [172]. PRL levels decrease by 55% in older men compared to younger men due to both a decreased basal secretion as well as the amount secreted with each secretory burst [171].

Changes in Prolactin Levels During the Menstrual Cycle

Some, but not all, women have higher levels at mid-cycle and lower levels in the follicular compared to the luteal phase [135,173,174]. In most of these studies, no correlations were found between PRL and estradiol, progesterone, LH and FSH levels. However, some studies have shown that PRL and LH secretion are often synchronous in the luteal phase and that very small doses of GnRH can cause the secretion of both PRL and LH at this time [175].

Changes in Prolactin Levels During Pregnancy

Basal PRL levels gradually increase throughout the course of pregnancy (Figure 5.6) [134,135]. This has generally been attributed to the stimulatory effect of the hormonal milieu of pregnancy, primarily estrogenic, on the pituitary lactotrophs. There is a gradual increase in the number of pituitary lactotrophs during pregnancy [8] and by term, PRL levels may be increased ten-fold to levels over 200 ng/ml [134,168]. These elevated PRL levels found at term prepare the breast for lactation.

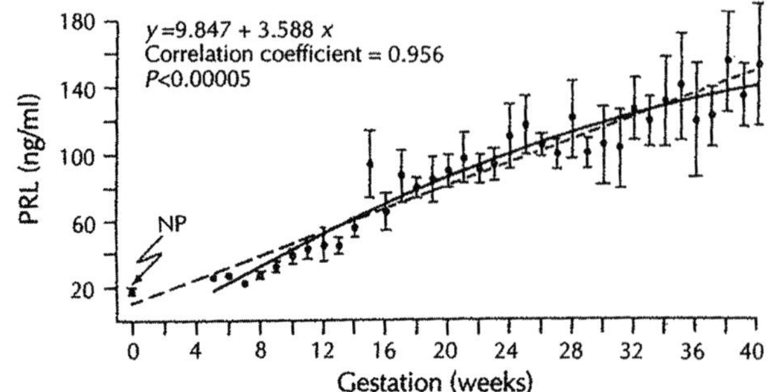

FIGURE 5.6 Serum prolactin (PRL) concentrations measured serially at weekly intervals as a function of gestation (n = 4). The dashed line represents the linear regression and the solid line represents the second-order regression. NP, nonpregnant PRL values. *Adapted from Rigg et al. [134].*

Changes in Prolactin Levels with Postpartum Lactation

Within the first 4–6 weeks postpartum basal PRL levels remain elevated in lactating women and each suckling episode triggers a rapid release of pituitary PRL resulting in a 3–5-fold increase in serum PRL levels, peaking about 10 minutes after the end of suckling [135,176]. Following termination of suckling PRL levels gradually fall to reach prenursing levels by about 3 hours after the beginning of the suckling episode [176]. Over the next 4–12 weeks, basal PRL levels gradually fall to normal and the PRL increase which occurs with each suckling episode decreases [176,177]. Eventually there is little or no rise in PRL with suckling despite continued milk production [135].

The decreases in basal and stimulated PRL levels between 3 and 6 months postpartum are largely the result of decreased breast-feeding as formula is introduced into the baby's diet. If intense nursing behavior is maintained, basal PRL levels remain elevated and postpartum amenorrhea persists [178]. Eighty minutes of nursing per day with a minimum of six nursing episodes will usually result in persistent hyperprolactinemia and amenorrhea [178]. However, the delay in the onset of menses is more associated with high suckling duration and frequency than with a particular level of PRL [178]. High-intensity lactation-induced failure to ovulate and menstruate has been used as a method of contraception in a number of developing countries for many years [178].

Breast stimulation may cause an increase in PRL levels in some nonbreast-feeding normal women but not in men [179] except for one study showing PRL increases in men after breast stimulation by their wives

[180]. Chronic nipple stimulation with nipple rings has been reported to cause sustained galactorrhea [181].

PRL is also produced directly by human breast glandular and adipose tissue [182]. Although progesterone inhibits the glandular PRL production, it has no effect on the adipocyte PRL production [182]. It is unclear whether the PRL present in breast milk is of local or systemic origin.

Changes in Prolactin Secretion with Stress

PRL has long been known to be one of the pituitary hormones released by stress, along with adrenocorticotropic hormone (ACTH) and GH [183]. The stress-induced rise in PRL generally consists of a doubling or tripling of PRL levels and lasts less than 1 hour. In humans, prolonged critical illness does not cause a sustained elevation of PRL; rather there is a reduction in the pulsatile secretion with an overall lowering of levels [184]. The teleological significance for these stress-induced changes in PRL is not clear.

The neuroendocrine mediation of the acute stress response is probably multifactorial but does not include a decrease in DA [185]. Corenblum and Taylor attempted to dissect out the neurotransmitter regulation of the PRL stress response in humans by administering various blocking agents immediately prior to surgery [186]. Blockade of histamine H_1 receptors using chlorpheniramine, serotonin receptors using cyproheptadine, and DA receptors using pimozide had little effect on the peak PRL level reached during surgery. Blockade of opiate receptors with high-dose naloxone resulted in a significant blunting, but not complete inhibition of the PRL response. These studies imply that the endogenous opiate-like peptidergic pathways may play a role in the PRL stress response. On the other hand, in humans naloxone has generally not been found to be able to block the PRL response to hypoglycemia [187]. Abe et al. found that VIP antisera inhibited the ether-induced PRL rise in rats [188].

Hypoglycemia has been regarded as a form of stress but whether it acts as a nonspecific stressor or has more specific effects is not clear. Among their tests of various types of stress, Noel et al. showed that PRL did indeed rise with hypoglycemia [183]. Acute exercise has also been regarded as a form of stress and results in an acute, transient increase in PRL levels [183]. Although chronic, high-level exercise often results in menstrual disturbance, it is not associated with sustained hyperprolactinemia [189].

NEUROENDOCRINE REGULATION

The hypothalamus exerts a predominantly inhibitory influence on PRL secretion through one or more PRL inhibitory factors (PIF) that reach the pituitary via the hypothalamic–pituitary portal vessels (Figure 5.7). There are PRL-releasing factors (PRF) as well. Disruption of the pituitary stalk leads to a moderate increase in PRL secretion as well as to decreased secretion of the other pituitary hormones.

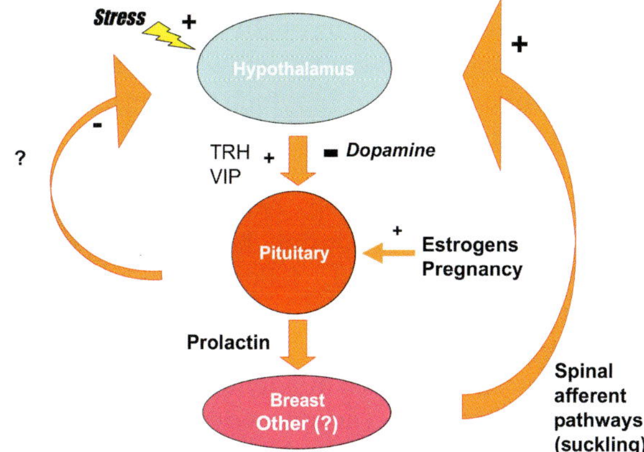

FIGURE 5.7 Neuroendocrine regulation of prolactin secretion. TRH, thyrotropin-releasing hormone; VIP, vasoactive intestinal peptide.

Prolactin-inhibiting Factors

Dopamine

In 1954, Everett demonstrated that the luteotropic properties of the pituitary (due to PRL) were increased when pituitaries were transplanted to beneath the renal capsule, a site away from the regulation by the hypothalamus, thus demonstrating the predominance of the inhibitory component of hypothalamic regulation of PRL secretion [190]. In the 1960s it was demonstrated that tuberoinfundibular DA released into the hypothalamic–pituitary portal vessels in the median eminence was the physiologic PIF with direct action on the pituitary [191].

A number of experiments firmly established that DA is the predominant, physiologic PIF, including the findings that the concentration of DA found in the pituitary stalk plasma (about 6 ng/ml) was sufficient to decrease PRL levels in rats and that stimuli which result in an acute release of PRL usually also result in an acute decrease in portal vessel DA levels [191]. However, in many experiments it was found that the PRL increase obtained by simply reducing DA was considerably less than the elevation of PRL achieved by simultaneous stimulation by a PRF; similarly, the PRL level achieved with the simultaneous stimulation by a PRF with the reduction in DA is usually greater than that achieved by a PRF alone [192]. It is likely that in most physiologic circumstances that cause a PRL rise, such as lactation, there is a simultaneous fall in DA along with a rise in a PRF, such as VIP, although there may well be circumstances in which various PRFs may stimulate PRL release with no concomitant lowering of DA levels or DA may be lowered with no concomitant increase in a PRF.

Newer work with mice in which the D_2 receptor or DA transporter has been "knocked out" (KO) has confirmed these earlier studies that employed pharmacologic methods or lesioning. Thus, mice with the D_2 receptor KO develop lactotroph hyperplasia and sustained hyperprolactinemia, followed by lactotroph adenomas in aged mice, demonstrating that a chronic loss of neurohormonal DA inhibition promotes a hyperplasia–neoplasia sequence in adenohypophyseal lactotrophs [193,194]. DA action within the synapse terminates by DA reuptake by the DA-secreting neurons via the DA transporter. In contrast to the findings with the DA receptor KO, DA transporter KO mice have increased dopaminergic tone and lactotroph hypoplasia [195]. Although such mice have normal circulating levels of PRL, they cannot increase these levels with various stimuli and are unable to lactate [195].

Although much of the direct work demonstrating DA in hypothalamic–pituitary portal vessels and the effects of DA on PRL release in vitro has been done in animals, it is clear that DA is the primary PIF in humans as well. Infusion of DA causes a rapid suppression of basal PRL levels that can be reversed by metoclopramide, a DA receptor blocker [196]. Dopamine also blocks the PRL increments induced by various stimuli [197]. Studies with low-dose DA infusions in humans have shown that DA blood concentrations similar to those found in rat and monkey hypothalamic–pituitary portal blood are able to suppress PRL secretion [198]. Blockade of endogenous DA receptors by a variety of drugs, including phenothiazines, butyrophenones, metoclopramide and domperidone causes a rise in PRL [199].

The axons responsible for the release of DA into the median eminence originate in perikarya in the dorsomedial portion of the arcuate nucleus and inferior portion of the ventromedial nucleus of the hypothalamus [109]. This pathway is known as the tubero–infundibular DA (TIDA) pathway. The DA that traverses the TIDA pathway binds to the class of DA receptors referred to as D_2 receptors on the lactotroph cell membrane [191]. As discussed above, activation of this receptor results in [1] an inhibition of adenyl cyclase with lowered intracellular cAMP levels, [2] inhibition of phosphoinositide metabolism, and [3] decreased intracellular calcium mobilization and inhibition of calcium transport through calcium channels. It has been proposed that these different actions of DA may actually be mediated by multiple similar D_2 receptors that are produced by alternative RNA splicing [191].

The inhibitory action of DA on PRL secretion is partially blocked by estrogen administration. This may be largely due to the direct action of estrogen on the estrogen response element of the PRL gene (see above). However, there may also be other mechanisms but with considerable interspecies differences. Estradiol is able to block the inhibitory action of DA on PRL release from rat lactotroph cells in vitro [200]. In studies in humans, the same dose of infused DA results in a greater suppression of PRL during the early follicular phase, when estrogen levels are low, compared to the late follicular or periovulatory phases, when estrogen levels are higher [201]. Estrogens result in a decrease in DA receptor numbers in rats [202] but the DA receptor population showed no sex-related differences in a limited number of human pituitaries [203].

Gonadotropin-associated Peptide (GAP)

Whether DA alone can account for all of the PIF activity of the hypothalamus has long been questioned. In 1985 Nikolics et al. [204] reported the PRL-inhibiting ability of a 56-amino acid polypeptide that is in the carboxyterminal region of the precursor to gonadotropin-releasing hormone (GnRH) and which they termed GAP. However, the GAP sequences in human and rat have 17-amino acid differences [205] and subsequent studies showed that GAP has no PRL-suppressing activity when tested against human prolactinomas cultured in vitro [206]. At this point, there is no evidence that GAP has any physiologic significance in humans as a PIF.

γ-Aminobutyric Acid (GABA)

GABA has an inhibitory effect on PRL secretion in vivo and in vitro in rats and high-affinity GABA receptors are present on lactotrophs [207,208]. A tuberoinfundibular GABAergic system has been described with perikarya located in the arcuate nucleus and nerve endings demonstrated in the median eminence, and GABA has been demonstrated to be present in portal blood [209].

Studies of the GABA system in humans have yielded conflicting results in studies of widely differing experimental designs. GABA itself causes a modest decrease in PRL levels when given to humans for several days [210] and activation of the endogenous GABAergic system with sodium valproate causes a suppression in the PRL rise induced by mechanical breast stimulation in puerperal women [211]. The physiologic role of GABA remains to be fully elucidated in the human.

Prolactin-releasing Factors

Thyrotropin-releasing Hormone

Shortly after its initial isolation and characterization, TRH was demonstrated to cause a rapid release of PRL from rat pituitary cell cultures [212] and in humans after intravenous injection [213]. Release of PRL is biphasic, the initial peak being mediated by activation of intracellular phosphoinositide pathways with IP_3 generation and mobilization of intracellular calcium causing release of stored hormone; the second, more sustained phase is mediated influx of extracellular calcium through calcium channels which causes sustained secretion and synthesis of new hormone [214].

A number of different experimental approaches have failed to clarify the physiologic role of TRH as a PRF. The smallest dose of TRH that releases TSH also releases PRL in humans [176]. Immunoneutralization of endogenous TRH with TRH antisera causes a 50% suppression of basal PRL levels in rats in some studies [215] but not in others. In the mouse with targeted disruption of the TRH gene (TRH KO), mice became hypothyroid with elevated levels of TSH with reduced biological activity but had normal PRL levels [216], further casting doubt on the essential role of TRH in PRL regulation.

If TRH mediates the PRL response to suckling, even in part, it ought to be accompanied by an increase in TSH, unless there were a concomitant increase in somatostatin. Studies in humans failed to show any elevations of TSH [217,218] with suckling. Very small doses of TRH given systemically were effective in releasing PRL and TSH in lactating rats and women in those studies, however, it is unlikely that failure to show a rise in TSH was due to an increase in somatostatin [218].

In hypothyroidism, TRH synthesis is increased [219], portal vessel TRH levels are increased [220], and there is an increased number of TRH receptors [221]. In human hypothyroidism, basal TSH and PRL levels are increased as are their responses to injected TRH [222]. Correction of the hypothyroidism with thyroid hormone corrects both the elevated TSH and PRL levels and their responses to TRH [223]. Conversely, in hyperthyroidism in humans, PRL levels are not low basally but the PRL response to TRH is markedly blunted and returns to normal with correction of the hyperthyroidism [223].

The above conflicting data from passive immunization studies, TRH KO mice, observation of TSH levels during lactation and examination of PRL levels in various thyroid states support a role for TRH as a physiologic PRF, albeit not the primary one or even one of major importance.

VIP and Peptide Histidine Methionine (PHM)/PHI

VIP stimulates PRL release [224] and is found in neuronal perikarya in the parvocellular region of the paraventricular nucleus with axons terminating in the external zone of the median eminence [225]. Its effects are selective for PRL and additive to TRH in causing PRL release [226] at concentrations found in hypothalamic–pituitary portal blood [227]. The effects of VIP appear to be mediated by stimulation of adenyl cyclase, although recent evidence suggests that transport of calcium through membrane calcium channels may also be important. In addition to stimulating PRL release, VIP also stimulates pituitary PRL mRNA content and PRL synthesis [228]. In conditions of increased PRL synthesis, such as lactation, hypothalamic VIP mRNA levels are also increased [229]. In addition to these studies in rats, intravenously administered VIP has also been shown to increase PRL levels in humans [224] at serum levels similar to those demonstrated in rat portal blood.

A number of experiments have been performed using passive immunoneutralization techniques to determine the physiologic role of VIP as a PRF. Anti-VIP antisera administered to rats have been shown to partially inhibit the PRL responses to suckling and ether-induced stress [188].

Part of the 20-kDa 170-amino acid VIP precursor is another similarly sized peptide known as PHM [230]. PHM and VIP colocalize in the hypothalamus and median eminence [231]. PHM given to humans has caused a PRL increment in some experiments [231] but not others [232].

Further complicating the role of VIP as a PRF is the finding that VIP is actually synthesized by anterior pituitary tissue [233]. Antisera to VIP inhibit basal PRL secretion from dispersed pituitary cells in vitro [234], suggesting a local "autocrine" role for VIP in PRL regulation within the pituitary.

The physiologic role of VIP as a PRF appears to be warranted by the experimental data. The precise roles of VIP vs. PHM and hypothalamic VIP vs. pituitary VIP still are not clear. How VIP/PHM interact with other PRFs, such as TRH, are additional areas requiring clarification.

Serotonin

A considerable number of experiments have demonstrated a role for serotonin as a neurotransmitter involved in the release of PRL. Most serotoninergic neuronal perikarya are in the dorsal and median raphe nuclei and their axons project forward to the hypothalamus and other limbic and cortical areas. Lesions of the dorsal but not the median raphe nuclei decrease forebrain serotonin levels and basal and stimulated serum PRL levels [235].

Studies in humans also suggest a role for serotonin in PRL secretion. Infusion of the serotonin precursor, 5-hydroxytryptophan, results in a prompt increase in PRL levels [236]. Nocturnal PRL secretion is inhibited by cyproheptadine [237]. On the other hand, pizotifen, a specific, non-ergot serotonin antagonist, had no effect on the suckling-induced PRL rise in postpartum women [238].

Whether serotonin's effects are mediated solely through brain pathways or whether it has direct effects on the pituitary is controversial. One possibility is that serotonin causes a decrease in hypothalamic DA generation. Synaptic junctions between serotoninergic nerve terminals and dopaminergic perikarya in the arcuate nucleus have been demonstrated [239]. Furthermore, intraventricular injections of serotonin decrease portal vessel DA concentrations [240]. It has also been proposed that serotonin acts by increasing VIP and oxytocin via effects at the paraventricular nucleus [241].

Serotonin has been found within the anterior pituitary serotoninergic nerve terminals that have been demonstrated within the median eminence [242]. High-affinity S_2 serotonin receptors have been found in the anterior pituitary [243] as well as uptake of labeled serotonin into cells of the pituitary [244]. In direct tests of the effects of serotonin on pituitary PRL release, serotonin has been found to increase basal and stimulated PRL secretion from pituitaries in vitro [245,246] and this appears to be mediated by the serotonin subtype 4 receptor [246].

Thus, although it is possible that serotonin is a direct secretagogue for PRL, via transport from the hypothalamus by the portal vessels or through an autocrine action within the pituitary, its role in this regard is still uncertain. It may mediate the nocturnal surge of PRL and may well participate in the suckling-induced rise in PRL via the ascending serotoninergic pathways from the dorsal raphe nucleus and mediated by activation of VIP release. Serotonin reuptake inhibitors (SSRIs) are widely prescribed antidepressants but only rarely have cases been reported of hyperprolactinemia due to their use [199,241].

Opioid Peptides

A detailed description of the various opioid peptides, their receptors and their neuronal pathways is beyond the scope of this discussion. Approaches to determining the roles of the opioid peptides and pathways in the regulation of PRL secretion have focused on using opioid agonists and antagonists in experimental animals and humans.

In rats, morphine, Met- and Leu-enkephalin, β-endorphin, dynorphin and leumorphin injected systemically or intracerebroventricularly have all been shown to cause release of PRL [247,248]. Subsequent studies employing specific agonists and antagonists operative on the μ, δ and κ opioid receptors and antibodies directed against several opioid peptides have shown that it is the μ receptor that is the predominant one involved in PRL release, the κ receptor is involved to a lesser extent, and the δ receptor is not involved at all [249]. Most evidence suggests that the opioid peptides do not have a direct effect on the pituitary and stimulate PRL release by inhibiting DA turnover and release by the TIDA pathway [250]. Orphanin FQ (also called nociceptin), which binds to an opioid-like orphan receptor, also causes an increase in PRL levels in rats when administered intracerebroventricularly [251].

In humans, morphine and morphine analogues increase PRL release acutely [252] and chronically [253]. However, blockade of the μ receptor with naloxone has minimal to no effect on PRL levels either basally or with stimulation by hypoglycemia, exercise, sleep, TRH, or physical stress [254]. Overall, it appears that the endogenous opioid pathways play at most only a minor role in the regulation of PRL secretion, especially in humans.

Growth-hormone-releasing Hormone (GHRH)

A number of studies have found GHRH to have PRL-releasing properties. The initial clue to this effect of GHRH was the finding that many of the patients with acromegaly due to GHRH-secreting tumors were hyperprolactinemic and PRL levels fell in parallel with GH following excision of the GHRH-secreting tumor [255]. Large doses of GHRH have been reported to release PRL in vivo in normal humans [256]. Chronic therapy with GHRH in children with GH neurosecretory dysfunction results in a sustained elevation of PRL levels [257]. In rat pituitary cell cultures, GHRH causes PRL and GH release but an increase only in GH mRNA and not PRL mRNA, indicating no stimulation of PRL synthesis [258]. The similarity of GH and PRL responses to a variety of stimuli, such as exercise, stress, hypoglycemia, arginine infusion and sleep, and the pathological conditions of renal failure and hepatic cirrhosis suggest but do not prove that GHRH may serve as a physiologic PRF under some circumstances.

Posterior Pituitary, Oxytocin, and Vasopressin

Studies in animals have shown that oxytocin, in doses found in the hypothalamic–pituitary portal vessels can stimulate PRL release when added to the medium of pituitary cell cultures or incubations or when given intravenously, but it lowers PRL levels when directly injected into the third ventricle [259]. Studies in which endogenous oxytocin was eliminated by passive immunization with oxytocin antisera or by oxytocin antagonists show a reduction and a delay in the suckling and cervical-stimulation-induced PRL surges in some but not all studies [260]. Experimental data also support the possibility that the oxytocin-induced PRL increase in these experimental paradigms is mediated by a decrease in DA [260]. Very limited studies in humans suggest that oxytocin administered intravenously has no effect on basal PRL levels and causes only a minimal increase in TRH-stimulated PRL levels [261]. It is likely that oxytocin plays at most a minimal role even in suckling-induced PRL secretion in humans [109].

Vasopressin also has PRL-releasing properties when injected intravenously into normal rats and sheep and rats with pituitaries transplanted to the renal capsule but not sheep with hypothalamic–pituitary disconnection [262]. The neurophysin portions of the precursors to oxytocin and vasopressin also stimulate PRL secretion in rats [263]. There are no studies to date of the effects of vasopressin on PRL secretion in humans.

Whether there are other PRFs in the posterior pituitary in addition to oxytocin, vasopressin, and their respective neurophysins has been a matter of controversy but isolation of such substances has not been successful [109]. Overall, it is felt that the posterior pituitary may play only a minor role in the regulation of PRL secretion [109].

Gonadotropin-releasing Hormone (GnRH)

GnRH was initially found to release PRL from rat pituitary cells in vitro [264]. Subsequently, GnRH has been found to cause a release of PRL in anovulatory women [265]. Postmenopausal women also have a PRL response to GnRH that is augmented with estrogen supplementation [266]. There is no PRL release in response to GnRH in normal, eugonadal males but such a release does occur with high doses of estrogen pretreatment (given to transsexual men) [267]. Analysis of PRL and LH secretory pulses suggests a high degree of concordance in women [175], thereby arguing for a physiologic role for GnRH in PRL secretion. A subset of human prolactinomas that also contain the glycoprotein α subunit has been shown to bind GnRH specifically and with high affinity and to release PRL in response to GnRH in vitro [268].

Renin–angiotensin System

Angiotensin-converting enzyme (ACE) and angiotensin II receptors and activity have been identified in the rat pituitary and median eminence of the hypothalamus [269–271]. In the human pituitary, renin, ACE and angiotensinogen have been detected in normal lactotroph cells and in PRL-secreting adenomas [272]. Angiotensin II incubated with rat pituitary cells stimulates release of PRL, an effect blocked by AT_1 but not AT_2 antagonists [273]. However, in humans, blockade of ACE with enalapril results in no change in basal PRL levels [274,275], no change in the TRH and metoclopramide-induced PRL rises [274], and only a minimal decrease in the PRL response to hypoglycemia [275]. It is unlikely, therefore, that the endogenous renin–angiotensin system of the hypothalamus and pituitary has significant physiologic effects on PRL regulation.

PRL-releasing Peptide

Hinuma et al. [47] discovered a 31-amino acid peptide capable of releasing PRL, termed PrRP31, by looking for endogenous ligands for an orphan receptor present in the human pituitary termed hGR3. In pituitary cell preparations, PrRP31 released PRL with a potency equal to that of TRH [47]. However, although PrRP31 is found in neuronal perikarya in the paraventricular and supraoptic nuclei, PrRP31-immunoreactive nerve fibers are not found in the external zone of the median eminence [276]. In human pituitaries, PrRP receptors are found only on corticotroph cells and not lactotroph cells [276]. At present, it is not thought that PrRP plays a significant role in PRL regulation in humans or any other species [276].

Other Neuroactive Peptides and Neurotransmitters

Somatostatin receptors have been found on human PRL- as well as GH-secreting adenomas [277]. Somatostatin has been found to inhibit adenyl cyclase activity of rat anterior pituitary homogenates and spontaneous and stimulated PRL release [278]. Furthermore, administration of somatostatin antiserum to rats causes a rise in PRL levels, implying a physiologic inhibitory action of somatostatin basally [277]. In humans, however, somatostatin administered exogenously has no effect on the TRH-induced PRL release [279].

A number of other peptides (neurotensin, substance P, cholecystokin, bombesin, calcitonin, endothelin, galanin, gastrin, transforming growth factor β) and bioamines such as glutamine have been found to have varying effects on PRL levels in rats in different experimental paradigms, but very limited studies in humans have shown no effect.

Histamine plays an uncertain role in PRL regulation [280]. Histamine neuronal perikarya are present in the posterior hypothalamic region and axons project to almost all of the nuclei of the hypothalamus [280]. Although some experiments show an effect of histamine via hypothalamic mechanisms, it has no effect on PRL release from pituitaries in vitro or in stalk-sectioned rats [281]. In humans, intravenous H_2 but not H_1 blockers cause a rise in PRL levels [282], but prolonged oral administration of H_2 blockers does not result in sustained PRL elevation [283]. The fact that the administration of high doses of H_2 blockers causes an increase in PRL levels in humans, that histamine cannot cross the blood–brain barrier, and that histamine has no effect on pituitaries in vitro suggests that histamine may play a physiologic facilatory role within the median eminence in PRL secretion.

The roles of other bioamines in the regulation of PRL secretion are even less well established. Central adrenergic α_2 agonists such as clonidine usually have no effect on PRL secretion although both increases and decreases have been reported, the differences being due to the doses used [284]. α-Methyl dopa, another central adrenergic agonist, causes a sustained elevation of PRL [285] but this may be due to inhibition of the synthesis of norepinephrine or DA centrally by inhibiting the enzyme l-aromatic acid decarboxylase, which is responsible for conversion of dopa to DA and by acting as a false neurotransmitter to decrease DA secretion or synthesis by a local feedback inhibitory action. However, monoamine oxidase inhibitors cause an increase in PRL levels [286]. Such an elevation is unexpected, since these drugs should increase the levels of norepinephrine and DA in the synapse.

Acetylcholine inhibits adenyl cyclase and cAMP accumulation, lowers intracellular free calcium levels, and decreases PRL release from pituitary cell cultures, acting through muscarinic and not nicotinic receptors [287]. Although atropine, a muscarinic receptor antagonist, blocks this acetylcholine inhibition of PRL in vitro [287], it had no effect on basal or TRH-induced PRL release in humans [288] and pirenzepine, another muscarinic receptor blocker, actually caused a modest decrease in PRL levels in humans in vivo [289]. The widespread presence of acetylcholine as a neurotransmitter in the CNS and the possibility that pituitary tissue itself may synthesize acetylcholine [290] makes interpretation of studies testing this system difficult and the true role of acetylcholine in the regulation of PRL secretion is uncertain.

Prolactin Short-loop Feedback

Considerable evidence in rats suggests that PRL is able to feedback negatively on its own secretion (short-loop feedback or autofeedback) [291]. Most evidence suggests that such feedback occurs via augmentation of hypothalamic TIDA turnover, including direct measurements of DA in portal vessels [291]. Studies using mice with targeted disruption of the *PRL* gene show that they have markedly decreased DA in TIDA neurons along with hyperplasia of lactotrophs that do not make PRL [292,293].

Direct evidence for such PRL short-loop feedback in the human has not been demonstrated. In a number of reports, however, it has been suggested that altered regulation of gonadotropin and TSH secretion in hyperprolactinemic patients may constitute indirect evidence of PRL-induced augmented TIDA activity [196,294,295]. In hyperprolactinemic patients, decreases in gonadotropin pulse amplitude and frequency are usually found, being attributed to altered gonadotropin-releasing hormone secretion (see below). Such an alteration of GnRH secretion has been postulated to be due, in part, to PRL-induced DA increase [296,297]. In a direct test of this hypothesis, however, no evidence was found of suppression of TSH, LH, or FSH levels with short-term administration of human PRL which resulted in a 2–3-fold elevation of PRL levels [298]. However, these acute studies do not rule out the possibility that such feedback may occur with more prolonged states of hyperprolactinemia. Alternatively, such feedback might occur via other mechanisms, such as a decrease in a PRF such as VIP [299].

PROLACTIN ACTION

Prolactin has a great diversity of actions in many species of animals from fish and birds to mammals, including osmoregulation, growth and developmental effects, metabolic effects, actions on ectodermal and integumentary structures, and actions related to reproduction [291]. However, in humans it has as its primary physiologic action the preparation of the breast for lactation in the postpartum period. A number of effects of increased levels of PRL may be seen on many tissues. Although the roles of physiologic levels of PRL in such tissues are quite speculative, considerable clarification of these roles has been elucidated from studies in PRL-KO and PRL receptor KO mice.

Prolactin Receptor

The prolactin receptor (PRLR) belongs to the class I cytokine receptor superfamily, a family of single-pass transmembrane proteins that transduce signals following phosphorylation by cytoplasmic kinases. The human PRLR (hPRLR) gene is located on chromosome 5p14-p13.2 and consists of eight or nine coding exons and two noncoding exons, which constitute the 5′ UTR. Six alternative forms of the first exon ($hE1_{N1}$–$hE1_{N5}$) are expressed in a tissue-specific manner, and are spliced into the noncoding exon 2. Exons 3–10 encode the full-length activating long form of the receptor. Multiple PRLR transcripts, resulting from alternative splicing and transcriptional start sites, give rise to intermediate and short forms of the receptor (described below). Transcripts from exon 11 are only present in the short forms of the receptor [300]. The entire hPRLR locus spans a region that exceeds 200 kb. The hPRLR cDNA is 1869 nucleotides long and encodes a protein of 622 amino acids, 24 of which represent the signal peptide.

The PRLR is ubiquitously expressed. Regulation of PRLR protein levels occurs at both transcriptional and post-transcriptional levels. Transcription of hPRLR is controlled by multiple promoters, with each of the alternative noncoding exons 1 utilizing a separate promoter [301,302]. The preferentially utilized, generic promoter 1/exon-1 (PIII/hE13) contains functional Sp1 and C/EBP sites that bind transcription factors Sp1/Sp3 and C/EBPβ, respectively [302,303]. Estradiol, operating through a nonclassical ERα signaling mechanism, activates the hPRLR hPIII promoter in breast cancer cells through ERα-mediated recruitment of Sp1 and C/EBPβ, and assembly of a coactivator complex consisting of p300, SRC-1 and pCAF [304]. PRLR levels are negatively regulated at a post-translational level by proteolytic degradation via receptor ubiquitination, facilitated by the SCF β-Trcp E3 ubiquitin ligase, and targeting to the lysosomal complex [305,306]. Alterations in PRLR degradation may contribute to transformation of breast cells [307].

The PRLR contains an extracellular domain (ECD) required for ligand binding, a transmembrane domain, and an intracellular domain (ICD) required for signal transduction (Figure 5.8). The hPRLR exists as at least nine recognized isoforms, which have different signaling properties. Mice and rats also express multiple PRLR isoforms. Within a species, the ECDs of most PRLR isoforms are identical, whereas the ICDs are of variable length and composition. The long PRLR serves as the canonical sequence, and is the only isoform that signals properly. The intermediate form results from a frameshift, and leads to absence of a portion of the ICD. The ΔS_1 isoform lacks exons 4 and 5, and has reduced affinity for hormone, but displays effective signal transduction. Short forms of the hPRLR known as S_{1a}, S_{1b} and $\Delta 4\text{-}S_{1b}$ are derived from alternative splicing. These forms have similar binding affinity for PRL as the long form, but cannot transduce signal and exhibit dominant negative activity when co-expressed with the long form. In addition to membrane anchored receptor, a soluble, freely circulating form of the receptor, prolactin receptor-binding protein (PRLRBP), is generated by proteolytic cleavage of the long hPRLR [308].

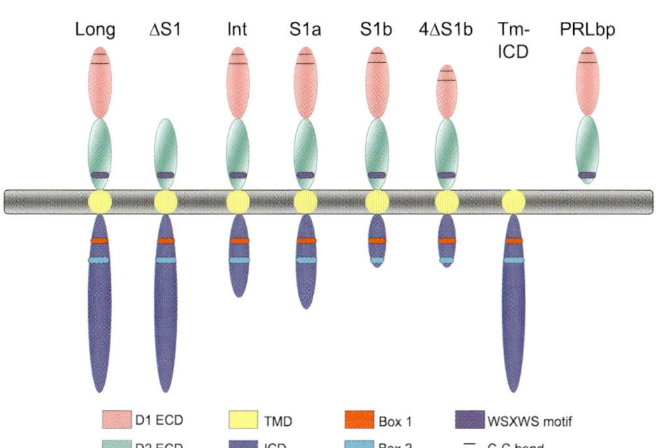

FIGURE 5.8 Schematic illustration of eight of the most common human prolactin receptor (PRLR) isoforms. The PRLR gene (not depicted) undergoes alternative splicing to yield several transcripts, and subsequently proteins, of variable length. In general, the extracellular and transmembrane domains are nearly identical, whereas the intracellular domains vary in length and composition. Motifs such as the disulfide bonds, WSXWS, box 1 and box 2 are highly conserved.

The functional significance of the various isoforms has not been determined conclusively, but some insights into their function have been gained through the phenotypic analysis of genetic mouse models in which a short PRLR isoform is overexpressed on a long *Prlr* null background ($Prlr^{-/-};rs^{tg}$) [309]. These mice display premature ovarian follicular development followed by massive follicular cell death. On a molecular level, PRL signaling through this particular short PRLR isoform in ovarian tissue represses transcription of several genes, including *FOXO3* and *Galt*, which are important for normal follicular development. Moreover, this short PRLR isoform does not activate JAK/Stat, but instead utilizes a unique intracellular signaling pathway involving calmodulin-dependent protein kinase (CamK) [310]. The phenotypic alterations demonstrated in $Prlr^{-/-};rs^{tg}$ ovaries are reversed by the reco-expression of the long PRLR, suggesting that the two isoforms inhibit the activity of each other, and the proper ratio of their expression is important for the normal physiological development of ovarian follicles. Whether improper ovarian PRLR isoform expression occurs in humans and contributes to ovarian failure is not known, but remains an important question. The short PRLR isoforms also appear to inhibit long PRLR function through heterodimerization with long PRLR isoforms resulting in dominant negative activity, and by enhancing PRLR degradation [311,312]. Alterations in the expression of PRLR isoforms and ratio of short to long PRLR isoforms have been observed in breast tumor tissue and cancer cell lines compared with the normal breast and control mammary cells [313]. Accordingly, abnormal signaling as a consequence of these changes could theoretically contribute to breast tumor development and/or progression.

The PRLR has three defining domains, two within the ECD and one in the ICD. The ECD contains two signature motifs: an amino-terminal region (S_1) and a membrane-proximal region (S_2). Two pairs of disulfide bonds in S_1 are highly conserved and critical for tertiary receptor folding of the ligand-binding domain. A highly conserved WSXWS motif constitutes the S2 motif and may be involved in receptor trafficking. The PRLR ECD, as resolved by X-ray crystallography, contains two subdomains, which are related to the type III repeats of fibronectin. Each domain is composed of seven β-strands folded into two antiparallel β-sheets [314]. The third defining motif, which lies in the ICD of the PRLR, is referred to as "box 1" and consists of an 8-amino acid proline-rich hydrophobic sequence that directly interacts with intracellular tyrosine kinases. Mutations in residues of box 1 completely disrupt JAK/Stat PRLR signaling [315,316]. Several additional structural domains within the ICD have been identified but are uncharacterized.

The active PRL/PRLR complex has a stochiometry of one hormone bound to two receptors (Figure 5.9). As such, two ECDs of the PRLR interact with two asymmetric ligand-binding sites located opposite each other within the receptor core. The formation of 1:2 complexes is an essential first step for subsequent signal transduction. Two different mechanisms of PRL binding to PRLR have been proposed. The conventional view holds that binding of PRL to a monomeric first receptor induces the sequential recruitment and dimerization of a second receptor [314,317]. This leads to activating changes in the ICD and initiates signal transduction. Recent data garnered from coimmunoprecipitation and bioluminescence resonance energy transfer (BRET1) analyses support an alternative model in which the PRLR dimerizes independently of ligand binding [311,318]. In this mode, PRLRs reside in dimeric form at the cell membrane, facilitated by interactions within the transmembrane domains. The receptors are held in an inactive state until PRL binding to the preformed dimers induces conformational changes in the receptor complex that lead to signal initiation. This latter ligand-independent model of PRLR dimerization is consistent with reports identifying receptor predimerization of the growth hormone and erythropoietin receptors [319,320], and thus may represent a common feature of cytokine receptors. For the GHR, GH binding to the preformed GHR dimer complex appears to activate the receptor through a specific structural mechanism that involves a relative rotation of receptor subunits within the transmembrane domain [319]. Although a similar conformational rearrangement may also occur with respect to PRLR activation, the exact mechanism by which PRL initiates activation of preformed PRLR dimeric complexes has not been formally determined.

PRLR Signal Transduction

Ligand binding to the PRLR results in rapid activation of janus kinase 2 (Jak2) tyrosine kinase, which is constitutively associated with box 1 of the PRLR. Jak2 activation is the most proximal event in the intracellular events that occur after ligand binding [321] (Figure 5.10). Jak2 phosphorylates tyrosine residues on the PRLR ICD and autophosphorylates residues within itself [322]. Receptor-associated Jak2 also phosphorylates cytoplasmic signal transducer and activator of transcription [323] proteins [324]. Four STAT family members (Stat 1, Stat 2, Stat 5a, Stat 5b) serve as the central transducer molecules of the signal transduction pathways initiated

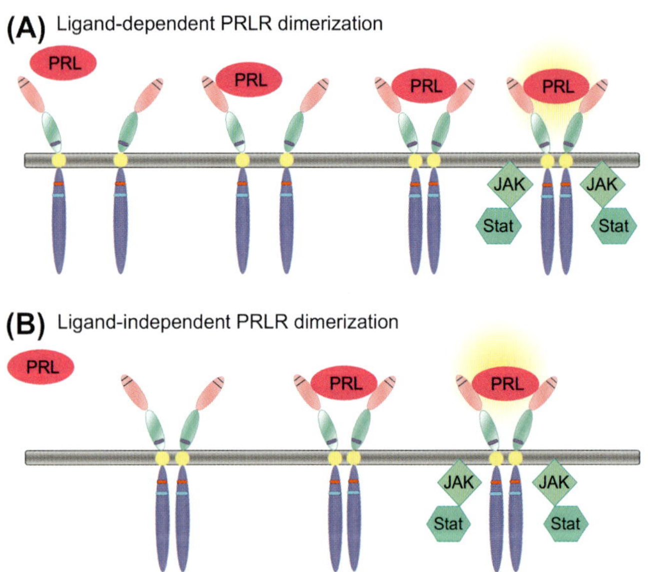

FIGURE 5.9 Schematic illustration demonstrating two models for prolactin receptor (PRLR) activation. (A) In the ligand-dependent dimerization model, one molecule of PRL binds to a PRLR monomer at binding site 1, which leads to the recruitment of the second PRLR monomer to bind PRL at site 2. Dimerization of the two PRLRs leads to phosphorylation of Janus kinase [513] and signal transducer and activator of transcription 5a (stat5). (B) In the ligand-independent dimerization model, the PRLRs exist as preformed dimers at the cell membrane in the absence of ligand. PRL binding to the dimeric PRLR receptor induces conformational changes that subsequently activate the receptor.

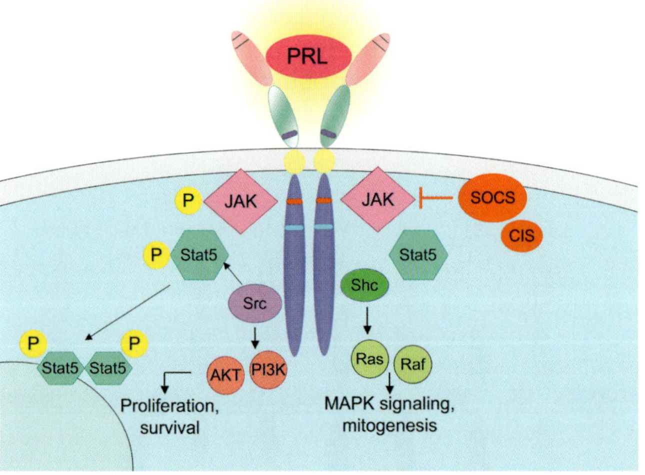

FIGURE 5.10 Schematic illustration depicting intracellular signal transduction pathways downstream of the prolactin receptor (PRL). Following activation of the PRLR, Janus kinase 2 [513] tyrosine kinase becomes activated through auto- or transphosphorylation. This triggers association with signal transducer and activator of transcription protein 5a (Stat5) followed by Stat5 phosphorylation, dimerization and nuclear translocation. Association with adaptor proteins such as Shc leads to signaling through the mitogen-activated protein kinase (MAPK) pathway to stimulate mitogenesis. Association with Src family kinases triggers phosphoinositide 3-kinase (PI3K) and Akt (protein kinase B) signaling to affect cell proliferation and survival. Members of the suppressors of cytokine signaling (SOCS) and cytokine-inducible inhibitor of signaling (CIS) proteins attenuate the actions of Jak.

by PRLR activation, but Stat 5a and, to a lesser extent, Stat 5b, are especially important for mammary gland development and lactogenesis [325,326]. A phosphorylated tyrosine residue of the activated PRLR interacts with the SH2 domain of a STAT protein. Following phosphorylation by activated Jak2, STAT proteins hetero- or homodimerize, translocate to the nucleus, and transactivate γ-interferon activation sequence (GAS) consensus elements on target genes [324]. The tyrosine phosphatase short heterodimer partner (Shp)-2 promotes PRL-stimulated assembly of the Jak-PRLR complex, and is a required component for Stat 5a activation during pregnancy and lactation [327]. Jak2-STAT signaling is attenuated through an intracellular negative-feedback system involving the action of several negative regulators, including: (1) suppressor of cytokine signaling (SOCS) proteins, which inhibit Jak2 kinases; (2) cytokine-inducible SH2-containing (CIS) proteins, which compete with STAT proteins for docking sites on the PRLR; and (3) protein tyrosine phosphatases, PTP1B1 and TC-PTP, which dephosphorylate PRL-activated STATs [328–331].

Although the Jak/STAT pathway mediates most physiological actions of PRL in mammary development and lactation, binding of PRL to its receptor also activates several additional intracellular cascades to promote specific cellular responses [332,333]. Effectors of these cascades engage in signaling cross-talk, and likely operate as a complex network rather than hierarchically depending upon cell type and context. Phosphotyrosine residues of the PRLR can serve as docking sites for adapter proteins (Shc/Grb2/SOS) connecting the receptor to the Ras/Raf/MAPK cascade [334,335]. This pathway appears to mediate at least some PRL mitogenic effects. Activation of PRLR also facilitates docking of Src family kinases, which couple to multiple signaling effectors, including phosphatidylinositol (PI) 3′-kinase/AKT and Erk 1/2, linking PRLR activation to cell survival and proliferation [336,337]. The requirement of Src as an essential mediator of PRLR signaling in normal mammary tissue is underscored by findings in female *Src*$^{-/-}$ mice, which demonstrate lactation failure and precocious mammary gland involution [338]. As they become available, detailed characterization of mouse genetic models lacking components of PRLR-signaling cascades should provide information on their physiologic roles and relevance.

Female Reproductive Tissues

PRL Effects on Breast

PRL plays a dominant role in several aspects of the breast, including growth and development of the mammary gland (mammogenesis), synthesis of milk (lactogenesis) and maintenance of milk secretion (galactopoiesis). Development of the mammary gland is a tightly coordinated process involving several hormones, in addition to PRL, that occurs in defined stages that include embryonic, prepubertal, pubertal and pregnancy [339]. During puberty, the epithelial cell compartment, which consists of a branched ductal system, expands while during pregnancy, the lobuloalveolar compartment differentiates and develops. Mammary gland development during the embryonic and prepubertal stages occurs independently of the actions of PRL, and PRL plays only a minor role in the pubertal stage. However PRL, together with ovarian steroids, local growth factors and cytokines, is essential for the morphological changes that occur in the mammary gland during pregnancy and lactation [340].

The combination of experimental mouse genetics and transcriptomic profiling has been useful for confirming the roles of genes and identifying PRL-dependent signaling pathways that control mammary development. At the onset of puberty, the ovarian steroids estradiol and progesterone and pituitary GH initiate and drive ductal morphogenesis [341]. Mammary gland development in *Prl*$^{-/-}$ and *Prlr*$^{-/-}$ mice is arrested at the stage of ductal elongation and these mice completely lack lobuloalveolar units, indicating that it is at this stage and beyond that PRL exerts developmental influences [293,342]. PRL indirectly influences the process of ductal side branching during puberty by promoting ovarian progesterone synthesis [343,344]. In contrast to these relatively minor effects, PRL plays a major role in the morphological and functional changes that occur in the breast during pregnancy. During pregnancy, high concentrations of estradiol and progesterone, produced by the placenta, coupled with high levels of PRL and hPL, promotes proliferation of the lobuloalveolar epithelium. During and after parturition, progesterone, estradiol and hPL levels decline, whereas PRL levels rise. These hormonal changes, together with the effects of local growth factors such as RANK-ligand and insulin-like growth factor 2 (IGF-2) induce the lobuloalveolar epithelium to convert into secretory acini [345–347]. Epithelial PRLRs are required for this process, as *Prlr*$^{-/-}$ mammary transplants fail to develop lobuloalveoli and cannot produce milk proteins during pregnancy [344]. PRL also acts in concert with insulin and hydrocortisone to induce differentiation of pluripotent mammary epithelial cells that produce progeny that subsequently grow into alveolar structures [348]. Members of the PRLR signaling pathway whose functions are essential for mediating PRL effects on alveolar morphogenesis include the transcription factors Stat5a, Id2, Socs-2, Gata-3 and Elf5 [325,349–352].

Both lactogenesis and galactopoiesis require pituitary PRL, since hypophysectomy during pregnancy prevents or stops, respectively, lactation [353]. *Prl*$^{-/-}$ and *Prlr*$^{-/-}$

mice cannot produce milk as a result of defective mammogenesis. PRL is also essential to maintain sustained lactation [354]. During lactation, PRL regulates the synthesis of milk proteins, including β-casein, lactoglobulin, lactalbumin and whey acidic protein [355]. PRL also regulates the synthesis of enzymes involved in lipid metabolism, including lactose synthetase, lipoprotein lipase, and fatty acid synthase [355].

Galactorrhea

Clinically, nonpuerperal galactorrhea has been regarded as being a sign of possible hyperprolactinemia. The presence of even minute amounts of milk expressible from one or both breasts indicates a diagnosis of galactorrhea. Its persistence for more than 1 year after normal delivery and cessation of breast-feeding or its occurrence in the absence of pregnancy generally is regarded as a definition of inappropriate lactation. If the material expressible from the nipple looks like milk, it probably is milk; if there is any uncertainty, examination of the breast secretion by staining of fat globules with Sudan IV is diagnostic.

The incidence of galactorrhea has been variously reported in normal women as ranging from 1 to 45% of subjects tested [356–359]. This variability is probably due to differences in the techniques used to express milk from the breast and the way in which nonmilky secretions are classified. The volume of milk expressed does not correlate with PRL levels. However, in individuals with hyperprolactinemia, lowering the blood PRL level to normal almost always will lead to a marked decrease in or abolition of lactation. Inappropriate lactation may be an important clue to the presence of pituitary–hypothalamic disease, especially if accompanied by amenorrhea. In a series of 70 women with galactorrhea, 19 (27%) had normal menses [360]. Of those with normal menses, only one had elevated PRL levels. Clinical experience suggests that galactorrhea may be present in about 5–10% of normally menstruating women and basal PRL levels are normal in more than 90% of these women.

PRL and Breast Cancer

The role of PRL and its receptor in the promotion or progression of human breast cancer remains an active area of debate. A wide range of studies has attempted to address the possible contribution of PRL to breast cancer through epidemiological analyses, cellular and molecular studies, and transgenic mouse models. Overall, epidemiological studies examining the relationship between serum PRL levels and the risk of breast cancer in women have shown conflicting results. The Nurses' Health Study, the largest prospective cohort study reported, found a significantly (34%) increased risk of breast cancer when comparing top to bottom quartiles of serum PRL in postmenopausal women [361] and a nonsignificant 30% increase in risk comparing top to bottom PRL quartiles in premenopausal women [362]. These findings are similar to results of previously reported smaller studies that found nonsignificant increases in breast cancer risk [363]. The number of studies investigating associations between genetic variability in the PRL or PRLR genes and the risk of breast cancer are limited, but favor lack of association. Analysis of high-density single-nucleotide polymorphism (SNP) data from the Multiethnic Cohort Study which included 1600 cases of breast cancer and 1900 controls, did not find a significant association between PRL and PRLR haplotypes or individual SNPs in relation to breast cancer risk [364].

Recent attention has turned to the question as to whether local production of PRL within breast tissue plays an autocrine or paracrine role in the etiology or progression of breast cancer [109,332]. Accumulating data from in vitro and animal studies have suggested that PRL and/or actions of the PRLR may be involved in mammary tumorigenesis by promoting cell proliferation and survival [365–367], increasing cell motility [368], supporting tumor vascularization [369] and/or contributing to cell transformation [307]. Transgenic mice that permanently overexpress PRL systemically [370] or locally within the mammary epithelia [371] develop mammary carcinomas at a long latency, whereas transient overexpression of PRL in differentiated, lactating mammary tissue leads to the development of benign mammary adenomas [372]. By contrast, genetic ablation of the PRLR delays, but does not prevent or reduce the incidence of, the development of SV40 large T-antigen-induced breast carcinomas [373]. Taken together, findings from these murine models support a modulatory role for PRLR function in mammary neoplasia. In humans, a substantial percentage of primary human breast carcinomas express PRL and PRLR [374–376], but immunostaining for the receptor does not correlate well with clinicopathological stage or disease-free survival. A heterozygous missense mutation in the PRLR (I146L substitution in the ECD) characterized by high levels of constitutive signaling has been identified in a small percentage (~7%) of human benign breast tumors [377,378]. Neither this mutation nor others have been identified in breast carcinomas, and the mechanistic nature of the relationship between the I146L PRLR mutation and the development of breast tumors has not been specified.

In light of the above listed observations that have suggested a role for PRL or PRLR in promoting mammary tumor growth, efforts have been initiated to investigate the potential usefulness of pharmacologic inhibition of the PRLR for the treatment of breast neoplasms or other conditions associated with hyperprolactinemia [379,380]. Preclinical studies using competitive PRLR antagonists have demonstrated proof-of-principal PRLR antagonism and inhibition of cell proliferation, but have been associated with unfavorable pharmacokinetics [381], and the potential adverse effects of PRLR inhibition, as observed in PRLR null mice, have not been ascertained.

PRL Effects on Gonadotropin Secretion

The effects of normal circulating PRL levels on gonadotropin secretion are not known. *Prl*$^{-/-}$ and *Prlr*$^{-/-}$ female mice are sterile, and both types have disordered estrous cycles, but whether the sterility in these cases is due to cell-autonomous effects in the gonads, altered gonadotropin secretion, or to a combination of these is not clear from these global knockout mice (see PRL effects on the ovary and PRL effects on the testes, below) [293,342]. Male mice deficient for PRL have reduced plasma LH levels; gonadotropin levels in male mice deficient for the PRLR are not altered. In normal women treated with short-term bromocriptine to lower PRL levels to about 5 ng/ml, there is no change in the pulsatile secretion of LH and FSH but estradiol levels are higher during the last 3 days of the follicular cycle, and progesterone levels lower during the luteal phase [382].

Hyperprolactinemia, on the other hand, has a number of effects on various steps in the reproductive axis (Figure 5.11). Hyperprolactinemia has been found in most studies to suppress LH pulsatile secretion by decreasing pulse amplitude and frequency [296,297]. At the menopausal transition in humans, hyperprolactinemia can prevent the expected rise in gonadotropins; normalization of PRL levels with bromocriptine results in a rise in gonadotropin levels and hot flushes [383].

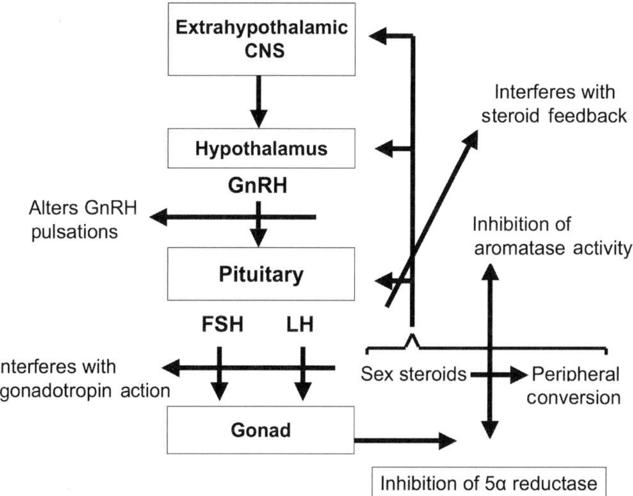

FIGURE 5.11 Diagram demonstrating how hyperprolactinemia produces hypogonadism. Schematic representation of sites where hyperprolactinemia interferes with the reproductive system and sex steroid action. CNS, central nervous system; FSH, follicle-stimulating hormone; LH, luteinizing hormone. *From Malarkey et al. [226].*

Hyperprolactinemia inhibits pulsatile gonadotropin secretion by a number of mechanisms. It had been postulated that the pulsatile gonadotropin secretion was directed by the hypothalamic GnRH pulse generator and that alteration of pulsatile secretion necessarily meant a direct hypothalamic action. However, direct measurement of portal vessel GnRH levels in rats showed a marked inhibitory effect of hyperprolactinemia in one study [299] but not in another [384]. The pituitary gonadotroph response to GnRH in hyperprolactinemia has generally been found to be normal, increased and decreased in humans [385–387]. In our own series of hyperprolactinemic women, the gonadotropin response to GnRH was normal in 22 of 25 patients and decreased in the remaining three [360]. GnRH plays a major role in the regulation of the number of its own receptors on the gonadotroph cell. The number of GnRH receptors on gonadotroph cells in hyperprolactinemic rats is reduced [388] even when endogenous GnRH is replaced with intra-arterial pulses of GnRH [389]. In addition to these effects, hyperprolactinemia in women has been associated with loss of positive estrogen feedback on gonadotropin secretion [390].

PRL Effects on the Ovary and Fertility

The effects of PRL on ovarian function and fertility are complex and to some extent species-specific. PRL is an essential luteotropic hormone in rodents, but not in humans. Instead, in humans, pituitary LH supports luteal development and steroidogenesis during the menstrual cycle, and the embryonic trophoblast sustains the corpus luteum during pregnancy. The action of PRL on the ovaries has been fairly well-characterized in rats, but the role of PRL in normal ovarian physiology is not well-defined in humans. A comparison of PRL profiles across the estrous and menstrual cycles in rodents and humans, respectively, reveals marked differences, supporting the notion that the function of PRL during these cycles differs between the two species. In humans, serum PRL levels remain relatively stable throughout the menstrual cycle, except for a slight increase during the luteal phase, the functional significance of which is not known [391]. By contrast, in rats, PRL levels rise in a triphasic manner showing a sharp rise just prior to ovulation, followed by a plateau and an extended termination phase [109]. The PRLR is expressed in human granulosa cells [392,393] and the human ovary produces its own PRL [392,394], but the specific roles of circulating versus autocrine-derived PRL on ovarian function are unknown. PRL is found in human follicular fluid where it has been shown to stimulate ovarian endothelial cell proliferation [395,396].

Although the role(s) of normal physiologic levels of PRL on ovarian function and female fertility are not fully known in humans, it is well established that the actions of PRL and the activity of its receptor are essential for fertility in female mice. Both $Prl^{-/-}$ and $Prlr^{-/-}$ female mice are completely infertile [293,342]. Mating of $Prl^{-/-}$ and $Prlr^{-/-}$ female mice with males of established fertility does not produce offspring. Moreover, female $Prl^{-/-}$ mice have irregular estrous cycles. Whether this is due to an ovarian or hypothalamic defect is not known for certain, but obvious histological defects in the ovaries are not observed. $Prlr^{-/-}$ female mice, on the other hand, display multiple reproductive abnormalities, including reduced rates of mating, fertilization and ovulation, as compared to wild-type mice. PRLR-deficient ovaries contain fewer primary follicles and those eggs that do become fertilized develop poorly, as oocyte development is arrested almost immediately after fertilization. In these mice, the corpus luteum regresses, and is unable to support implantation and placental development [397]. Administration of progesterone to $Prl^{-/-}$ and $Prlr^{-/-}$ females rescues implantation and early embryonic development [343,398]. Thus, regulation of sustained progesterone production, permitting the proper expression of progesterone-dependent genes, is the essential function of prolactin that is required for normal implantation in $Prl^{-/-}$ and $Prlr^{-/-}$ mice in early pregnancy. The cause of late embryonic lethality is not known for certain, but may be a result of the absence of local decidual PRL production, leading to de-repression of two genes, *IL-6* and *20α-HSD*, whose expression is detrimental for the normal progress of pregnancy [398]. The phenotypic differences between the $Prl^{-/-}$ and $Prlr^{-/-}$ mouse models could reflect compensatory action by numerous murine PRL-like proteins that are capable of activating the PRLR, whereas PRLR-deficient mice cannot respond to any of the PRL family members. Mice that overexpress a short PRLR isoform on a $Prlr^{-/-}$ background exhibit accelerated follicular recruitment and development, followed by early follicular cell death leading to premature ovarian failure [309]. Thus, signaling events that occur downstream of the long PRLR in the ovary are essential for follicular survival, at least in mice.

The major mechanism by which PRL performs its luteotropic action in rodents is through stimulation of progesterone production by luteal cells [399]. Specifically, PRL down-regulates the expression of 20α-hydroxysteroid dehydrogenase, which prevents the catabolism of progesterone to an inactive metabolite [400,401]. This serves to increase progesterone secretion from the corpus luteum. Paradoxically, in some experimental settings, PRL can induce luteolysis [402,403].

In human granulosa cells, PRL stimulates expression of type II 3β-hydroxysteroid dehydrogenase, the enzyme responsible for catalyzing the final step in progesterone biosynthesis, and increases IGF-2 secretion [404,405]. Perfusion studies of human ovaries in vitro show that PRL directly suppresses progesterone and estrogen secretion [406]. PRL inhibits estrogen formation by [1] antagonizing the stimulatory effects of FSH on aromatase activity [407] and [2] directly inhibiting aromatase synthesis itself [408]. In fact, PRL is required at low doses (<20 ng/ml) for progesterone production by granulosa cell cultures, but at higher concentrations (i.e., those that correlate with hyperprolacinemia in women), PRL inhibits progesterone production. These in vitro findings are in line with in vivo studies of luteal function in women where treatment with bromocriptine to lower normal PRL levels to hypoprolactinemic levels resulted in lowered progesterone levels and shorter luteal phases [382,409,410].

As noted above, during pregnancy, human maternal PRL secretion rises gradually beginning at 6–8 weeks gestation until term. In the human fetal circulation, PRL rises slightly starting at around 10 weeks, plateaus, and then rises again very sharply at 30 weeks until term. The decidual produces and secretes copious amounts of PRL into the amniotic fluid beginning at 12 weeks, peaking at around 20 weeks and then gradually declining until term. The exact function of decidual or amniotic fluid PRL is not known, although several functions of decidual PRL have been postulated. Results of investigations in PRL and PRLR knockout mice suggest that decidual PRL is a physiological repressor of IL-6 and 20α-HSD, the inhibition of which is necessary to temper the inflammatory response of pregnancy and to prevent catabolism of progesterone [398]. Other putative functions of decidual PRL, such as facilitation of trophoblast growth, inhibition of myometrial contractility and regulation of angiogenesis, have been suggested but limited data are available to support these theories [411]. Human placental lactogen (PL) shows a similar pattern of rise to that of PRL, only on a larger scale, such that by 30 weeks PL levels exceed PRL levels by ten-fold.

Clinical Effects of Hyperprolactinemia on Menstrual Function

Elevated serum PRL levels (hyperprolactinemia) in women causes oligoamenorrhea or amenorrhea. The amenorrhea caused by hyperprolactinemia is typically secondary, but primary amenorrhea can occur if the disorder begins before the usual age of puberty. Of 33 patients in two series presenting with primary amenorrhea and low gonadotropin levels, nine (27%) were found to have hyperprolactinemia [412,413]. However, in a third series of 38 patients with primary amenorrhea, PRL levels were normal in all [414]. In patients with primary amenorrhea due to hyperprolactinemia, estrogen deficiency and failure to develop normal secondary sexual characteristics may be the presenting problem. Galactorrhea is variable in this setting because the breast may not have been exposed to appropriate priming with estrogen and progesterone. Patients with primary amenorrhea tend to have macroadenomas more commonly than those with secondary amenorrhea, for uncertain reasons (see Prolactinoma, Chapter 15).

When amenorrhea or oligoamenorrhea is associated with galactorrhea, it is usually a manifestation of hyperprolactinemia. In our series of 51 women with galactorrhea-oligo/amenorrhea, 84% had hyperprolactinemia [360]. In combined series totaling 471 patients with galactorrhea-amenorrhea, 75.4% were found to have hyperprolactinemia [415].

Hyperprolactinemia is found in many women with a short luteal phase. It is likely that a short luteal phase is the first evidence of interference in the normal cycle by hyperprolactinemia [416]. Infertility also may be a presenting symptom of patients with hyperprolactinemia and is invariable when gonadotropin levels are suppressed with anovulation. In three series of women (combined number of 367 cases) studied for infertility, one-third were found to have hyperprolactinemia [415]. Most of these women presented with amenorrhea and galactorrhea as well, but hyperprolactinemia without other symptoms was found in five of the 22 hyperprolactinemic women in one series of 113 cases of infertility [417]. That PRL excess may be important in this type of patient is suggested by the finding that treatment of similar patients with bromocriptine restored fertility [418]. In some infertile women, transient hyperprolactinemia lasting for 1–2 days during the cycle can be documented; this subset usually responds to bromocriptine with increased progesterone during the luteal phase and improved fertility [419].

Reduced libido and orgasmic dysfunction are found in most hyperprolactinemic amenorrheic women when such complaints are specifically elicited [360]. Reduction of PRL levels to normal restores normal libido and sexual function in most of these women [420].

PRL levels may be elevated in 13–50% of women with polycystic ovary syndrome (PCOS) [421,422]. Bromocriptine treatment of hyperprolactinemic patients with PCOS usually results in a reduction of testosterone and LH levels and resumption of ovulatory cycles. Why many patients with PCOS have hyperprolactinemia is not clear. Del Pozo and Falaschi have hypothesized that the increased estrogen levels found in PCO stimulate increased PRL secretion; however, no correlation has been found between estrone levels and PRL levels in these patients [421].

Male Reproductive Tissues

While PRL clearly plays an essential reproductive role in females, the role of PRL in male reproductive function is less defined. A conclusive determination regarding the involvement of PRL in male fertility has not emerged from genetically engineered mouse models where PRL or the PRLR has been disrupted. In the original report of PRLR knockout mice, the absence of functional PRLR was associated with infertility or reduced fertility in ~50% of males [342]. Subsequent studies of PRLR knockout mice on different genetic backgrounds have produced divergent results. On a pure 129/Sv background, deletion of the PRLR does not alter fertility parameters, sperm reserves, plasma gonadotropin levels, testosterone levels, or weight or histology of the testes or epididymides [423]. However, on a predominantly 129/Sv Pas genetic background, the rate of total infertility in *Prlr*$^{-/-}$ mice is five-fold higher and the latency to produce a first pregnancy significantly increased, as compared to wild-type mice [424]. Deficiency of PRL itself in *Prl*$^{-/-}$ mice is associated with reduced plasma LH levels, but not with effects on male fertility parameters or basal plasma testosterone levels [425].

In other rodents and humans, indirect evidence supports the view that PRL plays a subtle role in testes and/or germ cell function. PRL promotes Leydig cell proliferation and differentiation in prepubertal hypophysectomized rats [426] and is involved in the maintenance of Leydig cell morphology, up-regulation of LH receptor expression and potentiation of LH-induced steroidogenesis [427–429]. In humans, PRLRs are expressed in germ cells undergoing spermatogenesis in seminiferous tubules, and in Leydig cells, vas deferens, epididymis, prostate and seminal vesicles [430]. Human semen contains significant quantities of PRL [431]. The functional significance of PRL or PRLR expression at many of these sites is still unclear. However, the presence of PRLR in differentiating germ cells in the testes is supportive of data that PRL acts as a prosurvival factor for human spermatozoa by preserving motility, suppressing sperm capacitation and enhancing vitality by inhibiting entry into the cell death pathway [432,433]. Moreover, reduction of normal PRL levels through the administration of bromocriptine in men results in suppression of basal and hCG-stimulated testosterone levels, implying a physiologic role for PRL in testosterone production in humans [434].

A substantial body of data from in vitro and in vivo studies supports mitogenic or prosurvival roles for PRL in the prostate. PRL and PRL isoforms are expressed and functional in normal human prostate epithelia and malignant human prostate tissue [435]. Some studies in human prostate cancer cell lines have shown that autocrine-derived PRL promotes prostate cancer cell growth [436,437]; others show that exogenous PRL inhibits apoptosis [438]. In rodents, elevated levels of PRL are associated with increased growth of the prostate [439,440]. Ubiquitous transgenic overexpression of PRL in mice leads to prostatic hyperplasia with elevated serum testosterone levels [441,442]. Prostate-specific transgenic overexpression of PRL leads to stromal hyperplasia, ductal dilatation, focal epithelial dysplasia, but without changes in serum androgen levels, indicating that the abnormal prostate findings are not consequential to hyperandrogenemia, and that autocrine-derived PRL is at least a contributing factor to these effects. By contrast, the prostate glands of PRL-deficient mice are ~30% smaller than those of wild-type mice [425], and, as found in murine models in the breast, PRLR deficiency reduces the incidence of SV40 T-antigen-induced prostate carcinoma [424]. Thus, these studies, which support pro-proliferative and/or anti-apoptotic properties for PRL in the prostate, suggest potential (patho-) physiological roles for PRL in human prostate development and/or disease, possibly elaborated at an autocrine level. However, data on the frequency of prostate hyperplasia or carcinoma in humans with sustained systemic hyperprolactinemia are lacking.

Clinical Effects of PRL in Males

Chronic hyperprolactinemia in males results in impotence and decreased libido in over 90% of cases [443–447]. Other findings of hypogonadism, such as decreased beard growth and strength are less common [445,446]. Galactorrhea in men is reported in 10–20% of cases of hyperprolactinemia, and is virtually pathognomonic of a prolactinoma [444–446]. The frequency of hyperprolactinemia among men with complaints of impotence or infertility as assessed by surveys ranges between 2 and 25% among various series [418,443,448]. However, only 1–5% of men with infertility have been found to be hyperprolactinemic [449].

Hyperprolactinemia in men is associated with decreased pulsatile secretion of LH and FSH (as noted above), and low or low-normal testosterone levels [443–447]. The testosterone response to stimulation with hCG has been reported to be both decreased [443,450] and normal [444,451]; in those with decreased responses there is improvement in the response when PRL levels are lowered with bromocriptine [443,447,452]. If there is sufficient normal pituitary tissue, reduction of elevated PRL levels to normal usually results in a return of normal testosterone levels [447,452]. Although some studies have suggested that drug-induced hyperprolactinemia partially inhibits the enzyme 5-alpha reductase, resulting in reduced dihydrotestosterone (DHT) levels [453], hyperprolactinemia in men with prolactinomas is not associated with this effect [450]. Hyperprolactinemia has an effect on impotence that is independent of testosterone levels; testosterone therapy of hyperprolactinemic men does not always correct the impotence until PRL levels are brought down to normal [444]. Whether this is due to a decrease in DHT levels has not been verified directly. Elevated PRL levels have adverse effects on male germ cell and testes function. Sperm counts and motility are decreased with an increase in abnormal forms [451,454]. Histology of the testes reveals abnormal seminiferous tubule walls and altered Sertoli cell ultrastructure [455]. Hyperprolactinemia may have a sustained effect on male reproductive function, as the semen analysis does not always return to normal despite therapy that successfully normalizes testosterone and prolactin levels [454].

Carbohydrate Metabolism and Adiposity

PRL functions as a metabolic regulator in two chief areas: (1) pancreatic β cell development and function; (2) appetite regulation and adiposity. The phenotypic assessment of *Prlr*$^{-/-}$ mice indicates that signaling through the PRLR, which serves as a common receptor for both PL and PRL, is important to fully attain normal β cell mass, insulin content and insulin secretory capacity [456]. The PRLR plays a particularly central role in the adaptation of islets to pregnancy, as illustrated by studies in heterozygous *Prlr*$^{+/-}$ female mice. Pregnant female mice haploinsufficient for PRLR exhibit impaired glucose clearance, reduced glucose-stimulated insulin release and lower insulin levels as a result of impaired islet expansion [457]. In support of the critical role of PRLR for islet expansion during gestation, it has been shown that Stat 5, PI3 kinase, MAPK and pathways involving the endocrine tumor suppressor menin all collaborate to mediate the proliferative effects of PRL and PL on pancreatic islets during pregnancy [458–460]. Treatment of mice with PRL also increases feeding behavior, raising the possibility that PRLRs both in the islet and the brain contribute to islet adaptation to pregnancy [461]. Although studies in humans are limited, in vitro experiments confirm that PRL increases β cell number and stimulates insulin secretion in cultured human islets [462,463].

With regard to appetite regulation and adiposity, in vivo studies in rodents and humans support a modest orexigenic effect of PRL. In rats, higher PRL levels are associated with greater food intake and body weight, while suppression of PRL levels leads to the opposite effects [323,464]. Likewise, injection of PRL into the paraventricular nucleus of the hypothalamus increases food intake [465]. PRLR-deficient mice exhibit a subtle reduction in parametrial and subcutaneous adipose tissue mass as compared to wild-type littermates, although no differences are observed in overall body weight [466]. PRL-deficient mice exhibit normal body weight and adiposity [467], suggesting that PLs or other ligands act in conjunction with PRL to influence adiposity. In humans, normal circulating PRL levels do not appear to modulate energy homeostasis; however, hyperprolactinemia has been shown to be associated with mild glucose intolerance, increases in body weight and insulin resistance [468,469]. Treatment with a DA agonist to normalize prolactin lowers glucose levels and induces weight loss in these individuals [468,469]. In contrast to these results, suppression of PRL levels with bromocriptine has no effect on glycemic control in normoprolactinemic subjects with insulin-dependent diabetes [470]. A new preparation of bromocriptine, which has been approved in the US for the treatment of diabetes [471], has been shown to cause a modest reduction in plasma glucose and hemoglobin A1c levels. However, the safety of lowering normal PRL levels to subnormal levels, with respect to fertility and sexual function, has not been proven.

Other in vitro studies suggest a possible role for PRL in adipogenesis. PRL itself is produced in small amounts by human adipocytes, including sources from the breast, visceral and subcutaneous adipose tissue [472]. The PRLR is expressed in both brown and white adipose tissue [472,473]. PRL up-regulates the mRNA expression of its receptor and two transcription factors that are principally involved in adipocyte differentiation, CEBP/β and PPARγ [474], and it also stimulates the conversion of NIH-3T3 fibroblasts into adipocytes. Complex interactions between PRL and several adipokines, such as leptin and adiponectin, have been described. However, the data regarding the effects of exogeneous PRL, transgenic overexpression of PRL, and PRL deficiency on leptin levels in vivo are inconsistent and preclude reliable conclusions [475]. Studies addressing the relationship between PRL and adiponectin levels have mostly shown inhibitory effects. PRL injections into mice inhibit adiponectin release [476,477], and treatment of human subcutaneous adipose tissue explants with PRL also suppresses adiponectin release [475].

Adrenal Cortex

Although PRL receptors are found on cells of the adrenal cortex, the physiologic role of PRL in adrenal steroidogenesis is unknown. Plasma dehydroepiandrosterone (DHEA) and DHEA sulfate (DHEAS) levels have been found to be mildly elevated in about 50% of women with hyperprolactinemia in some series [478–480]. In most of these studies, however, the investigators did not try to correlate the androgen levels with the presence of hirsutism or other indices of virilization. Glickman et al. [479] found low plasma sex-hormone-binding globulin and elevated free testosterone levels in 43% of hyperprolactinemic patients but increased DHEAS levels in only 19%. When the patients studied by Glickman et al. [479] were divided into those who were hirsute and those who were not, the hirsute patients had higher free testosterone levels but not higher DHEAS levels, although both groups had patients with elevated levels of both hormones. The abnormal androgen levels return to normal with correction of the hyperprolactinemia by bromocriptine [480].

Calcium and Bone Metabolism

PRL may have a physiologic role in calcium and bone metabolism. PRL has been shown to increase intestinal calcium absorption even in vitamin D-deficient rats [481] and can stimulate 1-α hydroxylation of 25 hydroxyvitamin D in the kidney, resulting in increased plasma levels of 1,25 $(OH)_2$ D [482]. In humans, however, plasma 1,25 $(OH)_2$D levels and intestinal calcium absorption are normal in hyperprolactinemic subjects [483]. The PRL receptor KO mouse has a decrease in bone formation rate and bone mineral density in association with increased parathyroid hormone levels, but decreased estradiol and progesterone levels so that it is difficult to say how much is due to the lack of PRL [484].

The initial observation by Klibanski et al. that hyperprolactinemic women have a decreased bone mineral density [485] was confirmed by others [486,487], but whether this effect is mediated by estrogen deficiency [488] or is a direct effect of the hyperprolactinemia [487] has been controversial. Correction of the hyperprolactinemia results in an increase in bone mass [488,489]. Studies of hyperprolactinemic women who were not amenorrheic and hypoestrogenemic have shown that their bone mineral density is normal [488,489], confirming the initial hypothesis that it is the estrogen deficiency that mediates the bone mineral loss. A similar, androgen-dependent loss of bone mineral is found in hyperprolactinemic men that is reversible with reversal of the hypoandrogenic state [488–490].

Immune System

Hypophysectomized rats evince thymic involution and decreased cell-mediated immune function, both of which are reversed by the administration of ovine PRL [491]. Similarly, hypoprolactinemia induced in animals by bromocriptine or anti-PRL antibodies has been shown to lead to impaired lymphocyte proliferation and macrophage-activating factor production, again reversed by ovine PRL [492]. In the murine model of systemic lupus erythematosus, bromocriptine was shown to suppress immunoglobulin levels, autoantibodies and immune-complex glomerulonephritis, and to improve survival rates [491]. Interestingly, however, PRL and PRL-receptor knockout animals have shown that prolactin is not essential for normal immunity, as they have normal development, distribution and function of T-lymphocytes, B-lymphocytes and NK cells [491]. It has been suggested that other cytokines may be compensating for the lack of prolactin in these knockout models or that prolactin has significant effects on the immune system only under conditions of stress [491].

Studies of patients with hyperprolactinemia of various etiologies have suggested an increased rate of autoantibodies (including antithyroid, anti-dsDNA, anti-ro, anticardiolipin and antinuclear antibodies [ANA]) without clinical evidence of autoimmune disease [491]. Conversely, elevated levels of prolactin have been found in patients with lupus, rheumatoid arthritis, psoriatic arthritis, multiple sclerosis, Reiter's syndrome, primary Sjögren's syndrome, psoriasis and uveitis, leading to hypothesized causal relationships and a possible therapeutic target [491]. Multiple trials of varying designs with DA agonists, primarily bromocriptine, have shown some clinical improvement in some of these disorders. However, it has not been firmly established in humans that there is a definitive role for PRL in immunomodulation and whether DA agonists have therapeutic utility in some of these disorders [491].

PATHOLOGIC STATES OF PROLACTIN SECRETION

Population studies of normal individuals reveal that PRL levels are not "normally" distributed and better fit a log-normal distribution contaminated by a small number of abnormally high measurements. Several studies have suggested that "elevated" PRL levels may be found in 1–10% of a random sample of individuals without evidence of endocrine abnormality [493–495]. When the frequency of abnormality in such a randomly sampled population is so high, it makes it difficult to determine what indeed is the upper limit of normal for that population and a number of mathematical formulations have been tried (for more complete discussions of this problem, see [493] and [496]). Furthermore, in a normal population, the frequency of macroprolactinemia as a cause of the hyperprolactinemia is likely to be much higher (see above).

As discussed previously, PRL is secreted episodically, resulting in varying blood PRL levels throughout the day. Therefore, a PRL level in a single sample that is in the upper part of the normal range should be confirmed with one or two repeated tests before considering it to be abnormal.

Hypoprolactinemia

As noted above, female mice with the PRL gene and PRL receptor KO are infertile [293,342]. Mice with the PRL gene KO have normal fertility but those with the PRL receptor KO have minimally impaired fertility [342,425].

Idiopathic PRL deficiency has been described in only a single case [497]. This was a 30-year-old woman who had had a minimally delayed puberty (thelarche, age 15 and menarche, age 17), regular menses and normal body hair and breast development who conceived but was unable to lactate postpartum. Her basal PRL levels were all <3 ng/ml, during pregnancy her highest PRL level was 7.8 ng/ml and during the first few days postpartum her highest PRL level was 11.7 ng/ml. Her pituitary function was otherwise normal. PRL levels in her two children and other family members were normal. The ability of this woman to develop primary and secondary sexual characteristics normally and then conceive and deliver a child speak of the minimal, if any, importance of PRL in normal reproductive function save that of postpartum lactation.

PRL deficiency may occur in the setting of panhypopituitarism, generally as a result of pituitary infarction or following ablative therapy for a pituitary adenoma. In Sheehan's peripartum necrosis, PRL levels are usually low [498], resulting in an inability to lactate postpartum along with other symptoms of hypopituitarism.

As discussed above, the new use of bromocriptine for the treatment of diabetes likely causes low PRL levels, but specific data in this regard and safety data regarding reproductive function are lacking.

Hyperprolactinemia

The differential diagnosis of sustained hyperprolactinemia is broad (Table 5.1). In this section, we discuss those causes of hyperprolactinemia other than prolactinomas, which are discussed in Chapter 15.

Medications (Table 5.2)

ANTIPSYCHOTICS

The antipsychotic agents (phenothiazines and butyrophenones) result in substantially elevated PRL levels (28–150 ng/ml) within a few hours of starting therapy and these levels fall to lower, though still elevated, levels after long-term treatment [199]. These drugs raise PRL levels by blocking DA receptors, both on the pituitary lactotrophs and in the hypothalamus. PRL levels usually fall to normal within 48–96 hours of discontinuation of neuroleptic drug therapy [199].

Of the newer atypical antipsychotics, risperidone and molindone are the ones most commonly associated with hyperprolactinemia [199]. Clozapine, olanzapine, quetiapine, ziprasidone and aripiprazole much less commonly elevate PRL levels [199]. The lack of effect of these last atypical agents is thought to be due to their being only transiently and weakly bound to the tuberoinfundibular D_2 receptor and to their having agonist as well as antagonist activity at the D_2 receptor [199]. The hyperprolactinemia caused by these drugs is frequently

TABLE 5.1 Etiologies of Hyperprolactinemia

Pituitary Disease
Prolactinomas
Acromegaly
"Empty Sella syndrome"
Lymphocytic hypophysitis
Cushing's disease
Hypothalamic Disease
Craniopharyngiomas
Meningiomas
Dysgerminomas
Nonsecreting pituitary adenomas
Other tumors
Sarcoidosis
Histiocytosis X
Neuraxis irradiation
Vascular
Pituitary stalk section
Neurogenic
Chest wall lesions
Spinal cord lesions
Breast stimulation
Medications
Phenothiazines
Haloperidol
Monoamine-oxidase inhibitors
Tricyclic antidepressants
Reserpine
Methyldopa
Metoclopramide
Amoxepin
Cocaine
Verapamil
Serotonin reuptake inhibitors
Other
Pregnancy
Hypothyroidism
Chronic renal failure
Cirrhosis
Adrenal insufficiency
Pseudocyesis
Idiopathic

TABLE 5.2 Effects of Psychotropic Medications on Prolactin Levels

Antipsychotics	**Increase in Prolactin**[1]
Typical	
Phenothiazines	+++
Butyrophenones	+++
Thioxanthenes	+++
Atypical	
Risperidone	+++
Molindone	++
Clozapine	0
Quetiapine	+
Ziprasidone	0
Aripiprazole	0
Olanzapine	+
Antidepressants	**Increase in Prolactin**
Tricyclics	
Amitriptyline	+
Desipramine	+
Clomipramine	+++
Nortriptyline	–
Imipramine	CR
Maprotiline	CR
Amoxapine	CR
Monoamine Oxidase Inhibitors	
Pargyline	+++
Clorgyline	+++
Tranylcypromine	±
SSRIs	
Fluoxetine	CR
Paroxetine	±
Citalopram	±
Fluvoxamine	±
Other	
Nefazodone	0
Bupropion	0
Venlaflaxine	0
Trazodone	0

[1] *0, no effect; ±, minimal increase but not to abnormal levels; +, increase to abnormal levels in small percentage of patients; ++, increase to abnormal levels in 25–50% of patients; +++, increase to abnormal levels in >50% of patients; CR, isolated case reports of hyperprolactinemia but generally no increase in prolactin levels.*

accompanied by decreased libido, erectile dysfunction in men, and galactorrhea and amenorrhea in women [199]. In one study, of all premenopausal women with antipsychotic-induced hyperprolactinemia, 31.6% had estradiol levels <73 pmol/L [499] and there are some data that show there may be an increased risk of osteopenia [500]. Studies in children treated with risperidone, however, have shown no delay in maturation [501] but gynecomastia and breast tenderness in boys and galactorrhea and irregular menses in girls have been reported [502]. Interestingly, when the D_2 receptor was genotyped in children receiving risperidone, the TaqIA A1 and the A-241G alleles were associated with higher PRL concentrations but the −141C Ins/Del and C957T variants had no significant effect [502]. Furthermore, carriers of the TaqIA A1 allele were four times more likely to experience PRL-related adverse effects [502].

ANTIDEPRESSANTS

Tricyclic antidepressants cause modest hyperprolactinemia in about 25% of patients [199]. Monoamine oxidase (MAO) inhibitors, when used chronically, may also cause a minimal elevation of PRL levels [199]. The mechanisms by which these drugs cause increased PRL levels are not certain and they likely facilitate several possible stimulatory pathways and their effects on portal vessel DA are uncertain. Serotonin reuptake inhibitors, by increasing synaptic serotonin levels, commonly cause a minimal increase in PRL to levels still within the normal range and such increases are asymptomatic; rarely does symptomatic hyperprolactinemia occur [199].

OPIATES AND COCAINE

Chronic opiate abuse is associated with mild hyperprolactinemia and menstrual dysfunction (see above). Cocaine abuse has also been associated with chronic, mild hyperprolactinemia [503].

ANTIHYPERTENSIVE DRUGS

Older drugs, such as alpha-methyldopa and reserpine, caused moderate hyperprolactinemia by altering central catecholaminergic mechanisms, while ACE inhibitors facilitate PRL release in some individuals but sustained hyperprolactinemia causing symptoms has not been reported with their use [199].

Verapamil in most studies has been found to increase basal PRL secretion and the PRL response to TRH [504] and patients have been described with galactorrhea associated with sustained hyperprolactinemia due to verapamil [505]. In a survey of patients taking verapamil, PRL levels were found to be elevated in 8.5% of patients [506]. Verapamil blocks the hypothalamic generation of DA itself rather than having a direct effect on the lactotroph [507]. Interestingly, other calcium channel blockers such as the dihydropyridines and benzothiazepines have no action on PRL section, implying that the action of the phenlalkylamine, verapamil, likely is acting on the neuronal N-type calcium channel [507].

OTHER MEDICATIONS

Metoclopramide and domperidone, two drugs commonly used to increase gastrointestinal motility and help stomach emptying in patients with gastroparesis diabetocorum, are D_2 receptor blockers. These drugs cause hyperprolactinemia in over 50% of patients and commonly cause symptoms of amenorrhea and galactorrhea in women and erectile dysfunction in men [199]. Although there are isolated case reports of hyperprolactinemia being associated with H_2 blockers and protease inhibitors, more systematic studies of these classes of medications have failed to support an etiologic role for them [199].

Stress

As noted previously, physical stress such as physical discomfort, exercise and hypoglycemia causes an acute, transient rise in PRL levels (see above). Chronic hyperprolactinemia due to prolonged physical stress has not been reported. Psychological stress may cause minimal elevations of PRL [508] but chronic hyperprolactinemia has not been reported with any chronic psychiatric state except that of pseudocyesis, in which PRL levels fall with psychotherapy [509].

Renal Disease

Hyperprolactinemia occurs in 73–91% of women and 25–57% of men with end-stage renal disease [510–512]. Although metabolic breakdown of PRL is delayed in renal failure, there is also increased production [159]. About one-quarter of individuals with renal insufficiency not requiring dialysis (serum creatinine 2.0–12.0 ng/ml) have PRL levels in the 25–100 ng/ml range [511] (Figure 5.12). When such patients take medications known to alter hypothalamic regulation of PRL, such as methyldopa or metoclopramide, PRL levels may rise to over 2000 ng/ml [511]. Correction of the renal failure with transplantation causes a return of PRL levels to normal [511,512].

Hyperprolactinemia plays a role in the hypogonadism of chronic renal failure, but probably does not explain all of the abnormalities in every case. Return of normal menses has occurred in some women treated with bromocriptine [510] but reports of restored ovulation are rare [512].

Cirrhosis

Basal PRL levels are increased in patients with alcoholic cirrhosis in frequencies varying from 16 to 100%

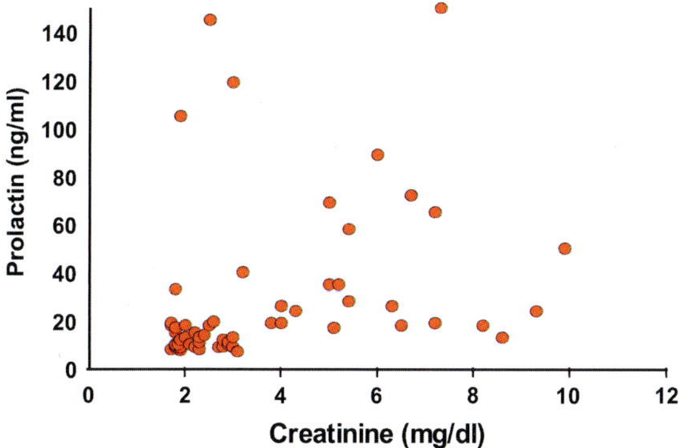

FIGURE 5.12 Prolactin levels in patients with renal insufficiency, including patients on medications (M, metoclopramide; all others designated receiving medications were taking methyldopa). *From Hou et al. [511].*

[513,514] and in patients with nonalcoholic cirrhosis from 5% [515] to 13% [514]. In women without cirrhosis, acute alcohol withdrawal is associated with hyperprolactinemia in 50% [516].

Hypothyroidism

Primary hypothyroidism is associated with a modest increase in the level of PRL in 40% of patients, but levels greater than 25 ng/ml are reached in only 10% [517]. The mechanisms involved probably include increased TRH production, increased sensitivity of lactotrophs to TRH and possibly increased pituitary VIP generation (see above). Because many patients with longstanding hypothyroidism may have evidence of pituitary enlargement on imaging, the finding of hyperprolactinemia, galactorrhea, and/or amenorrhea associated with an enlarged pituitary seen in hypothyroidism may be easily confused with a prolactinoma. Therapy with *l*-thyroxine will cause the PRL levels to return to normal and can even result in a regression of pituitary size [518].

Adrenal Insufficiency

As discussed above, glucocorticoids have a suppressive effect on PRL gene transcription and PRL release. Adrenalectomy has been reported to cause hyperprolactinemia in animals [519]. Rare cases in humans have been reported of hyperprolactinemia occurring in patients with adrenal insufficiency in whom the PRL levels return to normal with glucocorticoid replacement [520].

Neurogenic

As discussed above, sexual breast stimulation and suckling cause a reflex release of PRL that is mediated, in part, by afferent neural pathways going through the spinal cord. Chest wall and cervical cord lesions have been reported to result in elevated PRL levels and galactorrhea through stimulation of these afferent neural pathways [521]. Similar chronic elevations of PRL have been reported after mastectomy and thoracotomy [522], spinal cord injury [523] and nipple rings [181].

Ectopic Prolactin Secretion

Ectopic production of PRL is exceedingly rare. In a careful evaluation of 215 patients with a variety of malignancies, we found PRL elevations in only 15, and in 12 of these the elevations could be explained by the use of phenothiazines, opiates, or prior irradiation to the chest wall or head [524]. In one of the remaining three patients subsequent samples all had normal PRL measurements and in the other two, the cancer (lung and breast) could also have cause the modest hyperprolactinemia by stimulation of chest wall afferent nerves. However, in another series of patients with uterine cervical carcinoma, 229 of 743 patients had elevated serum PRL levels; surgery in 86 of these patients resulted in normalization of PRL levels [525]. In this same study, 22 out of 49 cervical carcinomas stained positively for PRL by immunohistochemistry and five out of eight carcinomas produced PRL when cultured [525]. In none of these cases were all of these aspects put together, i.e., elevated serum PRL levels that normalized after surgery and whose tumors either stained for PRL or produced PRL in vitro. However, symptomatic hyperprolactinemia due to well-documented PRL production from a renal cell carcinoma [526], a gonadoblastoma [527] and ectopic pituitary tissue in two ovarian teratomas [528,529] has been reported. More recently, a patient with probable ectopic production of PRL by a perivascular epithelioid cell tumor has been reported, although tumor staining for PRL was negative [530]. Given the great frequency of prolactinomas, "idiopathic hyperprolactinemia" and other causes of hyperprolactinemia, a search for an ectopic source of PRL secretion is not warranted unless some other tumor shows up coincidentally.

Hypothalamic/pituitary Stalk Disease

Hyperprolactinemia caused by lesions of the hypothalamus and of the pituitary stalk is due to disturbance of the neuroendocrine mechanisms that control PRL secretion. From hypothalamic lesion work in animals, it has been assumed that this PRL elevation is due to disinhibition of the tonic PIF (dopamine) acting at the level of the pituitary lactotrophs. PRL secretory dynamics were studied systematically in a group of such patients with hypothalamic hyperprolactinemia (six with hypothalamic lesions such as craniopharyngiomas, eosinophilic granuloma), eight with large "nonfunctioning" pituitary adenomas with marked suprasellar extension, and seven with partially empty sellas [531]. Basal PRL levels were <100 ng/ml in all but one (Figure 5.13). However, in one patient with a Rathke's cleft cyst preoperative PRL

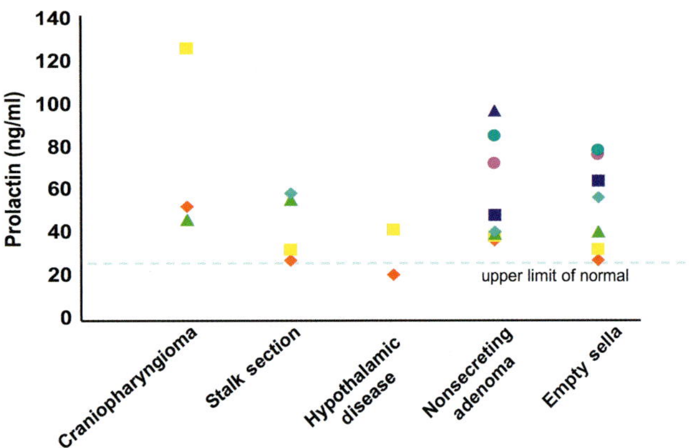

FIGURE 5.13 Basal prolactin levels in patients with hypothalamic disease. *From Molitch and Reichli [531].*

levels ranged between 93 and 148 ng/ml and she had normal TSH and ACTH function but following transsphenoidal resection she developed diabetes insipidus and panhypopituitarism, indicating high stalk section, and PRL levels fell to 25–28 ng/ml. Interestingly, of seven of these patients tested with insulin-induced hypoglycemia, three had normal PRL responses and seven of 12 showed a significant inhibition in response to L-dopa even after peripheral conversion to DA was blocked by carbidopa pretreatment. Furthermore, most of these patients had normal TSH and ACTH function. These results imply that there is still significant transmission of hypothalamic releasing factors to the pituitary in most of these cases despite increased PRL levels. The fall in PRL levels in the patient with the Rathke's cleft cyst along with the development of a true stalk section syndrome implies that there is a difference in patients with total stalk section in whom the PRL rise is due solely to DA deficiency and those with partial stalk/hypothalamic dysfunction who have DA deficiency plus continued PRF activity, resulting in higher PRL levels. In addition to this case with a Rathke's cleft cyst with a basal PRL level of 122 ng/ml a number of cases have been reported in the literature by others with PRL levels between 104 and 219 ng/ml [222,532,533]. Karavitaki et al. reported on 226 patients with pituitary adenomas, which were documented not to be prolactinomas by immunohistochemistry, finding that all but one patient had PRL levels less than 100 ng/mL [534].

It is also possible that some cases of hyperprolactinemia due to hypothalamic disease could be due to increased PRF activity with normal PIF activity. Anterior hypothalamic lesions that are irritative could potentially stimulate PRF pathways, similar to findings in experimental animals [535,536]. The finding of normal suppression of PRL with L-dopa alone and combined with carbidopa in two of our patients supports the concept of an intact TIDA system in these two patients [531].

Idiopathic Hyperprolactinemia

When no specific cause is found with the evaluation outlined below, the hyperprolactinemia is of uncertain etiology and has been designated to be idiopathic. It is recognized that in many such cases small prolactinomas may be present that are too small to be detected by current radiological techniques. In other cases the hyperprolactinemia is due to presumed hypothalamic regulatory dysfunction, but no dysfunction specific to idiopathic hyperprolactinemia has been definitively elucidated. Long-term follow-up of such patients has found that in about one-third, PRL levels return to normal, in 10–15% there is a rise in PRL levels to >50% over baseline, and in the remaining patients PRL levels remain stable [537,538]. Over a 2–6-year follow-up of 199 patients, only 23 developed evidence of microadenomas and none developed macroadenomas [537–541].

References

[1] O. Riddle, W.R. Bates, W.S. Dykshorn, A new hormone of the anterior pituitary, Proc Soc Exptl Biol Med 29 (1932) 1211–1212.

[2] O. Riddle, W.R. Bates, W.S. Dykshorn, The preparation, identification and assay of prolactin – a hormone of the anterior pituitary, Am J Physiol 105 (1933) 191–216.

[3] O. Riddle, F.P. Braucher, Studies on the physiology of reproduction in birds, Am J Physiol 97 (1931) 614–625.

[4] A.G. Frantz, D.L. Kleinberg, Prolactin: Evidence that it is separate from growth hormone in human blood, Science 170 (959) (1970) 745–747.

[5] B. Shome, A.F. Parlow, Human pituitary prolactin (hPRL): The entire linear amino acid sequence, J Clin Endocrinol Metab 45 (5) (1977) 1112–1115.

[6] N.E. Cooke, D. Coit, J. Shine, J.D. Baxter, J.A. Martial, Human prolactin. cDNA structural analysis and evolutionary comparisons, J Biol Chem 256 (8) (1981) 4007–4016.

[7] N.S. Halmi, J.A. Parsons, S.L. Erlandsen, T. Duello, Prolactin and growth hormone cells in the human hypophysis: A study with immunoenzyme histochemistry and differential staining, Cell Tissue Res 158 (4) (1975) 497–507.

[8] B.W. Scheithauer, T. Sano, K.T. Kovacs, W.F. Young Jr., N. Ryan, R.V. Randall, The pituitary gland in pregnancy: A clinicopathologic and immunohistochemical study of 69 cases, Mayo Clin Proc 65 (4) (1990) 461–474.

[9] A.S. Gleiberman, T. Michurina, J.M. Encinas, J.L. Roig, P. Krasnov, F. Balordi, et al., Genetic approaches identify adult pituitary stem cells, Proc Nat Acad Sci USA 105 (17) (2008) 6332–6337.

[10] S. Vidal, E. Horvath, K. Kovacs, R.V. Lloyd, H.S. Smyth, Reversible transdifferentiation: Interconversion of somatotrophs and lactotrophs in pituitary hyperplasia, Mod Pathol 14 (1) (2001) 20–28.

[11] D. Kelberman, K. Rizzoti, R. Lovell-Badge, I.C. Robinson, M.T. Dattani, Genetic regulation of pituitary gland development in human and mouse, Endocr Rev 30 (7) (2009) 790–829.

[12] S. Li, E.B. Crenshaw 3rd, E.J. Rawson, D.M. Simmons, L.W. Swanson, M.G. Rosenfeld, Dwarf locus mutants lacking three pituitary cell types result from mutations in the POU-domain gene pit-1, Nature 347 (6293) (1990) 528–533.

[13] J.W. Voss, M.G. Rosenfeld, Anterior pituitary development: Short tales from dwarf mice, Cell 70 (4) (1992) 527–530.

[14] R.M. Luque, G. Amargo, S. Ishii, C. Lobe, R. Franks, H. Kiyokawa, et al., Reporter expression, induced by a growth hormone promoter-driven Cre recombinase (rGHp-Cre) transgene, questions the developmental relationship between somatotropes and lactotropes in the adult mouse pituitary gland, Endocrinology 148 (5) (2007) 1946–1953.

[15] F. Schaufele, Regulation of estrogen receptor activation of the prolactin enhancer/promoter by antagonistic activation function-2-interacting proteins, Mol Endocrinol 13 (6) (1999) 935–945.

[16] A.T. Truong, C. Duez, A. Belayew, A. Renard, R. Pictet, G.I. Bell, et al., Isolation and characterization of the human prolactin gene, EMBO J 3 (2) (1984) 429–437.

[17] E.M. Prager, A.C. Wilson, J.M. Lowenstein, V.M. Sarich, Mammoth albumin, Science 209 (4453) (1980) 287–289.

[18] E.B. Crenshaw 3rd, K. Kalla, D.M. Simmons, L.W. Swanson, M.G. Rosenfeld, Cell-specific expression of the prolactin gene in transgenic mice is controlled by synergistic interactions between promoter and enhancer elements, Genes Dev 3 (7) (1989) 959–972.

[19] M. Berwaer, P. Monget, B. Peers, M. Mathy-Hartert, E. Bellefroid, J.R. Davis, et al., Multihormonal regulation of the human prolactin gene expression from 5000 bp of its upstream sequence, Mol Cell Endocrinol 80 (1–3) (1991) 53–64.

[20] M. Berwaer, J.A. Martial, J.R. Davis, Characterization of an up-stream promoter directing extrapituitary expression of the human prolactin gene, Mol Endocrinol 8 (5) (1994) 635–642.

[21] B. Gellersen, R. Kempf, R. Telgmann, G.E. DiMattia, Non-pituitary human prolactin gene transcription is independent of Pit-1 and differentially controlled in lymphocytes and in endometrial stroma, Mol Endocrinol 8 (3) (1994) 356–373.

[22] S. Gerlo, J.R. Davis, D.L. Mager, R. Kooijman, Prolactin in man: A tale of two promoters, Bioessays 28 (10) (2006) 1051–1055.

[23] L.K. Larsen, E.Z. Amri, S. Mandrup, C. Pacot, K. Kristiansen, Genomic organization of the mouse peroxisome proliferator-activated receptor beta/delta gene: Alternative promoter usage and splicing yield transcripts exhibiting differential translational efficiency, Biochem J 366 (Pt 3) (2002) 767–775.

[24] L. Pontrelli, K.G. Sidiropoulos, K. Adeli, Translational control of apolipoprotein B mRNA: Regulation via cis elements in the 5′ and 3′ untranslated regions, Biochemistry 43 (21) (2004) 6734–6744.

[25] L. Beltran, M.N. Fahie-Wilson, T.J. McKenna, L. Kavanagh, T.P. Smith, Serum total prolactin and monomeric prolactin reference intervals determined by precipitation with polyethylene glycol: Evaluation and validation on common immunoassay platforms, Clin Chem 54 (10) (2008) 1673–1681.

[26] C.A. Dunn, P. Medstrand, D.L. Mager, An endogenous retroviral long terminal repeat is the dominant promoter for human beta1,3-galactosyltransferase 5 in the colon, Proc Nat Acad Sci USA 100 (22) (2003) 12841–12846.

[27] L.N. van de Lagemaat, J.R. Landry, D.L. Mager, P. Medstrand, Transposable elements in mammals promote regulatory variation and diversification of genes with specialized functions, Trends Genet 19 (10) (2003) 530–536.

[28] R. Telgmann, E. Maronde, K. Tasken, B. Gellersen, Activated protein kinase A is required for differentiation-dependent transcription of the decidual prolactin gene in human endometrial stromal cells, Endocrinology 138 (3) (1997) 929–937.

[29] A.P. Bradford, K.S. Brodsky, S.E. Diamond, L.C. Kuhn, Y. Liu, A. Gutierrez-Hartmann, The Pit-1 homeodomain and beta-domain interact with Ets-1 and modulate synergistic activation of the rat prolactin promoter, J Biol Chem 275 (5) (2000) 3100–3106.

[30] A.P. Bradford, K.E. Conrad, P.H. Tran, M.C. Ostrowski, A. Gutierrez-Hartmann, GHF-1/Pit-1 functions as a cell-specific integrator of Ras signaling by targeting the Ras pathway to a composite Ets-1/GHF-1 response element, J Biol Chem 271 (40) (1996) 24639–24648.

[31] A.P. Bradford, K.E. Conrad, C. Wasylyk, B. Wasylyk, A. Gutierrez-Hartmann, Functional interaction of c-Ets-1 and GHF-1/Pit-1 mediates Ras activation of pituitary-specific gene expression: Mapping of the essential c-Ets-1 domain, Mol Cell Biol 15 (5) (1995) 2849–2857.

[32] A.P. Bradford, C. Wasylyk, B. Wasylyk, A. Gutierrez-Hartmann, Interaction of Ets-1 and the POU-homeodomain protein GHF-1/Pit-1 reconstitutes pituitary-specific gene expression, Mol Cell Biol 17 (3) (1997) 1065–1074.

[33] J.S. Dasen, S.M. O'Connell, S.E. Flynn, M. Treier, A.S. Gleiberman, D.P. Szeto, et al., Reciprocal interactions of Pit1 and GATA2 mediate signaling gradient-induced determination of pituitary cell types, Cell 97 (5) (1999) 587–598.

[34] R.N. Day, S. Koike, M. Sakai, M. Muramatsu, R.A. Maurer, Both Pit-1 and the estrogen receptor are required for estrogen responsiveness of the rat prolactin gene, Mol Endocrinol 4 (12) (1990) 1964–1971.

[35] A.M. Nalda, J.A. Martial, M. Muller, The glucocorticoid receptor inhibits the human prolactin gene expression by interference with Pit-1 activity, Mol Cell Endocrinol 134 (2) (1997) 129–137.

[36] F. Pernasetti, L. Caccavelli, C. Van de Weerdt, J.A. Martial, M. Muller, Thyroid hormone inhibits the human prolactin gene promoter by interfering with activating protein-1 and estrogen stimulations, Mol Endocrinol 11 (7) (1997) 986–996.

[37] J.W. Voss, L. Wilson, M.G. Rosenfeld, POU-domain proteins Pit-1 and Oct-1 interact to form a heteromeric complex and can cooperate to induce expression of the prolactin promoter, Genes Dev 5 (7) (1991) 1309–1320.

[38] S.E. Diamond, A. Gutierrez-Hartmann, The Pit-1beta domain dictates active repression and alteration of histone acetylation of the proximal prolactin promoter, J Biol Chem 275 (40) (2000) 30977–30986.

[39] K.M. Scully, E.M. Jacobson, K. Jepsen, V. Lunyak, H. Viadiu, C. Carriere, et al., Allosteric effects of Pit-1 DNA sites on long-term repression in cell type specification, Science 290 (5494) (2000) 1127–1131.

[40] T.C. Voss, I.A. Demarco, C.F. Booker, R.N. Day, Functional interactions with Pit-1 reorganize corepressor complexes in the living cell nucleus, J Cell Sci 118 (Pt 15) (2005) 3277–3288.

[41] L. Xu, R.M. Lavinsky, J.S. Dasen, S.E. Flynn, E.M. McInerney, T.M. Mullen, et al., Signal-specific coactivator domain requirements for Pit-1 activation, Nature 395 (6699) (1998) 301–306.

[42] K. Zanger, L.E. Cohen, K. Hashimoto, S. Radovick, F.E. Wondisford, A novel mechanism for cyclic adenosine 3′,5′-monophosphate regulation of gene expression by CREB-binding protein, Mol Endocrinol 13 (2) (1999) 268–275.

[43] S.E. Diamond, M. Chiono, A. Gutierrez-Hartmann, Reconstitution of the protein kinase A response of the rat prolactin promoter: Differential effects of distinct Pit-1 isoforms and functional interaction with Oct-1, Mol Endocrinol 13 (2) (1999) 228–238.

[44] C.J. Chen, Z. Deng, A.Y. Kim, G.A. Blobel, P.M. Lieberman, Stimulation of CREB binding protein nucleosomal histone acetyltransferase activity by a class of transcriptional activators, Mol Cell Biol 21 (2) (2001) 476–487.

[45] D. Gourdji, J.N. Laverriere, The rat prolactin gene: A target for tissue-specific and hormone-dependent transcription factors, Mol Cell Endocrinol 100 (1–2) (1994) 133–142.

[46] M.H. Quentien, A. Barlier, J.L. Franc, I. Pellegrini, T. Brue, A. Enjalbert, Pituitary transcription factors: From congenital deficiencies to gene therapy, J Neuroendocrinol 18 (9) (2006) 633–642.

[47] S. Hinuma, Y. Habata, R. Fujii, Y. Kawamata, M. Hosoya, S. Fukusumi, et al., A prolactin-releasing peptide in the brain, Nature 393 (6682) (1998) 272–276.

[48] D.L. Duval, A. Jean, A. Gutierrez-Hartmann, Ras signaling and transcriptional synergy at a flexible Ets-1/Pit-1 composite DNA element is defined by the assembly of selective activation domains, J Biol Chem 278 (41) (2003) 39684–39696.

[49] M. Kishimoto, Y. Okimura, K. Yagita, G. Iguchi, M. Fumoto, K. Iida, et al., Novel function of the transactivation domain of a pituitary-specific transcription factor, Pit-1, J Biol Chem 277 (47) (2002) 45141–45148.

[50] K. Zanger, S. Radovick, F.E. Wondisford, CREB binding protein recruitment to the transcription complex requires growth factor-dependent phosphorylation of its GF box, Mol Cell 7 (3) (2001) 551–558.

[51] L.E. Theill, J.L. Castrillo, D. Wu, M. Karin, Dissection of functional domains of the pituitary-specific transcription factor GHF-1, Nature 342 (6252) (1989) 945–948.

[52] D.L. Duval, M.D. Jonsen, S.E. Diamond, P. Murapa, A. Jean, A. Gutierrez-Hartmann, Differential utilization of transcription activation subdomains by distinct coactivators regulates Pit-1 basal and Ras responsiveness, Mol Endocrinol 21 (1) (2007) 172–185.

[53] A.E. Morris, B. Kloss, R.E. McChesney, C. Bancroft, L.A. Chasin, An alternatively spliced Pit-1 isoform altered in its ability to trans-activate, Nucleic Acids Res 20 (6) (1992) 1355–1361.

[54] M.D. Jonsen, D.L. Duval, A. Gutierrez-Hartmann, The 26-amino acid beta-motif of the Pit-1beta transcription factor is a dominant and independent repressor domain, Mol Endocrinol 23 (9) (2009) 1371–1384.

[55] S.E. Diamond, A.A. Gutierrez-Hartmann, 26-amino acid insertion domain defines a functional transcription switch motif in Pit-1beta, J Biol Chem 271 (46) (1996) 28925–28932.

[56] A.L. Ferry, D.M. Locasto, L.B. Meszaros, J.C. Bailey, M.D. Jonsen, K. Brodsky, et al., Pit-1beta reduces transcription and CREB-binding protein recruitment in a DNA context-dependent manner, J Endocrinol 185 (1) (2005) 173–185.

[57] R.A. Sporici, J.S. Hodskins, D.M. Locasto, L.B. Meszaros, A.L. Ferry, A.M. Weidner, et al., Repression of the prolactin promoter: A functional consequence of the heterodimerization between Pit-1 and Pit-1 beta, J Mol Endocrinol 35 (2) (2005) 317–331.

[58] E.M. Jacobson, P. Li, A. Leon-del-Rio, M.G. Rosenfeld, A.K. Aggarwal, Structure of Pit-1 POU domain bound to DNA as a dimer: Unexpected arrangement and flexibility, Genes Dev 11 (2) (1997) 198–212.

[59] R.N. Cohen, T. Brue, K. Naik, C.A. Houlihan, F.E. Wondisford, S. Radovick, The role of CBP/p300 interactions and Pit-1 dimerization in the pathophysiological mechanism of combined pituitary hormone deficiency, J Clin Endocrinol Metab 91 (1) (2006) 239–247.

[60] J.M. Holloway, D.P. Szeto, K.M. Scully, C.K. Glass, M.G. Rosenfeld, Pit-1 binding to specific DNA sites as a monomer or dimer determines gene-specific use of a tyrosine-dependent synergy domain, Genes Dev 9 (16) (1995) 1992–2006.

[61] C. Caelles, H. Hennemann, M. Karin, M-phase-specific phosphorylation of the POU transcription factor GHF-1 by a cell cycle-regulated protein kinase inhibits DNA binding, Mol Cell Biol 15 (12) (1995) 6694–6701.

[62] M.S. Kapiloff, Y. Farkash, M. Wegner, M.G. Rosenfeld, Variable effects of phosphorylation of Pit-1 dictated by the DNA response elements, Science 253 (5021) (1991) 786–789.

[63] A. Jean, A. Gutierrez-Hartmann, D.L. Duval, A Pit-1 threonine 220 phosphomimic reduces binding to monomeric DNA sites to inhibit Ras and estrogen stimulation of the prolactin gene promoter, Mol Endocrinol 24 (1) (2010) 91–103.

[64] N.A. Mitchner, C. Garlick, N. Ben-Jonathan, Cellular distribution and gene regulation of estrogen receptors alpha and beta in the rat pituitary gland, Endocrinology 139 (9) (1998) 3976–3983.

[65] M.A. Shupnik, L.K. Pitt, A.Y. Soh, A. Anderson, M.B. Lopes, E.R. Laws Jr., Selective expression of estrogen receptor alpha and beta isoforms in human pituitary tumors, J Clin Endocrinol Metab 83 (11) (1998) 3965–3972.

[66] K.F. Koehler, L.A. Helguero, L.A. Haldosen, M. Warner, J.A. Gustafsson, Reflections on the discovery and significance of estrogen receptor beta, Endocr Rev 26 (3) (2005) 465–478.

[67] G. Pelletier, S. Li, D. Phaneuf, C. Martel, F. Labrie, Morphological studies of prolactin-secreting cells in estrogen receptor alpha and estrogen receptor beta knockout mice, Neuroendocrinology 77 (5) (2003) 324–333.

[68] E. Brailoiu, S.L. Dun, G.C. Brailoiu, K. Mizuo, L.A. Sklar, T.I. Oprea, et al., Distribution and characterization of estrogen receptor G protein-coupled receptor 30 in the rat central nervous system, J Endocrinol 193 (2) (2007) 311–321.

[69] J. Isensee, L. Meoli, V. Zazzu, C. Nabzdyk, H. Witt, D. Soewarto, et al., Expression pattern of G protein-coupled receptor 30 in LacZ reporter mice, Endocrinology 150 (4) (2009) 1722–1730.

[70] K.M. Scully, A.S. Gleiberman, J. Lindzey, D.B. Lubahn, K.S. Korach, M.G. Rosenfeld, Role of estrogen receptor-alpha in the anterior pituitary gland, Mol Endocrinol 11 (6) (1997) 674–681.

[71] J.F. Couse, M.M. Yates, V.R. Walker, K.S. Korach, Characterization of the hypothalamic–pituitary–gonadal axis in estrogen receptor (ER) Null mice reveals hypergonadism and endocrine sex reversal in females lacking ERalpha but not ERbeta, Mol Endocrinol 17 (6) (2003) 1039–1053.

[72] B.E. Nowakowski, R.A. Maurer, Multiple Pit-1-binding sites facilitate estrogen responsiveness of the prolactin gene, Mol Endocrinol 8 (12) (1994) 1742–1749.

[73] J.J. Watters, T.Y. Chun, Y.N. Kim, P.J. Bertics, J. Gorski, Estrogen modulation of prolactin gene expression requires an intact mitogen-activated protein kinase signal transduction pathway in cultured rat pituitary cells, Mol Endocrinol 14 (11) (2000) 1872–1881.

[74] A.D. Adamson, S. Friedrichsen, S. Semprini, C.V. Harper, J.J. Mullins, M.R. White, et al., Human prolactin gene promoter regulation by estrogen: Convergence with tumor necrosis factor-alpha signaling, Endocrinology 149 (2) (2008) 687–694.

[75] B. Gellersen, R. Kempf, R. Telgmann, G.E. DiMattia, Pituitary-type transcription of the human prolactin gene in the absence of Pit-1, Mol Endocrinol 9 (7) (1995) 887–901.

[76] S. Friedrichsen, C.V. Harper, S. Semprini, M. Wilding, A.D. Adamson, D.G. Spiller, et al., Tumor necrosis factor-alpha activates the human prolactin gene promoter via nuclear factor-kappaB signaling, Endocrinology 147 (2) (2006) 773–781.

[77] P.W. Howard, R.A. Maurer, A composite Ets/Pit-1 binding site in the prolactin gene can mediate transcriptional responses to multiple signal transduction pathways, J Biol Chem 270 (36) (1995) 20930–20936.

[78] R.E. Schweppe, A.A. Frazer-Abel, A. Gutierrez-Hartmann, A.P. Bradford, Functional components of fibroblast growth factor (FGF) signal transduction in pituitary cells. Identification of FGF response elements in the prolactin gene, J Biol Chem 272 (49) (1997) 30852–30859.

[79] Y.H. Wang, R.A. Maurer, A role for the mitogen-activated protein kinase in mediating the ability of thyrotropin-releasing hormone to stimulate the prolactin promoter, Mol Endocrinol 13 (7) (1999) 1094–1104.

[80] R.N. Day, J. Liu, V. Sundmark, M. Kawecki, D. Berry, H.P. Elsholtz, Selective inhibition of prolactin gene transcription by the ETS-2 repressor factor, J Biol Chem 273 (48) (1998) 31909–31915.

[81] R.E. Schweppe, A.A. Melton, K.S. Brodsky, L.D. Aveline, K.A. Resing, N.G. Ahn, et al., Purification and mass spectrometric identification of GA-binding protein (GABP) as the functional pituitary Ets factor binding to the basal transcription element of the prolactin promoter, J Biol Chem 278 (19) (2003) 16863–16872.

[82] B.A. Amendt, L.B. Sutherland, A.F. Russo, Multifunctional role of the Pitx2 homeodomain protein C-terminal tail, Mol Cell Biol 19 (10) (1999) 7001–7010.

[83] M.H. Quentien, F. Pitoia, G. Gunz, M.P. Guillet, A. Enjalbert, I. Pellegrini, Regulation of prolactin, GH, and Pit-1 gene expression in anterior pituitary by Pitx2: An approach using Pitx2 mutants, Endocrinology 143 (8) (2002) 2839–2851.

[84] D.P. Szeto, A.K. Ryan, S.M. O'Connell, M.G. Rosenfeld, P-OTX: A PIT-1-interacting homeodomain factor expressed during anterior pituitary gland development, Proc Nat Acad Sci USA 93 (15) (1996) 7706–7710.

[85] J.J. Tremblay, C. Lanctot, J. Drouin, The pan-pituitary activator of transcription, Ptx1 (pituitary homeobox 1), acts in synergy with SF-1 and Pit1 and is an upstream regulator of the Lim-homeodomain gene Lim3/Lhx3, Mol Endocrinol 12 (3) (1998) 428–441.

[86] R.N. Day, R.A. Maurer, Thyroid hormone-responsive elements of the prolactin gene: Evidence for both positive and negative regulation, Mol Endocrinol 3 (6) (1989) 931–938.

[87] K.K. Jacob, F.M. Stanley, CCAAT/enhancer-binding protein alpha is a physiological regulator of prolactin gene expression, Endocrinology 140 (10) (1999) 4542–4550.

[88] I.A. Demarco, T.C. Voss, C.F. Booker, R.N. Day, Dynamic interactions between Pit-1 and C/EBPalpha in the pituitary cell nucleus, Mol Cell Biol 26 (21) (2006) 8087–8098.

[89] S.W. Davis, S.A. Camper, Noggin regulates Bmp4 activity during pituitary induction, Dev Biol 305 (1) (2007) 145–160.

[90] M. Paez-Pereda, D. Giacomini, D. Refojo, A.C. Nagashima, U. Hopfner, Y. Grubler, et al., Involvement of bone morphogenetic protein 4 (BMP-4) in pituitary prolactinoma pathogenesis through a Smad/estrogen receptor crosstalk, Proc Nat Acad Sci USA 100 (3) (2003) 1034–1039.

[91] D. Giacomini, M. Paez-Pereda, J. Stalla, G.K. Stalla, E. Arzt, Molecular interaction of BMP-4, TGF-beta, and estrogens in lactotrophs: Impact on the PRL promoter, Mol Endocrinol 23 (7) (2009) 1102–1114.

[92] S. Yu, S.L. Asa, S. Ezzat, Fibroblast growth factor receptor 4 is a target for the zinc-finger transcription factor Ikaros in the pituitary, Mol Endocrinol 16 (5) (2002) 1069–1078.

[93] S. Yu, L. Zheng, S.L. Asa, S. Ezzat, Fibroblast growth factor receptor 4 (FGFR4) mediates signaling to the prolactin but not the FGFR4 promoter, Am J Physiol Endocrinol Metab 283 (3) (2002) E490–E495.

[94] S. Ezzat, S. Yu, S.L. Asa, The zinc finger Ikaros transcription factor regulates pituitary growth hormone and prolactin gene expression through distinct effects on chromatin accessibility, Mol Endocrinol 19 (4) (2005) 1004–1011.

[95] H.P. Elsholtz, A.M. Lew, P.R. Albert, V.C. Sundmark, Inhibitory control of prolactin and Pit-1 gene promoters by dopamine. Dual signaling pathways required for D2 receptor-regulated expression of the prolactin gene, J Biol Chem 266 (34) (1991) 22919–22925.

[96] M. Ishida, T. Mitsui, K. Yamakawa, N. Sugiyama, W. Takahashi, H. Shimura, et al., Involvement of cAMP response element-binding protein in the regulation of cell proliferation and the prolactin promoter of lactotrophs in primary culture, Am J Physiol Endocrinol Metab 293 (6) (2007) E1529–E1537.

[97] R.A. Maurer, Transcriptional regulation of the prolactin gene by ergocryptine and cyclic AMP, Nature 294 (5836) (1981) 94–97.

[98] R.A. Maurer, Adenosine 3',5'-monophosphate derivatives increase prolactin synthesis and prolactin messenger ribonucleic acid levels in ergocryptine-treated pituitary cells, Endocrinology 110 (6) (1982) 1957–1963.

[99] L. Swennen, C. Denef, Physiological concentrations of dopamine decrease adenosine 3',5'-monophosphate levels in cultured rat anterior pituitary cells and enriched populations of lactotrophs: Evidence for a causal relationship to inhibition of prolactin release, Endocrinology 111 (2) (1982) 398–405.

[100] C.A. Keech, S.M. Jackson, S.K. Siddiqui, K.W. Ocran, A. Gutierrez-Hartmann, Cyclic adenosine 3',5'-monophosphate activation of the rat prolactin promoter is restricted to the pituitary-specific cell type, Mol Endocrinol 6 (12) (1992) 2059–2070.

[101] P. Kievit, J.D. Lauten, R.A. Maurer, Analysis of the role of the mitogen-activated protein kinase in mediating cyclic-adenosine 3',5'-monophosphate effects on prolactin promoter activity, Mol Endocrinol 15 (4) (2001) 614–624.

[102] J. Liang, K.E. Kim, W.E. Schoderbek, R.A. Maurer, Characterization of a non-tissue-specific, 3',5'-cyclic adenosine monophosphate-responsive element in the proximal region of the rat prolactin gene, Mol Endocrinol 6 (6) (1992) 885–892.

[103] J.C. Liu, R.E. Baker, C. Sun, V.C. Sundmark, H.P. Elsholtz, Activation of Go-coupled dopamine D2 receptors inhibits ERK1/ERK2 in pituitary cells. A key step in the transcriptional suppression of the prolactin gene, J Biol Chem 277 (39) (2002) 35819–35825.

[104] J. Hayakawa, M. Ohmichi, K. Tasaka, Y. Kanda, K. Adachi, Y. Nishio, et al., Regulation of the PRL promoter by Akt through cAMP response element binding protein, Endocrinology 143 (1) (2002) 13–22.

[105] A. Kimura, M. Ohmichi, K. Tasaka, Y. Kanda, H. Ikegami, J. Hayakawa, et al., Prolactin-releasing peptide activation of the prolactin promoter is differentially mediated by extracellular signal-regulated protein kinase and c-Jun N-terminal protein kinase, J Biol Chem 275 (5) (2000) 3667–3674.

[106] A.I. Castillo, R.M. Tolon, A. Aranda, Insulin-like growth factor-1 stimulates rat prolactin gene expression by a Ras, ETS and phosphatidylinositol 3-kinase dependent mechanism, Oncogene 16 (15) (1998) 1981–1991.

[107] T.A. Jackson, D.M. Koterwas, M.A. Morgan, A.P. Bradford, Fibroblast growth factors regulate prolactin transcription via an atypical Rac-dependent signaling pathway, Mol Endocrinol 17 (10) (2003) 1921–1930.

[108] D. Romano, K. Magalon, A. Ciampini, C. Talet, A. Enjalbert, C. Gerard, Differential involvement of the Ras and Rap1 small GTPases in vasoactive intestinal and pituitary adenylyl cyclase activating polypeptides control of the prolactin gene, J Biol Chem 278 (51) (2003) 51386–51394.

[109] N. Ben-Jonathan, C.R. LaPensee, E.W. LaPensee, What can we learn from rodents about prolactin in humans? Endocr Rev 29 (1) (2008) 1–41.

[110] S. Chen, M.L. Bangaru, L. Sneade, J.A. Dunckley, N. Ben-Jonathan, S. Kansra, Epidermal growth factor receptor cross-talks with ligand-occupied estrogen receptor-alpha to modulate both lactotroph proliferation and prolactin gene expression, Am J Physiol Endocrinol Metab 297 (2) (2009) E331–E339.

[111] N. Ben-Jonathan, S. Chen, J.A. Dunckley, C. LaPensee, S. Kansra, Estrogen receptor-alpha mediates the epidermal growth factor-stimulated prolactin expression and release in lactotrophs, Endocrinology 150 (2) (2009) 795–802.

[112] Y.N. Sinha, Structural variants of prolactin: Occurrence and physiological significance, Endocr Rev 16 (3) (1995) 354–369.

[113] F.E. Utama, M.J. LeBaron, L.M. Neilson, A.S. Sultan, A.F. Parlow, K.U. Wagner, et al., Human prolactin receptors are insensitive to mouse prolactin: Implications for xenotransplant modeling of human breast cancer in mice, J Endocrinol 188 (3) (2006) 589–601.

[114] C. Keeler, P.S. Dannies, M.E. Hodsdon, The tertiary structure and backbone dynamics of human prolactin, J Mol Biol 328 (5) (2003) 1105–1121.

[115] P.T. Tuazon, M.Y. Lorenson, A.M. Walker, J.A. Traugh, p21-activated protein kinase gamma-PAK in pituitary secretory granules phosphorylates prolactin, FEBS Lett 515 (1–3) (2002) 84–88.

[116] N. Hattori, K. Ikekubo, Y. Nakaya, K. Kitagawa, C. Inagaki, Immunoglobulin G subclasses and prolactin (PRL) isoforms in macroprolactinemia due to anti-PRL autoantibodies, J Clin Endocrinol Metab 90 (5) (2005) 3036–3044.

[117] E.J. Schenck, J.M. Canfield, C.L. Brooks, Functional relationship of serine 90 phosphorylation and the surrounding putative salt bridge in bovine prolactin, Mol Cell Endocrinol 204 (1–2) (2003) 117–125.

[118] Y.F. Wang, J.W. Liu, M. Mamidi, A.M. Walker, Identification of the major site of rat prolactin phosphorylation as serine 177, J Biol Chem 271 (5) (1996) 2462–2469.

[119] A.M. Walker, S179D prolactin: Antagonistic agony! Mol Cell Endocrinol 276 (1–2) (2007) 1–9.

[120] W. Wu, D. Coss, M.Y. Lorenson, C.B. Kuo, X. Xu, A.M. Walker, Different biological effects of unmodified prolactin and a molecular mimic of phosphorylated prolactin involve different signaling pathways, Biochemistry 42 (24) (2003) 7561–7570.

[121] T.W. Ho, F.S. Leong, C.H. Olaso, A.M. Walker, Secretion of specific nonphosphorylated and phosphorylated rat prolactin isoforms at different stages of the estrous cycle, Neuroendocrinology 58 (2) (1993) 160–165.

[122] V.L. Williams, A. DeGuzman, H. Dang, M. Kawaminami, T.W. Ho, D.G. Carter, et al., Common and specific effects of the two major forms of prolactin in the rat testis, Am J Physiol Endocrinol Metab 293 (6) (2007) E1795–E1803.

[123] T. Hoffmann, C. Penel, C. Ronin, Glycosylation of human prolactin regulates hormone bioactivity and metabolic clearance, J Endocrinol Invest 16 (10) (1993) 807–816.

[124] M. Guitelman, M.E. Colombani-Vidal, C.C. Zylbersztein, L. Fiszlejder, M. Zeller, O. Levalle, et al., Hyperprolactinemia in asymptomatic patients is related to high molecular weight posttranslational variants or glycosylated forms, Pituitary 5 (4) (2002) 255–260.

[125] Y.N. Sinha, T.A. Gilligan, D.W. Lee, D. Hollingsworth, E. Markoff, Cleaved prolactin: Evidence for its occurrence in human pituitary gland and plasma, J Clin Endocrinol Metab 60 (2) (1985) 239–243.

[126] C.A. Powers, Anterior pituitary glandular kallikrein: A putative prolactin processing protease, Mol Cell Endocrinol 90 (2) (1993) C15–C20.

[127] G. Ge, C.A. Fernandez, M.A. Moses, D.S. Greenspan, Bone morphogenetic protein 1 processes prolactin to a 17-kDa antiangiogenic factor, Proc Nat Acad Sci USA 104 (24) (2007) 10010–10015.

[128] C. Clapp, C. Gonzalez, Y. Macotela, J. Aranda, J.C. Rivera, C. Garcia, et al., Vasoinhibins: A family of N-terminal prolactin fragments that inhibit angiogenesis and vascular function, Front Horm Res 35 (2006) 64–73.

[129] D. Piwnica, P. Touraine, I. Struman, S. Tabruyn, G. Bolbach, C. Clapp, et al., Cathepsin D processes human prolactin into multiple 16K-like N-terminal fragments: Study of their antiangiogenic properties and physiological relevance, Mol Endocrinol 18 (10) (2004) 2522–2542.

[130] N. Hattori, Macroprolactinemia: A new cause of hyperprolactinemia, J Pharmacol Sci 92 (3) (2003) 171–177.

[131] J.A. Schlechte, The macroprolactin problem, J Clin Endocrinol Metab 87 (12) (2002) 5408–5409.

[132] D.I. Linzer, S.J. Fisher, The placenta and the prolactin family of hormones: Regulation of the physiology of pregnancy, Mol Endocrinol 13 (6) (1999) 837–840.

[133] M.J. Soares, H. Muller, K.E. Orwig, T.J. Peters, G. Dai, The uteroplacental prolactin family and pregnancy, Biol Reprod 58 (2) (1998) 273–284.

[134] L.A. Rigg, A. Lein, S.S. Yen, Pattern of increase in circulating prolactin levels during human gestation, Am J Obstet Gynecol 129 (4) (1977) 454–456.

[135] J.E. Tyson, H.G. Friesen, Factors influencing the secretion of human prolactin and growth hormone in menstrual and gestational women, Am J Obstet Gynecol 116 (3) (1973) 377–387.

[136] A. Golander, T. Hurley, J. Barrett, A. Hizi, S. Handwerger, Prolactin synthesis by human chorion-decidual tissue: A possible source of prolactin in the amniotic fluid, Science 202 (4365) (1978) 311–313.

[137] K. Tomita, J.A. McCoshen, H.G. Friesen, J.E. Tyson, Quantitative comparison between biological and immunological activities of prolactin derived from human fetal and maternal sources, J Clin Endocrinol Metab 55 (2) (1982) 269–271.

[138] B. Gellersen, G.E. DiMattia, H.G. Friesen, H.G. Bohnet, Prolactin (PRL) mRNA from human decidua differs from pituitary PRL mRNA but resembles the IM-9-P3 lymphoblast PRL transcript, Mol Cell Endocrinol 64 (1) (1989) 127–130.

[139] J.R. Huang, L. Tseng, P. Bischof, O.A. Janne, Regulation of prolactin production by progestin, estrogen, and relaxin in human endometrial stromal cells, Endocrinology 121 (6) (1987) 2011–2017.

[140] I.A. Maslar, R. Ansbacher, Effect of short-duration progesterone treatment on decidual prolactin production by cultures of proliferative human endometrium, Fertil Steril 50 (2) (1988) 250–254.

[141] K.M. Thrailkill, A. Golander, L.E. Underwood, R.G. Richards, S. Handwerger, Insulin stimulates the synthesis and release of prolactin from human decidual cells, Endocrinology 124 (6) (1989) 3010–3014.

[142] D.F. Horrobin, Prolactin as a regulator of fluid and electrolyte metabolism in mammals, Fed Proc 39 (8) (1980) 2567–2570.

[143] E.A. Stewart, P. Jain, M.D. Penglase, A.J. Friedman, R.A. Nowak, The myometrium of postmenopausal women produces prolactin in response to human chorionic gonadotropin and alpha-subunit in vitro, Fertil Steril 64 (5) (1995) 972–976.

[144] G.E. DiMattia, B. Gellersen, H.G. Bohnet, H.G. Friesen, A human B-lymphoblastoid cell line produces prolactin, Endocrinology 122 (6) (1988) 2508–2517.

[145] B. Gellersen, G.E. DiMattia, H.G. Friesen, H.G. Bohnet, Regulation of prolactin secretion in the human B-lymphoblastoid cell line IM-9-P3 by dexamethasone but not other regulators of pituitary prolactin secretion, Endocrinology 125 (6) (1989) 2853–2861.
[146] K.C. Swearingen, Heterogeneous turnover of adenohypophysial prolactin, Endocrinology 89 (6) (1971) 1380–1388.
[147] A.M. Walker, M.G. Farquhar, Preferential release of newly synthesized prolactin granules is the result of functional heterogeneity among mammotrophs, Endocrinology 107 (4) (1980) 1095–1104.
[148] L.S. Jacobs, M.Y. Lorenson, Cysteamine, zinc, and thiols modify detectability of rat pituitary prolactin: A comparison with effects on bovine prolactin suggests differences in hormone storage, Metabolism 35 (3) (1986) 209–215.
[149] A. Glezer, C.R. Soares, J.G. Vieira, D. Giannella-Neto, M.T. Ribela, V. Goffin, et al., Human macroprolactin displays low biological activity via its homologous receptor in a new sensitive bioassay, J Clin Endocrinol Metab 91 (3) (2006) 1048–1055.
[150] A. Leanos-Miranda, G. Cardenas-Mondragon, R. Rivera-Leanos, A. Ulloa-Aguirre, V. Goffin, Application of new homologous in vitro bioassays for human lactogens to assess the actual bioactivity of human prolactin isoforms in hyperprolactinaemic patients, Clin Endocrinol (Oxf) 65 (2) (2006) 146–153.
[151] F.F. Casanueva, M.E. Molitch, J.A. Schlechte, R. Abs, V. Bonert, M.D. Bronstein, et al., Guidelines of the Pituitary Society for the diagnosis and management of prolactinomas, Clin Endocrinol (Oxf) 65 (2) (2006) 265–273.
[152] E. St-Jean, F. Blain, R. Comtois, High prolactin levels may be missed by immunoradiometric assay in patients with macroprolactinomas, Clin Endocrinol (Oxf) 44 (3) (1996) 305–309.
[153] T.P. Smith, L. Kavanagh, M.L. Healy, T.J. McKenna, Technology insight: Measuring prolactin in clinical samples, Nat Clin Pract Endocrinol Metab 3 (3) (2007) 279–289.
[154] J. Chahal, J. Schlechte, Hyperprolactinemia, Pituitary 11 (2) (2008) 141–146.
[155] T.J. McKenna, Should macroprolactin be measured in all hyperprolactinaemic sera? Clin Endocrinol (Oxf) 71 (4) (2009) 466–469.
[156] L. Kavanagh, T.P. Smith, T.J. McKenna, Bioactivity of macroprolactin in the Nb2 bioassay may be explained by dissociation yielding bioactive monomeric prolactin, Clin Endocrinol (Oxf) 67 (6) (2007) 954.
[157] S. Vallette-Kasic, I. Morange-Ramos, A. Selim, G. Gunz, S. Morange, A. Enjalbert, et al., Macroprolactinemia revisited: A study on 106 patients, J Clin Endocrinol Metab 87 (2) (2002) 581–588.
[158] D.S. Cooper, E.C. Ridgway, B. Kliman, R.N. Kjellberg, F. Maloof, Metabolic clearance and production rates of prolactin in man, J Clin Invest 64 (6) (1979) 1669–1680.
[159] G.D. Sievertsen, V.S. Lim, C. Nakawatase, L.A. Frohman, Metabolic clearance and secretion rates of human prolactin in normal subjects and in patients with chronic renal failure, J Clin Endocrinol Metab 50 (5) (1980) 846–852.
[160] I.R. Falconer, A.T. Vacek, Degradation of 125I-labelled prolactin in the rabbit: Effect of nephrectomy and prolactin infusion, J Endocrinol 99 (3) (1983) 369–377.
[161] J.K. Stewart, D.K. Clifton, D.J. Koerker, A.D. Rogol, T. Jaffe, C.J. Goodner, Pulsatile release of growth hormone and prolactin from the primate pituitary in vitro, Endocrinology 116 (1) (1985) 1–5.
[162] J.D. Veldhuis, M.L. Johnson, Operating characteristics of the hypothalamo–pituitary–gonadal axis in men: Circadian, ultradian, and pulsatile release of prolactin and its temporal coupling with luteinizing hormone, J Clin Endocrinol Metab 67 (1) (1988) 116–123.
[163] M.H. Samuels, P. Henry, B. Kleinschmidt-Demasters, K. Lillehei, E.C. Ridgway, Pulsatile prolactin secretion in hyperprolactinemia due to presumed pituitary stalk interruption, J Clin Endocrinol Metab 73 (6) (1991) 1289–1293.
[164] D.C. Parker, L.G. Rossman, T.M. Siler, J. Rivier, S.S. Yen, R. Guillemin, Inhibition of the sleep-related peak in physiologic human growth hormone release by somatostatin, J Clin Endocrinol Metab 38 (3) (1974) 496–499.
[165] J.F. Sassin, A.G. Frantz, S. Kapen, E.D. Weitzman, The nocturnal rise of human prolactin is dependent on sleep, J Clin Endocrinol Metab 37 (3) (1973) 436–440.
[166] J.M. Stern, S. Reichlin, Prolactin circadian rhythm persists throughout lactation in women, Neuroendocrinology 51 (1) (1990) 31–37.
[167] H.E. Carlson, J.T. Miglietta, M.S. Roginsky, L.D. Stegink, Stimulation of pituitary hormone secretion by neurotransmitter amino acids in humans, Metabolism 38 (12) (1989) 1179–1182.
[168] A.N. Poindexter, V.C. Buttram, P.K. Besch, B. Lash, Circulating prolactin levels. I. Normal females, Int J Fertil 22 (1) (1977) 1–5.
[169] L.A. Balint-Peric, G.M. Prelevic, Changes in prolactin levels with the menopause: The effects of estrogen/androgen and calcitonin treatment, Gynecol Endocrinol 11 (4) (1997) 275–280.
[170] D. Foth, T. Romer, Prolactin serum levels in postmenopausal women receiving long-term hormone replacement therapy, Gynecol Obstet Invest 44 (2) (1997) 124–126.
[171] A. Iranmanesh, T. Mulligan, J.D. Veldhuis, Mechanisms subserving the physiological nocturnal relative hypoprolactinemia of healthy older men: Dual decline in prolactin secretory burst mass and basal release with preservation of pulse duration, frequency, and interpulse interval – a General Clinical Research Center study, J Clin Endocrinol Metab 84 (3) (1999) 1083–1090.
[172] P. Touraine, C. Deneux, G. Plu-Bureau, P. Mauvais-Jarvis, F. Kuttenn, Hormonal replacement therapy in menopausal women with a history of hyperprolactinemia, J Endocrinol Invest 21 (11) (1998) 732–736.
[173] P. Franchimont, C. Dourcy, J.J. Legros, A. Reuter, Y. Vrindts-Gevaert, J.R. Van Cauwenberge, et al., Prolactin levels during the menstrual cycle, Clin Endocrinol (Oxf) 5 (6) (1976) 643–650.
[174] A.S. McNeilly, T. Chard, Circulating levels of prolactin during the menstrual cycle, Clin Endocrinol (Oxf) 3 (2) (1974) 105–112.
[175] W. Braund, D.C. Roeger, S.J. Judd, Synchronous secretion of luteinizing hormone and prolactin in the human luteal phase: neuroendocrine mechanisms, J Clin Endocrinol Metab 58 (2) (1984) 293–297.
[176] G.L. Noel, R.C. Dimond, L. Wartofsky, J.M. Earll, A.G. Frantz, Studies of prolactin and TSH secretion by continuous infusion of small amounts of thyrotropin-releasing hormone (TRH), J Clin Endocrinol Metab 39 (1) (1974) 6–17.
[177] J.M. Johnston, J.A. Amico, A prospective longitudinal study of the release of oxytocin and prolactin in response to infant suckling in long term lactation, J Clin Endocrinol Metab 62 (4) (1986) 653–657.
[178] J.M. Stern, M. Konner, T.N. Herman, S. Reichlin, Nursing behaviour, prolactin and postpartum amenorrhoea during prolonged lactation in American and Kung mothers, Clin Endocrinol (Oxf) 25 (3) (1986) 247–258.

[179] G.L. Noel, H.K. Suh, A.G. Frantz, Prolactin release during nursing and breast stimulation in postpartum and non-postpartum subjects, J Clin Endocrinol Metab 38 (3) (1974) 413–423.
[180] R.C. Kolodny, L.S. Jacobs, W.H. Daughaday, Mammary stimulation causes prolactin secretion in non-lactating women, Nature 238 (5362) (1972) 284–286.
[181] G.A. Modest, J.J. Fangman, Nipple piercing and hyperprolactinemia, N Engl J Med 347 (20) (2002) 1626–1627.
[182] M. Zinger, M. McFarland, N. Ben-Jonathan, Prolactin expression and secretion by human breast glandular and adipose tissue explants, J Clin Endocrinol Metab 88 (2) (2003) 689–696.
[183] G.L. Noel, H.K. Suh, J.G. Stone, A.G. Frantz, Human prolactin and growth hormone release during surgery and other conditions of stress, J Clin Endocrinol Metab 35 (6) (1972) 840–851.
[184] G. Van den Berghe, F. de Zegher, R. Bouillon, Clinical review 95: Acute and prolonged critical illness as different neuroendocrine paradigms, J Clin Endocrinol Metab 83 (6) (1998) 1827–1834.
[185] R.R. Gala, The physiology and mechanisms of the stress-induced changes in prolactin secretion in the rat, Life Sci 46 (20) (1990) 1407–1420.
[186] B. Corenblum, P.J. Taylor, Mechanisms of control of prolactin release in response to apprehension stress and anesthesia-surgery stress, Fertil Steril 36 (6) (1981) 712–715.
[187] I.J. Spiler, M.E. Molitch, Lack of modulation of pituitary hormone stress response by neural pathways involving opiate receptors, J Clin Endocrinol Metab 50 (3) (1980) 516–520.
[188] H. Abe, D. Engler, M.E. Molitch, J. Bollinger-Gruber, S. Reichlin, Vasoactive intestinal peptide is a physiological mediator of prolactin release in the rat, Endocrinology 116 (4) (1985) 1383–1390.
[189] F.E. Chang, S.R. Richards, M.H. Kim, W.B. Malarkey, Twenty-four-hour prolactin profiles and prolactin responses to dopamine in long distance running women, J Clin Endocrinol Metab 59 (4) (1984) 631–635.
[190] J.W. Everett, Luteotrophic function of autografts of the rat hypophysis, Endocrinology 54 (6) (1954) 685–690.
[191] N. Ben-Jonathan, R. Hnasko, Dopamine as a prolactin (PRL) inhibitor, Endocr Rev 22 (6) (2001) 724–763.
[192] R.J. Mogg, W.K. Samson, Interactions of dopaminergic and peptidergic factors in the control of prolactin release, Endocrinology 126 (2) (1990) 728–735.
[193] S.L. Asa, M.A. Kelly, D.K. Grandy, M.J. Low, Pituitary lactotroph adenomas develop after prolonged lactotroph hyperplasia in dopamine D2 receptor-deficient mice, Endocrinology 140 (11) (1999) 5348–5355.
[194] M.A. Kelly, M. Rubinstein, S.L. Asa, G. Zhang, C. Saez, J.R. Bunzow, et al., Pituitary lactotroph hyperplasia and chronic hyperprolactinemia in dopamine D2 receptor-deficient mice, Neuron 19 (1) (1997) 103–113.
[195] R. Bosse, F. Fumagalli, M. Jaber, B. Giros, R.R. Gainetdinov, W.C. Wetsel, et al., Anterior pituitary hypoplasia and dwarfism in mice lacking the dopamine transporter, Neuron 19 (1) (1997) 127–138.
[196] M.E. Quigley, S.J. Judd, G.B. Gilliland, S.S. Yen, Functional studies of dopamine control of prolactin secretion in normal women and women with hyperprolactinemic pituitary microadenoma, J Clin Endocrinol Metab 50 (6) (1980) 994–998.
[197] W.F. Leebaw, L.A. Lee, P.D. Woolf, Dopamine affects basal and augmented pituitary hormone secretion, J Clin Endocrinol Metab 47 (3) (1978) 480–487.
[198] P.D. Levinson, D.S. Goldstein, P.J. Munson, J.R. Gill Jr., H.R. Keiser, Endocrine, renal, and hemodynamic responses to graded dopamine infusions in normal men, J Clin Endocrinol Metab 60 (5) (1985) 821–826.
[199] M.E. Molitch, Drugs and prolactin, Pituitary 11 (2) (2008) 209–218.
[200] V. Raymond, M. Beaulieu, F. Labrie, J. Boissier, Potent antidopaminergic activity of estradiol at the pituitary level on prolactin release, Science 200 (4346) (1978) 1173–1175.
[201] S.J. Judd, J.S. Rakoff, S.S. Yen, Inhibition of gonadotropin and prolactin release by dopamine: Effect of endogenous estradiol levels, J Clin Endocrinol Metab 47 (3) (1978) 494–498.
[202] C. Pasqualini, F. Bojda, B. Kerdelhue, Direct effect of estradiol on the number of dopamine receptors in the anterior pituitary of ovariectomized rats, Endocrinology 119 (6) (1986) 2484–2489.
[203] S.M. Foord, J.R. Peters, C. Dieguez, M.F. Scanlon, R. Hall, Dopamine receptors on intact anterior pituitary cells in culture: Functional association with the inhibition of prolactin and thyrotropin, Endocrinology 112 (5) (1983) 1567–1577.
[204] K. Nikolics, A.J. Mason, E. Szonyi, J. Ramachandran, P.H. Seeburg, A prolactin-inhibiting factor within the precursor for human gonadotropin-releasing hormone, Nature 316 (6028) (1985) 511–517.
[205] J.P. Adelman, A.J. Mason, J.S. Hayflick, P.H. Seeburg, Isolation of the gene and hypothalamic cDNA for the common precursor of gonadotropin-releasing hormone and prolactin release-inhibiting factor in human and rat, Proc Nat Acad Sci USA 83 (1) (1986) 179–183.
[206] M. Ishibashi, T. Yamaji, F. Takaku, A. Teramoto, T. Fukushima, M. Toyama, et al., Effect of GnRH-associated peptide on prolactin secretion from human lactotrope adenoma cells in culture, Acta Endocrinol (Copenh) 116 (1) (1987) 81–84.
[207] L. Grandison, A. Guidotti, gamma-Aminobutyric acid receptor function in rat anterior pituitary: Evidence for control of prolactin release, Endocrinology 105 (3) (1979) 754–759.
[208] A.V. Schally, T.W. Redding, A. Arimura, A. Dupont, G.L. Linthicum, Isolation of gamma-amino butyric acid from pig hypothalami and demonstration of its prolactin release-inhibiting (PIF) activity in vivo and in vitro, Endocrinology 100 (3) (1977) 681–691.
[209] J.J. Mulchahey, J.D. Neill, Gamma amino butyric acid (GABA) levels in hypophyseal stalk plasma of rats, Life Sci 31 (5) (1982) 453–456.
[210] F. Cavagnini, G. Benetti, C. Invitti, G. Ramella, M. Pinto, M. Lazza, et al., Effect of gamma-aminobutyric acid on growth hormone and prolactin secretion in man: Influence of pimozide and domperidone, J Clin Endocrinol Metab 51 (4) (1980) 789–792.
[211] G.B. Melis, F. Fruzzetti, A.M. Paoletti, V. Mais, A. Kemeny, F. Strigini, et al., Pharmacological activation of gamma-aminobutyric acid-system blunts prolactin response to mechanical breast stimulation in puerperal women, J Clin Endocrinol Metab 58 (1) (1984) 201–205.
[212] A.H. Tashjian Jr., N.J. Barowsky, D.K. Jensen, Thyrotropin releasing hormone: Direct evidence for stimulation of prolactin production by pituitary cells in culture, Biochem Biophys Res Commun 43 (3) (1971) 516–523.
[213] L.S. Jacobs, P.J. Snyder, J.F. Wilber, R.D. Utiger, W.H. Daughaday, Increased serum prolactin after administration of synthetic thyrotropin releasing hormone (TRH) in man, J Clin Endocrinol Metab 33 (6) (1971) 996–998.
[214] R. Ashworth, P.M. Hinkle, Thyrotropin-releasing hormone-induced intracellular calcium responses in individual rat lactotrophs and thyrotrophs, Endocrinology 137 (12) (1996) 5205–5212.

[215] Y. Koch, G. Goldhaber, I. Fireman, U. Zor, J. Shani, E. Tal, Suppression of prolactin and thyrotropin secretion in the rat by antiserum to thyrotropin-releasing hormone, Endocrinology 100 (5) (1977) 1476–1478.
[216] M. Yamada, Y. Saga, N. Shibusawa, J. Hirato, M. Murakami, T. Iwasaki, et al., Tertiary hypothyroidism and hyperglycemia in mice with targeted disruption of the thyrotropin-releasing hormone gene, Proc Nat Acad Sci USA 94 (20) (1997) 10862–10867.
[217] K.M. Gautvik, A.H. Tashjian Jr., I.A. Kourides, B.D. Weintraub, C.T. Graeber, F. Maloof, et al., Thyrotropin-releasing hormone is not the sole physiologic mediator of prolactin release during suckling, N Engl J Med 290 (21) (1974) 1162–1165.
[218] S. Jeppsson, K.O. Nilsson, G. Rannevik, L. Wide, Influence of suckling and of suckling followed by TRH or LH-RH on plasma prolactin, TSH, GH and FSH, Acta Endocrinol (Copenh) 82 (2) (1976) 246–253.
[219] T.P. Segerson, J. Kauer, H.C. Wolfe, H. Mobtaker, P. Wu, I.M. Jackson, et al., Thyroid hormone regulates TRH biosynthesis in the paraventricular nucleus of the rat hypothalamus, Science 238 (4823) (1987) 78–80.
[220] J.M. Rondeel, W.J. de Greef, P. van der Schoot, B. Karels, W. Klootwijk, T.J. Visser, Effect of thyroid status and paraventricular area lesions on the release of thyrotropin-releasing hormone and catecholamines into hypophysial portal blood, Endocrinology 123 (1) (1988) 523–527.
[221] M.H. Perrone, P.M. Hinkle, Regulation of pituitary receptors for thyrotropin-releasing hormone by thyroid hormones, J Biol Chem 253 (14) (1978) 5168–5173.
[222] P.J. Snyder, L.S. Jacobs, M.M. Rabello, F.H. Sterling, R.N. Shore, R.D. Utiger, et al., Diagnostic value of thyrotrophin-releasing hormone in pituitary and hypothalamic diseases. Assessment of thyrotrophin and prolactin secretion in 100 patients, Ann Intern Med 81 (6) (1974) 751–757.
[223] M. L'Hermite, C. Robyn, J. Golstein, G. Rothenbuchner, J. Birk, U. Loos, et al., Prolactin and thyrotropin in thyroid diseases: Lack of evidence for a physiological role of thyrotropin-releasing hormone in the regulation of prolactin secretion, Horm Metab Res 6 (3) (1974) 190–195.
[224] Y. Kato, Y. Iwasaki, J. Iwasaki, H. Abe, N. Yanaihara, H. Imura, Prolactin release by vasoactive intestinal polypeptide in rats, Endocrinology 103 (2) (1978) 554–558.
[225] E. Mezey, J.Z. Kiss, Vasoactive intestinal peptide-containing neurons in the paraventricular nucleus may participate in regulating prolactin secretion, Proc Nat Acad Sci USA 82 (1) (1985) 245–247.
[226] W.B. Malarkey, T.M. O'Dorisio, M. Kennedy, S. Cataland, The influence of vasoactive intestinal polypeptide and cholecystokinin on prolactin release in rat and human monolayer cultures, Life Sci 28 (22) (1981) 2489–2495.
[227] S.I. Said, J.C. Porter, Vasoactive intestinal polypeptide: Release into hypophyseal portal blood, Life Sci 24 (3) (1979) 227–230.
[228] A.J. Carrillo, T.B. Pool, Z.D. Sharp, Vasoactive intestinal peptide increases prolactin messenger ribonucleic acid content in GH3 cells, Endocrinology 116 (1) (1985) 202–206.
[229] I. Gozes, Y. Shani, Hypothalamic vasoactive intestinal peptide messenger ribonucleic acid is increased in lactating rats, Endocrinology 119 (6) (1986) 2497–2501.
[230] N. Itoh, K. Obata, N. Yanaihara, H. Okamoto, Human preprovasoactive intestinal polypeptide contains a novel PHI-27-like peptide, PHM-27, Nature 304 (5926) (1983) 547–549.
[231] A. Sasaki, S. Sato, M.G. Go, Y. Shimizu, O. Murakami, K. Hanew, et al., Distribution, plasma concentration, and in vivo prolactin-releasing activity of peptide histidine methionine in humans, J Clin Endocrinol Metab 65 (4) (1987) 683–688.
[232] Y. Yiangou, J.S. Gill, B.J. Chrysanthou, J. Burrin, S.R. Bloom, Infusion of prepro-VIP derived peptides in man: Effect on secretion of prolactin, Neuroendocrinology 48 (6) (1988) 615–618.
[233] M.A. Arnaout, T.L. Garthwaite, D.R. Martinson, T.C. Hagen, Vasoactive intestinal polypeptide is synthesized in anterior pituitary tissue, Endocrinology 119 (5) (1986) 2052–2057.
[234] T.C. Hagen, M.A. Arnaout, W.J. Scherzer, D.R. Martinson, T.L. Garthwaite, Antisera to vasoactive intestinal polypeptide inhibit basal prolactin release from dispersed anterior pituitary cells, Neuroendocrinology 43 (6) (1986) 641–645.
[235] L.D. Van de Kar, C.L. Bethea, Pharmacological evidence that serotonergic stimulation of prolactin secretion is mediated via the dorsal raphe nucleus, Neuroendocrinology 35 (4) (1982) 225–230.
[236] Y. Kato, Y. Nakai, H. Imura, K. Chihara, S. Ogo, Effect of 5-hydroxytryptophan (5-HTP) on plasma prolactin levels in man, J Clin Endocrinol Metab 38 (4) (1974) 695–697.
[237] J. Golstein, L. Vanhaelst, O.D. Bruno, M. L'Hermite, Effect of cyproheptadine on thyrotrophin and prolactin secretion in normal man, Acta Endocrinol (Copenh) 92 (2) (1979) 205–213.
[238] I. Lancranjan, A. Wirz-Justice, W. Puhringer, E. Del Pozo, Effect of 1-5 hydroxytryptophan infusion on growth hormone and prolactin secretion in man, J Clin Endocrinol Metab 45 (3) (1977) 588–593.
[239] J. Kiss, B. Halasz, Synaptic connections between serotoninergic axon terminals and tyrosine hydroxylase-immunoreactive neurons in the arcuate nucleus of the rat hypothalamus. A combination of electron microscopic autoradiography and immunocytochemistry, Brain Res 364 (2) (1986) 284–294.
[240] N.S. Pilotte, J.C. Porter, Dopamine in hypophysial portal plasma and prolactin in systemic plasma of rats treated with 5-hydroxytryptamine, Endocrinology 108 (6) (1981) 2137–2141.
[241] A.B. Emiliano, J.L. Fudge, From galactorrhea to osteopenia: Rethinking serotonin-prolactin interactions, Neuropsychopharmacology 29 (5) (2004) 833–846.
[242] R.S. Piezzi, F. Larin, R.J. Wurtman, Serotonin, 5-hydroxyindoleacetic acid (5-HIAA), and monoamide oxidase in the bovine median eminence and pituitary gland, Endocrinology 86 (6) (1970) 1460–1462.
[243] E.B. De Souza, Serotonin and dopamine receptors in the rat pituitary gland: Autoradiographic identification, characterization, and localization, Endocrinology 119 (4) (1986) 1534–1542.
[244] M.A. Johns, E.C. Azmitia, D.T. Krieger, Specific in vitro uptake of serotonin by cells in the anterior pituitary of the rat, Endocrinology 110 (3) (1982) 754–760.
[245] M.E. Apfelbaum, Effect of serotonin on basal and TRH-induced release of prolactin from rat pituitary glands in vitro, Acta Endocrinol (Copenh) 114 (4) (1987) 565–571.
[246] A. Papageorgiou, C. Denef, Estradiol induces expression of 5-hydroxytryptamine (5-HT) 4, 5-HT5, and 5-HT6 receptor messenger ribonucleic acid in rat anterior pituitary cell aggregates and allows prolactin release via the 5-HT4 receptor, Endocrinology 148 (3) (2007) 1384–1395.
[247] Y. Kato, Y. Iwasaki, H. Abe, S. Ohgo, H. Imura, Effects of endorphins on prolactin and growth hormone secretion in rats, Proc Soc Exp Biol Med 158 (3) (1978) 431–436.
[248] C. Rivier, M. Brown, W. Vale, Effect of neurotensin, substance P and morphine sulfate on the secretion of prolactin and growth hormone in the rat, Endocrinology 100 (3) (1977) 751–754.
[249] C.A. Leadem, S.V. Yagenova, Effects of specific activation of mu-, delta- and kappa-opioid receptors on the secretion of luteinizing hormone and prolactin in the ovariectomized rat, Neuroendocrinology 45 (2) (1987) 109–117.

[250] D.A. Van Vugt, P.W. Sylvester, C.F. Aylsworth, J. Meites, Comparison of acute effects of dynorphin and beta-endorphin on prolactin release in the rat, Endocrinology 108 (5) (1981) 2017–2018.
[251] W. Bryant, J. Janik, M. Baumann, P. Callahan, Orphanin FQ stimulates prolactin and growth hormone release in male and female rats, Brain Res 807 (1–2) (1998) 228–233.
[252] G. Tolis, J. Hickey, H. Guyda, Effects of morphine on serum growth hormone, cortisol, prolactin and thyroid stimulating hormone in man, J Clin Endocrinol Metab 41 (4) (1975) 797–800.
[253] V. Chan, C. Wang, R.T. Yeung, Effects of heroin addiction on thyrotrophin, thyroid hormones and porlactin secretion in men, Clin Endocrinol (Oxf) 10 (6) (1979) 557–565.
[254] J.B. Martin, G. Tolis, I. Woods, H. Guyda, Failure of naloxone to influence physiological growth hormone and prolactin secretion, Brain Res 168 (1) (1979) 210–215.
[255] M.O. Thorner, R.L. Perryman, M.J. Cronin, A.D. Rogol, M. Draznin, A. Johanson, et al., Somatotroph hyperplasia. Successful treatment of acromegaly by removal of a pancreatic islet tumor secreting a growth hormone-releasing factor, J Clin Invest 70 (5) (1982) 965–977.
[256] J.A. Goldman, M.E. Molitch, M.O. Thorner, W. Vale, J. Rivier, S. Reichlin, Growth hormone and prolactin responses to bolus and sustained infusions of GRH-1-40-OH in man, J Endocrinol Invest 10 (4) (1987) 397–406.
[257] J. Fragoso, R. Barrio, S. Donnay, M. Hernandez, Chronic stimulation of basal prolactin (PRL) secretion by growth hormone releasing hormone (GHRH) in children with GH neurosecretory dysfunction, Horm Metab Res 22 (1) (1990) 53–54.
[258] M. Barinaga, G. Yamonoto, C. Rivier, W. Vale, R. Evans, M.G. Rosenfeld, Transcriptional regulation of growth hormone gene expression by growth hormone-releasing factor, Nature 306 (5938) (1983) 84–85.
[259] M. Mori, S. Vigh, A. Miyata, T. Yoshihara, S. Oka, A. Arimura, Oxytocin is the major prolactin releasing factor in the posterior pituitary, Endocrinology 126 (2) (1990) 1009–1013.
[260] D.T. McKee, M.O. Poletini, R. Bertram, M.E. Freeman, Oxytocin action at the lactotroph is required for prolactin surges in cervically stimulated ovariectomized rats, Endocrinology 148 (10) (2007) 4649–4657.
[261] V. Coiro, A. Gnudi, R. Volpi, C. Marchesi, G. Salati, P. Caffarra, et al., Oxytocin enhances thyrotropin-releasing hormone-induced prolactin release in normal menstruating women, Fertil Steril 47 (4) (1987) 565–569.
[262] F. Petraglia, W. Vale, C. Rivier, Beta-endorphin and dynorphin participate in the stress-induced release of prolactin in the rat, Neuroendocrinology 45 (5) (1987) 338–342.
[263] A.E. Panerai, F. Petraglia, P. Sacerdote, A.R. Genazzani, Mainly mu-opiate receptors are involved in luteinizing hormone and prolactin secretion, Endocrinology 117 (3) (1985) 1096–1099.
[264] D.C. Herbert, E.G. Rennels, Effect of synthetic luteinizing hormone releasing hormone on prolactin secretion from clonal pituitary cells, Biochem Biophys Res Commun 79 (1) (1977) 133–138.
[265] R.F. Casper, S.S. Yen, Simultaneous pulsatile release of prolactin and luteinizing hormone induced by luteinizing hormone-releasing factor agonist, J Clin Endocrinol Metab 52 (5) (1981) 934–936.
[266] E. Christiansen, J.D. Veldhuis, A.D. Rogol, P. Stumpf, W.S. Evans, Modulating actions of estradiol on gonadotropin-releasing hormone-stimulated prolactin secretion in postmenopausal individuals, Am J Obstet Gynecol 157 (2) (1987) 320–325.
[267] L.J. Gooren, W. Harmsen-Louman, L. van Bergeyk, H. van Kessel, Studies on the prolactin-releasing capacity of luteinizing hormone releasing hormone in male subjects, Exp Clin Endocrinol 86 (3) (1985) 300–304.
[268] A.M. Brandi, G. Barrande, N. Lahlou, M. Crumeyrolle, M. Berthet, P. Leblanc, et al., Stimulatory effect of gonadotropin-releasing hormone (GnRH) on in vitro prolactin secretion and presence of GnRH specific receptors in a subset of human prolactinomas, Eur J Endocrinol 132 (2) (1995) 163–170.
[269] C.F. Deschepper, C.D. Seidler, M.K. Steele, W.F. Ganong, Further studies on the localization of angiotensin-II-like immunoreactivity in the anterior pituitary gland of the male rat, comparing various antisera to pituitary hormones and their specificity, Neuroendocrinology 40 (6) (1985) 471–475.
[270] A. Mukherjee, P. Kulkarni, S.M. McCann, A. Negro-Vilar, Evidence for the presence and characterization of angiotensin II receptors in rat anterior pituitary membranes, Endocrinology 110 (2) (1982) 665–667.
[271] J.M. Saavedra, J. Fernandez-Pardal, C. Chevillard, Angiotensin-converting enzyme in discrete areas of the rat forebrain and pituitary gland, Brain Res 245 (2) (1982) 317–325.
[272] J.P. Saint-Andre, V. Rohmer, F. Alhenc-Gelas, J. Menard, J.C. Bigorgne, P. Corvol, Presence of renin, angiotensinogen, and converting enzyme in human pituitary lactotroph cells and prolactin adenomas, J Clin Endocrinol Metab 63 (1) (1986) 231–237.
[273] G. Diaz-Torga, A. Gonzalez Iglesias, R. Achaval-Zaia, C. Libertun, D. Becu-Villalobos, Angiotensin II-induced Ca^{2+} mobilization and prolactin release in normal and hyperplastic pituitary cells, Am J Physiol 274 (3 Pt 1) (1998) E534–E540.
[274] P.W. Anderson, W.B. Malarkey, J. Salk, O.A. Kletsky, W.A. Hsueh, The effect of angiotensin-converting enzyme inhibition on prolactin responses in normal and hyperprolactinemic subjects, J Clin Endocrinol Metab 69 (3) (1989) 518–522.
[275] L.M. Winer, A. Molteni, M.E. Molitch, Effect of angiotensin-converting enzyme inhibition on pituitary hormone responses to insulin-induced hypoglycemia in humans, J Clin Endocrinol Metab 71 (1) (1990) 256–259.
[276] S.H. Lin, Prolactin-releasing peptide, Results Probl Cell Differ 46 (2008) 57–88.
[277] A. Enjalbert, P. Bertrand, M. Le Dafniet, J. Epelbaum, J.N. Hugues, C. Kordon, et al., Somatostatin and regulation of prolactin secretion, Psychoneuroendocrinology 11 (2) (1986) 155–165.
[278] W. Vale, C. Rivier, P. Brazeau, R. Guillemin, Effects of somatostatin on the secretion of thyrotropin and prolactin, Endocrinology 95 (4) (1974) 968–977.
[279] D. Carr, A. Gomez-Pan, D.R. Weightman, V.C. Roy, R. Hall, G.M. Besser, et al., Growth hormone release inhibiting hormone: Actions on thyrotrophin and prolactin secretion after thyrotrophinreleasing hormone, Br Med J 3 (5975) (1975) 67–69.
[280] U.P. Knigge, Histaminergic regulation of prolactin secretion, Dan Med Bull 37 (2) (1990) 109–124.
[281] U. Knigge, S. Matzen, J. Warberg, Histaminergic stimulation of prolactin secretion mediated via H1- or H2-receptors: Dependence on routes of administration, Neuroendocrinology 44 (1) (1986) 41–48.
[282] H.E. Carlson, A.F. Ippoliti, Cimetidine, an H2-antihistamine, stimulates prolactin secretion in man, J Clin Endocrinol Metab 45 (2) (1977) 367–370.
[283] A. Masala, S. Alagna, R. Faedda, A. Satta, P.P. Rovasio, Prolactin secretion in man following acute and long-term cimetidine administration, Acta Endocrinol (Copenh) 93 (4) (1980) 392–395.

[284] L.C. Terry, J.B. Martin, Evidence for alpha-adrenergic regulation of episodic growth hormone and prolactin secretion in the undisturbed male rat, Endocrinology 108 (5) (1981) 1869–1873.
[285] J. Steiner, J. Cassar, K. Mashiter, I. Dawes, T.R. Fraser, A. Breckenridge, Effects of methyldopa on prolactin and growth hormone, Br Med J 1 (6019) (1976) 1186–1188.
[286] S.L. Slater, S. Lipper, D.J. Shiling, D.L. Murphy, Elevation of plasma-prolactin by monoamine-oxidase inhibitors, Lancet 2 (8032) (1977) 275–276.
[287] P. Onali, C. Eva, M.C. Olianas, J.P. Schwartz, E. Costa, In GH3 pituitary cells, acetylcholine and vasoactive intestinal peptide antagonistically modulate adenylate cyclase, cyclic AMP content, and prolactin secretion, Mol Pharmacol 24 (2) (1983) 189–194.
[288] F.F. Casanueva, L. Villanueva, Y. Diaz, J. Devesa, A. Fernandez-Cruz, A.V. Schally, Atropine selectively blocks GHRH-induced GH secretion without altering LH, FSH, TSH, PRL and ACTH/cortisol secretion elicited by their specific hypothalamic releasing factors, Clin Endocrinol (Oxf) 25 (3) (1986) 319–323.
[289] A. Masala, S. Alagna, L. Devilla, P.P. Rovasio, S. Rassa, R. Faedda, et al., Muscarinic receptor blockade by pirenzepine: Effect on prolactin secretion in man, J Endocrinol Invest 5 (1) (1982) 53–55.
[290] P. Carmeliet, C. Denef, Immunocytochemical and pharmacological evidence for an intrinsic cholinomimetic system modulating prolactin and growth hormone release in rat pituitary, Endocrinology 123 (2) (1988) 1128–1139.
[291] D.R. Grattan, I.C. Kokay, Prolactin: A pleiotropic neuroendocrine hormone, J Neuroendocrinol 20 (6) (2008) 752–763.
[292] M.E. Cruz-Soto, M.D. Scheiber, K.A. Gregerson, G.P. Boivin, N.D. Horseman, Pituitary tumorigenesis in prolactin gene-disrupted mice, Endocrinology 143 (11) (2002) 4429–4436.
[293] N.D. Horseman, W. Zhao, E. Montecino-Rodriguez, M. Tanaka, K. Nakashima, S.J. Engle, et al., Defective mammopoiesis, but normal hematopoiesis, in mice with a targeted disruption of the prolactin gene, EMBO J 16 (23) (1997) 6926–6935.
[294] C. Dieguez, J.R. Peters, M.D. Page, R. John, R. Hall, M.F. Scanlon, Thyroid function in patients with hyperprolactinaemia: Relationship to dopaminergic inhibition of TSH release, Clin Endocrinol (Oxf) 25 (4) (1986) 435–440.
[295] M.F. Scanlon, M.D. Rodriguez-Arnao, A.M. McGregor, D. Weightman, M. Lewis, D.B. Cook, et al., Altered dopaminergic regulation of thyrotrophin release in patients with prolactinomas: Comparison with other tests of hypothalamic-pituitary function, Clin Endocrinol (Oxf) 14 (2) (1981) 133–143.
[296] S.E. Sauder, M. Frager, G.D. Case, R.P. Kelch, J.C. Marshall, Abnormal patterns of pulsatile luteinizing hormone secretion in women with hyperprolactinemia and amenorrhea: Responses to bromocriptine, J Clin Endocrinol Metab 59 (5) (1984) 941–948.
[297] S.J. Winters, P. Troen, Altered pulsatile secretion of luteinizing hormone in hypogonadal men with hyperprolactinaemia, Clin Endocrinol (Oxf) 21 (3) (1984) 257–263.
[298] M.E. Molitch, R.W. Rebar, C.P. Barsano, Effect of human prolactin administration on gonadotropin and thyrotropin secretion in normal men, J Endocrinol Invest 16 (8) (1993) 559–564.
[299] D.K. Sarkar, Evidence for prolactin feedback actions on hypothalamic oxytocin, vasoactive intestinal peptide and dopamine secretion, Neuroendocrinology 49 (5) (1989) 520–524.
[300] Z.Z. Hu, J. Meng, M.L. Dufau, Isolation and characterization of two novel forms of the human prolactin receptor generated by alternative splicing of a newly identified exon 11, J Biol Chem 276 (44) (2001) 41086–41094.
[301] Z.Z. Hu, L. Zhuang, J. Meng, M. Leondires, M.L. Dufau, The human prolactin receptor gene structure and alternative promoter utilization: The generic promoter hPIII and a novel human promoter hP(N), J Clin Endocrinol Metab 84 (3) (1999) 1153–1156.
[302] Z.Z. Hu, L. Zhuang, J. Meng, C.H. Tsai-Morris, M.L. Dufau, Complex 5′ genomic structure of the human prolactin receptor: Multiple alternative exons 1 and promoter utilization, Endocrinology 143 (6) (2002) 2139–2142.
[303] Z.Z. Hu, L. Zhuang, J. Meng, M.L. Dufau, Transcriptional regulation of the generic promoter III of the rat prolactin receptor gene by C/EBPbeta and Sp1, J Biol Chem 273 (40) (1998) 26225–26235.
[304] J. Dong, C.H. Tsai-Morris, M.L. Dufau, A novel estradiol/estrogen receptor alpha-dependent transcriptional mechanism controls expression of the human prolactin receptor, J Biol Chem 281 (27) (2006) 18825–18836.
[305] G. Swaminathan, B. Varghese, C. Thangavel, C.J. Carbone, A. Plotnikov, K.G. Kumar, et al., Prolactin stimulates ubiquitination, initial internalization, and degradation of its receptor via catalytic activation of Janus kinase 2, J Endocrinol 196 (2) (2008) R1–R7.
[306] B. Varghese, H. Barriere, C.J. Carbone, A. Banerjee, G. Swaminathan, A. Plotnikov, et al., Polyubiquitination of prolactin receptor stimulates its internalization, post-internalization sorting, and degradation via the lysosomal pathway, Mol Cell Biol 28 (17) (2008) 5275–5287.
[307] A. Plotnikov, B. Varghese, T.H. Tran, C. Liu, H. Rui, S.Y. Fuchs, Impaired turnover of prolactin receptor contributes to transformation of human breast cells, Cancer Res 69 (7) (2009) 3165–3172.
[308] J.B. Kline, C.V. Clevenger, Identification and characterization of the prolactin-binding protein in human serum and milk, J Biol Chem 276 (27) (2001) 24760–24766.
[309] J. Halperin, S.Y. Devi, S. Elizur, C. Stocco, A. Shehu, D. Rebourcet, et al., Prolactin signaling through the short form of its receptor represses forkhead transcription factor FOXO3 and its target gene galt causing a severe ovarian defect, Mol Endocrinol 22 (2) (2008) 513–522.
[310] Y.S. Devi, A. Shehu, C. Stocco, J. Halperin, J. Le, A.M. Seibold, et al., Regulation of transcription factors and repression of Sp1 by prolactin signaling through the short isoform of its cognate receptor, Endocrinology 150 (7) (2009) 3327–3335.
[311] A.M. Qazi, C.H. Tsai-Morris, M.L. Dufau, Ligand-independent homo- and heterodimerization of human prolactin receptor variants: Inhibitory action of the short forms by heterodimerization, Mol Endocrinol 20 (8) (2006) 1912–1923.
[312] D. Tan, A.M. Walker, Short form 1b human prolactin receptor down-regulates expression of the long form, J Mol Endocrinol 44 (3) (2010) 187–194.
[313] J. Meng, C.H. Tsai-Morris, M.L. Dufau, Human prolactin receptor variants in breast cancer: Low ratio of short forms to the long-form human prolactin receptor associated with mammary carcinoma, Cancer Res 64 (16) (2004) 5677–5682.
[314] I. Broutin, J.B. Jomain, E. Tallet, J. van Agthoven, B. Raynal, S. Hoos, et al., Crystal structure of an affinity-matured prolactin complexed to its dimerized receptor reveals the topology of hormone binding site 2, J Biol Chem 285 (11) (2010) 8422–8433.
[315] J.J. Lebrun, S. Ali, A. Ullrich, P.A. Kelly, Proline-rich sequence-mediated Jak2 association to the prolactin receptor is required but not sufficient for signal transduction, J Biol Chem 270 (18) (1995) 10664–10670.

[316] A. Pezet, H. Buteau, P.A. Kelly, M. Edery, The last proline of Box 1 is essential for association with JAK2 and functional activation of the prolactin receptor, Mol Cell Endocrinol 129 (2) (1997) 199–208.
[317] A.A. Kossiakoff, The structural basis for biological signaling, regulation, and specificity in the growth hormone-prolactin system of hormones and receptors, Adv Protein Chem 68 (2004) 147–169.
[318] S.L. Gadd, C.V. Clevenger, Ligand-independent dimerization of the human prolactin receptor isoforms: Functional implications, Mol Endocrinol 20 (11) (2006) 2734–2746.
[319] R.J. Brown, J.J. Adams, R.A. Pelekanos, Y. Wan, W.J. McKinstry, K. Palethorpe, et al., Model for growth hormone receptor activation based on subunit rotation within a receptor dimer, Nat Struct Mol Biol 12 (9) (2005) 814–821.
[320] N. Seubert, Y. Royer, J. Staerk, K.F. Kubatzky, V. Moucadel, S. Krishnakumar, et al., Active and inactive orientations of the transmembrane and cytosolic domains of the erythropoietin receptor dimer, Mol Cell 12 (5) (2003) 1239–1250.
[321] G.S. Campbell, L.S. Argetsinger, J.N. Ihle, P.A. Kelly, J.A. Rillema, C. Carter-Su, Activation of JAK2 tyrosine kinase by prolactin receptors in Nb2 cells and mouse mammary gland explants, Proc Nat Acad Sci USA 91 (12) (1994) 5232–5236.
[322] H. Rui, J.J. Lebrun, R.A. Kirken, P.A. Kelly, W.L. Farrar, JAK2 activation and cell proliferation induced by antibody-mediated prolactin receptor dimerization, Endocrinology 135 (4) (1994) 1299–1306.
[323] J.C. Byatt, N.R. Staten, W.J. Salsgiver, J.G. Kostelc, R.J. Collier, Stimulation of food intake and weight gain in mature female rats by bovine prolactin and bovine growth hormone, Am J Physiol 264 (6 Pt 1) (1993) E986–E992.
[324] C. Bole-Feysot, V. Goffin, M. Edery, N. Binart, P.A. Kelly, Prolactin (PRL) and its receptor: Actions, signal transduction pathways and phenotypes observed in PRL receptor knockout mice, Endocr Rev 19 (3) (1998) 225–268.
[325] X. Liu, G.W. Robinson, K.U. Wagner, L. Garrett, A. Wynshaw-Boris, L. Hennighausen, Stat5a is mandatory for adult mammary gland development and lactogenesis, Genes Dev 11 (2) (1997) 179–186.
[326] K. Miyoshi, J.M. Shillingford, G.H. Smith, S.L. Grimm, K.U. Wagner, T. Oka, et al., Signal transducer and activator of transcription (Stat) 5 controls the proliferation and differentiation of mammary alveolar epithelium, J Cell Biol 155 (4) (2001) 531–542.
[327] Y. Ke, J. Lesperance, E.E. Zhang, E.A. Bard-Chapeau, R.G. Oshima, W.J. Muller, et al., Conditional deletion of Shp2 in the mammary gland leads to impaired lobulo-alveolar outgrowth and attenuated Stat5 activation, J Biol Chem 281 (45) (2006) 34374–34380.
[328] N. Aoki, T. Matsuda, A nuclear protein tyrosine phosphatase TC-PTP is a potential negative regulator of the PRL-mediated signaling pathway: Dephosphorylation and deactivation of signal transducer and activator of transcription 5a and 5b by TC-PTP in nucleus, Mol Endocrinol 16 (1) (2002) 58–69.
[329] F. Dif, E. Saunier, B. Demeneix, P.A. Kelly, M. Edery, Cytokine-inducible SH2-containing protein suppresses PRL signaling by binding the PRL receptor, Endocrinology 142 (12) (2001) 5286–5293.
[330] A. Pezet, H. Favre, P.A. Kelly, M. Edery, Inhibition and restoration of prolactin signal transduction by suppressors of cytokine signaling, J Biol Chem 274 (35) (1999) 24497–24502.
[331] A. Yoshimura, T. Ohkubo, T. Kiguchi, N.A. Jenkins, D.J. Gilbert, N.G. Copeland, et al., A novel cytokine-inducible gene CIS encodes an SH2-containing protein that binds to tyrosine-phosphorylated interleukin 3 and erythropoietin receptors, EMBO J 14 (12) (1995) 2816–2826.
[332] C.V. Clevenger, P.A. Furth, S.E. Hankinson, L.A. Schuler, The role of prolactin in mammary carcinoma, Endocr Rev 24 (1) (2003) 1–27.
[333] J.H. Gutzman, D.E. Rugowski, M.D. Schroeder, J.J. Watters, L.A. Schuler, Multiple kinase cascades mediate prolactin signals to activating protein-1 in breast cancer cells, Mol Endocrinol 18 (12) (2004) 3064–3075.
[334] R. Das, B.K. Vonderhaar, Involvement of SHC, GRB2, SOS and RAS in prolactin signal transduction in mammary epithelial cells, Oncogene 13 (6) (1996) 1139–1145.
[335] R.A. Erwin, R.A. Kirken, M.G. Malabarba, W.L. Farrar, H. Rui, Prolactin activates Ras via signaling proteins SHC, growth factor receptor bound 2, and son of sevenless, Endocrinology 136 (8) (1995) 3512–3518.
[336] J.J. Acosta, R.M. Munoz, L. Gonzalez, A. Subtil-Rodriguez, M.A. Dominguez-Caceres, J.M. Garcia-Martinez, et al., Src mediates prolactin-dependent proliferation of T47D and MCF7 cells via the activation of focal adhesion kinase/Erk1/2 and phosphatidylinositol 3-kinase pathways, Mol Endocrinol 17 (11) (2003) 2268–2282.
[337] M.A. Dominguez-Caceres, J.M. Garcia-Martinez, A. Calcabrini, L. Gonzalez, P.G. Porque, J. Leon, et al., Prolactin induces c-Myc expression and cell survival through activation of Src/Akt pathway in lymphoid cells, Oncogene 23 (44) (2004) 7378–7390.
[338] H. Watkin, M.M. Richert, A. Lewis, K. Terrell, J.P. McManaman, S.M. Anderson, Lactation failure in Src knockout mice is due to impaired secretory activation, BMC Dev Biol 8 (2008) 6.
[339] L. Hennighausen, G.W. Robinson, Signaling pathways in mammary gland development, Dev Cell 1 (4) (2001) 467–475.
[340] H.L. LaMarca, J.M. Rosen, Minireview: Hormones and mammary cell fate – what will I become when I grow up? Endocrinology 149 (9) (2008) 4317–4321.
[341] G.J. Allan, E. Tonner, M.C. Barber, M.T. Travers, J.H. Shand, R.G. Vernon, et al., Growth hormone, acting in part through the insulin-like growth factor axis, rescues developmental, but not metabolic, activity in the mammary gland of mice expressing a single allele of the prolactin receptor, Endocrinology 143 (11) (2002) 4310–4319.
[342] C.J. Ormandy, A. Camus, J. Barra, D. Damotte, B. Lucas, H. Buteau, et al., Null mutation of the prolactin receptor gene produces multiple reproductive defects in the mouse, Genes Dev 11 (2) (1997) 167–178.
[343] N. Binart, C. Helloco, C.J. Ormandy, J. Barra, P. Clement-Lacroix, N. Baran, et al., Rescue of preimplantatory egg development and embryo implantation in prolactin receptor-deficient mice after progesterone administration, Endocrinology 141 (7) (2000) 2691–2697.
[344] C. Brisken, S. Kaur, T.E. Chavarria, N. Binart, R.L. Sutherland, R.A. Weinberg, et al., Prolactin controls mammary gland development via direct and indirect mechanisms, Dev Biol 210 (1) (1999) 96–106.
[345] C. Brisken, A. Ayyannan, C. Nguyen, A. Heineman, F. Reinhardt, J. Tan, et al., IGF-2 is a mediator of prolactin-induced morphogenesis in the breast, Dev Cell 3 (6) (2002) 877–887.
[346] R.C. Hovey, J. Harris, D.L. Hadsell, A.V. Lee, C.J. Ormandy, B.K. Vonderhaar, Local insulin-like growth factor-II mediates prolactin-induced mammary gland development, Mol Endocrinol 17 (3) (2003) 460–471.
[347] S. Srivastava, M. Matsuda, Z. Hou, J.P. Bailey, R. Kitazawa, M.P. Herbst, et al., Receptor activator of NF-kappaB ligand induction via Jak2 and Stat5a in mammary epithelial cells, J Biol Chem 278 (46) (2003) 46171–46178.

[348] B.W. Booth, C.A. Boulanger, G.H. Smith, Alveolar progenitor cells develop in mouse mammary glands independent of pregnancy and lactation, J Cell Physiol 212 (3) (2007) 729–736.
[349] Y.S. Choi, R. Chakrabarti, R. Escamilla-Hernandez, S. Sinha, Elf5 conditional knockout mice reveal its role as a master regulator in mammary alveolar development: Failure of Stat5 activation and functional differentiation in the absence of Elf5, Dev Biol 329 (2) (2009) 227–241.
[350] J. Harris, P.M. Stanford, K. Sutherland, S.R. Oakes, M.J. Naylor, F.G. Robertson, et al., Socs2 and elf5 mediate prolactin-induced mammary gland development, Mol Endocrinol 20 (5) (2006) 1177–1187.
[351] S. Mori, S.I. Nishikawa, Y. Yokota, Lactation defect in mice lacking the helix-loop-helix inhibitor Id2, EMBO J 19 (21) (2000) 5772–5781.
[352] S.R. Oakes, M.J. Naylor, M.L. Asselin-Labat, K.D. Blazek, M. Gardiner-Garden, H.N. Hilton, et al., The Ets transcription factor Elf5 specifies mammary alveolar cell fate, Genes Dev 22 (5) (2008) 581–586.
[353] W.O. Nelson, R. Gaunt, Initiation of lactation in the hypophysectomized guinea pig, Proc Soc Exp Biol Med 34 (1936) 671–673.
[354] A.T. Cowie, P.E. Hartmann, A. Turvey, The maintenance of lactation in the rabbit after hypophysectomy, J Endocrinol 43 (4) (1969) 651–662.
[355] M.C. Neville, T.B. McFadden, I. Forsyth, Hormonal regulation of mammary differentiation and milk secretion, J Mammary Gland Biol Neoplasia 7 (1) (2002) 49–66.
[356] M.T. Buckman, G.T. Peake, Prolactin in clinical practice, JAMA 236 (7) (1976) 871–874.
[357] S. Friedman, A. Goldfien, Breast secretions in normal women, Am J Obstet Gynecol 104 (6) (1969) 846–849.
[358] J.R. Jones, G.P. Gentile, Incidence of galactorrhea in ovulatory and anovulatory females, Obstet Gynecol 45 (1) (1975) 13–14.
[359] M.V. Lavric, Breast secretion in nulligravid women, Am J Obstet Gynecol 112 (8) (1972) 1139–1140.
[360] B.J. Biller, A.E. Boyd, M.E. Molitch, Galactorrhea syndromes, in: K.D. Post, I.M.D. Jackson, S. Reichlin (Eds.), The Pituitary Adenoma, Plenum Medical Book Company, New York, 1980, pp. 65–90.
[361] S.S. Tworoger, A.H. Eliassen, B. Rosner, P. Sluss, S.E. Hankinson, Plasma prolactin concentrations and risk of postmenopausal breast cancer, Cancer Res 64 (18) (2004) 6814–6819.
[362] S.S. Tworoger, A.H. Eliassen, P. Sluss, S.E. Hankinson, A prospective study of plasma prolactin concentrations and risk of premenopausal and postmenopausal breast cancer, J Clin Oncol 25 (12) (2007) 1482–1488.
[363] J. Manjer, R. Johansson, G. Berglund, L. Janzon, R. Kaaks, A. Agren, et al., Postmenopausal breast cancer risk in relation to sex steroid hormones, prolactin and SHBG (Sweden), Cancer Causes Control 14 (7) (2003) 599–607.
[364] S.A. Lee, C.A. Haiman, N.P. Burtt, L.C. Pooler, I. Cheng, L.N. Kolonel, et al., A comprehensive analysis of common genetic variation in prolactin (PRL) and PRL receptor (PRLR) genes in relation to plasma prolactin levels and breast cancer risk: The multiethnic cohort, BMC Med Genet 8 (2007) 72.
[365] P. Chakravarti, M.K. Henry, F.W. Quelle, Prolactin and heregulin override DNA damage-induced growth arrest and promote phosphatidylinositol-3 kinase-dependent proliferation in breast cancer cells, Int J Oncol 26 (2) (2005) 509–514.
[366] K. Liby, B. Neltner, L. Mohamet, L. Menchen, N. Ben-Jonathan, Prolactin overexpression by MDA-MB-435 human breast cancer cells accelerates tumor growth, Breast Cancer Res Treat 79 (2) (2003) 241–252.
[367] C.M. Perks, A.J. Keith, K.L. Goodhew, P.B. Savage, Z.E. Winters, J.M. Holly, Prolactin acts as a potent survival factor for human breast cancer cell lines, Br J Cancer 91 (2) (2004) 305–311.
[368] S.L. Miller, G. Antico, P.N. Raghunath, J.E. Tomaszewski, C.V. Clevenger, Nek3 kinase regulates prolactin-mediated cytoskeletal reorganization and motility of breast cancer cells, Oncogene 26 (32) (2007) 4668–4678.
[369] I. Struman, F. Bentzien, H. Lee, V. Mainfroid, G. D'Angelo, V. Goffin, et al., Opposing actions of intact and N-terminal fragments of the human prolactin/growth hormone family members on angiogenesis: An efficient mechanism for the regulation of angiogenesis, Proc Nat Acad Sci USA 96 (4) (1999) 1246–1251.
[370] H. Wennbo, M. Gebre-Medhin, A. Gritli-Linde, C. Ohlsson, O.G. Isaksson, J. Tornell, Activation of the prolactin receptor but not the growth hormone receptor is important for induction of mammary tumors in transgenic mice, J Clin Invest 100 (11) (1997) 2744–2751.
[371] T.A. Rose-Hellekant, L.M. Arendt, M.D. Schroeder, K. Gilchrist, E.P. Sandgren, L.A. Schuler, Prolactin induces ERalpha-positive and ERalpha-negative mammary cancer in transgenic mice, Oncogene 22 (30) (2003) 4664–4674.
[372] C. Manhes, C. Kayser, P. Bertheau, B. Kelder, J.J. Kopchick, P.A. Kelly, et al., Local over-expression of prolactin in differentiating mouse mammary gland induces functional defects and benign lesions, but no carcinoma, J Endocrinol 190 (2) (2006) 271–285.
[373] S.R. Oakes, F.G. Robertson, J.G. Kench, M. Gardiner-Garden, M.P. Wand, J.E. Green, et al., Loss of mammary epithelial prolactin receptor delays tumor formation by reducing cell proliferation in low-grade preinvasive lesions, Oncogene 26 (4) (2007) 543–553.
[374] S. Gill, D. Peston, B.K. Vonderhaar, S. Shousha, Expression of prolactin receptors in normal, benign, and malignant breast tissue: An immunohistological study, J Clin Pathol 54 (12) (2001) 956–960.
[375] K. McHale, J.E. Tomaszewski, R. Puthiyaveettil, V.A. Livolsi, C.V. Clevenger, Altered expression of prolactin receptor-associated signaling proteins in human breast carcinoma, Mod Pathol 21 (5) (2008) 565–571.
[376] C. Reynolds, K.T. Montone, C.M. Powell, J.E. Tomaszewski, C.V. Clevenger, Expression of prolactin and its receptor in human breast carcinoma, Endocrinology 138 (12) (1997) 5555–5560.
[377] R.L. Bogorad, C. Courtillot, C. Mestayer, S. Bernichtein, L. Harutyunyan, J.B. Jomain, et al., Identification of a gain-of-function mutation of the prolactin receptor in women with benign breast tumors, Proc Nat Acad Sci USA 105 (38) (2008) 14533–14538.
[378] C. Courtillot, Z. Chakhtoura, R. Bogorad, C. Genestie, S. Bernichtein, Y. Badachi, et al., Characterization of two constitutively active prolactin receptor variants in a cohort of 95 women with multiple breast fibroadenomas, J Clin Endocrinol Metab 95 (1) (2010) 271–279.
[379] C.V. Clevenger, J. Zheng, E.M. Jablonski, T.L. Galbaugh, F. Fang, From bench to bedside: Future potential for the translation of prolactin inhibitors as breast cancer therapeutics, J Mammary Gland Biol Neoplasia 13 (1) (2008) 147–156.
[380] V. Goffin, P. Touraine, M.D. Culler, P.A. Kelly, Drug insight: Prolactin-receptor antagonists, a novel approach to treatment of unresolved systemic and local hyperprolactinemia? Nat Clin Pract Endocrinol Metab 2 (10) (2006) 571–581.
[381] S. Bernichtein, C. Kayser, K. Dillner, S. Moulin, J.J. Kopchick, J.A. Martial, et al., Development of pure prolactin receptor antagonists, J Biol Chem 278 (38) (2003) 35988–35999.

[382] A. Kauppila, H. Martikainen, U. Puistola, M. Reinila, L. Ronnberg, Hypoprolactinemia and ovarian function, Fertil Steril 49 (3) (1988) 437–441.

[383] B. Scoccia, A.B. Schneider, E.L. Marut, A. Scommegna, Pathological hyperprolactinemia suppresses hot flashes in menopausal women, J Clin Endocrinol Metab 66 (4) (1988) 868–871.

[384] C.Y. Cheung, Prolactin suppresses luteinizing hormone secretion and pituitary responsiveness to luteinizing hormone-releasing hormone by a direct action at the anterior pituitary, Endocrinology 113 (2) (1983) 632–638.

[385] H.G. Bohnet, H.G. Dahlen, W. Wuttke, H.P. Schneider, Hyperprolactinemic anovulatory syndrome, J Clin Endocrinol Metab 42 (1) (1976) 132–143.

[386] A. Klibanski, I.Z. Beitins, N.T. Zervas, J.W. McArthur, E.C. Ridgway, alpha-Subunit and gonadotropin responses to luteinizing hormone-releasing hormone in hyperprolactinemic women before and after bromocriptine, J Clin Endocrinol Metab 56 (4) (1983) 774–780.

[387] J. van Campenhout, S. Papas, P. Blanchet, H. Wyman, M. Somma, Pituitary responses to synthetic luteinizing hormone-releasing hormone in thirty-four cases of amenorrhea or oligomenorrhea associated with galactorrhea, Am J Obstet Gynecol 127 (7) (1977) 723–728.

[388] B. Marchetti, F. Labrie, Prolactin inhibits pituitary luteinizing hormone-releasing hormone receptors in the rat, Endocrinology 111 (4) (1982) 1209–1216.

[389] J.A. Duncan, A. Barkan, L. Herbon, J.C. Marshall, Regulation of pituitary gonadotropin-releasing hormone (GnRH) receptors by pulsatile GnRH in female rats: Effects of estradiol and prolactin, Endocrinology 118 (1) (1986) 320–327.

[390] M.R. Glass, R.W. Shaw, W.R. Butt, R.L. Edwards, D.R. London, An abnormality of oestrogen feedback in amenorrhoea-galactorrhoea, Br Med J 3 (5978) (1975) 274–275.

[391] J.R. Brumsted, D.H. Riddick, Prolactin and the human menstrual cycle, Semin Reprod Med 10 (1992) 220–227.

[392] C.M. Perks, P.V. Newcomb, M. Grohmann, R.J. Wright, H.D. Mason, J.M. Holly, Prolactin acts as a potent survival factor against C2-ceramide-induced apoptosis in human granulosa cells, Hum Reprod 18 (12) (2003) 2672–2677.

[393] N.P. Vlahos, E.M. Bugg, M.J. Shamblott, J.Y. Phelps, J.D. Gearhart, H.A. Zacur, Prolactin receptor gene expression and immunolocalization of the prolactin receptor in human luteinized granulosa cells, Mol Hum Reprod 7 (11) (2001) 1033–1038.

[394] J.Y. Phelps, E.M. Bugg, M.J. Shamblott, N.P. Vlahos, J. Whelan, H.A. Zacur, Prolactin gene expression in human ovarian follicular cells, Fertil Steril 79 (1) (2003) 182–185.

[395] A. Castilla, C. Garcia, M. Cruz-Soto, G. Martinez de la Escalera, S. Thebault, C. Clapp, Prolactin in ovarian follicular fluid stimulates endothelial cell proliferation, J Vasc Res 47 (1) (2010) 45–53.

[396] C. Mendoza, E. Ruiz-Requena, E. Ortega, N. Cremades, F. Martinez, R. Bernabeu, et al., Follicular fluid markers of oocyte developmental potential, Hum Reprod 17 (4) (2002) 1017–1022.

[397] I. Grosdemouge, A. Bachelot, A. Lucas, N. Baran, P.A. Kelly, N. Binart, Effects of deletion of the prolactin receptor on ovarian gene expression, Reprod Biol Endocrinol 1 (2003) 12.

[398] L. Bao, C. Tessier, A. Prigent-Tessier, F. Li, O.L. Buzzio, E.A. Callegari, et al., Decidual prolactin silences the expression of genes detrimental to pregnancy, Endocrinology 148 (5) (2007) 2326–2334.

[399] M. Cecim, J. Kerr, A. Bartke, Infertility in transgenic mice overexpressing the bovine growth hormone gene: Luteal failure secondary to prolactin deficiency, Biol Reprod 52 (5) (1995) 1162–1166.

[400] C.T. Albarracin, T.G. Parmer, W.R. Duan, S.E. Nelson, G. Gibori, Identification of a major prolactin-regulated protein as 20 alpha-hydroxysteroid dehydrogenase: Coordinate regulation of its activity, protein content, and messenger ribonucleic acid expression, Endocrinology 134 (6) (1994) 2453–2460.

[401] L. Zhong, T.G. Parmer, M.C. Robertson, G. Gibori, Prolactin-mediated inhibition of 20alpha-hydroxysteroid dehydrogenase gene expression and the tyrosine kinase system, Biochem Biophys Res Commun 235 (3) (1997) 587–592.

[402] C. Martel, D. Gagne, J. Couet, Y. Labrie, J. Simard, F. Labrie, Rapid modulation of ovarian 3 beta-hydroxysteroid dehydrogenase/delta 5-delta 4 isomerase gene expression by prolactin and human chorionic gonadotropin in the hypophysectomized rat, Mol Cell Endocrinol 99 (1) (1994) 63–71.

[403] C. Martel, C. Labrie, E. Dupont, J. Couet, C. Trudel, E. Rheaume, et al., Regulation of 3 beta-hydroxysteroid dehydrogenase/delta 5-delta 4 isomerase expression and activity in the hypophysectomized rat ovary: Interactions between the stimulatory effect of human chorionic gonadotropin and the luteolytic effect of prolactin, Endocrinology 127 (6) (1990) 2726–2737.

[404] F.A. Feltus, B. Groner, M.H. Melner, Stat5-mediated regulation of the human type II 3beta-hydroxysteroid dehydrogenase/delta5-delta4 isomerase gene: Activation by prolactin, Mol Endocrinol 13 (7) (1999) 1084–1093.

[405] K. Ramasharma, C.H. Li, Human pituitary and placental hormones control human insulin-like growth factor II secretion in human granulosa cells, Proc Nat Acad Sci USA 84 (9) (1987) 2643–2647.

[406] R. Demura, M. Ono, H. Demura, K. Shizume, H. Oouchi, Prolactin directly inhibits basal as well as gonadotropin-stimulated secretion of progesterone and 17 beta-estradiol in the human ovary, J Clin Endocrinol Metab 54 (6) (1982) 1246–1250.

[407] J.H. Dorrington, R.E. Gore-Langton, Antigonadal action of prolactin: Further studies on the mechanism of inhibition of follicle-stimulating hormone-induced aromatase activity in rat granulosa cell cultures, Endocrinology 110 (5) (1982) 1701–1707.

[408] J.S. Krasnow, G.J. Hickey, J.S. Richards, Regulation of aromatase mRNA and estradiol biosynthesis in rat ovarian granulosa and luteal cells by prolactin, Mol Endocrinol 4 (1) (1990). 13–12.

[409] D. Muhlenstedt, H.G. Bohnet, J.P. Hanker, H.P. Schneider, Short luteal phase and prolactin, Int J Fertil 23 (3) (1978) 213–218.

[410] K.D. Schulz, W. Geiger, E. del Pozo, H.J. Kunzig, Pattern of sexual steroids, prolactin, and gonadotropic hormones during prolactin inhibition in normally cycling women, Am J Obstet Gynecol 132 (5) (1978) 561–566.

[411] H.N. Jabbour, H.O. Critchley, Potential roles of decidual prolactin in early pregnancy, Reproduction 121 (2) (2001) 197–205.

[412] E. Kemmann, J.R. Jones, Hyperprolactinemia and primary amenorrhea, Obstet Gynecol 54 (6) (1979) 692–694.

[413] C.A. Mashchak, O.A. Kletzky, V. Davajan, D.R. Mishell Jr., Clinical and laboratory evaluation of patients with primary amenorrhea, Obstet Gynecol 57 (6) (1981) 715–721.

[414] R.J. Pepperell, Prolactin and reproduction, Fertil Steril 35 (3) (1981) 267–274.

[415] M.E. Molitch, S. Reichlin, Hyperprolactinemic disorders, Dis Mon 28 (9) (1982) 1–58.

[416] M. Seppala, T. Ranta, E. Hirvonen, Hyperprolactinaemia and luteal insufficiency, Lancet 1 (7953) (1976) 229–230.

[417] J.V. Kredentser, C.F. Hoskins, J.Z. Scott, Hyperprolactinemia – a significant factor in female infertility, Am J Obstet Gynecol 139 (3) (1981) 264–267.

[418] P. Skrabanek, D. McDonald, E. de Valera, O. Lanigan, D. Powell, Plasma prolactin in amenorrhoea, infertility, and other disorders: A retrospective study of 608 patients, Ir J Med Sci 149 (6) (1980) 236–245.

[419] K.E. Huang, T.A. Bonfiglio, E.K. Muechler, Transient hyperprolactinemia in infertile women with luteal phase deficiency, Obstet Gynecol 78 (4) (1991) 651–655.

[420] K.D. Post, B.J. Biller, L.S. Adelman, M.E. Molitch, S.M. Wolpert, S. Reichlin, Selective transsphenoidal adenomectomy in women with galactorrhea-amenorrhea, JAMA 242 (2) (1979) 158–162.

[421] P. Falaschi, E. del Pozo, A. Rocco, V. Toscano, E. Petrangeli, P. Pompei, et al., Prolactin release in polycystic ovary, Obstet Gynecol 55 (5) (1980) 579–582.

[422] R.B. Filho, L. Domingues, L. Naves, E. Ferraz, A. Alves, L.A. Casulari, Polycystic ovary syndrome and hyperprolactinemia are distinct entities, Gynecol Endocrinol 23 (5) (2007) 267–272.

[423] N. Binart, N. Melaine, C. Pineau, H. Kercret, A.M. Touzalin, P. Imbert-Bollore, et al., Male reproductive function is not affected in prolactin receptor-deficient mice, Endocrinology 144 (9) (2003) 3779–3782.

[424] F.G. Robertson, J. Harris, M.J. Naylor, S.R. Oakes, J. Kindblom, K. Dillner, et al., Prostate development and carcinogenesis in prolactin receptor knockout mice, Endocrinology 144 (7) (2003) 3196–3205.

[425] R.W. Steger, V. Chandrashekar, W. Zhao, A. Bartke, N.D. Horseman, Neuroendocrine and reproductive functions in male mice with targeted disruption of the prolactin gene, Endocrinology 139 (9) (1998) 3691–3695.

[426] D. Dombrowicz, B. Sente, J. Closset, G. Hennen, Dose-dependent effects of human prolactin on the immature hypophysectomized rat testis, Endocrinology 130 (2) (1992) 695–700.

[427] W.J. Huang, J.Y. Yeh, S.C. Tsai, H. Lin, Y.C. Chiao, J.J. Chen, et al., Regulation of testosterone secretion by prolactin in male rats, J Cell Biochem 74 (1) (1999) 111–118.

[428] P.R. Manna, T. El-Hefnawy, J. Kero, I.T. Huhtaniemi, Biphasic action of prolactin in the regulation of murine Leydig tumor cell functions, Endocrinology 142 (1) (2001) 308–318.

[429] R.R. Maran, J. Arunakaran, M.M. Aruldhas, Prolactin and Leydig cells: Biphasic effects of prolactin on LH-, T3- and GH-induced testosterone/oestradiol secretion by Leydig cells in pubertal rats, Int J Androl 24 (1) (2001) 48–55.

[430] W.M. Hair, O. Gubbay, H.N. Jabbour, G.A. Lincoln, Prolactin receptor expression in human testis and accessory tissues: Localization and function, Mol Hum Reprod 8 (7) (2002) 606–611.

[431] M.L. Smith, W.A. Luqman, Prolactin in seminal fluid, Arch Androl 9 (2) (1982) 105–113.

[432] G.F. Gonzales, M. Garcia-Hjarles, G. Velazquez, J. Coyotupa, Seminal prolactin and its relationship to sperm motility in men, Fertil Steril 51 (3) (1989) 498–503.

[433] D.A. Pujianto, B.J. Curry, R.J. Aitken, Prolactin exerts a pro-survival effect on human spermatozoa via mechanisms that involve the stimulation of Akt phosphorylation and suppression of caspase activation and capacitation, Endocrinology 151 (3) (2010) 1269–1279.

[434] F. Oseko, A. Nakano, K. Morikawa, J. Endo, A. Taniguchi, T. Usui, Effects of chronic bromocriptine-induced hypoprolactinemia on plasma testosterone responses to human chorionic gonadotropin stimulation in normal men, Fertil Steril 55 (2) (1991) 355–357.

[435] M.T. Nevalainen, E.M. Valve, P.M. Ingleton, M. Nurmi, P.M. Martikainen, P.L. Harkonen, Prolactin and prolactin receptors are expressed and functioning in human prostate, J Clin Invest 99 (4) (1997) 618–627.

[436] A. Dagvadorj, S. Collins, J.B. Jomain, J. Abdulghani, J. Karras, T. Zellweger, et al., Autocrine prolactin promotes prostate cancer cell growth via Janus kinase-2-signal transducer and activator of transcription-5a/b signaling pathway, Endocrinology 148 (7) (2007) 3089–3101.

[437] T. Janssen, F. Darro, M. Petein, G. Raviv, J.L. Pasteels, R. Kiss, et al., In vitro characterization of prolactin-induced effects on proliferation in the neoplastic LNCaP, DU145, and PC3 models of the human prostate, Cancer 77 (1) (1996) 144–149.

[438] A. Ruffion, K.A. Al-Sakkaf, B.L. Brown, C.L. Eaton, F.C. Hamdy, P.R. Dobson, The survival effect of prolactin on PC3 prostate cancer cells, Eur Urol 43 (3) (2003) 301–308.

[439] A. Nakamura, T. Shirai, K. Ogawa, S. Wada, N.A. Fujimoto, A. Ito, et al., Promoting action of prolactin released from a grafted transplantable pituitary tumor (MtT/F84) on rat prostate carcinogenesis, Cancer Lett 53 (2–3) (1990) 151–157.

[440] F. Van Coppenolle, C. Slomianny, F. Carpentier, X. Le Bourhis, A. Ahidouch, D. Croix, et al., Effects of hyperprolactinemia on rat prostate growth: Evidence of androgeno-dependence, Am J Physiol Endocrinol Metab 280 (1) (2001) E120–E129.

[441] J. Kindblom, K. Dillner, L. Sahlin, F. Robertson, C. Ormandy, J. Tornell, et al., Prostate hyperplasia in a transgenic mouse with prostate-specific expression of prolactin, Endocrinology 144 (6) (2003) 2269–2278.

[442] H. Wennbo, J. Kindblom, O.G. Isaksson, J. Tornell, Transgenic mice overexpressing the prolactin gene develop dramatic enlargement of the prostate gland, Endocrinology 138 (10) (1997) 4410–4415.

[443] B. Ambrosi, M. Gaggini, P. Travaglini, P. Moriondo, R. Elli, G. Faglia, Hypothalamic–pituitary–testicular function in men with PRL-secreting tumors, J Endocrinol Invest 4 (3) (1981) 309–315.

[444] J.N. Carter, J.E. Tyson, G. Tolis, S. Van Vliet, C. Faiman, H.G. Friesen, Prolactin-screening tumors and hypogonadism in 22 men, N Engl J Med 299 (16) (1978) 847–852.

[445] R.H. Goodman, M.E. Molitch, K.D. Post, I.M.D. Jackson, Prolactin-secreting adenomas in the male, in: K.D. Post, I.M.D. Jackson, S. Reichlin (Eds.), The Pituitary Adenoma, Plenum Medical Book Co, New York, 1980, pp. 91–108.

[446] R.L. Perryman, M.O. Thorner, The effects of hyperprolactinemia on sexual and reproductive function in men, J Androl 5 (1981) 233–242.

[447] R.W. Prescott, D.G. Johnston, P. Kendall-Taylor, A. Crombie, K. Hall, A. McGregor, et al., Hyperprolactinaemia in men – response to bromocriptine therapy, Lancet 1 (8266) (1982) 245–248.

[448] M.F. Schwartz, J.E. Bauman, W.H. Masters, Hyperprolactinemia and sexual disorders in men, Biol Psychiatry 17 (8) (1982) 861–876.

[449] T.B. Hargreave, J.D. Richmond, J. Liakatas, R.A. Elton, N.S. Brown, Searching for the infertile man with hyperprolactinemia, Fertil Steril 36 (5) (1981) 630–632.

[450] H.M. Heshmati, G. Turpin, K. Nahoul, A. Carayon, D. Salmon, A. Gueguen, et al., Testicular response to human chorionic gonadotrophin in chronic hyperprolactinaemia, Acta Endocrinol (Copenh) 108 (4) (1985) 565–569.

[451] R. Luboshitzky, E. Rosen, S. Trestian, I.M. Spitz, Hyperprolactinaemia and hypogonadism in men: Response to exogenous gonadotrophins, Clin Endocrinol (Oxf) 11 (2) (1979) 217–223.

[452] M.E. Molitch, R.L. Elton, R.E. Blackwell, B. Caldwell, R.J. Chang, R. Jaffe, et al., Bromocriptine as primary therapy for prolactin-secreting macroadenomas: Results of a prospective multicenter study, J Clin Endocrinol Metab 60 (4) (1985) 698–705.

[453] B. Magrini, J.R. Ebiner, P. Burckhardt, J.P. Felber, Study on the relationship between plasma prolactin levels and androgen metabolism in man, J Clin Endocrinol Metab 43 (4) (1976) 944–947.

[454] M. De Rosa, A. Ciccarelli, S. Zarrilli, E. Guerra, M. Gaccione, A. Di Sarno, et al., The treatment with cabergoline for 24 months normalizes the quality of seminal fluid in hyperprolactinaemic males, Clin Endocrinol (Oxf) 64 (3) (2006) 307–313.

[455] D.F. Cameron, F.T. Murray, D.D. Drylie, Ultrastructural lesions in testes from hyperprolactinemic men, J Androl 5 (4) (1984) 283–293.

[456] M. Freemark, I. Avril, D. Fleenor, P. Driscoll, A. Petro, E. Opara, et al., Targeted deletion of the PRL receptor: Effects on islet development, insulin production, and glucose tolerance, Endocrinology 143 (4) (2002) 1378–1385.

[457] C. Huang, F. Snider, J.C. Cross, Prolactin receptor is required for normal glucose homeostasis and modulation of beta-cell mass during pregnancy, Endocrinology 150 (4) (2009) 1618–1626.

[458] M.E. Amaral, D.A. Cunha, G.F. Anhe, M. Ueno, E.M. Carneiro, L.A. Velloso, et al., Participation of prolactin receptors and phosphatidylinositol 3-kinase and MAP kinase pathways in the increase in pancreatic islet mass and sensitivity to glucose during pregnancy, J Endocrinol 183 (3) (2004) 469–476.

[459] S.K. Karnik, H. Chen, G.W. McLean, J.J. Heit, X. Gu, A.Y. Zhang, et al., Menin controls growth of pancreatic beta-cells in pregnant mice and promotes gestational diabetes mellitus, Science 318 (5851) (2007) 806–809.

[460] J.Y. Lee, O. Gavrilova, B. Davani, R. Na, G.W. Robinson, L. Hennighausen, The transcription factors Stat5a/b are not required for islet development but modulate pancreatic beta-cell physiology upon aging, Biochim Biophys Acta 1773 (9) (2007) 1455–1461.

[461] R.L. Sorenson, M.G. Johnson, J.A. Parsons, J.D. Sheridan, Decreased glucose stimulation threshold, enhanced insulin secretion, and increased beta cell coupling in islets of prolactin-treated rats, Pancreas 2 (3) (1987) 283–288.

[462] L. Labriola, W.R. Montor, K. Krogh, F.H. Lojudice, T. Genzini, A.C. Goldberg, et al., Beneficial effects of prolactin and laminin on human pancreatic islet-cell cultures, Mol Cell Endocrinol 263 (1–2) (2007) 120–133.

[463] J.A. Parsons, T.C. Brelje, R.L. Sorenson, Adaptation of islets of Langerhans to pregnancy: Increased islet cell proliferation and insulin secretion correlates with the onset of placental lactogen secretion, Endocrinology 130 (3) (1992) 1459–1466.

[464] T. Gerardo-Gettens, B.J. Moore, J.S. Stern, B.A. Horwitz, Prolactin stimulates food intake in a dose-dependent manner, Am J Physiol 256 (1 Pt 2) (1989) R276–R280.

[465] D. Sauve, B. Woodside, Neuroanatomical specificity of prolactin-induced hyperphagia in virgin female rats, Brain Res 868 (2) (2000) 306–314.

[466] D.J. Flint, N. Binart, S. Boumard, J.J. Kopchick, P. Kelly, Developmental aspects of adipose tissue in GH receptor and prolactin receptor gene disrupted mice: Site-specific effects upon proliferation, differentiation and hormone sensitivity, J Endocrinol 191 (1) (2006) 101–111.

[467] C.R. LaPensee, N.D. Horseman, P. Tso, T.D. Brandebourg, E.R. Hugo, N. Ben-Jonathan, The prolactin-deficient mouse has an unaltered metabolic phenotype, Endocrinology 147 (10) (2006) 4638–4645.

[468] Y. Greenman, K. Tordjman, N. Stern, Increased body weight associated with prolactin secreting pituitary adenomas: Weight loss with normalization of prolactin levels, Clin Endocrinol (Oxf) 48 (5) (1998) 547–553.

[469] R. Landgraf, M.M. Landraf-Leurs, A. Weissmann, R. Horl, K. von Werder, P.C. Scriba, Prolactin: A diabetogenic hormone, Diabetologia 13 (2) (1977) 99–104.

[470] I.N. Scobie, C.M. Kesson, J.G. Ratcliffe, A.C. Maccuish, The effects of prolonged bromocriptine administration on PRL secretion GH and glycaemic control in stable insulin-dependent diabetes mellitus, Clin Endocrinol (Oxf) 18 (2) (1983) 179–185.

[471] R. Scranton, A. Cincotta, Bromocriptine – unique formulation of a dopamine agonist for the treatment of type 2 diabetes, Expert Opin Pharmacother 11 (2) (2010) 269–279.

[472] E.R. Hugo, T.D. Brandebourg, C.E. Comstock, K.S. Gersin, J.J. Sussman, N. Ben-Jonathan, LS14: A novel human adipocyte cell line that produces prolactin, Endocrinology 147 (1) (2006) 306–313.

[473] C. Ling, L. Svensson, B. Oden, B. Weijdegard, B. Eden, S. Eden, et al., Identification of functional prolactin (PRL) receptor gene expression: PRL inhibits lipoprotein lipase activity in human white adipose tissue, J Clin Endocrinol Metab 88 (4) (2003) 1804–1808.

[474] R. Nanbu-Wakao, Y. Fujitani, Y. Masuho, M. Muramatu, H. Wakao, Prolactin enhances CCAAT enhancer-binding protein-beta (C/EBP beta) and peroxisome proliferator-activated receptor gamma (PPAR gamma) messenger RNA expression and stimulates adipogenic conversion of NIH-3T3 cells, Mol Endocrinol 14 (2) (2000) 307–316.

[475] T. Brandebourg, E. Hugo, N. Ben-Jonathan, Adipocyte prolactin: Regulation of release and putative functions, Diabetes Obes Metab 9 (4) (2007) 464–476.

[476] T.P. Combs, A.H. Berg, M.W. Rajala, S. Klebanov, P. Iyengar, J.C. Jimenez-Chillaron, et al., Sexual differentiation, pregnancy, calorie restriction, and aging affect the adipocyte-specific secretory protein adiponectin, Diabetes 52 (2) (2003) 268–276.

[477] L. Nilsson, N. Binart, Y.M. Bohlooly, M. Bramnert, E. Egecioglu, J. Kindblom, et al., Prolactin and growth hormone regulate adiponectin secretion and receptor expression in adipose tissue, Biochem Biophys Res Commun 331 (4) (2005) 1120–1126.

[478] J.N. Carter, J.E. Tyson, G.L. Warne, A.S. McNeilly, C. Faiman, H.G. Friesen, Adrenocortical function in hyperprolactinemic women, J Clin Endocrinol Metab 45 (5) (1977) 973–980.

[479] S.P. Glickman, R.L. Rosenfield, R.M. Bergenstal, J. Helke, Multiple androgenic abnormalities, including elevated free testosterone, in hyperprolactinemic women, J Clin Endocrinol Metab 55 (2) (1982) 251–257.

[480] R.A. Lobo, O.A. Kletzky, E.M. Kaptein, U. Goebelsmann, Prolactin modulation of dehydroepiandrosterone sulfate secretion, Am J Obstet Gynecol 138 (6) (1980) 632–636.

[481] D.N. Pahuja, H.F. DeLuca, Stimulation of intestinal calcium transport and bone calcium mobilization by prolactin in vitamin D-deficient rats, Science 214 (4524) (1981) 1038–1039.

[482] E. Spanos, D.J. Brown, J.C. Stevenson, I. MacIntyre, Stimulation of 1,25-dihydroxycholecalciferol production by prolactin and related peptides in intact renal cell preparations in vitro, Biochim Biophys Acta 672 (1) (1981) 7–15.

[483] R. Kumar, C.F. Abboud, B.L. Riggs, The effect of elevated prolactin levels on plasma 1,25-dihydroxyvitamin D and intestinal absorption of calcium, Mayo Clin Proc 55 (1) (1980) 51–53.

[484] P. Clement-Lacroix, C. Ormandy, L. Lepescheux, P. Ammann, D. Damotte, V. Goffin, et al., Osteoblasts are a new target for prolactin: Analysis of bone formation in prolactin receptor knockout mice, Endocrinology 140 (1) (1999) 96–105.

[485] A. Klibanski, R.M. Neer, I.Z. Beitins, E.C. Ridgway, N.T. Zervas, J.W. McArthur, Decreased bone density in hyperprolactinemic women, N Engl J Med 303 (26) (1980) 1511–1514.

[486] M.C. Koppelman, D.W. Kurtz, K.A. Morrish, E. Bou, J.K. Susser, J.R. Shapiro, et al., Vertebral body bone mineral content in hyperprolactinemic women, J Clin Endocrinol Metab 59 (6) (1984) 1050–1053.

[487] J.A. Schlechte, B. Sherman, R. Martin, Bone density in amenorrheic women with and without hyperprolactinemia, J Clin Endocrinol Metab 56 (6) (1983) 1120–1123.

[488] A. Klibanski, B.M. Biller, D.I. Rosenthal, D.A. Schoenfeld, V. Saxe, Effects of prolactin and estrogen deficiency in amenorrheic bone loss, J Clin Endocrinol Metab 67 (1) (1988) 124–130.

[489] E. Ciccarelli, L. Savino, V. Carlevatto, A. Bertagna, G.C. Isaia, F. Camanni, Vertebral bone density in non-amenorrhoeic hyperprolactinaemic women, Clin Endocrinol (Oxf) 28 (1) (1988) 1–6.

[490] S.L. Greenspan, D.S. Oppenheim, A. Klibanski, Importance of gonadal steroids to bone mass in men with hyperprolactinemic hypogonadism, Ann Intern Med 110 (7) (1989) 526–531.

[491] E. Chuang, M.E. Molitch, Prolactin and autoimmune diseases in humans, Acta Biomed 78 (Suppl 1) (2007) 255–261.

[492] E.W. Bernton, M.S. Meltzer, J.W. Holaday, Suppression of macrophage activation and T-lymphocyte function in hypoprolactinemic mice, Science 239 (4838) (1988) 401–404.

[493] J.B. Josimovich, M.A. Lavenhar, M.M. Devanesan, H.J. Sesta, S.A. Wilchins, A.C. Smith, Heterogeneous distribution of serum prolactin values in apparently healthy young women, and the effects of oral contraceptive medication, Fertil Steril 47 (5) (1987) 785–791.

[494] K. Miyai, K. Ichihara, K. Kondo, S. Mori, Asymptomatic hyperprolactinaemia and prolactinoma in the general population – mass screening by paired assays of serum prolactin, Clin Endocrinol (Oxf) 25 (5) (1986) 549–554.

[495] A. Miyake, M. Ikegami, C.F. Chen, N. Arita, T. Aono, O. Tanizawa, et al., Mass screening for hyperprolactinemia and prolactinoma in men, J Endocrinol Invest 11 (5) (1988) 383–384.

[496] S.L. Jeffcoate, Diagnosis of hyperprolactinaemia, Lancet 2 (8102) (1978) 1245–1247.

[497] A. Kauppila, P. Chatelain, P. Kirkinen, S. Kivinen, A. Ruokonen, Isolated prolactin deficiency in a woman with puerperal alactogenesis, J Clin Endocrinol Metab 64 (2) (1987) 309–312.

[498] M. Shahmanesh, Z. Ali, M. Pourmand, I. Nourmand, Pituitary function tests in Sheehan's syndome, Clin Endocrinol (Oxf) 12 (3) (1980) 303–311.

[499] B.J. Kinon, J.A. Gilmore, H. Liu, U.M. Halbreich, Hyperprolactinemia in response to antipsychotic drugs: Characterization across comparative clinical trials, Psychoneuroendocrinology 28 (Suppl 2) (2003) 69–82.

[500] M. Misra, G.I. Papakostas, A. Klibanski, Effects of psychiatric disorders and psychotropic medications on prolactin and bone metabolism, J Clin Psychiatry 65 (12) (2004) 1607–1618, quiz 590, 760–761.

[501] F. Dunbar, V. Kusumakar, D. Daneman, M. Schulz, Growth and sexual maturation during long-term treatment with risperidone, Am J Psychiatry 161 (5) (2004) 918–920.

[502] C.A. Calarge, V.L. Ellingrod, L. Acion, D.D. Miller, J. Moline, M.J. Tansey, et al., Variants of the dopamine D2 receptor gene and risperidone-induced hyperprolactinemia in children and adolescents, Pharmacogenet Genomics 19 (5) (2009) 373–382.

[503] J.H. Mendelson, N.K. Mello, S.K. Teoh, J. Ellingboe, J. Cochin, Cocaine effects on pulsatile secretion of anterior pituitary, gonadal, and adrenal hormones, J Clin Endocrinol Metab 69 (6) (1989) 1256–1260.

[504] T.J. Kamal, M.E. Molitch, Effects of calcium channel blockade with verapamil on the prolactin responses to TRH, L-dopa, and bromocriptine, Am J Med Sci 304 (5) (1992) 289–293.

[505] L.E. Gluskin, B. Strasberg, J.H. Shah, Verapamil-induced hyperprolactinemia and galactorrhea, Ann Intern Med 95 (1) (1981) 66–67.

[506] J.H. Romeo, R. Dombrowski, Y.S. Kwak, S. Fuehrer, D.C. Aron, Hyperprolactinaemia and verapamil: Prevalence and potential association with hypogonadism in men, Clin Endocrinol (Oxf) 45 (5) (1996) 571–575.

[507] S.R. Kelley, T.J. Kamal, M.E. Molitch, Mechanism of verapamil calcium channel blockade-induced hyperprolactinemia, Am J Physiol 270 (1 Pt 1) (1996) E96–E100.

[508] S. Miyabo, T. Hisada, T. Asato, N. Mizushima, K. Ueno, Growth hormone and cortisol responses to psychological stress: Comparison of normal and neurotic subjects, J Clin Endocrinol Metab 42 (6) (1976) 1158–1162.

[509] S.S. Yen, R.W. Rebar, W. Quesenberry, Pituitary function in pseudocyesis, J Clin Endocrinol Metab 43 (1) (1976) 132–136.

[510] F. Gomez, F.I. Reyes, C. Faiman, Nonpuerperal galactorrhea and hyperprolactinemia. Clinical findings, endocrine features and therapeutic responses in 56 cases, Am J Med 62 (5) (1977) 648–660.

[511] S.H. Hou, S. Grossman, M.E. Molitch, Hyperprolactinemia in patients with renal insufficiency and chronic renal failure requiring hemodialysis or chronic ambulatory peritoneal dialysis, Am J Kidney Dis 6 (4) (1985) 245–249.

[512] V.S. Lim, S.C. Kathpalia, L.A. Frohman, Hyperprolactinemia and impaired pituitary response to suppression and stimulation in chronic renal failure: Reversal after transplantation, J Clin Endocrinol Metab 48 (1) (1979) 101–107.

[513] M.Y. Morgan, A.W. Jakobovits, M.B. Gore, M.R. Wills, S. Sherlock, Serum prolactin in liver disease and its relationship to gynaecomastia, Gut 19 (3) (1978) 170–174.

[514] D.H. Van Thiel, C.J. McClain, M.K. Elson, M.J. McMillan, R. Lester, Evidence for autonomous secretion of prolactin in some alcoholic men with cirrhosis and gynecomastia, Metabolism 27 (12) (1978) 1778–1784.

[515] V. Nunziata, G. Ceparano, G. Mazzacca, G. Budillon, Prolactin secretion in nonalcoholic liver cirrhosis, Digestion 18 (3–4) (1978) 157–161.

[516] M. Valimaki, R. Pelkonen, M. Harkonen, P. Tuomala, P. Koistinen, R. Roine, et al., Pituitary-gonadal hormones and adrenal androgens in non-cirrhotic female alcoholics after cessation of alcohol intake, Eur J Clin Invest 20 (2) (1990) 177–181.

[517] K.S. Honbo, A.J. van Herle, K.A. Kellett, Serum prolactin levels in untreated primary hypothyroidism, Am J Med 64 (5) (1978) 782–787.

[518] R.C. Smallridge, Thyrotropin-secreting pituitary tumors, Endocrinol Metab Clin North Am 16 (3) (1987) 765–792.

[519] M. Ben-David, A. Danon, R. Benveniste, C.P. Weller, F.G. Sulman, Results of radioimmunoassays of rat pituitary and serum prolactin after adrenalectomy and perphenazine treatment in rats, J Endocrinol 50 (4) (1971) 599–606.

[520] T.D. Stryker, M.E. Molitch, Reversible hyperthyrotropinemia, hyperthyroxinemia, and hyperprolactinemia due to adrenal insufficiency, Am J Med 79 (2) (1985) 271–276.

[521] A.E. Boyd 3rd, S. Spare, B. Bower, S. Reichlin, Neurogenic galactorrhea–amenorrhea, J Clin Endocrinol Metab 47 (6) (1978) 1374–1377.

[522] V. Herman, W.J. Kalk, N.G. de Moor, J. Levin, Serum prolactin after chest wall surgery: Elevated levels after mastectomy, J Clin Endocrinol Metab 52 (1) (1981) 148–151.

[523] Y.H. Wang, T.S. Huang, I.N. Lien, Hormone changes in men with spinal cord injuries, Am J Phys Med Rehabil 71 (6) (1992) 328–332.

[524] M.E. Molitch, S. Schwartz, B. Mukherji, Is prolactin secreted ectopically? Am J Med 70 (4) (1981) 803–807.

[525] C.T. Hsu, M.H. Yu, C.Y. Lee, H.L. Jong, M.Y. Yeh, Ectopic production of prolactin in uterine cervical carcinoma, Gynecol Oncol 44 (2) (1992) 166–171.

[526] T.H. Stanisic, J. Donovan, Prolactin secreting renal cell carcinoma, J Urol 136 (1) (1986) 85–86.

[527] W.H. Hoffman, R.R. Gala, K. Kovacs, M.G. Subramanian, Ectopic prolactin secretion from a gonadoblastoma, Cancer 60 (11) (1987) 2690–2695.

[528] G.A. Kallenberg, C.M. Pesce, B. Norman, R.E. Ratner, S.G. Silvergerg, Ectopic hyperprolactinemia resulting from an ovarian teratoma, JAMA 263 (18) (1990) 2472–2474.

[529] P.E. Palmer, S. Bogojavlensky, A.K. Bhan, R.E. Scully, Prolactinoma in wall of ovarian dermoid cyst with hyperprolactinemia, Obstet Gynecol 75 (3 Pt 2) (1990) 540–543.

[530] E. Proust-Lemoine, V. Mitchell, P. Deruelle, A. Lamblin, B. Neraud, X. Leroy, et al., Ectopic hyperprolactinaemia in a woman with a mesocolic perivascular epithelioid cell tumor ("PEComa"), Ann Endocrinol (Paris) 69 (3) (2008) 240–243.

[531] M.E. Molitch, S. Reichlin, Hypothalamic hyperprolactinemia: Neuroendocrine regulation of prolactin secretion in patients with lesions of the hypothalamus and pituitary stalk, in: R.M. MacLeod, M.O. Thorner, U. Scapagnini (Eds.), Prolactin Basic and Clinical Correlates, Liviana Press, Padova, 1985, pp. 709–719.

[532] J.S. Bevan, C.W. Burke, M.M. Esiri, C.B. Adams, Misinterpretation of prolactin levels leading to management errors in patients with sellar enlargement, Am J Med 82 (1) (1987) 29–32.

[533] O.B. Leramo, J.D. Booth, B. Zinman, C. Bergeron, A.A. Sima, T.P. Morley, Hyperprolactinemia, hypopituitarism, and chiasmal compression due to carcinoma metastatic to the pituitary, Neurosurgery 8 (4) (1981) 477–480.

[534] N. Karavitaki, G. Thanabalasingham, H.C. Shore, R. Trifanescu, O. Ansorge, N. Meston, et al., Do the limits of serum prolactin in disconnection hyperprolactinaemia need re-definition? A study of 226 patients with histologically verified non-functioning pituitary macroadenoma, Clin Endocrinol (Oxf) 65 (4) (2006) 524–529.

[535] P.V. Malven, Prolactin release induced by electrical stimulation of the hypothalamic preoptic area in unanesthetized sheep, Neuroendocrinology 18 (1) (1975) 65–71.

[536] J.S. Tindal, G.S. Knaggs, Pathways in the forebrain of the rat concerned with the release of prolactin, Brain Res 119 (1) (1977) 211–221.

[537] T.L. Martin, M. Kim, W.B. Malarkey, The natural history of idiopathic hyperprolactinemia, J Clin Endocrinol Metab 60 (5) (1985) 855–858.

[538] A.V. Sluijmer, R.E. Lappohn, Clinical history and outcome of 59 patients with idiopathic hyperprolactinemia, Fertil Steril 58 (1) (1992) 72–77.

[539] A.E. Pontiroli, L. Falsetti, Development of pituitary adenoma in women with hyperprolactinaemia: Clinical, endocrine, and radiological characteristics, Br Med J (Clin Res Ed) 288 (6416) (1984) 515–518.

[540] H.K. Rjosk, R. Fahlbusch, K. von Werder, Spontaneous development of hyperprolactinaemia, Acta Endocrinol (Copenh) 100 (3) (1982) 333–336.

[541] J. Schlechte, K. Dolan, B. Sherman, F. Chapler, A. Luciano, The natural history of untreated hyperprolactinemia: A prospective analysis, J Clin Endocrinol Metab 68 (2) (1989) 412–418.

CHAPTER

6

Thyroid-stimulating Hormone

Virginia D. Sarapura [1], David F. Gordon [1], Mary H. Samuels [2]

[1] University of Colorado Denver, Aurora, CO, USA [2] Oregon Health and Science University, Portland, OR, USA

INTRODUCTION

Thyroid-stimulating hormone (TSH) is a glycoprotein produced by the thyrotrope cells of the anterior pituitary gland. TSH, luteinizing hormone (LH) and follicle-stimulating hormone (FSH), as well as the placental hormone chorionic gonadotropin (CG), consist of a heterodimer of two noncovalently linked subunits, α and β. The β subunit is unique to each and confers specificity of action while the α-subunit is common to all four glycoprotein hormones. Each TSH subunit is encoded by a separate gene located on a different chromosome and is transcribed in a coordinated manner responsive mainly to the stimulatory effect of hypothalamic thyrotropin-releasing hormone (TRH) and the inhibitory effect of thyroid hormone. Production of bioactive TSH involves a process of cotranslational glycosylation and folding that enables combination between the nascent α and β subunits. TSH is stored in secretory granules and released into the circulation in a regulated manner responsive mainly to the stimulatory effect of TRH. Circulating TSH binds to specific cell-surface receptors on the thyroid gland where it stimulates the production of thyroid hormones, L-thyroxine (T_4) and L-triiodothyronine (T_3), which act on multiple organs and tissues to modulate many metabolic processes as well as result in a negative inhibition of TSH output. The introduction of sensitive TSH assays has allowed accurate measurement of the level of circulating TSH and has led to the recognition of abnormal production of TSH related with abnormal function of the thyroid gland reflecting in a wide range of metabolic derangements.

ONTOGENY OF THYROTROPE CELLS

Thyrotropes comprise only 5% of the cells in the anterior pituitary gland, yet these cells are solely responsible for synthesizing the α- and β-subunits of TSH, the key pituitary hormone that circulates in serum and controls the growth and function of the thyroid gland. The distinct cell types of the anterior and intermediate lobes of the pituitary are defined by the hormone they produce and secrete, these include thyrotropes (TSH), gonadotropes (LH, FSH), corticotropes (ACTH), somatotropes (GH), lactotropes (PRL) and melanotropes (MSH). The anterior pituitary develops from Rathke's pouch, an invagination of oral ectoderm located at the anterior neural ridge, directly contacting the emerging infundibulum [1]. The close association between these tissues suggests that inductive interactions are apt to be very important [2]. Pituitary organogenesis involves the proliferation of common progenitor cells and their subsequent differentiation by a series of precisely controlled extrinsic and intrinsic signals that regulate cell proliferation, lineage commitment and terminal cell differentiation [3]. Many of the key genes initiating and regulating these developmental pathways continue to be uncovered and include transcription factors, signaling molecules and cell surface receptors. Many of these factors act transiently during pituitary development while expression of others persists in the mature differentiated cell. Signals derived from Rathke's pouch and the adjacent infundibulum at embryonic day 9.5 (e9.5) in the mouse initiate the temporal and spatial organization of the different pituitary cell types. The key factors involved in this initial phase include sonic hedgehog (Shh) and members of fibroblast growth factor (FGF), bone morphogenetic protein (BMP), Notch and Wnt families of morphogens/growth factors [4]. These factors themselves are not specific to the pituitary but play additional roles in the patterning of other organ systems. Expression of dorsal factors such as FGF8/10/18 act by opposing the developmental actions of the ventral BMP2/Shh signals [3]. Several of the genes critical for regulating pituitary development have been

The Pituitary, Third Edition, DOI: 10.1016/B978-0-12-380926-1.10006-9

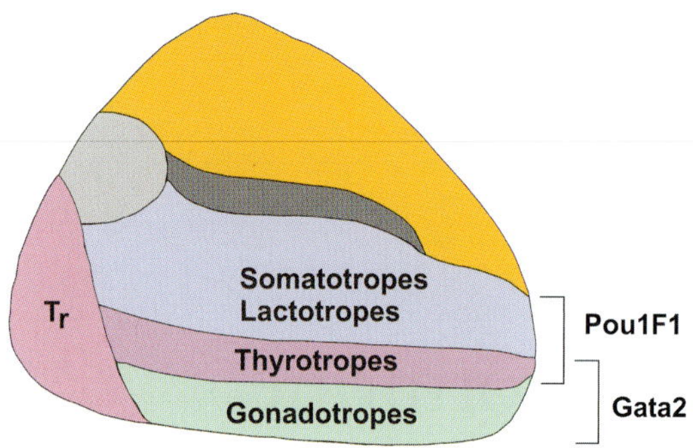

FIGURE 6.1 Thyrotrope cell origin during anterior pituitary development. Schematic representation of the regions of the pituitary where Pou1F1 and GATA-2 transcripts are detected. Somatotropes and lactotropes evolve from Pou1F1(+)/GATA-2(−) cells, gonadotropes from POU1F1(−)/GATA-2(+) cells and thyrotropes from Pou1F1(+)/GATA-2(+) cells. The thyrotropes in the rostral tip (Tr) appear at an earlier stage in the region where TEF is expressed, but do not persist in the adult. *Modified from Dasen JS, O'Connell SM, Flynn SE, Treier M, Gleiberman AS, Szeto DP, Hooshmand F, Aggarwal AK, Rosenfeld MG. Reciprocal interactions of Pit1 and GATA2 mediate signaling gradient-induced determination of pituitary cell types. Cell 97:587–598, 1999 [6].*

identified through the characterization of hereditary mouse and human pituitary endocrine deficiencies [5]. Distinct cell lineages emerge as a result of signaling gradients of transcription factors formed in a spatially and temporally specific fashion (Figure 6.1) [6]. The end result is overlapping programs of transcription factor expression [7]. The stereotypic pattern of activation of these early transcription factors as well as an assemblage of other tissue-restricted factors are critical for determination of the cells that produce the glycoprotein hormone α-subunit (αGSU), which is common to the dimeric pituitary hormones TSH, LH and FSH.

The glycoprotein hormone α-subunit (αGSU, CGA) is the first pituitary hormone gene expressed during early development [8] at mouse e10.5. Wnt5a and BPM4, which are expressed in the adjacent neuroepithelium, provide the initiating signals followed by expression of Hesx1, Ptx1/2 and Lhx3/4 [2]. TSHβ expression begins in the rostral tip of the pituitary at mouse e12.5 and correlates with expression of thyrotrope embryonic factor (TEF) which is restricted to the pituitary at this embryonic stage [9]. By birth, TSHβ expression in the rostral tip has disappeared and another population of thyrotropes arises by e15.5 in the caudomedial region, following expression of Pou1F1 (Pit-1), a POU-homeodomain transcription factor restricted to thyrotropes, somatotropes and lactotropes [10]. Both POU1F1 and TSH β-subunit expression are present in the wild-type but not in the Snell dwarf mouse, which has a POU1F1 gene mutation that renders it inactive [11]. These data suggest that the second population of thyrotropes, associated with Pou1F1, is likely the source of mature thyrotropes. In addition, Pou1F1 mutations have also been reported in humans [12,13] and are associated with a lack of thyrotropes, somatotropes and lactotropes, analogous to the Snell dwarf mouse phenotype. Pou1F1 synergizes with Lhx3 to activate the TSH α-subunit promoter [14]. Pou1F1 expression, in turn, depends on the expression of another transcription factor, Prophet of Pou1F1 (Prop1). Mutations in this factor have been associated with many cases of combined pituitary hormone deficiency in humans, affecting not only thyrotrope, somatotrope and lactotrope but also gonadotrope expression [15]. Mutations in the Prop1 gene were also found in the Ames dwarf mouse that exhibits a similar phenotype [16]. When complexed with β-catenin it acts as a transcriptional activator of Pou1F1 and can also work to repress Hesx1. An additional enhancing factor, Atbf1, also activates early Pou1F1 expression along with Prop1 [17]. Of note, both Atbf1 and Prop1 only persist in the pituitary for a limited time period between e10.5 and e14.5. Thus precise temporal regulation is critical for proper pituitary development [3].

However, other cell-type-restricted factors must be involved in the initiation of thyrotrope-specific gene expression, since the presence of both Pou1F1 and Lhx3 in somatotropes and lactotropes does not result in TSH production by these cells. Mechanisms exist that establish combinatorial codes which specify distinct cell phenotypes. In many cases, such a code involves reciprocal synergistic or inhibitory protein–protein interactions between two or more cell-type-restricted transcription factors. Recent studies have suggested that a zinc finger transcription factor, Gata2, plays a critical role in thyrotrope differentiation [6]. Gata2 is transcribed in the developing anterior pituitary as early as e10.5 and persists in an expression pattern coincident with the glycoprotein hormone α-subunit. Gata2 binds and transactivates the αGSU promoter [18] and acts synergistically with Pou1F1 to activate the TSHβ gene [19]. A ventral–dorsal gradient of Gata2 occurs early in development in response to BMP-2: the intermediate cells that express both Gata2 and Pou1F1 activate the thyrotrope-specific genes, whereas the more ventral cells that express Gata2 and not Pou1F1 become gonadotropes and the more dorsal cells that express Pou1F1 and not Gata2 become somatotropes and lactotropes [6]. The in vivo function of Gata2 in pituitary development has recently been examined by targeted inactivation of Gata2 in a transgenic mouse model using Cre recombinase directed by the αGSU promoter/enhancer [20], which is active early in pituitary development. The Gata2 knockout mice in the pituitary have a decreased thyrotrope cell population at birth and lower levels of circulating TSH and FSH in the serum of adults. This demonstrated the role of Gata2 in the production of both TSHβ and αGSU subunits. Thyroid ablation and castration studies demonstrated a decreased capacity of mutant thyrotropes and gonadotropes to mount the appropriate response to the loss of negative feedback by thyroid hormones and steroid hormones, respectively. These studies showed that Gata2 is important for optimal thyrotrope and gonadotrope function but not for thyrotrope and gonadotrope cell fate specification [20].

A recent study has uncovered the existence of a population of multipotent stem cells in the adult pituitary [21,22] that are distinct from the embryonic precursor cells. These nestin- and Sox2-containing stem cells reside in a localized niche within the perilumenal region of the gland, have the capacity to expand into all of the terminally differentiated pituitary cell types after birth, and may contribute to pituitary tumors [21]. These newly discovered cells may, in fact, contribute to the dynamic changes in cell growth that occur in the pituitary gland under certain physiologic or pathologic states, such as the marked thyrotrope hyperplasia/hypertrophy seen following severe hypothyroidism [23].

TSH SUBUNIT GENES

The TSH α- and β-subunits are encoded by two separate genes located on different chromosomes. Since the isolation and characterization of these genes, much information has been gained regarding the molecular events that result in the regulated production of TSH α- and β-subunit mRNAs and protein. Most of this information has been obtained from studies performed in mouse thyrotropic tumors and rodent pituitary glands. Thyrotrope cells are believed to contain specific transcription factors that bind to the regulatory regions of the genes and interact with ubiquitous factors to initiate transcription. The identification of those specific factors is an active area of investigation. Regulation of TSH subunit gene transcription, mainly activation by TRH or inhibition by thyroid hormone, is achieved by modulating the activity of the specific and ubiquitous factors. Extensive biochemical studies show that activation and/or repression of these genes within thyrotropes is fundamentally determined by modifications of the chromatin state at each TSH subunit gene. Following an activating or inhibitory stimulus to the cell, factors bind to the promoter, recruit specific chromatin-modifying enzymes, and initiate transcription when the DNA is in an accessible state or silence the gene if inaccessible to the transcriptional machinery.

TSH β-subunit Gene Structure

The human TSH β-subunit gene has been isolated and its structure characterized [24]. The gene is 4527 base pairs (bp) in size, and is located on the short arm of chromosome 1 at position 13.2 [25]. The gene structure consists of three exons and two introns (Figure 6.2, top panel). The first exon of 37 bp contains the 5′ untranslated region of the gene. It is separated from the second exon by a large first intron of 3.9 kb. The coding region is contained in the second (163 bp) and third (326 bp) exons, which are separated by a 0.45 kb intron, while the 3′ untranslated region is contained in the third exon.

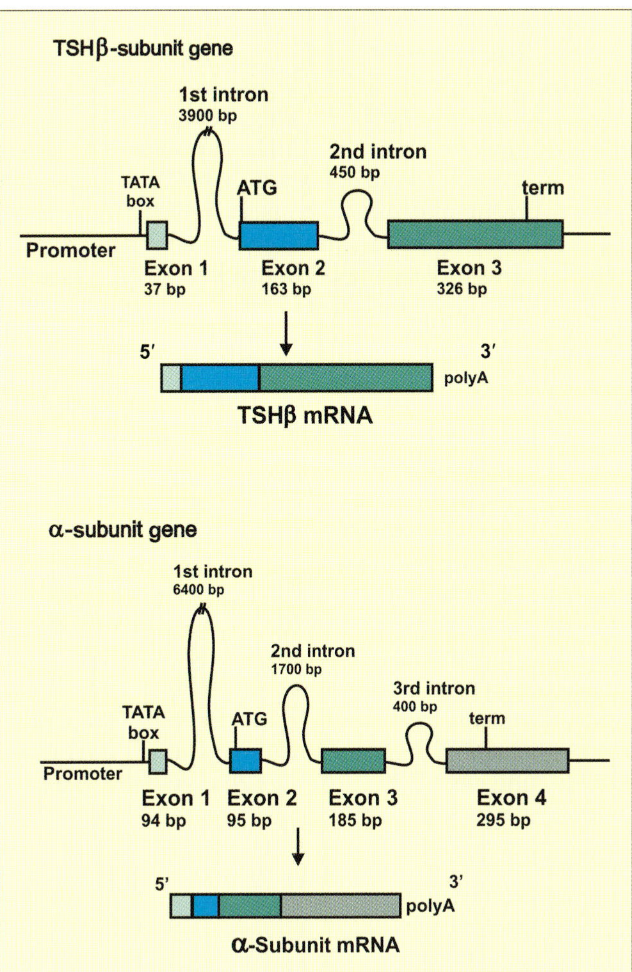

FIGURE 6.2 Structural organization of the human TSH subunit genes and mRNAs. The two panels show the TSH β- (top) and α-subunit (bottom) genes. Shown are the relative locations and sizes of the exons and introns. The TATA box important for positioning the RNA transcriptional start is located in the promoter close to exon 1. Following transcription, introns are spliced out, exons precisely joined, and a polyA tail added to the 3′ end of the mature mRNA. *From L.J. De Groot and J.L. Jameson (Eds), Endocrinology, 6th edn, Elsevier. Chapter 73 Thyroid-stimulating hormone: Physiology and secretion, Figure 1.*

DNA sequences close to the transcriptional start site in the promoter of the TSHβ gene reporter contain elements responsible for initiating transcription and regulating expression. A consensus TATA box, a sequence that is important for positioning RNA polymerase II activity, is located 28 bp upstream of the transcriptional start site and is important for the accurate initiation of RNA transcripts. In contrast to the human gene, both the mouse and the rat genes have two transcriptional start sites. The human exon 1 is 10 bp longer than that of the mouse and rat, presumably due to an insertion that displaces the TATA box 9 bp further upstream relative to the TATA box in the mouse and rat genes. Progressive 5′ deletions of the mouse TSHβ promoter linked to a luciferase reporter following expression into thyrotrope cells defined the *cis*-acting sequences required for expression to the first 270 bp of the promoter [26,27]. While these sequences defined the minimal promoter, other studies have shown that enhancer sequences located more than 6 kb upstream are also required for the promoter to express in pituitary thyrotropes in transgenic mice [28]. However, the mouse TSHβ promoter region from −271 to −80 is sufficient to confer thyrotrope-specific activity [26] and thyrotrope transcription factors can bind to these DNA sequences [29]. Within this broad area, four regions of protein interaction have been identified by DNase footprint analysis using nuclear extracts from thyrotrope cells [27]. Two transcription factors, Pou1F1 and Gata2, bind to adjacent sequences located within a composite *cis*-acting region on the proximal TSHβ promoter from the region −135 to −88 relative to the major transcriptional start site (Figure 6.3, top panel). This composite DNA element has a 5′ Pou1F1 site and a 3′ Gata2 site. Between these two sites are 16 bp that include overlapping putative Pou1F1 and Gata2 sites. This 16 bp intervening sequence is critical for high promoter activity, independent of the actual spacing between the flanking Pou1F1 and Gata-2 sites [19]. Mechanistically, binding of Pou1F1 may provide stabilizing effects through direct contacts with Gata2, it may induce stabilizing contacts between Gata2 and DNA, or it may alter DNA conformation. It is currently unknown whether other thyrotrope-specific genes are regulated by such a unique composite element. The DNA behaves as a docking platform which recruits multiple components of a fundamental regulatory assembly initiated by binding of Pou1F1 and Gata2 to facilitate thyrotrope-specific transcription. An additional transcription factor, Med1 (TRAP220, PBP), was shown to be recruited to the TSHβ proximal promoter and play a role in transcriptional activation [30]. Med1 was originally defined as part of a transcriptional mediator complex that interacts with hormone-occupied thyroid/steroid hormone receptors in a ligand-dependent manner [31]. The physiological relevance of these studies originated with the observation that mice with one half the genetic complement encoding this factor were hypothyroid with a pituitary phenotype characterized by reduced levels of TSHβ gene expression [32]. Med1 is recruited to the TSHβ gene by virtue of its physical interaction with both Pou1F1 and Gata2 since the protein itself does not possess a DNA-binding domain. Cotransfections in nonpituitary CV-1 cells showed that Pou1F1, Gata2, or Med1 alone do not markedly stimulate the TSHβ promoter. However, Pou1F1 plus Gata2 resulted in a ten-fold activation, demonstrating synergistic cooperativity, and addition of Med1 resulted in a further dose-dependent stimulation up to 25-fold that was promoter-specific [33]. Interaction studies showed that Med1 or Gata2 each bound the homeodomain of

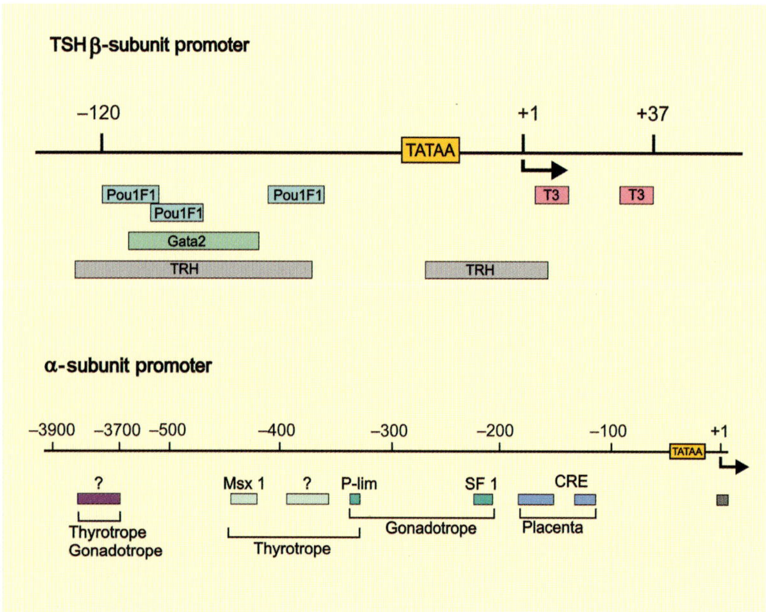

FIGURE 6.3 Schematic representation of the human TSH β-subunit (top) and the glycoprotein hormone α-subunit (bottom) promoters. The transcriptional start site is indicated by the arrow and the TATA box is shown. The numbers above the line denote the position of the nucleotides relative to the transcriptional start site set at +1. The boxes under the line indicate the regions important for the responses to the various factors that regulate transcription, as shown (top panel). The Gata2 binding sites have only been described in the mouse TSH β-subunit gene (bottom panel). The placental-specific, gonadotrope-specific and thyrotrope-specific activities of the glycoprotein hormone α-subunit are shown. The thyrotrope-specific regions other than the P-LIM-binding region have only been described in the mouse α-subunit gene.

Pou1F1, whereas Med1 interacted independently with each zinc finger of Gata2, and Med1 interacted with Gata2 and Pou1F1 over a broad region of its N terminus. These regions of interaction were also important for maximal function. Chromatin immunoprecipitation assays have shown in vivo occupancy on the proximal TSHβ promoter [30]. Thus, the TSHβ gene is activated by a unique combination of transcription factors present in pituitary thyrotropes, including those that act via binding to the proximal promoter as well as others recruited to the promoter via protein–protein interactions.

α-Subunit Gene Structure

The human glycoprotein hormone α-subunit gene is located on chromosome 6 at position 6q12-q21 [34]. The gene is 9635 bp in size and consists of four exons and three introns. It contains a consensus TATA box located 26 bp upstream of the transcriptional start site [35]. The first exon (94 bp) contains virtually all of the 5′ untranslated sequence and is separated from the second exon by a 6.4 kb intron. The second exon contains 7 bp of 5′ untranslated sequence and 88 bp of the coding region. The coding sequence continues in the third (185 bp) and fourth (75 bp) exons and the 3′ untranslated region (220 bp) is contained completely in the fourth exon (Figure 6.2, bottom panel). The second and third introns are 1.7 kb and 0.4 kb, respectively. The genomic organization of the mouse (located on chromosome 4), rat and cow α-subunit genes are similar, except that in the rat and cow the second intron is located 12 bp downstream, resulting in a peptide sequence that is four amino acids longer. There are also differences in the length of the 5′ untranslated sequence, which is 10 bp longer in the mouse, apparently due to a 10 bp insertion between the TATA box and the transcriptional start site [19].

The elements responsible for initiating transcription and regulating the expression are located in the 5′ flanking region of the α-subunit gene (Figure 6.3, bottom panel). The human α-subunit gene contains a consensus TATA box located 26 bp upstream of the transcriptional start site. A single transcriptional start site has been found in the glycoprotein hormone α-subunit genes of all the species that have been studied. Analysis of the mouse α-subunit promoter in transgenic mice showed that 381 bp of the 5′ flanking region is sufficient for expression of a β-galactosidase reporter gene in both thyrotropes and gonadotropes, although hormonally and temporally regulated high levels of expression are achieved when longer promoter fragments of 4.6 kb were included [36,37]. This indicates that an enhancer region of the promoter located several thousand base pairs upstream of the transcriptional start site is required along with key *cis*-acting proximal promoter elements for maximal in vivo expression of the glycoprotein hormone α-subunit gene in pituitary thyrotropes and gonadotropes. There have been a number of proximal *cis*-acting elements identified by gene transfer and DNA-binding studies that have been shown to be important for α-subunit expression in pituitary and placental cells. These elements interact with cell-specific and/or ubiquitous *trans*-acting factors to allow regulated expression in the appropriate cell type.

The glycoprotein hormone α-subunit gene is unique in that it is expressed in thyrotropes (thyrotropin, TSH), gonadotropes (lutropin/follicotropin, LH/FSH) and placental cells (chorionic gonadotropin, CG), and in each of these cell types it is differentially regulated. Studies from several laboratories using the human and mouse genes have demonstrated that the cell-specific expression in each cell type is dependent on vastly different regions of the promoter (Figure 6.3, bottom panel). Whereas the region downstream of −200 is sufficient for placental expression [38], gonadotropes require sequences between −225 and −200 [39], and regions further upstream appear to be critical for thyrotrope expression [40]. The elements involved in human placental α-subunit expression extend from −177 to −84 and include the upstream regulatory element (URE), also called trophoblast-specific element (TSE), that binds the placental-specific protein TSEB [41], two cAMP response elements (CREs) that bind the ubiquitous protein CREB [42], the junctional regulatory element (JRE) that binds a 50-kDa protein [43], the CCAAT-box that binds a 53-kDa α-subunit binding factor (α CBF) [44], and a Gata motif that interacts with Gata-binding proteins [18]. Some of these regions binding to similar factors may also play a role in pituitary α-subunit expression. A region from −225 to −200 that binds the orphan nuclear receptor SF-1 appears to be critical for gonadotrope expression of the α-subunit gene [45], but this region has no effect on thyrotrope expression [46]. Basic helix-loop-helix E-box-binding proteins [47] and GATA-binding proteins [18] also appear to play a role in α-subunit expression in gonadotropes. Transgenic mouse studies have shown that 313 bp of the bovine α-subunit 5′ flanking DNA, which contain the SF-1-binding region, targeted expression to gonadotropes but not thyrotropes [48], suggesting that this region was sufficient for expression in gonadotropes. It was then shown that 480 bp of the mouse α-subunit 5′ flanking DNA was able to target transgenic expression to both gonadotropes and thyrotropes [37], in agreement with in vitro transfection studies which showed that the same promoter region mediates a high level of expression in thyrotrope and gonadotrope cells. Several sequences within the region from −480 to −300 appear to be important for mouse α-subunit expression in thyrotropes but not gonadotropes [49]. Among these is the sequence from −434 to −421 that interacts with the developmental homeodomain transcription factor Msx1 [50]. This factor was found to be expressed in mature thyrotropes, but its role in α-subunit expression has not been elucidated. Another important sequence is the pituitary glycoprotein hormone basal element, or PGBE, extending from −342 to −329, that is critical for both thyrotrope and gonadotrope expression [51]. The PGBE interacts with P-LIM (mLIM3, Lhx3), a pituitary-specific LIM-homeodomain transcription factor [52], that is important not only for thyrotrope and gonadotrope cell specification but is also important for somatotropes and lactotropes [53]. In gonadotropes, gonadotropin-releasing hormone regulates expression of the α-subunit via two elements in the proximal promoter, PGBE and a second element recognized by an ETS factor which is activated by mitogen-activated protein kinase (MAPK) [54]. Other sequences within the 480 bp promoter have been found to interact with the pituitary-specific homeodomain factor Ptx-1 [49], and a synergism between Ptx-1 and P-LIM, mediated by the co-activator C-LIM, has recently been described [55]. Studies with the mouse promoter also showed that an upstream DNA element located between −4.6 and −3.7 kb further enhanced transgenic expression in both thyrotropes and gonadotropes, by interacting with proximal sequences [36]. The active region was localized to 125 nucleotides upstream of −3700, and this same region was shown to mediate inhibition of expression in GH_3 somatotropic cells where α-subunit is not endogenously expressed [56]. The upstream 125 bp enhancer element harbors consensus-binding sites for GATA, SF1, Sp1, ETS, bHLH factors, and suggests cooperativity between factors binding both to proximal *cis*-acting elements and to the distal enhancer. In spite of significant advances in this area, thyrotrope-specific factors that determine α-subunit gene expression have not yet been completely identified.

BIOSYNTHESIS OF TSH

The intact TSH molecule is a heterodimeric glycoprotein with a molecular weight of 28-kDa that is composed of the noncovalently linked α- and β-subunits. The common α-subunit contains 92 amino acids while the specific TSH β-subunit has 118 amino acids. TSH biosynthesis and secretion by thyrotrope cells of the anterior pituitary are precisely regulated events. This section examines our understanding of the biosynthesis of TSH, including the processes of transcription, translation, glycosylation, folding, combination and storage.

Transcription of TSH Subunit Genes

The TSH β- and α-subunit genes are transcribed into a precursor RNA by a series of enzymatic steps as directed by each of their promoters with the participation of both ubiquitous and specific transcription factors. The transcribed RNAs undergo a precise series of splicing events at the exon–intron junctions that lead to the production of the mature messenger RNA (mRNA). This mRNA then exits the nucleus and is translated into protein within the cytoplasm prior to post-translational modification, subunit association, storage and finally secretion. Transcription of the TSH β- and α-subunit genes is coordinated under the influence of physiologic regulators, the most important of which are TRH and T_3.

Translation of TSH Subunits

The next steps in TSH biosynthesis are summarized in Figure 6.4 [57]. The mRNAs for TSHβ- and α-subunit are independently translated by ribosomes in the cytoplasm. The first peptide sequences consist of "signal" peptides of 20 amino acids for TSH β and 24 amino acids for α [58]. These signal peptides are hydrophobic, allowing insertion through the lipid bilayer of the membrane of the rough endoplasmic reticulum. Translation into TSH β-subunit and α-pre-subunits continues into the lumen of the rough endoplasmic reticulum, and cleavage of the signal peptide occurs before translation is completed. This results in the formation of a 118-amino acid TSH β-subunit [59] and a 92-amino acid α-subunit. Cleavage of TSH β to a protein of 112 amino acids appears to be an artifact of purification. Synthesis of recombinant TSH β-subunit has resulted in two products of 112 and 118 amino acids, both of which are similarly active in vitro [60].

Glycosylation of TSH

Glycosylation of TSH has a significant impact on its biological activity [61]. The TSH β-subunit has a single glycosylation site, the asparagine residue at position 23, whereas the α-subunit is glycosylated in two sites, the asparagine residues at positions 52 and 78 [62] (Figure 6.4). Excess free α-subunit is glycosylated at an additional site, the threonine residue at position 39 [63]. This residue is located in a region believed to be important for combination with the TSH β-subunit. It is not known whether glycosylation at this residue is a regulated step that inhibits combination with the TSH β-subunit or whether it occurs in excess free α-subunits because this site is exposed.

Extensive studies on the processes of TSH subunit glycosylation have been carried out. Glycosylation of the TSH β- and α-subunits begins before translation is

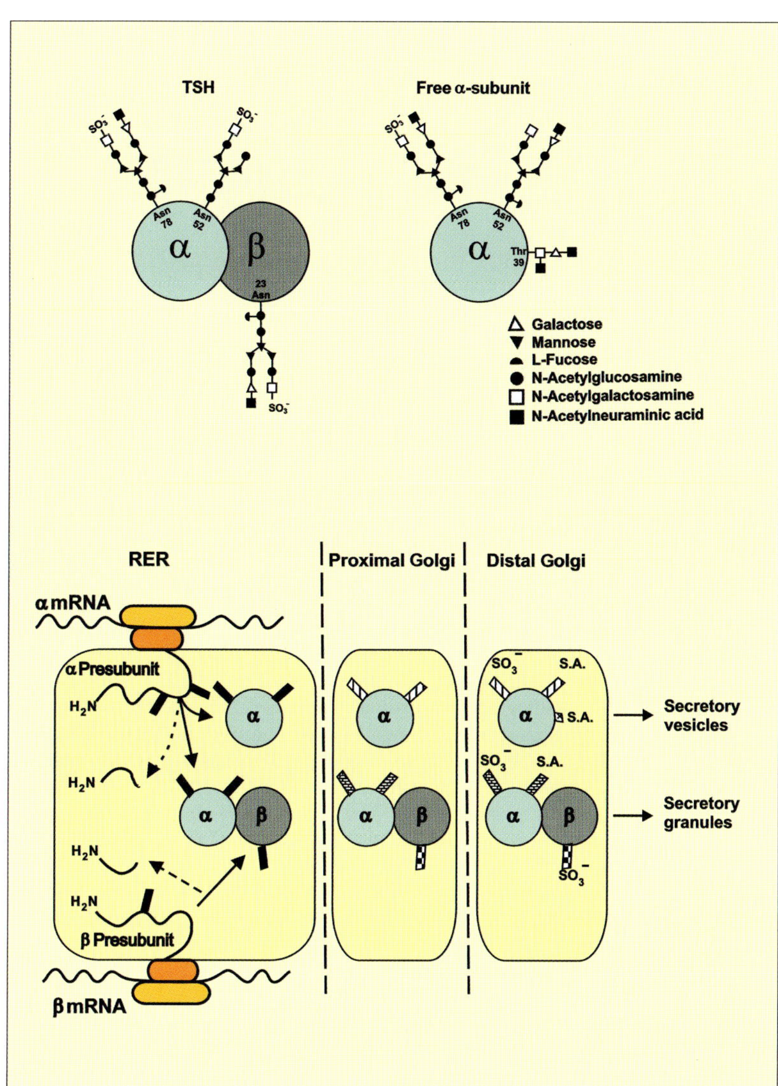

FIGURE 6.4 (Top panel) Oligosaccharide chains of thyroid-stimulating hormone (TSH). Shown are typical oligosaccharide chains present on the TSH heterodimer and the free α-subunit. Glycosylated asparagine (Asp) and threonine (Thr) residues are indicated. Symbols represent the oligosaccharide chain residues as indicated in the key (bottom panel). Biosynthesis of thyroid-stimulating hormone (TSH). (Schematic) Shown are the processes of translation and glycosylation within the rough endoplasmic reticulum (RER) and Golgi apparatus, divided into proximal and distal. Cleavage of the aminoterminal (H_2N) signal peptide and early addition of high mannose chains (black boxes) as well as combination of α- and β-subunits occur in the RER. In the proximal Golgi, oligosaccharide chains are modified and the final steps of sulfation and sialation occur in the distal Golgi apparatus. *Adapted from: Weintraub BD, Gesundheit N, Thyroid-stimulating hormone synthesis and glycosylation: Clinical implications. Thyroid Today 10:1–11, 1987 [57].*

completed (cotranslational glycosylation), while addition of the second oligosaccharide in the α-subunit occurs after translation is completed (post-translational glycosylation). The first step in this process involves the assembly of a 14-residue oligosaccharide, $(glucose)_3$-$(mannose)_9$-$(N\text{-acetylglucosamine})_2$ on a dolichol-phosphate carrier. This oligosaccharide is then transferred to asparagine residues by the enzyme oligosaccharyl transferase that recognizes the tripeptide sequence (asparagine)-(X)-(serine or threonine). This mannose-rich oligosaccharide is progressively cleaved in the rough endoplasmic reticulum and Golgi apparatus. An intermediate with only six residues is produced, and then other residues are added resulting in complex oligosaccharides [64]. The residues added include N-acetylglucosamine, fucose, galactose and N-acetylgalactosamine. Oligosaccharides prior to the six-residue intermediate are termed high-mannose and are sensitive to endoglycosidase H that releases the oligosaccharide from the protein, whereas the intermediate and the complex oligosaccharides are endoglycosidase H-resistant. Complex oligosaccharides usually consist of two branches (biantennary) but sometimes three or four branches are seen, as well as hybrid oligosaccharides consisting of one complex and another high-mannose branch. Sulfation and sialation occur late in the pathway, within the distal Golgi apparatus. Sulfate is bound to N-acetylgalactosamine residues, and sialic acid, or its precursor N-acetylneuraminic acid, is bound to galactoside residues [65]. Thus, the activation of the enzymes sulfotransferase and N-acetylgalactosamine transferase may be important regulatory steps that impact the ratio of sulfate to sialic acid. As demonstrated with LH, it appears that sulfation increases and sialylation decreases the bioactivity of TSH [65], since the exclusively sialylated recombinant glycoprotein produced in Chinese hamster ovary cells has been found to have attenuated activity in vitro [66].

Processing of complex oligosaccharides appears to occur at a slower rate for secreted glycoproteins, such as TSH, when compared to nonsecreted glycoproteins. For example, after an 11-minute pulse labeling with [^{35}S]methionine and a 30-minute chase only a few α-subunits were endoglycosidase H-resistant and only 76% reached this stage after an 18-hour chase [67]. Secretion was observed after a 60-minute chase and the secreted products – TSH, free α-subunit, but no free β-subunit – had mostly complex oligosaccharides associated with them [62]. It may be important to note that many of the studies described were carried out in thyrotropic tumor tissue obtained from hypothyroid mice, and glycosylation may differ in the euthyroid as compared to the hypothyroid state. In addition, differences between species have been noted, such as the human TSH containing more sialic acid than the bovine TSH [59].

Folding, Combination, and Storage of TSH

The elucidation of the crystal structure of human CG (hCG) [68] allowed the construction of a model of human TSH (Figure 6.5), supported by other evidence [69,70]. This model has greatly facilitated the interpretation of structure–function studies of the protein backbone. However, crystallization was only achieved with partly deglycosylated hCG, so it is likely that the conformation of the glycosylated protein may differ to some extent, although nuclear magnetic resonance studies suggest that the α-subunit carbohydrate moieties project outward and may be freely mobile [71]. Nevertheless, this model predicts that the tertiary structure of each TSH subunit consists of two hairpin loops on one side of a central knot formed by three disulfide bonds and a long loop on the opposite side. In this tertiary structure, the glycoprotein hormones share features in common with transforming growth factor β, nerve growth factor, platelet-derived growth factor, vascular endothelial growth factor, inhibin and activin, all of which are now grouped in the family of "cystine knot" growth factors [72].

Folding of nascent peptides begins before translation is completed. It has been shown that proper folding is dependent on glycosylation, since the drug tunicamycin that prevents the initial oligosaccharide transfer to the asparagine residue results in a peptide that does not fold properly and is degraded intracellularly [73]. Site-directed mutagenesis of a single glycosylation site also disrupted processing and decreased TSH secretion in transfected Chinese hamster ovary cells [74]. Folding is a critical step that allows correct internal disulfide bonding that stabilizes the tertiary structure of the protein allowing subunit combination.

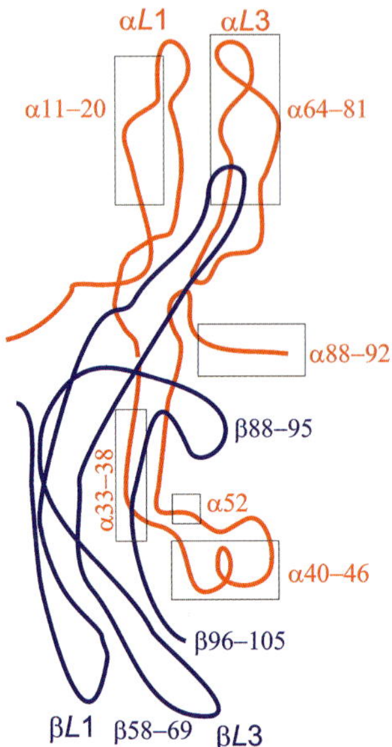

FIGURE 6.5 Human thyroid-stimulating hormone (TSH) ribbon homology model showing domains important for activity. The schematic drawing is based on a molecular homology model built on the template of the human chorionic gonadotropin (hCG) model derived from crystallographic coordinates obtained from the Brookhave Data Bank. The α-subunit is shown as a red line, and the TSH β-subunit as a blue line. The two hairpin loops (L1, L3) in each subunit are marked. The long loops (L2) in each subunit extend from the opposite side of the central cystine knot. The functionally important α-subunit domains are boxed: α11–20, α33–38, α40–46 ("α-helix"), α52, α64–81 and α88–92. The functionally important β-subunit domains are indicated within the line drawing: β58–69, β88–95 – the "determinant loop" or N-terminal segment of the seatbelt – and β96–105 – C-terminal segment of the seatbelt –. The β-subunit beyond 106 is not drawn because the corresponding region of hCG was not traceable. The oligosaccharide chains are not shown because hCG was deglycosylated before crystallization. *Adapted from: Grossmann M, Weintraub BD, Szkudlinski MW, Novel insights into the molecular mechanisms of human thyrotropin action: Structural, physiological, and therapeutic implications for the glycoprotein hormone family. Endocr Rev 18:476–501, 1997 [77].*

Combination of TSH β- and α-subunits begins soon after translation is completed in the rough endoplasmic reticulum, and continues in the Golgi apparatus [62]. Subunit combination then accelerates and modifies oligosaccharide processing of the α-subunit [75]. In fact, studies have suggested that the conformation of the α-subunit differs after combination with each type of β-subunit [76,77], and this may affect subsequent processing. The rate of combination of TSH β- and α-subunits has been examined in mouse thyrotropic tumors. After a 20-minute pulse labeling with [^{35}S] methionine, 19% of TSH β-subunits were combined with α-subunits, and this percentage increased to 61% after an additional 60-minute chase incubation [62]. Recent studies have shown that the combination of the TSH β- and α-subunits, as is also the case with other glycoprotein hormones, occurs after the "latching" of the disulfide "seat belt" of the β-subunit, with subsequent "threading" of loop 2 and the attached oligosaccharide of the α-subunit beneath that "seatbelt" [78].

The sequence of the TSH β-subunit from amino acid 27 to 31 (CAGYC) is highly conserved among species and is thought to be important for combination with the α-subunit. In a case of congenital hypothyroidism, a point mutation in the CAGYC region (see Disorders of TSH production) results in the synthesis of altered TSH β-subunits that are unable to associate with α-subunits, with consequent lack of intact TSH production [79]. A lack of free-circulating TSH β-subunit was also observed, suggesting that combination with α-subunit is necessary for TSH β-subunit secretion. This phenomenon was also demonstrated in studies where synthesis of wild type recombinant TSH β-subunit was carried out in the presence or absence of recombinant α-subunit [80]. Using site-directed mutagenesis, another study showed that a mutation at residue 25 in the glycosylation recognition site that substitutes a serine for a threonine does not alter glycosylation but decreases TSH production by 70%, possibly because of disruption of the nearby CAGYC region [81].

After TSH and free α-subunit are processed in the distal Golgi apparatus they are transported into secretory granules or vesicles [82]. The secretory granules constitute a regulated secretory pathway, mainly influenced by TRH and other hypothalamic factors. These granules contain mostly TSH, whereas free α-subunit is contained in the secretory vesicles that constitute a nonregulated secretory pathway.

REGULATION OF TSH BIOSYNTHESIS

TSH biosynthesis is regulated by coordinated signals from the central nervous system and feedback from the peripheral circulation. The most important positive input for TSH biosynthesis is hypothalamic TRH and the most powerful negative regulator is circulating thyroid hormone levels. However, additional hypothalamic factors and circulating hormones have important modifying effects. Most of these factors have independent effects on the biosynthesis of the two subunits of TSH.

Hypothalamic Regulation of TSH β-subunit Transcription

Thyrotropin-releasing hormone (TRH) is a tripeptide secreted from the hypothalamus, transported to the pituitary via the hypothalamic–hypophyseal portal system, and is a major activator of TSH production with a significant 3–5-fold increase in the transcription of both TSH β- and α-subunit mRNAs [83]. TRH from maternal or fetal sources is not required for normal thyrotrope development during ontogeny and TRH-deficient mice are not hypothyroid at birth. However, TRH is required for the postnatal maintenance of TSH activation [84].

TRH binding to its cell surface receptor initiates a cascade of intracellular events. In GH_3 cells, the TRH–receptor complex interacts with a guanine nucleotide-binding regulatory protein (G) that then binds and activates GTP (G′). G′ binds to phospholipase C (C) and activates it (C′). C′ catalyzes the hydrolysis of phosphatidylinositol 4,5 bisphosphate, which results in the formation of two intracellular "second messengers," inositol triphosphate ($InsP_3$) and 1,2-diacylglycerol (1,2-DG). $InsP_3$ diffuses from the cell surface membrane to the endoplasmic reticulum, where it causes the release of sequestered Ca^{2+}. This activates the movement of secretory granules to the cell surface and their exocytosis. Simultaneously with these events, there is a parallel activation of protein kinase C by 1,2-DG that also leads to phosphorylation of proteins involved in exocytosis. TRH has been shown to stimulate a nuclear protein, Islet-brain-1 (IB1)/JIP-1, in the anterior pituitary gland and in cultured rat GH_3 cells [85] and has been implicated in the action of TRH in stimulating the TSH β gene in thyrotropes. Studies in somatomammotrope cells, where TRH stimulates prolactin production, have suggested that phosphatidylinositol, protein kinase C and calcium-dependent pathways may be involved [86], while TRH stimulation of the TSH β-subunit promoter may be mediated by AP1 [87].

Two TRH-response regions are located from −128 to −61 and from −28 to +8 of the human TSH β promoter [88]. The upstream region contains binding sites for the pituitary-specific transcription factor, Pou1F1, suggesting a role for this or a similar factor in the regulation of the TSH β-subunit gene by TRH. In the rat TSH β-subunit gene, responsiveness to TRH has been localized to regions upstream of −204, where Pou1F1 binding sites are also found [89]. Furthermore, it has been shown that both protein kinase C and protein kinase A pathways can phosphorylate Pou1F1 at two sites in response to phorbol esters and cAMP [90], and alters the binding to Pou1F1 transactivation elements on the human TSHβ gene [91].

Dopamine acting via DA2 dopamine receptors inhibits TSH α- and β-subunit gene transcription by decreasing the intracellular levels of cAMP [83]. Studies of the TSH β-subunit gene have localized two regions of the promoter necessary for cAMP stimulation, from −128 to −61 bp and from +3 to +8 bp. The upstream region coincides with the TRH-responsive region and contains Pou1F1-binding sites. The downstream region resides within the regions responsive to T_3 (+3 to +37) and TRH (−28 to +8). The downstream region also overlaps with an AP1-binding site (−1 to +6). The sequence from −1 to +6 appears to cooperate with Pou1F1 in mediating responses to cAMP and TRH [87]. Thus, multiple interactions between transcription factors and hormonal regulators appear to converge on sequences close to the transcriptional start site.

Peripheral Regulation of TSH β-subunit Transcription

Thyroid hormone is thought to act predominantly through a classical thyroid receptor-mediated genomic model. T_4 serves as a minimally active prohormone that is converted into a metabolically active T_3 by a family of tissue deiodinases termed D1, D2 and D3. These selenoprotein enzymes are membrane bound and can activate or inactivate substrate in a time- and tissue-specific manner [92]. D2 is the major T_4-activating deiodinase. It is present on the endoplasmic reticulum close to the nucleus, and produces 3,5,3′-triiodothyronine (T_3), by the removal of an iodine residue from the outer ring of thyroxine. D2 activity is rapidly lost in the presence of its substrate T_4 by a ubiquitin proteasomal mechanism [93]. Rat pituitary thyrotropes co-express D2 RNA and protein and both are increased in hypothyroidism. Murine thyrotropes in TtT-97 tumors or the TαT1 cell line have extremely high levels of D2 which accounts for the sustained production of T_3 by thyrotropes even in the presence of supraphysiological T_4 levels [94]. Serum TSH levels in normal mice are suppressed by administration of either T_4 or T_3, although only T_3 was effective in the mouse with targeted disruption of the D2 gene. The observed phenotype of pituitary resistance to T_4 demonstrated the critical importance of D2 in controlling negative thyroid hormone regulation of TSH in thyrotropes.

T_4 can also act, in some cases, via nongenomic mechanisms that do not involve classical nuclear TR mechanisms. T_4 can bind to a cell surface integrin αVβ3 receptor followed by activation of a mitogen-activated protein kinase cascade that transduces the signal into a complex series of cellular and nuclear actions. These nongenomic hormone actions are likely to be contributors to basal rate-setting of transcription of some genes as well as control of complex cellular events [95].

TSH β- and α-subunit gene transcription rates are markedly inhibited by treatment with triiodothyronine (T_3). Studies using mouse TtT-97 thyrotropic tumors have demonstrated that suppression of TSH β- and α-subunit mRNA transcription rates measured by nuclear run-on assays is evident by 30 minutes after treatment and is maximal by 4 hours [96]. This effect was seen in the presence of the protein synthesis inhibitor cycloheximide, indicating that it did not require an intermediary protein. Other studies using mouse and rat pituitaries along with mouse thyrotropic tumors have demonstrated that steady-state mRNA levels of TSH β- and α-subunit are dramatically decreased by T_3 [97]. The mechanism of action of T_3 involves interaction with nuclear receptors that act mainly at the transcriptional level. The transcriptional response to T_3 is proportional to the nuclear receptor occupancy [98], and the time course of T_3 nuclear binding and transcriptional inhibition are also in agreement (Figure 6.6) [99].

The T_3 inhibitory effect on the TSH β gene requires ligand occupied T_3 receptor (TR), specifically the TRβ1 or TRβ2 isoform, since patients with thyroid hormone resistance and inappropriate secretion of TSH have abnormalities only in the TRβ, not the TRα gene [100]. TRβ interacts with specific *cis*-acting DNA sequences close to the transcriptional start. T_3 response elements have been reported to be located between +3 and +37 of the human TSHβ gene [101]. There are two T_3 receptor-binding sites, from +3 to +13 and +28 to +37 that may mediate T_3 inhibition. T_3 responses can be mediated through receptor monomers, homodimers, or heterodimers involving retinoid X receptors (RXR) [102]. An RXR-selective ligand was shown in vitro to inhibit TSHβ expression in TtT-97 thyrotropic tumor cells [103] and in cultured TαT1 thyrotropes [104]. This finding has been confirmed in vivo and resulted in central hypothyroidism (low T_4 and low TSH) in cancer

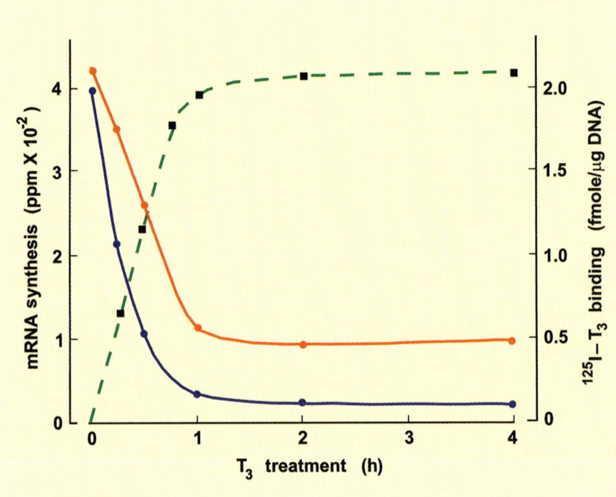

FIGURE 6.6 The effect of thyroid hormone on the transcription of the thyroid-stimulating hormone (TSH) β- (blue circles) and α-subunit (red circles) genes. Murine thyrotropic tumor explants were incubated for up to 4 hours with 5 nmol T_3 for transcription measurements or with 5 nmole ^{125}I T_3, with or without 1000-fold excess of unlabeled T_3 for binding measurements. Transcription rates were measured in pools of isolated nuclei. There is an inverse relationship between T_3 binding and TSH β- and α-subunit mRNA synthesis. *Adapted from: Shupnik MA, Ridgway EC, Triiodothyronine rapidly decreases transcription of the thyrotropin subunit genes in thyrotropic tumor explants. Endocrinology 117:1940–1946, 1985 [99].*

patients treated with the retinoid bexarotene [105]. The RXR-selective retinoid (LG 268) decreased circulating TSH and T_4 levels in mice with marked lowering of pituitary TSHβ mRNA without decreasing TRH suggesting a direct effect on thyrotropes [104].

Other, more recent studies have disputed the requirement of the negative response element located in exon 1 of the human gene since its deletion did not eliminate T_3 suppression of TSHβ promoter activity in a reconstitution system [106]. These studies showed that liganded TRβ can associate with Gata2 in vitro and in vivo via direct interaction between the zinc fingers of Gata2 and the DNA-binding domain of TRβ. In addition, T_3 occupied TR can physically interact with Med1/Trap220. Thus, interference with the transactivation function of the Pou1F1/Gata2/Med1 complex on the proximal TSHβ promoter likely plays an important role in T_3-negative regulation.

Abundant information exists as to the mechanisms involved in positive gene regulation by T_3. In the absence of T_3, unliganded TRs bind to NCoR/SMRT (nuclear receptor corepressor and silencing mediator for retinoic and thyroid hormone receptors) within a complex containing transducing β-like protein (TBL1) and histone deacetylase 3 (HDAC3) to mediate basal transcription [107]. When T_3 is added corepressor complexes are released from hormone-occupied TR that then associate with coactivator complexes containing steroid receptor coactivator (SRC), cAMP response element-binding protein (CREB) and P/CAF, resulting in histone acetylation in the proximity of the α-promoter TRE. Further chromating remodeling complexes containing Brahma-related gene 1 [108] are recruited along with Mediator complex protein (Med1, Trap220) that recruits RNA polymerase II to allow transcription [109]. Generally, TRs bind to *cis*-acting DNA response elements (TRE) in the absence of ligand, interact with a family of nuclear receptor corepressor molecules that recruit histone deacetylases, and locally modify chromatin structure to result in repression of the target gene [110]. In the presence of T_3 the corepressor complexes rapidly dissociate and are replaced by coactivator complexes that bind to TRs, increase histone methylation and acetylation locally on the chromosomal DNA, which unwinds the chromatin into an open configuration [111]. Other activating transcription factors such as Med1 are then recruited to the TR, via protein–protein interactions, which then activate RNA polymerase II-mediated transcription.

In contrast, the molecular mechanisms involved in negative T_3 regulation, such as the TSH subunit genes, have not been completely characterized. Liganded TRβ has been reported to recruit histone deacetylase 3 and reduce histone H4 acetylation that modify histones and result in a fully repressed chromosomal state of TSH subunit genes [111]. Using chromatin immunoprecipitation assays with the α-subunit promoter it was shown that T_3 decreased transcription and increased histone acetylation of the promoter, mediated directly by TRs. Overexpression of nuclear receptor corepressor (NCoR) and histone deacylase 3 (HDAC3) increased ligand-independent basal transcription. T_3 caused release of a corepressor complex, composed of NCoR, HDAC3 and a transducin β-like protein. Unexpectedly, histone acetylation was increased and coincided with lowered rates of αTSH transcription. These data show the participation of similar complexes and overlapping epigenetic changes can participate in both positive and negative T_3 regulation of the αGSU promoter [112].

Several recent studies have demonstrated the requirement for an intact DNA-binding domain of TRβ in the negative regulation of the TSHβ gene in vitro [113] and in vivo [114]. In one study, a combination of Pou1F1 and Gata2 activated a human TSHβ (−128/+37) reporter construct along with vectors containing TRβ1 constructs in the absence or presence of T_3. These investigators found that unliganded TRβ1 did not stimulate promoter activity, whereas a mutation lacking the N-terminus and DNA-binding domain of TRβ1 lost the ability of T_3-treated cells to negatively regulate TSHβ promoter activity. This demonstrated the importance of various modular domains constituting the molecular structure of TRs. Moreover, using a gene-targeting approach in transgenic mice, replacement of the wild-type TRβ gene with a mutant that abolished DNA binding in vitro did not alter ligand and cofactor interactions [114]. Homozygous mutant mice demonstrated central thyroid hormone resistance with 20-fold higher serum TSH in the face of 2–3-fold higher T_3 and T_4 levels that were similar to those of TRβ homozygous null mice.

Although thyrotrope cells contain all TRs: TRα1, TRβ1 and TRβ2, as well as non-T_3 binding variant α2, it is TRβ2 that is expressed predominantly in the pituitary and T_3-responsive TRH neurons and is most critical for the regulation of TSH [115]. Moreover, TRβ2-deficient mice had a phenotype consistent with pituitary resistance to thyroid hormone, with increased TSH and thyroid hormone levels, even in the presence of TRβ1 and TRα1 showing the lack of compensation between TR isoforms [116]. However, TRβ1 and TRα1 may still play a role, since they are able to form heterodimers with TRβ2. Heterodimers of a TR and a TR accessory protein, such as RXR, may also bind to DNA [117], constituting heterodimeric complexes that may have different affinities for specific DNA sequences and different functional activities. A particular RXR isoform, RXRγ1, is uniquely expressed in thyrotropes and appears to mediate the inhibition by 9-*cis*-retinoic acid through a region extending from −200 to −149 of the mouse TSH β-subunit promoter, an area upstream and distinct from that mediating negative regulation by thyroid hormone [103]. Other proteins that interact with TR include the coactivators, such as the glucocorticoid-receptor-interacting protein-1 (GRIP-1) and the steroid receptor coactivator-1 (SRC-1) [118], and corepressors, such as the silencing mediator for retinoid receptors and thyroid hormone receptors (SMRT) and the nuclear receptor corepressor (NCoR) [119]. These coactivators and corepressors modulate the effect of many members of the steroid–thyroid hormone receptor superfamily. Their role in the regulation of the TSH subunit promoters by thyroid hormone remains to be elucidated in detail. Studies with genetic knockout mouse models where both TRH and TRβ genes were removed have recently shown an unexpected dominant role for TRH in vivo in regulating the hypothalamic–pituitary–thyroid axis. It appears that the presence of both TRβ and TRH is necessary for a normal thyrotroph response during hypothyroidism, suggesting that unliganded TRβ stimulates TSH subunit gene expression [120].

Post-transcriptional effects of T_3 have also been described. T_3 decreases the halflife of TSH β-subunit mRNA and decreases the size of the poly(A) tail [121]. The shortening of the poly(A) tail is thought to cause mRNA instability. They also showed that T_3 increased the binding of an RNA-binding protein present in rat pituitary to the 3′ untranslated region of the rat TSHβ mRNA and also induced a shortening of the poly(A) tail of the mouse TSHβ mRNA from 160 to 30 nucleotides [122].

Steroid hormones, specifically glucocorticoids, inhibit TSH production but TSH subunit mRNA levels do not change significantly [123]. Their major effect may be at the secretory level. Estrogens mildly reduce both α- and TSHβ-subunit mRNA in hypothyroid rats compared with euthyroid controls [124]. In this study, estrogen also abolished the early rise in subunit mRNA levels seen following T_3 replacement. Other studies showed that E_2 inhibits the up-regulation of αGSU and TSHβ mRNA levels in the pituitary of hypothyroid rats [125] and that ovariectomy increased pituitary TSHβ mRNA levels [126]. In the thyrotroph cell line, TαT1, estrogen treatment reduced TSHβ mRNA levels as measured by reverse transcription PCR and suggested that Gata2 may be prevented from gene activation by an interaction with liganded ERα [127]. Finally, testosterone has been shown to increase TSH β-subunit mRNA in castrated rat pituitary and mouse thyrotropic tumor [128].

Leptin and neuropeptide-Y (NPY) have opposite effects on TSH biosynthesis. Leptin is the product of the ob gene, found mainly in adipose tissue that regulates body weight and energy expenditure [129]. NPY is a neuropeptide synthesized in the arcuate nucleus of the hypothalamus that plays many roles in neuroendocrine function [130]. In dispersed rat pituitary cells, leptin stimulated and NPY inhibited TSHβ mRNA levels in a dose-related manner [131]. In contrast, both agents increased α-subunit steady-state mRNA levels.

Hypothalamic Regulation of α-subunit Transcription

TRH stimulates α-subunit biosynthesis through a novel mechanism. A CRE-binding protein that binds to the region from −151 to −135 of the human α-subunit promoter appears to be important for TRH regulation, as well as a Pou1F1-like protein that binds to a more distal region from −223 to −190 [132]. The CRE of the human glycoprotein hormone α-subunit gene promoter consists of an 18 bp repeat and extends from −146 to −111 [133]. The mechanisms involved in TRH stimulation of the α-subunit gene appear to involve two transcription factors, P-Lim and CREB-binding protein (CBP). When stimulated with TRH, both of these factors transcriptionally cooperate to activate α-subunit promoter activity due to direct protein–protein interactions [134]. Both of these factors synergistically activated the α-subunit gene promoter during TRH stimulation and interact in a TRH-dependent manner. P-Lim binds to the α-subunit promoter directly but CBP does not possess a DNA-binding domain so it must be recruited to the promoter via interacting with another factor. The P-Lim/CBP binding is formed in a TRH signaling-specific manner, in contrast to forskolin, which mimics the protein kinase A signaling, and dissociates both the binding and the transcriptional synergy. α-Subunit gene expression in thyrotropes is inhibited by dopamine in coordination with the expression of the TSH β-subunit gene. Its action is mediated by decreases in intracellular cAMP levels.

Peripheral Regulation of α-subunit Transcription

Thyroid hormone inhibition of α-subunit gene transcription is observed in thyrotropes in coordination with that of the TSH β-subunit (Figure 6.6). The T_3 response element of the human α-subunit gene promoter has been reported to be located from −22 to −7 [135]. Similar to the TSH β-subunit gene, the T_3 response elements of the human as well as the mouse [40] and rat [136] α-subunit genes are located close to the transcriptional start. T_3 inhibition may be mediated by different isoforms of the T_3 receptor [137] in combination with the corepressors SMRT and NCoR [138]. Studies have suggested that mutations of the T_3 response element of the human α-subunit promoter that eliminate TR binding do not abrogate the inhibitory effect of T_3, suggesting that protein–protein interactions may be more important than protein–DNA binding [139].

Steroid hormone regulation of α-subunit gene transcription is probably of limited importance. Androgen inhibition and androgen receptor (AR) binding has been localized to a region from −120 to −100. Negative regulation by estrogen was described in the gonadotropes of transgenic mice expressing a reporter gene under the control of both human and bovine promoters, but no binding of these regions to the estrogen receptor (ER) was detected suggesting an indirect effect [140]. However, other studies using rat somatomammotropes have found positive regulation by estrogen localized to the proximal 98 bp of 5′ flanking DNA of the human α-subunit gene and binding of the ER to the T_3 response element from −22 to −7 [141]. Transcriptional inhibition by glucocorticoids may be mediated by binding of the glucocorticoid receptor to sequences between −122 and −93 of the human α-subunit gene. However, no direct binding was detected in other studies suggesting that the GR inhibits transcription by interfering with other transactivating proteins [142].

Regulation of TSH Glycosylation

Glycosylation is a regulated process that is primarily modulated by TRH and thyroid hormone [143]. Primary hypothyroidism [144] and TRH administration have been found to increase oligosaccharide addition that results in an increased bioactivity of TSH. The same was noted in patients with resistance to thyroid hormone. TSH glycosylation patterns were also found to differ in several pathological states, such as central hypothyroidism, TSH-producing pituitary adenomas and euthyroid sick syndrome [145]. Also observed were changes in the sulfation and sialylation of the oligosaccharide residues, which modulates bioactivity [144,146,147]. Recently, thyroid hormone was shown to increase TSH bioactivity, and this was correlated with decreased sialylation [148].

TSH SECRETION

In euthyroid humans, the production rate of TSH is between 100 and 400 mU/day, the plasma halflife is approximately 50 minutes, and the plasma clearance rate is approximately 50 ml/min [149,150]. The distribution space of TSH is slightly greater than the plasma volume. In hypothyroid subjects, TSH secretion rates increase by 10–15 times normal rates, while the clearance rates decrease slightly. In hyperthyroid subjects, TSH secretion is suppressed and metabolic clearance is accelerated.

Ontogeny of TSH Levels

At 8–10 weeks of gestation in the human, TRH is measurable in the hypothalamus, with progressive increases in TRH levels until term. By 12 weeks of gestation, immunoreactive TSH cells are present in the human pituitary gland, and TSH is detectable in the pituitary and the serum [151]. Serum and pituitary TSH levels remain low until week 18, when TSH levels increase rapidly, followed by increases in serum T_4 and T_3 concentrations. Fetal serum TSH and T_4 concentrations continue to increase between 20 and 40 weeks of gestation. Pituitary TSH begins to respond to exogenous TRH early in the third trimester, while negative feedback control of TSH secretion develops during the last half of gestation and the first 1–2 months of life [152].

An abrupt rise in serum TSH levels occurs within 30 minutes of birth in term infants. This is followed by an increase in serum T_3 concentrations within 4 hours and a lesser increase in T_4 levels within the first 24–36 hours. The initial increase in serum TSH levels appears to be stimulated by cooling in the extrauterine environment. Serum TSH levels fall to the adult range by 3–5 days after birth, and serum thyroid hormone levels stabilize by 1–2 months. Serum TSH levels in healthy premature infants (less than 37 weeks gestational age) are quite variable, but tend to be lower at birth compared to term infants. TSH levels decrease slightly during the first week of life, followed by a gradual increase to normal term levels. Serum TSH levels are even lower in ill premature infants, but rise towards normal levels during recovery [152,153,154].

Patterns of TSH Secretion

TSH is secreted from the pituitary gland in a dual fashion, with secretory bursts (pulses) superimposed upon basal (apulsatile) secretion [155] (Figure 6.7, upper panel). Basal TSH secretion accounts for 30–40% of the total amount released into the circulation, and secretory bursts account for the remaining 60–70%. TSH pulses occur approximately every 2–3 hours, although there is considerable variability among individuals [156]. TSH pulses appear to directly stimulate T_3 secretion from the thyroid gland, as cross-correlation analysis has shown that a free T_3 peak occurs between 0.5 and 2.5 hours after a TSH peak. However, changes in free T_3 levels from nadir to peak are only 11% of mean free T_3 levels, probably because T_3 has a long serum halflife, and most T_3 does not arise from the thyroid gland [157].

In healthy euthyroid subjects, TSH is secreted in a circadian pattern, with nocturnal levels increasing up to twice daytime levels [156] (Figure 6.7, upper panel). Peak TSH levels occur between 23:00 and 05:00 hours in subjects with normal sleep–wake cycles, and nadir

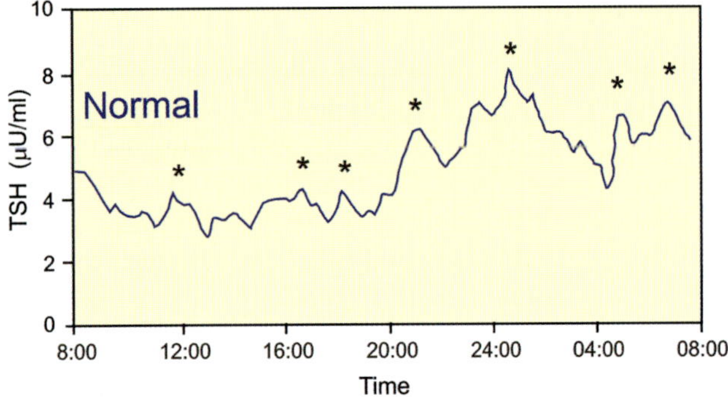

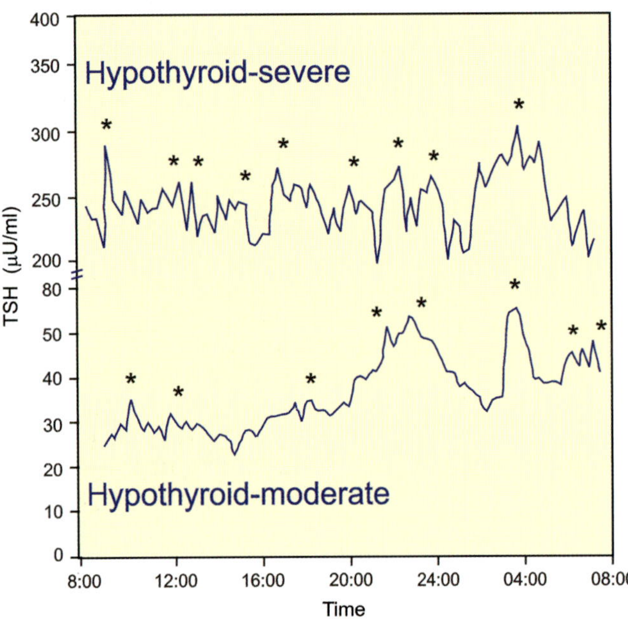

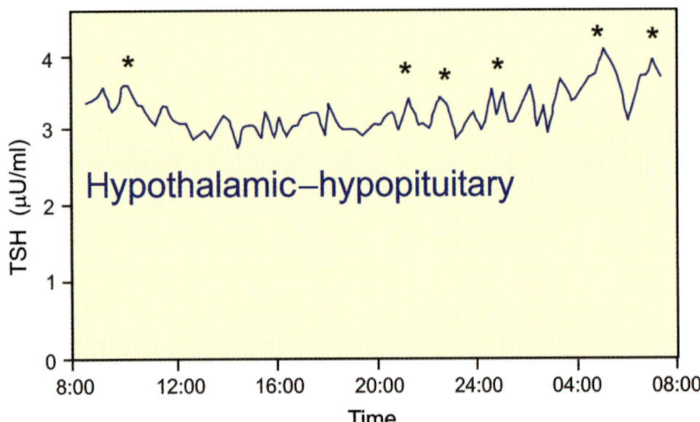

FIGURE 6.7 Serum thyroid-stimulating hormone (TSH) levels measured every 15 minutes in a healthy subject (upper panel), in two subjects with primary hypothyroidism (middle panel) and in a subject with hypothyroidism due to a craniopharyngioma (lower panel). Significant TSH pulses were located by Cluster analysis, a computerized pulse detection program, and are indicated by asterisks *Adapted from: Samuels MH, Veldhuis JD, Henry P, Ridgway EC, Pathophysiology of pulsatile and copulsatile release of thyroid-stimulating hormone, luteinizing hormone, follicle-stimulating hormone, and α-subunit. J Clin Endocrinol Metab 71:425–432, 1990 [155].*

levels occur at about 11:00 hours. The TSH circadian rhythm emerges between 1 and 2 months of life, and is well-established in healthy children [158]. TSH pulsatile and circadian secretion is then maintained throughout adulthood, increasing slightly with age, at least in women [156]. The circadian variation in TSH levels is due to increased mass of TSH secreted per burst at night, as well as slight increased frequency of bursts and more rapid increase to maximal TSH secretion within a burst [156]. The nocturnal increase in TSH levels can precede the onset of sleep, and sleep deprivation enhances TSH secretion. Therefore, in contrast to other pituitary hormones with a circadian variation, the nocturnal rise in TSH levels is not sleep entrained. Instead, there is a sleep-related inhibition of TSH release that is of insufficient magnitude to counteract the nocturnal TSH surge.

Subjects with primary hypothyroidism have increased TSH pulse amplitude with attenuation of the circadian variation in TSH levels [159]. In contrast, patients with hypothalamic–pituitary causes of hypothyroidism secrete less TSH over a 24-hour period, with loss of the nocturnal TSH surge in pulse amplitude (Figure 6.7, lower panel) [160]. A similar pattern of reduced 24-hour TSH secretion occurs in critical illness [161].

The origin of pulsatile and circadian TSH secretion is not known. Thyroid hormones alter TSH pulse amplitude, but have little effect on pulse frequency, and therefore are unlikely to participate in TSH pulse generation. The TSH pulse generator may reside in the hypothalamus, with TRH neurons acting in concert to stimulate a burst of TSH secretion from the pituitary gland. However, constant TRH infusions do not change TSH pulse frequency in humans, which casts doubt on this theory [162]. Somatostatin and dopamine suppress TSH pulse amplitude, but neither agent has any major effect on TSH pulse frequency, and therefore somatostatin and dopamine do not appear to control pulsatile TSH secretion. There is a diurnal variation in the activity of anterior pituitary 5′-monodeiodinase in the rat, which may control circadian TSH secretion [163]. However, this has not been confirmed in the human.

Physiologic serum cortisol levels affect circadian TSH secretion, although cortisol does not appear to affect TSH pulse frequency. When subjects with adrenal insufficiency were studied under conditions of glucocorticoid withdrawal, daytime TSH levels were increased, and the usual TSH circadian rhythm was abolished. When these subjects were given physiologic doses of hydrocortisone in a pattern that mimicked normal pulsatile and circadian cortisol secretion, daytime TSH levels were decreased, and the normal TSH circadian rhythm was re-established. Hydrocortisone infusions at the same dose given as pulses of constant amplitude throughout the 24-hour period also decreased 24-hour TSH levels, but there was no circadian variation [164]. Similarly, when healthy subjects were given metyrapone (an inhibitor of endogenous cortisol synthesis), TSH levels increased during the day, leading to abolition of the usual TSH circadian variation [165]. These data suggest that the normal early morning increase in endogenous serum cortisol levels decreases serum TSH levels and leads to the observed normal circadian variation in TSH.

REGULATION OF TSH SECRETION

TSH secretion is a result of complex interactions between central (hypothalamic) and peripheral hormones (Figure 6.8).

Hypothalamic Regulation of TSH Secretion

TRH directly affects TSH secretion in vivo and in vitro at concentrations that exist in the pituitary portal blood [165,166]. Immunoneutralization of TRH in animals leads to a decline in thyroid function [167], and TRH knockout mice have a reduced postnatal TSH surge, followed by impaired baseline thyroid function with a poor TSH response to hypothyroidism. Lesions of the PVN decrease circulating TRH and TSH levels in normal or hypothyroid animals and cause hypothyroidism [168], while electrical stimulation of this area causes TSH release. Although baseline levels of TSH are reduced in animals with lesions of the PVN, TSH levels still show appropriate responses to changes in circulating thyroid hormone levels. Thus, TRH likely determines the set point of feedback control by thyroid hormones.

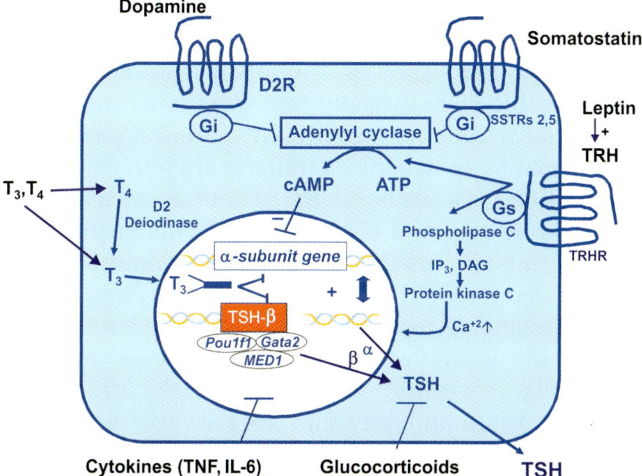

FIGURE 6.8 Neuroendocrine and peripheral control of thyroid-stimulating hormone (TSH) secretion. T_4, thyroxine; T_3, triiodothyronine; TRH, thyrotropin-releasing hormone; TRHR, TRH receptor; SSTRs, somatostatin receptors; D2R, dopamine receptor type 2; D2, deiodinase type II; TNF, tumor necrosis factor; IL-6, interleukin 6.

Acute intravenous administration of TRH to human subjects causes a dose-related release of TSH from the pituitary. This occurs within 5 minutes and is maximal at 20–30 minutes. Serum TSH levels return to basal levels by 2 hours [169]. More prolonged (2–4-hour) infusions of TRH lead to biphasic increases in serum TSH levels in humans and animals [170]. The early phase may reflect release of stored TSH, while the later phase may reflect release of newly synthesized TSH. Interpretation of TSH responses to even more prolonged TRH infusions is complicated by the increase in serum T_3 levels, which feed back to suppress further TSH release [161]. Continuous TRH administration in vitro also causes desensitization of TSH responses, which may further explain decreased TSH levels with long-term TRH exposure [171].

Somatostatin (SS) in humans and animals inhibits basal and TRH-stimulated TSH secretion in vivo and in vitro at concentrations that exist in the pituitary portal blood [172]. In the hypothalamus, the highest concentrations of SS occur in the anterior paraventricular region. From this region, axonal processes of SS-containing neurons project to the median eminence. Animals that have undergone sectioning of these fibers have depletion of SS content of the median eminence and increased serum TSH levels [172]. Similarly, immunoneutralization of SS in animals increases basal TSH levels and TSH responses to TRH [173]. In humans, SS infusions suppress TSH pulse amplitude, slightly decrease TSH pulse frequency and abolish the nocturnal TSH surge [174]. Thus, TSH secretion is probably regulated through a simultaneous dual-control system of TRH stimulation and SS inhibition from the hypothalamus.

SS binds to specific, high-affinity receptors in the anterior pituitary gland. SS receptor subtypes (SST) 1 and 5 have been localized to thyrotropes [175]. Binding of SS to its receptor inhibits adenylate cyclase via the inhibitory subunit of the guanine nucleotide regulatory protein, which lowers protein kinase A activity and decreases TSH secretion. SS may also exert some effects by cAMP-independent actions on intracellular calcium levels. Hypothyroidism reduces the efficacy of SS in decreasing TSH secretion in vitro, which is reversed by thyroid hormone administration [176]. Further studies in mouse thyrotropic tumors indicate that both SST1 and 5 are markedly down-regulated in hypothyroidism and are induced by thyroid hormone [175]. Although short-term infusions of SS lead to pronounced suppression of TSH secretion in humans, long-term treatment with SS or its analogues does not cause hypothyroidism [177]. This probably reflects compensatory mechanisms in the thyroid hormone feedback loop. GH deficiency is associated with increased TSH responses to TRH, while GH administration or endogenous GH excess (acromegaly) decrease basal, pulsatile and TRH-stimulated TSH secretion [178,179], possibly due to GH stimulation of hypothalamic SS release.

Dopamine also inhibits basal and TRH-stimulated TSH secretion in vivo and in vitro at concentrations that exist in the pituitary portal blood [180]. In humans, dopamine infusions rapidly suppress TSH pulse amplitude, do not affect TSH pulse frequency and abolish the nocturnal TSH surge [174], while administration of a dopamine antagonist has the opposite effect [181]. Dopamine also has direct effects on hypothalamic hormone secretion that may indirectly impact TSH secretion. For example, dopamine and dopamine-agonist drugs stimulate both TRH and SS release from rat hypothalami [182].

In the hypothalamus, dopamine is secreted by neurons in the arcuate nucleus. From the arcuate nucleus, neuronal processes project to the median eminence. Dopamine acts by binding to type 2 dopamine receptors (DA_2) on thyrotrope cells [183]. This leads to inhibition of adenylate cyclase, which decreases the synthesis and secretion of TSH. The inhibitory effects of dopamine on TSH secretion vary according to sex steroids, body mass and thyroid status. Dopamine antagonist drugs cause greater increases in serum TSH levels in women than in men. Recent studies show that obesity is associated with enhanced TSH secretion, which may be mediated via blunted central dopaminergic tone [184]. Dopamine inhibition of TSH release is greater in patients with mild hypothyroidism than in normal subjects, although subjects with severe hypothyroidism may be less responsive [185]. Although short-term infusions of dopamine lead to pronounced suppression of TSH secretion, long-term treatment with dopamine agonists does not cause hypothyroidism. This probably reflects compensatory mechanisms in the thyroid hormone feedback loop.

Adrenergic effects have also been reported in vivo and in vitro. α-Adrenergic activation stimulates TSH release directly from the rat pituitary gland at physiologic concentrations of catecholamines [186]. α-Adrenergic agonists stimulate TSH release in rats, while blockade of norepinephrine synthesis or treatment with adrenergic receptor blockers decrease TSH levels [187]. It is unclear whether these effects are mediated via changes in TRH and/or SS levels. In humans, there are limited data regarding adrenergic effects on TSH secretion. α-Adrenergic blockade diminishes serum TSH responses to TRH [188]. However, administration of epinephrine does not alter TRH-stimulated TSH secretion [189]. These data suggest that endogenous adrenergic pathways do not have a major role in TSH secretion. Noradrenergic stimulation of TSH secretion is mediated by high-affinity α_1-adrenoreceptors linked to adenylate cyclase [188]. Therefore, dopamine and epinephrine appear to exert opposing actions on thyrotropes by opposite effects on cAMP generation.

Opioid administration to rats suppresses basal or stimulated TSH levels, and the opioid receptor antagonist naloxone reverses these effects [190]. Acute opiate administration in humans may slightly stimulate TSH levels, while acute naloxone administration has little effect [191]. In contrast to these acute studies, when naloxone is given over 24 hours, the 24-hour TSH secretion decreases, primarily due to a decrease in nocturnal TSH pulse amplitude [192]. TSH responses to TRH are also decreased. Serum T_3 levels are decreased as well, suggesting that the magnitude of TSH suppression is sufficient to affect thyroid gland function. These findings suggest that endogenous opioids may play a role in tonic stimulation of TSH secretion.

Peripheral Regulation of TSH Secretion

Thyroid hormones directly block pituitary secretion of TSH. Acute administration of T_3 suppresses TSH levels within hours, while chronic administration leads to further suppression. Slight changes in serum thyroid hormone levels within the normal range alter basal and TRH-stimulated TSH levels, confirming the sensitivity of the pituitary gland to thyroid hormone feedback. Recent genetic studies have suggested that genetic variations that influence thyroid hormone production and the conversion of T_4 to T_3 may affect these endogenous TSH levels in humans [193,194]. Thyroid hormones alter tonic TSH secretion and TSH pulse amplitude without affecting pulse frequency, since subjects with primary hypothyroidism have a near-normal number of TSH pulses, and T_4 replacement leads to a decrease in TSH pulse amplitude without much change in pulse frequency [159]. In addition to direct effects on TSH secretion, thyroid hormones have other actions that impact on TSH secretion. In particular, recent studies in transgenic animals show that there is a central role for feedback inhibition of TRH by thyroid hormones in the normal hypothalamic–pituitary–thyroid axis [195]. In addition, hypothalamic SS content is decreased in hypothyroid rats, and is restored by T_3 treatment [196]. These combined effects of thyroid hormones on TRH and SS decrease TRH release from the hypothalamus, and indirectly decrease TSH secretion.

Glucocorticoids at pharmacologic doses or high endogenous cortisol levels (Cushing's syndrome) suppress basal and pulsatile TSH levels, blunt TSH responses to TRH, and diminish the nocturnal TSH surge in humans and animals [197–199]. Glucocorticoid-induced changes in TSH levels are due to decreased TSH pulse amplitude without alteration in TSH pulse frequency, with more profound suppression of nocturnal TSH secretion and abolition of the TSH surge.

Physiologic glucocorticoid levels also affect TSH secretion [164,165]. Untreated patients with adrenocortical insufficiency can have elevated serum TSH levels that resolve with steroid replacement. Complementary studies of metyrapone (an inhibitor of cortisol synthesis) administration to healthy subjects confirm that endogenous cortisol levels suppress TSH secretion, and physiologic hydrocortisone replacement in patients with adrenal insufficiency decreases daytime TSH levels back to those seen in healthy subjects.

Glucocorticoid suppression of TSH levels may occur directly at the pituitary gland. Animal studies suggest that glucocorticoids exert direct effects on thyrotropes to impair TSH secretion, although these appear to be highly dependent on dose and time-course of administration [200,201]. Glucocorticoids do not appear to directly affect TSH gene transcription. In humans, TSH pulse frequency is maintained during glucocorticoid administration, while TSH pulse amplitude is reduced and TSH responses to exogenous TRH are attenuated, suggesting a direct effect on TSH secretion. In addition to direct pituitary effects, it appears that glucocorticoids may have hypothalamic actions that affect TSH levels. Dexamethasone increases hypothalamic TRH levels, while circulating TRH levels are decreased [202].

Patients with Cushing's syndrome or subjects receiving prolonged courses of glucocorticoids may have low serum T_4 as well as TSH levels. Whether such patients have true hypothyroidism and whether they should be treated with thyroid hormone, is unclear; however, patients with acute or chronic illnesses and similar abnormalities in thyroid hormone levels do not appear to benefit from thyroid hormone therapy.

Leptin is primarily a product of adipocytes, although it is also located in thyrotrophs. It regulates food intake and energy expenditure, decreasing acutely with fasting in animals and humans [129]. Exogenous leptin administration to fed rats raises serum TSH levels, probably by increasing TRH gene expression and TRH release [203]. Similarly, leptin administration to fasted rats or humans reverses fasting-induced decrements in TSH levels, also by increasing TRH gene expression and release [204]. This suggests that fasting-related reductions in leptin levels play a role in suppressing TSH secretion. However, immunoneutralization of leptin increases TSH levels, and therefore endogenous leptin may inhibit TSH release, at least in rats.

Sex steroids may account for higher serum and pituitary TSH concentrations in male compared to female rats. TSH content is reduced by castration and is restored by androgen administration [129], which also increases basal and TRH-stimulated serum TSH levels [205]. In contrast, androgen administration to intact female rats does not alter serum or pituitary levels of TSH [206]. Estrogen administration to euthyroid rats does not alter serum TSH levels. In euthyroid humans, most studies suggest that changes in endogenous or exogenous sex steroid levels do not affect basal or TRH-stimulated TSH levels [207]. There is no significant gender difference in the basal mean and pulsatile secretion of TSH [156]. Therefore, sex steroids do not appear to play a major regulatory role in TSH secretion in humans.

Cytokines are circulating mediators of the inflammatory response that are produced by many cells and have systemic effects on the hypothalamic–pituitary–thyroid axis [208–210]. Administration of tumor necrosis factor (TNF) or interleukin-6 (IL-6) decreases serum TSH levels in healthy human subjects, and TNF and interleukin-1 (IL-1) decrease TSH levels in animals. Administration of these cytokines recapitulates the alterations in thyroid hormone and TSH levels seen in acute nonthyroidal illness. In rats, TNF reduces hypothalamic TRH content and pituitary TSH gene transcription. IL-1 stimulates type II 5′-deiodinase activity in rat brain, which may decrease TSH secretion by increasing intrapituitary T_3 levels.

Autocrine and paracrine peptides may alter regulatory pathways within the pituitary gland for TSH secretion, acting in concert with the central and peripheral factors described above [211]. Peptides that have been implicated in this role include neurotensin, opioid-related peptides, galanin, substance P, epidermal growth factor (EGF), fibroblast growth factor (FGF), IL-1 and IL-6. Of particular interest is neuromedin B, a mammalian peptide structurally and functionally related to the amphibian peptide bombesin [212]. Neuromedin B is present in high concentrations in thyrotrope cells, with levels that change according to thyroid status. Administration of neuromedin B to rodents decreases TSH levels, while intrathecal administration of neuromedin B antiserum increases TSH levels. Therefore, neuromedin B appears to act as an autocrine factor that exerts a tonic inhibitory effect on TSH secretion. Further data suggest that neuromedin B may modulate the action of other TSH secretagogues and release inhibitors, including TRH and thyroid hormones.

ACTION OF TSH

TSH acts on the thyroid gland by binding to the TSH receptor. An excellent review of this subject has been published [213]. This receptor is located on the plasma membranes of thyroid cells and consists of a long extracellular domain, a transmembrane domain and a short intracellular domain. Knowledge of the molecular structure of the receptor has allowed a better understanding of the mechanism of action of TSH that results in the production of thyroid hormone.

TSH Receptor Gene

The human TSH receptor gene is located on chromosome 14 locus q31 and spans a region greater than 60 kb in size containing ten exons [214]. Exons one through nine have 327, 72, 75, 75, 75, 78, 69, 78 and 189 bp, respectively, and encode part of the extracellular domain, whereas exon ten is greater than 1412 bp and encodes the rest of the extracellular domain as well as all of the transmembrane and the intracellular domains. The promoter region of the human TSH receptor gene has also been partially characterized [214]. The major transcriptional start site, designated as +1, is located 157 bp upstream of the translation initiation codon ATG. There are no consensus CAAT or TATA boxes but there are degenerate CAAGGAAAGT and TAGGGAA boxes located at positions −86 and −43, respectively. The regions of the promoter important for tissue-specific expression and those responsive to TSH and cAMP, the two main regulators that have been shown to inhibit the rat TSH receptor gene expression [215], are yet to be defined. Northern blot analysis has revealed two major transcripts of the human TSH receptor of 3.9 and 4.6 kb in size that differ only in the length of the 3′ untranslated region [216,217].

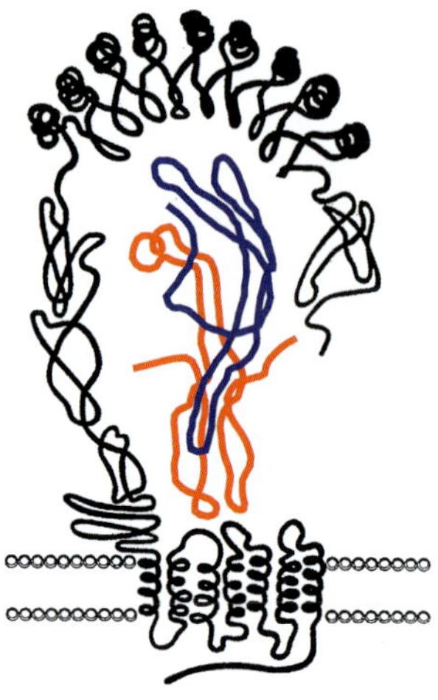

FIGURE 6.9 Schematic model of the human thyroid-stimulating hormone (TSH)−TSH receptor complex. The receptor (black) is depicted in accordance with models based on the leucine-rich repeats (LRR)-containing ribonuclease inhibitor (203k) and G-protein-coupled rhodopsin (203n). In the center, the α-subunit (red ribbon) and TSH β-subunit (blue ribbon) are shown folded and combined, with the α hairpin loops oriented toward the extracellular loops of the transmembrane domain of the receptor, and the β hairpin loops toward the concave surface of the LRR. *Adapted from: Grossmann M, Weintraub BD, Szkudlinski MW, Novel insights into the molecular mechanisms of human thyrotropin action: Structural, physiological, and therapeutic implications for the glycoprotein hormone family. Endocr Rev 18:476−501, 1997 [77].*

TSH Receptor Structure

The TSH receptor is synthesized as a single polypeptide chain of 764 amino acids that includes a 20-amino acid signal peptide [218]. However, the TSH receptor has been found to exist on the cell surface as a single chain and also as a two-subunit form, produced by internal cleavage apparently at two sites, releasing a potentially immunogenic 5−7-kDa peptide [219,220]. Cleavage of the TSH receptor has been found to depend on cell−cell contacts [221]. The amino-terminal half of the protein contains 16 hydrophilic leucine-rich repeats (LRR) that form the extracellular domain and include six potential glycosylation sites. The asparagine-linked oligosaccharides appear to be important for correct folding, membrane targeting and receptor function [222,223]. The LRR are the common feature of the superfamily of LRR proteins. One of these, the ribonuclease inhibitor, has been co-crystallized with its ligand [224], and this has allowed the construction of a model of the extracellular domain of the TSH receptor bound to TSH [225], as shown in Figure 6.9. The carboxyl-terminal half of the protein was modeled after the structure of the G-protein-coupled receptors, based on rhodopsin [226]. This region contains seven hydrophobic transmembrane segments, three extracellular loops, three cytoplasmatic loops and a short cytoplasmatic tail of 82 amino acids.

Determinants of TSH Binding to its Receptor

The entire extracellular domain and parts of the transmembrane domain of the TSH receptor contribute to TSH binding. However, two regions, from residue 201 to 211 and 222 to 230, are particularly important in TSH-specific binding [227]. Inactivating TSH receptor mutations, a rare cause of congenital hypothyroidism in humans [228], frequently map to the aminoterminal extracellular domain [229]. In contrast, a different region of the extracellular domain, called the hinge region, from residue 287 to 404, appears to be more important for binding of TSH receptor antibodies [230]. Other authors have reported considerable overlap of TSH-binding regions and antibody epitopes [231], although binding to the hinge region was studied using bovine TSH and was found to be dependent on positive-charged residues [232], which are less common in human TSH [233]. Interestingly, studies using rat FRTL-5 cells have shown that thyroid-stimulating autoantibodies (TSAbs or TSI) stimulate whereas TSH-binding inhibitory antibodies (TBIAbs) inhibit TSH-mediated gene expression, suggesting that these antibodies must act on different epitopes of the receptor that differ in their signal transduction mechanism [215]. Recently the crystal structure of the extracellular domain of the TSH receptor bound to a stimulating TSH receptor monoclonal antibody was determined to be similar to the LH-FSH receptor crystal structure, but the hinge region of the TSH receptor was not included [234]. The transmembrane domain of the TSH receptor also appears to be important in ligand binding. A point mutation in the fourth transmembrane domain of the TSH receptor gene has been described in the *hyt/hyt* congenitally hypothyroid mouse that abolishes TSH binding [235].

Specificity of TSH binding is conferred by the TSH β-subunit. It appears that amino acid residues from 58 to 69, within the βL3 loop, and from 88 to 105, the "seat-belt" region of the TSH β-subunit [236] play an important role in binding to and activation of the TSH receptor. The carboxyl-terminal end of TSHβ contains multiple lysine residues (positions 101, 107 and 110) and a cysteine at position 105 that are critical for the ability to bind to the receptor [237]. Congenital hypothyroidism due to biologically inactive TSH was found to result from a frameshift mutation with loss of β-cysteine^{105} [238] (see Disorders of TSH production). Several regions of the α-subunit are also important for TSH activity, particularly the residues α11–20 and α88–92 [69,74]. In addition, the oligosaccharide chain at position α-asparagine^{52} plays an important role in both binding affinity and receptor activation. A mutant TSH lacking the α-asparagine^{52} oligosaccharide showed increased in vitro activity, although this same mutation had the opposite effect on CG binding to its native receptor [74]. However, such a mutation also increased TSH clearance and this decreased in vivo activity [74]. In addition, the oligosaccharide chains on the TSH subunits are critically important for signal transduction [61,239]. In this regard, the α-subunit oligosaccharides are important for all the pathways activated by the receptor, whereas the TSH β-subunit oligosaccharide only influences the adenylate cyclase pathway [240]. The mechanism by which the oligosaccharides influence signal transduction is not known. A model for the action of the glycoprotein hormones has been proposed that suggests a role for the oligosaccharides in directly modulating the influx of calcium into the target cell [241].

The ability of chorionic gonadotropin to bind to the TSH receptor was demonstrated in rat thyroid cells [242] and confirmed in studies using recombinant human TSH receptor [243,244]. The activity of CG was estimated to be less than 0.1% compared to TSH. LH was found to have a ten-fold higher potency for activation of the TSH receptor when compared to CG, but a mutant of CG that lacks the carboxyl-terminal region of CGβ from amino acid residues 115 to 145 showed a potency equivalent to that of LH [244]. This truncated form of CG is one of the forms in the heterogeneous population of CG molecules produced in normal pregnancy and in trophoblastic tumors and may be present in amounts sufficient to cause significant thyroid gland stimulation [245,246]. The occurrence of gestational hyperthyroidism due to a mutation in the TSH receptor that increases its sensitivity to CG has also been described [247].

Signal Transduction at the TSH Receptor

The three intracytoplasmatic loops of the transmembrane domain appear to be important for signal transduction [248]. The TSH receptor is coupled to the G_s protein cascade probably through the carboxyl-terminus of the third cytoplasmic loop [249]. Binding of G_s is dependent on TSH receptor cleavage [250] by the metalloprotease ADAM 10 [251]. Thus, binding of TSH activates adenylate cyclase to produce cAMP [252,253]. The G_q/phospholipase C/inositol phosphate/Ca^{2+} pathway is also activated and appears to play a role in TSH synthesis, particularly in regulating iodination [254], but this pathway is slower and requires a higher concentration of TSH [252]. Specific amino acids in the third cytoplasmic loop have been identified that are important for the phosphatidylinositol pathway but do not appear to play a role in the adenylate cyclase pathway [253]. TSH is also able to signal through the JAK/STAT [255] and mTOR/S6K1 [256] pathways, with important roles in thyroid cell growth.

The unliganded TSH receptor has been found to have significant constitutive activity [257,258], suggesting that regulation may involve the release of an inhibitory restraint. This would explain the relatively high frequency of activating mutations of the TSH receptor compared to inactivating mutations. In cases of congenital hyperthyroidism [257,259,260], the mutations were located in the extracellular domain and the second, fourth, fifth and sixth transmembrane domains, while in hyperfunctioning adenomas the mutations were found to localize to the carboxyl terminus of the third cytoplasmic loop and adjacent sixth transmembrane domain. Recently, an activating mutation was described that localized to the intracellular C-terminal region [261]. All these mutations resulted in constitutive activation of adenylate cyclase [262]. Germline mutations of the cytoplasmatic tail of the TSH receptor have been described in 33.3% of patients with toxic multinodular goiter and 16.3% with Graves' disease, and this mutation was found to result in an exaggerated cAMP response to TSH [263].

Effects of TSH

TSH action on the receptor results in activation of the adenylate cyclase pathway and to some extent the phosphatidylinositol pathway, as described above, and leads to the activation of multiple proteins, including JAK/STAT [255], mTOR/S6K1 [256] and cell cycle-related proteins [264]. Proteins phosphorylated by the protein kinase C pathway appear to be different from those phosphorylated by protein kinase A [265]. In addition, phosphoprotein phosphatases are activated and lead to the dephosphorylation of another set of proteins [266]. The effects of TSH on the thyroid gland include changes in thyroid gland growth, cell morphology, iodine metabolism and synthesis of thyroid hormone.

Effects of TSH on Thyroid Gland Development and Growth

Embryologic development of the thyroid gland appears to be independent of TSH, as shown by experiments using knock out mice deficient in TSH and TSH receptor in which the size and follicular structure, as well as thyroid-specific transcription factor expression and thyroglobulin production, were similar to wild-type [265]. However, expression of thyroperoxidase and sodium/iodine symporter and maintenance of thyroid gland architecture after birth is severely affected in these mice. In the adult thyroid gland, TSH is the main regulator of thyroid gland growth. After long-term stimulation by TSH, the thyroid gland enlarges as a result of hyperplasia and hypertrophy. Acutely, TSH has a rapid mitogenic effect on the thyroid gland that is evident within 5 minutes [267]. It increases DNA synthesis through the adenylate cyclase pathway [268], specifically through activation of protein kinase A type I [269]. TSH may also regulate growth by cAMP-independent pathways [270], such as the mTOR/S6K1 pathway [256], and interactions with the action of the growth factors epidermal growth factor (EGF) and insulin-like growth factor-I (IGF-I) [271,272]. It has been found that TSH increases the transcription of specific immediate early genes in rat thyroid cells [273]. TSH also inhibits apoptosis [274], perhaps by regulating p53 and bcl-2, as shown for gonadotropins [275,276]. Mutations within the α33–44 region were found to reduce growth stimulation but not affect cAMP production [277], although a clear dissociation of the various actions by TSH analogues has not yet been achieved.

Effects of TSH on Thyroid Cell Morphology

TSH causes dramatic changes in the morphology of the thyroid [278]. The initial response to TSH is the incorporation of exocytotic vesicles into the cell membrane at the apical pole of the follicular cells that is quickly followed by formation of cytoplasmatic projections and microvilli. The number of cytoplasmatic projections has been correlated with the level of TSH [279]. After stimulation, the follicular cells become columnar and filled with colloid droplets and luminal colloid is nearly depleted, collapsing the follicles. Lysosomes migrate from the basal pole toward the apical pole where they fuse with the colloid droplets and then migrate toward the basal pole, becoming smaller and denser. The cytoskeletal system, that includes myosin, actin, tropomyosin, calmodulin, profilin and tubulin, has been implicated in this process [278,280].

Effects of TSH on Iodine Metabolism

As stated above, TSH is necessary for sodium/iodide symporter and thyroid peroxidase espression both during embryogenesis and after birth [265]. TSH primarily regulates post-transcriptional activation of the sodium–iodide symporter via the adenylate cyclase pathway [281]. Thyroid peroxidase transcription and mRNA stability are increased by TSH also through the adenylate cyclase pathway [282]. However, generation of peroxide and iodide organification appear to be mediated by a phosphatidylinositol pathway independent of protein kinase C [283].

Effects of TSH on the Synthesis of Thyroid Hormone

The end-point of TSH action is the production of thyroid hormone by the thyroid gland. The process begins with thyroglobulin gene transcription, which in itself is able to occur independently of TSH [284]. However, the transcriptional rate and possibly the mRNA stability are increased by TSH [285]. TSH regulates the expression and activation of Rab5a and Rab7, which are rate-limiting catalysts of thyroglobulin internalization and transfer to lysosomes [286]. TSH stimulates iodide uptake and organification, as described above. TSH then acts on the iodinated thyroglobulin stored in the luminal colloid and stimulates its hydrolysis resulting in the release of the constituent amino acids, including the iodothyronines T_3 and T_4.

TSH-induced Receptor Desensitization

The phenomenon of desensitization, whereby prior TSH stimulation leads to a decrease in the subsequent cAMP response to TSH stimulation, is mediated by cAMP [215]. Studies using recombinant TSH receptor have shown that desensitization does not occur when the receptor is expressed in nonthyroidal cells, suggesting that this phenomenon requires a cell-specific factor [287].

Extrathyroidal Actions of TSH

The occurrence of precocious puberty in cases of severe juvenile primary hypothyroidism has suggested that high levels of TSH are able to cross-activate the gonadotropin receptors. This interaction has now been demonstrated using recombinant human TSH, which has been found to be capable of activating the FSH [288] but not the CG/LH receptor [289].

Expression of thyrotropin receptor has been reported in the brain [290] and pituitary gland [291]. In the brain, both astrocytes and neuronal cells were found to express TSH receptor mRNA and protein [290], and stimulated arachidonic acid release and type II 5′-iodothyronine-deiodinase activity [292]. In the pituitary gland, the TSH receptor was localized to folliculo-stellate cells and may be involved in paracrine feedback inhibition of TSH secretion that may also occur in response to TSH receptor autoantibodies [291,293].

Expression of both TSH and its receptor has been reported in lymphocytes [294], erythrocytes [295], adipose tissue [296], bone [297], hair follicle [298], liver [299], ovary [300] and thyroid C cells [301]. Interestingly, a recently identified glycoprotein hormone, thyrostimulin, has been found to be produced in a variety of tissues and to be able to activate the TSH receptor [302,303], and this may suggest a paracrine mechanism of regulation. More studies are needed to determine the physiological significance of the extrathyroidal effects mediated by the TSH receptor, as this may impact the safety of future treatment modalities for thyroid cancer that may attempt to target radioisotopes to the TSH receptor [304].

TSH MEASUREMENTS

Accurate and specific measurements of serum TSH concentrations have become the most important method for diagnosing and treating the vast majority of thyroid disorders. Initially, the radioimmunoassays were very insensitive and could only detect high levels seen in primary hypothyroidism [305]. Modifications subsequently led to improved sensitivity and specificity enabling detection of TSH levels as low as 0.5−1.0 mU/L. These were called "first-generation assays." One hundred percent of primary hypothyroid subjects had elevated TSH levels but these "first-generation assays" could not accurately quantitate values within the normal range and there was considerable overlap with the values found in euthyroid and hyperthyroid subjects. The subsequent development of monoclonal antibody technology allowed two or more antibodies with precise epitope specificity to be used in sandwich-type assays that were subsequently called immunometric assays [306,307]. One or more of the monoclonal antibodies are labeled and are called the "signal antibodies." The signal may be isotopic, chemiluminescent, or enzymatic. Another monoclonal antibody with completely different epitope specificity is attached to a solid support and is called the "capture antibody." All antibodies are used in excess and therefore all TSH molecules in a sample are captured and the signal generated is directly proportional to the level of TSH.

These modifications in the measurement of TSH resulted in important changes. First, the assays were highly specific with no crossreaction to the other human glycoprotein hormones. Second, 100% of euthyroid controls have detectable and quantifiable levels of TSH. Third, there is little or no overlap in TSH values in patients with hyperthyroidism compared to euthyroid controls. The degree to which a given assay can separate undetectable TSH levels found in hyperthyroid subjects from normal values in euthyroid controls has improved steadily [305]. These improvements have resulted in progressively lower functional detection limits, defined as the lowest TSH value detected with an interassay coefficient of variation $\leq$20%. Thus, first-generation assays (usually radioimmunoassays) have functional detection limits of 0.5−1.0 mU/L, second-generation assays 0.1−0.2 mU/L, third-generation assays 0.01−0.02 mU/L and fourth-generation assays 0.001−0.002 mU/L. At the present time, the most sensitive commercially available TSH assays are third-generation assays.

In commercially available TSH assays, the normal range is typically reported as between approximately 0.3 and 4.0−5.0 mU/L. Recent data cast doubts on this broad normal range, suggesting that the upper normal range is skewed by the inclusion of subjects with incipient thyroid dysfunction [308,309]. This leads to the conclusion that the true normal range is narrower, with an upper limit of normal of 3.0−4.0 mU/L. However, this assumption is controversial, with other data suggesting that TSH levels rise with age, thereby explaining the skewed upper limit of normal [310].

Although the population normal range for serum TSH levels is relatively broad, within an individual subject TSH levels are more tightly regulated around an endogenous set-point. In a recent study of monthly sampling over a year in healthy euthyroid subjects, the significant difference in serum TSH levels on repeated testing was only 0.75 mU/L, far less than the population normal range [311]. It is not clear what determines this individual set-point, although studies of monozygotic and dizygotic twins suggest that it is primarily genetically determined [312]. Genetic analysis has revealed a number of significant linkage peaks, but no single gene appears to have a major regulatory influence, and the regulation of the TSH set-point is likely polygenic [194,313]. The main environmental factor that affects TSH levels in healthy euthyroid subjects appears to be iodine intake [314].

Free TSH β- and α-subunit Measurements

TSH β- and α-subunits were purified in 1974 from human TSH and specific antibodies to them developed [315]. Radioimmunoassays were first developed and then immunometric assays for the free α-subunit. In general, free TSHβ levels are detectable only in primary hypothyroidism and therefore are of limited utility. Free α-subunit levels have been useful in the evaluation of pituitary and placental disease. Free α-subunit is detectable and measurable in both euthyroid and eugonadal human subjects [316]. Elevated values of free α-subunit are found in the sera of patients with TSH-secreting or gonadotropin-secreting pituitary tumors [317], choriocarcinoma [318], and in a variety of nonpituitary and nonplacental malignancies including cancers of the lung, pancreas, stomach, prostate and ovary [319,320].

Provocative Testing of TSH

TRH directly stimulates TSH biosynthesis and secretion. Given intravenously, intramuscularly, or orally, TRH causes a reproducible rise in serum TSH levels in euthyroid subjects [169]. In euthyroid subjects, there is an immediate release of TSH rising to peak levels approximately 20–30 min after TRH injection, usually reaching values 5–10-fold higher than basal (Figure 6.10). In hyperthyroid subjects undetectable basal serum TSH levels correlate with absent TSH responses to TRH. Patients with low basal serum TSH levels secondary to pituitary or hypothalamic insufficiency have absent or attenuated TSH responses to TRH [322]. Patients with elevated TSH levels due to primary hypothyroidism have exuberant responses to TRH stimulation, while elevated TSH levels in patients with pituitary TSH-secreting tumors respond less than two-fold to TRH stimulation.

Drugs and TSH Levels

Among the most common causes of abnormal TSH levels are pharmacological interventions which alter TSH production. These can be divided into those that directly affect hypothalamic–pituitary function, those that affect thyroid gland function, and those that alter the distribution of thyroid hormones between the free and protein-bound thyroid hormones in plasma. Only the drugs that directly affect TSH synthesis and/or secretion will be considered further here.

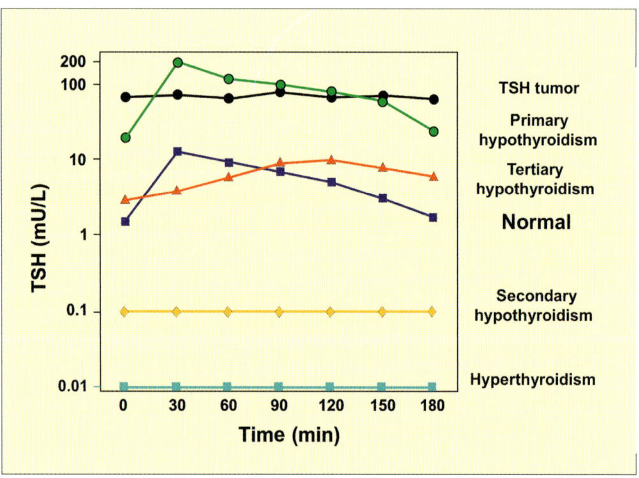

FIGURE 6.10 Schematic representation of thyrotropin-releasing hormone (TRH) stimulation tests in patients with a variety of thyroid disorders. TRH was administered at time 0. Serum samples of TSH were collected at baseline and every 30 minutes for 3 hours. Subjects with different disorders are indicated on the right. *From L.J. De Groot and J.L. Jameson (Eds), Endocrinology, 6th edn, Elsevier. Chapter 73 Thyroid-stimulating hormone: Physiology and secretion, Figure 7.*

Drugs that Decrease Serum TSH Levels

Clinically, the most important drug that results in decreased serum TSH levels is exogenously administered thyroid hormone. Twenty to thirty percent of patients treated with thyroid hormone have low serum TSH levels, most fitting the diagnostic criteria for subclinical hyperthyroidism. Thyroid hormone analogues such as TRIAC have the same effect in decreasing TSH secretion [323]. An interesting recent finding has been the discovery that RXR analogues such as bexaroten, used in the treatment of cutaneous lymphoma, can decrease TSHβ transcription, serum TSH and T_4 levels with resultant central hypothyroidism [105]. Exogenous glucocorticoids, somatostatin and its analogues, and dopamine and its analogues all directly lower TSH production, as discussed in more detail in previous sections. Interestingly, although these drugs acutely decrease TSH production, chronic administration usually results in compensatory mechanisms that prevent clinical hypothyroidism from developing. Growth hormone administration stimulating IGF-1 production may decrease TSH levels by stimulation of endogenous hypothalamic somatostatin production [178]. Exogenous leptin administration can stimulate hypothalamic TRH production resulting in higher TSH levels [202,204]. Cytokine administration (interferon and interleukins) commonly suppresses TSH levels, which has been thought to be mediated through stimulation of endogenous glucocorticoids. However, a novel alternative mechanism postulates that cytokines stimulate hypothalamic NfκB production and this protein directly increases deiodinase 2 gene transcription in astrocytes leading to increased T_4 to T_3 conversion, TRH suppression and central hypothyroidism [208–210]. Drugs affecting the serotonin pathway (the serotonin receptor antagonist cyproheptadine and the serotonin reuptake inhibitors sertraline and fluoxetine) have been reported to decrease TSH production in animal studies, but in human studies these drugs have not been shown to have a significant effect on TSH levels [324,325]. A similar lack of effect on the TSH level was found after administration of histamine receptor blockers (cimetidine and ranitidine) and benzodiazepines [326,327]. In contrast, the α-adrenergic blocker thymoxamine, used topically as an ophthalmologic agent, has been found to decrease TSH secretion when administered systemically [328].

Drugs that Increase Serum TSH Levels

A sustained increase in TSH production by direct stimulation of either the hypothalamus or pituitary is very unusual. TRH administration is the most potent but can be completely attenuated by subsequent rises in circulating thyroid hormones. The opioid class of drugs, including morphine, apomorphine, heroin, buprenorphine and pentazocine, have all been associated with increases in TSH levels [191]. Theophylline and amphetamines may directly stimulate hypothalamic TRH or pituitary TSH production [329,330]. The dopamine receptor antagonist metochlopramide increases TSH release by decreasing dopaminergic tone and thereby inhibiting tonic suppression of TSH by endogenous dopamine [181]. Certain neuroleptics, such as chlorpromazine, have been reported to increase TSH levels, although the circulating thyroid hormone levels are lower, suggesting a secondary effect [331].

DISORDERS OF TSH PRODUCTION

Acquired TSH Deficiency

TSH deficiency resulting in hypothyroidism ("central hypothyroidism") can occur due to destructive processes in the anterior pituitary ("secondary hypothyroidism") or hypothalamus ("tertiary hypothyroidism") (Table 6.1). These destructive processes include infiltrative or infectious disorders, compressive neoplastic processes, and ischemic or hemorrhagic processes. The most common causes of acquired pituitary TSH deficiency are compression of normal anterior pituitary cells by a pituitary neoplasm, craniopharyngioma, or metastatic tumor. These processes can also extend into the hypothalamus and interrupt normal TRH production. Multiple pituitary deficiencies are present, including LH, FSH, GH and usually ACTH deficiency. Central hypothyroidism is manifested by low serum free T_4 and T_3 levels, generally in association with a low or normal basal TSH level, although in tertiary hypothyroidism the TSH may be minimally elevated [322], in which case the circulating TSH is biologically defective [332]. The 24-hour secretory profile of TSH in patients with tertiary hypothyroidism is also abnormal [160]. The frequency of the TSH pulses is the same as euthyroid controls, but the amplitude of the pulses is decreased, particularly at nighttime, resulting in a loss of the normal nocturnal surge (Figure 6.7, bottom panel).

TABLE 6.1 Causes of Central Hypothyroidism

NEOPLASTIC
Pituitary adenoma
Craniopharyngioma
Metastatic tumor
Dysgerminoma
Meningioma
INFILTRATIVE
Sarcoidosis
Histiocytosis X
Eosinophilic granuloma
TRAUMATIC
Radiation
Head injury
Post surgical
INFECTIOUS
Tuberculosis
Fungus
Virus
VASCULAR
Stalk interruption
Necrosis
CONGENITAL
Midline defects
Rathke's pouch cysts
Genetic mutations

Congenital TSH Deficiency

Congenital causes of TSH deficiency (Table 6.1) include developmental abnormalities, such as midline defects and Rathke's pouch cysts, which will not be discussed in this chapter, and genetic mutations. The latter may result in isolated TSH deficiency or may affect other pituitary hormones. Isolated TSH deficiency is generally inherited as an autosomal recessive disorder, and individuals affected with congenital hypothyroidism have severe mental and growth retardation. The molecular basis for isolated TSH deficiency has usually involved mutations in the TSHβ gene (Table 6.2). For example, a single base substitution in one family at nucleotide position 145 of the TSHβ gene altered the CAGYC region [333], a critically important contact point for the noncovalent combination of the TSH β- and α-subunits. In other kindreds, a single base substitution introduced a premature stop codon resulting in a truncated TSH β-subunit which included only the first 11 [334] amino acids. Another type of mutation involves a nonsense 25-amino acid protein resulting from mutation of a donor splice site and a new out-of-frame

TABLE 6.2 Congenital Hypothyroidism: Isolated TSH β Defects

	I	II	III	IV	V	VI
Inheritance	Autosomal recessive	Autosomal recessive	Autosomal recessive	Autosomal recessive	Autosomal recessive	Autosomal recessive
Syndrome	Cretinism	Cretinism	Cretinism	Cretinism	Cretinism	Cretinism, with phenotypic variability
Serum T_4	↓	↓	↓	↓	↓	↓
Serum TSH	None detected	None detected	Normal, ↓ or none	↓ or none	None detected	↓
Response to TRH	None detected	None detected	Impaired or none	Impaired or none	None detected	Impaired or none
Nucleotide change	Exon 2,Missense, G85A	Exon 2,Nonsense, G34T	Exon 3,Deletion, T313del	Exon 3,Nonsense,C145T	Exon 3,Missense, T256C	Intron 2 donor splice site variant IVS2 +5G→A
Protein defect	G29R Altered CAGYC region, No combination with α	E12 X Premature stop (βL1 loop region) Truncated TSHβ (11 amino acids)	C105Vfs114X Altered seat-belt region & frameshift with premature stop codon (114 amino acids)	Q49X Truncated TSHβ (48 amino acids)	C85R Unstable or no combination with α	Nonsense protein of 25 amino acids
Reported cases	5 families in Japan [79,333]	2 families in Greece [358]	Over 10 families, in Brazil [238], Germany [361,362,338,363,364], Belgium [365], Switzerland [336], Argentina [366], Portugal [361], France * [336] and USA [337,367]	Families in Egypt [359] Turkey [335], Greece [335] and France * [361]	One case in Greece [335]	3 families in Turkey [359,360]

** Compound heterozygozity for T313del (C105Vfs114X) and C145T (Q49X) in one infant.*

translational start point [335]. In other cases, the disorder involves the production of biologically inactive TSH with loss of cysteine[105] that disrupts the disulfide bridge formation important in the "seat belt" stability [336,337], and is perhaps the most common of the TSH β mutations, and the less common mutation at cysteine[85] that disrupts the cysteine knot that is important for heterodimer formation and TSH receptor binding [335,338], resulting in a similar phenotype, except that in some of these cases circulating TSH was detectable. TRH receptor mutations have also been described [339].

A more common cause of congenital TSH deficiency arises not as a result of a mutation in the TSHβ gene, but defective production of a key transcription factor necessary for TSHβ gene expression. This occurs in the syndrome known as combined pituitary hormone deficiency (CPHD). There are several types of CPHD. The first one was described in subjects with congenital hypothyroidism and growth retardation secondary to TSH and GH deficiencies [340,341]. Mutations in the coding region of the *Pou1F1* (*Pit-1*) gene alter the function of the Pou1F1 protein or completely disrupt its structure. The absence of Pou1F1 prevents normal pituitary development resulting in hypoplasia of the pituitary and deficiency of TSH, GH and prolactin that are dependent on the pituitary-specific transcription factor Pou1F1 for their expression. In heterozygotes, where a normal allele is present, the abnormal Pou1F1 protein can bind to DNA but is not able to effect transactivation, interfering with the function of the normal Pou1F1 (dominant negative mechanism). Interestingly, a similar combined hormone deficiency syndrome has been reported in two murine models in which the *POU1F1* gene is defective: a point mutation found in the Snell dwarf (dw) [11] and a major deletion in the Jackson dwarf (dwJ) [342]. The second and more frequent type of CPHD is associated to mutations in the pituitary-specific transcription factor called "prophet of Pou1F1" (PROP-1) [343,344]. Mutation of this paired-like homeodomain protein in the murine species causes the Ames dwarf (df) mouse phenotype [16]. Over 50% of families with CPHD have been shown to contain mutations in the PROP-1 gene [15], exceeding the prevalence of mutations in the *POU1F1* gene. The mutations are all found in the homeodomain region of the molecule. Interestingly, the phenotype of patients with PROP-1 mutations includes deficiencies not only of GH, prolactin and TSH, but also of LH and FSH. Furthermore, the hormone deficiencies may not be present at birth but rather progressively occur up to the age of adolescence. ACTH deficiency has also been reported as a late consequence in patients with PROP-1 mutations [345]. Finally, mutations in other early developmental genes, including *HESX1*, *SOX2*, *SOX3*, *LHX3*, *LHX4* and *OTX2* [346,347] have also been associated with the CPHD syndrome.

Acquired TSH Excess

Most cases of elevated serum TSH levels result from primary thyroid disease rather than primary pituitary disease. However, an important, although uncommon, cause is the TSH-secreting pituitary tumor. TSHomas comprise less than 1% of all pituitary tumors [348]. The patients have high levels of thyroid hormones in association with normal or high levels of TSH. The tumor cells are quite differentiated but synthesize the α-subunit in excess of the TSH β-subunit [349], so that the molar ratio of α-subunit:TSH (ng/ml of α-subunit divided by μU/ml of TSH multiplied by 10) of greater than 1 supports the diagnosis of a TSH-secreting pituitary tumor when found in a hyperthyroid and eugonadal patient. This ratio is not accurate in menopausal women, who have high gonadotropins and high free α-subunit levels. TSH-secreting tumors fail to respond to TRH stimulation and suppression by dopamine (Figure 6.11). Another characteristic of these tumors is their failure to respond to thyroid hormone by the normal negative feedback of thyroid hormone on TSH production. In contrast, inhibition of TSH release in response to somatostatin is preserved in these tumors (Figure 6.11).

Congenital TSH Excess

Two interesting disorders resulting in elevated levels of serum TSH are thyroid hormone resistance (RTH) [350,351] and resistance to TSH (RTSH) [352]. In 1967, Refetoff et al. [353] were the first to describe RTH in three siblings who were clinically euthyroid or hypothyroid with goiters, stippled epiphyses and deaf mutism. Each of the children had elevated levels of protein-bound iodide which were subsequently shown to be associated with high serum total and free thyroid hormone levels, elevated TSH levels and peripheral tissue responses that were refractory to not only the endogenous high levels of thyroid hormone, but also to exogenously administered supraphysiological levels of thyroid hormone [350]. RTH was found to be linked to the TRβ gene locus on chromosome 3, and was then localized to point mutations in the ninth and tenth exons of the TRβ gene which encode for the T_3-binding and adjacent hinge domains. These mutations usually disrupt normal T_3 binding without altering DNA binding. Most cases of RTH are heterozygotes and inherited as autosomal dominant traits, with only half of the TRβ receptors being abnormal. The overwhelming majority of mutations are single-nucleotide substitutions which change a single amino acid or introduce a stop codon. Since 1967 over 1000 cases of RTH belonging to 372 families have been identified [351]. Mutations have been found in 343 of these families and many families have the same mutation since only

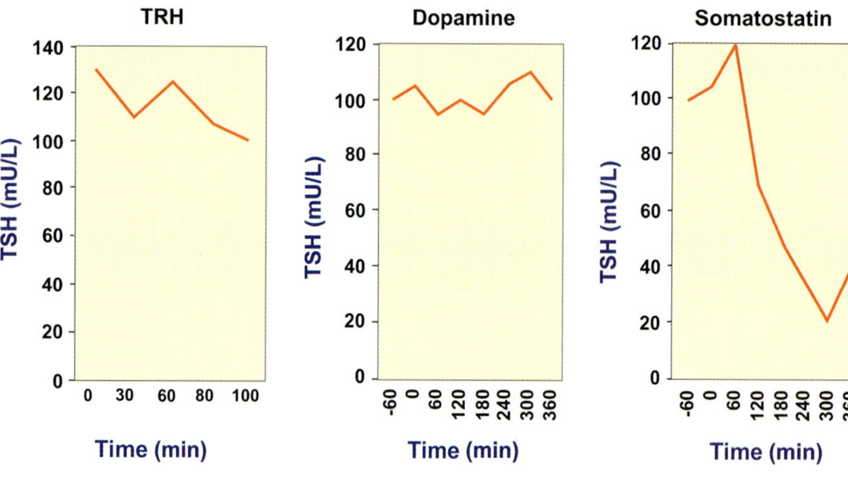

FIGURE 6.11 Thyroid-stimulating hormone (TSH) responses to various stimulation and suppression tests in a patient with a TSH pituitary tumor. Thyrotropin-releasing hormone (TRH) (500 μg intravenously) gave no response, dopamine (4 μg/minute for 4 hours) resulted in no suppression, somatostatin (500 μg bolus followed by 250 μg/minute for 4 hours) resulted in significant suppression of serum TSH levels. *From L.J. De Groot and J.L. Jameson (Eds), Endocrinology, 6th edn, Elsevier. Chapter 73 Thyroid-stimulating hormone: Physiology and secretion, Figure 8.*

124 different mutations have been identified. In about 8% of the families with RTH, a TRβ mutation has not been identified. TRα gene mutations have not been reported in RTH.

RTSH was first described by Sunthornthepvarakui et al. [352] in three siblings with very high TSH levels, normal T_4 and T_3 levels and thyroid glands of normal size. After excluding RTH with a normal response to T_3 administration, sequencing of the TSH receptor revealed compound heterozygous mutations, with a different abnormal allele from each parent. Other mutations in the TSH receptor have since been found [254,355,356], with a prevalence of 29% in a group of 38 children with nonautoimmune subclinical hypothyroidism who were normal at neonatal screening [357].

References

[1] T. Kouki, H. Imai, K. Aoto, K. Eto, S. Shioda, K. Kawamura, et al., Developmental origin of the rat adenohypophysis prior to the formation of Rathke's pouch, Development 128 (2001) 959–963.

[2] M. Treier, A.S. Gleiberman, S.M. O'Connell, D.P. Szeto, J.A. McMahon, A.P. McMahon, et al., Multistep signaling requirements for pituitary organogenesis in vivo, Genes Dev 12 (1998) 1691–1704.

[3] X. Zhu, A.S. Gleiberman, M.G. Rosenfeld, Molecular physiology of pituitary development: Signaling and transcriptional networks, Physiol Rev 87 (2007) 933–963.

[4] J.S. Dasen, M.G. Rosenfeld, Signaling and transcriptional mechanisms in pituitary development, Annu Rev Neurosci 24 (2001) 327–355.

[5] L.T. Raetzman, R. Ward, S.A. Camper, Lhx4 and Prop1 are required for cell survival and expansion of the pituitary primordia, Development 129 (2002) 4229–4239.

[6] J.S. Dasen, S.M. O'Connell, S.E. Flynn, M. Treier, A.S. Gleiberman, D.P. Szeto, et al., Reciprocal interactions of Pit1 and GATA2 mediate signaling gradient-induced determination of pituitary cell types, Cell 97 (1999) 587–598.

[7] J. Ericson, S. Norlin, T.M. Jessell, T. Edlund, Integrated FGF and BMP signaling controls the progression of progenitor cell differentiation and the emergence of pattern in the embryonic anterior pituitary, Development 125 (1998) 1005–1015.

[8] J.W. Voss, M.G. Rosenfeld, Anterior pituitary development: short tales from dwarf mice, Cell 70 (1992) 527–530.

[9] D.W. Drolet, K.M. Scully, D.M. Simmons, M. Wegner, K. Chu, L.W. Swanson, et al., TEF, a transcription factor expressed specifically in the anterior pituitary during embryogenesis, defines a new class of leucine zipper proteins, Genes and Development 5 (1991) 1739–1753.

[10] D.M. Simmons, J.W. Voss, J.M. Holloway, R.S. Broide, M.G. Rosenfeld, L.W. Swanson, Pituitary cell phenotypes involve cell-specific Pit-1 mRNA translation and synergistic interactions with other classes of transcription factors, Genes and Development 4 (1990) 695–711.

[11] S.A. Camper, T.L. Saunders, R.W. Katz, R.H. Reeves, The Pit-1 transcription factor gene is a candidate for the murine Snell dwarf mutation, Genomics 8 (1990) 586–590.

[12] K. Tatsumi, K. Miyai, T. Notomi, K. Kaibe, N. Amino, Y. Mizuno, et al., Cretinism with combined hormone deficiency caused by a mutation in the PIT1 gene, Nat Genet 1 (1992) 56–58.

[13] S. Radovick, M. Nations, Y. Du, L.A. Berg, B.D. Weintraub, F.E. Wondisford, A mutation in the POU-homeodomain of Pit-1 responsible for combined pituitary hormone deficiency, Science 257 (1992) 1115–1118.

[14] K.W. Sloop, B.C. Meier, J.L. Bridwell, G.E. Parker, A.M. Schiller, S.J. Rhodes, Differential activation of pituitary hormone genes by human Lhx3 isoforms with distinct DNA binding properties, Mol Endocrinol 13 (1999) 2212–2225.

[15] J. Deladoey, C. Fluck, A. Buyukgebiz, B.V. Kuhlmann, A. Eble, P.C. Hindmarsh, et al., "Hot spot" in the PROP1 gene responsible for combined pituitary hormone deficiency, J Clin Endocrinol Metab 84 (1999) 1645–1650.

[16] M.W. Sornson, W. Wu, J.S. Dasen, S.E. Flynn, D.J. Norman, S.M. O'Connell, et al., Pituitary lineage detemination by the Prophet of Pit-1 homeodomain factor defective in Ames dwarfism, Nature 384 (1996) 327–333.

[17] Y. Qi, J.A. Ranish, X. Zhu, A. Krones, J. Zhang, R. Aebersold, et al., Atbf1 is required for the Pit1 gene early activation, Proc Nat Acad Sci USA 105 (2008) 2481–2486.

[18] D.J. Steger, J.H. Hecht, P.L. Mellon, GATA-binding proteins regulate the human gonadotropin alpha-subunit gene in the placenta and pituitary gland, Mol Cell Biol 14 (1994) 5592–5602.

[19] D.F. Gordon, W.M. Wood, E.C. Ridgway, Organization and nucleotide sequence of the mouse alpha-subunit gene of the pituitary glycoprotein hormones, DNA 7 (1988) 679–690.

[20] M.A. Charles, T.L. Saunders, W.M. Wood, K. Owens, A.F. Parlow, S.A. Camper, et al., Pituitary-specific gata2 knockout: Effects on gonadotrope and thyrotrope function, Mol Endocrinol 20 (2006) 1366–1377.

[21] A.S. Gleiberman, T. Michurina, J.M. Encinas, J.L. Roig, P. Krasnov, F. Balordi, et al., Genetic approaches identify adult pituitary stem cells, Proc Nat Acad Sci USA 105 (2008) 6332–6337.

[22] T. Fauquier, K. Rizzoti, M. Dattani, R. Lovell-Badge, I.C. Robinson, SOX2-expressing progenitor cells generate all of the major cell types in the adult mouse pituitary gland, Proc Nat Acad Sci USA 105 (2008) 2907–2912.

[23] M.L. Brinkmeier, J.H. Stahl, D.F. Gordon, B.D. Ross, V.D. Sarapura, J.M. Dowding, et al., Thyroid hormone-responsive pituitary hyperplasia independent of somatostatin receptor 2, Mol Endocrinol 15 (2001) 2129–2136.

[24] F.E. Wondisford, S. Radovick, J.M. Moates, S.J. Usala, B.D. Weintraub, Isolation and characterization of the human thyrotropin beta-subunit gene: Differences in gene structure and promoter function from murine species, J Biol Chem 263 (1988) 12538–12542.

[25] N.C. Dracopoli, W.J. Rettig, G.K. Whitfield, G.J. Darlington, B.A. Spengler, J.L. Biedler, et al., Assignment of the gene for the beta subunit of thyroid-stimulating hormone to the short arm of human chromosome 1, Proc Nat Acad Sci USA 83 (1986) 1822–1826.

[26] W.M. Wood, M.Y. Kao, D.F. Gordon, E.C. Ridgway, Thyroid hormone regulates the mouse thyrotropin beta subunit gene promoter in transfected primary thyrotropes, J Biol Chem 264 (1989) 14840–14847.

[27] B.R. Haugen, M.T. McDermott, D.F. Gordon, C.L. Rupp, W.M. Wood, E.C. Ridgway, Determinants of thyrotrope-specific TSH-beta promoter activation: Cooperation of Pit-1 with another factor, J Biol Chem 271 (1996) 385–389.

[28] S.A. Camper, T.L. Saunders, S.K. Kendall, R.A. Keri, A.F. Seasholtz, D.F. Gordon, et al., Implementing transgenic and embryonic stem cell technology to study gene expression, cell–cell interactions and gene function, Biol Reprod 52 (1995) 246–257.

[29] W.M. Wood, K.W. Ocran, M.Y. Kao, D.F. Gordon, L.M. Alexander, A. Gutierrez-Hartmann, et al., Protein factors in thyrotropic tumor nuclear extracts bind to a region of the mouse thyrotropin beta-subunit promoter essential for expression in thyrotropes, Mol Endocrinol 4 (1990) 1897–1904.

[30] D.F. Gordon, E.A. Tucker, K. Tundwal, H. Hall, W.M. Wood, E.C. Ridgway, MED220/thyroid receptor-associated protein 220 functions as a transcriptional coactivator with Pit-1 and GATA-2 on the thyrotropin-beta promoter in thyrotropes, Mol Endocrinol 20 (2006) 1073–1089.

[31] C.X. Yuan, M. Ito, J.D. Fondell, Z.Y. Fu, R.G. Roeder, The TRAP220 component of a thyroid hormone receptor-associated protein (TRAP) coactivator complex interacts directly with nuclear receptors in a ligand-dependent fashion, Proc Nat Acad Sci USA 95 (1998) 7939–7944.

[32] M. Ito, C.X. Yuan, H.J. Okano, R.B. Darnell, R.G. Roeder, Involvement of the TRAP220 component of the TRAP/SMCC coactivator complex in embryonic development and thyroid hormone action, Mol Cell 5 (2000) 683–693.

[33] D.F. Gordon, E.A. Tucker, K. Tundwal, H. Hall, W.M. Wood, E.C. Ridgway, MED220/thyroid receptor-associated protein 220 functions as a transcriptional coactivator with Pit-1 and GATA-2 on the thyrotropin-beta promoter in thyrotropes, Mol Endocrinol 20 (2003) 1073–1089.

[34] S.L. Naylor, W.W. Chin, H.M. Goodman, P.A. Lalley, K.H. Grzeshik, A.Y. Sakaguchi, Chromosomal assignment of genes encoding the alpha and beta subunits of glycoprotein hormones in man and mouse, Somat Cell Genet 9 (1983) 757–770.

[35] J.C. Fiddes, H.M. Goodman, The gene encoding the common alpha subunit of the four human glycoprotein hormones, J Mol Appl Genet 1 (1981) 3–18.

[36] M.L. Brinkmeier, D.F. Gordon, J.M. Dowding, T.L. Saunders, S.K. Kendall, V.D. Sarapura, et al., Cell specific expression of the mouse glycoprotein hormone alpha-subunit gene requires multiple interacting DNA elements in transgenic mice and cultured cells, Mol Endocrinol 12 (1998) 622–633.

[37] S.K. Kendall, D.F. Gordon, T.S. Birkmeier, D. Petrey, V.D. Sarapura, K.S. O'Shea, et al., Enhancer-mediated high level expression of mouse pituitary glycoprotein hormone alpha-subunit transgene in thyrotropes, gonadotropes, and developing pituitary gland, Mol Endocrinol 8 (1994) 1420–1433.

[38] J.L. Jameson, R.C. Jaffe, P.J. Deutsch, C. Albanese, J.F. Habener, The gonadotropin alpha-gene contains multiple protein binding domains that interact to modulate basal and cAMP-responsive transcription, J Biol Chem 263 (1988) 9879–9886.

[39] F. Horn, J.J. Windle, K.M. Barnhart, P.L. Mellon, Tissue-specific gene expression in the pituitary: The glycoprotein hormone alpha-subunit gene is regulated by a gonadotrope-specific protein, Mol Cell Biol 12 (1992) 2143–2153.

[40] V.D. Sarapura, W.M. Wood, D.F. Gordon, K.W. Ocran, M.Y. Kao, E.C. Ridgway, Thyrotrope expression and thyroid hormone inhibition map to different regions of the mouse glycoprotein hormone alpha-subunit promoter, Endocrinology 127 (1990) 1352–1361.

[41] A.M. Delegeane, L.H. Ferland, P.L. Mellon, Tissue-specific enhancer of the human glycoprotein alpha-subunit gene: Dependence on cyclic AMP-inducible elements, Mol Cell Biol 7 (1987) 3994–4002.

[42] J.P. Hoeffler, T.E. Meyer, Y. Yun, J.L. Jameson, J.F. Habener, Cyclic AMP-responsive DNA-binding protein: Structure based on a cloned placental cDNA, Science 242 (1988) 1430–1433.

[43] B. Andersen, G.C. Kennedy, J.H. Nilson, A cis-acting element located between the cAMP response elements and CCAAT box augments cell-specific expression of the glycoprotein hormone alpha subunit gene, J Biol Chem 265 (1990) 21874–21880.

[44] G.C. Kennedy, B. Andersen, J.H. Nilson, The human alpha subunit glycoprotein hormone gene utilizes a unique CCAAT binding factor, J Biol Chem 265 (1990) 6279–6285.

[45] K.M. Barnhart, P.L. Mellon, The orphan nuclear receptor, steroidogenic factor-1, regulates the glycoprotein hormone alpha-subunit gene in pituitary gonadotropes, Mol Endocrinol 8 (1994) 878–885.

[46] W.M. Wood, J.M. Dowding, V.D. Sarapura, M.T. McDermott, D.F. Gordon, E.C. Ridgway, Functional interactions of an upstream enhancer of the mouse glycoprotein hormone alpha-subunit gene with proximal promoter sequences, Mol Cell Endocrinol 142 (1998) 141–152.

[47] S.M. Jackson, A. Gutierrez-Hartmann, J.P. Hoeffler, Upstream stimulatory factor, a basic-helix-loop-helix-zipper protein, regulates the activity of the alpha-glycoprotein hormone subunit gene in pituitary cells, Mol Endocrinol 9 (1995) 278–291.

[48] S.K. Kendall, T.L. Saunders, L. Jin, R.V. Lloyd, L.M. Glode, T.M. Nett, et al., Targeted ablation of pituitary gonadotropes in transgenic mice, Mol Endocrinol 5 (1991) 2025–2036.

[49] V.D. Sarapura, H.L. Strouth, W.M. Wood, D.F. Gordon, E.C. Ridgway, Activation of the glycoprotein hormone alpha-subunit gene promoter in thyrotropes, Mol Cell Endocrinol 146 (1998) 77–86.

[50] V.D. Sarapura, D.F. Gordon, H.L. Strouth, WM, E.C. Ridgway, Msx1 is present in thyrotropic cells and binds to a consensus site on the glycoprotein hormone alpha-subunit promoter, Mol Endocrinol 11 (1997) 1782–1794.

[51] M.S. Roberson, W.E. Schoderbek, G. Tremml, R.A. Maurer, Activation of the glycoprotein hormone alpha-subunit promoter by a LIM-homeodomain transcription factor, Mol Cell Biol 14 (1994) 2985–2993.
[52] I. Bach, S.J. Rhodes, Pearse II, T. Heinzel, B. Gloss, K.M. Scully, et al., P-Lim, a LIM homeodomain factor, is expressed during pituitary organ and cell commitment and synergizes with Pit-1, Proc Nat Acad Sci USA 92 (1995) 2720–2724.
[53] H.Z. Sheng, A.B. Zhadanov, B. Mosinger, T. Fujii, S. Bertuzzi, A. Grinberg, et al., Specification of pituitary cell lineages by the lim homeobox gene Lhx3, Science 272 (1996) 1004–1007.
[54] M.S. Roberson, A. Misra-Press, M.E. Laurance, P.J. Stork, R.A. Maurer, A role for mitogen-activated protein kinase in mediating activation of the glycoprotein hormone alpha-subunit promoter by gonadotropin-releasing hormone, Mol Cell Biol 15 (1995) 3531–3539.
[55] I. Bach, C. Carriere, H.P. Ostendorff, B. Andersen, M.G. Rosenfeld, A family of LIM domain-associated cofactors confer transcriptional synergism between LIM and Otx homeodomain proteins, Genes and Development 11 (1997) 1370–1380.
[56] W.M. Wood, J.M. Dowding, D.F. Gordon, E.C. Ridgway, An upstream regulator of the glycoprotein hormone alpha-subunit gene mediates pituitary cell type activation and repression by different mechanisms, J Biol Chem 274 (1999) 15526–15532.
[57] B.D. Weintraub, N. Gesundheit, Thyroid-stimulating hormone synthesis and glycosylation: Clinical implications, Thyroid Today 10 (1987) 1–11.
[58] J.C. Fiddes, K. Talmadge, Structure, expression and evolution of the genes for the human glycoprotein hormones, Recent Prog Horm Res 40 (1984) 43–78.
[59] J.G. Pierce, T.F. Parsons, Glycoprotein hormones: Structure and function, Annu Rev Biochem 50 (1981) 465–495.
[60] K. Takata, S. Watanabe, M. Hirono, M. Tamaki, H. Teraoka, Y. Hayashizaki, The role of the carboxyl-terminal 6 amino acid extension of human TSH-beta subunit, Biochem Biophys Res Commun 165 (1989) 1035–1042.
[61] N.R. Thotakura, L. LiCalzi, B.D. Weintraub, The role of carbohydrate in thyrotropin action assessed by a novel method of enzymatic deglycosylation, J Biol Chem 265 (1990) 11527–11534.
[62] J.A. Magner, B.D. Weintraub, Thyroid-stimulating hormone subunit processing and combination in microsomal subfractions of mouse pituitary tumor, J Biol Chem 257 (1982) 6709–6715.
[63] T.F. Parsons, G.A. Bloomfield, J.G. Pierce, Purification of an alternative form of the alpha subunit of the glycoprotein hormones from bovine pituitaries and identification of its O-linked oligosaccharides, J Biol Chem 258 (1983) 240–244.
[64] R. Kornfeld, S. Kornfeld, Assembly of asparagine-linked oligosaccharides, Annu Rev Biochem 54 (1985) 631–664.
[65] J.A. Magner, Thyroid stimulating hormone: Biosynthesis, cell biology, and bioactivity, Endoc Rev 11 (1990) 354–385.
[66] N.R. Thotakura, R.K. Desai, L.G. Bates, E.S. Cole, B.M. Pratt, B.D. Weintraub, Biological activity and metabolic clearance of a recombinant human thyrotropin produced in Chinese hamster ovary cells, Endocrinology 128 (1991) 341–348.
[67] B.D. Weintraub, B.S. Stannard, L. Meyers, Glycosylation of thyroid-stimulating hormone in pituitary cells: Influence of high mannose oligosaccharide units on subunit aggregation, combination, and intracellular degradation, Endocrinology 112 (1983) 1331–1345.
[68] A.J. Lapthorn, D.C. Harris, A. Littlejohn, J.W. Lustbader, R.E. Canfield, K.J. Machin, et al., Crystal structure of human chorionic gonadotropin, Nature 369 (1994) 455–461.
[69] M.W. Szkudlinski, N.G. Teh, M. Grossmann, J.E. Tropea, B.D. Weintraub, Engineering human glycoprotein hormone superactive analogs, Nat Biotechnol 14 (1996) 1257–1263.
[70] W.D. Fairlie, P.G. Stanton, M.T.W. Hearn, The disulphide bond structure of thyroid-stimulating hormone beta-subunit, Biochem J 314 (1996) 449–455.
[71] C.T. Weller, J. Lustbader, K. Seshadri, J.M. Brown, C.A. Chadwick, C.E. Kolthoff, et al., Structural and conformational analysis of glycan moieties in situ on isotopically 13C,15N-enriched human chorionic gonadotropin, Biochemistry 35 (1996) 8815–8823.
[72] P.D. Sun, D.R. Davies, The cystine-knot growth factor superfamily, Ann Rev Biophys Biomol Struct 24 (1995) 269–291.
[73] B.D. Weintraub, B.S. Stannard, D. Linnekin, M. Marshall, Relationship of glycosylation to de novo thyroid-stimulating hormone biosynthesis and secretion by mouse pituitary tumor cells, J Biol Chem 255 (1980) 5715–5723.
[74] M. Grossmann, M.W. Szkudlinski, J.E. Tropea, L.A. Bishop, N.R. Thotakura, P.R. Schofield, et al., Expression of human thyrotropin in cell lines with different glycosylation patterns combined with mutagenesis of specific glycosylation sites. Characterization of a novel role for the oligosaccharides in the in vitro and in vivo bioactivity, J Biol Chem. 270 (1995) 29378–29385.
[75] J.A. Magner, E. Papagiannes, Structures of high-mannose oligosaccharides of mouse thyrotropin: Differential processing of alpha- versus beta-subunits of the heterodimer, Endocrinology 120 (1987) 10–17.
[76] R.S. Weiner, J.A. Dias, Biochemical analyses of proteolytic nicking of the human glycoprotein hormone alpha-subunit and its effect on conformational epitopes, Endocrinology 131 (1992) 1026–1036.
[77] M. Grossmann, B.D. Weintraub, M.W. Szkudlinski, Novel Insights into the Molecular Mechanisms of human thyrotropin action: Structural, physiological, and therapeutic implications for the glycoprotein hormone family, Endocr Rev 18 (1997) 476–501.
[78] Y. Xing, R.V. Myers, D. Cao, W. Lin, M. Jiang, M.P. Bernard, et al., Glycoprotein hormone assembly in the endoplasmic reticulum. I. The glycosylated end of human alpha-subunit loop 2 is threaded through a beta-subunit hole, J Biol Chem 279 (2004) 35426–35436.
[79] Y. Hayashizaki, Y. Hiraoka, Y. Endo, K. Miyai, K. Matsubara, Thyroid-stimulating hormone (TSH) deficiency caused by a single base substitution in the CAGYC region of the beta-subunit, EMBO J 8 (1989) 2291–2296.
[80] M.M. Matzuk, C.M. Kornmeier, G.K. Whitfield, I.A. Kourides, I. Boime, The glycoprotein hormone alpha-subunit is critical for secretion and stability of the human thyrotropin beta-subunit, Mol Endocrinol 2 (1988) 95–100.
[81] R.W. Lash, R.K. Desai, C.A. Zimmerman, M.R. Flack, T. Yoshida, F.E. Wondisford, et al., Mutations of the human thyrotropin beta-subunit glycosylation site reduce thyrotropin synthesis independent of changes in glycosylation status, J Endocrinol Invest 15 (1992) 255–263.
[82] R.B. Kelly, Pathways of protein secretion in eukaryotes, Science 230 (1985) 25–32.
[83] M.A. Shupnik, S.L. Greenspan, E.C. Ridgway, Transcriptional regulation of thyrotropin subunit genes by thyrotropin-releasing hormone and dopamine in pituitary cell cultures, J Biol Chem 261 (1986) 12675–12679.
[84] N. Shibusawa, M. Yamada, J. Hirato, T. Monden, T. Satoh, M. Mori, Requirement of thyrotropin-releasing hormone for the postnatal functions of pituitary thyrotrophs: Ontogeny study of congenital tertiary hypothyroidism in mice, Mol Endocrinol 14 (2000) 137–146.

[85] H. Abe, K. Murao, H. Imachi, W.M. Cao, X. Yu, K. Yoshida, et al., Thyrotropin-releasing hormone-stimulated thyrotropin expression involves islet-brain-1/c-Jun N-terminal kinase interacting protein-1, Endocrinology 145 (2004) 5623–5628.
[86] M.A. Shupnik, J. Weck, P.M. Hinkle, Thyrotropin (TSH)-releasing hormone stimulates TSH beta promoter activity by two distinct mechanisms involving calcium influx through L type Ca^{2+} channels and protein kinase C, Mol Endocrinol 10 (1996) 90–99.
[87] M.K. Kim, J.H. McClaskey, D.L. Bodenner, B.D. Weintraub, An AP-1-like factor and the pituitary-specific factor Pit-1 are both necessary to mediate hormonal induction of human thyrotropin beta gene expression, J Biol Chem 268 (1993) 23366–23375.
[88] B.D. Weintraub, F.E. Wondisford, E.A. Farr, H.J. Steinfelder, S. Radovick, N. Gesundheit, et al., Pre-translational and post-translational regulation of TSH synthesis in normal and neoplastic thyrotrophs, Horm Res 32 (1989) 22–24.
[89] M.A. Shupnik, B.A. Rosenzweig, M.O. Showers, Interactions of thyrotropin-releasing hormone, phorbol ester, and forskolin-sensitive regions of the rat thyrotropin-beta gene, Mol Endocrinol 4 (1990) 829–836.
[90] M.S. Kapiloff, Y. Farkash, M. Wegner, M.G. Rosenfeld, Variable effects of phosphorylation of Pit-1 dictated by the DNA response elements, Science 253 (1991) 786–789.
[91] H.J. Steinfelder, S. Radovick, F.E. Wondisford, Hormonal regulation of the thyrotropin beta-subunit gene by phosphorylation of the pituitary-specific transcription factor Pit-1, Proc Nat Acad Sci USA 89 (1992) 5942–5945.
[92] D.L. St Germain, V.A. Galton, The deiodinase family of selenoproteins, Thyroid 7 (1997) 655–668.
[93] A.C. Bianco, D. Salvatore, B. Gereben, M.J. Berry, P.R. Larsen, Biochemistry, cellular and molecular biology, and physiological roles of the iodothyronine selenodeiodinases, Endocr Rev 23 (2002) 38–89.
[94] M.A. Christoffolete, R. Ribeiro, P. Singru, C. Fekete, W.S. da Silva, D.F. Gordon, et al., Atypical expression of type 2 iodothyronine deiodinase in thyrotrophs explains the thyroxine-mediated pituitary thyrotropin feedback mechanism, Endocrinology 147 (2006) 1735–1743.
[95] P.J. Davis, J.L. Leonard, F.B. Davis, Mechanisms of nongenomic actions of thyroid hormone, Front Neuroendocrinol 29 (2008) 211–218.
[96] M.A. Shupnik, W.W. Chin, J.F. Habener, E.C. Ridgway, Transcriptional regulation of the thyrotropin subunit genes by thyroid hormone, J Biol Chem 260 (1985) 2900–2903.
[97] M.A. Shupnik, E.C. Ridgway, Thyroid hormone control of thyrotropin gene expression in rat anterior pituitary cells, Endocrinology 121 (1987) 619–624.
[98] M.A. Shupnik, L.J. Ardisson, M.J. Meskell, J. Bornstein, E.C. Ridgway, Triiodothyronine (T3) regulation of thyrotropin subunit gene transcription is proportional to T3 nuclear receptor occupancy, Endocrinology 118 (1986) 367–371.
[99] M.A. Shupnik, E.C. Ridgway, Triiodothyronine rapidly decreases transcription of the thyrotropin subunit genes in thyrotropic tumor explants, Endocrinology 117 (1985) 1940–1946.
[100] S. Refetoff, Resistance to thyroid hormone, Curr Ther Endocrinol Metab 6 (1997) 132–134.
[101] D.L. Bodenner, M.A. Mroczynski, B.D. Weintraub, S. Radovick, F.E. Wondisford, A detailed functional and structural analysis of a major thyroid hormone inhibitory element in the human thyrotropin beta-subunit gene, J Biol Chem 266 (1991) 21666–21673.
[102] C.K. Glass, M.G. Rosenfeld, The coregulator exchange in transcriptional functions of nuclear receptors, Genes Dev 14 (2000) 121–141.
[103] B.R. Haugen, N.S. Brown, W.M. Wood, D.F. Gordon, E.C. Ridgway, The thyrotrope-restricted isoform of the retinoid X receptor (gamma 1) mediates 9-cis retinoic acid suppression of thyrotropin beta promoter activity, Mol Endocrinol 11 (1997) 481–489.
[104] V. Sharma, W.R. Hays, W.M. Wood, U. Pugazhenthi, D.L. St Germain, A.C. Bianco, et al., Effects of rexinoids on thyrotrope function and the hypothalamic–pituitary–thyroid axis, Endocrinology 147 (2006) 1438–1451.
[105] S.I. Sherman, J. Gopal, B.R. Haugen, A.C. Chiu, K. Whaley, P. Nowlakha, et al., Central hypothyroidism associated with retinoid X receptor-selective ligands, N Engl J Med 340 (1999) 1075–1079.
[106] A. Matsushita, S. Sasaki, Y. Kashiwabara, K. Nagayama, K. Ohba, H. Iwaki, et al., Essential role of GATA2 in the negative regulation of thyrotropin beta gene by thyroid hormone and its receptors, Mol Endocrinol 21 (2007) 865–884.
[107] T. Ishizuka, M.A. Lazar, The N-CoR/histone deacetylase 3 complex is required for repression by thyroid hormone receptor, Mol Cell Biol 23 (2003) 5122–5131.
[108] B. Lemon, C. Inouye, D.S. King, R. Tjian, Selectivity of chromatin remodeling cofactors for ligand activated transcription, Nature 414 (2001) 924–928.
[109] S.W. Park, G. Li, Y.P. Lin, M.J. Barrero, K. Ge, R.G. Roeder, et al., Thyroid hormone-induced juxtaposition of regulatory elements/factors and chromatin remodeling of Crabp1 dependent on MED1/TRAP220, Mol Cell 19 (2005) 643–653.
[110] P. Ordentlich, M. Downes, R.M. Evans, Corepressors and nuclear hormone receptor function, Curr Top Microbiol Immunol 254 (2001) 101–116.
[111] Y. Liu, X. Xia, J.D. Fondell, P.M. Yen, Thyroid hormone regulated target genes have distinct patterns of coactivator recruitment and histone acetylation, Mol Endocrinol 20 (2006) 483–490.
[112] D. Wang, X. Xia, Y. Liu, A. Oetting, R.L. Walker, Y. Zhu, et al., Negative regulation of TSHalpha target gene by thyroid hormone involves histone acetylation and corepressor complex dissociation, Mol Endocrinol 23 (2009) 600–609.
[113] K. Nakano, A. Matsushita, S. Sasaki, H. Misawa, K. Nishiyama, Y. Kashiwabara, et al., Thyroid-hormone-dependent negative regulation of thyrotropin beta gene by thyroid hormone receptors: Study with a new experimental system using CV1 cells, Biochem J 378 (2004) 549–557.
[114] N. Shibusawa, K. Hashimoto, A.A. Nikrodhanond, M.C. Liberman, M.L. Applebury, X.H. Liao, et al., Thyroid hormone action in the absence of thyroid hormone receptor DNA-binding in vivo, J Clin Invest 112 (2003) 588–597.
[115] M.F. Langlois, K. Zanger, T. Monden, J.D. Safer, A.N. Hollenberg, F.E. Wondisford, A unique role of the beta-2 thyroid hormone receptor isoform in negative regulation by thyroid hormone. Mapping of a novel amino-terminal domain important for ligand-independent activation, J Biol Chem 272 (1997) 24927–24933.
[116] E.D. Abel, H.C. Kaulbach, A. Campos-Barros, R.S. Ahima, M.E. Boers, K. Hashimoto, et al., Novel insight from transgenic mice into thyroid hormone resistance and the regulation of thyrotropin, J Clin Invest 103 (1999) 271–279.
[117] P.L. Hallenbeck, M. Phyillaier, V. Nikodem, Divergent effects of 9-cis-retinoic acid receptor on positive and negative thyroid hormone receptor-dependent gene expression, J Biol Chem 268 (1993) 3825–3828.

[118] R.E. Weiss, J. Xu, G. Ning, J. Pohlenz, B.W. O'Malley, S. Refetoff, Mice deficient in the steroid receptor co-activator 1 (SRC-1) are resistant to thyroid hormone, EMBO J 18 (1999) 1900–1904.

[119] T. Tagami, W.X. Gu, P.T. Peairs, B.L. West, J.L. Jameson, A novel natural mutation in the thyroid hormone receptor defines a dual functional domain that exchanges nuclear receptor corepressors and coactivators, Mol Endocrinol 12 (1998) 1888–1902.

[120] A.A. Nikrodhanond, T.M. Ortiga-Carvalho, N. Shibusawa, K. Hashimoto, X.H. Liao, S. Refetoff, et al., Dominant role of thyrotropin-releasing hormone in the hypothalamic–pituitary–thyroid axis, J Biol Chem 281 (2006) 5000–5007.

[121] I.M. Krane, E.R. Spindel, W.W. Chin, Thyroid hormone decreases the stability and the poly(A) tract length of rat thyrotropin beta-subunit messenger RNA, Mol Endocrinol 5 (1991) 469–475.

[122] P.J. Leedman, A.R. Stein, W.W. Chin, Regulated specific protein binding to a conserved region of the 3'-untranslated region of thyrotropin beta-subunit mRNA, Mol Endocrinol 9 (1995) 375–387.

[123] D.S. Ross, M.F. Ellis, P. Milbury, E.C. Ridgway, A comparison of changes in plasma thyrotropin beta- and alpha-subunits, and mouse thyrotropic tumor thyrotropin beta- and alpha-subunit mRNA concentrations after in vivo dexamethasone or T3 administration, Metabolism 36 (1987) 799–803.

[124] J.A. Ahlquist, J.A. Franklyn, D.F. Wood, N.J. Balfour, K. Docherty, M.C. Sheppard, et al., Hormonal regulation of thyrotrophin synthesis and secretion, Horm Metab Res Suppl 17 (1987) 86–89.

[125] J.A. Franklyn, D.F. Wood, N.J. Balfour, D.B. Ramsden, K. Docherty, M.C. Sheppard, Modulation by oestrogen of thyroid hormone effects on thyrotrophin gene expression, J Endocrinol 115 (1987) 53–59.

[126] M Bottner, J. Christoffel, G. Rimoldi, W. Wuttke, Effects of long-term treatment with resveratrol and subcutaneous and oral estradiol administration on the pituitary–thyroid axis, Exp Clin Endocrinol Diabetes 114 (2006) 82–90.

[127] K. Nakamura, S. Sasaki, A. Matsushita, K. Ohba, H. Iwaki, H. Matsunaga, et al., Inhibition of GATA2-dependent transactivation of the TSHβ gene by ligand-bound estrogen receptor alpha, J Endocrinol 199 (2008) 113–125.

[128] D.S. Ross, Testosterone increases TSH-beta mRNA, and modulates alpha-subunit mRNA differentially in mouse thyrotropic tumor and castrate rat pituitary, Horm Metab Res 22 (1990) 163–169.

[129] J.M. Friedman, J.L. Halaas, Leptin and the regulation of body weight in mammals, Nature 395 (1998) 763–770.

[130] C. Fekete, J. Kelly, E. Mihaly, S. Sarkar, W.M. Rand, G. Legradi, et al., Neuropeptide Y has a central inhibitory action on the hypothalamic–pituitary–thyroid axis, Endocrinology 142 (2001) 2606–2613.

[131] I. Chowdhury, J.T. Chien, A. Chatterjee, J.Y. Yu, Effects of leptin and neuropeptide-Y on transcript levels of thyrotropin beta and common alpha subunits of rat pituitary cells in vitro, Life Sci 75 (2004) 2897–2909.

[132] D.S. Kim, J.H. Yoon, S.K. Ahn, K.E. Kim, R.H. Seong, S.H. Hong, et al., A 33kDa Pit-1-like protein binds to the distal region of the human thyrotrophin alpha-subunit gene, J Mol Endocrinol 14 (1995) 313–322.

[133] P.J. Deutsch, J.L. Jameson, J.F. Habener, Cyclic AMP responsiveness of human gonadotropin-alpha gene transcription is directed by a repeated 18-base pair enhancer, J Biol Chem 262 (1987) 12169–12174.

[134] K. Hashimoto, K. Zanger, A.N. Hollenberg, L.E. Cohen, S. Radovick, F.E. Wondisford, cAMP response element-binding protein-binding protein mediates thyrotropin-releasing hormone signaling on thyrotropin subunit genes, J Biol Chem 275 (2000) 33365–33372.

[135] V.K. Chatterjee, J.K. Lee, A. Rentoumis, J.L. Jameson, Negative regulation of the thyroid-stimulating hormone alpha gene by thyroid hormone: Receptor interaction adjacent to the TATA box, Proc Nat Acad Sci USA 86 (1989) 9114–9118.

[136] J. Burnside, D.S. Darling, F.E. Carr, W.W. Chin, Thyroid hormone regulation of the rat glycoprotein hormone alpha-subunit gene promoter activity, J Biol Chem 264 (1989) 6886–6891.

[137] V.D. Sarapura, W.M. Wood, T.M. Bright, K.W. Ocran, D.F. Gordon, E.C. Ridgway, Reconstitution of triiodothyronine inhibition in non-triiodothyronine responsive thyrotropic tumor cells using transfected thyroid hormone receptor isoforms, Thyroid 7 (1997) 453–461.

[138] T. Tagami, L.D. Madison, T. Nagaya, J.L. Jameson, Nuclear receptor corepressors activate rather than suppress basal transcription of genes that are negatively regulated by thyroid hormone, Mol Cell Biol 17 (1997) 2642–2648.

[139] L.D. Madison, J.A. Ahlquist, S.D. Rogers, J.L. Jameson, Negative regulation of the glycoprotein hormone alpha gene promoter by thyroid hormone: Mutagenesis of a proximal receptor binding site preserves transcriptional repression, Mol Cell Endocrinol 94 (1993) 129–136.

[140] R.A. Keri, B. Andersen, G.C. Kennedy, D.L. Hamernik, C.M. Clay, A.D. Brace, et al., Estradiol inhibits transcription of the human glycoprotein hormone alpha-subunit gene despite the absence of a high affinity binding site for estrogen receptor, Mol Endocrinol 5 (1991) 725–733.

[141] N.J. Yarwood, J.A. Gurr, M.C. Sheppard, J.A. Franklyn, Estradiol modulates thyroid hormone regulation of the human glycoprotein hormone alpha subunit gene, J Biol Chem 268 (1993) 21984–21989.

[142] V.K. Chatterjee, L.D. Madison, S. Mayo, J.L. Jameson, Repression of the human glycoprotein hormone alpha-subunit gene by glucocorticoids: Evidence for receptor interactions with limiting transcriptional activators, Mol Endocrinol 5 (1991) 100–110.

[143] L. Persani, Hypothalamic thyrotropin-releasing hormone and thyrotropin biological activity, Thyroid 8 (1998) 941–946.

[144] L. Persani, S. Borgato, R. Romoli, C. Asteria, A. Pizzocaro, P. Beck-Peccoz, Changes in the degree of sialylation of carbohydrate chains modify the biological properties of circulating thyrotropin isoforms in various physiological and pathological states, J Clin Endocrinol Metab 83 (1998) 2486–2492.

[145] M.J. Papandreou, L. Persani, C. Asteria Ronin, P. Beck-Peccoz, Variable carbohydrate structures of circulating thyrotropin as studied by lectin affinity chromatography in different clinical conditions, J Clin Endocrinol Metab 77 (1993) 393–398.

[146] J. Trojan, M. Theodoropoulou, K.H. Usadel, G.K. Stalla, L. Schaaf, Modulation of human thyrotropin oligosaccharide structures – enhanced proportion of sialylated and terminally galactosylated serum thyrotropin isoforms in subclinical and overt primary hypothyroidism, J Endocrinol 158 (1998) 359–365.

[147] L. Persani, E. Ferretti, S. Borgato, G. Faglia, P. Beck-Peccoz, Circulating thyrotropin bioactivity in sporadic central hypothyroidism, J Clin Endocrinol Metab 85 (2000) 3631–3635.

[148] J.H.A. Oliveira, E.R. Barbosa, T. Kasamatsu, J. Abucham, Evidence for thyroid hormone as a positive regulator of serum thyrotropin bioactivity, J Clin Endocrinol Metab 92 (2007) 3108–3113.

[149] W.D. Odell, R.D. Utiger, J.F. Wilber, P.G. Condliffe, Estimation of the secretion rate of thyrotropin in man, J Clin Invest 46 (1967) 953–959.

[150] E.C. Ridgway, B.D. Weintraub, F. Maloof, Metabolic clearance and production rates of human thyrotropin, J Clin Invest 53 (1974) 895–903.

[151] D.A. Fisher, D.H. Polk, Development of the thyroid, Ballieres Clin Endocrinol Metab 3 (1989) 67–80.

[152] E. Roti, Regulation of thyroid stimulating hormone (TSH) secretion in the fetus and neonate, J Endocrinol Invest 11 (1988) 145–155.

[153] L.M. Adams, J.R. Emery, S. Clark, E.I. Carlton, J.C. Nelson, Reference ranges for newer thyroid function tests in premature infants, J Pediatr 126 (1995) 122–127.

[154] A.G. Van Wassenaer, J.H. Kolk, F.W. Dekker, J.J.M. De Vijlder, Thyroid function in very preterm infants: Influences of gestational age and disease, Pediatr Res 42 (1997) 604–609.

[155] M.H. Samuels, J.D. Veldhuis, P. Henry, E.C. Ridgway, Pathophysiology of pulsatile and copulsatile release of thyroid-stimulating hormone, luteinizing hormone, follicle-stimulating hormone, and alpha-subunit, J Clin Endocrinol Metab 71 (1990) 425–432.

[156] F. Roelfsema, A.M. Pereira, J.D. Veldhuis, R. Adriaanse, E. Endert, E. Fliers, et al., Thyrotropin secretion profiles are not different in men and women, J Clin Endocrinol Metab 94 (2009) 3964–3967.

[157] W. Russell, R.F. Harrison, N. Smith, K. Darzy, S. Shalet, A.P. Weetman, et al., Free triiodothyronine has a distinct circadian rhythm that is delayed but parallels thyrotropin levels, J Clin Endocrinol Metab 93 (2008) 2300–2306.

[158] S. Mantagos, A. Koulouris, M. Makri, A.G. Bagenakis, Development of thyrotropin circadian rhythm in infancy, J Clin Endocrinol Metab 74 (1992) 71–74.

[159] F. Roelfsema, A.M. Pereira, R. Adriaanse, E. Endert, E. Fliers, J.A. Romijn, et al., Thyrotropin secretion in mild and severe primary hypothyroidism is distinguished by amplified burst mass and basal secretion with increased spikiness and approximate entropy, J Clin Endocrinol Metab 95 (2010) 928–934.

[160] M.H. Samuels, K. Lillehei, B.K. Kleinschmidt-Demasters, J. Stears, E.C. Ridgway, Patterns of pulsatile pituitary glycoprotein secretion in central hypothyroidism and hypogonadism, J Clin Endocrinol Metab 70 (1990) 391–395.

[161] G. Van Den Barghe, F. de Zegher, J.D. Veldhuis, P. Wouters, S. Gouwy, W. Stockman, et al., Thyrotrophin and prolactin release in prolonged critical illness: Dynamics of spontaneous secretion and effects of growth hormone-secretagogues, Clin Endocrinol (Oxf) 47 (1997) 599–612.

[162] M.H. Samuels, P. Henry, M. Luther, E.C. Ridgway, Pulsatile TSH secretion during 48-hour continuous TRH infusions, Thyroid 3 (1993) 201–206.

[163] M. Murakimi, K. Tanaka, M.A. Greer, There is a nyctohemeral rhythm of type II iodothyronine 5′-deiodinase activity in rat anterior pituitary, Endocrinology 123 (1988) 1631–1635.

[164] M.H. Samuels, Effects of variations in physiological cortisol levels on thyrotropin secretion in subjects with adrenal insufficiency: A clinical research center study, J Clin Endocrinol Metab 85 (2000) 1388–1393.

[165] M.H. Samuels, Effects of metyrapone administration on thyrotropin secretion in healthy subjects – a clinical research center study, J Clin Endocrinol Metab 85 (2000) 3049–3052.

[166] W.J. Sheward, A.J. Harmar, H.M. Fraser, G. Fink, TRH in rat pituitary stalk blood and hypothalamus. Studies with high performance liquid chromatography, Endocrinology 113 (1983) 1865–1869.

[167] H.M. Fraser, A.S. McNeilly, Effect of chronic immunoneutralisation of thyrotropin-releasing hormone on the hypothalamic–pituitary thyroid axis, prolactin and reproductive function in the ewe, Endocrinology 111 (1982) 1964–1971.

[168] T. Aizawa, M. Green, Delineation of the hypothalamic area controlling thyrotropin secretion in the rat, Endocrinology 109 (1981) 1731–1738.

[169] C.A. Spencer, D. Schwarzbein, R.B. Guttler, J.S. LoPresti, J.T. Nicoloff, Thyrotropin (TSH)-releasing hormone stimulation test responses employing third and fourth generation TSH assays, J Clin Endocrinol Metab 76 (1993) 494–498.

[170] V. Chan, C. Wang, R.T. Yeung, Thyrotropin: Alpha- and beta-subunits of thyrotropin, and prolactin responses to four-hour constant infusions of thyrotropin-releasing hormone in normal subjects and patients with pituitary–thyroid disorders, J Clin Endocrinol Metab 49 (1979) 127–133.

[171] M.C. Sheppard, K.I. Shennan, Desensitisation of rat anterior pituitary gland to thyrotrophin releasing hormone, Endocrinology 101 (1984) 101–105.

[172] S. Urman, V. Critchlow, Long-term elevations in plasma thyrotropin, but not growth hormone, concentrations associated with lesion-induced depletion of median eminence somatostatin, Endocrinology 112 (1983) 659–664.

[173] A. Arima, A.V. Schally, Increase in basal and thyrotropin-releasing hormone stimulated secretion of thyrotropin by passive immunization with antiserum to somatostatin, Endocrinology 98 (1976) 1069–1075.

[174] M.H. Samuels, P. Henry, E.C. Ridgway, Effects of dopamine and somatostatin on pulsatile pituitary glycoprotein secretion, J Clin Endocrinol Metab 74 (1992) 217–222.

[175] R.A. James, V.D. Sarapura, C. Bruns, F. Raulf, J.M. Dowding, D.F. Gordon, et al., Thyroid hormone-induced expression of specific somatostatin receptor subtypes correlates with involution of the TtT-97 murine thyrotrope tumor, Endocrinology 138 (1997) 719–724.

[176] E.C. Ridgway, A. Klibanski, M.A. Martorana, P. Milbury, J.D. Kieffer, W.W. Chin, The effect of somatostatin on the release of thyrotropin and its subunits from bovine anterior pituitary cells in vitro, Endocrinology 112 (1983) 1937–1942.

[177] M.D. Page, M.E. Millward, A. Taylor, M. Preece, M. Hourihan, R. Hall, et al., Long-term treatment of acromegaly with a long-acting analogue of somatostatin, octreotide, Q J Med 74 (1990) 189–201.

[178] B.M. Lippe, A.J. Van Herle, S.H. La Franchi, R.P. Uller, N. Lavin, S.A. Kaplan, Reversible hypothyroidism in growth hormone-deficient children treated with human growth hormone, J Clin Endocrinol Metab 40 (1975) 612–618.

[179] F. Roelfsema, N.R. Beirmasz, M. Frolich, D.M. Keenan, J.D. Veldhuis, J.A. Romijn, Diminished and irregular thyrotropin secretion with preserved diurnal rhythm in patients with active acromegaly, J Clin Endocrinol Metab 94 (2009) 1945–1950.

[180] D.S. Cooper, A. Klibanski, E.C. Ridgway, Dopaminergic modulation of TSH and its subunits: In vivo and in vitro studies, Clin Endocrinol (Oxf) 18 (1983) 265–272.

[181] M.H. Samuels, P. Kramer, Effects of metoclopramide on fasting-induced TSH suppression, Thyroid 6 (1996) 85–89.

[182] B.M. Lewis, C. Dieguez, M.D. Lewis, M.F. Scanlon, Dopamine stimulates release of thyrotrophin-releasing hormone from perfused intact rat hypothalamus via hypothalamic D2 receptors, J Endocrinol 115 (1987) 419–424.

[183] S.M. Foord, J.R. Peters, C. Dieguez, M.F. Scanlon, R. Hall, Dopamine receptors on intact anterior pituitary cells in culture: Functional association with the inhibition of prolactin and thyrotropin, Endocrinology 112 (1983) 1567–1571.

[184] P. Kok, F. Roelfsema, M. Frolich, A.E. Meinders, H. Pijl, Spontaneous diurnal thyrotropin secretion is enhanced in proportion to circulating leptin in obese premenopausal women, J Clin Endocrinol Metab 90 (2005) 6185–6191.

[185] M.F. Scanlon, V. Chan, M. Heath, M. Pourmand, M.D. Rodriguez-Arnao, D.R. Weightman, et al., Dopaminergic control of thyrotropin, alpha-subunit and prolactin in euthyroidism and hypothyroidism: Dissociated responses to dopamine receptor blockade with metoclopramide in euthyroid and hypothyroid subjects, J Clin Endocrinol Metab 53 (1981) 360–365.

[186] A. Klibanski, P.E. Milbury, W.W. Chin, E.C. Ridgway, Direct adrenergic stimulation of the release of thyrotropin and its subunits from the thyrotrope in vitro, Endocrinology 113 (1983) 1244–1250.

[187] L. Krulich, M.A. Mayfield, M.K. Steele, B.A. McMillen, S.M. McCann, J.I. Koenig, Differential effects of pharmacological manipulations of central alpha 1- and alpha 2-adrenergic receptors on the secretion of thyrotropin and growth hormone in male rats, Endocrinology 35 (1982) 139–145.

[188] S. Zgliczynski, M. Kaniewski, Evidence for alpha-adrenergic receptors mediated TSH release in men, Acta Endocrinol (Copenh) 95 (1980) 172–179.

[189] A.D. Rogol, G.D. Reeves, M.M. Varma, R.M. Blizzard, Thyroid stimulating hormone and prolactin response to thyrotropin-releasing hormone during infusion of epinephrine and propranolol in man, Neuroendocrinol 29 (1979) 413–420.

[190] T.A. Howlett, L.H. Rees, Endogenous opioid peptides and hypothalamo–pituitary function, Ann Rev Physiol 48 (1986) 527–536.

[191] J.E. Morley, N.G. Baranetsky, T.D. Wingert, H.E. Carlson, J.M. Hershman, S. Melmed, et al., Endocrine effects of naloxone-induced opiate receptor blockade, J Clin Endocrinol Metab 50 (1980) 251–257.

[192] M.H. Samuels, P. Kramer, D. Wilson, G. Sexton, Effects of naloxone infusions on pulsatile thyrotropin secretion, J Clin Endocrinol Metab 78 (1994) 1249–1252.

[193] M. Torlontano, C. Durante, I. Torrente, U. Crocetti, G. Augello, G. Ronga, et al., Type 2 deiodinase polymorphism (threonine 92 alanine) predicts L-thyroxine dose to achieve target thyrotropin levels in thyroidectomized patients, J Clin Endocrinol Metab 93 (2008) 910–913.

[194] L. Arnaud-Lopez, G. Usala, G. Ceresini, B.D. Mitchell, M.G. Pilia, M.G. Piras, et al., Phosphodiesterase 8B gene variants are associated with serum TSH levels and thyroid function, Am J Hum Genet 82 (2008) 1270–1280.

[195] M.I. Chiamolera, F.E. Wondisford, Minireview: Thyrotropin-releasing hormone and the thyroid hormone feedback mechanism, Endocrinology 150 (2009) 1091–1096.

[196] M. Berelowitz, K. Maefa, S. Harris, L.A. Frohmman, The effect of alterations in the pituitary–thyroid axis on hypothalamic content and in vitro release of somatostatin-like immunoreactivity, Endocrinology 107 (1980) 24–29.

[197] F. Roelfsema, A.M. Pereira, N.R. Biermasz, M. Frolich, D.M. Keenan, J.D. Veldhuis, et al., Diminished and irregular TSH secretion with delayed acrophase in patients with Cushing's syndrome, Eur J Endocrinol 161 (2009) 695–703.

[198] M.H. Samuels, M. Luther, P. Henry, E.C. Ridgway, Effects of hydrocortisone on pulsatile pituitary glycoprotein secretion, J Clin Endocrinol Metab 78 (1994) 211–215.

[199] M.H. Samuels, P.A. McDaniel, Thyrotropin levels during hydrocortisone infusions that mimic fasting-induced cortisol elevations – a clinical research center study, J Clin Endocrinol Metab 82 (1997) 3700–3704.

[200] T. Mitsuma, T. Nogimori, Effects of dexamethasone on the hypothalamic–pituitary–thyroid axis in rats, Acta Endocrinol (Copenh) 100 (1982) 51–56.

[201] T. Mitsuma, Y. Hirooka, T. Nogimori, Effects of dexamethasone on TRH, TRH-glycine and pre-pro-TRH (178-199) levels in various rat organs, Endocr Regul 27 (1993) 49–55.

[202] T. Mitsuma, Y. Hirooka, T. Nogimori, Effects of dexamethasone on TRH and TRH precursor peptide (lys-arg-gln-his-pro-gly-arg-arg) levels in various rat organs, Endocr Regul 26 (1992) 29–34.

[203] T.M. Ortiga-Carvalho, K.J. Oliveira, B.A. Soares, C.C. Pazos-Moura, The role of leptin in the regulation of TSH secretion in the fed state: In vivo and in vitro studies, J Endocrinol 174 (2002) 121–125.

[204] S. Schurgin, B. Canavan, P. Koutkia, A.M. Depaoli, S. Grinspoon, Endocrine and metabolic effects of physiologic r-metHuLeptin administration during acute caloric deprivation in normal-weight women, J Clin Endocrinol Metab 89 (2004) 5402–5409.

[205] L. Farbota, C. Hofman, R. Oslapas, E. Paloyan, Sex hormone modulation of serum TSH levels, Surgery 102 (1987) 1081–1087.

[206] J.A. Ahlquist, J.A. Franklyn, D.B. Ramsden, M.C. Sheppard, Regulation of alpha and thyrotrophin-beta subunit mRNA levels by androgens in the female rat, J Mol Endocrinol 5 (1990) 1–6.

[207] E.M. Erfurth, U.B. Ericsson, The role of estrogen in the TSH and prolactin responses to thyrotropin-releasing hormone in postmenopausal as compared to premenopausal women, Horm Metab Res 24 (1992) 528–531.

[208] R.M. Hermus, C.G. Sweep, M.J. van der Meer, H.A. Ross, A.G. Smals, T.J. Benraad, et al., Continuous infusion of interleukin-1 induces a nonthyroidal illness syndrome in the rat, Endocrinology 131 (1992) 2139–2146.

[209] T. Van der Poll, J.A. Romijn, W.M. Wiersinga, H.P. Sauerwein, Tumor necrosis factor: A putative mediator of the sick euthyroid syndrome in man, J Clin Endocrinol Metab 71 (1990) 1567–1572.

[210] D.J. Torpy, C. Tsigos, A.J. Lotsikas, R. Defensor, G.P. Chrousos, D.A. Papanicolaou, Acute and delayed effects of a single-dose injection of interleukin-6 on thyroid function in healthy humans, Metabolism 47 (1998) 1289–1293.

[211] C.C. Pazos-Moura, T.M. Ortiga-Carvalho, E. Gaspar de Moura, The autocrine/paracrine regulation of thyrotropin secretion, Thyroid 13 (2003) 167–175.

[212] K.J. Oliveira, T.M. Ortiga-Carvalho, A. Cabanelas, M.A. Veiga, K. Aoki, H. Ohki-Hamazaki, et al., Disruption of neuromedin B receptor gene results in dysregulation of the pituitary–thyroid axis, J Mol Endocrinol 36 (2006) 73–80.

[213] N.R. Farid, M.W. Szkudlinski, Minireview: Structural and functional evolution of the thyrotropin receptor, Endocrinology 145 (2004) 4048–4057.

[214] B. Gross, M. Misrahi, S. Sar, E. Milgram, Composite structure of the human thyrotropin receptor gene, Biochem Biophys Res Commun 177 (1991) 679–687.

[215] T. Akamizu, S. Ikuyama, M. Saji, S. Kosugi, C. Kozak, O.W. McBride, et al., Cloning, chromosomal assignment, and regulation of the rat thyrotropin receptor: Expression of the gene is regulated by thyrotropin agents that increase cAMP levels, and thyroid autoantibodies, Proc Nat Acad Sci USA 87 (1990) 5677–5681.

[216] F. Libert, A. Lefort, C. Gerard, M. Parmentier, J. Perret, M. Ludgate, et al., Cloning, sequencing and expression of the human thyrotropin (TSH) receptor: Evidence for binding of autoantibodies, Biochem Biophys Res Commun 165 (1989) 1250–1255.

[217] M. Misrahi, H. Loosfelt, M. Atger, S. Sar, A. Guiochon-Mantel, E. Milgram, Cloning, sequencing and expression of human TSH receptor, Biochem Biophys Res Commun 166 (1990) 394–403.

[218] Y. Nagayama, K.D. Kaufman, P. Seto, B. Rapoport, Molecular cloning, sequence and functional expression of the cDNA for the human thyrotropin receptor, Biochem Biophys Res Commun 165 (1989) 1184–1190.

[219] B. Rapoport, G.D. Chazenbalk, J.C. Jaume, M. McLachlan, The thyrotropin (TSH)-releasing hormone receptor: Interaction with TSH and autoantibodies, Endocr Rev 19 (1998) 673–716.

[220] K. Tanaka, G.D. Chazenbalk, S.M. McLachlan, B. Rapoport, Subunit structure of thyrotropin receptors expressed on the cell surface, J Biol Chem 274 (1999) 33979–33984.

[221] M.T. Hai, A. Radu, N. Ghinea, The cleavage of thyroid-stimulating hormone receptor is dependent on cell–cell contacts and regulates the hormonal stimulation of phospholipase C, J Cell Mol Med 13 (2009) 2253–2260.

[222] D. Russo, G.D. Chazenbalk, Y. Nagayama, H.L. Wadsworth, B. Rapoport, Site-directed mutagenesis of the human thyrotropin receptor: Role of asparagine-linked oligosaccharides in the expression of a functional receptor, Mol Endocrinol 5 (1991) 29–33.

[223] Y. Nagayama, H. Namba, N. Yokoyama, S. Yamashita, M. Niwa, Role of asparagine-linked oligosaccharides in protein folding, membrane targetting, and thyrotropin and autoantibody binding of the human thyrotropin receptor, J Biol Chem 273 (1998) 33423–33428.

[224] B. Kobe, J. Deisenhofer, A structural basis of the interactions between leucine-rich repeats and protein ligands, Nature 374 (1995) 183–186.

[225] A.V. Kajava, G. Vassart, S.J. Wodak, Modeling of the three-dimensional structure of proteins with the typical leucine-rich repeats, Structure 3 (1995) 867–877.

[226] J.M. Baldwin, The probable arrangement of the helices in G protein-coupled receptors, EMBO J 12 (1993) 1693–1703.

[227] Y. Nagayama, D. Russo, H.L. Wadsworth, G.D. Chazenbalk, B. Rapoport, Eleven amino acids (Lys-201 to Lys-211) and 9 amino acids (Gly-222 to Leu-230) in the human thyrotropin receptor are involved in ligand binding, J Biol Chem 266 (1991) 14926–14930.

[228] S. LaFranchi, Congenital hypothyroidism: Etiologies, diagnosis, and management, Thyroid 9 (1999) 735–740.

[229] S. Refetoff, Resistance to thyrotropin, J Endocrinol Invest 26 (2003) 770–779.

[230] S. Kosugi, T. Ban, T. Akamizu, L.D. Kohn, Site-directed mutagenesis of a portion of the extracellular domain of the rat thyrotropin receptor important in autoimmune thyroid disease and nonhomologous with gonadotropin receptors. Relationship of functional and immunogenic domains, J Biol Chem 266 (1991) 19413–19418.

[231] P.N. Graves, T.F. Davies, New insights into the thyroid-stimulating hormone receptor: The major antigen of Graves' disease, Endocrinol Metab Clin North Am 29 (2000) 267–286.

[232] Y. Mizutori, C.-R. Chen, S.M. McLachlan, B. Rapoport, The thyrotropin receptor hinge region is not simply a scaffold for the leucine-rich domain but contributes to ligand binding and signal transduction, Mol Endocrinol 22 (2008) 1171–1182.

[233] S. Mueller, G. Kleinau, H. Jaeschke, R. Paschke, G. Krause, Extended hormone binding site of the human thyroid stimulating hormone receptor: Distinctive acidic residues in the hinge region are involved in bovine stimulating hormone binding and receptor activation, J Biol Chem 283 (2008) 18048–18055.

[234] J. Sanders, D.Y. Chirgadze, P. Sanders, S. Baker, A. Sullivan, A. Bhardwaja, et al., Crystal structure of the TSH receptor in complex with a thyroid-stimulating autoantibody, Thyroid 17 (2007) 395–410.

[235] S.A. Stein, E.L. Oates, C.R. Hall, R.M. Grumbles, L.M. Fernandez, N.A. Taylor, et al., Identification of a point mutation in the thyrotropin receptor of the *hyt/hyt* hypothyroid mouse, Mol Endocrinol 8 (1994) 129–138.

[236] M. Grossmann, M.W. Szkudlinski, R. Wong, J.A. Dias, T.H. Ji, B.D. Weintraub, Substitution of the seat-belt region of the thyroid-stimulating hormone (TSH) beta-subunit with the corresponding regions of choriogonadotropin or follitropin confers luteotropic but not follitropic activity to chimeric TSH, J Biol Chem 272 (1997) 15532–15540.

[237] M.C. Leinung, E.R. Bergert, D.J. McCormick, J.C. Morris, Synthetic analogs of the carboxyl-terminus of beta-thyrotropin: The importance of basic amino acids in receptor binding activity, Biochemistry 31 (1992) 10094–10098.

[238] G. Medeiros-Neto, D.T. Herodotou, S. Rajan, S. Kommareddi, L. de Lacerda, R. Sandrini, et al., A circulating, biologically inactive thyrotropin caused by a mutation in the beta subunit gene, J Clin Invest 97 (1996) 1250–1256.

[239] M.W. Szkudlinski, N.R. Thotakura, B.D. Weintraub, Subunit-specific functions of N-linked oligosaccharides in human thyrotropin: Role of terminal residues of alpha- and beta-subunit oligosaccharides in metabolic clearance and bioactivity, Proc Nat Acad Sci USA 92 (1995) 9062–9066.

[240] N.R. Thotakura, R.K. Desai, M.W. Szkudlinski, B.D. Weintraub, The role of the oligosaccharide chains of thyrotropin alpha- and beta-subunits in hormone action, Endocrinology 131 (1992) 82–88.

[241] A. Renwick, P. Wiggin, An antipodean perception of the mode of action of glycoprotein hormones, FEBS Lett 297 (1992) 1–3.

[242] T.F. Davies, M. Platzer, hCG-induced receptor activation and growth acceleration in FRTL-5 thyroid cells, Endocrinology 118 (1986) 2149–2151.

[243] Y. Tomer, G.K. Huber, T.F. Davies, Human chorionic gonadotropin (hCG) interacts directly with recombinant human TSH receptors, J Clin Endocrinol Metab 74 (1992) 1477–1479.

[244] M. Yoshimura, J.M. Hershman, X.P. Pang, L. Berg, A.E. Pekary, Activation of the thyrotropin (TSH) receptor by human chorionic gonadotropin and luteinizing hormone in Chinese hamster ovary cells expressing functional human TSH receptors, J Clin Endocrinol Metab 77 (1993) 1009–1013.

[245] J.M. Hershman, Physiological and pathological aspects of the effect of human chorionic gonadotropin on the thyroid, Best Pract Res Clin Endocrinol Metab 18 (2004) 249–265.

[246] M. Yoshimura, J.M. Hershman, Thyrotropic action of human chorionic gonadotropin, Thyroid 5 (1995) 425–434.

[247] P. Rodien, C. Bremont, M.L. Sanson, J. Parma, J. Van Sande, S. Costagliola, et al., Familial gestational hyperthyroidism caused by a mutant thyrotropin receptor hypersensitive to human chorionic gonadotropin, N Engl J Med 339 (1998) 1823–1826.

[248] G.D. Chazenbalk, Y. Nagayama, D. Russo, H.L. Wadsworth, B. Rapoport, Functional analysis of the cytoplasmic domains of the human thyrotropin receptor by site-directed mutagenesis, J Biol Chem 265 (1990) 20970–20975.

[249] M. Parmentier, F. Libert, C. Maenhaut, A. Lefort, C. Gerard, J. Perret, et al., Molecular cloning of the thyrotropin receptor, Science 246 (1989) 1620–1622.

[250] I. Ciullo, R. Latif, P. Graves, T.F. Davies, Functional assessment of the thyrotropin receptor-beta subunit, Endocrinology 144 (2003) 3176–3181.

[251] V. Kaczur, L.G. Puskas, Z.U. Nagy, N. Miled, A. Rebai, F. Juhasz, et al., Cleavage of the human thyrotropin receptor by ADAM10 is regulated by thyrotropin, J Mol Recognit 20 (2007) 392–404.
[252] E. Laurent, J. Mockel, J. Van Sande, I. Graff, J.E. Dumont, Dual activation by thyrotropin of the phopholipase C and cyclic AMP cascades in human thyroid, Mol Cell Endocrinol 52 (1987) 273–278.
[253] S. Kosugi, F. Okajima, T. Ban, A. Hidaka, A. Shenker, L.D. Kohn, Mutation of alanine 623 in the third cytoplasmic loop of the rat thyrotropin (TSH) receptor results in a loss in the phosphoinositide but not cAMP signal induced by TSH and receptor autoantibodies, J Biol Chem 267 (1992) 24153–24156.
[254] H. Grasberger, J. Van Sande, A.H.-D. Mahameed, Y. Tenenbaum-Rakover, S. Refetoff, A familial thyrotropin (TSH) receptor mutation provides in vivo evidence that the inositol phosphates/Ca^{2+} cascade mediates TSH action on thyroid hormone synthesis, J Clin Endocrinol Metab 92 (2007) 2816–2820.
[255] E.S. Park, H. Kim, J.M. Suh, S.J. Park, S.H. You, H.K. Chung, et al., Involvement of JAK/STAT (Janus kinase/Signal transducer and activator of transcription) in the thyrotropin signaling pathway, Mol Endocrinol 14 (2000) 662–670.
[256] C. Brewer, N. Yeager, A. Di Cristofano, Thyroid-stimulating hormone-initiated proliferative signals converge in vivo on the mTOR kinase without activating AKT, Cancer Res 67 (2007) 8002–8006.
[257] J. Van Sande, J. Parma, M. Tonacchera, S. Swillens, J. Dumont, G. Vassart, Somatic and germline mutations of the TSH receptor gene in thyroid diseases, J Clin Endocrinol Metab 80 (1995) 2577–2585.
[258] G.D. Chazenbalk, A. Kakinuma, J.C. Jaume, S.M. McLachlan, B. Rapoport, Evidence of negative cooperativity among human thyrotropin receptors overexpressed in mammalian cells, Endocrinology 137 (1996) 4586–4591.
[259] C.T. Esapa, L. Duprez, M. Ludgate, M.S. Mustafa, P. Kendall-Taylor, G. Vassart, et al., A novel thyrotropin receptor mutation in an infant with severe thyrotoxicosis, Thyroid 9 (1999) 1005–1010.
[260] B.U. Nwosu, L. Gourgiotis, M.C. Gershengorn, S. Neumann, A novel activating mutation in transmembrane helix 6 of the thyrotropin receptor as cause of hereditary nonautoimmune hyperthyroidism, Thyroid 16 (2006) 505–512.
[261] Z. Liu, Y. Sun, Q. Dong, M. He, C.H.K. Cheng, F. Fan, A novel TSHR gene mutation (Ile691Phe) in a Chinese family causing autosomal dominant non-autoimmune hyperthyroidism, J Hum Genet 53 (2008) 475–478.
[262] J. Parma, L. Duprez, J. Van Sande, P. Cochaux, C. Gervy, J. Mockel, et al., Somatic mutations in the thyrotropin receptor gene cause hyperfunctioning thyroid adenomas, Nature 365 (1993) 649–651.
[263] E.M. Gabriel, E.R. Bergert, C.S. Grant, J.A. van Heerden, G.B. Thompson, J.C. Morris, Germline polymorphism of codon 727 of human thyroid-stimulating hormone receptor is associated with toxic multinodular goiter, J Clin Endocrinol Metab 84 (1999) 3328–3335.
[264] G. Colletta, A.M. Cirafici, TSH is able to induce cell cycle-related gene expression in rat thyroid cell, Biochem Biophys Res Commun 183 (1992) 265–272.
[265] M.P. Postiglione, R. Parlato, A. Rodriguez-Mallon, A. Rosica, P. Mithbaokar, M. Maresca, et al., Role of the thyroid-stimulating hormone receptor signaling in development and differentiation of the thyroid gland, Proc Nat Acad Sci USA 99 (2002) 15462–15467.
[266] L. Contor, F. Lamy, R. Lecocq, P.P. Roger, J.E. Dumont, Differential protein phosphorylation in induction of thyroid cell proliferation by thyrotropin, epidermal growth factor or phorbol ester, Mol Cell Biol 8 (1988) 2494–2503.
[267] A. Bybee, A.R. Tuffery, Rapid proliferative response of rat thyroid gland to a single injection of TSH in vivo, J Endocrinol 121 (1989) 27–30.
[268] P. Ealey, C.A. Ahene, J.M. Emmerson, N.J. Marshall, Forskolin and thyrotropin stimulation of rat FRTL-5 thyroid cell growth: The role of cyclic AMP, J Endocrinol 114 (1987) 199–205.
[269] J. Van Sande, A. Lefort, S. Beebe, Pairs of cyclic AMP analogues that are specifically synergistic for type I and type II cAMP dependent protein kinase mimic thyrotropin effects on the function, differentiation, expression and mitogenesis of dog thyroid cells, Eur J Biochem 183 (1989) 699–708.
[270] G. Karsenty, C. Alquier, C. Jelsema, B.D. Weintraub, Thyrotropin induces growth and iodothyronine production in a human thyroid cell line without affecting adenosine 3′5′ monophosphate production, Endocrinology 123 (1988) 1977–1983.
[271] D. Tramontano, A.C. Moses, B.M. Veneziani, S.H. Ingbar, Adenosine 3′5′-monophosphate mediates both the mitogenic effect of thyrotropin and its ability to amplify the response to insulin-like growth factor I in FRTL-5 cells, Endocrinology 122 (1988) 127–132.
[272] K. Westermark, B. Westermark, F.A. Karlsson, L.E. Ericson, Location of epidermal growth factor receptors in porcine thyroid follicle cells and receptor regulation by thyrotropin, Endocrinology 118 (1986) 1040–1046.
[273] T. Tominaga, J. Dela Cruz, G.N. Burrow, J.L. Meinkoth, Divergent patterns of immediate early gene expression in response to thyroid-stimulating hormone and insulin-like growth factor I in Wistar rat thyrocytes, Endocrinology 135 (1994) 1212–1219.
[274] A. Kawakami, K. Eguchi, N. Matsouka, M. Tsuboi, Y. Kawabe, N. Ishikawa, et al., Thyroid-stimulating hormone inhibits Fas antigen-mediated apoptosis of human thyrocytes in vitro, Endocrinology 137 (1996) 3163–3169.
[275] J.L. Tilly, K.I. Tilly, M.L. Kenton, A.L. Johnson, Expression of members of the Bcl-2 gene family in the immature rat ovary: Equine gonadotropin-mediated inhibition of granulosa cell apoptosis is associated with decreased Bax and constitutive Bcl-2 and Bcl-xlong messenger ribonucleic acid levels, Endocrinology 136 (1995) 232–241.
[276] K.I. Tilly, S. Banerjee, P.P. Banerjee, J.L. Tilly, Expression of the p53 and Wilms' tumor suppressor genes in the rat ovary: Gonadotropin repression in vivo and immunohistochemical localization of nuclear p53 protein to apoptotic granulosa cells of atretic follicles, Endocrinology 136 (1995) 1394–1402.
[277] M. Grossmann, M.W. Szkudlinski, J.A. Dias, H. Xia, R. Wong, D. Puett, et al., Site-directed mutagenesis of amino acids 33-44 of the common alpha-subunit reveals different structural requirements for heterodimer expression among the glycoprotein hormones and suggests that cAMP production and growth promotion are potentially dissociable functions of hTSH, Mol Endocrinol 10 (1996) 769–779.
[278] T.B. Nielsen, M.S. Ferdows, B.R. Brinkley, J.B. Field, Morphological and biochemical responses of cultured thyroid cells to thyrotropin, Endocrinology 116 (1985) 788–797.
[279] M. Nilsson, G. Engstrom, L.E. Ericson, Graded response in the individual thyroid follicle cell to increasing doses of TSH, Mol Cell Endocrinol 44 (1986) 165–169.

[280] P.P. Roger, F. Rukaert, F. Lamy, M. Authelot, J.E. Dumont, Actin stress fiber disruption and tropomyosin isoform switching in normal thyroid epithelial cells stimulated by thyrotropin and phorbol esters, Exp Cell Res 182 (1989) 1–13.
[281] C. Riedel, O. Levy, N. Carrasco, Post-transcriptional regulation of the sodium/iodide symporter by thyrotropin, J Biol Chem 276 (2001) 21458–21463.
[282] G. Damante, G. Chazenbalk, D. Russo, B. Rapoport, D. Foti, S. Filetti, Thyrotropin regulation of thyroid peroxidase messenger ribonucleic acid levels in cultured rat thyroid cells: Evidence for involvement of a non-transcriptional mechanism, Endocrinology 124 (1989) 2889–2894.
[283] D. Corda, L.D. Kohn, Phorbol myristate acetate inhibits adrenergically but not thyrotropin-regulated function in FRTL-5 rat thyroid cells, Endocrinology 120 (1987) 1152–1160.
[284] R.C. Marians, L. Ng, H.C. Blair, P. Unger, P.N. Graves, T.F. Davies, Defining thyrotropin-dependent and -independent steps of thyroid hormone synthesis by using thyrotropin receptor-null mice, Proc Nat Acad Sci USA 99 (2002) 15776–15781.
[285] Z. Tosta, O. Chabaud, J. Chebath, Identification of thyroglobulin mRNA sequences in the nucleus and cytoplasm of cultured thyroid cells: A fast transcriptional effect of thyrotropin, Biochem Biophys Res Commun 116 (1983) 54–61.
[286] M.-F. Van den Hove, K. Croizet-Berger, D. Tyteca, C. Selvais, P. de Diesbach, P.J. Courtoy, Thyrotropin activates guanosine 5'diphosphate/guanosine 5'-triphosphate exchange on the rate-limited endocytic catalyst, Rab5a, in human thyrocytes in vivo and in vitro, J Clin Endocrinol Metab 92 (2007) 2803–2810.
[287] G.D. Chazenbalk, Y. Nagayama, K.D. Kaufman, B. Rapoport, The functional expression of recombinant human thyrotropin receptors in non-thyroidal eukaryotic cells provides evidence that homologous desensitization to thyrotropin stimulation requires a cell-specific factor, Endocrinology 127 (1990) 1240–1244.
[288] J.N. Anasti, M.R. Flack, J. Froelich, L.M. Nelson, B.C. Nisula, A potential novel mechanism for precocious puberty in juvenile hypothyroidism, J Clin Endocrinol Metab 80 (1995) 276–279.
[289] Y. Nagayama, H. Yamasaki, A. Takeshita, H. Kimura, K. Ashizawa, N. Yokoyama, et al., Thyrotropin binding specificity for the thyrotropin receptor, J Endocrinol Invest 18 (1995) 283–287.
[290] P. Crisanti, B. Omri, E.J. Hughes, G. Meduri, C. Hery, E. Clauser, et al., The expression of thyrotropin receptor in the brain, Endocrinology 142 (2001) 812–822.
[291] M.F. Prummel, L.J.S. Brokken, G. Meduri, M. Misrahi, O. Bakker, W.M. Wiersinga, Expression of the thyroid-stimulating hormone receptor in the folliculo-stellate cells of human anterior pituitary, J Clin Endocrinol Metab 85 (2000) 4347–4353.
[292] B. Saunier, M. Pierre, C. Jacquemin, F. Courtin, Evidence of cAMP-independent thyrotropin effects on astroglial cells, Eur J Biochem 218 (1993) 1091–1094.
[293] M.F. Prummel, L.J. Brokken, W.M. Wiersinga, Ultra short-loop feedback control of thyrotropin secretion, Thyroid 14 (2004) 825–829.
[294] M.E. Peele, F.E. Carr, J.R. Baker, L. Wartofsky, K.D. Burman, TSH beta subunit gene expression in human lymphocytes, Am J Med Sci 305 (1993) 1–7.
[295] S. Balzan, G. Nicolini, F. Forini, G. Boni, R. Del Carratore, A. Nicolini, et al., Presence of a functional TSH receptor on human erythrocytes, Biomedicine and Pharmacotherapy 61 (2007) 463–467.
[296] T. Endo, K. Ohta, K. Haraguchi, T. Onaya, Cloning and functional expression of thyrotropin receptor cDNA from fat cells, J Biol Chem 270 (1995) 10833–10837.
[297] J.H.D. Bassett, G.R. Williams, Critical role of the hypothalamic–pituitary–thyroid axis in bone, Bone 43 (2008) 418–426.
[298] E. Bodó, A. Kromminga, T. Bíró, I. Borbíró, E. Gáspár, M.A. Zmijewski, et al., Human female hair follicles are a direct, nonclassical target for thyroid-stimulating hormone, J Invest Dermatol 129 (2009) 1126–1139.
[299] W. Zhang, L.M. Tian, Y. Han, H.Y. Ma, L.C. Wang, J. Guo, et al., Presence of thyrotropin receptor in hepatocytes: Not a case of illegitimate transcription, J Cell Mol Med 13 (2009) 4636–4642.
[300] L. Aghajanova, M. Lindeberg, I.B. Carlsson, A. Stavreus-Evers, P. Zhang, J.E. Scott, et al., Receptors for thyroid-stimulating hormone and thyroid hormones in human ovarian tissue, Reprod Biomed Online 18 (2009) 337–347.
[301] J. Morillo-Bernal, J.M. Fernández-Santos, J.C. Utrilla, M. de Miguel, R. García-Marín, I. Martín-Lacave, Functional expression of the thyrotropin receptor in C cells: New insights into their involvement in the hypothalamic–pituitary–thyroid axis, J Anat 215 (2009) 150–158.
[302] K. Nakabayashi, H. Matsumi, A. Bhalla, J. Bae, S. Mosselman, S.Y. Hsu, et al., Thyrostimulin, a heterodimer of two new human glycoprotein hormone subunits, activates the thyroid-stimulating hormone receptor, J Clin Invest 109 (2002) 1445–1452.
[303] S.C. Sun, P.J. Hsu, F.J. Wu, S.H. Li, C.H. Lu, C.W. Luo, Thyrostimulin, but not thyroid-stimulating hormone, acts as a paracrine regulator to activate thyroid-stimulating hormone receptor in the mammalian ovary, J Biol Chem 285 (2010) 3758–3765.
[304] J.C. Morris, Structure and function of the TSH receptor: Its suitability as a target for radiotherapy, Thyroid 7 (1997) 253–258.
[305] E.C. Ridgway, Thyrotropin radioimmunoassays: Birth, life and demise, Mayo Clin Proc 63 (10) (1988) 1028–1034.
[306] W.D. Odell, J. Griffin, R. Zahradnik, Two-monoclonal-antibody sandwich-type assay for thyrotropin, with use of an avidin-biotin separation technique, Clin Chem 32 (1986) 1873–1878.
[307] V. Van Heyningen, S.R. Abbott, S.G. Daniel, L.J. Ardisson, E.C. Ridgway, Development and utility of a monoclonal-antibody-based, highly sensitive immunoradiometric assay of thyrotropin, Clin Chem 33 (1987) 1387–1390.
[308] C.A. Spencer, J.G. Hollowell, M. Kazarosyan, L.E. Braverman, National Health and Nutrition Examination Survey III thyroid stimulating hormone (TSH)-thyroperoxidase antibody relationships demonstrate that TSH upper reference limits may be skewed by occult thyroid dysfunction, J Clin Endocrinol Metab 92 (2007) 4236–4240.
[309] T.E. Hamilton, S. Davis, L. Onstad, K.J. Kopecky, Thyrotropin levels in a population with no clinical, autoantibody, or ultrasonographic evidence of thyroid disease: Implications for the diagnosis of subclinical hypothyroidism, J Clin Endocrinol Metab 93 (2008) 1224–1230.
[310] M.I. Surks, J.G. Hollowell, Age-specific distribution of serum thyrotropin and antithyroid antibodies in the US population: Implications for the prevalence of subclinical hypothyroidism, J Clin Endocrinol Metab 92 (2007) 4575–4582.
[311] S. Andersen, K.M. Pedersen, N.H. Bruun, P. Laurberg, Narrow individual variations in serum T(4) and T(3) in normal subjects: A clue to the understanding of subclinical thyroid disease, J Clin Endocrinol Metab 87 (2002) 1068–1072.
[312] P.S. Hansen, T.H. Brix, T.I. Sørensen, K.O. Kyvik, L. Hegedüs, Major genetic influence on the regulation of the pituitary–thyroid axis: A study of healthy Danish twins, J Clin Endocrinol Metab 89 (2004) 1181–1187.
[313] V. Panicker, S.G. Wilson, T.D. Spector, S.J. Brown, B.S. Kato, P.W. Reed, et al., Genetic loci linked to pituitary–thyroid axis set points: A genome-wide scan of a large twin cohort, J Clin Endocrinol Metab 93 (2008) 3519–3523.

[314] H. Guan, Z. Shan, X. Teng, Y. Li, D. Teng, Y. Jin, et al., Influence of iodine on the reference interval of TSH and the optimal interval of TSH: Results of a follow-up study in areas with different iodine intakes, Clin Endocrinol (Oxf) 69 (2008) 136–141.

[315] I.A. Kourides, B.D. Weintraub, M.A. Levko, F. Maloof, Alpha and beta subunits of human thyrotropin: Purification and development of specific radioimmunoassays, Endocrinology 94 (1974) 1411–1421.

[316] I.A. Kourides, B.D. Weintraub, E.C. Ridgway, F. Maloof, Pituitary secretion of free alpha and beta-subunit of human thyrotropin in patients with thyroid disorders, J Clin Endocrinol Metab 40 (1975) 872–885.

[317] M.H. Samuels, E.C. Ridgway, Glycoprotein secreting pituitary adenomas, Baillieres Clin Endocrinol Metab 9 (1995) 337–358.

[318] M.R. Blackman, B.D. Weintraub, S.W. Rosen, I.A. Kourides, K. Steinwascher, M.H. Gail, Human placental and pituitary glycoprotein hormones and their subunits as tumor markers: A quantitative assessment, J Natl Cancer Inst 65 (1980) 81–93.

[319] C.R. Kahn, S.W. Rosen, B.D. Weintraub, S.S. Fajans, P. Gorden, Ectopic production of chorionic gonadotropin and its subunits by islet cell tumors: A specific marker for malignancy, N Engl J Med 197 (1977) 565–569.

[320] S.W. Rosen, B.D. Weintraub, S.A. Aaronson, Nonrandom ectopic protein production by malignant cells: Direct evidence in vitro, J Clin Endocrinol Metab 50 (1980) 834–841.

[321] M.R. Blackman, B.D. Weintraub, S.W. Rosen, S.M. Harmen, Comparison of the effects of lung cancer, benign lung disease, and normal aging on pituitary–gonadal function in men, J Clin Endocrinol Metab 66 (1988) 88–95.

[322] Y.C. Patel, H.G. Burger, Serum thyrotropin (TSH) in pituitary and/or hypothalamic hypothyroidism: Normal or elevated basal levels and paradoxical responses to thyrotropin-releasing hormone, J Clin Endocrinol Metab 37 (1973) 190–196.

[323] D. Bracco, O. Morin, Y. Schutz, H. Liang, E. Jéquier, A.G. Burger, Comparison of the metabolic and endocrine effects of 3,5,3′-triiodothyroacetic acid and thyroxine, J Clin Endocrinol Metab 77 (1993) 221–228.

[324] G.A. de Carvalho, S.C. Bahls, A. Boeving, H. Graf, Effects of selective serotonin reuptake inhibitors on thyroid function in depressed patients with primary hypothyroidism or normal thyroid function, Thyroid 19 (2009) 691–697.

[325] B.P. O'Malley, P.E. Jennings, N. Cook, D.B. Barnett, F.D. Rosenthal, The role of serotonin (5-HT) in the control of TSH and prolactin release in euthyroid subjects as assessed by the administration of ketanserin (5-HT2 antagonist) and zimelidine (5-HT re-uptake inhibitor), Psychoneuroendocrinology 9 (1984) 13–19.

[326] G. Perret, J.N. Hugues, M. Louchahi, O. Varoquaux, E. Modigliani, Effect of a short-term oral administration of cimetidine and ranitidine on the basal and thyrotropin-releasing hormone-stimulated serum concentrations of prolactin, thyrotropin and thyroid hormones in healthy volunteers. A double-blind cross-over study, Pharmacology 32 (1986) 101–108.

[327] T. Humbert, D. Pujalte, T. Bottaï, B. Hüe, R. Pouget, P. Petit, Pilot investigation of thyrotropin-releasing hormone-induced thyrotropin and prolactin release in anxious patients treated with diazepam, Clin Neuropharmacol 21 (1998) 80–85.

[328] R. Valcavi, C. Dieguez, C. Azzarito, C. Artioli, I. Portioli, M.F. Scanlon, Alpha-adrenoreceptor blockade with thymoxamine reduces basal thyrotrophin levels but does not influence circadian thyrotrophin changes in man, J Endocrinol 115 (1987) 187–191.

[329] K. Fukutani, Effects of long-term administration of theophylline on the pituitary–thyroid axis in asthmatics, Arerugi 40 (1991) 1176–1185.

[330] D. Jacobs, T. Silverstone, L. Rees, The role of dopaminergic and noradrenergic receptors in human TSH and LH release, Int Clin Psychopharmacol 4 (1989) 149–160.

[331] A. Martinos, P. Rinieris, D.N. Papachristou, A. Souvatzoglou, D.A. Koutras, C. Stefanis, Effects of six weeks' neuroleptic treatment on the pituitary–thyroid axis in schizophrenic patients, Neuropsychobiology 16 (1986) 72–77.

[332] P. Beck-Peccoz, S. Amr, N.M. Menezes-Ferreira, G. Faglia, B.D. Weintraub, Decreased receptor binding of biologically inactive thyrotropin in central hypothyroidism: Effect of treatment with thyrotropin-releasing hormone, N Engl J Med 312 (1985) 1085–1090.

[333] Y. Hayashizaki, Y. Hiraoka, K. Tatsumi, T. Hashimoto, J. Furuyama, K. Miyai, et al., DNA analyses of five families with familial inherited thyroid stimulating hormone (TSH) deficiency, J Clin Endocrinol Metab 71 (1990) 792–796.

[334] G. Borck, A.K. Topaloglu, E. Korsch, U. Martine, G. Wildhardt, N. Onenli-Mungan, et al., Four new cases of congenital secondary hypothyroidism due to a splice site mutation in the thyrotropin-beta gene: Phenotypic variability and founder effect, J Clin Endocrinol Metab 89 (2004) 4136–4141.

[335] A. Sertedaki, A. Papadimitriou, A. Voutetakis, M. Dracopoulou, M. Maniati-Christidi, C. Dacou-Voutetakis, Low TSH congenital hypothyroidism: Identification of a novel mutation of the TSH beta-subunit gene in one sporadic case (C85R) and of mutation Q49stop in two siblings with congenital hypothyroidism, Pediatr Res 52 (2002) 935–940.

[336] J. Deladoey, J.-M. Vuissoz, H.M. Domene, N. Malik, L. Gruneiro-Papendieck, A. Chiesa, et al., Congenital secondary hypothyroidism due to a mutation C105Vfs114X thyrotropin-beta mutation: Genetic study of five unrelated families from Switzerland and Argentina, Thyroid 13 (2003) 553–559.

[337] M.T. McDermott, B.R. Haugen, J.N. Black, W.M. Wood, D.F. Gordon, E.C. Ridgway, Congenital isolated central hypothyroidism caused by a "hot spot" mutation in the thyrotropin-beta gene, Thyroid 12 (2002) 1141–1146.

[338] J.-M. Vuissoz, J. Deladoey, A. Buyukgebiz, G.G. Cemeroglu, S. Gallati, P.E. Mullis, New autosomal recessive mutation of the TSH-beta subunit gene causing central isolated hypothyroidism, J Clin Endocrinol Metab 86 (2001) 4468–4471.

[339] R. Collu, J. Tang, J. Castagné, G. Lagacé, N. Masson, C. Huot, et al., A novel mechanism for isolated central hypothyroidism: Inactivating mutations in the thyrotropin-releasing hormone receptor gene, J Clin Endocrinol Metab 82 (1997) 1561–1565.

[340] A.D. Rogol, C.R. Kahn, Congenital hypothyroidism in a young man with growth hormone, thyrotropin, and prolactin deficiencies, J Clin Endocrinol Metab 39 (1976) 356–363.

[341] J.M. Wit, N.M. Drayer, M. Jansen, M.J. Walenkamp, W.H.L. Hackeng, J.H.H. Thijssen, et al., Total deficiency of GH and prolactin and partial deficiency of thyroid stimulating hormone in two Dutch families: A new variant of hereditary pituitary deficiency, Horm Res 32 (1989) 170–177.

[342] R.R. Behringer, L.S. Mathews, R.D. Palmiter, Dwarf mice produced by genetic ablation of growth hormone expressing cells, Genes & Dev 2 (1988) 453–461.

[343] W. Wu, J.D. Cogan, R.W. Pfaffle, J.S. Dasen, H. Frisch, S.M. O'Connell, et al., Mutations in PROP-1 cause familial combined pituitary hormone deficiency, Nature Genet 18 (1998) 147–149.

[344] C. Fluck, J. Deladoey, K. Rutishauser, A. Eble, U. Mrti, W. Wu, et al., Phenotypic variability in familial combined pituitary hormone deficiency caused by a PROP-1 gene mutation resulting in the substitution of Arg−>Cys at codon 120 (R120C), J Clin Endocrinol Metab 83 (1998) 3727−3734.
[345] C. Lamesch, S. Neumann, R. Pfäffle, W. Kiess, R. Paschke, Adrenocorticotrope deficiency with clinical evidence for late onset in combined pituitary hormone deficiency caused by a homozygous 301−302delAG mutation of the PROP1 gene, Pituitary 5 (2002) 163−168.
[346] D. Kelberman, M.T. Dattani, Hypopituitarism oddities: Congenital causes, Horm Res 68 (2007) 138−144.
[347] D. Diaczok, C. Romero, J. Zunich, I. Marshall, S. Radovick, A novel dominant negative mutation of OTX2 associated with combined pituitary hormone deficiency, J Clin Endocrinol Metab 93 (11) (2008) 4351−4359.
[348] P. Beck-Peccoz, L. Persani, Thyrotropinomas, Endocrinol Metab Clin North Am 37 (2008) 123−134.
[349] I.A. Kourides, E.C. Ridgway, B.D. Weintraub, S.T. Bigos, M.C. Gershengorn, F. Maloof, Thyrotropin-induced hyperthyroidism: Use of alpha and beta-subunit levels to identify patients with pituitary tumors, J Clin Endocrinol Metab 45 (1977) 534−543.
[350] S. Refetoff, R.E. Weiss, S.J. Usala, The syndromes of resistance to thyroid hormone, Endocr Rev 14 (1993) 348−399.
[351] S. Refetoff, Resistance to thyroid hormone: One of several defects causing reduced sensitivity to thyroid hormone, Nat Clin Pract Endocrinol Metab 4 (2008) 1.
[352] T. Sunthornthepvarakui, M.E. Gottschalk, Y. Hayashi, S. Refetoff, Brief report: Resistance to thyrotropin caused by mutations in the thyrotropin-receptor gene, N Engl J Med 332 (1995) 155−160.
[353] S. Refetoff, L.T. DeWind, L.J. DeGroot, Familial syndrome combining deaf-mutism, stippled epiphyses, goiter, and abnormally high PBI: Possible target organ refractoriness to thyroid hormone, J Clin Endocrinol Metab 27 (1967) 279−294.
[354] K. Tsunekawa, K. Onigata, T. Morimura, T. Kasahara, S. Nishiyama, T. Kamoda, et al., Identification and functional analysis of novel inactivating thyrotropin receptor mutations in patients with thyrotropin resistance, Thyroid 16 (2006) 471−479.
[355] M. Tonacchera, C. Di Cosmo, G. De Marco, P. Agretti, M. Banco, A. Perri, et al., Identification of TSH receptor mutations in three families with resistance to TSH, Clin Endocrinol (Oxf) 67 (2007) 712−718.
[356] S. Sura-Trueba, C. Aumas, A. Carre, S. Durif, J. Leger, M. Polak, et al., An inactivating mutation within the first extracellular loop of the thyrotropin receptor impedes normal post-translational maturation of the extracellular domain, Endocrinology 150 (2009) 1043−1050.
[357] A. Nicoletti, M. Bal, G. De Marco, L. Baldazzi, P. Agretti, S. Menabò, et al., Thyrotropin-stimulating hormone receptor gene analysis in pediatric patients with non-autoimmune subclinical hypothyroidism, J Clin Endocrinol Metab 94 (2009) 4187−4194.
[358] C. Dacou-Voutetakis, D.M. Feltquate, M. Drakopoulou, I.A. Kourides, N.C. Dracopoli, Familial hypothyroidism caused by a nonsense mutation in the thyroid-stimulating hormone beta-subunit gene, Am J Hum Genet 46 (1990) 988−993.
[359] M. Bonomi, M.C. Proverbio, G. Weber, G. Chiumello, P. Beck-Peccoz, L. Persani, Hyperplastic pituitary gland, high serum glycoprotein hormone alpha-subunit, and variable circulating thyrotropin (TSH) levels as hallmark of central hypothyroidism due to mutations of the TSH beta gene, J Clin Endocrinol Metab 86 (2001) 1600−1604.
[360] J. Pohlenz, A. Dumitrescu, U. Aumann, G. Koch, R. Melchior, D. Prawitt, et al., Congenital secondary hypothyroidism caused by exon skipping due to a homozygous donor splice site mutation in the TSH beta-subunit gene, J Clin Endocrinol Metab 87 (2002) 336−339.
[361] B. Karges, B. LeHeup, E. Schoenle, C. Castro-Correia, M. Fontoura, R. Pfaffle, et al., Compound heterozygous and homozygous mutations of the TSH beta gene as a cause of congenital central hypothyroidism in Europe, Horm Res 62 (2004) 149−155.
[362] B.M. Doeker, R.W. Pfaffle, J. Pohlenz, W. Andler, Congenital central hypothyroidism due to a homozygous mutation in the thyrotropin beta-subunit gene follows an autosomal recessive inheritance, J Clin Endocrinol Metab 83 (1998) 1762−1765.
[363] H. Brumm, A. Pfeufer, H. Biebermann, D. Schnabel, D. Deiss, A. Gruters, Congenital central hypothyroidism due to homozygous thyrotropin beta 313deltaT mutation is caused by a founder effect, J Clin Endocrinol Metab 87 (2002) 4811−4816.
[364] C.J. Partsch, F.G. Riepe, N. Krone, W.G. Sippell, J. Pohlenz, Initially elevated TSH and congenital central hypothyroidism due to a homozygous mutation of the TSH beta subunit gene: Case report and review of the literature, Exp Clin Endocrinol Diabetes 114 (2006) 227−234.
[365] C. Heinrichs, J. Parma, N.H. Scherberg, F. Delange, G. Van Vliet, L. Duprez, et al., Congenital central hypothyroidism caused by a homozygous mutation in the TSH-beta subunit gene, Thyroid 10 (2000) 387−391.
[366] H.M. Domene, L. Gruneiro-Papendieck, A. Chiesa, S. Iocansky, V.C. Herzovich, R. Papazian, et al., The C105fs114X is the prevalet thyrotropin beta-subunit gene mutation in Argentinean patients with congenital central hypothyroidism, Horm Res 61 (2004) 41−46.
[367] E.I. Felner, B.A. Dickson, P.C. White, Hypothyroidism in siblings due to a homozygous mutation of the TSH-beta subunit gene, J Pediatr Endocrinol Metab 17 (2004) 669−672.

CHAPTER

7

Gonadotropin Hormones

Ursula B. Kaiser

Brigham and Women's Hospital and Harvard Medical School, Boston, MA, USA

INTRODUCTION

The pituitary gonadotropin hormones, luteinizing hormone (LH) and follicle-stimulating hormone (FSH), are dimeric glycoprotein hormones that play an essential role in the mammalian reproductive process. Synthesized in the gonadotropes of the anterior pituitary, LH and FSH are secreted into the systemic circulation and act on the ovary and testis to direct steroidogenesis and the final steps of gametogenesis [1]. Because these hormones are responsible for sexual maturation and normal reproductive function, the regulation of their synthesis and secretion is essential for the preservation of a species. LH and FSH are each composed of two distinct carbohydrate-containing protein subunits in noncovalent association, a common alpha (α) subunit and a distinct beta (β) subunit that bestows biologic specificity (LHβ and FSHβ, for LH and FSH, respectively) [2]. Befitting their important roles in endocrine physiology, the synthesis and secretion of LH and FSH are under complex regulation by counterbalancing stimulatory hypothalamic inputs (e.g., gonadotropin-releasing hormone, or GnRH) and negative feedback from gonadal sex steroid and peptide hormones, with further paracrine modulation by local factors produced within the pituitary gland itself (e.g., activins, inhibins and follistatin) [3]. The integration of these signals results in the coordinated control of subunit gene expression, protein synthesis, and gonadotropin secretion to promote sexual maturation and control normal reproductive function.

DEVELOPMENT, EMBRYOLOGY AND HISTOLOGY

Gonadotrope Cells in the Pituitary

For details of the morphology of the gonadotrope, the reader is referred to several classical reviews [4–6]. The anterior pituitary cell types responsible for the synthesis and secretion of LH and FSH are known as gonadotropes and first appear in the anterior pituitary gland during early fetal development. Gonadotropes constitute about 7–15% of anterior pituitary cells. In the human pituitary, gonadotropes are dispersed throughout the pars distalis. Gonadotropes are composed of a heterogeneous population of cells that have been studied extensively by light and electron microscopy using antisera specific for intact LH and FSH or their subunits. Gonadotropes are medium-sized cells, oval or irregular in shape, with a prominent nucleus. Electron microscopy reveals a spherical and eccentric nucleus, prominent rough endoplasmic reticulum (RER) and Golgi complexes and several vesicles containing secretory granules. The secretory granules are electron-dense and are of two sizes, the larger ones measuring 350–450 nm and the smaller ones 150–250 nm. In studies of rat pituitary cells fractionated by elutriation, most of the gonadotropin-staining cells are among the largest cells [7]. However, a significant number of cells among the poorly granulated small cell fractions also secrete gonadotropins. Small gonadotrophs may represent the immature population that later give rise to the highly responsive large secretory cells.

Immunocytochemical studies have demonstrated the presence of both bihormonal and monohormonal groups of gonadotropes. About 70% of gonadotropes in the adult male rat pituitary contain both LH and FSH, 15% contain LH alone and 15% FSH alone [8]. However, the distribution of these three populations is dynamic and shifts in the number and proportion of bihormonal and monohormonal gonadotropes are observed under different physiological conditions, such as castration or throughout the estrous cycle. These findings suggest that monohormonal cells represent a similar cell type in different secretory phases [7], although they could also reflect the existence of

The Pituitary, Third Edition, DOI: 10.1016/B978-0-12-380926-1.10007-0

a precursor pool of gonadotropes or plasticity of this pituitary cell type. The coexistence of LH and FSH within the same pituitary cell type is consistent with the coupled secretion of LH and FSH, for example at the time of the midcycle ovulatory surge. On the other hand, monohormonal gonadotrope populations may underlie differential LH and FSH release under different physiological conditions. An alternative explanation for differential LH and FSH release is the known existence of gonadotrope secretory granules that selectively store LH or FSH.

Gonadotropes from male and female pituitary glands cannot be distinguished on morphologic grounds. Castration leads to an increase in size as well as number of gonadotropes that become morphologically distinct. These castration cells are characterized by large vacuoles in the cytoplasm due to dilation of the endoplasmic reticulum, which may displace the nucleus to one side. Gonadotrope hyperplasia and hypertrophy following removal of the gonad may lead to an increase in the size of the sella. On the other hand, studies in patients with idiopathic hypogonadotropic hypogonadism reveal only a few poorly developed gonadotropes.

Molecular Basis of Gonadotrope Development

Pituitary development is discussed in detail in Chapter 1. The focus here will be on gonadotrope development and differentiation. Advances in genetic and molecular techniques have greatly increased our understanding of the mechanisms underlying pituitary development, and genetic analyses of mutations associated with developmental disorders of the pituitary in humans have begun to reveal the molecular mechanisms of pituitary development and cell lineage determination [9,10]. The anterior pituitary gland arises from midline cells in the anterior neural ridge, which form Rathke's pouch, an oral ectodermal invagination, by the fourth to fifth weeks of gestation in response to inductive signaling from the ventral diencephalon. Coordinated spatiotemporal regulation of cell lineage-specific transcription factors expressed in pluripotential pituitary stem cells together with dynamic gradients of locally acting extrinsic signals regulate progenitor cell proliferation, lineage commitment and terminal differentiation. Neuroectodermal signals important for pituitary morphogenesis include BMP4, FGF8/10/18 and Wnt5. Ventral developmental patterning is dictated by BMP2 and Shh. Coordinated, temporal expression of a number of transcription factors directs the embryological development of the differentiated cell types. Mutations in transcription factors required for Rathke's pouch formation, cell proliferation, or the differentiation of multiple lineages are associated with combined pituitary hormone deficiency (CPHD), whereas mutations in transcription factors required for the differentiation of only one cell lineage are associated with a single hormone deficiency. The list of transcription factors implicated in gonadotrope development and differentiation is rapidly growing, and a few key factors will be mentioned here (Figure 7.1; Table 7.1).

During pituitary development, Notch signaling is active early in pituitary organogenesis, signaling through Hes family members [10]. Hesx1 is a paired-like homeodomain transcription factor that acts as a transcriptional repressor. It is one of the earliest markers of the pituitary primordium and also contributes to the development of the forebrain, the ventral diencephalon and the hypothalamus. Targeted disruption of Hesx1 in mice results in disruption of forebrain development, absent optic vesicles and microphthalmia. In humans, mutations in Hesx1 have been identified and are associated with variable septo-optic dysplasia and

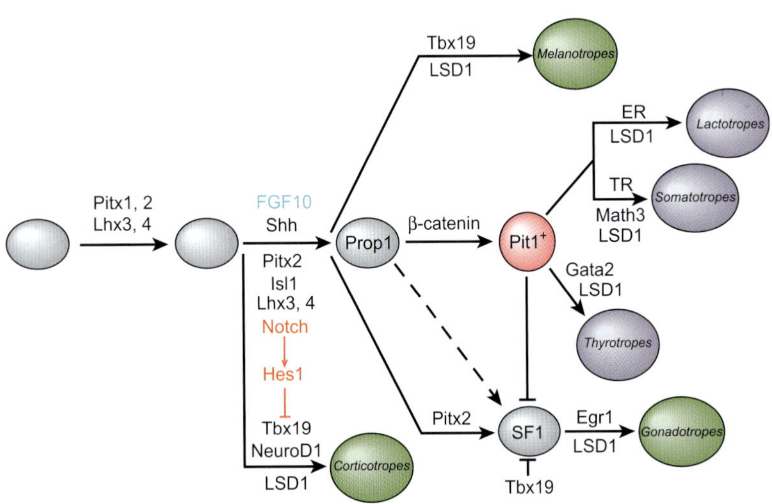

FIGURE 7.1 Model for development of the human anterior pituitary gland and cell lineage determination, including gonadotrope differentiation. *From Zhu [10].*

TABLE 7.1 Clinical Features Associated with Mutations in Genes Involved in Gonadotrope Development

Transcription Factor	Chr.	Inheritance	Hormone Deficiencies	Other Features
HESX1	3p21	AR, AD	CPHD, IGHD	Septo-optic dysplasia
PITX2	4q25	AD	CPHD	Rieger's syndrome
SOX2	3q27	AD (de novo)	HH, variable GHD	Anophthalmia/microphthalmia, oesophageal atresia, genital tract abnormalities, hypothalamic hamartoma, sensorineural hearing loss, diplegia
SOX3	Xq26	XL	CPHD, IGHD	Mental retardation
LHX3	9q34	AD	GH, TSH, LH, FSH, PRLACTH may be deficient	Limited neck rotation, short cervical spine, sensorineural deafness
LHX4	1q25	AD	CPHD (GH, TSH, ACTH deficiencies; variable gonadotrophin deficiency)	Cerebellar abnormalities
PROP1	5q35	AR	GH, TSH, LH, FSH, PRLEvolving ACTH deficiency	May show transient AP hyperplasia
OTX2	14q21	AD	IGHD or CPHD (GH, TSH, PRL, LH, FSH)	Bilateral anophthalmia, bilateral severe microphthalmia

AR, autosomal recessive; AD, autosomal dominant; XL, X-linked; CPHD, combined pituitary hormone deficiency; IGHD, isolated growth hormone deficiency; HH, hypogonadotropic hypogonadism; AP, anterior pituitary.

hypopituitarism, ranging from CPHD including gonadotropins to isolated growth hormone deficiency [11–13]. Mutations in Sox2 and Sox3, members of the Sry-related high-mobility group box (Sox) genes, are also associated with septo-optic dysplasia and anterior pituitary hypoplasia and hypogonadotropic hypogonadism [12].

Pitx1 and Pitx2, members of the class of bicoid homeodomain proteins, show a high degree of homology and are expressed in an overlapping pattern during pituitary development [9,14]. Pitx1 is expressed in all five anterior pituitary lineages in both the fetal and adult pituitary gland and is able to activate the expression of all six of the major anterior pituitary hormones, including LH and FSH, frequently acting in synergy with other pituitary transcription factors [15]. *Pitx1*$^{-/-}$ mice have mild defects and the loss of Pitx1 appears to be compensated by Pitx2 in pituitary development, whereas *Pitx2*$^{-/-}$ mice have arrested pituitary development, and studies of mice with a hypomorphic Pitx2 have revealed that Pitx2 is also required for gonadotrope differentiation [16]. Mutations in Pitx2 cause Rieger syndrome, characterized by defects in the eyes, teeth and heart as well as pituitary hormone deficiencies [17].

FGF8 activates two key regulatory genes, *Lhx3* and *Lhx4*, two LIM-type homeodomain transcription factors essential for pituitary development. Targeted deletion of either of these two genes in mice results in failure of pituitary gland morphogenesis and an aplastic or hypoplastic pituitary with reduced numbers of all cell types. Mutations in *Lhx3* and *Lhx4* have been identified in patients with CPHD including impaired gonadotropin release [9,11,12,18].

Mutations in *PROP1* (Prophet of Pit1) are the most common genetic cause of CPHD [19]. *PROP1* is a member of the paired-like family of homeodomain transcription factors, expressed early in Rathke's pouch. The well-known Ames dwarf mouse has GH, prolactin and TSH deficiency due to a homozygous missense mutation in the *PROP1* gene [20]. Gonadotrope differentiation is also impaired, and homozygous females and most males are infertile. Most patients with *PROP1* mutations develop GH and TSH deficiency in childhood, whereas the reproductive phenotype is more variable, with some presenting as pubertal failure in adolescence and others developing hypogonadism later in life. Corticotrope insufficiency can also develop later in life in some patients [9,11,12]. In contrast to *PROP1* mutations, mutations in *PIT1*, also a member of the POU homeodomain family, have pituitary deficiencies limited to GH, prolactin and TSH [9].

Steroidogenic factor-1 (SF-1) is a member of the nuclear receptor family that is expressed throughout the reproductive axis (hypothalamus, pituitary and gonads) and in the adrenal gland. It is a key transcriptional regulator of many genes involved in sexual differentiation, steroidogenesis and reproduction, including the pituitary gonadotropin α-subunit, LHβ, FSHβ and GnRHR genes [11,21]. SF-1 null mice show complete adrenal and gonadal agenesis as well as impaired development of the ventromedial hypothalamus and of gonadotropes [22]. Patients with mutations in SF-1 have been described with varying degrees of XY sex reversal, testicular dysgenesis, ovarian insufficiency, adrenal failure and impaired pubertal maturation [23]. DAX-1 is a related nuclear receptor transcription factor with a similar distribution pattern of expression. Mutations in this X-linked gene cause primary adrenal insufficiency and hypogonadotropic hypogonadism [24]. A role for DAX-1 in gonadotrope development has not been established; the major role for DAX-1 apears to be, paradoxically, as a repressor of SF-1-mediated transcription.

In addition to the genes discussed here, the list of transcription factors implicated in gonadotrope development and differentiation and in control of gonadotropin gene expression is growing. GATA-2 is one example; targeted deletion in the anterior pituitary is associated with reduced basal and castration-induced gonadotropin production, although it does not appear to be essential for gonadotrope cell fate, perhaps as a result of compensatory up-regulation of other GATA transcription family members [25].

The importance of epigenetic modification of DNA and histones in cellular differentiation during development is becoming increasingly recognized. Distinct cell types, arising from common progenitors, share an identical genetic composition, yet establish unique profiles of gene expression and cellular function [10]. The field of epigenetics has advanced greatly in recent years, with the identification of enzymes and protein complexes that catalyze DNA methylation and histone modifications, including acetylation, methylation, phosphorylation and ubiquitination [26,27]. LSD1 is a histone demethylase important for chromatin modification and transcriptional regulation as a component of the CtBP–CoREST corepressor complex [28]. It is expressed in the pituitary throughout development, and has recently been implicated in pituitary and gonadotope development [29]. A conditional targeted deletion of LSD1 in the pituitary was generated, revealing that LSD1 is required for late cell-lineage determination and terminal differentiation events. LSD1 interacts with Pit1 to regulate activation of Pit1 target genes, and also attenuates Notch1 signaling, thereby establishing LSD1 as a functional component of both coactivator and corepressor complexes to regulate activation and repression programs important for terminal differentiation. The targeted deletion of LSD1 from the pituitary resulted in reduced levels of GH, TSHβ, LHβ and POMC, markers of somatotrope, thyrotrope, gonadotrope and corticotrope differentiation, respectively, and implicating LSD1 in the terminal differentiation of all pituitary cell types [10, 29].

Stem cells and other progenitor cells were long thought to be restricted to embryonic tissues in most cell types. However, during the last two decades, stem cells are being identified in an ever increasing number of adult organs and tissues, including those long considered to be postmitotic with negligible regenerative potential such as neurons [30,31]. Childs et al. [7] have proposed that adenohypophyseal cells are derived from a common multipotential stem or progenitor cell. The existence of multipotent cells in the pituitary was first suggested 40 years ago, when chromophobes were purified from rat pituitaries and transplanted, giving rise to acidophils and basophils. Whether the endogenous pituitary cells have regenerative capacity is a contentious issue. Given the plasticity of the pituitary gland, the presence of the stem cell population would not be unexpected. Plasticity such as lactotrope hyperplasia during pregnancy or thyrotrope hyperplasia during primary hypothyroidism suggests at a minimum a population of multipotential reserve or progenitor cells that differentiate into the desired cell type depending on the physiological environment of the organism [32]. Stem cells have also been implicated in the pathogenesis of pituitary adenomas. Candidates for pituitary stem cells include chromophobes, folliculstellate cells. Expression of potential stem cell markers such as nestin in the marginal zone around Rathke's cleft has suggested that the stem cell population may exist in this marginal zone. Nonetheless, none of these cells has yet been unequivocally demonstrated to meet all of the criteria to be classified as stem cells.

BIOCHEMICAL STRUCTURE AND MOLECULAR BIOLOGY OF LH AND FSH

Hormone Structure

The gonadotropins belong to a family of dimeric glycoprotein hormones that includes LH, FSH, thyroid-stimulating hormone (TSH) and placental chorionic gonadotropin (CG) that share structural features. Each of these hormones is heterodimeric, consisting of two different noncovalently associated subunits, an α- and a β-subunit (Figure 7.2). Whereas the α-subunit of LH, FSH, TSH and CG is common to all members of this family of glycoprotein hormones and identical in primary polypeptide sequence, each β-subunit has a different amino acid sequence and confers biologic specificity [34]. The α- and β-subunits are encoded by different genes locate on separate chromosomes [2]. The common α-subunit contains 92 amino acids, while the β-subunits of FSH, LH and CG contain 111, 121 and 145 amino acids, respectively (Table 7.2) [35]. Both subunits are glycosylated at specific residues. Significant homology between the two subunits suggests that these subunits arose from a common ancestral gene [2]. Although the individual subunits can be found in the unassociated or "free" form in the pituitary and in the circulation, they have no known biological activity;

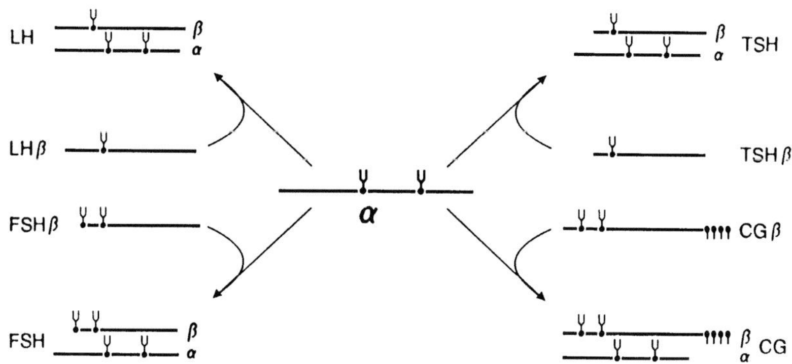

FIGURE 7.2 Schematic depiction of the subunit structure and glycosylation sites of the four human glycoprotein hormones and their subunits. Asn-linked oligosaccharides are depicted as Ү and Ser/Thr-linked oligosaccharides as ↑. *From Baenziger [37].*

heterodimerization is essential. Once association between an α- and a β-subunit occurs, the resulting heterodimers confer hormonal bioactivity, with the specific β-subunit imparting its unique biological specificity [34].

Each subunit is cysteine-rich and highly linked internally by disulfide bonds. Consequently, the location of the cysteines, to some degree, confers the three-dimensional structure of the glycoprotein by determining the folding [35]. The complex and elaborate folding results in multiple noncontiguous segments of the primary amino acid sequence that contribute to receptor binding and activation. The two subunits are noncovalently associated, dependent on a unique "seat-belt" arrangement provided by the disulfide pairing between highly conserved cysteine residues within each subunit. The regions of similarity between different β-subunits are felt to be involved in binding to the α-subunits and the variable regions in receptor binding. Each subunit also bears carbohydrate moieties that contribute to biologic activity and metabolic fate of the glycoprotein hormones.

The α-subunit

The α- and β-subunits of LH and FSH are encoded by separate genes [2,35]. A single gene codes for the α-subunit of the four glycoprotein hormones [36]. The human α-subunit gene is located on the short arm of chromosome 6 and consists of four exons and three introns (Figure 7.3; Table 7.2). The gene encodes for an mRNA species 0.73–0.8 kilobase (kb) length. This mRNA corresponds to a precursor peptide with a molecular mass of 14-kDa, comprising a 24-amino acid signal peptide followed by a 92-amino acid protein in humans. The gene is expressed in gonadotropes and thyrotropes of the anterior pituitary gland and in the placenta. A striking feature of the mature α-subunit is the presence of ten highly conserved cysteine residues, which are oxidized to form five disulfide bonds critical to the tertiary "cysteine knot" structure of the mature protein. This cystine knot motif identifies the glycoprotein hormones as members of the cystine knot growth factor (CKGF) superfamily, which also includes the nerve growth factor (NGF), platelet-derived growth factor (PDGF) and transforming growth factor (TGF)-β families. The resultant tertiary structure enables heterodimerization with β-subunit partners as well as ligand–receptor interaction. In addition to the cysteines, the mature α-subunit also bears two asparagine-linked oligosaccharides, at amino acid residues 56 and 83 [37].

TABLE 7.2 Structures of the Glycoprotein Hormone Alpha, Thyroid-stimulating Hormone Beta, Luteinizing Hormone Beta, Human Chorionic Gonadotropin Beta and Follicle-stimulating Hormone Beta Genes

Subunit	Locus	Gene Length (Kb)	Number of Exons (introns)	mRNA Length (Kb)	Number of Amino Acids	Number of Glycosylation Sites (location)[a]
Common α	6p21.1-23	9.4	4(3)	0.8	92	2 (N: 52, 78)[b]
TSHβ	1p22	4.9	3(2)	0.7	118[c]	1 (N: 23)
LHβ	19q13.3	1.5	3(2)	0.7	121	1 (N:30)
CGβ	19q13.3	1.9	3(2)	1.0	145	6 (N: 13, 30; S: 121, 127, 132, 138)
FSHβ	11p13	3.9	3(2)	1.8	117	2 (N: 7, 24)

[a] *Oligosaccharide chains are attached either to asparagine (N) (N-linked) or to serine (S) (O-linked). N or S residues are numbered according to their position in the respective sequence.*
[b] *Free α-subunit may also contain an additional site of O-glycosylation at threonine (T) 39.*
[c] *118-amino-acid coding region; six amino acids can be cleaved at the C-terminal end.*

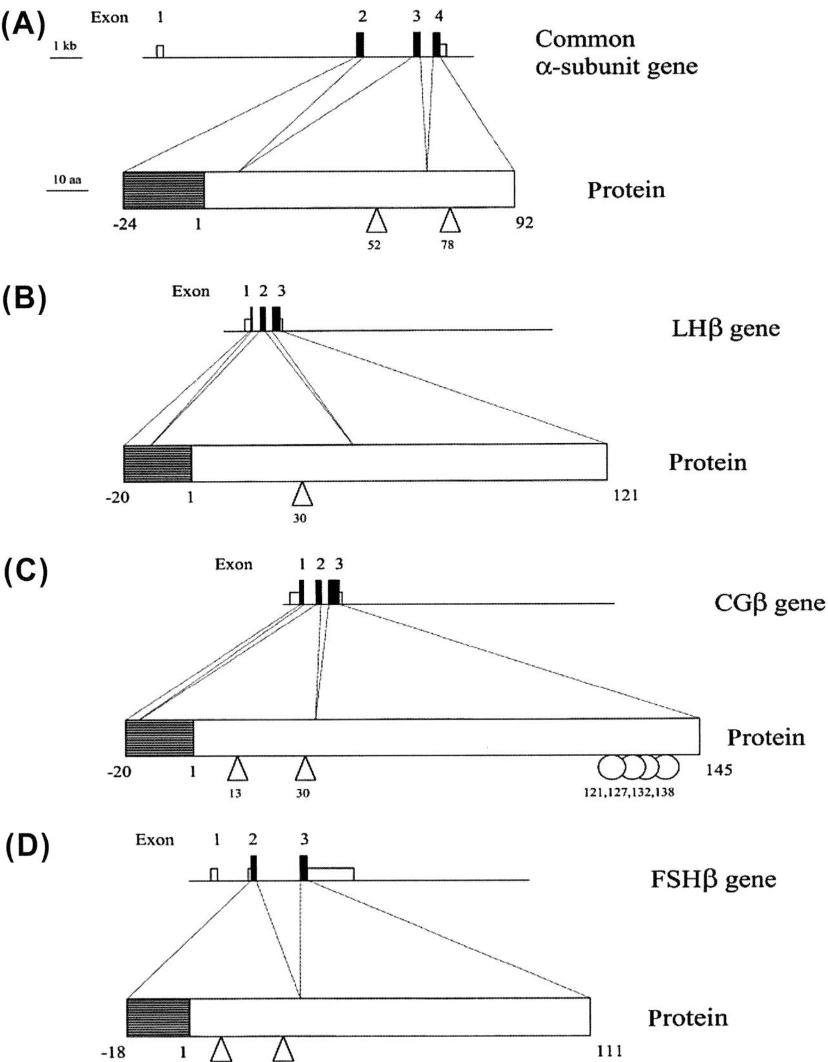

FIGURE 7.3 Schematic representation of the human gonadotropin subunit genes. The top part of each scheme depicts the gene structure. Open bars indicate noncoding sequences; solid bars indicate coding sequences. The bottom part of each scheme shows the protein structure. Signal peptides are shaded while the mature peptide is depicted by an open bar. The positions of N-linked glycosylation sites are depicted by triangles and O-linked glycosylation by circles. Amino acid positions are depicted by numbers. *From Themmen [35].*

The LHβ-subunit

The LH/CGβ-subunit genes form a cluster with a complex organization [38]. The human LHβ-subunit is encoded by a member of a cluster of seven different genes located on chromosome 19q13.3, which also includes the gene coding for the CGβ-subunit. This gene cluster is believed to have evolved by gene duplication, and the other five copies are thought to represent either pseudogenes or are expressed at very low levels. Studies suggest that LHβ and CGβ genes diverged only recently in evolution [38]. The LHβ gene is expressed in the pituitary gonadotrope with high specificity, whereas the CGβ gene is expressed primarily in the placenta, only in certain mammalian species such as horses, baboons and humans [38]. The LHβ gene is relatively small in size (~1.5 kb). The general organization of the LHβ gene (three exons and two introns) is similar to other glycoprotein hormone β-subunit genes (Table 7.2; Figure 7.3).

Several distinctions are notable between the LHβ and CGβ genes. First, the CGβ genes are present only in primate and equine species, whereas LHβ genes are present in all vertebrates that have been examined. Second, the LHβ gene encodes a 145-amino acid precursor protein of molecular mass 15–17-kDa, which is cleaved to produce a 24-amino acid signal peptide followed by a 121-amino acid mature LHβ-subunit. In contrast, the mature hCGβ protein is 145 amino acids in length and does not include a leader, but contains a 24-amino acid carboxyterminal extension [2,35,38]. Third, the LHβ and CGβ genes have different transcriptional start sites and utilize different promoters, accounting for their different tissue distribution patterns of expression [39]. Nonetheless, like all members of the glycoprotein hormone β-subunit family, the

LHβ-subunit bears a highly conserved backbone of 12 cysteine residues that are oxidized to form six disulfide bonds [35]. The LHβ-subunit also contains one glycosylation site (Asn30), whereas the hCGβ-subunit contains two (Asn13, Asn30). The hCGβ-subunit contains four additional serine O-linked oligosaccharide units in its carboxyterminal extension. This domain influences processing of the subunit and is important for maintaining the longer biologic half life of hCG. The amino acid sequences of the human LHβ- and CGβ-subunits share 82% homology, and when associated with the α-subunit, these two hormones activate the same receptor.

The FSHβ-subunit

The human FSHβ-subunit gene is encoded by a single gene located on the short arm of chromosome 11. The general organization of the FSHβ gene is similar to that of other glycoprotein hormone β genes in that it has three exons and two introns [2,35,40]. The first exon contains only 5′-untranslated sequences, while the second and third exons contain the entire coding sequence (Table 7.2; Figure 7.3). The third exon also contains a relatively long (1−1.5 kb) 3′-untranslated sequence. The human FSHβ-subunit includes a signal peptide of 19 amino acids followed by a mature peptide of 111 amino acids, with two glycosylation sites (Asn7 and Asn24). Like LHβ, the FSHβ gene is expressed only in pituitary gonadotropes.

Synthesis and Post-translational Processing of LH and FSH

Subunit precursors are processed by enzymatic removal of amino terminal leader peptides and also by addition of carbohydrates as they enter the lumen of the endoplasmic reticulum. The α-subunit contains two asparagine-linked carbohydrate chains, while the β-subunit chain contains one or two [34,37]. In addition, O-linked oligosaccharides are added to serine or threonine residues of the free α-subunit and the carboxyterminal extension of the hCGβ-subunit (see Figures 7.2, 7.3).

The glycosylation occurs cotranslationally in several steps [41]. First, oligosaccharide complexes are transferred to nascent proteins via lipid-linked intermediates or isoprenoid-dolichol-pyrophosphate carriers. The complexes are added to specific asparagine residues with sequences of the form Asn-X-Thr (Ser) [42]. The core carbohydrates are of the general structure: Glc−13 (α-Man4−6 Man β1−4 Glc), Ac β1−4 Glc NAc-Asn. Second, glucose residues are removed by glucose-specific glucosidases, leaving a high-mannose oligosaccharide [43]. The Asn-linked oligosaccharides undergo further remodeling in the Golgi with the addition of sugars to result in the formation of complex and heterogeneous branched carbohydrate structures, terminating with sialic acid, fucose, galactose, as well as sulfated N-acetylgalactosamine in the case of LH (but not FSH) [37]. Tissue- and protein-specific differences occur in the processing of glycoprotein hormones and variations can occur even for a given hormone. As a result, several isomeric forms of LH and FSH can be produced at any time in an individual. For example, shifts to more biologically active isoforms of circulating gonadotropins occur at the onset of puberty or at specific phases of the menstrual cycle.

The functional importance of these complex oligosaccharide side chains is reflected in their influence on hormone metabolic clearance rates and bioactivity [34,44]. Gonadotropin hormone clearance involves both liver metabolism and renal excretion. Predominantly sulfated oligosaccharides have shorter plasma half lives than those with sialylated oligosaccharides, likely contributing to the longer circulating half life of FSH (1-4 h) compared to LH (10−50 min). The carboxyterminal sequence of the hCGβ-subunit with its O-linked glycosylation prolongs the half life and in vivo bioactivity of hCG compared to the other glycoprotein hormones. Fusion of this sequence to the other subunits, such as LHβ or FSHβ, in a region that is not important for receptor binding or signal transduction, does not interfere with subunit folding or assembly, secretion, receptor binding or in vitro bioactivity of the dimers. Moreover, the presence of this sequence significantly increases the in vivo bioactivity and half lives of the engineered chimeras. These chimeras could serve as potent agonists for clinical use. Furthermore, this strategy could have broader applications for enhancing the in vivo half life of diverse proteins [34]. Glycosylation of gonadotropin subunits is not required for their heterodimerization or for receptor binding. However, studies have demonstrated that chemically deglycosylated glycoprotein hormones bind to the receptor but fail to induce cAMP production in target cells in the testis and ovary. Thus, the carbohydrate side-chains may be essential for transduction of biologic signals.

In parallel with cleavage of signal peptides and initiation of oligosaccharide moiety addition, the partially glycosylated α- and β-subunits undergo folding, formation of multiple intramolecular disulfide linkages and dimerization in the endoplasmic reticulum, followed by further processing of the oligosaccharides in the Golgi. The mature glycoprotein hormones are then packaged into secretory granules. The β-subunit is the rate-limiting factor in the biosynthesis of LH and FSH, and the α-subunit is present in excess. As a result, intact dimeric glycoprotein hormones and free α-subunits are present in the circulation, but free β-subunits are rarely found.

ONTOGENY AND PHYSIOLOGY OF LH AND FSH SECRETION

Fetal Life

GnRH is present in the fetal hypothalamus as early as 6 weeks of gestation [45,46]. The fetal pituitary contains measurable amounts of LH and FSH by 10 weeks, and gonadotropins are first detectable in the human fetal circulation by weeks 12–14 of gestation [47]. Their biosynthesis at this early stage of development appears to be at least partially dependent on GnRH, as reflected by the absence of LHβ and FSHβ in the pituitary glands of anencephalic infants who lack a hypothalamus and the ability of GnRH to induce LH and FSH synthesis and secretion in human fetal pituitary cells in vitro [48]. Serum levels of LH and FSH rise gradually to a peak at about 20 weeks [49]. In the second half of pregnancy, serum LH and FSH levels in the fetus decline progressively, likely the result of the rise in sex steroid secretion by the fetal gonad, rising maternal estrogen levels and the development of negative-feedback mechanisms [46,47,49].

Placental hCG plays a significant role in stimulating androgen production by the fetal testis in early pregnancy. High androgen levels are required for differentiation of Wolffian structures in the male. In addition, FSH stimulates differentiation and development of seminiferous tubules. These data are consistent with observations that patients with hypogonadotropic hypogonadism (HH) have normal differentiation of Wolffian structures and external genitalia because the placental hCG drives the fetal testis to produce sufficient androgen, even in the absence of pituitary LH and FSH. However, because of FSH deficiency, these patients have impaired development of seminiferous tubules. On the other hand, testicular descent is partially dependent on androgen levels during the later part of pregnancy, which, during this period of fetal life, are maintained by LH derived from the fetal pituitary. As a result, patients with HH often have associated cryptorchidism or undescended testes [47,50]. Thus a thorough understanding of the ontogenetic changes in gonadotropin secretion can be helpful in defining the pathophysiology of the disorders of sexual differentiation.

Postnatal Life and Childhood Years

After birth, serum LH and FSH levels rise again, and in the first 6 months of postnatal life, LH and FSH levels are measurable in blood. The pulsatile pattern of LH and FSH secretion is discernible during this brief period of reactivation of the hypothalamic–pituitary axis. Serum LH and FSH levels peak around 2–3 months of age and then decline to prepubertal levels by about 6 months of age in boys and 1–2 years of age in girls [46,47,50]. This brief period of postnatal life thus provides a unique, albeit narrow, window in which the integrity of the hypothalamic–pituitary–gonadal axis can be assessed before gonadotropin and sex steroid levels fall back to the low range.

During childhood years, the hypothalamic–pituitary–gonadal axis remains quiescent until the onset of puberty [46,47,50,51]. However, the pituitary and the testis retain the ability to respond to GnRH and to LH, respectively. The response of the prepubertal pituitary to a GnRH stimulus is relatively damped. In addition, the GnRH-induced rise in serum FSH in prepubertal humans is greater than that in LH. This is in contrast to an adult in whom a single dose of GnRH causes a greater rise in LH. During pubertal maturation, serum LH and FSH levels rise. It is generally believed that activation of FSH secretion precedes that of LH. Nocturnal, sleep-entrained pulsatile secretion of LH is characteristic of early stages of puberty. Reactivation of the hypothalamic GnRH pulse generator at the time of puberty results in progressive increases in the amplitude and frequency of gonadotropin pulses, initially nocturnally and then during the daytime as puberty progresses [46,47,51]. The quiescence of the GnRH pulse generator and of circulating LH and FSH levels during childhood and their reactivation at the time of puberty are independent of gonadal function, as reflected in the patterns observed in agonadal humans and monkeys (Figure 7.4) [52,53]. The preservation of this developmental pattern in agonadal monkeys and human subjects led to the rejection of the "gonadostat" hypothesis and the generation of a model of gonad-independent central inhibition or restraint to account for prepubertal reduction in pulsatile GnRH release, followed by a pubertal increase in GnRH resulting from either removal of an inhibitory input or development of a stimulatory signal to the GnRH neuronal network, or a combination of both [54,55].

Although the mean plasma gonadotropin levels increase only about two-fold during puberty with considerable overlap between prepubertal and pubertal levels [56], the increase in gonadotropin secretion is much higher, as reflected by rises in urinary gonadotropin secretion of ~4-fold in FSH and ~12-fold in LH. Furthermore, there is an increase in bioactivity of circulating gonadotropins. More recently, new methodologies have been applied using highly sensitive immunofluorometric (IFMA) and immunochemiluminometric (ICMA) LH and FSH assays. No overlap of basal LH levels as determined by ICMA was observed between prepubertal and pubertal males, but basal LH determined by IFMA overlapped in 11.8% of subjects. In girls, both methods yielded overlapping values (10.4%, ICMA and 84.6%, IFMA). This study indicated that ICMA is

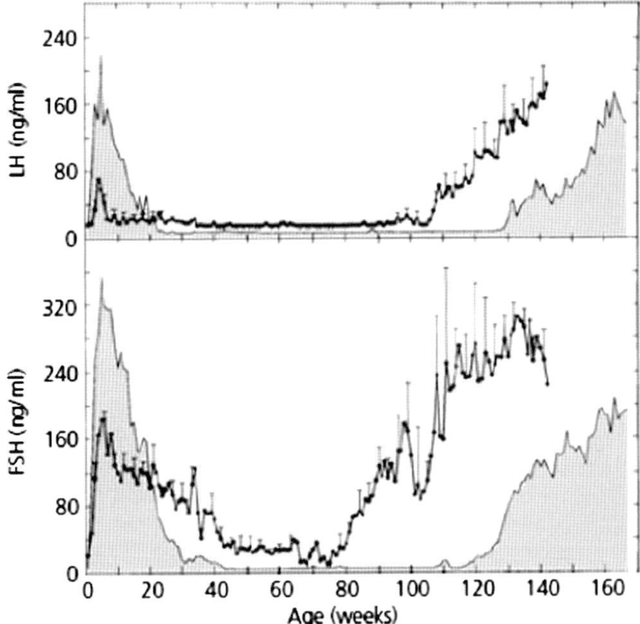

FIGURE 7.4 The on–off–on pattern of gonadotropin-releasing hormone pulse generator activity during postnatal development in agonadal male (stippled area) and female (closed data points ± error bars) rhesus monkeys as reflected by circulating mean LH (top panel) and FSH (bottom panel) concentrations from birth to 142–166 weeks of age. Note that in females, the intensity and duration of the prepubertal hiatus in the secretion of FSH, and to a lesser extent LH, is truncated in comparison to males. *Adapted from Plant [53].*

more sensitive and precise than IFMA, permitting differentiation of pubertal and prepubertal stages in boys under basal conditions which may be very useful in the diagnostic work-up of pubertal disorders. However, in girls the overlap of basal values was marked, indicating the need for a GnRH stimulation test to establish maturity of the hypothalamus–pituitary–gonadal axis [56].

Gonadotropin Secretion During the Menstrual Cycle

Both males and females secrete gonadotropins in a pulsatile fashion during adulthood but in very different patterns. In the adult male, wide variations in LH interpulse intervals have been reported, with an average 2-h frequency [47]. In the female, the reproductive axis is under more dynamic regulation, with a cyclical pattern of intricate changes in gonadotropin secretion, ovarian sex steroid secretion, and the responses of the endometrium and reproductive tract to these hormonal changes constituting the menstrual cycle (Figure 7.5). Menstrual bleeding serves as a useful clinical marker and, by tradition, the first day of the bleeding is designated day 1 of the human menstrual cycle. The cycle length is usually between 25 and 30 days. Extensive reviews of the hormonal and histologic changes during the menstrual cycle have been published. This section will focus primarily on the changes in the gonadotropins.

During the early follicular phase, serum FSH levels are relatively higher but LH, estradiol and progesterone levels are low [57]. This relative preponderance of FSH in the early part of the cycle is felt to be important in the recruitment and maturation of a cohort of ovarian follicles, one of which will eventually ovulate [58]. Suppression of plasma FSH during the early follicular phase delays the development of the dominant follicle in the non-human primate and prolongs the follicular phase [58]. Conversely, supraphysiologic doses of FSH can lead to simultaneous development of several follicles [58]. The mechanisms that lead to selection of the dominant follicle and atresia of all others are not fully understood.

FSH promotes follicular growth and estradiol production and induces LH receptors on granulosa cells [35]. Serum estradiol levels gradually rise as the follicular phase progresses and follicular growth occurs. Increasing estradiol levels suppress serum FSH levels. In the late follicular phase, serum estradiol levels begin to rise rapidly. The positive feedback effects of the high late follicular phase estradiol levels increase LH and FSH secretion and pituitary responsiveness to GnRH, resulting in the mid-cycle LH surge [59]. In some species, increased GnRH output in the periovulatory period has been demonstrated, although it remains unclear if in the human GnRH plays a permissive, essential, or nonessential role in the ovulatory LH surge [60]. The FSH peak at the mid-cycle is of a smaller magnitude than the LH peak. After ovulation, the FSH levels decrease and remain low during the luteal phase. On the other hand, LH is essential for maintaining corpus luteum function; LH stimulates the production of progesterone and estradiol by the luteinized follicle [61]. In the absence of fertilization, corpus luteum function declines as reflected by decreasing progesterone and estradiol levels during the latter part of the luteal phase. Serum FSH levels then begin to rise, partly in response to a decrease in serum levels of estradiol and progesterone levels, initiating events for the next cycle.

The pattern of LH pulses has been well characterized during different phases of the menstrual cycle and these data have been used to derive inferences about the hypothalamic GnRH secretion [62]. LH pulses are of higher frequency (interpulse interval of 1–2 hours) during the early follicular phase; the LH pulse amplitude tends to be more uniform. The LH pulse frequency increases during the late follicular phase. The pulse generator slows markedly during the luteal phase; the interpulse interval may range from 2–6 hours [47].

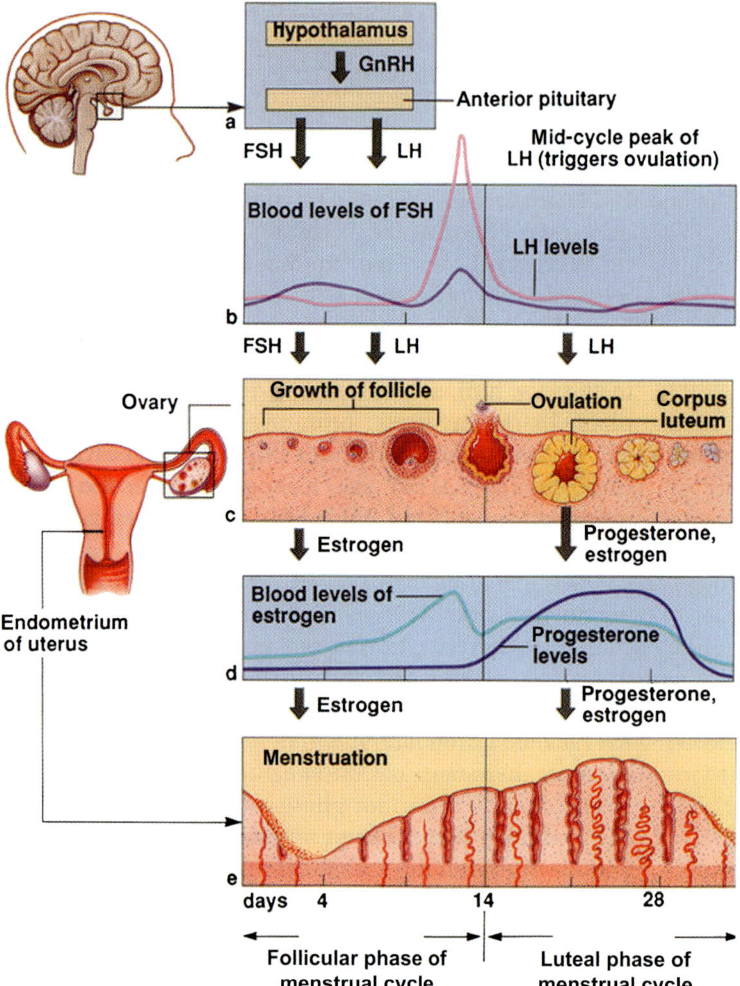

FIGURE 7.5 The menstrual cycle. Changes in serum levels of LH, FSH, estradiol and progesterone, in the ovarian follicle, and in the endometrial lining during the menstrual cycle. *From http://www.soc.ucsb.edu/sexinfo/article/the-menstrual-cycle.*

The pulse amplitude also varies considerably between pulses.

The changes in the expression of gonadotropin subunit genes have been examined during the rat estrous cycle [3]. In the female rat, the estrous cycle has a length of 4 days. Serum LH and FSH concentrations are low throughout the cycle except for the surge on the late afternoon and evening of proestrus. LHβ- and α-subunit mRNAs change little on the day of metestrus, but increase two-fold during diestrus. LHβ mRNA levels increase three-fold before the preovulatory rise in serum LH, but α-subunit mRNA levels remain unchanged during the proestrus gonadotropin surges. FSHβ mRNA levels increase during the metestrus morning, falling to basal levels by metestrus evening. On the afternoon of proestrus, FSHβ mRNA concentrations increase but the maximal expression of FSHβ mRNA is seen 2 hours after the proestrus FSH surge. Thus, the changes in the expression of the three gonadotropin subunit genes do not tightly correlate with the circulating LH and FSH levels [2].

Aging and Gonadotropins

Serum testosterone levels decline progressively in men with advancing age (Figure 7.6); almost 25% of men over the age of 70 have serum testosterone levels in the hypogonadal range [63]. The sex-hormone-binding globulin levels increase with age, resulting in a greater decrease in free and bioavailable testosterone than total testosterone. The diurnal rhythm of testosterone secretion, observed in younger men, may be attenuated or lost in older men. There is also an increase in circulating estradiol and estrone levels with age due, in part, to the increased peripheral aromatization of androgen to estrogen.

Aging-associated declines in testosterone levels occur due to defects at all levels of the hypothalamic–pituitary–gonadal axis. Androgen secretion by the testes of elderly men is decreased due to primary abnormalities at the gonadal level. This is supported by their higher basal LH and FSH levels, decreased testosterone response to hCG, and diminished Leydig

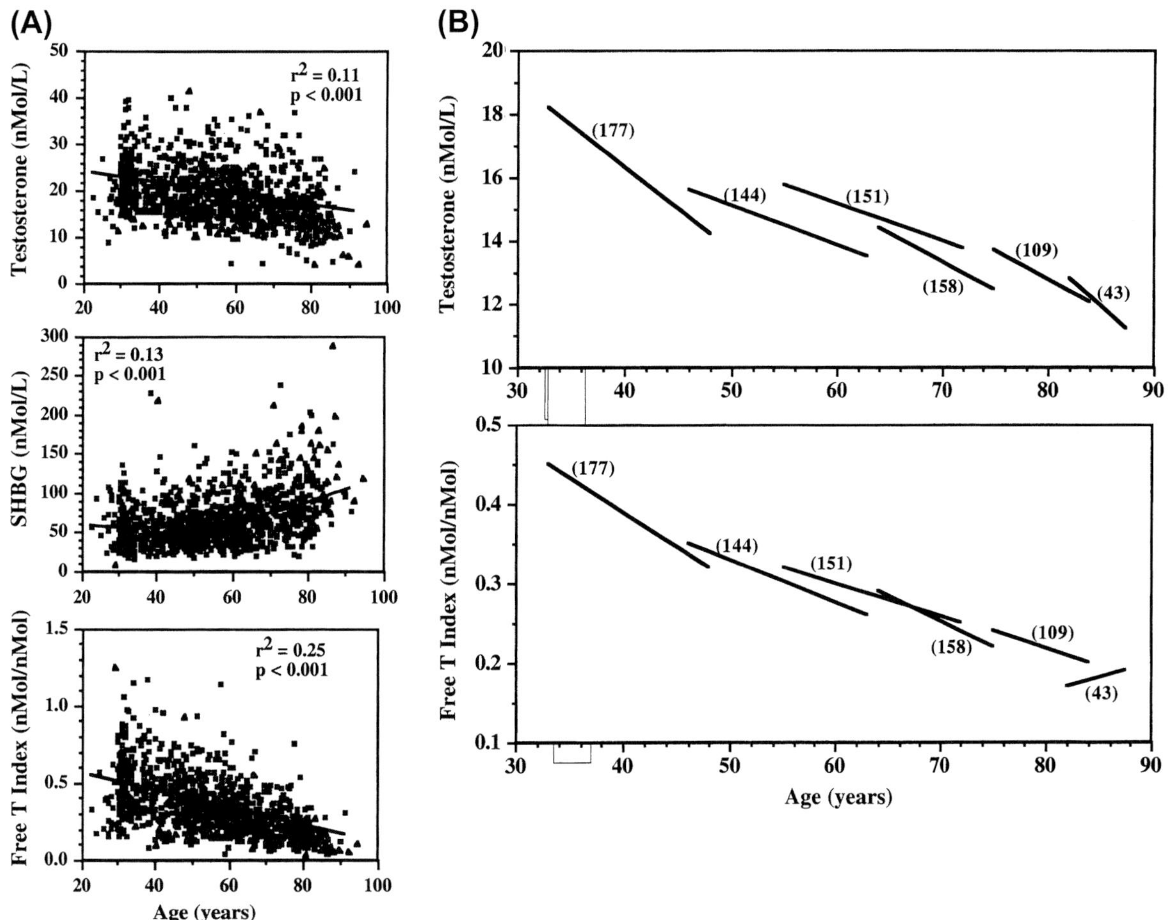

FIGURE 7.6 Age-related changes in testosterone secretion. (A) Effects of age on serum T, SHBG and free T index. Individual data points for T (upper panel), SHBG (middle panel) and free T index (lower panel) against age. Best-fit regression lines, r^2 and P values are shown. Total T concentrations and free T index values decreased linearly with increasing age, whereas SHBG exhibited a curvilinear increase with age, rising at a slightly greater rate in the older, than in younger, men. (B) Longitudinal effects of aging on T and free T index. Linear segment plots for total T and free T index vs. age are shown for men with T and SHBG values on at least two visits. Numbers in parentheses represent the number of men in each cohort. With the exception of free T index in the ninth decade, segments show significant downward progression at every age, with no significant change in slopes for T or free T index over the entire age range. *Adapted from Harman et al. [63].*

cell mass in aging men. In addition, secondary defects may exist at the hypothalamic–pituitary level, as indicated by the blunted LH and FSH responses of older men to GnRH, more irregular secretion of LH, and less synchronicity between LH and testosterone secretion than younger men. Therefore, aging is associated with abnormalities of the normal feedback control mechanisms that control the flow of information between different components of the hypothalamic–pituitary–testicular network, and a disruption of the orderly pattern of pulsatile hormonal secretion [64].

Aging has dramatic effects on the reproductive system in women [65,66]. The reproductive system is one of the first biological systems to show age-related decline. Certainly the most notable changes in the hypothalamic–pituitary–gonadal axis arise from the decline in ovarian function, and thus the loss of negative feedback effects on the hypothalamus and pituitary. Reproductive aging in women is related to the depletion of a fixed number of germ cells within the ovary. Women progress through the menopausal transition by a median age of 51.4 years. A progressive decrease in inhibins results in an early increase in FSH, which initially maintains folliculogenesis and estradiol secretion. Over time, regular ovulatory cycles give way to inconsistent folliculogenesis and ovulation, fluctuations in estradiol and gonadotropin levels, and irregular cycles. Most of the decrease in estradiol and increase in FSH associated with menopause is found to occur during the late menopausal transition. While depletion of ovarian follicles clearly relates to the end of reproductive function in females, evidence is accumulating that neuroendocrine changes can precede the decline in ovarian function and a hypothalamic defect is critical in the transition from cyclicity to acyclicity [67].

The central nervous system does not respond normally to estrogen and fails to produce preovulatory LH surges in women in the early menopausal transition. Changes in the sensitivity to estrogen positive feedback for the ovulatory LH surge may contribute to cycle disruption. Decreases of hypothalamic dopamine, norepinephrine, glutamate, VIP and IGF-1 have been reported [68]. In a middle-aged, regularly cycling rat model, GnRH neurons demonstrated dramatically decreased Fos activation during the proestrous LH surge, suggesting an age-associated loss of hypothalamic sensitivity to the E2 positive feedback required for GnRH/LH surge [68]. It has been postulated in humans that repercussions of anovulatory menstrual cycles, precipitated by loss of hypothalamic responsiveness to E2 during perimenopause, establish the dysregulation of ovarian trophic support by FSH, activin and inhibin that cascades into accelerated ovarian decline and menopause. Kisspeptin expressed in neurons in the hypothalamic anteroventral periventricular nucleus (AVPV) has been implicated as a mediator of E2 positive feedback [69]. Indeed, the age-related decline of the LH surge corresponds to the decreased sensitivity of AVPV kisspeptin neurons to E2 positive feedback [70,71]. Blunting of pituitary expression of the GnRH receptor and the gonadotropin subunits in middle-aged rats has also been reported, suggesting that age-related changes in pituitary physiology may also contribute to reproductive senescence [72].

Studies in older postmenopausal women also indicate that changes in the neuroendocrine axis occur with aging that are independent of the changing ovarian hormonal milieu of the menopausal transition. LH and FSH decrease progressively after the menopause, as does gonadotropin-releasing hormone (GnRH) pulse frequency [65]. Clinically, it is important to appreciate that the entire reproductive system, not just the ovary, is undergoing change across the transition [66].

BIOLOGIC FUNCTIONS OF LH AND FSH

Roles of LH and FSH in the Male

The target organs of LH and FSH are the gonads. In the male, the primary role of LH is to stimulate testosterone biosynthesis by Leydig cells (Figure 7.7). LH stimulates the activity of steroidogenic enzymes including CYP cholesterol-side-chain cleavage enzyme and CYP 17α-hydroxylase in Leydig cells, which are required for testosterone synthesis [73]. LH is required for maintaining the very high intratesticular levels of testosterone, essential for spermatogenesis. Circulating testosterone is also essential for maintaining sexual function, secondary sexual characteristics, and a number of other androgen-dependent physiologic processes such as bone, mineral and protein metabolism and muscle mass and function [35].

FSH in the male is responsible for the initiation of spermatogenesis (Figure 7.7). FSH binds to specific receptors on Sertoli cells and stimulates the production of a number of proteins including inhibins, transferrin, androgen-binding protein, androgen receptor and a glutamyl transpeptidase. The precise role of FSH in the spermatogenic process remains unclear [74]. The classical theory proposes that LH acts on Leydig cells to stimulate generation of high intratesticular levels of testosterone. Testosterone then acts on the spermatogonia and primary spermatocytes leading the germ cells through the meiotic division. FSH is felt to be essential for spermiogenesis, i.e., the maturation process by which spermatids develop into mature spermatozoa, through effects mediated on Sertoli cells.

In both rats and primates, testosterone alone can maintain spermatogenesis when administered shortly after hypophysectomy or stalk resection. However, if testosterone is given after a lapse of several weeks to months, it is much less effective in reinitiating spermatogenesis. It is also worth noting that spermatogenesis maintained by treatment of hypophysectomized male

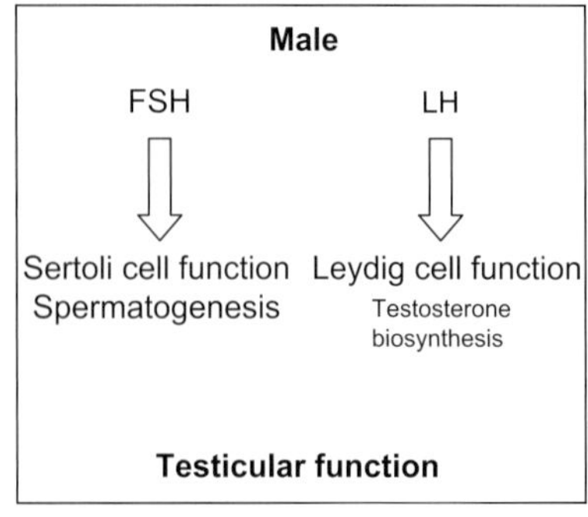

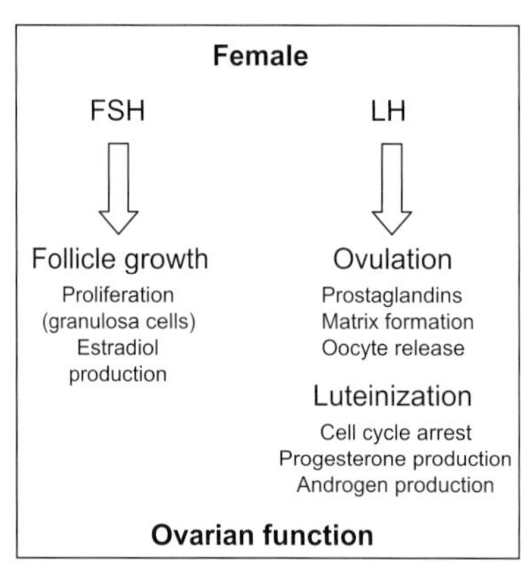

FIGURE 7.7 Functions of LH and FSH in the male and female. *Modified from Richards [76] and Layman [327].*

rodents or non-human primates by testosterone is qualitatively, but not quantitatively, normal. FSH is required for initiating the spermatogenic process but once this has occurred, testosterone in high doses can maintain spermatogenesis. Even though FSH and testosterone have independent roles in spermatogenesis, they also act in a cooperative manner to promote quantitative spermatogenesis presumably by modulation of post-receptor events within Sertoli cells. Both FSH and testosterone act in a stage-dependent manner and act at different cellular sites during spermatogenesis in order to optimize the spermatogenic process. Thus, the combination of testosterone and FSH is more effective than testosterone alone in spermatogenesis. Both FSH and testosterone are required for qualitatively, as well as quantitatively, normal spermatogenesis. The circulating concentration of FSH is proposed to provide the signal that sets the level of sperm production above the basal rate induced by intratesticular testosterone. The action of FSH on the germ cells is indirect and mediated by a paracrine signal(s) of Sertoli cell origin that amplifies a basal level of spermatogenesis that is maintained by testosterone [74,75].

The Roles of LH and FSH in the Female

The roles of LH and FSH in the ovary are better delineated (Figure 7.7). Although many of the early stages of follicle growth occur independently of pituitary gonadotropins, FSH is required for granulosa cell differentiation and these cells rely on FSH to facilitate follicular growth [76]. In the ovary, granulosa cells are the only target cells of FSH action. FSH receptors are acquired by granulosa cells in early stages of their cytodifferentiation and FSH is important in the cytodifferentiation of granulosa cells. FSH plays a critical role in follicle growth and is responsible for the development of a mature follicle, although a number of growth factors also play an important role in stimulating granulosa cell mitosis. The initiation of follicular growth can occur independently of gonadotropin stimulation, after which further maturation requires FSH. FSH receptor is only expressed from the primary follicle onward, and in the absence of FSH follicular growth can occur up to the stage of secondary recruitment. Only at more advanced stages of development do follicles become responsive to FSH and obtain the capacity to convert the theca-cell-derived substrate androstenedione to estradiol (E_2) by the induction of the aromatase enzyme activity [77]. FSH is, therefore, critical in regulating estrogen production in the ovary. During the later stages of follicular growth, activins and estradiol enhance the actions of FSH [78,79]. FSH also controls granulosa cell production of inhibin during the follicular phase, and also modulates LH receptor expression in granulosa cells. At the same time that FSH promotes the development of the dominant follicle, it also initiates the recruitment of the next generation of follicles that will enlarge during subsequent cycles [35,76].

LH is a major regulator of ovarian steroid synthesis. The midcycle LH surge stimulates resumption of oocyte meiosis and maturation in the preovulatory follicle, initiates the rupture of the ovulatory follicle and the processes of ovulation, oocyte meiosis, expansion of the cumulus cell oocyte complex and conversion of the follicle wall into the corpus luteum (luteinization) [76,77]. In the ovary, LH stimulates estrogen production by promoting synthesis of androgen precursors in theca cells, which then diffuse into neighboring granulosa cells where they are aromatized into estrogens under the control of FSH [35]. LH causes rapid increases in the amount of cholesterol available for steroidogenesis. The transfer of cholesterol from the outer to the inner membrane where it becomes available for steroidogenesis is mediated by steroidogenic acute regulatory protein (StAR) [80]. The StAR protein regulates this rate-limiting step in the steroidogenic process, and is in turn regulated by LH. In addition, LH causes an increase in the activity of the side-chain cleavage enzyme, a cytochrome P450-linked enzyme that converts cholesterol to pregnenolone. LH increases the delivery of cholesterol to the side-chain cleavage enzyme thus increasing its capacity to convert more cholesterol to pregnenolone. The long-term effects of LH include stimulation of gene expression and synthesis of a number of key enzymes in the steroid biosynthetic pathway, including not only the side-chain cleavage enzyme, but also 3-β-hydroxysteroid dehydrogenase, 17-α-hydroxylase and 17,20-lyase. LH stimulates the expression of progesterone receptors on the granulosa cells of the dominant follicle, which promotes luteinization. In addition, LH helps to sustain luteinization of the ruptured ovarian follicle, which then forms a corpus luteum during the second half of the ovulatory cycle by stimulating progesterone synthesis.

Taken together, LH and FSH play different but equally important roles in follicular development. FSH is important for early granulosa cell maturation, including the expression of LH receptors. LH, acting initially on theca cells, promotes androgen production to supply substrate for aromatization to estrogen. Although only FSH is required in early folliculogenesis, full ovarian steroidogenesis requires LH as well.

Gonadotropin Receptors

It has long been recognized that gonadotropins stimulate cAMP production in their target cells, suggesting that their receptors would be members of the G-protein-coupled receptor family. This was confirmed by the cloning of the receptors for LH/hCG [81,82] and FSH [83]. The gonadotropin receptors are present in the plasma membrane where they interact with hormones present in the extracellular fluid with high affinity and specificity. The interaction of the receptor with its ligand induces a conformational change in the receptor, which in turn activates a membrane-associated, G-protein-coupled signaling system. The LH/hCG receptor (LHR) can bind both LH and hCG, and this binding stimulates adenylate cyclase activity and intracellular cAMP production to lead to testosterone production. Activation of the LHR also stimulates several other intracellular second-messenger systems including the phospholipase A2, C and D pathways.

Both the LHR and FSHR consist of a large extracellular N-terminal domain, followed by the classical seven-transmembrane α-helical domains and a small intracytoplasmic C-terminal domain characteristic of G-protein-coupled receptors, sharing homology with other members of this family such as rhodopsin, adrenergic, muscarinic and serotonin receptors, as well as with the TSHR [84] and with each other (Figure 7.8). Their large extracellular hormone-binding domain at the N-terminus distinguishes this receptor subgroup among the larger family of G-protein-coupled receptors [35]. The LHR gene, located on human chromosome 2p21, encodes for a protein of up to 700 amino acids, including a 26-amino acid signal peptide and a mature protein with a predicted molecular mass of 75-kDa. The purified LHR has an apparent molecular mass of 93-kDa on SDS gel electrophoresis. The difference between the predicted (75-kDa) and observed (93-kDa) molecular weight is likely due to glycosylation of the receptor. In the case of the LHR, the N-terminal extracellular domain comprises 341 amino acid residues, with six potential sites for N-linked glycosylation and several leucine-rich segments [35,85]. This extracellular domain has been shown to be both necessary and sufficient for ligand binding, and the leucine repeat motifs are thought to be involved in receptor activation after formation of the hormone–receptor complex. Unlike most members of the G-protein-coupled receptor family, which are encoded by a single exon, the LH/CG receptor is comprised of 11 exons and ten introns. The largest of these exons (exon 11), encodes for the entire transmembrane and intracellular domains of the receptor, whereas the other exons encode for various sections of the N-terminal extracellular domain. The carboxyterminal cytoplasmic segment has several serines and threonines which may serve as putative sites for phosphorylation.

The FSH receptor gene, located on human chromosome 2p21-16, spans 85 kb and contains ten exons, nine of which encode the extracellular domain. The human

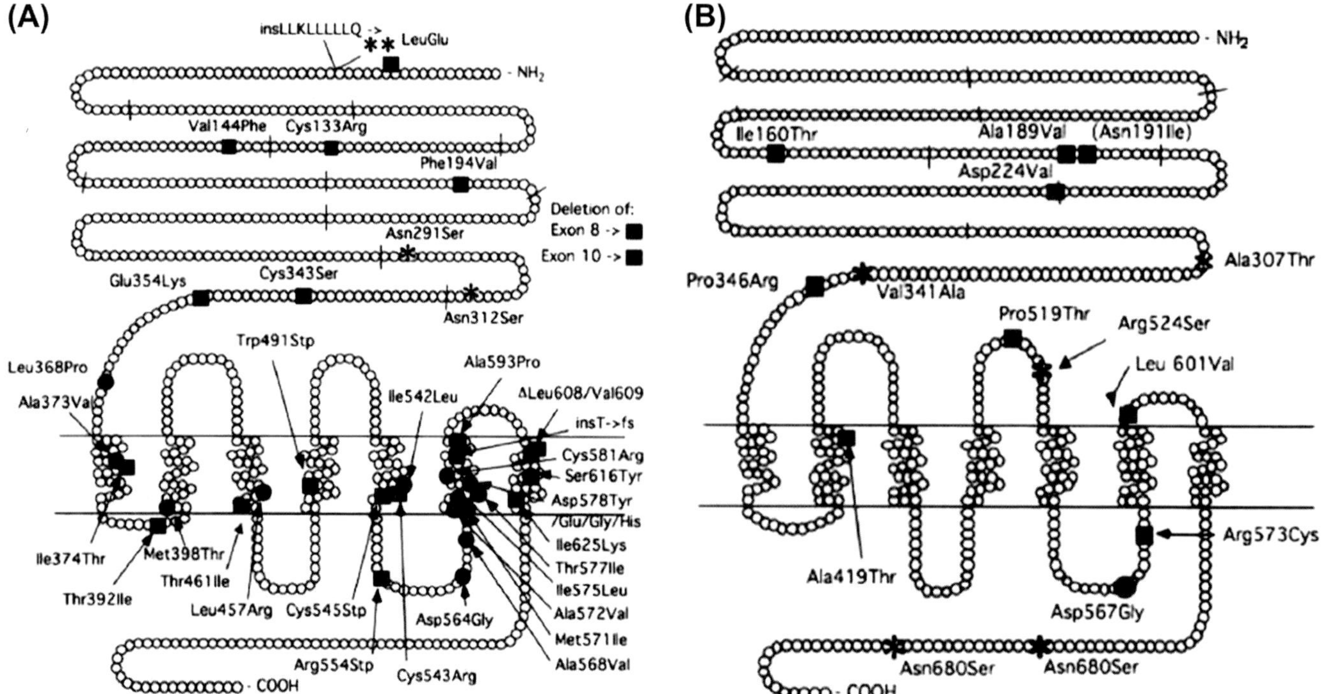

FIGURE 7.8 (A) Structure of the LH receptor. Schematic representation of the human LH/hCG receptor (LHR) with known mutations. Inactivating mutations are indicated by filled squares, whereas activating mutations are indicated by filled circles. Ins, insertion; fs, frameshift. (B) Structure of the FSH receptor. Schematic model of the human FSH receptor (FSHR) with currently known mutations. *From Huhtaneimi [328].*

FSHR contains 678 amino acids with 50% sequence homology to the LHR in their extracellular domains and 80% homology in the transmembrane segments. As for the LHR, the FSHR is also a G-protein-coupled receptor consisting of a large glycosylated N-terminal extracellular domain with a leucine-rich repeat region as well as four potential N-linked glycosylation sites. The extracellular domain again appears responsible for the recognition and binding of the hormone ligand. FSH action in stimulating estradiol production by the granulosa cells is mediated via the cAMP pathway.

Gonadotropin receptor expression is classically thought to be restricted to gonadal cell populations. Indeed, FSHR is restricted to granulosa cells of the ovary and Sertoli cells of the testes [74,75,86]. In the testis, LHR is primarily expressed on Leydig cells. Within the ovary, LHR is expressed on differentiated granulosa, luteal, theca and interstitial cells. Although LHR expression is nearly undetectable in the granulosa cells of preantral follicles, these levels are markedly increased with development to the preovulatory stage [76,77]. In ovarian theca cells, LHR is detectable in preantral follicles, with further induction during follicular maturation. Corpus luteum cells express high levels of LHR. Interestingly, LHR expression is not limited to the gonads, but has also been identified in human endometrium, myometrium, fallopian tubes and brain, suggesting possible extragonadal functions. Experimental and clinical evidence has shown low levels of expression of LHR in the normal human adrenal cortex [87,88]. Some human adrenal tumors ectopically express LHR and respond excessively to gonadotropic stimulation [89]. Such tumors often develop when gonadotropin secretion is chronically elevated, such as in postmenopausal women. Interestingly, the rare conditions of ACTH-independent and pregnancy-associated Cushing syndrome also demonstrate direct LH/hCG effects on the adrenal cortex.

ASSAY SYSTEMS FOR THE MEASUREMENT OF GONADOTROPINS

Two types of measurement systems are currently available for quantitation of LH and FSH in blood (Table 7.3). First are immunoassays which quantitate the mass of immunoreactive species; second are assays which measure biologic activity, including: (1) ligand-binding assays that quantitate receptor binding; and (2) bioassays that quantitate the net bioactivity of circulating LH and FSH species. Ideally, complete characterization of circulating LH and/or FSH status should include assessment of mass (by immunoassays) and biologic activity (by ligand binding and bioassays). However, because of their cumbersome nature, assays based on ligand binding and bioactivity are not widely used in clinical practice. As outlined elsewhere in this chapter, in several clinical situations, such as acute illness, some pituitary tumors, monitoring of GnRH agonist treatment, chronic renal failure and aging, the assessment of LH and/or FSH by radioimmunoassays (RIAs) may diverge significantly from that based on bioassays due, in part, to the problems inherent in one or both types of assay systems.

TABLE 7.3 Available Methods for Measurement of LH and FSH in Serum or Plasma

Method	Comments
MEASUREMENT OF MASS: IMMUNOASSAYS	
Traditional radioimmunoassay	Sensitivity limited
	α-subunit crossreactivity
Immunofluorometric assay	Sensitivity much better
	No α-subunit crossreactivity
	No radioactivity involved
Immunochemiluminescent assay	Sensitivity much better
	No α-subunit crossreactivity
	No radioactivity involved
MEASUREMENT OF BIOACTIVITY	
Receptor binding assays	Uses rat interstitial cells
Classical bioassays	Rat MA-1 cells
LH	
(i) Rat interstitial cell testosterone assay	Cumbersome Susceptible to serum effects
(ii) Mouse interstitial cell testosterone assay	
FSH	
(i) Granulosa cell aromatase assay	Sensitivity limited
(iii) Sertoli cell aromatase assay	

Radioimmunoassays for LH and FSH

The first RIAs for measurements of serum LH and FSH were described over 20 years ago [90,91]. These proved extremely useful in studying LH and FSH secretion and its regulation in health and disease. Antisera to hCG were initially used in assays for LH based on the close structural and immunologic similarities between these two hormones, but this assay was replaced by the use of antisera to purified LH. Radioimmunoassays using antisera against the hCGβ-subunit or its unique carboxyterminal sequence are highly specific for the measurement of hCG, even in the presence of high levels of LH. Subunit antisera are also available for the meaurement of glycoprotein hormone subunits present in the circulation, secreted by the pituitary, placenta, or ectopically by some neoplasms. However, the original RIAs for hLH and hFSH had a number of limitations.

While crossreactivity of other pituitary glycoprotein hormones has not been a significant problem in LH and FSH radioimmunoassays, the crossreactivity of the free α-subunit in the LH RIA is considerable. Another problem pertains to the microheterogeneity of circulating LH and FSH species. Post-translational modifications may contribute to heterogeneity of circulating isoforms and may also result in altered biologic activity [44]. A third problem was that most of the existing reference preparations of LH and FSH are not homogeneous and have varying degrees of impurities. Although potency estimates are available, direct comparisons of the data obtained by using different types of reference preparations may not always be valid because of the problems of microheterogeneity of circulating isoforms and different degrees of contamination of the reference material being used. Fourth, the sensitivities of the conventional LH and FSH RIAs are limited so that the serum concentrations of follicle-stimulating hormone in some normal men are close to or below the limit of assay sensitivity. This greatly limits their application in clinical and physiologic paradigms requiring measurements of low or suppressed levels, e.g., during the peripubertal period, in hypogonadotropic disorders, or during GnRH analogue-induced gonadotropin suppression.

Improvements in LH and FSH Immunoassays

A number of commercially available, two-site-directed immunoradiometric or nonisotopic methods (e.g., immunofluorometric assay, IFMA, or immunochemiluminescent assay, ICMA) have now overcome many of the limitations of the original RIAs. The sensitivity is much better – e.g., a time-resolved LH IFMA can measure serum LH levels down to 0.1 mIU/ml [56,92]. Furthermore, crossreactivity is no longer a problem in these two-site-directed assays, and correlation with bioassays is also much better than the original radioimmunoassays [92]. These more sensitive LH and FSH measurement systems have been extremely useful in studying physiologic events characterized by low LH and FSH levels [56]. For example, changes in the low serum LH and FSH levels in early puberty had been difficult to study due to the sensitivity problems of traditional RIAs. However, re-examination of gonadotropin levels using IFMA has now greatly clarified the issue.

Another instance when specificity of two-site-directed assays proved critical was in GnRH agonist studies [56]. For several years, it was known that serum LH levels in GnRH agonist-treated men, measured by conventional RIA, did not decrease in proportion to the far greater decline in serum testosterone levels. However, serum bioassayable LH concentrations markedly decreased during GnRH agonist treatment so that the bioassayable to immunoassayable (B/I) LH ratios decreased during treatment [93]. Subsequent studies revealed that the LH levels measured by IFMA decreased correspondingly with those measured by bioassay. These observations led to the recognition that the change in LH B/I ratios during GnRH agonist treatment were due, at least in part, to the crossreactivity of the free α-subunit.

Receptor-binding Assays

Two types of receptor-binding assay have been in use in research, but neither has yet attracted wide clinical applicability. The traditional assay uses ^{125}I-hCG/^{125}I-LH or ^{125}I-FSH as the ligand, and crude rat gonadal homogenates as the source of membrane receptors [94].

Bioassays for LH and FSH

Bioassays for LH are based on stimulation of testosterone secretion from dispersed Leydig cells. Two types of bioassay used for measurement of serum LH bioactivity include the mouse interstitial cell testosterone assay (MICT) or the rat interstitial cell testosterone assay (RICT) [95]. The free or unassociated subunits have no intrinsic biologic activity and, therefore, do not crossreact in the LH or FSH bioassay. Operationally, the MICT is somewhat easier to use than the RICT because mouse Leydig cells can be mechanically dispersed. However, both assays have been used by many laboratories worldwide.

Several in vitro bioassays have been developed for FSH [96]. These include the plasminogen activator production by rat granulosa cells, stimulation of aromatase activity in rat Sertoli cells, cAMP production by rat seminiferous tubules, and ^{3}H-thymidine incorporation into mouse ovaries. These assays, because of low sensitivity and serum interference, were not practical for measurement of circulating FSH bioactivity. However, two types of bioassay available were developed that are sufficiently sensitive for serum bioassayable FSH measurement. These include the granulosa cell aromatase bioassay (GAB), validated by Jia and Hsueh [97], and the Sertoli cell aromatase bioassay first described by Van Damme et al. [98]. For a long time, measurement of serum FSH by bioassay had been difficult because of unpredictable serum effects. Jia and Hsueh showed that these could be minimized by prior treatment of serum with polyethylene glycol. Although these assays allow measurement of bioassayable serum FSH down to about 2.5 mU/ml, they are cumbersome, time-consuming and require difficult cell culture procedures. Nonetheless, the availability of bioassays for LH and FSH in combination with radioimmunoassay permits calculation of bioactive/immunoactive ratios, which provide a useful index of qualitative changes in the gonadotropins.

HYPOTHALAMIC REGULATION OF LH AND FSH SECRETION

The biosynthesis and secretion of LH and FSH are tightly regulated throughout development and across the reproductive cycle. Gonadotropin expression and secretion are controlled by hypothalamic factors (primarily GnRH), paracrine intrapituitary factors (primarily activin and follistatin) and gonadal feedback (both gonadal sex steroids and gonadal peptide hormones) (Figure 7.9).

Hypothalamic control of gonadotropin secretion occurs primarily through actions of GnRH, a neuropeptide encoded by a gene on human chromosome 8p. During early research on the hypothalamic control of gonadotropin secretion, it was first postulated that there would be two distinctly different hypothalamic hypophysiotropic factors regulating LH and FSH. Thus, while GnRH was originally identified as the LH-releasing hormone, it stimulates the release of both LH and FSH, and a distinct hypothalamic FSH-releasing hormone has yet to be identified.

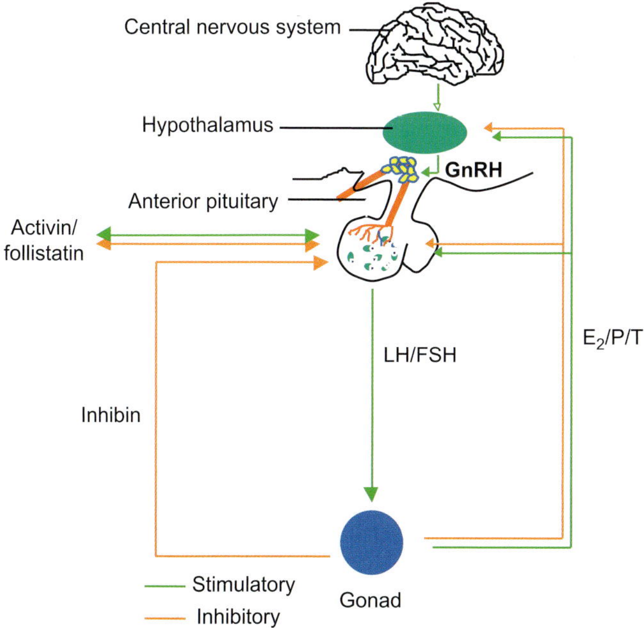

FIGURE 7.9 Schematic view of the hypothalamic–pituitary-gonadal axis.

Insights into the mechanisms that regulate activation of GnRH secretion have been provided by the identification and study of genetic abnormalities in patients with pubertal disorders or infertility as well as using animal models. These pathways have been reviewed extensively recently and will be discussed only briefly here in light of our focus on the pituitary [50,99,100]. Molecular defects that manifest as GnRH deficiency or hypogonadotropic hypogonadism (HH) can be classified as defects in GnRH neuronal development, defects in control of GnRH secretion and defects in GnRH action (Figure 7.10; Table 7.4).

GnRH Neuronal Development

During development, GnRH neurons originate in the region of the olfactory placode [101]. These neurons migrate, along with the olfactory and vomeronasal nerves, into the forebrain and then into their final location in the medial basal hypothalamus (MBH). This orderly migration of GnRH neurons requires the coordinated action of direction-finding molecules, adhesion proteins and enzymes that help the neuronal cells burrow their way through intercellular matrix. Mutations of any of these proteins can arrest the migratory process and result in GnRH deficiency. In at least a subset of patients, idiopathic hypogonadotropic hypogonadism (IHH) can thus be viewed as a developmental migratory disorder resulting from failure of the GnRH neurons to migrate into the hypothalamus. These patients frequently have an associated phenotype of anosmia, explained by the common embryonic origins and developmental pathways of GnRH and olfactory neurons. Impaired migration of GnRH and olfactory neurons is the underlying cause of Kallmann syndrome (HH associated with anosmia). Other associated neurological and somatic abnormalities such as synkinesia, cerebellar ataxia, sensorineural deafness, mental retardation, unilateral renal agenesis and cleft palate, may segregate with the Kallmann syndrome phenotype, which suggests a common genetic origin of these abnormalities [99,102,103].

The first gene identified to play a role in GnRH neuronal migration was *KAL1*, located on the X chromosome and encoding an extracellular adhesion protein, anosmin 1, essential for axonal guidance and migration of olfactory and GnRH neurons from the nasal placode to their final location in the brain [104]. Mutations in *KAL1* cause X-linked Kallmann syndrome. Anosmin-1 colocalizes with basic fibroblast growth factor receptor 1 (FGFR1) in the olfactory bulb during development,

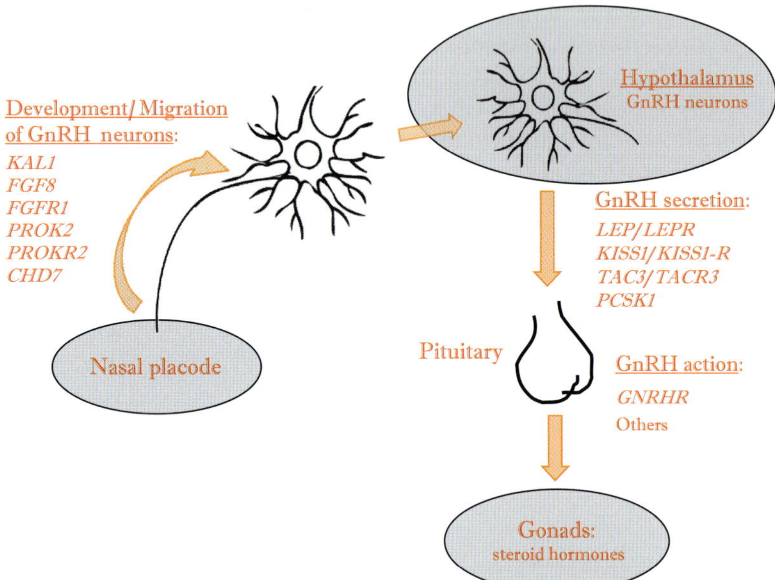

FIGURE 7.10 Genetic and molecular basis of GnRH neuronal development and migration, GnRH secretion, and GnRH action. *From Bianco [99].*

which suggests that this protein is a component of FGFR1 signaling [105]. FGFR1 is a member of the tyrosine kinase superfamily of receptors. In the presence of heparin sulfate, FGFs bind FGFR1 with high affinity, activating downstream signaling to regulate neuronal migration, differentiation and survival [106]. Kallmann syndrome caused by mutations in *FGFR1* is typically transmitted in an autosomal dominant fashion and can be associated with failed morphogenesis of the olfactory bulbs, cleft palate and dental agenesis. The severity of the hypogonadism and the presence of associated phenotypes have variable expressivity with incomplete penetrance, and *FGFR1* mutations have been reported in patients with normosmic IHH [107]. Reversal of hypogonadism has also been reported in patients with *FGFR1* mutations [108]. Mutations in *FGF8* have also been associated with Kallmann syndrome, suggesting that FGF8 is the FGFR1 ligand responsible for GnRH neuronal development and migration [109].

The inactivation of the prokineticin 2 system also leads to defective olfactory morphogenesis and hypogonadism in mice and humans [99,110]. Mice deficient in prokineticin-2 (Prok2) or its cognate G-protein-coupled receptor, prokineticin receptor-2 (Prokr2), have olfactory hypoplasia, hypogonadotropic hypogonadism and an absence of GnRH neurons in the hypothalamus [111,112]. Interestingly, GnRH neurons in $Prok2^{-/-}$ mice were able to cross the cribriform plate to enter the central nervous system during embryonic development, but the neurons did not migrate into and populate the hypothalamus. The phenotypic similarities between $Prokr2^{-/-}$ mice and Kallmann syndrome in humans inspired the hypothesis that inactivating mutations in the prokineticin system could lead to anosmia and hypogonadotropic hypogonadism in humans. Indeed, human mutations in *PROK2* and *PROKR2* have been found in the heterozygous, homozygous, or compound heterozygous state, suggesting a complex mode of inheritance [110,112–114]. A monogenic autosomal recessive mode of transmission has been demonstrated clearly, but in very few cases. Many of the heterozygous mutations of *PROKR2* have also been identified in clinically unaffected individuals, raising the question of their actual contribution to the hypogonadotropic hypogonadism phenotype. Potential digenic and oligogenic transmission or modulating influences of other genetic or environmental factors have been suggested, but further studies will be necessary to confirm the actual pathogenic role of heterozygous PROKR2 mutations. Interestingly, PROK2 is expressed in a rhythmic manner in the suprachiasmatic nucleus, PROKR2 is expressed in most primary target areas of the suprachiasmatic nucleus, and PROK2 expression/release is controlled by core clock genes, suggesting a role for the prokineticin 2 system in circadian rhythms. Indeed, *Prok2* and *Prokr2* null mice exhibit disruption of circadian rhythms, with reduced rhythmicity of locomotor activity, body temperature and sleep [115,116].

Recently, mutations in the gene *CHD7*, encoding chromodomain-helicase-DNA-binding protein 7 and thought to be involved in chromatin remodeling, have been identified in patients with CHARGE syndrome, a multisystem disorder that may include HH. CHD7 is expressed in olfactory epithelium, the hypothalamus and the pituitary. Mutations in CHD7 have now been identified in patients with normosmic HH or Kallmann

TABLE 7.4 Congenital and Acquired Causes of Hypogonadotropic Hypogonadism

CONGENITAL DISORDERS
Kallmann syndrome
Mutations of *KAL1*
Mutations of *FGFR1*
Mutations of *FGF8*
Mutations of *PROK2*
Mutations of *PROKR2*
Mutations of *CHD7*
Normosmic idiopathic hypogonadotropic hypogonadism
Mutations of *KISS1R*
Mutations of *TAC3*
Mutations of *TACR3*
Mutations of *LEP*
Mutations of *LEPR*
Mutations of *GNRH1*
Mutations in *PCSK1*
Mutations of *GNRHR*
Mutations of FSHβ
Mutations of LHβ
Prader-Willi syndrome
Laurence-Moon-Biedl syndrome
Mutations of pituitary transcription factors
Miscellaneous disorders
ACQUIRED DISORDERS
Hypothalamic amenorrhea
Chronic renal failure
Hemochromatosis
Hyperprolactinemia
Neoplastic
Inflammatory and infiltrative

syndrome without other manifestations of CHARGE syndrome [117].

GnRH Secretion

In primates, the majority of the GnRH neuronal cell bodies are located in the arcuate nucleus of the MBH, with additional cells in the preoptic area of the anterior hypothalamus. GnRH produced by these neurons is transported through axons in the tuberoinfundibular tract to the median eminence where it is released into the hypophyseal portal circulation and delivered to the anterior pituitary for action on gonadotropes via a highly specific, G-protein-coupled GnRH receptor. GnRH neurons also project to other CNS regions including the limbic system, amygdala, hippocampus and periaqueductal gray matter, where GnRH may influence reproductive behavior. However, only the GnRH neuronal projections to the median eminence significantly control gonadotropin secretion.

The hallmark of the hypothalamic secretion of GnRH is its pulsatile rather than continuous release into the hypophyseal portal circulation, resulting in episodic stimulation of the gonadotrope. In a series of pioneering studies, Knobil and his colleagues in the late 1970s demonstrated the absolute requirement for such a pulsatile stimulus to sustain LH and FSH secretion, whereas continuous infusion of GnRH was not effective (Figure 7.11) [118]. This observation has been confirmed in humans by the restoration of gonadotropin secretion in GnRH-deficient subjects after exogenous pulsatile GnRH treatment [119]. Conversely, after a transient stimulatory response, continuous GnRH exposure suppresses gonadotropin secretion. This inhibitory effect of continuous GnRH has been exploited in the treatment of sex-steroid-dependent disorders including precocious puberty, endometriosis, prostate cancer and breast cancer, as well as in infertility therapies [120].

Because of the short half life of GnRH and the large dilutional effect, levels of GnRH in the systemic circulation are too low to measure reliably. Measurement of hypophyseal portal GnRH concentrations has been performed in sheep and monkeys, confirming that GnRH secretion is pulsatile [121,122]. In humans, of course, such measurements are not feasible. Nonetheless, circulating LH levels have been shown to be highly correlated with GnRH release into the hypophyseal portal system, with each pulse of GnRH being followed by an LH pulse. Therefore, frequent blood sampling (i.e., every 10 minutes) for measurement of LH pulses can be used as an accurate indicator of GnRH secretion patterns. While FSH secretion is also correlated with GnRH secretion, it is less useful as a marker because of its longer half life [123].

Many neurotransmitter systems directly or indirectly modulate GnRH secretion. These include norepinephrine, dopamine, serotonin, GABA, glutamate, opiate peptides, neuropeptide Y (NPY) and galanin, among others. Glutamate and norepinephrine provide stimulatory drive to the reproductive axis, whereas GABA and opioid peptides are inhibitory. NPY acts at both hypothalamic and pituitary levels, by increasing GnRH release from the median eminence in the presence of gonadal steroids, and by facilitating GnRH-induced LH release at the level of the gonadotrope. Pituitary adenylate cyclase-activating polypeptide has also been implicated in the up-regulation of LH secretion, acting both as a hypothalamic hypophysiotropic factor and a pituitary paracrine factor [124].

New insights into pathways that regulate GnRH secretion have been provided by the identification and study of genetic abnormalities in patients with HH. The roles of kisspeptin and its G-protein-coupled

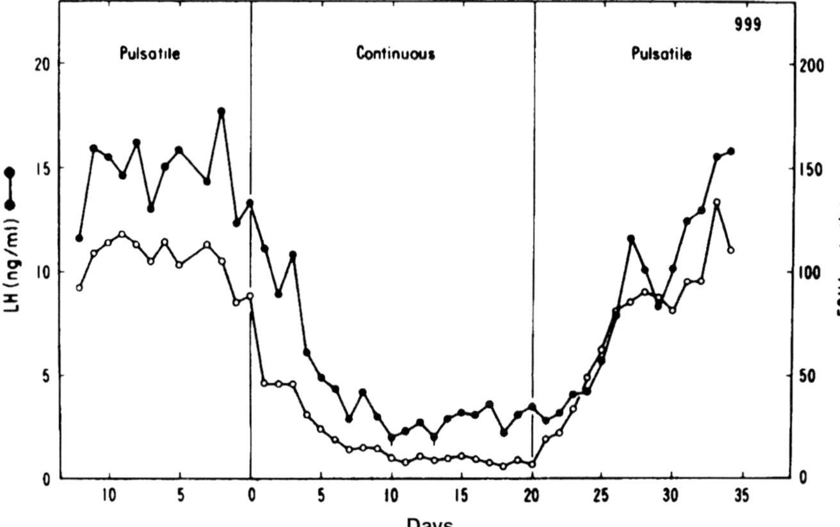

FIGURE 7.11 Knobil's experiments: pulsatile GnRH administration is essential for physiologic LH and FSH secretion. *From Belchetz [118].*

receptor, KISS1R (also known as GPR54) were revealed in 2003, when inactivating mutations in *KISS1R* were found in members of two large consanguineous families with a history of normosmic IHH [125,126]. Subsequent studies have shown that both kisspeptin and its receptor are expressed in areas of the hypothalamus involved in the control of reproduction [127]. Furthermore, centrally or peripherally injected kisspeptin-1 results in a robust stimulation of GnRH and gonadotropin secretion, and accelerates puberty in prepubertal rodents [99,128]. In rodents, the hypothalamic regions with the highest levels of kisspeptin-expressing neurons are the arcuate (ARC) and the anteroventral periventricular (AVPV) nuclei, each differentially regulated by gonadal steroids, acting through ERα and likely AR. Kisspeptin expression increases in the ARC following gonadectomy and decreases with gonadal steroid administration. Thus ARC kisspeptin neurons are predicted to play an important role in sex-steroid-negative feedback regulation of the reproductive axis [129]. Kisspeptin expression in the AVPV is sexually dimorphic, with 10–20-fold higher levels in females than males, and increases in response to gonadal steroids. AVPV kisspeptin expression has also been shown to vary during the estrous cycle, culminating with the highest levels of expression coincident with the ovulatory LH surge. These findings suggest a role for the AVPV kisspeptin neurons as effectors of the estrogen-positive feedback mechanism leading to the gonadotropin surge in females [99,128–130]. Inactivating mutations in *KISS1R* in human patients with HH show an autosomal recessive pattern of transmission. The key role of the KISS1R in the regulation of the onset of puberty was reinforced when the first identifiable genetic cause of central precocious puberty was recognized as a gain-of-function mutation, the result of a reduced rate of desensitization of this G-protein-coupled receptor [131]. Mutations in the *KISS1* gene encoding the ligand have also been reported recently in patients with central precocious puberty [132].

Interestingly, neurokinin B (NKB), a member of the substance-P-related tachykinin family encoded by *TAC3*, is co-expressed with kisspeptin in the ARC [133]. Its G-protein-coupled receptor, the NK3R, encoded by *TACR3*, is also expressed in the kisspeptin neurons [134]. The precise mechanisms of NKB action remain to be elucidated, as NKB agonists can have either an excitatory or inhibitory effect on GnRH-induced gonadotropin secretion in rodent models, depending on gender and sex steroid milieu [135]. Nonetheless, loss-of-function mutations have been identified in both *TAC3* and *TACR3* in patients with normosmic HH [136,137].

Additional genetic mutations that cause impaired GnRH secretion include mutations in the GnRH gene itself [138,139] and mutations in prohormone convertases that process the GnRH prohormone to the mature secreted biologically active decapeptide. Mutations in PCSK1 have been reported as a cause of normosic HH in association with obesity, hypoglycemia, hypocortisolemia, and evidence of impaired processing of POMC and proinsulin [140]. Another link between obesity and HH occurs in patients with mutations in the gene encoding leptin or its receptor. Leptin is a fat-derived hormone that regulates food intake, energy expenditure and reproduction, mediated through hypothalamic pathways. The central role of leptin in these cases is highlighted by the recovery of gonadotropin secretion and menstrual cyclicity following treatment with recombinant leptin in females with amenorrhea due to congenital letpin deficiency or hypothalamic amenorrhea [140]. Kisspeptin has been implicated as a mediator of the effects of leptin on GnRH secretion [141].

GnRH Action

The pattern of GnRH signal is important in determining the quantity and quality of gonadotropins secreted [142]. GnRH signaling begins with recognition by its receptor, GnRHR. The GnRHR is expressed in the pituitary as well as in additional minor sites of expression including hypothalamic GnRH neurons, testicular Leydig cells, ovarian granulosa and luteal cells, placental cells, and in endometrial, breast, and prostate cancers and cancer cell lines. The GnRHR was first cloned from the murine gonadotrope-derived αT3-1 cell line and subsequently from multiple other species, all composed of three exons and two introns and with a high degree of homology within their coding regions [59,143]. The GnRHR (encoded by *GNRHR*) is a 328-amino acid protein that belongs to the rhodopsin family of G-protein-coupled receptors [144]. Activation of the GnRHR increases calcium mobilization and stimulates influx of extracellular calcium. This increase in intracellular calcium induces pituitary LH and FSH secretion [145].

Mutations in *GNRHR* were among the first genetic mutations identified in patients with IHH [146,147]. Since then, more than 20 additional loss-of-function mutations in the GnRHR have been identified in patients with IHH (Figure 7.12) [148,149]. The cellular and molecular phenotypes of each mutation have been studied extensively in vitro, and mutations can be classified as partial or complete loss-of-function mutations. Amino acid substitutions have been identified in virtually every section of the receptor. All but two known *GNRHR* mutations are missense, leading to single amino acid substitutions. These mutations impair GnRH signaling due to loss of receptor expression, ligand binding, G protein coupling and/or abnormal intracellular trafficking of the receptor. Large-scale screening indicates that *GNRHR* mutations account for 3.5–16% of sporadic cases of normosmic IHH and up to 40% of familial cases of normosmic IHH [99,148]. Inheritance is autosomal recessive and most patients have compound heterozygous *GNRHR* mutations [99]. Functional responses and structure–function relationships of GnRH receptor mutations have been described in detail [148,149].

Before being trafficked to the cell membrane, receptors are first modified and folded at the site of synthesis within the endoplasmic reticulum. At this level, defective and misfolded proteins may be routed to pathways of degradation [150]. Recent evidence suggests that the human GnRHR is prone to such misrouting, and even a proportion of wild-type receptors never reach the plasma membrane [149,151]. Misfolding is not inevitable as cells naturally rely on molecular chaperones to help properly arrange nascent proteins [152]. This

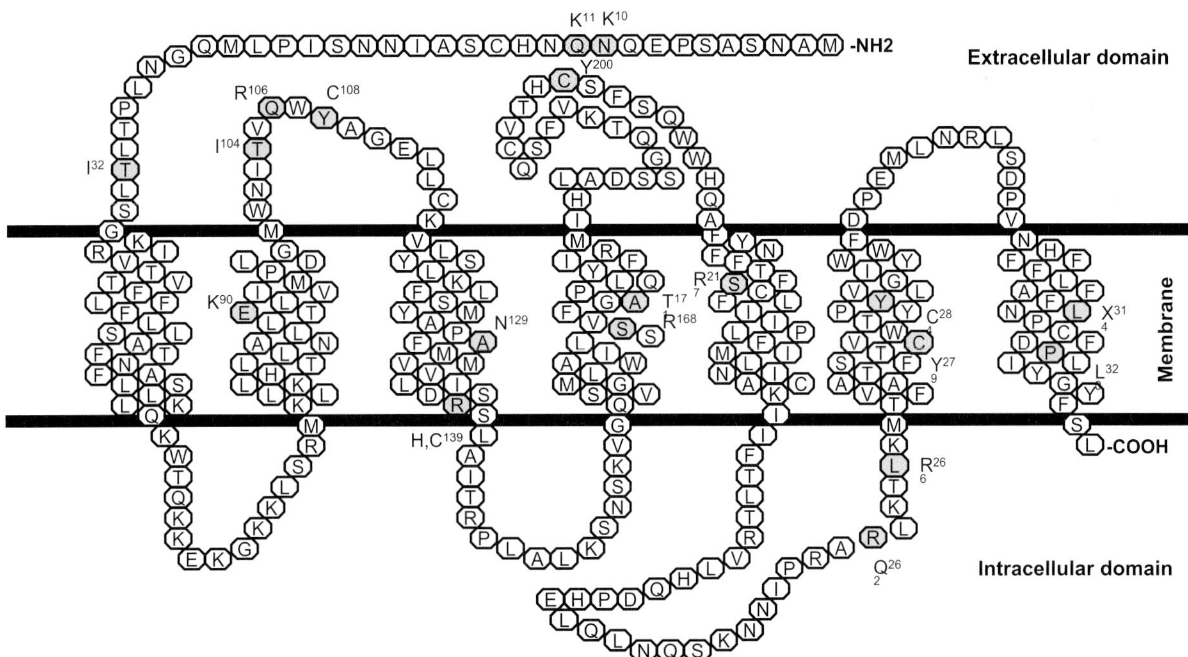

FIGURE 7.12 Schematic representation of the human GnRHR with reported mutations. This two-dimensional diagram shows the human GnRHR embedded in the cell membrane with its seven-transmembrane domains connected by three extra- and intracellular loops. Naturally occurring mutations reported to date are highlighted by shaded circles with the resulting "mutant" residue and its relative position listed next to each. *From Bedecarrats [148].*

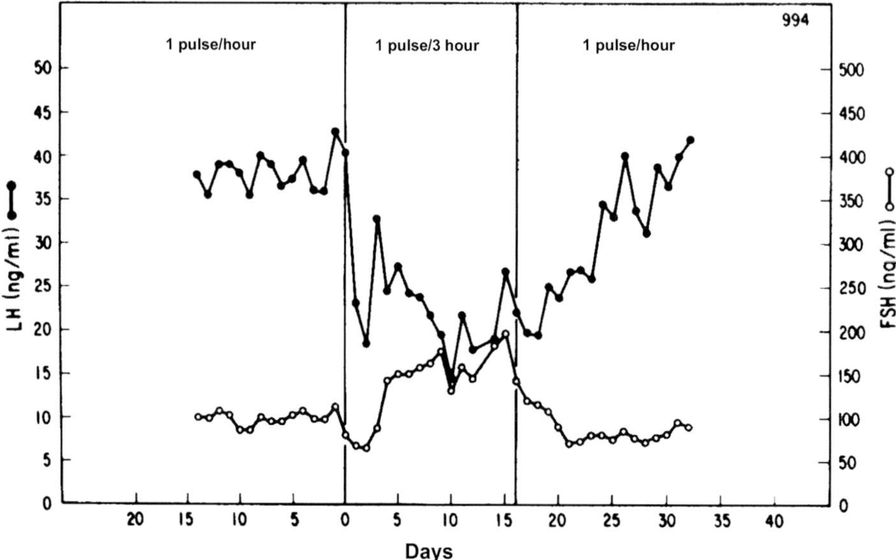

FIGURE 7.13 Knobil's experiments: the frequency of pulsatile GnRH administration has differential effects on gonadotropin secretion – more rapid GnRH pulse frequencies favor LH secretion, whereas slower pulse frequencies favor FSH. *From Wildt [159].*

has led to the development of "pharmacochaperones" (pharmacological compounds acting as chaperones). Pharmacochapperones are small molecules that enter cells, bind specifically to misfolded mutant proteins, correct their folding, and allow correct routing. Frequently, such molecules are identified as peptidomimetic antagonists from high-throughput screens [149]. Of interest, a non-peptidic cell-permeant GnRHR antagonist, IN3, has been shown to partially restore the function of several naturally occurring mutant human receptors [151]. As this compound was also able to enhance cell surface expression of the wild-type human receptor, it was proposed that IN3 could promote and/or rescue proper GnRHR folding. Thus the development of pharmacological chaperones to overcome receptor misrouting has the potential to lead to new therapeutic approaches for patients with IHH due to GnRHR mutations [148].

The phenotypic spectrum of IHH due to mutations in the GnRHR ranges from complete absence of any sexual maturation to partial phenotypes with some evidence of pubertal development, the fertile eunuch variant, and delayed puberty. The clinical phenotype generally correlates with biochemical LH pulsatility profiles and responses to exogenous GnRH. Complete IHH is typically associated with low levels of apulsatile LH, whereas some spontaneous LH pulses, albeit reduced in amplitude, may be seen in patients with partial IHH phenotypes. While patients with complete IHH due to inactive GnRHR variants are characterized by an absent response to exogenous GnRH, some patients with GnRHR mutations respond to exogenous GnRH administration, but with a reduced sensitivity to GnRH [153]. This partial resistance to GnRH can be overcome, as is evident from the successful use of pulsatile GnRH for ovulation induction and pregnancy in a patient with a compound heterozygous mutation in GnRHR [154]. Phenotype–genotype correlation studies indicate that the clinical phenotype is, in most cases, well correlated with the functional alteration of the GnRHR in vitro, with the phenotype and response to exogenous GnRH administration correlating best with the GnRHR variant with the less severe loss-of-function in compound heterozygotes. Spontaneous reversal of IHH has been reported in a male patient homozygous for $Gln^{2.69}$ $^{[106]}$Arg GnRHR, and similarly the occurrence of a spontaneous pregnancy has been reported in a female patient homozygous for this mutation [155,156]. A mild phenotype has also been reported for a patient homozygous for $Arg^{6.30}$ $^{[262]}$Gln GnRHR, who presented with delayed puberty [157]. Phenotypic variability has been observed in affected related subjects bearing the same mutations, suggesting that other factors may influence the phenotype. Potential modifying factors include gender (e.g., via sex steroid hormone effects), environmental factors, or modifier genes. The identification of digenic mutations in some pedigrees with IHH and GnRHR mutations may account for at least some such phenotypic heterogeneity [112,148].

Influence of Patterns of Pulsatile GnRH

The amplitude, frequency and contour of GnRH pulses can all vary and each of these characteristics can influence gonadotrope responses, providing a mechanism for the differential synthesis and secretion of the two gonadotropins, LH and FSH. GnRH pulse pattern varies across the female menstrual cycle. Studies have estimated that GnRH pulses occur every 94 minutes on average in the early follicular phase, increasing to every 71 minutes due to the effects of increasing circulating levels of estradiol in the late follicular phase, and slowing further to every 216 minutes under the influence of elevated levels of progesterone in the luteal phase [158]. In an extension of Knobil's pioneering studies, it was demonstrated that more rapid GnRH pulse frequencies favor LH secretion, whereas slower pulse frequencies favor FSH (Figure 7.13) [159]. These and other studies [160] established that the pulsatile release of GnRH at an optimum pulse frequency and amplitude is integral to optimum gonadotrope function, and variations in GnRH pulse frequency markedly influence both the absolute levels and the ratio of LH and FSH release [161]. In parallel rat models, as well as in in vitro systems, decreased frequency of GnRH pulses results in a differential increase in FSHβ transcription and FSH biosynthesis over LH [161–163]. Thus it is hypothesized that this builds up greater intracellular stores of FSH to allow for the greater FSH secretion. These alterations in GnRH pulse frequency are one mechanism by which two functionally distinct gonadotropins can be differentially regulated by a single hypothalamic-releasing hormone. The molecular mechanisms by which these differential regulatory effects occur have been the subject of considerable investigation (see section on Molecular biology of gonadotropin subunit genes, below).

FEEDBACK REGULATION OF LH AND FSH SECRETION

Estrogens

The gonadal steroid hormones include estrogens, progesterones and androgens. Effects on gonadotropins occur both directly at the level of the gonadotrope and indirectly via effects at the hypothalamus that modulate GnRH secretion. Estrogen, androgen and progesterone receptors have been identified in gonadotropes, consistent with direct actions. Within the hypothalamus, receptors for sex steroids have been identified in multiple neuronal cell types, suggesting that alterations in GnRH release can also occur indirectly through modulation of neuronal systems known to impinge on GnRH neurons [164].

The complexity of estradiol effects on gonadotropin secretion has been well reviewed [164–166]. In women, estrogens can exert dual-feedback effects on gonadotropin secretion, depending on the reproductive state. The negative-feedback effects of estrogens are clearly demonstrated by the elevation of LH and FSH levels that occur following ovariectomy or after menopause, that reverse with estrogen replacement. On the other hand, during the late follicular phase of the menstrual cycle, the feedback effects of estrogens shift from negative to positive, triggering the mid-cycle ovulatory surge of LH and FSH secretion.

We now know that ERs are present in many subcellular locations and signal through multiple pathways (Figure 7.14). In the classical genomic pathway, estradiol binds to ERs, and then the ER binds to estrogen response elements, resulting in changes in gene transcription. An alternate mechanism is the nonclassical genomic pathway, in which estradiol binds with ERα, which then binds to a transcription factor, potentially modifying in transcription of other genes. Finally, there is a nonclassical, nongenomic pathway, in which membrane receptors or receptors in other locations signal through protein kinase cascades, resulting in phosphorylation of transcription factors that then may result in transcription of yet other genes [164]. In addition to ERα, there is also a second nuclear receptor for estrogen, ERβ, and a putative G-protein-coupled receptor for estrogen, GPR30.

Negative feedback effects of estrogens are observed at the level of α-subunit, LHβ- and FSHβ-subunit mRNA levels through effects on gene transcription in addition to effects on LH and FSH secretion. Estrogen's negative feedback effects are thought to be mediated in part directly at the level of the pituitary gland. Estrogen has been shown to decrease GnRH-mediated LH secretion in vitro in cultured pituitary cells as well as in vivo in hypothalamic-lesioned monkeys given hourly GnRH pulses. Estrogen also likely has negative feedback effects at the levels of the hypothalamic pulse generator, as estradiol administration to monkeys leads to a decrease in LH pulse frequency. Similarly, estradiol inhibits LH pulse amplitude in normal men and in GnRH-deficient men maintained on GnRH [167]. Whether ERα and ERβ are expressed and functional in GnRH neurons has been controversial [166]. Increasing evidence suggests that kisspeptin neurons in the arcuate nucleus could be responsible for mediating the negative feedback effects of estrogen on GnRH secretion. These neurons contain ERα and gonadectomy increases arcuate kisspeptin expression whereas estrogen replacement restores expression to that observed in intact, untreated animals. The suppression of kisspeptin activity by sex steroids in the arcuate nucleus appears to be mediated by ERα in the female. These findings are consistent with a role for kisspeptins in mediating the negative feedback effects of gonadal steroids on GnRH secretion (Figure 7.15) [69,129].

Positive feedback effects of estrogen are mediated in large part at the level of the hypothalamus, as GnRH pulse frequency is increased at the time of the LH surge.

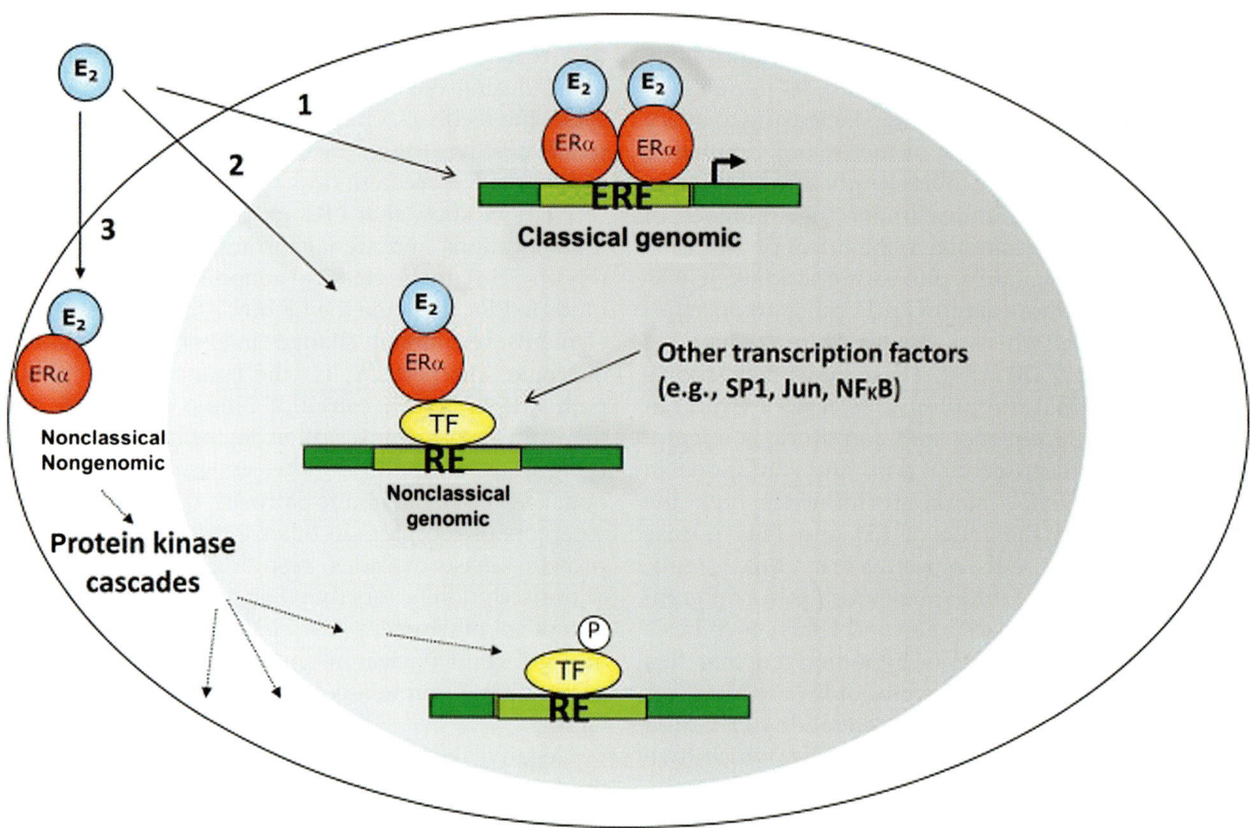

FIGURE 7.14 Estradiol signals through ERα via multiple pathways: (1) classical genomic pathway; (2) nonclassical genomic pathway; (3) nonclassical, nongenomic pathway. *From Blaustein [164].*

Direct positive effects of estrogens at the pituitary level may also contribute. In support of a pituitary site of action, estrogen increases LHβ mRNA synthesis in vitro in pituitary fragments [2]. Nonetheless, the major site of positive feedback appears to be at the hypothalamus, mediated through kisspeptin neurons in the AVPV of the rodent. Kisspeptin expression in the AVPV is positively regulated by sex steroids. Targeted disruption of the ERα gene blocks the ability of estradiol to induce the expression of kisspeptin in the AVPV [69,129]. The AVPV is thought to play a vital role in the generation of the preovulatory gonadotropin surge, so the current working model proposes that kisspeptin neurons in this region mediate positive feedback effects of estrogens on gonadotropin secretion (Figure 7.15). Evidence demonstrating that a blockade of kisspeptin signaling in the female rat abolishes the preovulatory LH surge is consonant with a role in positive feedback for kisspeptin in the female [168].

Recent evidence suggests that classical, estrogen response element (ERE)-dependent pathways mediate estradiol action on the LH surge mechanism in female mice, whereas nonclassical pathways are responsible for the effect of estradiol on negative feedback of LH [164,169,170]. These studies took advantage of the NERKI (nonclassical estrogen receptor knockin) mouse, which has a mutant ERα allele. This ERα does not bind to DNA and can signal only through membrane-initiated or ERE-independent genomic pathways. LH secretion remains normal in female mice with ovaries intact, indicating that negative feedback is functional. Therefore, the ERE-independent nonclassical genomic ERα signaling pathway is sufficient for rapid negative feedback on LH by estradiol, although it remains possible that classical, ERE-dependent mechanisms contribute to some aspects of negative feedback. The rescue of negative feedback in NERKI females appears to also reflect rapid, nongenotropic actions of E_2 originating at the plasma membrane [171]. Recent evidence has implicated GPR30 as a mediator of rapid actions of estrogen on GnRH neurons [172]. In terms of estrogen positive feedback, NERKI female mice do not exhibit an LH surge, spontaneous ovulation, or estrous cyclicity, indicating that they do not respond to the positive feedback actions of estradiol. These results suggest that while nonclassical ERα-signaling mechanisms are sufficient to restore estrogen negative feedback effects on LH, they are not sufficient to mediate estrogen stimulatory actions on the LH surge [169,170]. These classical and nonclassical mechanisms

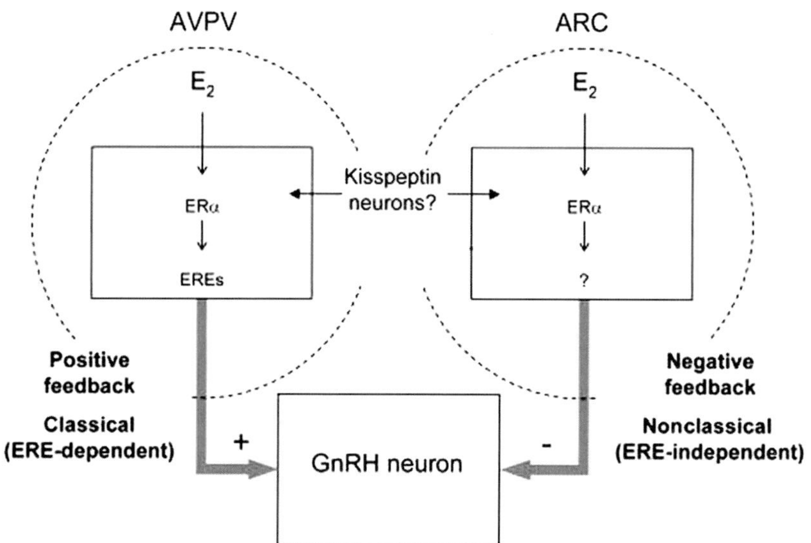

FIGURE 7.15 Proposed model for classical and nonclassical ERα signaling in estrogen positive and negative feedback. Negative feedback actions of estrogen on GnRH/LH secretion are mediated in part by nonclassical (ERE-independent) ERα signaling mechanisms. In contrast, positive feedback actions of estrogen on GnRH/LH surges are mediated by classical (ERE-dependent) ERα signaling mechanisms. These classical and nonclassical mechanisms appear to be mediated at least in part by kisspeptin neurons. *Adapted from McDevitt [170].*

appear to be mediated at least in part by kisspeptin neurons [173].

Progesterone

The principal effect of progesterone is to decrease the frequency of gonadotropin pulses, presumably mediated by hypothalamic effects on GnRH pulse frequency. During the luteal phase of the human menstrual cycle, when progesterone concentrations are at their highest, LH pulse frequency markedly slowed [174]. Progesterone effects on hypothalamic GnRH secretion appear to involve opioidergic pathways, since naloxone, an opioid antagonist, increases the LH pulse frequency during the luteal phase [175]. An additional direct pituitary effect of progesterone cannot be excluded, and progesterone can also augment the stimulatory effects of estrogen on LH secretion in the late follicular phase, when serum progesterone levels are rising along with estrogens, contributing to the ovulatory LH surge [176].

The majority of progesterone actions are currently believed to be dependent upon the binding and activation of its cognate nuclear receptors (nPRs). Bound nPRs recruit coactivator proteins and function as ligand-activated transcription factors that regulate transcription of target genes. Neuroendocrine assessments of PRKO mice have demonstrated involvement of nPRs in the generation of preovulatory gonadotropin surges. The relatively rapid effects of progesterone on gonadotropin secretion are suggestive of additional mechanisms that do not involve changes in gene transcription. A recent study in PRKO mice has demonstrated that progesterone can exert inhibitory effects on GnRH release that are manifest in the absence of nPRs and that these effects may be mediated by membrane receptors coupled to Gi protein involving the inhibition of intracellular cAMP formation [177].

Androgens

Testosterone and its aromatized derivative estradiol are the two steroid hormones that exert negative feedback effects on gonadotropin secretion in the male. Serum LH and FSH levels and α, LHβ and FSHβ mRNA levels rise after castration in a number of experimental animals [2]. The effects of testosterone on FSH synthesis and secretion are complex. The net in vivo effect of testosterone administration to normal men is inhibition of serum FSH levels [178]. It is, however, clear that the direct effects of testosterone on FSH output at the pituitary level are stimulatory [179]. In isolated pituitary cell cultures, testosterone increased FSHβ mRNA levels and FSH release [180]. The differential effects of testosterone on LHβ and FSHβ expression can be attributed to opposing effects on FSHβ between the hypothalamus and the pituitary.

Testosterone inhibits LH secretion when given to normal men and rats. Much like the effects of estrogen, these inhibitory effects are felt largely to be at the hypothalamic level [167]. The available evidence suggests that 5-α reduction of testosterone is not essential for the inhibitory effects of testosterone on LH. Administration of a potent 5-α reductase inhibitor, finasteride, to normal men did not result in elevated LH and FSH levels, consistent with direct inhibitory effects on LH by testosterone without obligatory 5-α reduction [181]. Much as the negative feedback effects of estrogen on GnRH secretion are mediated by kisspeptin neurons in the arcuate nucleus, these neurons also contain AR and the suppression of kisspeptin activity by testosterone in the arcuate nucleus appears to be mediated by both AR and ERα. These findings indicate a role for kisspeptins in mediating the negative feedback effects of gonadal steroids on GnRH secretion in the male as well [69,129].

Inhibins, Activins and Follistatins

The hypothesis that a peptide of gonadal origin selectively regulates FSH secretion dates back to at least 1932 [182]; it took over 50 years to isolate and characterize the structure of inhibin and its related peptides [183–187]. Inhibins are dimeric proteins covalently linked by a disulfide bridge and consisting of a common α-subunit and one of two highly homologous β-subunits, βA or βB (Figure 7.16A). The heterodimer of α:βA is called inhibin A and of α:βB heterodimer, inhibin B [188]. Whether inhibin A and inhibin B play similar or distinct roles in physiological settings is yet to be resolved, although some functional differences have been suggested [189]. In addition, βA subunits can form homodimers called activin A, βB subunits can form homodimers called activin B, or heterodimers of the two β-subunits can form activin AB. Activins stimulate FSH synthesis and secretion [186,187,190,191]. To date five β-subunits have been identified (βA to βE), although only dimers of the βA- and βB-subunits have been shown to have an effect on FSH secretion. A structurally unrelated glycosylated monomeric polypeptide hormone, follistatin, has also been identified, based on its ability to inhibit FSH [192]. Effects on LHβ gene expression and LH secretion are modest, and these three peptides (inhibins, activins and follistatin) are considered to be relatively selective for FSH in terms of their effects on gonadotropins.

Inhibin-related peptides are widely distributed in organ systems and have significant homology with members of the transforming growth factor-β family of proteins that also includes müllerian inhibiting substance, bone morphogenetic proteins and the decapentaplegic gene complex of *Drosophila* and other growth and differentiation factors. While inihibins appear to act primarily as classic circulating endocrine hormones,

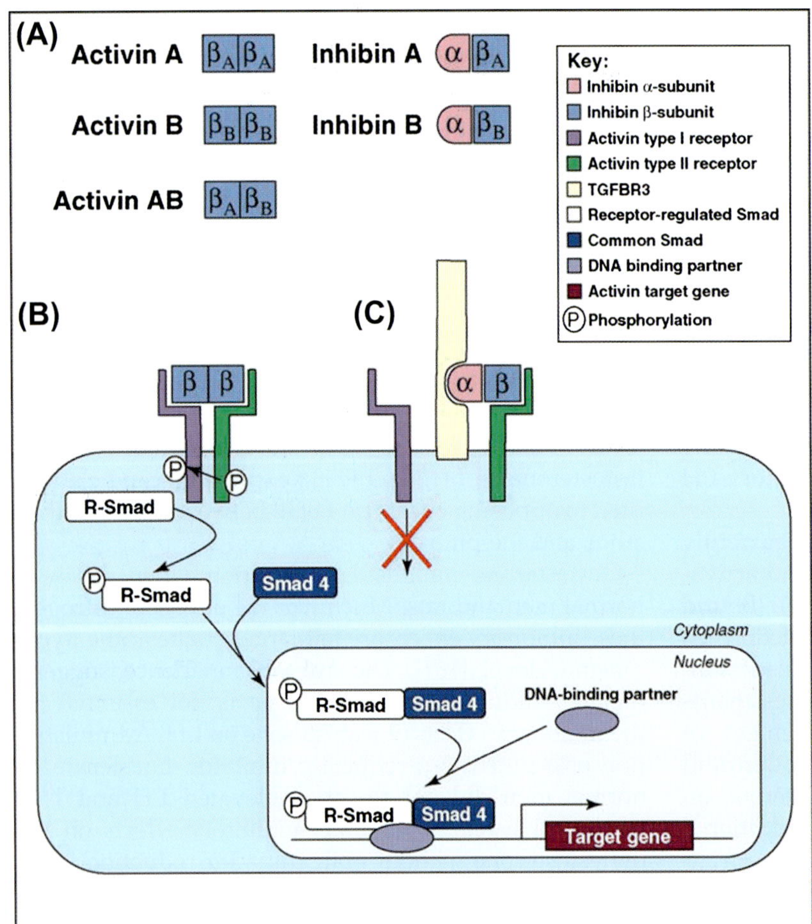

FIGURE 7.16 Activins and inhibins and their mechanism of action. (A) Inhibin and activins are dimeric proteins made up of two subunits. Inhibins are made up of an α-subunit linked to one of two β-subunits, whereas activins are made up by dimerization of two β-subunits. (B) Activin signaling pathway. Activins bind to specific sets of serine–threonine kinase type I and type II receptors on the cell surface. Upon ligand binding, the type II receptor phosphorylates and thereby activates the type I receptor, which in turn phosphorylates downstream signaling molecules, the receptor regulated (RSmads). Once phosphorylated, the R-Smads associate with the common co-Smad (Smad4) and translocate to the nucleus where, in combination with cell-type-specific binding partners, they bind to the promoter sequences of target genes to regulate gene transcription and cellular function. (C) Inhibins bind to activin type II receptors and block the recruitment of type I receptors, thereby blocking R-Smad activation and activin signaling. The presence of TGFBR3, a TGF-β superfamily accessory receptor also known as betaglycan, enhances the binding of inhibins to type II receptors, thereby enhancing the antagonistic actions of inhibins. *From Stenvers [189].*

activins play an important role as regulators of growth and differentiation in diverse tissues, acting locally as autocrine/paracrine factors. For example, activin has been shown to act in the ovary to regulate luteolysis, in the testis to stimulate Sertoli cell proliferation and spermatogenesis, and in the pancreas to enhance beta cell proliferation and insulin secretion [187].

Just as activin is a member of the TGF-β family, the activin receptor and signaling system is similar to the TGFβ receptor system. Activin receptors are heteromeric complexes comprising type I (Act-RI) and type II (Act-RII) serine-threonine kinase receptors (Figure 7.16B). Activin binds to the type II receptors, thereby increasing association with the type I receptor and stimulating its trans-phosphorylation, which in turn results in the activation by phosphorylation of intracellular signaling proteins, receptor-regulated Smad proteins. Activins, TGFβs and growth differentiation factor (GDF) 9 signal via Smad2 and Smad3, whereas BMPs generally signal via Smads 1, 5 and 8. These activated receptor Smads then interact with the common Smad4, resulting in translocation of the Smad complex to the nucleus, where it binds to gene-regulatory elements and interacts with other transcription factors and coactivators to regulate gene transcription, thereby influencing cell fate and function [189,193].

Activin is typically produced locally in multiple tissues where it acts as an autocrine/paracrine factor. Activin biosynthesis itself does not appear to be modulated to a significant degree. Local activity of activin is modulated through multiple modalities. Follistatin and inhibin act as extracellular modulators of activin through distinct mechanisms. These two extracellular proteins modulate activin signaling before activin binds its receptor (follistatin), or before signal transduction is fully activated (inhibin), thereby providing the first of several levels for regulating activin action.

Follistatin (FS) serves as an activin-binding protein and inhibits activin action by interfering with activin's ability to bind to its receptor. The high affinity of the activin–FS interaction approaches irreversibility due to its slow dissociation rate, rendering the bound activin unavailable for binding to its own receptor. The bound complex consists of two FS molecules for each activin β/β homodimer; the low affinity of inhibin for FS may be due to availability of only a single β-subunit in the β/α heterodimer [187].

Inhibins compete for binding to type II activin and BMP receptors through their β-subunits. In this manner, inhibins can antagonize the actions of activins, BMPs, and potentially other TGF-β superfamily members that utilize these type II receptors by preventing the recruitment of the respective type I receptors, thereby blocking R-Smad activation and activin signaling (Figure 7.16C). Since inhibins have significantly lower affinity for the activin and BMP type II receptors compared with the agonists themselves, additional inhibin-binding proteins that increase the affinity of inhibin for the type II receptors are thought to be involved in the antagonistic actions of inhibins. The type III TGF-β superfamily accessory receptor, TGFBR3 (also known as betaglycan), increases the binding affinities of inhibins to the activin and BMP type II receptors, thereby enhancing the antagonistic actions of inhibins [189,194].

At the intracellular level, the activin signal is modulated by inhibitory Smads. Inhibitory Smads form stable associations with type I receptors but cannot be activated, and thereby prevent activation of the receptor Smads. Smad7 inhibits signaling in the activin/TGFβ pathway by blocking phosphorylation of Smads 2 and 3. Smad6, on the other hand, represses the BMP pathway [186]. Another level of regulation occurs through membrane-bound modifiers like BMP and activin receptor membrane-bound inhibitor (BAMBI) and Cripto, a GPI-anchored membrane protein, which inhibits activin signaling by forming an active complex with activin and ActRIIA [186]. At the intracellular level, another mechanism of regulation of activin signaling is through a protein named SMAD anchor for receptor activation (SARA). SARA binds to unphosphorylated SMAD2 to mask its nuclear localization signal and maintain a cytoplasmic distribution. Following receptor activation, SARA interacts with the type I receptor to facilitate SMAD2 phosphorylation and activation. As a result, SMAD2 dissociates from SARA and complexes with SMAD4, after which the complex translocates to the nucleus [186].

While inhibin A does not seem to be a major endocrine regulator of FSH in the human male, inhibin B is stimulated by gonadotropins and circulates systemically to provide feedback inhibition of FSH. In women, inhibin A is secreted by dominant follicles and corpora lutea, contributing to high circulating levels during the late follicular and luteal phases. Inhibin B is reciprocally elevated during the late luteal and early follicular phases of the cycle [186,195]. Circulating inhibin levels drop abruptly after castration in animal models, supporting a primarily gonadal origin. The correlation between circulating inhibin levels and FSH secretion is consistent with a role for inhibin in the feedback regulation of FSH. Activin is detectable in the serum, but levels are low, do not change across the menstrual cycle, and are highly protein-bound to follistatin and α_2-macroglobulin. Therefore, while inhibin is thought to circulate in the bloodstream and act in a classical endocrine fashion, both activin and follistatin can be produced by extragonadal sources and may exert their effects via paracrine/autocrine mechanisms at or near their site of production [193].

Within the pituitary, the gonadotropes and other cell types produce the inhibin α- and β-subunits as well as follistatin. Activin B is produced locally and supports FSH production, as evidenced by a decrease in FSH secretion following treatment of pituitary cultures with an activin-blocking antibody. GnRH and gonadal steroid hormones have been shown to modulate inhibin subunit and follistatin gene expression, and so may modulate gonadotropin gene expression and secretion directly as well as via modulation of activin action [193]. Activin not only increases FSH secretion, but also induces FSHβ gene expression in gonadotrope cells [196]. Smad3 appears to be the principal regulator of activin-induced FSHβ transcription. This functional difference between Smad2 and Smad3 appears to be attributable to the second of the two loops in the Smad2 MH1 domain, which prevents Smad2 from directly binding to DNA [3,193,197–199]. Additional details of the molecular mechanisms underlying regulation of FSHβ transcription by activin are described below in the section on Molecular biology of LH and FSH subunit genes.

MOLECULAR BIOLOGY OF LH AND FSH SUBUNIT GENES

α-subunit

To date, the promoter regions of mouse and human α-subunit genes have been studied the most among species, and the *cis*-elements and *trans*-factors necessary for gonadotrope-specific gene expression are quite similar in these two species. The mouse α-subunit gene contains at least three types of sequences for transcription factor interaction within the proximal 5′-flanking region: cell-type-specific (gonadotropes vs. thyrotropes and/or trophoblasts), basal and hormone-responsive *cis*-elements. These include a GnRH-response element (GnRH-RE) at position −406 to −399, a pituitary homeobox-1 (Pitx-1) binding site at −398 to −385, a pituitary glycoprotein hormone basal element (PGBE) at −344 to −300 and a gonadotrope-specific element (GSE) at −215 to −207, relative to the major transcriptional start site α-subunit (Figure 7.17) [200].

The element in the mouse α-subunit promoter that has been best characterized as a basal, tissue-specific

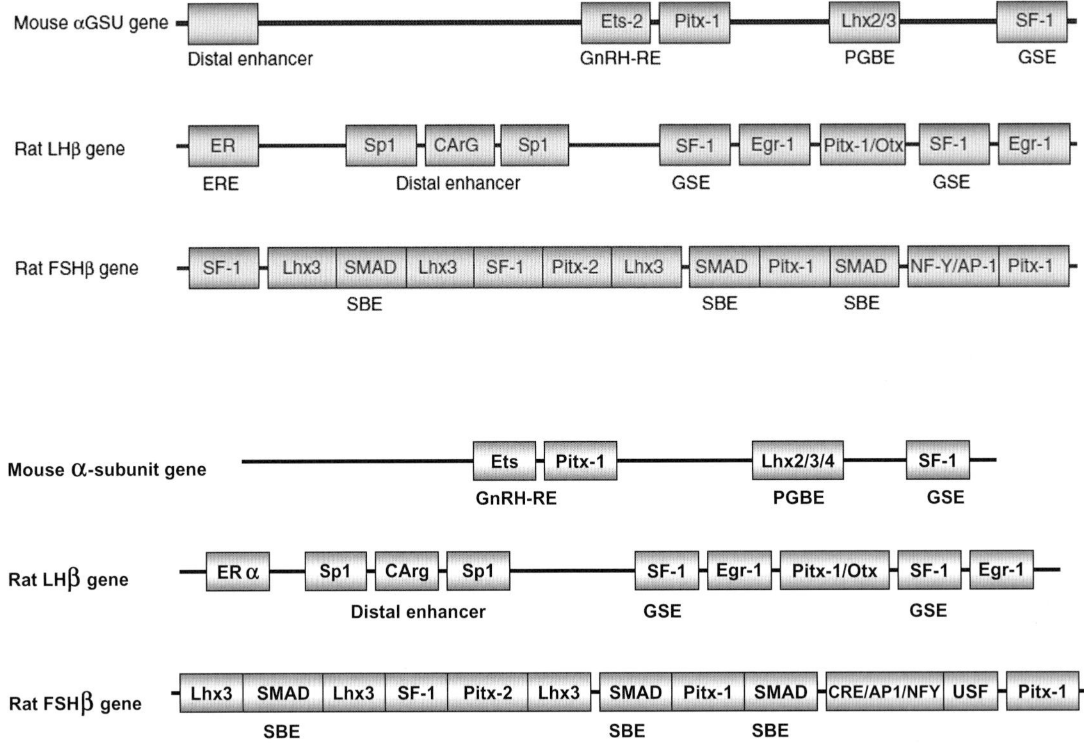

FIGURE 7.17 Schematic diagram of 5′-flanking regions of the rodent αGSU, LHβ and FSHβ genes which contain *cis*-acting elements and transcription factors important for cell-specific and GnRH-regulated expression of each gene. Note that this illustration is simplified for clarity. AP-1, activating protein-1; CArG, CC (A/T)$_6$GG factor; CRE, cAMP response element; CREB, CRE binding protein; DARE, downstream activin regulatory element; Egr-1, early growth response protein-1; ER, estrogen receptor; ERE, estrogen response element; FoxL2, forkhead/winged-helix family protein; GnRH-RE, GnRH-response element; GRAS, GnRHR activating sequence; GSE, gonadotrope-specific element; Lhx, LIM-homeodomain protein; NF-Y, nuclear transcription factor-Y; Oct-1, octamer-1; Otx, orthodenticle; PGBE, pituitary glycoprotein hormone basal element; Pitx, pituitary homeobox; SBE, SMAD binding element; SF-1, steroidogenic factor-1; SMAD, Sma/Mothers against decapentaplegic homolog; Sp1, specificity protein 1; SURG-1, sequence underlying responsiveness to GnRH.

enhancer is the GSE. The GSE sequence, TGACCTTGT, is highly conserved among species and is bound by steroidogenic factor-1 (SF-1). An orphan nuclear receptor, SF-1, was first identified by its ability to coordinately regulate the expression of genes encoding enzymes in the corticosteroid biosynthetic pathway. It is expressed in the ventromedial hypothalamus, pituitary gonadotropes, adrenal cortex and gonadal tissues, and is considered a defining factor for pituitary-specific expression of α-subunit gene. SF-1 deletion in mice precludes adrenal and gonadal development and also results in the selective loss of expression of gonadotrope-specific markers, including LHβ, FSHβ and GnRHR, and a reduction in α-subunit levels; a mutation in human SF-1 causes similar defects [21,22,24,201].

An additional putative basal enhancer of the mouse α-subunit gene is the PGBE [200]. A member of the LIM (lin-11, isl-1, mec-3 and Lmx-1)-homeodomain (HD) family of transcription factors, Lhx2, was shown to bind to this element. Lhx homeodomain transcription factors are important for pituitary development and differentiation as well as for transcriptional activation of the gonadotropin subunit genes [202]. Lhx3 is expressed in the mouse pituitary throughout development and in the adult, and can also bind to the PGBE. Targeted disruption of the *Lhx3* gene in mice leads to failure of growth and differentiation of the anterior and intermediate lobes of the pituitary, and the development of all pituitary cell lineages, except the corticotropes, was affected [203]. Similar phenotypes have been reported in human patients with combined pituitary hormone deficiency due to *Lhx3* gene mutations [18]. *Lhx4* has been shown to act with *Lhx3* for pituitary development, with *Lhx4*-deficient mice exhibiting a reduced number of all the anterior pituitary cell types [204].

A pan-pituitary *bicoid*-related HD protein, Pitx-1, has been shown to interact with a Pitx-1 binding site and has been implicated in cooperative function specifically with Lhx3 for the mouse α-subunit gene expression through protein–protein interaction [205]. Pitx-1-deficient mice exhibit a diminished number of gonadotropes and reduced expression of gonadotrope-specific genes, including the α-subunit [206]. These studies suggest Pitx-1 is important in α-subunit gene expression. Pitx-2 and Hesx1 have also been implicated in regulation of the α-subunit gene through the Pitx-1-binding site.

Like the mouse α-subunit gene, the human α-subunit gene also contains an array of *cis*-elements within the proximal 5′-flanking region. A PGBE is located at position −329 to −320, α-basal element 1 and 2 (αBE1 and 2) at −316 to −302 and −296 to −285, respectively, a GSE at −219 to −211, an α-activating element (αACT) at −161 to −141, two CREs at −146 to −111, a Pitx-1-responsive element at −80 to −65, and two E boxes at −51 to −45 and −21 to −16. These sequences serve as gonadotrope-specific *cis*-elements or as common *cis*-elements for expression in gonadotropes, thyrotropes and/or trophoblasts [200].

Two CREs have been identified within the 5′-flanking region of the human α-subunit gene and are the most important contributors to human promoter activity. These tandem CREs have been shown to regulate α-subunit gene transcription in a synergistic manner [200]. These two CREs play a role not only in regulation by cAMP but also in basal expression and tissue specificity. Unlike the human, the α-subunit genes of lower primates contain a single CRE, and the α-subunit genes of other mammalian species, including the mouse, also have a single CRE but with a one-base pair substitution from the primate CRE (TGATGTCA). This one-base pair substitution in these species has been shown to decrease the binding affinity for CREB, while heterodimers of c-Jun and ATF-2 bind to this nonprimate-variant CRE with much higher affinity than CREB [207]. Thus, α-subunit gene responsiveness to cAMP has diverged between primate and nonprimate species. In primates, CREB appears to play a central role, whereas in nonprimates, other nuclear proteins may mediate both tissue specificity and responsiveness to cAMP. ATF-3 has also been shown to play an important role in regulating α-subunit gene expression through this element [208].

The mouse α-subunit gene promoter confers a robust GnRH-induced activity compared with that of other species. An upstream element of the mouse α-subunit gene confers responsiveness to GnRH, as well as to PMA and to cAMP, and GnRH responsiveness requires the cooperative interaction of this GnRH-RE and the PGBE. The need for a complex response unit for the mediation of GnRH stimulation may provide a mechanism for the maintenance of appropriate, tissue-specific expression and regulation of the α-subunit gene. An Ets factor has been identified as a GnRH-RE binding factor, which appears to be important in mediating GnRH stimulation of α-subunit gene expression [209].

The nuclear androgen receptor (AR) has an important role in modulation of gonadotropin subunit gene expression, mediating feedback inhibition by testosterone [200]. Previous studies have shown that AR represses human α-subunit gene promoter activity by either directly or indirectly binding to the CRE and αBE region in a ligand-dependent manner, suggesting that activated AR may interfere with the binding of cognate factors, thereby leading to an attenuation in transcription of human α-subunit gene. In contrast, estrogen and ER do not have this effect. Subsequent studies have suggested that AR-mediated suppression of human α-subunit gene expression occurs through protein–protein interaction with c-Jun and ATF-2. Thus, as a common feature for both the mouse and human α-subunit genes, it has been suggested that, in the presence of testosterone, α-subunit gene expression is under repression due to the prevention of binding of cognate factors to the CREs, the PGBE and/or αBEs by activated AR, thereby interfering with functional and combinatorial interactions through a common co-activator or adapter complex. Moreover, GnRH stimulation, or the absence of testosterone, releases the AR bound to the c-Jun/ATF-2 heterodimer to allow interactions between these protein complexes and result in synergistic activation of α-subunit gene transcription.

Dominant negative mutant forms of Ras, ERK1 and ERK2 reduce expression of the human α-subunit gene, suggesting an involvement of MAPK cascade in the regulation. A mouse with a pituitary-specific deletion of ERK1/2 had reduced α-subunit gene expression and failure to induce expression in response to GnRH, supporting a key role for this signaling pathway in the regulation of α-subunit gene expression [210].

LHβ-subunit

Almost all the regulatory *cis*-elements identified from each species to date as important for LHβ gene expression are located in the 5′-flanking region, within 500 bp of the transcriptional start site. Within this region, the proximal 140 bp are conserved across species, implying their functional significance [211]. The rat LHβ gene contains two specificity protein 1 (Sp1)-binding sites located at positions −450 to −434 and −366 to −354, a CC $(A/T)_6$GG factor (CArG)-binding site at −443 to −434, two GSEs at −127 to −119 and −58 to −50, two early growth response protein-1 (Egr-1)-binding sites at −112 to −104 and −49 to −41, a Pitx-1-binding site at −99 to −94, and a TATA box at −30 to −26 [200]. Among them, five elements, namely the Pitx-1-binding site, two GSEs and two Egr-1-binding sites, where transcription factors Pitx-1, SF-1 and Egr-1 bind, respectively, form a proximal promoter core cassette. Two Sp1- and the CarG-binding sites, where the GC box-binding protein Sp1, a three-zinc finger transcription factor, and a serum response factor-related protein CArG bind, respectively, form a distal enhancer subunit (Figure 7.17). Proximal 5′-flanking regions of mouse and human LHβ genes also contain a similar set of proximal elements [212].

The zinc finger protein Egr-1 is an immediate-early serum response gene product expressed in various tissues in response to a range of physiological states. Egr-1 mRNA and protein levels are stimulated by GnRH in gonadotrope cell lines, and are critical in mediating GnRH-induced LHβ gene expression by binding to its cognate-binding sites [213]. Disruption of *Egr-1* in mice causes defects in reproductive function, as well as in growth [200]. In the pituitary, gonadotropes are normal in numbers, but specifically fail to express the LHβ-subunit, whereas FSHβ production is evident. These findings suggest that Egr-1 influences reproductive capacity through its regulation of LHβ gene transcription. On the other hand, SF-1 is critical for gonadotrope-specific or basal, but not for GnRH-induced, expression of the LHβ gene. Both Egr-1 and SF-1 interact with Pitx-1, forming a tripartite protein complex to synergistically activate the LHβ gene promoter. This functional synergism suggests the importance of interactions among these factors, directly and cooperatively, for both gonadotrope-specific and GnRH-induced expression of the LHβ gene.

The upstream Sp1-binding sites are also required for GnRH responsiveness. Mutations of these elements alone, preventing Sp1 binding, can reduce GnRH-induced and/or SF-1/Egr-1-mediated rat LHβ gene promoter activity, and combined mutations of the Sp-1-, GSE- and Egr-1-binding sites further eliminate GnRH responsiveness [214]. A transcriptional coactivator, small nuclear RING finger protein (SNURF), interacts with Sp1 and SF-1 to mediate interactions between the distal and proximal GnRH response regions of the LHβ promoter to stimulate transcription [215].

An Egr-1-binding protein (Nab1) is stimulated by GnRH. Nab1 suppresses Egr-1 activation of LHβ gene expression [216]. Nab1 is activated by low-frequency pulsatile GnRH stimulation, whereas Egr-1 is induced to a greater extent by high-frequency pulsatile GnRH stimulation, implicating the balance of Egr-1/Nab1 in the frequency-dependent differential regulation of LHβ by pulsatile GnRH to favor LHβ activation at higher GnRH pulse frequencies (Figure 7.18) [59,217].

The rat LHβ gene promoter region harbors an ERE between −1173 and −1159 which binds to ER and confers a direct stimulatory response to estradiol. This ERE contains a 15-base imperfect palindromic sequence, and ER binds to this region with high affinity [218]. The rat LHβ gene promoter also confers an inhibitory response to testosterone. This inhibitory response to testosterone suppresses GnRH stimulation of LHβ gene promoter activity, and this AR-mediated suppression appears to occur by disrupting the interaction of SNURF with the distal and proximal stimulatory elements of the LHβ promoter [215].

A PKC-mediated stimulatory effect of GnRH on LHβ gene transcription has been well characterized. ERK1 and 2, JNK and p38 all have been shown to be involved in mediating GnRH-induced LHβ gene expression, downstream of PKC, suggesting an involvement of a multitude of diverse and complex signaling pathways which may eventually participate in a complicated cross-talk network to maximize the signaling amplification. In support of the central role of ERK in mediating LHβ stimulation, targeted pituitary deficiency of ERK1/2 resulted in female infertility due to markedly reduced LHβ expression and LH biosynthesis [210].

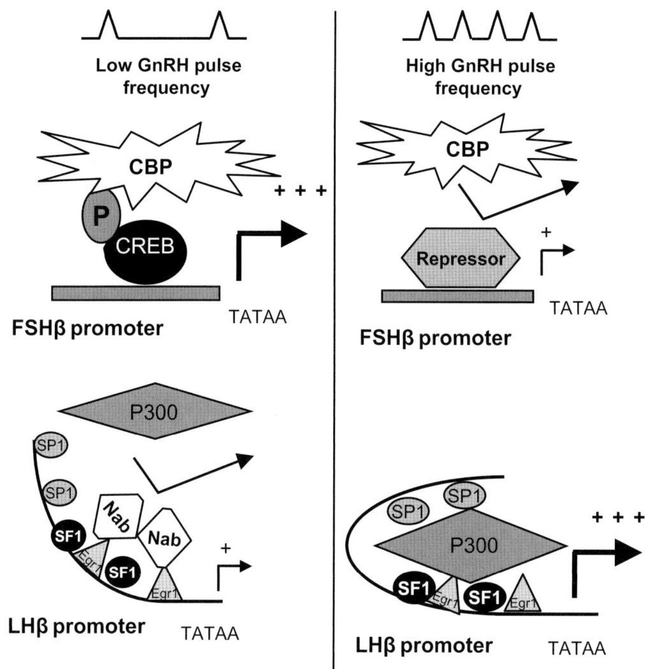

FIGURE 7.18 Low and high GnRH pulse frequencies differentially regulate FSHβ and LHβ transcription through induction or modification of transcription factors and recruitment of coactivators. *From Ciccone [222].*

FSH β-subunit

GnRH stimulates FSHβ expression in gonadotropes. Along with GnRH, activin from paracrine/autocrine sources is considered as a major regulator of FSHβ gene expression. Activin acts independently of GnRH and can induce FSH secretion in GnRH-desensitized pituitary cells. Activin also enhances GnRH responsiveness in gonadotrope cells and synergizes with GnRH in the stimulation of FSHβ gene transcriptional activity.

Rat FSHβ gene promoter *cis*-elements identified to date include a Pitx1/2-binding site in the proximal promoter (−54/−48 in rat, −53/−49 in mouse). This element is important not only for basal expression but also for synergy with GnRH in the activation of FSHβ transcription [219]. Lhx3 expression in gonadotrope cell lines (albeit at low levels) and binding of the protein to the proximal murine FSHβ promoter suggests a role in basal, cell-specific expression as well [220]. Given that Pitx-1 can interact with Lhx3 and that the rat FSHβ gene promoter contains both Pitx-1- and Lhx3-binding sites, a logical analogy is that these factors may interact with each other to synergize in the tissue-specific expression of the FSHβ gene. SF-1 and NF-Y are important basal regulators in many systems. Despite the observation that SF-1 alone has only a minimal effect on mouse FSHβ gene promoter activity, NF-YA and SF-1 functionally interact to regulate the mouse FSHβ gene expression in a cell-type-specific manner, which requires intact GSE and NF-Y-binding sites [221]. It is possible that SF-1 and NF-Y maintain and regulate basal and gonadotrope-specific expression of the mouse FSHβ gene (Figure 7.17) [220].

A major GnRH-responsive element within the proximal FSHβ promoter, which contains a partial cAMP response element (CRE)/AP1 site, has been characterized by several groups in the rat and mouse gene [222–225]. This GnRH-responsive element is fully conserved in the human. This site appears promiscuous with the ability to bind the bZIP transcription family member, CREB, as well as members of the AP1 family, such as c-Fos and c-Jun. A mechanism by which GnRH stimulates FSHβ transcription is by inducing phosphorylation of promoter-bound CREB, leading to the recruitment of the histone acetyltransferase CREB-binding protein (CBP).

The transcriptional repressor, inducible cAMP early repressor (ICER), is induced by pulsatile GnRH. High GnRH pulse frequencies preferentially induce ICER, which binds to the CRE/AP1 site to antagonize CREB-mediated FSHβ stimulation and thereby attenuate FSHβ expression [226]. These data suggest that ICER production antagonizes the stimulatory action of CREB to attenuate FSHβ transcription at high GnRH pulse frequencies, thereby playing a critical role in regulating cyclic reproductive function (Figure 7.18).

In contrast to the αGSU and LHβ genes, androgen has a stimulatory effect on the ovine FSHβ gene promoter activity [3]. This effect is mediated by direct interaction of the androgen receptor with the proximal FSHβ promoter. Progesterone has similar activating effects on FSHβ, mediated by the progesterone receptor. In contrast, estrogen did not appear to have direct positive or negative effects on FSHβ gene expression [227].

Activin is a potent inducer of FSHβ transcription. Intracellular signaling molecules SMAD2, 3 and 4 have all been shown to mediate activin-stimulated activity of the FSHβ promoter as well as FSHβ mRNA synthesis [199,228–231], although the role of SMAD2 is less clear [193,199,229–231]. Three activin response elements have been identified in the FSHβ promoter [3]. SMAD3 and 4 bind to the distal SBE (−266/−259) of the rat FSHβ gene promoter, and deletion of this SBE abolishes activin-mediated FSHβ gene transcriptional activity [193]. Pitx-2 has been shown to up-regulate basal and activin-mediated rat FSHβ gene promoter activity in a dose-dependent manner, and elimination of the Pitx-2-binding site results in a loss of activin-regulated FSHβ gene promoter activity [198,232].

Activin-regulated FSHβ gene expression is highly specific and selective compared with other gonadotropin genes. This signal specificity and selectivity is likely to be achieved by the interaction of SMADs with other tissue- and cell-specific partners or coregulators. For example, the activin-specific SMADs can interact with forkhead transcription factors, such as FoxL2, to bind to DNA [233,234]. The TALE homeodomain proteins, Pbx1 and Prep1, have also been shown to interact with Smad proteins to mediate activin induction of FSHβ transcription [229].

Synergy between activin and GnRH signaling pathways has been identified in both in vivo and in vitro studies [3,193]. Nuclear translocation of SMADs can be detected subsequent to GnRH treatment in αT3-1 and LβT2 cells, suggesting cross-talk between GnRH and activin signaling pathways and the ability of GnRH to stimulate activin signaling pathways in gonadotropes. Although there are several possible mechanisms by which activin and GnRH may interact, SMAD3 and 4 have been shown to interact with Jun/Fos proteins, and promoter activities for genes containing AP-1 sites are enhanced by activin, suggesting synergistic associations between SMADs and AP-1 proteins, especially upon concomitant activin and GnRH stimulation, possibly by sharing a common coactivator or adaptor complex.

DIAGNOSTIC TESTS

GnRH Stimulation Test

The effects of graded single doses of GnRH (25–100 μg) given intravenously on serum LH and FSH secretion in normal men and women have been extensively studied [235,236]. Rapid and dose-dependent increases in serum LH and FSH levels are seen, with peak levels of both hormones within 20–30 minutes. Increases in serum LH are greater than those in serum FSH levels. Mortimer et al. evaluated the utility of a 100 μg GnRH bolus as a diagnostic test in classifying 155 patients with disorders of the hypothalamic–pituitary–gonadal axis [237]. A wide range of LH responses was seen with peak values ranging from 8 to 34 mIU/ml. Patients with IHH have diminished LH responses and often exhibit a greater FSH than LH response. A similar prepubertal pattern of diminished LH and FSH response and reversal of the usual LH/FSH ratios after GnRH administration can be seen in patients with anorexia nervosa [238]. After repetitive administration of GnRH pulses, LH and FSH responses are normalized in both groups of patients indicating the intactness of the pituitary. The GnRH stimulation test has some utility in the diagnosis of pubertal disorders [239]. An alternative test is the measurement of LH 2–3 hours after administration of a GnRH agonist such as leuprolide [240]. However, the LH and FSH responses to GnRH also vary with the sex, age, degree of sexual maturation and the phase of menstrual cycle. Thus, the GnRH stimulation test has had limited usefulness in the diagnosis of hypothalamic–pituitary disorders in adults. In most instances, careful evaluation of baseline hormone levels (LH, FSH and testosterone) in the appropriate context of historical and radiological data is sufficient to arrive at the correct diagnosis. The GnRH stimulation test has also not generally been useful in differentiating delayed puberty from IHH [241,242]. While more difficult to administer, evaluation of LH responses to repetitive administration of graded doses of GnRH can be more informative [243].

Clomiphene Test

Clomiphene is an antiestrogen, but acts as a partial agonist in that it also has weak estrogenic activity at high doses. In adult men and women, its antiestrogenic action predominates in most tissues in vivo, resulting in increased secretion of GnRH and thereby LH and FSH. In prepubertal children with very low or negligible amounts of estrogen, it acts as an estrogen and inhibits LH and FSH. The usual protocol is to administer 100 mg clomiphene orally each day for 1–4 weeks. Serum LH levels generally increase by 100% or more, while FSH levels show about a 50% increase over baseline [244,245]. A normal response to clomiphene indicates normality of the hypothalamic–pituitary axis. However, an abnormal/absent response does not distinguish hypothalamic from pituitary disease. Clinical indications for the clomiphene test are limited; it has had some use as a research tool in establishing the normality and maturity of the hypothalamic–pituitary unit. Currently, the main clinical use is in the assessment of ovarian reserve. However, as it provides no additional information when the basal day 3 FSH is elevated, there is no reason to perform the test in those women [246].

Detection and Characterization of Gonadotropin Pulse Patterns

Soon after the introduction of LH and FSH radioimmunoassays, it became apparent that these hormones are secreted into the circulation in a pulsatile pattern. The ability to measure small amounts of hormones in serum samples led to recognition that secretion of many, if not all, hormones is episodic [247]. In light of this episodic hormone secretion, there was an interest in the development of discrete pulse-detection algorithms. Signal detection methods, including spectral analysis, cross-spectral analyses, and other procedures for smoothing and filtering data to enhance detection of a signal of interest have existed for a considerable time, but have limitations for the detection of biological hormone pulses. Several difficulties inherent in the biologic data confounded efforts to develop a single, ideal pulse-detection algorithm. As opposed to the highly episodic physical or mathematical events, LH pulse patterns in humans are characterized by a lack of absolute regularity in the frequency and amplitude of LH pulses, limitations of assay precision, and dependence of false-positive and false-negative rates on sampling intensity [247].

Santen and Bardin developed the first algorithm which defined a peak as a 20% increase in the hormone concentration in a single sample over the preceding sample [248]. Subsequent modifications of the method include selection of a chosen multiple (e.g., three-fold) of the assay coefficient of variation (CV) to define the pulse. The simplicity of use and apparent freedom from assumptions have made this a widely used program, and modified versions are still commonly used [126].

A number of refinements and alternative algorithms have been developed and readers are referred to a recent review [247]. Such refinements have enhanced the validity and applicability of pulse-detection algorithms. The development of highly sensitive and specific immunoassays for quantitation of LH and FSH have helped to clarify the nature and significance of low-amplitude pulses. Developments of conditional probability modeling methods and the adaptation and validation of cross-correlation methods for demonstrating coincidence of two or more hormone pulses have shown a high degree of concordance between LH, FSH, free α-subunit and testosterone pulses [247]. Type I (false-positive) and type II (false-negative) statistical errors have been better defined.

Application of deconvolution to pulse analysis made it possible to determine the instantaneous secretory rates of hormones [249]. Deconvolution techniques resolve the hormone series into appearance and disappearance curves. Current deconvolution models permit determination of: (1) identity and characterization of all secretory episodes; (2) production rates of the hormone; and (3) estimation of half-life of hormone disappearance.

CLINICAL DISORDERS AFFECTING THE GONADOTROPE

Disorders affecting gonadotropin secretion and action can be broadly classified into two categories: first, hypogonadotropic disorders, or those associated with decreased LH and/or FSH secretion; and second, hypergonadotropic disorders, or those characterized by excessive or physiologically inappropriate secretion of LH and/or FSH.

Hypogonadotropic Disorders

Because LH and FSH are trophic hormones for the testes and ovaries, impaired secretion of these gonadotropins (hypogonadotropism) results in hypogonadism. Clinically, patients with hypogonadotropic hypgonadism may present with symptoms and signs of sex steroid (androgen in male and estrogen in the female) deficiency, and/or infertility due to impaired germ cell development.

The symptoms and signs of androgen deficiency depend on its time of onset and the degree of gonadotropin deficiency. Androgen deficiency during fetal life may result in failure of the Wolffian structures to develop, ambiguity of external genitalia due to failure of fusion, hypospadias, microphallus, or a combination of these. In patients with isolated hypogonadotropism, placental hCG stimulates the fetal testis to produce sufficient androgen in early fetal life. Therefore, most patients with congenital GnRH deficiency have normal Wolffian structures and external genitalia. However, during the second half of pregnancy, the fetal gonad is under the control of fetal pituitary LH and FSH. Therefore, severe LH and FSH deficiency during this period may result in undescended testes and microphallus, since testicular descent is partly androgen-dependent. In addition, because of FSH deficiency, these patients have impaired development of seminiferous tubules [47,50]. The ovaries have little functional activity during fetal development, so LH and FSH deficiency during fetal development in females results in no significant clinical manifestation.

If androgen or estrogen deficiency occurs after birth but before puberty, sexual development is delayed or arrested; these children present with delayed or absent puberty. Other androgen- and estrogen-dependent events that occur in the peripubertal period, such as the epiphyseal fusion of long bones and calcification of laryngeal cartilages, are also delayed. Delay in the fusion of the epiphyses results in continued growth of long bones causing increased height and reversal of the upper segment to lower segment ratios, and eunuchoidal proportions (span greater than height by more than 2 cm). Men with prepubertal androgen deficiency retain their high-pitched voice and do not develop the male pattern temporal recession of the hairline.

Androgen deficiency acquired after completion of puberty is characterized by regression of the secondary sex characteristics, impairment of libido and sexual function, loss of muscle mass, increased fat mass and infertility. However, these changes often occur insidiously so that many years might elapse before these patients seek medical attention. This may partly explain why men with hypogonadism resulting from prolactin-secreting pituitary adenomas usually have large tumors (macroadenomas) at the time of initial presentation. Early interruption of the menstrual cycle by hyperprolactinemia in women, on the other hand, alerts them to seek medical advice earlier, leading to an earlier diagnosis of their pituitary adenoma and detection when the tumor is still small (microadenomas).

Disorders associated with hypogonadotropic hypogonadism can be classified into congenital and acquired disorders (Table 7.4). Acquired disorders are much more common than congenital disorders and may result from functional abnormalities in GnRH or gonadotropin secretion or from organic diseases such as neoplastic, inflammatory, or infiltrative diseases.

Congenital Hypogonadotropic Disorders

Heterogeneity of Pulsatile Gonadotropin Secretion in Patients with Idiopathic Hypogonadotropic Hypogonadism

There is considerable heterogeneity in the clinical presentation of IHH. The phenotype, to a large degree, is determined by the severity of GnRH deficiency. Those with the most severe deficiency may present with complete absence of pubertal development, sexual infantilism, and in some cases with varying degrees of hypospadias and undescended testes. Male patients may have complete absence of secondary sex characteristics, infantile testes and azoospermia, while female patients may present with primary amenorrhea. Patients with partial GnRH deficiency may have varying degrees of delay in sexual development in proportion to the severity of gonadotropin deficiency.

Patients with IHH are quite heterogeneous in their LH-secretory profiles [47,126,250,251]. Patients with the most severe GnRH deficiency typically display no pulsatile LH secretion at all. Others may display low-amplitude pulses or reduced frequency. A subset is characterized by sleep-entrained pulses reminiscent of the pattern seen in the early stages of puberty.

Two variants of IHH are particularly interesting. The term "fertile eunuch syndrome" has been used to describe patients with eunuchoidal proportions and delayed sexual development but who have normal-sized testes. Such individuals appear to have sufficient gonadotropins to stimulate high intratesticular testosterone levels and to initiate spermatogenesis, but not enough testosterone secretion into the blood to adequately virilize the peripheral tissues; they are, in fact, partially gonadotropin-deficient [156]. Another variant with predominantly FSH deficiency has also been described, although these patients are rare [252].

Nonreproductive Phenotypes Associated with Kallmann Syndrome and Hypogonadotropic Hypogonadism

Kallman first described a syndrome characterized by delayed or arrested sexual development associated with anosmia [253]. These patients have selective gonadotropin deficiency resulting from an isolated defect in GnRH secretion. The primary pathogenic defect in these patients is hypothalamic and the impaired gonadotropin secretion is secondary to the hypothalamic abnormality in GnRH secretion [47]. Details of the genetics and pathogenesis of this syndrome were described earlier (see section on GnRH neuronal development); here we will focus on the distinctive clinical manifestations [47,50,102,103,254]. Although anosmia and hyposmia are the most well-known and the first associations described in this syndrome, a number of other somatic abnormalities have been recorded. Synkinesia is found in about 80% of patients with Kallmann syndrome due to mutations in the X-linked *KAL1* gene. Unilateral renal agenesis or horseshoe-shaped kidneys are present in approximately 30% of males with *KAL1* mutations. This is often asymptomatic, and must be evaluated by ultrasound examination. Other manifestations include sensorineural hearing loss, high-arched palate, cleft lip and palate, color blindness, cryptorchidism and optic atrophy. Nonreproductive phenotypes associated with Kallmann syndrome due to *FGFR1* mutations include synkinesia in about 10% of affected individuals, cleft lip and/or palate, dental agenesis, digit malformations (brachydactyly, syndactyly) and agenesis of the corpus callosum, which can be seen on brain MRI. Nonreproductive phenotypes associated with mutations in *PROK2* or *PROKR2* have been less well characterized, but some that have been reported include obesity, pectus excavatum, seizures, synkinesia, high-arched palate, pes planus, hyperlaxity of digits and hearing loss. Whether these manifestations are all truly linked to the genetic mutation remains to be determined. Mutations in *CHD7* have also been identified in patients with Kallmann syndrome. This gene has been implicated in CHARGE syndrome, a multisystem disorder consisting of eye coloboma, heart defects, choanal atresia, retardation of growth and development, genito-urinary anomalies and ear abnormalities (vestibular and auditory). *CHD7* mutations in patients with Kallmann syndrome without the full CHARGE syndrome are thought to represent milder allelic variants, but some of the features of CHARGE syndrome may be present. In particular, high-arched or cleft palate, dental agenesis, auricular dysplasia, deafness and hypoplasia of semicircular canals, coloboma and short stature have been associated phenotypic features [117,255].

The genetic causes of hypogonadotropic hypogonadism due to defects in GnRH secretion (rather than developmental defects in GnRH neuronal migration) are not typically associated with anosmia and also usually have fewer nonreproductive phenotypes. These disorders are often termed isolated or normosmic hypogonadotropic hypogonadism. For example, patients with inactivating mutations in *KISS1R* have isolated HH with hypogonadism but no other identified distinctive phenotypic features. Some male patients with *KISS1R* mutations have been reported to have cryptorchidism [256]. On the other hand, mutations in *TAC3* or *TACR3* are more commonly associated with microphallus in males and absent spontaneous thelarche in females, yet these patients had evidence for reversibility of their hypogonadotropism later in life. These phenotypic manifestations suggest that the neurokinin B pathway plays an important role during early sexual development, but its importance in sustaining the integrity of the hypothalamic–pituitary–gonadal axis appears attenuated over time [250]. Mutations in the GnRH and GnRHR genes also cause isolated normosmic hypogonadotropic hypogonadism, with the clinical severity determined in large part by the degree of loss-of-function caused by the mutation [138,139,148]. On the other hand, mutations in the genes encoding leptin or leptin receptor cause normosmic HH associated with morbid obesity, and mutations in PCSK1, a prohormone convertase that processes the GnRH prohormone to the mature secreted biologically active decapeptide, is also associated with obesity, as well as hypoglycemia and hypocortisolemia and impaired processing of POMC and proinsulin [140].

Mutations in the Genes Encoding LHβ- and FSHβ-subunits

Hypogonadism Associated with Mutations in the FSHβ Gene

Inherited mutations of the *FSHβ* gene are uncommon, but have been reported to produce hypogonadism and delayed puberty in both males and females. Four inactivating FSHβ mutations have been characterized in women, which resulted in a similar phenotype of delayed puberty, absent or incomplete breast development, primary amenorrhea and infertility, with low levels of E2 and P, high LH and undetectable FSH [257–260]. A detailed study of ovarian function from one of these FSH-deficient women showed no effects of LH excess. Ovarian synthesis of sex steroids occurs according to a two-cell model involving collaborative actions of theca and granulosa cells. LH acts on theca cells to stimulate the synthesis of androgens, which diffuse into adjacent granulosa cells. FSH acts on granulosa cells to mediate follicular development and the expression of aromatase, converting androgens derived from theca cells to estrogens. In other conditions involving increased ratios of LH to FSH, such as polycystic ovary syndrome, hyperandrogenism occurs. In contrast, our patient had a low serum testosterone concentration despite a high serum luteinizing hormone concentration, suggesting that FSH-induced follicular recruitment and development are necessary for increased androgen production. This finding is consistent with studies showing that FSH enhances the production of androgen by theca cells. These findings provide supportive evidence that FSH is not necessary for the development of small preantral follicles readily responsive to FSH. Female mice deficient in FSHβ are infertile with a block in folliculogenesis prior to antral follicle formation [261].

Four men with inactivating *FSHβ* mutations have been described. All of them were azoospermic, but two had normal puberty associated with normal to low-normal testosterone levels and high LH levels, whereas the third presented with a low testosterone concentration and absent puberty [257,259,260,262]. FSH-deficient male mice, on the other hand, are fertile although they have small testes and subnormal spermatogenesis, indicating that FSH is not absolutely essential for spermatogenesis in mice [261].

Hypogonadism Associated with Mutations of the LHβ Gene

Mutations that abolish the activity of luteinizing hormone are rare; they have been reported in six men and one woman [260,263–265]. The phenotypes of the men suggest that LH is not required for male sexual differentiation but is critical to the proliferation and function of Leydig cells and to the induction of puberty. Infertility and very low levels of spermatogenesis persist in the affected men, despite long-term exposure to human chorionic gonadotropin, suggesting that the absence of perinatal exposure to luteinizing hormone alters Leydig cells' proliferation and maturation, impairing the onset of normal spermatogenesis, which is thought to be critically dependent on a high level of intratesticular testosterone. In one case involving a partial loss of LH function, despite undetectable circulating LH and a low serum testosterone level, the patient had a small population of mature Leydig cells expressing the steroidogenic enzymes necessary for androgen synthesis and producing sufficient levels of intratesticular testosterone to trigger and maintain complete and quantitatively normal spermatogenesis [263]. The one case reported in a female revealed a phenotype characterized by normal pubertal development and menarche, secondary amenorrhea and infertility.

Inactivating Mutations of LH and FSH Receptor Genes

Inactivating Mutations of the LH Receptor Gene

In genetic males, homozygous inactivating mutations of *LHR* cause 46,XY disorders of sexual development and differentiation, previously referred to as complete male pseudohermaphroditism, whereas mutations that cause only partial loss of function result in hypospadias and/or micropenis and hypogonadism (Figure 7.8A)

[35,266]. hCG and LH bind to the same LHR on testicular Leydig cells. Early in gestation, hCG, acting through the LHR, is fundamental for secretion of testosterone and development of the male external and internal genitalia. Inactivating mutations of *LHR* result in reduced or absent testosterone secretion and consequent impairment of masculinization of the external genitalia. In the absence of androgen action during human fetal development, the external genitalia remain female, irrespective of chromosomal or gonadal sex. Interestingly, a deletion of exon 10 of *LHR* has been described, resulting in a phenotype of hypogonadism in a man with normal male external genitalia. In vitro, the *LHR* with this deletion responded normally to hCG, but not to LH, explaining the phenotype while revealing that exon 10 of the *LHR* is responsible for specificity of LH binding [266,267]. The clinical findings of LH-deficient hypogonadal men with *LHβ* mutations contrast with the feminization of the external genitalia in 46,XY subjects harboring inactivating mutations in the *LHR*.

Four unrelated women with different mutations in *LHR* have been reported [35,266]. All patients were identified because they were sisters of probands with 46,XY disorders of sexual development. All had female external genitalia, normal development of secondary sex characteristics, increased LH levels, primary or secondary amenorrhea and infertility. In contrast to the 46,XY subjects, the phenotypes of 46,XX patients with *LHβ* and *LHR* mutations were very similar, with the exception of the difference in circulating LH levels. Accordingly, women with *LHβ* mutations may be treated with exogenous LH or hCG, whereas women with *LHR* mutations are resistant to LH and, at present, no treatment is effective in rescuing their fertility.

Inactivating Mutations of FSH Receptor Gene

The first inactivating *FSHR* mutation in females was found in association with features of hypergonadotropic hypogonadism, primary amenorrhea, variable pubertal development, high gonadotropin and low estrogen levels [35,268,269]. Ovaries were hypoplastic with impaired follicle growth. No functional responses were observed after treatment with high doses of recombinant FSH. This first identified mutation was only partially inactivating. Identification and characterization of a patient with a completely inactivating *FSHR* mutant showed delayed puberty, primary amenorrhea, elevated gonadotrophins, low estradiol and inhibin B levels and testosterone levels in the lower/normal range [270]. She had osteoporosis, a hypoplastic uterus and ovaries, and follicles were at the primordial stage with absent secondary follicles. Thus, FSH appears to be critical for follicular maturation beyond the primary stage in humans. FSH resistance causes infertility, which is associated with the persistence of a large number of small follicles in the ovaries, probably due to a low follicular recruitment, as observed in prepubertal ovaries (Figure 7.8B) [35,268,270].

Male family members harboring the first identified inactivating FSHR mutation had normal pubertal development but moderately or slightly decreased testicular volume, and were fertile. They had normal plasma testosterone, normal to elevated LH levels, but high FSH. None of the patients had azoospermia, but they showed variable spermatogenic abnormalities with reduced sperm counts or low volumes of seminal fluid. Studies of these individuals showed that FSH action is required for normal spermatogenesis but is not critical for male fertility [35,268,269].

Other Congenital Hypogonadotropic Disorders

Prader-Willi Syndrome

Prader-Willi syndrome is a multisystemic disorder associated with dysfunction of the hypothalamic–pituitary axis. It is characterized by a range of mental and physical symptoms mostly related to hypothalamic deficiency, including short stature, muscular hypotonia, excessive appetite with progressive obesity, hypogonadism, growth hormone deficiency, mental retardation, behavioral abnormalities, sleep disturbances, respiratory disease and dysmorphic features [271]. Prader-Willi syndrome is a disorder of genomic imprinting that arises from the lack of expression of paternally inherited imprinted genes on chromosome 15q11-q13. These genes are imprinted and silenced on the maternally inherited chromosome, presumably by DNA methylation. Therefore, the deletion of the paternally derived copy of the normally active genes produces the disease. In 70–75% of affected individuals there is a deletion of that segment of the paternally derived chromosome 15; 20–25% of patients exhibit maternal disomy of the same region of chromosome 15 (inheritance of both copies of this region of chromosome 15 from the mother, rather than one from each parent); 2–5% have sporadic or inherited microdeletion in the imprinting center; and 1% have translocations. Three paternally derived intronless genes (*MKRN3, MAGEL2* and *NDN*) have been identified in the 15q11-q13 region, as well as the small nuclear ribonucleoprotein polypeptide N (SNRPN) gene encoding for SNURF [271].

Laurence-Moon-Biedl Syndrome

Laurence-Moon-Biedl or Bardet-Biedl syndrome (BBS) is an autosomal recessive disorder characterized by obesity, hypogonadism, mental retardation, polydactyly and retinitis pigmentosa. Renal abnormalities are common, and speech disorders, brachydactyly, polyuria and polydipsia, ataxia, poor coordination/clumsiness, diabetes mellitus, left ventricular hypertrophy and hepatic fibrosis can also occur. Twelve genes are known to be associated with Bardet-Biedl syndrome: *BBS1, BBS2, ARL6/BBS3, BBS4, BBS5, MKKS/BBS6, BBS7, TTC8/BBS8, B1/BBS9, BBS10, TRIM32/BBS11* and *BBS12*. Molecular genetic testing is available on a clinical basis for some of the most common mutations. However, despite the identification of 12 BBS genes, the molecular basis of the disorder remains elusive. All of the known BBS proteins are components of the centrosome and/or basal body and have an impact on ciliary transport [272].

Miscellaneous Congenital Hypogonadotropic Disorders

A large number of congenital defects and syndromes have been decribed in association with hypogonadotropic hypogonadism. An extensive list of these disorders can be found in textbooks of genetic disorders.

Hypogonadotropic Hypogonadism Associated with Developmental Disorders of the Pituitary Due to Mutations of Transcription Factors

Mutations in pituitary transcription factors associated with hypogonadotropic hypogonadism were discussed earlier (see section on Molecular basis of pituitary development) (Figure 7.1; Table 7.1). For example, human mutations in *Hesx1* have been identified and are associated with variable septo-optic dysplasia and hypopituitarism, ranging from CPHD including gonadotropins to isolated growth hormone deficiency [11–13]. Mutations in *Sox2* and *Sox3* are also associated with septo-optic dysplasia, anterior pituitary hypoplasia and hypogonadotropic hypogonadism [12]. Mutations in *Pitx2* cause Rieger syndrome, characterized by defects in the eyes, teeth and heart, as well as pituitary hormone deficiencies [17]. Mutations in *Lhx3* and *Lhx4* have been identified in patients with CPHD including impaired gonadotropin release [9,11,12,18]. Mutations in *PROP1* are the most common genetic cause of CPHD [19]. Gonadotrope differentiation is also impaired, and homozygous females and most males are infertile. In contrast to *PROP1* mutations, mutations in *PIT1*, also a member of the POU homeodomain family, have pituitary deficiencies limited to GH, prolactin and TSH [9].

Steroidogenic factor-1 (SF-1) is a member of the nuclear receptor family expressed throughout the reproductive axis (hypothalamus, pituitary and gonads) and in the adrenal gland. It is a key transcriptional regulator of many genes involved in sexual differentiation, steroidogenesis and reproduction, including the pituitary gonadotropin α-subunit, *LHβ, FSHβ* and *GnRHR* genes [11,21]. SF-1 null mice show complete adrenal and gonadal agenesis as well as impaired development of the ventromedial hypothalamus and of gonadotropes [22]. Patients with mutations in SF-1 have been described with varying degrees of XY sex reversal, testicular dysgenesis, ovarian insufficiency, adrenal failure and impaired pubertal maturation [23].

DAX-1 (***d***osage-sensitive sex-reversal ***a***drenal hypoplasia critical region on the ***X*** chromosome protein 1) is a nuclear receptor transcription factor related to SF-1 with a similar distribution pattern of expression. Mutations in *NR0B1*, the X-linked gene encoding DAX-1, are associated with X-linked hypogonadotropic hypogonadism and adrenal hypoplasia congenita [24,201,273,274]. To date more than 100 different mutations in *NR0B1* have been identified, the majority causing truncations or frameshifts rendering the protein nonfunctional. Hypogonadotropic hypogonadism is often mild, revealing itself as failure to undergo puberty or incomplete puberty. The role of DAX-1 in the hypothalamus and pituitary glands has not been studied extensively, although the hypogonadism appears to be a mixed defect of hypothalamic and pituitary function. DAX-1 is a transcriptional repressor, and paradoxically has been shown to inhibit SF1-mediated transcription of an array of target genes, including LHβ. How the loss of function in these two opposing genes, *SF-1* and *DAX-1*, results in similar phenotypes is not well understood. The hypogonadism is likely due to a developmental defect of the hypothalamus and pituitary, suggesting a role for DAX-1 in proper development of these organs.

Acquired Hypogonadotropic Disorders

Hypothalamic Amenorrhea

Hypothalamic amenorrhea (HA) is a reversible disorder in which no anatomic or organic abnormalities of the hypothalamic–pituitary–ovarian (H–P–O) axis can be identified [275,276]. It is the most common cause of secondary amenorrhea, responsible for approximately 35% of cases. HA is associated mainly with conditions of stress or energy deficits. Dieting, robust psychological stress, acute or chronic medical illness, or excessive exercise can lead to disruption of hypothalamic–pituitary activity controlling ovarian function. All such stressors negatively affect the reproductive axis by acting on hypothalamic regulatory pathways.

The key finding in HA is the reduction in central gonadotropin-releasing hormone (GnRH) release from the medial basal hypothalamus, leading to a reduction in GnRH pulse frequency, amplitude, or both, which in turn results in lower levels of LH and FSH secretion by the pituitary gland [277]. The resulting gonadotropin deficiency fails to provide adequate stimulation to the ovarian follicles so that the normal sequence of follicular growth, maturation, follicular selection and ovulation becomes attenuated. As a result, ovarian estradiol production is low and endometrial growth is reduced, resulting in prolonged intervals of amenorrhea. The transition from normal menstrual cycles to anovulation and amenorrhea can take place gradually and may be characterized by inadequate luteal phases, irregular menses and ultimately complete amenorrhea [275,276]. HA is of particular clinical importance as the associated hypoestrogenism has been correlated with decreased bone density [277].

Diagnostic criteria for hypothalamic amenorrhea include amenorrhea for at least 6 months with low serum LH and FSH levels. Hypothalamic amenorrhea is associated with eating disorders such as bulimia and anorexia nervosa and with exercise-associated amenorrhea [275,276]. There is a high prevalence of amenorrhea, anovulatory cycles and other menstrual irregularities in adult female athletes, particularly long-distance runners, dancers and swimmers [278,279]. The athletes tend to weigh less and have a lower percentage of body fat. Serum estradiol levels and the frequency of LH pulses are lower in athletes who are amenorrheic than in nonexercising controls. If intense exercise or an eating disorder manifests prior to the onset of puberty, then the onset and progression of puberty can be markedly delayed. Periods of rest or reduction in exercise intensity due to injury are associated with rapid sexual development and the occurrence of menses.

Hypogonadism in critical illness is well documented. The degree of suppression of the hypothalamic–pituitary–gonadal axis correlates with the severity of illness [280]. In men, serum testosterone levels fall at the onset of illness and recover during recuperation. Although the magnitude of gonadotropin suppression is generally correlated to the severity of illness, there is considerable heterogeneity in serum gonadotropin profiles in acutely ill patients. The pathophysiology of reproductive dysfunction that accompanies the course of acute illness is unknown. Malnutrition, cytokines and other mediators and products of systemic inflammatory response, and drugs may all contribute to the suppression at multiple levels of the reproductive axis. Similarly, in many chronic illnesses such as that associated with the human immunodeficiency virus, end-stage renal disease, chronic obstructive lung disease and some types of cancer, there is a high frequency of hypothalamic amenorrhea, suppression of gonadotropins and low testosterone levels [281].

In addition to taking a history and excluding pregnancy, a thorough evaluation of individuals presenting with HA requires baseline studies of FSH, prolactin, estradiol and an MRI study of the hypothalamic–pituitary region to rule out other etiologies of amenorrhea. A progestin challenge test will usually result in scant or no menstrual bleeding; however, addition of combined estrogen with progestin will result in endometrial growth followed by menses because the uterine compartment remains functionally normal [275,276].

Numerous neurotransmitters and neuromodulators modulate GnRH pulsatile secretion. These substances are released in the cerebral cortex, suprahypothalamic centers and hypothalamus. Most of them, for example neuropeptide Y (NPY), corticotropin-releasing hormone (CRH), leptin, ghrelin and β-endorphin, act directly on the GnRH pulse generator as well as on the appetite and food intake center [275,276].

It has been hypothesized that maintenance of normal reproductive function in women requires a minimum fat to body mass ratio. The circulating leptin level is a gauge for energy reserves and directs the central nervous system to adjust food intake and energy expenditure accordingly. Through leptin receptor-mediated pathways in the hypothalamus, leptin activates neural circuits involving an array of neuropeptides to control food intake and energy expenditure. In response to fasting, leptin levels decrease rapidly before and out of proportion to any changes in fat mass, and reproductive hormone levels decrease. Women with anorexia nervosa and exercise-induced hypothalamic amenorrhea are chronically energy-deprived and these conditions are associated with low circulating levels of leptin. Leptin treatment in replacement doses in women with hypothalamic amenorrhea improves or fully normalizes gonadal function and restores ovulatory menstruation [195,282].

Kisspeptin is emerging as an important player in mediating the reproductive effects of leptin. Leptin receptors have been found in kisspeptin neurons in the arcuate nucleus of rodents. Compared with wild-type mice, leptin-deficient *ob/ob* male mice show decreased kisspeptin expression in the arcuate nucleus, which is restored by leptin treatment [129]. Fasting is associated with reduced kisspeptin expression, and central injections of kisspeptin reverse the fasting-induced inhibition of GnRH secretion [283]. The specific hypothalamic sites where leptin acts to stimulate KiSS-1 in this paradigm are not yet known. These studies are consistent with a model whereby leptin and perhaps other adiposity and satiety factors trigger production of kisspeptin and stimulation of GnRH release. It is tempting to speculate that reproductive deficits associated with leptin-deficient states may be attributable to diminished kisspeptin. Nevertheless, it is likely that additional peripheral and central regulators cooperate with leptin and kisspeptin for the integration of energy balance and reproductive function [284–286].

Whereas abnormalities of GnRH secretion and menstrual function are well documented in female athletes, similar reproductive abnormalities have not been widely reported in male athletes or men with nutritional deficits. Although it is possible that the signs and symptoms of androgen deficiency in men may be subtle and, therefore, remain undetected, clinically important hypogonadism does not appear to be common in male endurance athletes. Serum testosterone and LH concentrations are usually normal or low-normal in male endurance athletes [287]. Nonetheless, it would not be unexpected for similar perturbations in GnRH secretion to occur in men under conditions of stress, exercise and malnutrition, and it is likely that they are underdiagnosed.

Chronic Renal Failure and Gonadal Dysfunction

Hypogonadism is very common in patients with end-stage renal disease [288]. Abnormalities at multiple levels of the hypothalamic–pituitary–gonadal axis contribute to hypogonadism. Sperm concentrations and semen quality are usually depressed; steroidogenesis is also suppressed to varying degrees. Depression of libido and potency is common in uremic men, and menstrual irregularities and infertility are common in premenopausal women. Reproductive dysfunction in uremic patients is usually multifactorial in nature; atherosclerotic disease, neuropathy, malnutrition, chronic illness, hypertension, diabetes mellitus and drugs all contribute. Hypogonadism usually does not improve after initiation of dialysis. However, restoration of normal kidney function after transplantation will often, although not always, lead to improvement.

Hemochromatosis

This is an iron-storage disorder in which parenchymal iron deposition results in damage to a number of tissues especially liver, pancreas, heart and pituitary [289]. Hypogonadism and testicular atrophy are common in men with hemochromatosis. Both the pituitary and the testis can be involved by excessive iron deposition. However, the pituitary defect is the predominant lesion in a majority of patients with hemochromatosis and hypogonadism. Thus, hypogonadotropic hypogonadism is by far the more common defect. Diagnosis of hemochromatosis is suggested by the association of diabetes mellitus, hepatic enlargement, heart disease, characteristic skin pigmentation, arthritis and hypogonadism. Excessive parenchymal iron stores can be demonstrated by determination of high transferrin saturation, very high serum ferritin concentrations, high chelatable iron stores using the agent desferrioxamine and liver biopsy.

Hyperprolactinemia and Hypogonadotropism

Elevated levels of prolactin are often associated with suppression of LH and FSH secretion, resulting in menstrual cycle dysfunction and amenorrhea in women and reduced testosterone levels in men [290,291]. In fact, the clinical presentations of a small prolactinoma may be primarily related to the associated hypogonadotropic hypogonadism. Gonadotropin deficiency in hyperprolactinemic disorders may result from one or more mechanisms. Prolactin can inhibit hypothalamic GnRH secretion either directly or through modulation of tuberoinfundibular dopaminergic pathways [292]. Second, a prolactin-secreting tumor may destroy the surrounding gonadotrophs in the pituitary gland by direct invasion, compression, or interference with vascular supply. Third, a pituitary tumor may cause compression of the pituitary infundibulum resulting both in hyperprolactinemia through interference with hypothalamic dopamine delivery to lactotropes and in hypogonadotropism through interference with GnRH delivery to gonadotropes. The function of the HPG axis is typically restored to normal after normalization of serum prolactin levels.

Space-occupying Lesions

Neoplastic and non-neoplastic lesions in the region of the hypothalamus and pituitary can directly or indirectly affect gonadotrope function. Lesions involving the hypothalamus or the hypothalamic–pituitary connection may arise primarily in the hypothalamus, in the suprasellar structures, or within the sella itself and extend upwards.

Pituitary tumors are discussed elsewhere in this book. In the adult human, pituitary adenomas constitute the largest single category of space-occupying lesions affecting gonadotrope function.

Hypothalamic Syndromes

The tumors in the suprasellar region that affect hypothalamic function can often be distinguished from those localized within the sella by the presence or absence of several unique clinical features.

1. Diabetes insipidus is distinctly unusual with lesions contained within the sella turcica. Its presence usually indicates a suprasellar lesion affecting the hypothalamic arginine vasopressin (AVP)-secreting nuclei in the preoptic and paraventricular region, or compressing the hypothalamic–pituitary stalk connection. The association of diabetes insipidus in patients with pituitary adenomas is usually indicative of suprasellar extension.
2. Visual field deficits indicate a suprasellar location. Pituitary adenomas can extend suprasellarly and compress the optic chiasm from below, resulting initially in superior temporal field defects. However, depending upon the origin and location of the suprasellar mass, a variety of visual field defects can result.

3. The presence of neurologic and/or neuropsychiatric syndromes should also alert the physician to the possibility of hypothalamic lesions.
4. Thermoregulatory and sleep defects also favor hypothalamic lesions.
5. Autonomic dysregulation characterized by extreme perspiration, sinus tachycardia and low blood pressure are seen only in hypothalamic lesions.
6. Disturbances of appetite and energy homeostasis favor hypothalamic involvement.

Lesions in different regions of the hypothalamus may also present some unique clinical features that can assist in anatomic and functional localization. For examples, lesions in or around the median eminence and ventromedial area, or those resulting in stalk compression, often lead to panhypopituitarism, hyperprolactinemia and diabetes insipidus. Lesions of the lateral hypothalamus may present with anorexia and weight loss, perhaps related to destruction of the feeding center. Lesions of the ventromedial area lead to hyperphagia and obesity. Lesions of the caudal hypothalamus may cause sexual precocity. The neoplastic lesions may also compress or erode a number of contiguous structures so that the clinical picture is often more complex.

TABLE 7.5 Disorders Characterized by Excessive or Physiologically Inappropriate Gonadotropin Secretion

EXCESSIVE GONADOTROPIN PRODUCTION
Gonadotropin-secreting adenomas
Ectopic hCG secretion
Ectopic LH or FSH secretion
Polycystic ovarian syndrome
PREMATURE GONADOTROPIN SECRETION
Idiopathic precocious puberty
Constitutional sexual precocity
Mutations in *KISS1*
Mutations in *KISS1R*
Hypothalamic hamartoma
Central nervous system tumors
Other central nervous system lesions such as hydrocephalus, granulomas, cysts, head trauma
True sexual precocity in children with congenital adrenal hyperplasia or androgen-secreting tumors
Miscellaneous
McCune-Albright syndrome

Hypergonadotropic Disorders: Excessive or Nonphysiologic Secretion of Gonadotropins

Physiologically inappropriate secretion of gonadotropins may occur in several clinical disorders (Table 7.5). Autonomous secretion of LH, FSH and/or free α-subunit may characterize pituitary gonadotrope adenomas (see Chapter 18). Ectopic LH and FSH secretion is uncommon but does occur [293]. Premature reactivation of the hypothalamic–pituitary–gonadal axis because of premature GnRH secretion can present with the clinical syndrome of precocious puberty.

Ectopic Gonadotropin Secretion

Ectopic production of hCG has been described from a number of neoplasms of trophoblastic and nontrophoblastic origin [294]. These neoplasms include malignant melanoma, adrenocortical carcinoma, breast cancer, renal carcinoma, lung cancer, pancreas, stomach and colon cancer, and a variety of teratocarcinomas [573–575]. Some carcinomas appear to glycosylate this protein resulting in detectable blood levels and biologic activity (due to retarded clearance).

Ectopic LH- and FSH-secreting tumors are exceedingly rare, likely reflecting the need for highly tissue-specific factors for the transcription of the subunit genes, together with the need for subunit glycosylation and heterodimerization for functional activity. A patient with a neuroendocrine thoracic carcinoid secreting functional FSH, presenting with symptoms of relapsing ovarian hyperstimulation syndrome, was recently reported [293]. A few cases of ectopic LH secretion in association with pancreatic tumors, adrenocortical tumors, or urogenital tumors have been described, presenting with hyperandrogenism and elevated serum androgen and LH levels leading to hyperthecosis and luteinized granulosa-thecal cell tumors of the ovaries [293,295,296].

Precocious Gonadotropin-dependent Puberty

Puberty results when pulsatile secretion of gonadotropin-releasing hormone (GnRH) is reinitiated and the hypothalamo–pituitary–gonadal axis is activated. The onset of puberty is marked by breast development in girls (Tanner stage 2 breast development, best assessed by both inspection and palpation) and testicular enlargement in boys (Tanner stage 2 genital development, assessed as testicular volume greater than 4 ml or testicular length greater than 25 mm) [297]. Pubertal onset is considered precocious if a boy develops secondary sex characteristics before the age of 9 years, or a girl before the age of 8 years [297]. True or central sexual precocity is gonadotropin-dependent and results from premature activation of GnRH secretion. The prevalence of central precocious puberty (CPP) is about ten times higher in girls than in boys [298]. In many such patients, no definable cause can be found and the condition is referred to as idiopathic CPP. The timing of the onset of puberty is normally distributed; consequently, some children who are quite normal will start pubertal development at an earlier age simply due to the nature of the Gaussian curve. There may be a familial predisposition towards earlier onset of puberty in some patients.

Genetic factors play a fundamental role in the timing of pubertal onset, as illustrated by the similar age at menarche among members of an ethnic group and in mother–daughter, monozygotic-twin and sibling pairs [299]. A 27.5% prevalence of familial central precocious puberty has been reported; segregation analysis in these families suggested autosomal dominant transmission with incomplete sex-dependent penetrance [300]. These studies support a genetic contribution to CPP. Indeed, an autosomal dominant *KISS1R* mutation was identified in a girl with idiopathic CPP. In vitro studies showed that the mutant receptor leads to prolonged activation of intracellular signaling pathways in response to kisspeptin [131]. Furthermore, two *KISS1* mutations were identified in unrelated patients with idiopathic CPP, one of which was shown to result in higher kisspeptin resistance to degradation in comparison with wild-type kisspeptin, suggesting a role for this mutation in the precocious puberty phenotype [132].

Several tumors, mostly intracranial, can cause precocious sexual development [297]. Central nervous system tumors, both benign and malignant, are found more often in boys than in girls. Although hypothalamic hamartomas have been shown to express GnRH, the expression of GnRH did not differ between hamartomas associated and not associated with CPP. The majority of these tumors probably cause sexual precocity by removing inhibitory influences on the GnRH-secreting nuclei, resulting in their premature activation. Hypothalamic hamartomas associated with CPP were more likely to contact the infundibulum or tuber cinereum and were larger than hamartomas not associated with CPP. Thus, anatomic features rather than expression patterns of candidate molecules seem to distinguish hypothalamic hamartomas that are associated with CPP from those that are not [301]. Astrocytomas, ependymomas and gliomas of the optic nerve or hypothalamus have all been reported in association with central sexual precocity. The availability of computed tomography (CT) and magnetic resonance imaging (MRI) scanning has made it easier to diagnose CNS tumors. Some germinomas secrete hCG and may result in premature androgen production; others are associated with premature gonadotropin secretion and true sexual precocity. Besides intracranial tumors, a variety of other intracranial lesions can cause sexual precocity. These include granulomas, suprasellar cysts, hydrocephalus and head trauma.

In some patients with congenital adrenal hyperplasia who have premature virilization due to excessive androgen production by the adrenal gland, institution of glucocorticoid therapy may trigger the onset of true gonadotropin-dependent sexual precocity [302]. Similar events may occur in children with virilizing tumors after removal of the tumor.

Patients with McCune-Albright syndrome (cafe-au-lait spots, fibrous dysplasia of bones and sexual precocity) often have autonomously functioning follicular cysts in the ovary, which may produce estrogens. However, some children with this syndrome have true gonadotropin-dependent sexual precocity.

Activating Mutations of LH and FSH Receptor Genes

Activating Mutations of the LH Receptor

Activating or gain-of-function mutations of the LHR are associated with gonadotropin-independent sexual precocity in boys, but do not produce a discernible phenotype in females [303]. This is referred to as familial male-limited precocious puberty, also called testotoxicosis, and is an autosomal-dominant disease caused by constitutive activating mutations in the human LHR (Figure 7.8A). The disease generally presents at around 2–4 years of age with signs of pubertal onset, accelerated virilization and excessive growth velocity ultimately leading to short stature in adulthood due to precocious closure of the epiphyses. Testosterone levels are high despite low levels of basal gonadotropins and a prepubertal response to the exogenous GnRH stimulation test. Treatment consists of drugs that block adrenal and testicular synthesis of androgens (ketoconazole) and/or androgenic receptor blockage (cyproterone acetate), estrogen receptor blockers and aromatase inhibitors [304]. Most activating mutations are situated in the cytoplasmic halves of the transmembrane segments or in the third intracellular loop, and may involve increased or activating interactions with the Gs protein [35]. Activating LH receptor mutations appear to have no phenotype in the female, which may be explained by the absence of LHR expression in prepubertal girls [35].

Activating Mutations of FSH Receptor

The first case of an activating mutation of the FSHR was reported in a male patient who was hypophysectomized because of a pituitary tumor and continued to have normal spermatogenesis despite undetectable serum levels of gonadotropins [35,305]. The mutation was able to cause ligand-independent constitutive activation of FSHR in vitro. In transgenic mice expressing this mutant FSHR, the constitutive activation of the receptor could completely compensate for the absence of FSH, with normal spermatogenesis and normal fertility (Figure 7.8B) [306].

Subsequent changes in the FSHR were identified in women in association with ovarian hyperstimulation syndrome (OHSS) [307–309]. OHSS is a common complication of IVF, appearing after administration of exogenous FSH followed by hCG administration in the presence of high estradiol levels. Spontaneous OHSS, appearing in the absence of exogenous hormonal stimulation of follicular growth, is rare, but can occur due to the presence of elevated circulating endogenous hCG or TSH levels (mimicking FSH action on granulosa cells); for example, in case of a hydatiform mole, spontaneous multiple pregnancy, or hypothyroidism. Isolated cases of spontaneous OHSS have been described in women with FSHR variants having an increased sensitivity to normal TSH and/or hCG levels. These mutations confer to the receptor the ability to respond to hCG or TSH because of a conformational change that leads to a loss of specificity. As a result, these mutations increase the risk for OHSS during IVF therapy and predispose to spontaneous OHSS in women during pregnancy or in women with hypothyroidism (Figure 7.19) [307–309].

Polycystic Ovarian Syndrome

Polycystic ovarian syndrome (PCOS) can be considered a disorder of gonadotropin excess resulting from a state of increased GnRH secretion with an increased GnRH pulse frequency. Patients with PCOS have elevated serum concentrations of LH with normal or low FSH. The high LH/FSH ratio may contribute to defective ovulation by causing a cycle initiation defect, since a relative deficiency of FSH during the follicular phase is associated with impaired follicle maturation and inadequate luteinization. The high mean LH concentrations are due to an increase in LH pulse frequency and/or pulse amplitude, reflecting the increase in pusatile secretion of hypothalamic GnRH [310].

PCOS is one of the most common endocrine disorders in reproductive-age women, affecting 7–10% of premenopausal women. PCOS is characterized by hyperandrogenism, and oligo- or amenorrhea, classically with a peripubertal onset. The ovaries typically appear polycystic on ultrasound. The syndrome is often associated with obesity, insulin resistance and metabolic syndrome [311]. Women with PCOS are at increased risk for obesity, insulin resistance, type 2 diabetes and cardiovascular disease.

The pathophysiologic basis of PCOS is unknown. Increased LH pulsatility and reduced FSH levels lead to increased androgen production and anovulation. Hyperandrogenemia and impaired luteinization, in turn, impair hypothalamic sensitivity to progesterone and prevent the slowing of GnRH pulses [312]. An increase in LH pulsatility has been observed in girls by late puberty [313]. Whereas LH regulates androgen synthesis by theca cells, FSH regulates aromatase activity in granulosa cells. When the concentration of LH increases relative to FSH, the ovaries preferentially synthesize androgen [310]. Furthermore, it has been demonstrated that insulin stimulates ovarian synthesis of androgens. Insulin acts synergistically with LH in stimulating ovarian androgen production and also upregulates LH receptors, thus increasing ovarian responsiveness to circulating LH. Insulin also inhibits hepatic synthesis of sex-hormone-binding globulin (SHBG), the key circulating protein that binds to testosterone, and thereby increases the proportion of testosterone that circulates in the unbound, biologically available state (Figure 7.20) [310].

Both PCOS and the accompanying insulin resistance appear to have major genetic components. There is evidence for familial aggregation of PCOS that is consistent with a genetic contribution to the disease. However, to date, there is no consensus regarding any proposed PCOS candidate gene, despite the publication of numerous association studies. Many findings have not been replicated or confirmed in follow-up studies. The most promising candidate so far has been a PCOS candidate region surrounding D19S884, a microsatellite marker in intron 55 of fibrillin 3 (*FBN3*), located on chromosome 19p13.2 about 800 kb centromeric to the insulin receptor (*INSR*) gene. Fibrillin 3 is an extracellular matrix protein, and is expressed in the human ovary. Other members of the fibrillin family of proteins are known to bind members of the TGFβ family, which play significant roles in controlling ovarian follicular development as well as muscle and adipocyte development and differentiation, all processes that can be impaired in PCOS [314]. It is likely that PCOS is a complex multigenic disorder.

Obesity alone, without PCOS, impacts on reproductive function. Excess body fat has been associated with an increased risk of oligo- or anovulation. Obesity is associated with an increased risk of hyperandrogenism and anovulatory cycles in women. In men with mild to moderate obesity, alterations in total testosterone levels are due to reduction in testicular testosterone production, exacerbated by changes in circulating levels of sex-hormone-binding globulin (SHBG). Because SHBG levels decrease in inverse proportion to the degree of obesity, serum total testosterone levels decrease as body weight increases. The decrease in SHBG levels in obese men is believed to be due, in part, to the increase in circulating insulin concentrations that attend weight gain. Insulin is an inhibitor of SBHG production and plasma insulin levels correlate inversely with SHBG levels [315].

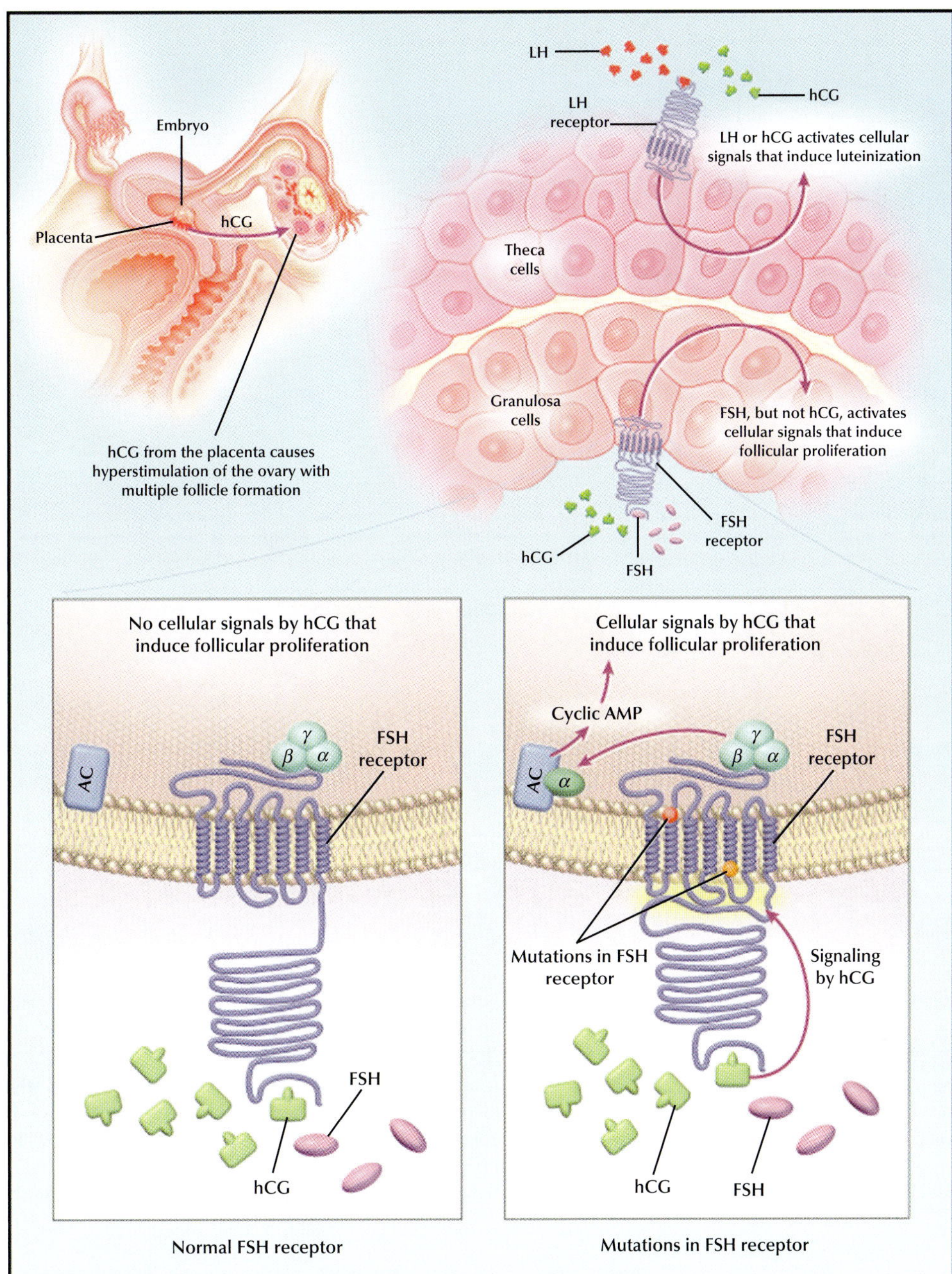

FIGURE 7.19 Pathogenesis of familial gestational spontaneous ovarian hyperstimulation syndrome. hCG synthesized by the syncytiotrophoblast cells of the developing placenta in pregnancy circulates to act at the level of the ovary. In a normal pregnancy, its activity is limited to LH receptors. Stimulation of LH receptors in the corpus luteum results in continued progesterone production to allow the maintenance of pregnancy. Either of two mutations (depicted in red and orange) in the FSH receptor allow activation of downstream signaling events by hCG (modeled as a change in the conformation of the mutant FSH receptor, so that the low-affinity binding of hCG to the receptor ectodomain leads to activation of the serpentine domain). This conformational change results in the stimulation of FSH receptors by hCG in the granulosa cells of developing follicles, leading in turn to excessive follicular recruitment and enlargement. AC, adenylyl cyclase; α, β and γ, G-protein subunits. *From Kaiser [307].*

TREATMENT OF HYPOGONADOTROPIC DISORDERS

When a neoplasm or other mass lesion is responsible for hypogonadotropic hypogonadism, therapy should be directed at the underlying cause when possible, to evoke a cure. In many instances of macroadenomas, cure by resection is not possible and adjunct treatment directed at shrinking the tumor and lowering hormone secretion is desirable. If

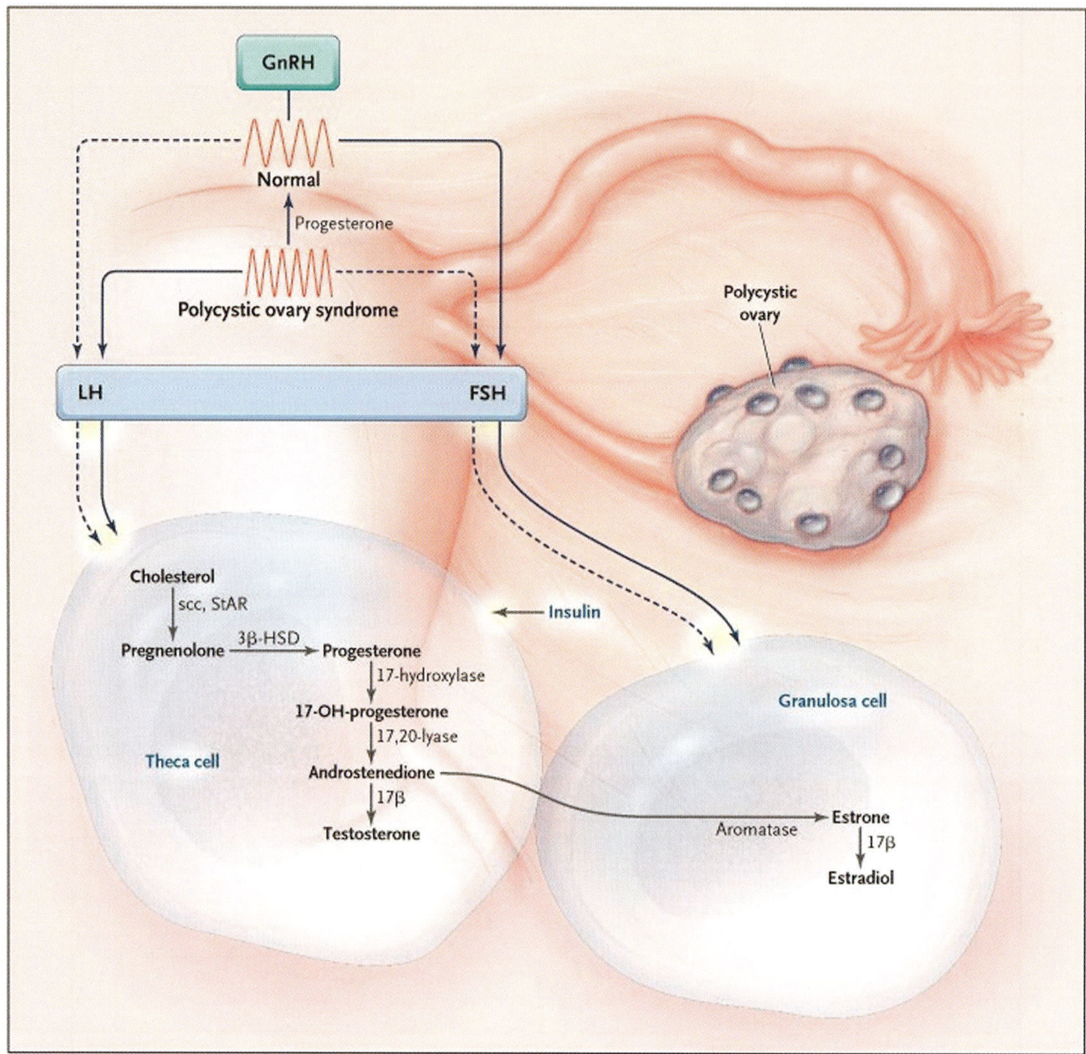

FIGURE 7.20 The hypothalamic–pituitary–ovarian axis and the role of insulin. Increased ovarian androgen biosynthesis in PCOS results from abnormalities at all levels of the hypothalamic–pituitary–ovarian axis. The increased frequency of GnRH pulses leads to increased frequency of LH pulses, favoring the production of LH over FSH. The relative increase in LH leads to an increase in ovarian theca cell androgen production. Insulin acts synergistically with LH to enhance androgen production. Scc, side-chain cleavage enzyme; StAR, steroidogenic acute regulatory protein; 3β-HSD, 3β-hydroxysteroid dehydrogenase. Solid arrows denote a higher degree of stimulation than dashed arrows. *From Ehrmann [310].*

gonadotropins are normalized, the resultant hypogonadism is usually corrected.

The goals of therapy are to induce and maintain normal reproductive function, gonadal sex steroid hormone production and stimulation of gametogenesis in those desiring fertility. If fertility is not an immediate objective, sex steroid hormone replacement is usually sufficient. For induction of spermatogenesis, therapy with gonadotropins or GnRH is usually required.

Gonadotropin Treatment of Hypogonadotropic Hypogonadism

hCG and human menopausal gonadotropin (hMG) preparations have been commercially available for four decades. hCG is purified from the urine of pregnant women, being secreted primarily by the human placenta during pregnancy. hMG is derived from the urine of postmenopausal women. While hCG primarily interacts with LH/hCG receptors, hMG contains LH and FSH activities in almost equal proportions. Since their introduction into clinical practice in 1961, gonadotropins extracted from the urine of postmenopausal women have played a central role in ovulation induction therapy. This initially crude preparation was refined to make available purified urinary FSH. Since 1996, recombinant human FSH (rhFSH), expressed in Chinese hamster ovary cell lines and purified to homogeneity, has been available, and recombinant hCG (rhCG) is also available [316].

For ovulation induction, rhFSH is administered subcutaneously starting on day 3 of spontaneous or induced uterine withdrawal bleeding. Doses are increased incrementally until serum estradiol concentrations begin to increase, reflecting induction of follicle maturation. The dose is then maintained and the ovarian response to gonadotropin therapy is monitored by measuring serum estradiol levels and using transvaginal ultrasonography to measure follicular diameter. Criteria for follicle maturity include a follicle diameter of 18 mm and/or a serum estradiol concentration of 200 pg/mL per dominant follicle. Complications of ovulation induction therapy with gonadotropins include multiple pregnancies, OHSS and increased spontaneous miscarriage rates. Multiple pregnancy and OHSS rates can be kept to a minimum by using lower doses of rhFSH. If more than two follicles larger than 15 mm are present, stimulation should be stopped to prevent multiple pregnancies and OHSS. Once a dominant follicle is identified, follicle rupture is induced by either urinary or recombinant hCG administration [1].

For induction of spermatogenesis in men with hypogonadotropic hypogonadism, the traditional approach is the administration of hCG to induce full steroidogenesis from Leydig cells and hMG or rhFSH to induce spermatogenesis [317]. A variety of treatment regimens have been used and there is no consensus on what constitutes the optimum dose and schedule of gonadotropin administration. Published data and empiric clinical experience indicate that a dose of 1500–2000 IU given intramuscularly three times weekly is a reasonable starting dose [318]. Doses are adjusted based on serum testosterone levels with the goal of achieving serum testosterone levels in the mid-normal range. Higher testosterone concentrations tend to be associated with more elevated serum estrogen concentrations and an increased incidence of gynecomastia. Sperm counts should be monitored on a monthly basis. It may take several months for spermatogenesis to be restored. If spermatogenesis is not restored after 6 months of therapy with hCG alone with serum testosterone levels in the mid-normal range, then it is recommended to add FSH. Men with initial testes of less than 5 ml almost always require the addition of FSH, whereas spermatogenesis often can be induced with hCG alone in men with larger testicular volumes. FSH doses are guided by testicular size and seminal fuid analysis. It may occasionally take 18–24 months or longer for spermatogenesis to be restored.

Pulsatile GnRH Therapy

Pioneering studies by Knobil's group had predicted that pulsatile administration of GnRH would be required to maintain normal LH and FSH output from the pituitary. As discussed earlier in this chapter, continuous infusion of GnRH in monkeys made hypogonadotropic by radiofrequency lesions of the hypothalamic GnRH-secreting nuclei, down-regulates LH and FSH secretion [118,159].

Pulsatile administration of exogenous GnRH using an infusion pump is an effective therapy for the stimulation of endogenous LH and FSH secretion, follicle development and ovulation in women with GnRH deficiency [319]. The resulting serum FSH and LH concentrations remain within the normal range and the chances of multiple pregnancies and OHSS are therefore low. However, success of GnRH therapy assumes normal pituitary and gonadal function. A pulse interval is 60–90 minutes and a dose of 2.5–10 μg per pulse is typically used, using the lowest dose required to induce ovulation to minimize the likelihood of multiple pregnancies. The agonist analogues of GnRH are not useful for restoring gonadotropin secretion, because after an initial short-lived stimulatory phase, GnRH agonists down-regulate pituitary LH and FSH output [320].

Successful induction of puberty by pulsatile administration of low doses of GnRH has been achieved in boys with Kallmann syndrome or IHH [321,322]. Therapy is usually started with an initial dose of 25 ng/kg per pulse administered subcutaneously every 2 hours by a portable infusion pump. Serum testosterone, LH and FSH levels are monitored, and the dose of GnRH is progressively increased until serum testosterone levels in the mid-normal range are reached. There is considerable variability in GnRH dose requirements and doses ranging from 25 to 200 ng/kg may be required to induce virilization. Once pubertal changes have been initiated, the dose of GnRH can often be reduced without adverse effects on serum testosterone, LH and FSH levels. Development of anti-GnRH antibodies is an uncommon occurrence, but can be a cause of treatment failure. Treatment failure can also occur in patients with pituitary disease as their etiology of the hypogonadotropic hypogonadism. Pulsatile GnRH therapy is an effective but currently unapproved treatment for GnRH-deficient men seeking fertility and is used primarily in research studies. While induction of virilization by pulsatile GnRH administration in patients with IHH has provided important insights into the mechanisms of puberty and regulation of gonadotropin secretion by GnRH, this approach has no particular advantage over the traditional gonadotropin therapy [318]. In fact, wearing a portable infusion device can be quite cumbersome and follow-up of these patients often requires considerable physician supervision and laboratory monitoring. GnRH is currently not commercially available.

GnRH Analogues

A large number of GnRH analogues are currently available for therapeutic use [632,636]. The primary structure of GnRH was determined in 1971. The half life of GnRH is very short (2–4 minutes) as it is degraded rapidly by peptidases in the hypothalamus and pituitary. These peptidases cleave bonds between amino acids 5 and 6, 6 and 7, and 9 and 10. Analogues have been synthesized by changing the amino acids at these positions. Over 2000 synthetic analogues have been synthesized and tested, which can be broadly divided into two classes: GnRH agonist analogues and GnRH antagonist analogues. Agonist analogues bind to the GnRH receptors and initiate the same series of post-receptor events that underlie LH release by native GnRH. However, chronic administration of GnRH agonists leads to paradoxical decrease in LH and FSH secretion and inhibition of gonadal function, a phenomenon referred to as desensitization or down-regulation. The antagonist analogues of GnRH, on the other hand, bind to GnRH receptors and block the action of GnRH. The antagonist analogues thus have no intrinsic ability to trigger the post-receptor events usually attributable to GnRH.

GnRH Agonists

Comparison of the amino acid sequences of GnRH across species reveals a remarkable conservation in the N-terminus (pGlu-His-Trp-Ser) and C-terminus (Pro-Gly-NH_2), supporting an important role for these residues in receptor binding and activation. The Arg at position 8 is critical for binding, and substitutions at this position result in loss of binding affinity. Several key aspects of the structure–activity relationships are important in the design of GnRH agonists [323,324]. Replacement of the Gly residue at position 6 with D-alanine increases the potency and also increases the peptide stability. Replacement of the C-terminal glycinamide residue by an ethylamide group is a key modification that has formed the basis of many subsequent structural modifications, increasing receptor binding affinity and also prolonging the duration of action. When these two modifications are combined the biological potency of the resulting compound is further amplified. GnRH agonists can be administered subcutaneously, intranasally, or intramuscularly. These compounds have an initial agonistic response with an increase in circulating levels of LH and FSH, followed by desensitization and down-regulation to produce hypogonadotropic hypogonadism, due to desensitization and uncoupling of the receptor from its signaling pathways and down-regulation of receptors on the plasma membrane, as well as post-receptor events [323].

The wide clinical applicability of GnRH agonists has spurred development and testing of a large number of agonist analogues by the pharmaceutical industry and the Contraceptive Development Branch of the NICHD. GnRH agonists have been found to be effective therapeutic agents in many sex steroid- (androgen or estrogen)-dependent clinical disorders [325]. Their lack of systemic toxicity has been striking. Most side effects have been related to the decrease in androgens or estrogens due to the desired down-regulation of gonadotropin secretion. The main pharmacologic difference among the currently approved GnRH agonists is the method of administration. Leuprolide is the most commonly used GnRH agonist and can be administered as a daily subcutaneous injection or as a monthly depot injection. Osmotic pump implants are also available that deliver leuprolide acetate at a controlled rate for up to 12 months. Long-acting agonists are utilized therapeutically to suppress gonadotropins in several conditions, including endometriosis, uterine fibroids, central gonadotropin-dependent precocious puberty [297] and androgen-dependent prostate cancer. Their main drawback is that gonadotropin suppression does not occur immediately; instead, there is a transient (several days) increase ("flare") in sex hormone levels, followed by a lasting suppression of hormone synthesis and secretion.

GnRH Antagonists

More recently, several antagonist analogues of GnRH have become available; these have several advantages over the agonist analogues. Antagonist analogues are far more potent in inhibiting gonadotropin secretion in men and experimental animals than agonist analogues. In addition, the antagonist analogues have the potential advantage of rapid onset of inhibitory action and do not have the initial stimulatory effects that characterize GnRH agonists. Changes in the conserved N-terminal residues of GnRH result in analogues with antagonistic properties. This modification, together with the substitution of the Gly at position 6 with a D-amino acid, forms the basis of all antagonists [323,326].

The GnRH antagonists cetrorelix and ganirelix are sometimes used in assisted reproduction; in the early to mid-follicular phase of the menstrual cycle they suppress an early surge in LH, resulting in improved rates of implantation and pregnancy. GnRH antagonists also have applications for palliation of metastatic prostate cancer. In this situation, a direct GnRH antagonist has the advantage of avoiding the initial surge in testosterone seen with GnRH agonists [326].

Acknowledgments

I acknowledge Drs Shalendar Bhasin, Charles Fisher and Ronald Swerdloff, the authors of the corresponding chapter in the previous edition of this textbook, for the use of some of the material in this chapter.

References

[1] K.H. Burns, M.M. Matzuk, Minireview: Genetic models for the study of gonadotropin actions, Endocrinology 143 (8) (2002) 2823–2835.

[2] S.D. Gharib, M.E. Wierman, M.A. Shupnik, W.W. Chin, Molecular biology of the pituitary gonadotropins, Endocr Rev 11 (1) (1990) 177–199.

[3] V.G. Thackray, P.L. Mellon, D. Coss, Hormones in synergy: Regulation of the pituitary gonadotropin genes, Mol Cell Endocrinol 314 (2) (2010) 192–203.

[4] G.V. Childs, Cytochemical studies of multifunctional gonadotropes, Microsc Res Tech 39 (2) (1997) 114–130.

[5] K. Kovacs, E. Horvath, Morphology of adenohypophyseal cells and pituitary adenomas, in: L. Martini (Ed.), The Pituitary Gland, Raven Press, New York, 1985, pp. 25–56.

[6] G.C. Moriarty, Adenohypophysis: Ultrastructural cytochemistry. A review, J Histochem Cytochem 21 (10) (1973) 855–894.

[7] G.V. Childs, G.U. D.G. E, Functional differentiation of gonadotropes and thyrotropes, in: W.W. Chin, I. Boime (Eds.), Glycoprotein Hormones, Serono Symposia, Norwell, 1990, pp. 1–10.

[8] G.C. Moriarty, Immunocytochemistry of the pituitary glycoprotein hormones, J Histochem Cytochem 24 (7) (1976) 846–863.

[9] X. Zhu, C.R. Lin, G.G. Prefontaine, J. Tollkuhn, M.G. Rosenfeld, Genetic control of pituitary development and hypopituitarism, Curr Opin Genet Dev 15 (3) (2005) 332–340.

[10] X. Zhu, J. Wang, B.G. Ju, M.G. Rosenfeld, Signaling and epigenetic regulation of pituitary development, Curr Opin Cell Biol 19 (6) (2007) 605–611.

[11] J.C. Achermann, J. Weiss, E.J. Lee, J.L. Jameson, Inherited disorders of the gonadotropin hormones, Mol Cell Endocrinol 179 (1–2) (2001) 89–96.

[12] K.S. Alatzoglou, M.T. Dattani, Genetic forms of hypopituitarism and their manifestation in the neonatal period, Early Hum Dev 85 (11) (2009) 705–712.

[13] M.T. Dattani, J.P. Martinez-Barbera, P.Q. Thomas, J.M. Brickman, R. Gupta, I.L. Martensson, et al., Mutations in the homeobox gene HESX1/Hesx1 associated with septo-optic dysplasia in human and mouse, Nat Genet 19 (2) (1998) 125–133.

[14] M.H. Quentien, A. Barlier, J.L. Franc, I. Pellegrini, T. Brue, A. Enjalbert, Pituitary transcription factors: From congenital deficiencies to gene therapy, J Neuroendocrinol 18 (9) (2006) 633–642.

[15] J.J. Tremblay, C. Lanctot, J. Drouin, The pan-pituitary activator of transcription, Ptx1 (pituitary homeobox 1), acts in synergy with SF-1 and Pit1 and is an upstream regulator of the Lim-homeodomain gene Lim3/Lhx3, Mol Endocrinol 12 (3) (1998) 428–441.

[16] H. Suh, P.J. Gage, J. Drouin, S.A. Camper, Pitx2 is required at multiple stages of pituitary organogenesis: Pituitary primordium formation and cell specification, Development 129 (2) (2002) 329–337.

[17] I. Saadi, A. Kuburas, J.J. Engle, A.F. Russo, Dominant negative dimerization of a mutant homeodomain protein in Axenfeld-Rieger syndrome, Mol Cell Biol 23 (6) (2003) 1968–1982.

[18] R.D. Mullen, S.C. Colvin, C.S. Hunter, J.J. Savage, E.C. Walvoord, A.P. Bhangoo, et al., Roles of the LHX3 and LHX4 LIM-homeodomain factors in pituitary development, Mol Cell Endocrinol 265-266 (2007) 190–195.

[19] S. Mody, M.R. Brown, J.S. Parks, The spectrum of hypopituitarism caused by PROP1 mutations, Best Pract Res Clin Endocrinol Metab 16 (3) (2002) 421–431.

[20] M.W. Sornson, W. Wu, J.S. Dasen, S.E. Flynn, D.J. Norman, S.M. O'Connell, et al., Pituitary lineage determination by the Prophet of Pit-1 homeodomain factor defective in Ames dwarfism, Nature 384 (6607) (1996) 327–333.

[21] B.P. Schimmer, P.C. White, Minireview: Steroidogenic Factor 1: Its roles in differentiation, development, and disease, Mol Endocrinol 24 (2010) 1322–1337.

[22] Y. Ikeda, X. Luo, R. Abbud, J.H. Nilson, K.L. Parker, The nuclear receptor steroidogenic factor 1 is essential for the formation of the ventromedial hypothalamic nucleus, Mol Endocrinol 9 (4) (1995) 478–486.

[23] B. Kohler, L. Lin, B. Ferraz-de-Souza, P. Wieacker, P. Heidemann, V. Schroder, et al., Five novel mutations in steroidogenic factor 1 (SF1, NR5A1) in 46,XY patients with severe underandrogenization but without adrenal insufficiency, Hum Mutat 29 (1) (2008) 59–64.

[24] J.C. Achermann, J.J. Meeks, J.L. Jameson, Phenotypic spectrum of mutations in DAX-1 and SF-1, Mol Cell Endocrinol 185 (1–2) (2001) 17–25.

[25] M.A. Charles, T.L. Saunders, W.M. Wood, K. Owens, A.F. Parlow, S.A. Camper, et al., Pituitary-specific Gata2 knockout: effects on gonadotrope and thyrotrope function, Mol Endocrinol 20 (6) (2006) 1366–1377.

[26] A.D. Goldberg, C.D. Allis, E. Bernstein, Epigenetics: A landscape takes shape, Cell 128 (4) (2007) 635–638.

[27] T. Kouzarides, Chromatin modifications and their function, Cell 128 (4) (2007) 693–705.

[28] Y. Shi, F. Lan, C. Matson, P. Mulligan, J.R. Whetstine, P.A. Cole, et al., Histone demethylation mediated by the nuclear amine oxidase homolog LSD1, Cell 119 (7) (2004) 941–953.

[29] J. Wang, K. Scully, X. Zhu, L. Cai, J. Zhang, G.G. Prefontaine, et al., Opposing LSD1 complexes function in developmental gene activation and repression programmes, Nature 446 (7138) (2007) 882–887.

[30] F.H. Gage, Mammalian neural stem cells, Science 287 (5457) (2000) 1433–1438.

[31] T.A. Rando, Stem cells, ageing and the quest for immortality, Nature 441 (7097) (2006) 1080–1086.

[32] H. Vankelecom, Stem cells in the postnatal pituitary? Neuroendocrinology 85 (2) (2007) 110–130.

[33] J.G. Pierce, T.F. Parsons, Glycoprotein hormones: Structure and function, Annu Rev Biochem 50 (1981) 465–495.

[34] F. Fares, The role of O-linked and N-linked oligosaccharides on the structure-function of glycoprotein hormones: Development of agonists and antagonists, Biochim Biophys Acta 1760 (4) (2006) 560–567.

[35] A.P.N. Themmen, I.T. Huhtaniemi, Mutations of gonadotropins and gonadotropin receptors: Elucidating the physiology and pathophysiology of pituitary-gonadal function, Endocr Rev 21 (5) (2000) 551–583.

[36] J.C. Fiddes, K. Talmadge, Structure, expression, and evolution of the genes for the human glycoprotein hormones, Recent Prog Horm Res 40 (1984) 43–78.

[37] J. Baenziger, The asparagine-linked oligosaccharides of the glycoprotein hormones, in: W.W. Chin, I. Boime (Eds.), Glycoprotein Hormones, Serono Symposia, Norwell, 1990, pp. 1–18.

[38] K. Talmadge, N.C. Vamvakopoulos, J.C. Fiddes, Evolution of the genes for the beta subunits of human chorionic gonadotropin and luteinizing hormone, Nature 307 (5946) (1984) 37–40.

[39] C. Albanese, I.M. Colin, W.F. Crowley, M. Ito, R.G. Pestell, J. Weiss, et al., The gonadotropin genes: Evolution of distinct mechanisms for hormonal control, Recent Prog Horm Res 51 (1996) 23–58 discussion 9–61.
[40] P.C. Watkins, R. Eddy, A.K. Beck, V. Vellucci, B. Leverone, R.E. Tanzi, et al., DNA sequence and regional assignment of the human follicle-stimulating hormone beta-subunit gene to the short arm of human chromosome 11, DNA 6 (3) (1987) 205–212.
[41] R. Kornfeld, S. Kornfeld, Comparative aspects of glycoprotein structure, Annu Rev Biochem 45 (1976) 217–237.
[42] C.J. Waechter, W.J. Lennarz, The role of polyprenol-linked sugars in glycoprotein synthesis, Annu Rev Biochem 45 (1976) 95–112.
[43] L.A. Hunt, J.R. Etchison, D.F. Summers, Oligosaccharide chains are trimmed during synthesis of the envelope glycoprotein of vesicular stomatitis virus, Proc Nat Acad Sci USA 75 (2) (1978) 754–758.
[44] L. Wide, K. Eriksson, P.M. Sluss, J.E. Hall, The common genetic variant of luteinizing hormone has a longer serum half-life than the wild type in heterozygous women, J Clin Endocrinol Metab 95 (1) (2010) 383–389.
[45] J.A. Clements, F.I. Reyes, J.S. Winter, C. Faiman, Ontogenesis of gonadotropin-releasing hormone in the human fetal hypothalamus, Proc Soc Exp Biol Med 163 (3) (1980) 437–444.
[46] M.M. Grumbach, A window of opportunity: The diagnosis of gonadotropin deficiency in the male infant, J Clin Endocrinol Metab 90 (5) (2005) 3122–3127.
[47] S.B. Seminara, F.J. Hayes, W.F. Crowley Jr., Gonadotropin-releasing hormone deficiency in the human (idiopathic hypogonadotropic hypogonadism and Kallmann's syndrome): Pathophysiological and genetic considerations, Endocr Rev 19 (5) (1998) 521–539.
[48] R.H. Castillo, R.L. Matteri, D.A. Dumesic, Luteinizing hormone synthesis in cultured fetal human pituitary cells exposed to gonadotropin-releasing hormone, J Clin Endocrinol Metab 75 (1) (1992) 318–322.
[49] P. Lee, Pubertal neuroendocrine maturation: Early differentiation and stages of development, Adolesc Pediatr Gynecol 1 (1988) 3–14.
[50] F. Brioude, J. Bouligand, S. Trabado, B. Francou, S. Salenave, P. Kamenicky, et al., Non-syndromic congenital hypogonadotropic hypogonadism: Clinical presentation and genotype-phenotype relationships, Eur J Endocrinol 162 (5) (2010) 835–851.
[51] M.M. Grumbach, The neuroendocrinology of human puberty revisited, Horm Res 57 (Suppl 2) (2002) 2–14.
[52] F.A. Conte, M.M. Grumbach, S.L. Kaplan, A diphasic pattern of gonadotropin secretion in patients with the syndrome of gonadal dysgenesis, J Clin Endocrinol Metab 40 (4) (1975) 670–674.
[53] T.M. Plant, Hypothalamic control of the pituitary–gonadal axis in higher primates: Key advances over the last two decades, J Neuroendocrinol 20 (6) (2008) 719–726.
[54] S.R. Ojeda, A. Lomniczi, C. Mastronardi, S. Heger, C. Roth, A.S. Parent, et al., Minireview: The neuroendocrine regulation of puberty: Is the time ripe for a systems biology approach? Endocrinology 147 (3) (2006) 1166–1174.
[55] E. Terasawa, D.L. Fernandez, Neurobiological mechanisms of the onset of puberty in primates, Endocr Rev 22 (1) (2001) 111–151.
[56] E.A. Resende, B.H. Lara, J.D. Reis, B.P. Ferreira, G.A. Pereira, M.F. Borges, Assessment of basal and gonadotropin-releasing hormone-stimulated gonadotropins by immunochemiluminometric and immunofluorometric assays in normal children, J Clin Endocrinol Metab 92 (4) (2007) 1424–1429.
[57] C.M. Cargille, G.T. Ross, T. Yoshimi, Daily variations in plasma follicle stimulating hormone, luteinizing hormone and progesterone in the normal menstrual cycle, J Clin Endocrinol Metab 29 (1) (1969) 12–19.
[58] G.S. diZerega, G.D. Hodgen, Folliculogenesis in the primate ovarian cycle, Endocr Rev 2 (1) (1981) 27–49.
[59] R. Tsutsumi, N.J. Webster, GnRH pulsatility, the pituitary response and reproductive dysfunction, Endocr J 56 (6) (2009) 729–737.
[60] M.M. Martin, S.M. Wu, A.L. Martin, O.M. Rennert, W.Y. Chan, Testicular seminoma in a patient with a constitutively activating mutation of the luteinizing hormone/chorionic gonadotropin receptor, Eur J Endocrinol 139 (1) (1998) 101–106.
[61] C. Stocco, C. Telleria, G. Gibori, The molecular control of corpus luteum formation, function, and regression, Endocr Rev 28 (1) (2007) 117–149.
[62] N. Reame, S.E. Sauder, R.P. Kelch, J.C. Marshall, Pulsatile gonadotropin secretion during the human menstrual cycle: evidence for altered frequency of gonadotropin-releasing hormone secretion, J Clin Endocrinol Metab 59 (2) (1984) 328–337.
[63] S.M. Harman, E.J. Metter, J.D. Tobin, J. Pearson, M.R. Blackman, Longitudinal effects of aging on serum total and free testosterone levels in healthy men. Baltimore Longitudinal Study of Aging, J Clin Endocrinol Metab 86 (2) (2001) 724–731.
[64] S. Bhasin, O.M. Calof, T.W. Storer, M.L. Lee, N.A. Mazer, R. Jasuja, et al., Drug insight: Testosterone and selective androgen receptor modulators as anabolic therapies for chronic illness and aging, Nat Clin Pract Endocrinol Metab 2 (3) (2006) 146–159.
[65] J.E. Hall, Neuroendocrine changes with reproductive aging in women, Semin Reprod Med 25 (5) (2007) 344–351.
[66] N. Santoro, The menopausal transition, Am J Med 118 (Suppl. 12B) (2005) 8–13.
[67] D.W. Brann, V.B. Mahesh, The aging reproductive neuroendocrine axis, Steroids 70 (4) (2005) 273–283.
[68] J.L. Downs, P.M. Wise, The role of the brain in female reproductive aging, Mol Cell Endocrinol 299 (1) (2009) 32–38.
[69] H.M. Dungan, D.K. Clifton, R.A. Steiner, Minireview: Kisspeptin neurons as central processors in the regulation of gonadotropin-releasing hormone secretion, Endocrinology 147 (3) (2006) 1154–1158.
[70] M.A. Lederman, D. Lebesgue, V.V. Gonzalez, J. Shu, Z.O. Merhi, A.M. Etgen, et al., Age-related LH surge dysfunction correlates with reduced responsiveness of hypothalamic anteroventral periventricular nucleus kisspeptin neurons to estradiol positive feedback in middle-aged rats, Neuropharmacology 58 (1) (2010) 314–320.
[71] G. Neal-Perry, D. Lebesgue, M. Lederman, J. Shu, G.D. Zeevalk, A.M. Etgen, The excitatory peptide kisspeptin restores the luteinizing hormone surge and modulates amino acid neurotransmission in the medial preoptic area of middle-aged rats, Endocrinology 150 (8) (2009) 3699–3708.
[72] W. Zheng, M. Jimenez-Linan, B.S. Rubin, L.M. Halvorson, Anterior pituitary gene expression with reproductive aging in the female rat, Biol Reprod 76 (6) (2007) 1091–1102.
[73] X. Wu, S. Wan, M.M. Lee, Key factors in the regulation of fetal and postnatal Leydig cell development, J Cell Physiol 213 (2) (2007) 429–433.
[74] T.M. Plant, G.R. Marshall, The functional significance of FSH in spermatogenesis and the control of its secretion in male primates, Endocr Rev 22 (6) (2001) 764–786.
[75] S.M. Ruwanpura, R.I. McLachlan, S.J. Meachem, Hormonal regulation of male germ cell development, J Endocrinol 205 (2) (2010) 117–131.

[76] J.S. Richards, S.A. Pangas, The ovary: Basic biology and clinical implications, J Clin Invest 120 (4) (2010) 963–972.
[77] N.S. Macklon, R.L. Stouffer, L.C. Giudice, B.C. Fauser, The science behind 25 years of ovarian stimulation for in vitro fertilization, Endocr Rev 27 (2) (2006) 170–207.
[78] B.J. Deroo, K.F. Rodriguez, J.F. Couse, K.J. Hamilton, J.B. Collins, S.F. Grissom, et al., Estrogen receptor beta is required for optimal cAMP production in mouse granulosa cells, Mol Endocrinol 23 (7) (2009) 955–965.
[79] M. Hunzicker-Dunn, E.T. Maizels, FSH signaling pathways in immature granulosa cells that regulate target gene expression: Branching out from protein kinase A, Cell Signal 18 (9) (2006) 1351–1359.
[80] M. Jamnongjit, S.R. Hammes, Ovarian steroids: the good, the bad, and the signals that raise them, Cell Cycle 5 (11) (2006) 1178–1183.
[81] M. Ascoli, D.L. Segaloff, On the structure of the luteinizing hormone/chorionic gonadotropin receptor, Endocr Rev 10 (1) (1989) 27–44.
[82] K.C. McFarland, R. Sprengel, H.S. Phillips, M. Kohler, N. Rosemblit, K. Nikolics, et al., Lutropin-choriogonadotropin receptor: An unusual member of the G protein-coupled receptor family, Science 245 (4917) (1989) 494–499.
[83] R. Sprengel, T. Braun, K. Nikolics, D.L. Segaloff, P.H. Seeburg, The testicular receptor for follicle stimulating hormone: Structure and functional expression of cloned cDNA, Mol Endocrinol 4 (4) (1990) 525–530.
[84] M. Parmentier, F. Libert, C. Maenhaut, A. Lefort, C. Gerard, J. Perret, et al., Molecular cloning of the thyrotropin receptor, Science 246 (4937) (1989) 1620–1622.
[85] B. Kobe, J. Deisenhofer, A structural basis of the interactions between leucine-rich repeats and protein ligands, Nature 374 (6518) (1995) 183–186.
[86] J.S. Richards, Maturation of ovarian follicles: Actions and interactions of pituitary and ovarian hormones on follicular cell differentiation, Physiol Rev 60 (1) (1980) 51–89.
[87] S. Bernichtein, H. Peltoketo, I. Huhtaniemi, Adrenal hyperplasia and tumours in mice in connection with aberrant pituitary–gonadal function, Mol Cell Endocrinol 300 (1–2) (2009) 164–168.
[88] J.E. Pabon, X. Li, Z.M. Lei, J.S. Sanfilippo, M.A. Yussman, C.V. Rao, Novel presence of luteinizing hormone/chorionic gonadotropin receptors in human adrenal glands, J Clin Endocrinol Metab 81 (6) (1996) 2397–2400.
[89] A. Lacroix, N. Ndiaye, J. Tremblay, P. Hamet, Ectopic and abnormal hormone receptors in adrenal Cushing's syndrome, Endocr Rev 22 (1) (2001) 75–110.
[90] W.D. Odell, A.F. Parlow, C.M. Cargille, G.T. Ross, Radioimmunoassay for human follicle-stimulating hormone: Physiological studies, J Clin Invest 47 (12) (1968) 2551–2562.
[91] W.D. Odell, G.T. Ross, P.L. Rayford, Radioimmunoassay for luteinizing hormone in human plasma or serum: Physiological studies, J Clin Invest 46 (2) (1967) 248–255.
[92] T. Jaakkola, Y.Q. Ding, P. Kellokumpu-Lehtinen, R. Valavaara, H. Martikainen, J. Tapanainen, et al., The ratios of serum bioactive/immunoreactive luteinizing hormone and follicle-stimulating hormone in various clinical conditions with increased and decreased gonadotropin secretion: Reevaluation by a highly sensitive immunometric assay, J Clin Endocrinol Metab 70 (6) (1990) 1496–1505.
[93] S. Bhasin, R.S. Swerdloff, Mechanisms of gonadotropin-releasing hormone agonist action in the human male, Endocr Rev 7 (1) (1986) 106–114.
[94] V. Kalia, A.N. Jadhav, K.K. Bhutani, Luteinizing hormone estimation, Endocr Res 30 (1) (2004) 1–17.
[95] M.L. Dufau, I.Z. Beitins, J.W. McArthur, K.J. Catt, Effects of luteinizing hormone releasing hormone (LHRH) upon bioactive and immunoreactive serum LH levels in normal subjects, J Clin Endocrinol Metab 43 (3) (1976) 658–667.
[96] C. Wang, Bioassays of follicle stimulating hormone, Endocr Rev 9 (3) (1988) 374–377.
[97] X.C. Jia, A.J. Hsueh, Granulosa cell aromatase bioassay for follicle-stimulating hormone: Validation and application of the method, Endocrinology 119 (4) (1986) 1570–1577.
[98] M.P. Van Damme, D.M. Robertson, R. Marana, E.M. Ritzen, E. Diczfalusy, A sensitive and specific in vitro bioassay method for the measurement of follicle-stimulating hormone activity, Acta Endocrinol (Copenh) 91 (2) (1979) 224–237.
[99] S.D. Bianco, U.B. Kaiser, The genetic and molecular basis of idiopathic hypogonadotropic hypogonadism, Nat Rev Endocrinol 5 (10) (2009) 569–576.
[100] G.P. Sykiotis, N. Pitteloud, S.B. Seminara, U.B. Kaiser, W.F. Crowley Jr., Deciphering genetic disease in the genomic era: The model of GnRH deficiency, Sci Transl Med 2 (32) (2010) 32rv2.
[101] M. Schwanzel-Fukuda, D.W. Pfaff, Origin of luteinizing hormone-releasing hormone neurons, Nature 338 (6211) (1989) 161–164.
[102] S.M. Cadman, S.H. Kim, Y. Hu, D. Gonzalez-Martinez, P.M. Bouloux, Molecular pathogenesis of Kallmann's syndrome, Horm Res 67 (5) (2007) 231–242.
[103] A. Cariboni, R. Maggi, Kallmann's syndrome, a neuronal migration defect, Cell Mol Life Sci 63 (21) (2006) 2512–2526.
[104] R. Legouis, J.P. Hardelin, J. Levilliers, J.M. Claverie, S. Compain, V. Wunderle, et al., The candidate gene for the X-linked Kallmann syndrome encodes a protein related to adhesion molecules, Cell 67 (2) (1991) 423–435.
[105] B. Ayari, N. Soussi-Yanicostas, FGFR1 and anosmin-1 underlying genetically distinct forms of Kallmann syndrome are co-expressed and interact in olfactory bulbs, Dev Genes Evol 217 (2) (2007) 169–175.
[106] R.T. Bottcher, C. Niehrs, Fibroblast growth factor signaling during early vertebrate development, Endocr Rev 26 (1) (2005) 63–77.
[107] S. Salenave, P. Chanson, H. Bry, M. Pugeat, S. Cabrol, J.C. Carel, et al., Kallmann's syndrome: A comparison of the reproductive phenotypes in men carrying KAL1 and FGFR1/KAL2 mutations, J Clin Endocrinol Metab 93 (3) (2008) 758–763.
[108] N. Pitteloud, J.S. Acierno Jr., A.U. Meysing, A.A. Dwyer, F.J. Hayes, W.F. Crowley Jr., Reversible Kallmann syndrome, delayed puberty, and isolated anosmia occurring in a single family with a mutation in the fibroblast growth factor receptor 1 gene, J Clin Endocrinol Metab 90 (3) (2005) 1317–1322.
[109] J. Falardeau, W.C. Chung, A. Beenken, T. Raivio, L. Plummer, Y. Sidis, et al., Decreased FGF8 signaling causes deficiency of gonadotropin-releasing hormone in humans and mice, J Clin Invest 118 (8) (2008) 2822–2831.
[110] A.P. Abreu, U.B. Kaiser, A.C. Latronico, The role of prokineticins in the pathogenesis of hypogonadotropic hypogonadism, Neuroendocrinology 91 (2010) 283–290.
[111] S. Matsumoto, C. Yamazaki, K.H. Masumoto, M. Nagano, M. Naito, T. Soga, et al., Abnormal development of the olfactory bulb and reproductive system in mice lacking prokineticin receptor PKR2, Proc Nat Acad Sci USA 103 (11) (2006) 4140–4145.
[112] N. Pitteloud, C. Zhang, D. Pignatelli, J.D. Li, T. Raivio, L.W. Cole, et al., Loss-of-function mutation in the prokineticin 2 gene causes Kallmann syndrome and normosmic idiopathic hypogonadotropic hypogonadism, Proc Nat Acad Sci USA 104 (44) (2007) 17447–17452.

[113] A.P. Abreu, E.B. Trarbach, M. de Castro, E.M. Frade Costa, B. Versiani, M.T. Matias Baptista, et al., Loss-of-function mutations in the genes encoding prokineticin-2 or prokineticin receptor-2 cause autosomal recessive Kallmann syndrome, J Clin Endocrinol Metab 93 (10) (2008) 4113–4118.

[114] C. Dode, L. Teixeira, J. Levilliers, C. Fouveaut, P. Bouchard, M.L. Kottler, et al., Kallmann syndrome: Mutations in the genes encoding prokineticin-2 and prokineticin receptor-2, PLoS Genet 2 (10) (2006) e175.

[115] M.Y. Cheng, E.L. Bittman, S. Hattar, Q.Y. Zhou, Regulation of prokineticin 2 expression by light and the circadian clock, BMC Neurosci 6 (2005) 17.

[116] J.D. Li, W.P. Hu, L. Boehmer, M.Y. Cheng, A.G. Lee, A. Jilek, et al., Attenuated circadian rhythms in mice lacking the prokineticin 2 gene, J Neurosci 26 (45) (2006) 11615–11623.

[117] H.G. Kim, I. Kurth, F. Lan, I. Meliciani, W. Wenzel, S.H. Eom, et al., Mutations in CHD7, encoding a chromatin-remodeling protein, cause idiopathic hypogonadotropic hypogonadism and Kallmann syndrome, Am J Hum Genet 83 (4) (2008) 511–519.

[118] P.E. Belchetz, T.M. Plant, Y. Nakai, E.J. Keogh, E. Knobil, Hypophysial responses to continuous and intermittent delivery of hypothalamic gonadotropin-releasing hormone, Science 202 (4368) (1978) 631–633.

[119] W.F. Crowley Jr., J.W. McArthur, Simulation of the normal menstrual cycle in Kallman's syndrome by pulsatile administration of luteinizing hormone-releasing hormone (LHRH), J Clin Endocrinol Metab 51 (1) (1980) 173–175.

[120] J.B. Engel, A.V. Schally, Drug insight: Clinical use of agonists and antagonists of luteinizing-hormone-releasing hormone, Nat Clin Pract Endocrinol Metab 3 (2) (2007) 157–167.

[121] J.E. Levine, V.D. Ramirez, In vivo release of luteinizing hormone-releasing hormone estimated with push-pull cannulae from the mediobasal hypothalami of ovariectomized, steroid-primed rats, Endocrinology 107 (6) (1980) 1782–1790.

[122] J.D. Neill, J.M. Patton, R.A. Dailey, R.C. Tsou, G.T. Tindall, Luteinizing hormone releasing hormone (LHRH) in pituitary stalk blood of rhesus monkeys: Relationship to level of LH release, Endocrinology 101 (2) (1977) 430–434.

[123] W.F. Crowley Jr., M. Filicori, D.I. Spratt, N.F. Santoro, The physiology of gonadotropin-releasing hormone (GnRH) secretion in men and women, Recent Prog Horm Res 41 (1985) 473–531.

[124] C.M. Grafer, R. Thomas, L. Lambrakos, I. Montoya, S. White, L.M. Halvorson, GnRH stimulates expression of PACAP in the pituitary gonadotropes via both the PKA and PKC signaling systems, Mol Endocrinol 23 (7) (2009) 1022–1032.

[125] N. de Roux, E. Genin, J.C. Carel, F. Matsuda, J.L. Chaussain, E. Milgrom, Hypogonadotropic hypogonadism due to loss of function of the KiSS1-derived peptide receptor GPR54, Proc Nat Acad Sci USA 100 (19) (2003) 10972–10976.

[126] S.B. Seminara, S. Messager, E.E. Chatzidaki, R.R. Thresher, J.S. Acierno Jr., J.K. Shagoury, et al., The GPR54 gene as a regulator of puberty, N Engl J Med 349 (17) (2003) 1614–1627.

[127] M.L. Gottsch, M.J. Cunningham, J.T. Smith, S.M. Popa, B.V. Acohido, W.F. Crowley, et al., A role for kisspeptins in the regulation of gonadotropin secretion in the mouse, Endocrinology 145 (9) (2004) 4073–4077.

[128] A.K. Roseweir, R.P. Millar, The role of kisspeptin in the control of gonadotrophin secretion, Hum Reprod Update 15 (2) (2009) 203–212.

[129] J.T. Smith, M.J. Cunningham, E.F. Rissman, D.K. Clifton, R.A. Steiner, Regulation of Kiss1 gene expression in the brain of the female mouse, Endocrinology 146 (9) (2005) 3686–3692.

[130] J. Clarkson, A.E. Herbison, Postnatal development of kisspeptin neurons in mouse hypothalamus; sexual dimorphism and projections to gonadotropin-releasing hormone neurons, Endocrinology 147 (12) (2006) 5817–5825.

[131] M.G. Teles, S.D. Bianco, V.N. Brito, E.B. Trarbach, W. Kuohung, S. Xu, et al., A GPR54-activating mutation in a patient with central precocious puberty, N Engl J Med 358 (7) (2008) 709–715.

[132] L.G. Silveira, S.D. Noel, A.P. Silveira-Neto, A.P. Abreu, V.N. Brito, M.G. Santos, et al., Mutations of the KISS1 gene in disorders of puberty, J Clin Endocrinol Metab 95 (5) (2010) 2276–2280.

[133] R.L. Goodman, M.N. Lehman, J.T. Smith, L.M. Coolen, C.V. de Oliveira, M.R. Jafarzadehshirazi, et al., Kisspeptin neurons in the arcuate nucleus of the ewe express both dynorphin A and neurokinin B, Endocrinology 148 (12) (2007) 5752–5760.

[134] Y. Wakabayashi, T. Nakada, K. Murata, S. Ohkura, K. Mogi, V.M. Navarro, et al., Neurokinin B and dynorphin A in kisspeptin neurons of the arcuate nucleus participate in generation of periodic oscillation of neural activity driving pulsatile gonadotropin-releasing hormone secretion in the goat, J Neurosci 30 (8) (2010) 3124–3132.

[135] V.M. Navarro, M.L. Gottsch, C. Chavkin, H. Okamura, D.K. Clifton, R.A. Steiner, Regulation of gonadotropin-releasing hormone secretion by kisspeptin/dynorphin/neurokinin B neurons in the arcuate nucleus of the mouse, J Neurosci 29 (38) (2009) 11859–11866.

[136] A.K. Topaloglu, F. Reimann, M. Guclu, A.S. Yalin, L.D. Kotan, K.M. Porter, et al., TAC3 and TACR3 mutations in familial hypogonadotropic hypogonadism reveal a key role for Neurokinin B in the central control of reproduction, Nat Genet 41 (3) (2009) 354–358.

[137] E. Gianetti, C. Tusset, S.D. Noel, M.G. Au, A.A. Dwyer, V.A. Hughes, et al., TAC3/TACR3 mutations reveal preferential activation of gonadotropin-releasing hormone release by Neurokinin B in neonatal life followed by reversal in adulthood, J Clin Endocrinol Metab (2010) in press.

[138] J. Bouligand, C. Ghervan, J.A. Tello, S. Brailly-Tabard, S. Salenave, P. Chanson, et al., Isolated familial hypogonadotropic hypogonadism and a GNRH1 mutation, N Engl J Med 360 (26) (2009) 2742–2748.

[139] Y.M. Chan, A. de Guillebon, M. Lang-Muritano, L. Plummer, F. Cerrato, S. Tsiaras, et al., GNRH1 mutations in patients with idiopathic hypogonadotropic hypogonadism, Proc Nat Acad Sci USA 106 (28) (2009) 11703–11708.

[140] S. Farooqi, S. O'Rahilly, Genetics of obesity in humans, Endocr Rev 27 (7) (2006) 710–718.

[141] M. Tena-Sempere, Kisspeptins and the metabolic control of reproduction: Physiologic roles and physiopathological implications, Ann Endocrinol (Paris) 71 (3) (2010) 201–202.

[142] J.D.C.D. Veldhuis, W.F. Crowley, et al., Preferred attributes of objective pulse analysis methods, in: W.F. Crowley (Ed.), Episodic Hormone Secretion, John Wiley and Sons, New York, 1988.

[143] J. Reinhart, L.M. Mertz, K.J. Catt, Molecular cloning and expression of cDNA encoding the murine gonadotropin-releasing hormone receptor, J Biol Chem 267 (30) (1992) 21281–21284.

[144] W.C. Probst, L.A. Snyder, D.I. Schuster, J. Brosius, S.C. Sealfon, Sequence alignment of the G-protein coupled receptor superfamily, DNA Cell Biol 11 (1) (1992) 1–20.

[145] Z. Naor, Signaling by G-protein-coupled receptor (GPCR): Studies on the GnRH receptor, Front Neuroendocrinol 30 (1) (2009) 10–29.

[146] N. de Roux, J. Young, M. Misrahi, R. Genet, P. Chanson, G. Schaison, et al., A family with hypogonadotropic hypogonadism and mutations in the gonadotropin-releasing hormone receptor, N Engl J Med 337 (22) (1997) 1597–1602.

[147] L.C. Layman, D.P. Cohen, M. Jin, J. Xie, Z. Li, R.H. Reindollar, et al., Mutations in gonadotropin-releasing hormone receptor gene cause hypogonadotropic hypogonadism, Nat Genet 18 (1) (1998) 14–15.

[148] G.Y. Bedecarrats, U.B. Kaiser, Mutations in the human gonadotropin-releasing hormone receptor: Insights into receptor biology and function, Semin Reprod Med 25 (5) (2007) 368–378.

[149] P.M. Conn, A. Ulloa-Aguirre, Trafficking of G-protein-coupled receptors to the plasma membrane: Insights for pharmacoperone drugs, Trends Endocrinol Metab 21 (3) (2010) 190–197.

[150] M.D. Thompson, W.M. Burnham, D.E. Cole, The G protein-coupled receptors: Pharmacogenetics and disease, Crit Rev Clin Lab Sci 42 (4) (2005) 311–392.

[151] P.M. Conn, A. Ulloa-Aguirre, J. Ito, J.A. Janovick, G protein-coupled receptor trafficking in health and disease: Lessons learned to prepare for therapeutic mutant rescue in vivo, Pharmacol Rev 59 (3) (2007) 225–250.

[152] F.U. Hartl, M. Hayer-Hartl, Molecular chaperones in the cytosol: From nascent chain to folded protein, Science 295 (5561) (2002) 1852–1858.

[153] M. Beranova, L.M. Oliveira, G.Y. Bedecarrats, E. Schipani, M. Vallejo, A.C. Ammini, et al., Prevalence, phenotypic spectrum, and modes of inheritance of gonadotropin-releasing hormone receptor mutations in idiopathic hypogonadotropic hypogonadism, J Clin Endocrinol Metab 86 (4) (2001) 1580–1588.

[154] S.B. Seminara, M. Beranova, L.M. Oliveira, K.A. Martin, W.F. Crowley Jr., J.E. Hall, Successful use of pulsatile gonadotropin-releasing hormone (GnRH) for ovulation induction and pregnancy in a patient with GnRH receptor mutations, J Clin Endocrinol Metab 85 (2) (2000) 556–562.

[155] D. Dewailly, A. Boucher, C. Decanter, J.P. Lagarde, R. Counis, M.L. Kottler, Spontaneous pregnancy in a patient who was homozygous for the Q106R mutation in the gonadotropin-releasing hormone receptor gene, Fertil Steril 77 (6) (2002) 1288–1291.

[156] N. Pitteloud, P.A. Boepple, S. DeCruz, S.B. Valkenburgh, W.F. Crowley Jr., F.J. Hayes, The fertile eunuch variant of idiopathic hypogonadotropic hypogonadism: Spontaneous reversal associated with a homozygous mutation in the gonadotropin-releasing hormone receptor, J Clin Endocrinol Metab 86 (6) (2001) 2470–2475.

[157] L. Lin, W.X. Gu, G. Ozisik, W.S. To, C.J. Owen, J.L. Jameson, et al., Analysis of DAX1 (NR0B1) and steroidogenic factor-1 (NR5A1) in children and adults with primary adrenal failure: Ten years' experience, J Clin Endocrinol Metab 91 (8) (2006) 3048–3054.

[158] M. Filicori, N. Santoro, G.R. Merriam, W.F. Crowley Jr., Characterization of the physiological pattern of episodic gonadotropin secretion throughout the human menstrual cycle, J Clin Endocrinol Metab 62 (6) (1986) 1136–1144.

[159] L. Wildt, A. Hausler, G. Marshall, J.S. Hutchison, T.M. Plant, P.E. Belchetz, et al., Frequency and amplitude of gonadotropin-releasing hormone stimulation and gonadotropin secretion in the rhesus monkey, Endocrinology 109 (2) (1981) 376–385.

[160] A.C. Dalkin, D.J. Haisenleder, G.A. Ortolano, T.R. Ellis, J.C. Marshall, The frequency of gonadotropin-releasing-hormone stimulation differentially regulates gonadotropin subunit messenger ribonucleic acid expression, Endocrinology 125 (2) (1989) 917–924.

[161] U.B. Kaiser, A. Jakubowiak, A. Steinberger, W.W. Chin, Differential effects of gonadotropin-releasing hormone (GnRH) pulse frequency on gonadotropin subunit and GnRH receptor messenger ribonucleic acid levels in vitro, Endocrinology 138 (3) (1997) 1224–1231.

[162] D.J. Haisenleder, A.C. Dalkin, G.A. Ortolano, J.C. Marshall, M.A. Shupnik, A pulsatile gonadotropin-releasing hormone stimulus is required to increase transcription of the gonadotropin subunit genes: Evidence for differential regulation of transcription by pulse frequency in vivo, Endocrinology 128 (1) (1991) 509–517.

[163] H.A. Ferris, M.A. Shupnik, Mechanisms for pulsatile regulation of the gonadotropin subunit genes by GNRH1, Biol Reprod 74 (6) (2006) 993–998.

[164] J.D. Blaustein, The year in neuroendocrinology, Mol Endocrinol 24 (1) (2010) 252–260.

[165] J. Clarkson, A.E. Herbison, Oestrogen, kisspeptin, GPR54 and the pre-ovulatory luteinising hormone surge, J Neuroendocrinol 21 (4) (2009) 305–311.

[166] L.Z. Krsmanovic, L. Hu, P.K. Leung, H. Feng, K.J. Catt, The hypothalamic GnRH pulse generator: Multiple regulatory mechanisms, Trends Endocrinol Metab 20 (8) (2009) 402–408.

[167] J.S. Finkelstein, L.S. O'Dea, R.W. Whitcomb, W.F. Crowley Jr., Sex steroid control of gonadotropin secretion in the human male. II. Effects of estradiol administration in normal and gonadotropin-releasing hormone-deficient men, J Clin Endocrinol Metab 73 (3) (1991) 621–628.

[168] S. Adachi, S. Yamada, Y. Takatsu, H. Matsui, M. Kinoshita, K. Takase, et al., Involvement of anteroventral periventricular metastin/kisspeptin neurons in estrogen positive feedback action on luteinizing hormone release in female rats, J Reprod Dev 53 (2) (2007) 367–378.

[169] C. Glidewell-Kenney, L.A. Hurley, L. Pfaff, J. Weiss, J.E. Levine, J.L. Jameson, Nonclassical estrogen receptor alpha signaling mediates negative feedback in the female mouse reproductive axis, Proc Nat Acad Sci USA 104 (19) (2007) 8173–8177.

[170] M.A. McDevitt, C. Glidewell-Kenney, M.A. Jimenez, P.C. Ahearn, J. Weiss, J.L. Jameson, et al., New insights into the classical and non-classical actions of estrogen: Evidence from estrogen receptor knock-out and knock-in mice, Mol Cell Endocrinol 290 (1–2) (2008) 24–30.

[171] Z. Zhao, C. Park, M.A. McDevitt, C. Glidewell-Kenney, P. Chambon, J. Weiss, et al., p21-Activated kinase mediates rapid estradiol-negative feedback actions in the reproductive axis, Proc Nat Acad Sci USA 106 (17) (2009) 7221–7226.

[172] S.D. Noel, K.L. Keen, D.I. Baumann, E.J. Filardo, E. Terasawa, Involvement of G protein-coupled receptor 30 (GPR30) in rapid action of estrogen in primate LHRH neurons, Mol Endocrinol 23 (3) (2009) 349–359.

[173] M.L. Gottsch, V.M. Navarro, Z. Zhao, C. Glidewell-Kenney, J. Weiss, J.L. Jameson, et al., Regulation of Kiss1 and dynorphin gene expression in the murine brain by classical and nonclassical estrogen receptor pathways, J Neurosci 29 (29) (2009) 9390–9395.

[174] M.R. Soules, R.A. Steiner, D.K. Clifton, N.L. Cohen, S. Aksel, W.J. Bremner, Progesterone modulation of pulsatile luteinizing hormone secretion in normal women, J Clin Endocrinol Metab 58 (2) (1984) 378–383.

[175] J.F. Ropert, M.E. Quigley, S.S. Yen, Endogenous opiates modulate pulsatile luteinizing hormone release in humans, J Clin Endocrinol Metab 52 (3) (1981) 583–585.

[176] W.D. Odell, R.S. Swerdloff, Progestogen-induced luteinizing and follicle-stimulating hormone surge in postmenopausal women: A simulated ovulatory peak, Proc Nat Acad Sci USA 61 (2) (1968) 529–536.

[177] N. Sleiter, Y. Pang, C. Park, T.H. Horton, J. Dong, P. Thomas, et al., Progesterone receptor A (PRA) and PRB-independent effects of progesterone on gonadotropin-releasing hormone release, Endocrinology 150 (8) (2009) 3833–3844.

[178] S.J. Winters, J.J. Janick, D.L. Loriaux, R.J. Sherins, Studies on the role of sex steroids in the feedback control of gonadotropin concentrations in men. II. Use of the estrogen antagonist, clomiphene citrate, J Clin Endocrinol Metab 48 (2) (1979) 222–227.

[179] S. Bhasin, T.J. Fielder, R.S. Swerdloff, Testosterone selectively increases serum follicle-stimulating hormone (FSH) but not luteinizing hormone (LH) in gonadotropin-releasing hormone antagonist-treated male rats: Evidence for differential regulation of LH and FSH secretion, Biol Reprod 37 (1) (1987) 55–59.

[180] M.E. Wierman, C. Wang, Androgen selectively stimulates follicle-stimulating hormone-beta mRNA levels after gonadotropin-releasing hormone antagonist administration, Biol Reprod 42 (3) (1990) 563–571.

[181] G.J. Gormley, Chemoprevention strategies for prostate cancer: The role of 5 alpha-reductase inhibitors, J Cell Biochem Suppl 16H (1992) 113–117.

[182] D.R. McCullagh, Dual endocrine activity of the testes, Science 1932 (76) (1957) 19–20.

[183] F.S. Esch, S. Shimasaki, K. Cooksey, M. Mercado, A.J. Mason, S.Y. Ying, et al., Complementary deoxyribonucleic acid (cDNA) cloning and DNA sequence analysis of rat ovarian inhibins, Mol Endocrinol 1 (5) (1987) 388–396.

[184] N. Ling, S.Y. Ying, N. Ueno, F. Esch, L. Denoroy, R. Guillemin, Isolation and partial characterization of a Mr 32,000 protein with inhibin activity from porcine follicular fluid, Proc Nat Acad Sci USA 82 (21) (1985) 7217–7221.

[185] A.J. Mason, J.S. Hayflick, N. Ling, F. Esch, N. Ueno, S.Y. Ying, et al., Complementary DNA sequences of ovarian follicular fluid inhibin show precursor structure and homology with transforming growth factor-beta, Nature 318 (6047) (1985) 659–663.

[186] C. Welt, Y. Sidis, H. Keutmann, A. Schneyer, Activins, inhibins, and follistatins: From endocrinology to signaling. A paradigm for the new millennium, Exp Biol Med (Maywood) 227 (9) (2002) 724–752.

[187] Y. Xia, A.L. Schneyer, The biology of activin: Recent advances in structure, regulation and function, J Endocrinol 202 (1) (2009) 1–12.

[188] S.Y. Ying, Inhibins, activins, and follistatins: Gonadal proteins modulating the secretion of follicle-stimulating hormone, Endocr Rev 9 (2) (1988) 267–293.

[189] K.L. Stenvers, J.K. Findlay, Inhibins: From reproductive hormones to tumor suppressors, Trends Endocrinol Metab 21 (3) (2010) 174–180.

[190] N. Ling, S.Y. Ying, N. Ueno, S. Shimasaki, F. Esch, M. Hotta, et al., Pituitary FSH is released by a heterodimer of the beta-subunits from the two forms of inhibin, Nature 321 (6072) (1986) 779–782.

[191] W. Vale, J. Rivier, J. Vaughan, R. McClintock, A. Corrigan, W. Woo, et al., Purification and characterization of an FSH releasing protein from porcine ovarian follicular fluid, Nature 321 (6072) (1986) 776–779.

[192] N. Ueno, N. Ling, S.Y. Ying, F. Esch, S. Shimasaki, R. Guillemin, Isolation and partial characterization of follistatin: A single-chain Mr 35,000 monomeric protein that inhibits the release of follicle-stimulating hormone, Proc Nat Acad Sci USA 84 (23) (1987) 8282–8286.

[193] S.J. Gregory, C.T. Lacza, A.A. Detz, S. Xu, L.A. Petrillo, U.B. Kaiser, Synergy between activin A and gonadotropin-releasing hormone in transcriptional activation of the rat follicle-stimulating hormone-beta gene, Mol Endocrinol 19 (1) (2005) 237–254.

[194] K.A. Lewis, P.C. Gray, A.L. Blount, L.A. MacConell, E. Wiater, L.M. Bilezikjian, et al., Betaglycan binds inhibin and can mediate functional antagonism of activin signalling, Nature 404 (6776) (2000) 411–414.

[195] C.K. Welt, J.L. Chan, J. Bullen, R. Murphy, P. Smith, A.M. DePaoli, et al., Recombinant human leptin in women with hypothalamic amenorrhea, N Engl J Med 351 (10) (2004) 987–997.

[196] J. Weiss, M.J. Guendner, L.M. Halvorson, J.L. Jameson, Transcriptional activation of the follicle-stimulating hormone beta-subunit gene by activin, Endocrinology 136 (5) (1995) 1885–1891.

[197] P. Lamba, M.M. Santos, D.P. Philips, D.J. Bernard, Acute regulation of murine follicle-stimulating hormone beta subunit transcription by activin A, J Mol Endocrinol 36 (1) (2006) 201–220.

[198] M.I. Suszko, D.M. Balkin, Y. Chen, T.K. Woodruff, Smad3 mediates activin-induced transcription of follicle-stimulating hormone beta-subunit gene, Mol Endocrinol 19 (7) (2005) 1849–1858.

[199] M.I. Suszko, D.J. Lo, H. Suh, S.A. Camper, T.K. Woodruff, Regulation of the rat follicle-stimulating hormone beta-subunit promoter by activin, Mol Endocrinol 17 (3) (2003) 318–332.

[200] J.S. Jorgensen, C.C. Quirk, J.H. Nilson, Multiple and overlapping combinatorial codes orchestrate hormonal responsiveness and dictate cell-specific expression of the genes encoding luteinizing hormone, Endocr Rev 25 (4) (2004) 521–542.

[201] J.C. Achermann, W.X. Gu, T.J. Kotlar, J.J. Meeks, L.P. Sabacan, S.B. Seminara, et al., Mutational analysis of DAX1 in patients with hypogonadotropic hypogonadism or pubertal delay, J Clin Endocrinol Metab 84 (12) (1999) 4497–4500.

[202] J.A. Bridwell, J.R. Price, G.E. Parker, A. McCutchan Schiller, K.W. Sloop, S.J. Rhodes, Role of the LIM domains in DNA recognition by the Lhx3 neuroendocrine transcription factor, Gene 277 (1–2) (2001) 239–250.

[203] H.Z. Sheng, A.B. Zhadanov, B. Mosinger Jr., T. Fujii, S. Bertuzzi, A. Grinberg, et al., Specification of pituitary cell lineages by the LIM homeobox gene Lhx3, Science 272 (5264) (1996) 1004–1007.

[204] L.T. Raetzman, R. Ward, S.A. Camper, Lhx4 and Prop1 are required for cell survival and expansion of the pituitary primordia, Development 129 (18) (2002) 4229–4239.

[205] I. Bach, C. Carriere, H.P. Ostendorff, B. Andersen, M.G. Rosenfeld, A family of LIM domain-associated cofactors confer transcriptional synergism between LIM and Otx homeodomain proteins, Genes Dev 11 (11) (1997) 1370–1380.

[206] D.P. Szeto, C. Rodriguez-Esteban, A.K. Ryan, S.M. O'Connell, F. Liu, C. Kioussi, et al., Role of the bicoid-related homeodomain factor Pitx1 in specifying hindlimb morphogenesis and pituitary development, Genes Dev 13 (4) (1999) 484–494.

[207] L.L. Heckert, K. Schultz, J.H. Nilson, The cAMP response elements of the alpha subunit gene bind similar proteins in trophoblasts and gonadotropes but have distinct functional sequence requirements, J Biol Chem 271 (49) (1996) 31650–31656.

[208] J. Xie, S.P. Bliss, T.M. Nett, B.J. Ebersole, S.C. Sealfon, M.S. Roberson, Transcript profiling of immediate early genes reveals a unique role for activating transcription factor 3 in mediating activation of the glycoprotein hormone alpha-subunit promoter by gonadotropin-releasing hormone, Mol Endocrinol 19 (10) (2005) 2624–2638.

[209] M.S. Roberson, A. Misra-Press, M.E. Laurance, P.J. Stork, R.A. Maurer, A role for mitogen-activated protein kinase in mediating activation of the glycoprotein hormone alpha-subunit promoter by gonadotropin-releasing hormone, Mol Cell Biol 15 (7) (1995) 3531–3539.

[210] S.P. Bliss, A. Miller, A.M. Navratil, J. Xie, S.P. McDonough, P.J. Fisher, et al., ERK signaling in the pituitary is required for female but not male fertility, Mol Endocrinol 23 (7) (2009) 1092–1101.

[211] J.J. Tremblay, J. Drouin, Egr-1 is a downstream effector of GnRH and synergizes by direct interaction with Ptx1 and SF-1 to enhance luteinizing hormone beta gene transcription, Mol Cell Biol 19 (4) (1999) 2567–2576.

[212] G.B. Call, M.W. Wolfe, Species differences in GnRH activation of the LHbeta promoter: Role of Egr1 and Sp1, Mol Cell Endocrinol 189 (1–2) (2002) 85–96.

[213] L.M. Halvorson, U.B. Kaiser, W.W. Chin, The protein kinase C system acts through the early growth response protein 1 to increase LHbeta gene expression in synergy with steroidogenic factor-1, Mol Endocrinol 13 (1) (1999) 106–116.

[214] U.B. Kaiser, L.M. Halvorson, M.T. Chen, Sp1, steroidogenic factor 1 (SF-1), and early growth response protein 1 (egr-1) binding sites form a tripartite gonadotropin-releasing hormone response element in the rat luteinizing hormone-beta gene promoter: An integral role for SF-1, Mol Endocrinol 14 (8) (2000) 1235–1245.

[215] D. Curtin, H.A. Ferris, M. Hakli, M. Gibson, O.A. Janne, J.J. Palvimo, et al., Small nuclear RING finger protein stimulates the rat luteinizing hormone-beta promoter by interacting with Sp1 and steroidogenic factor-1 and protects from androgen suppression, Mol Endocrinol 18 (5) (2004) 1263–1276.

[216] M.W. Wolfe, G.B. Call, Early growth response protein 1 binds to the luteinizing hormone-beta promoter and mediates gonadotropin-releasing hormone-stimulated gene expression, Mol Endocrinol 13 (5) (1999) 752–763.

[217] H. Kanasaki, G.Y. Bedecarrats, K.Y. Kam, S. Xu, U.B. Kaiser, Gonadotropin-releasing hormone pulse frequency-dependent activation of extracellular signal-regulated kinase pathways in perifused LbetaT2 cells, Endocrinology 146 (12) (2005) 5503–5513.

[218] M.A. Shupnik, B.A. Rosenzweig, Identification of an estrogen-responsive element in the rat LH beta gene. DNA-estrogen receptor interactions and functional analysis, J Biol Chem 266 (26) (1991) 17084–17091.

[219] M.M. Zakaria, K.H. Jeong, C. Lacza, U.B. Kaiser, Pituitary homeobox 1 activates the rat FSHbeta (rFSHbeta) gene through both direct and indirect interactions with the rFSHbeta gene promoter, Mol Endocrinol 16 (8) (2002) 1840–1852.

[220] D.J. Bernard, J. Fortin, Y. Wang, P. Lamba, Mechanisms of FSH synthesis: What we know, what we don't, and why you should care, Fertil Steril 93 (8) (2010) 2465–2485.

[221] S.B. Jacobs, D. Coss, S.M. McGillivray, P.L. Mellon, Nuclear factor Y and steroidogenic factor 1 physically and functionally interact to contribute to cell-specific expression of the mouse follicle-stimulating hormone-beta gene, Mol Endocrinol 17 (8) (2003) 1470–1483.

[222] N.A. Ciccone, U.B. Kaiser, The biology of gonadotroph regulation, Curr Opin Endocrinol Diabetes Obes 16 (4) (2009) 321–327.

[223] N.A. Ciccone, C.T. Lacza, M.Y. Hou, S.J. Gregory, K.Y. Kam, S. Xu, et al., A composite element that binds basic helix-loop-helix and basic leucine zipper transcription factors is important for gonadotropin-releasing hormone regulation of the follicle-stimulating hormone beta gene, Mol Endocrinol 22 (8) (2008) 1908–1923.

[224] D. Coss, S.B. Jacobs, C.E. Bender, P.L. Mellon, A novel AP-1 site is critical for maximal induction of the follicle-stimulating hormone beta gene by gonadotropin-releasing hormone, J Biol Chem 279 (1) (2004) 152–162.

[225] Y. Wang, J. Fortin, P. Lamba, M. Bonomi, L. Persani, M.S. Roberson, et al., Activator protein-1 and smad proteins synergistically regulate human follicle-stimulating hormone beta-promoter activity, Endocrinology 149 (11) (2008) 5577–5591.

[226] N.A. Ciccone, S. Xu, C.T. Lacza, R.S. Carroll, U.B. Kaiser, Frequency-dependent regulation of follicle-stimulating hormone beta by pulsatile gonadotropin-releasing hormone is mediated by functional antagonism of bZIP transcription factors, Mol Cell Biol 30 (4) (2010) 1028–1040.

[227] V.G. Thackray, S.M. McGillivray, P.L. Mellon, Androgens, progestins, and glucocorticoids induce follicle-stimulating hormone beta-subunit gene expression at the level of the gonadotrope, Mol Endocrinol 20 (9) (2006) 2062–2079.

[228] J. Dupont, J. McNeilly, A. Vaiman, S. Canepa, Y. Combarnous, C. Taragnat, Activin signaling pathways in ovine pituitary and LbetaT2 gonadotrope cells, Biol Reprod 68 (5) (2003) 1877–1887.

[229] J.S. Bailey, N. Rave-Harel, S.M. McGillivray, D. Coss, P.L. Mellon, Activin regulation of the follicle-stimulating hormone beta-subunit gene involves Smads and the TALE homeodomain proteins Pbx1 and Prep1, Mol Endocrinol 18 (5) (2004) 1158–1170.

[230] D.J. Bernard, Both SMAD2 and SMAD3 mediate activin-stimulated expression of the follicle-stimulating hormone beta subunit in mouse gonadotrope cells, Mol Endocrinol 18 (3) (2004) 606–623.

[231] S.J. Gregory, U.B. Kaiser, Regulation of gonadotropins by inhibin and activin, Semin Reprod Med 22 (3) (2004) 253–267.

[232] M.I. Suszko, M. Antenos, D.M. Balkin, T.K. Woodruff, Smad3 and Pitx2 cooperate in stimulation of FSHbeta gene transcription, Mol Cell Endocrinol 281 (1–2) (2008) 27–36.

[233] P.S. Corpuz, L.L. Lindaman, P.L. Mellon, D. Coss, FoxL2 is required for activin induction of the mouse and human follicle-stimulating hormone beta-subunit genes, Mol Endocrinol 24 (5) (2010) 1037–1051.

[234] P. Lamba, J. Fortin, S. Tran, Y. Wang, D.J. Bernard, A novel role for the forkhead transcription factor FOXL2 in activin A-regulated follicle-stimulating hormone beta subunit transcription, Mol Endocrinol 23 (7) (2009) 1001–1013.

[235] R. Rebar, H.L. Judd, S.S. Yen, J. Rakoff, G. Vandenberg, F. Naftolin, Characterization of the inappropriate gonadotropin secretion in polycystic ovary syndrome, J Clin Invest 57 (5) (1976) 1320–1329.

[236] D.I. Spratt, W.F. Crowley Jr., J.P. Butler, A.R. Hoffman, P.M. Conn, T.M. Badger, Pituitary luteinizing hormone responses to intravenous and subcutaneous administration of gonadotropin-releasing hormone in men, J Clin Endocrinol Metab 61 (5) (1985) 890–895.

[237] C.H. Mortimer, G.M. Besser, A.S. McNeilly, J.C. Marshall, P. Harsoulis, W.M. Tunbridge, et al., Luteinizing hormone and follicle stimulating hormone-releasing hormone test in patients with hypothalamic–pituitary–gonadal dysfunction, Br Med J 4 (5884) (1973) 73–77.

[238] N. Santoro, M. Filicori, W.F. Crowley Jr., Hypogonadotropic disorders in men and women: Diagnosis and therapy with pulsatile gonadotropin-releasing hormone, Endocr Rev 7 (1) (1986) 11–23.

[239] V.N. Brito, M.C. Batista, M.F. Borges, A.C. Latronico, M.B. Kohek, A.C. Thirone, et al., Diagnostic value of fluorometric assays in the evaluation of precocious puberty, J Clin Endocrinol Metab 84 (10) (1999) 3539–3544.

[240] V.N. Brito, A.C. Latronico, I.J. Arnhold, B.B. Mendonca, A single luteinizing hormone determination 2 hours after depot leuprolide is useful for therapy monitoring of gonadotropin-dependent precocious puberty in girls, J Clin Endocrinol Metab 89 (9) (2004) 4338–4342.

[241] J.C. Job, P.E. Garnier, J.L. Chaussain, G. Milhaud, Elevation of serum gonadotropins (LH and FSH) after releasing hormone (LH-RH) injection in normal children and in patients with disorders of puberty, J Clin Endocrinol Metab 35 (3) (1972) 473–476.

[242] J.C.K.R. Roth, S.L. Kaplan, M.M. Grumbach, Patterns of LH, FSH and testosterone release stimulated by synthetic LRH in prepubertal, pubertal and adult subjects and in patients with hypogonadotropic and hypergonadotropic hypogonadism, J Clin Endocrinol Metab 35 (1972) 926–930.

[243] V.A. Hughes, P.A. Boepple, W.F. Crowley Jr., S.B. Seminara, Interplay between dose and frequency of GnRH administration in determining pituitary gonadotropin responsiveness, Neuroendocrinology 87 (3) (2008) 142–150.

[244] E. Loumaye, J.M. Billion, J.M. Mine, I. Psalti, M. Pensis, K. Thomas, Prediction of individual response to controlled ovarian hyperstimulation by means of a clomiphene citrate challenge test, Fertil Steril 53 (2) (1990) 295–301.

[245] R.J. Santen, J.M. Leonard, R.J. Sherins, H.M. Gandy, C.A. Paulsen, Short- and long-term effects of clomiphene citrate on the pituitary–testicular axis, J Clin Endocrinol Metab 33 (6) (1971) 970–979.

[246] D.J. Hendriks, B.W. Mol, L.F. Bancsi, E.R. te Velde, F.J. Broekmans, The clomiphene citrate challenge test for the prediction of poor ovarian response and nonpregnancy in patients undergoing in vitro fertilization: A systematic review, Fertil Steril 86 (4) (2006) 807–818.

[247] J.D. Veldhuis, D.M. Keenan, S.M. Pincus, Motivations and methods for analyzing pulsatile hormone secretion, Endocr Rev 29 (7) (2008) 823–864.

[248] R.J. Santen, C.W. Bardin, Episodic luteinizing hormone secretion in man. Pulse analysis, clinical interpretation, physiologic mechanisms, J Clin Invest 52 (10) (1973) 2617–2628.

[249] J.D. Veldhuis, M.L. Carlson, M.L. Johnson, The pituitary gland secretes in bursts: Appraising the nature of glandular secretory impulses by simultaneous multiple-parameter deconvolution of plasma hormone concentrations, Proc Nat Acad Sci USA 84 (21) (1987) 7686–7690.

[250] E. Gianetti, C. Tusset, S.D. Noel, M.G. Au, A.A. Dwyer, V.A. Hughes, et al., TAC3/TACR3 mutations reveal preferential activation of gonadotropin-releasing hormone release by Neurokinin B in neonatal life followed by reversal in adulthood, J Clin Endocrinol Metab 95 (6) (2010) 2857–2867.

[251] D.I. Spratt, D.B. Carr, G.R. Merriam, R.E. Scully, P.N. Rao, W.F. Crowley Jr., The spectrum of abnormal patterns of gonadotropin-releasing hormone secretion in men with idiopathic hypogonadotropic hypogonadism: Clinical and laboratory correlations, J Clin Endocrinol Metab 64 (2) (1987) 283–291.

[252] J. Waldstreicher, S.B. Seminara, J.L. Jameson, A. Geyer, L.B. Nachtigall, P.A. Boepple, et al., The genetic and clinical heterogeneity of gonadotropin-releasing hormone deficiency in the human, J Clin Endocrinol Metab 81 (12) (1996) 4388–4395.

[253] F.S.W. Kallman, S. Barrera, The genetic aspects of primary eunuchoidism, Am J Mental Def 48 (1944) 203–236.

[254] J.C. Pallais, M. Caudill, N. Pitteloud, S. Seminara, W.F. Crowley, Hypogonadotropic Hypogonadism Overview, in: R.A. Pagon, T.C. Bird, C.R. Dolan, K. Stephens (Eds.), GeneReviews [Internet] Seattle (WA), University of Washington, Seattle, May 23, 2007, pp. 1993–2007.

[255] M.C. Jongmans, C.M. van Ravenswaaij-Arts, N. Pitteloud, T. Ogata, N. Sato, H.L. Claahsen-van der Grinten, et al., CHD7 mutations in patients initially diagnosed with Kallmann syndrome – the clinical overlap with CHARGE syndrome, Clin Genet 75 (1) (2009) 65–71.

[256] Y. Tenenbaum-Rakover, M. Commenges-Ducos, A. Iovane, C. Aumas, O. Admoni, N. de Roux, Neuroendocrine phenotype analysis in five patients with isolated hypogonadotropic hypogonadism due to a L102P inactivating mutation of GPR54, J Clin Endocrinol Metab 92 (3) (2007) 1137–1144.

[257] L.C. Layman, E.J. Lee, D.B. Peak, A.B. Namnoum, K.V. Vu, B.L. van Lingen, et al., Delayed puberty and hypogonadism caused by mutations in the follicle-stimulating hormone beta-subunit gene, N Engl J Med 337 (9) (1997) 607–611.

[258] K. Berger, H. Souza, V.N. Brito, C.B. d'Alva, B.B. Mendonca, A.C. Latronico, Clinical and hormonal features of selective follicle-stimulating hormone (FSH) deficiency due to FSH beta-subunit gene mutations in both sexes, Fertil Steril 83 (2) (2005) 466–470.

[259] L.C. Layman, A.L. Porto, J. Xie, L.A. da Motta, L.D. da Motta, W. Weiser, et al., FSH beta gene mutations in a female with partial breast development and a male sibling with normal puberty and azoospermia, J Clin Endocrinol Metab 87 (8) (2002) 3702–3707.

[260] A. Lofrano-Porto, L.A. Casulari, P.P. Nascimento, L. Giacomini, L.A. Naves, L.D. da Motta, et al., Effects of follicle-stimulating hormone and human chorionic gonadotropin on gonadal steroidogenesis in two siblings with a follicle-stimulating hormone beta subunit mutation, Fertil Steril 90 (4) (2008) 1169–1174.

[261] T.R. Kumar, Y. Wang, N. Lu, M.M. Matzuk, Follicle stimulating hormone is required for ovarian follicle maturation but not male fertility, Nat Genet 15 (2) (1997) 201–204.

[262] M. Phillip, J.E. Arbelle, Y. Segev, R. Parvari, Male hypogonadism due to a mutation in the gene for the beta-subunit of follicle-stimulating hormone, N Engl J Med 338 (24) (1998) 1729–1732.

[263] C. Achard, C. Courtillot, O. Lahuna, G. Meduri, J.C. Soufir, P. Liere, et al., Normal spermatogenesis in a man with mutant luteinizing hormone, N Engl J Med 361 (19) (2009) 1856–1863.

[264] H. Valdes-Socin, R. Salvi, A.F. Daly, R.C. Gaillard, P. Quatresooz, P.M. Tebeu, et al., Hypogonadism in a patient with a mutation in the luteinizing hormone beta-subunit gene, N Engl J Med 351 (25) (2004) 2619–2625.

[265] J. Weiss, L. Axelrod, R.W. Whitcomb, P.E. Harris, W.F. Crowley, J.L. Jameson, Hypogonadism caused by a single amino acid substitution in the beta subunit of luteinizing hormone, N Engl J Med 326 (3) (1992) 179–183.

[266] I.J. Arnhold, A. Lofrano-Porto, A.C. Latronico, Inactivating mutations of luteinizing hormone beta-subunit or luteinizing hormone receptor cause oligo-amenorrhea and infertility in women, Horm Res 71 (2) (2009) 75–82.

[267] T. Muller, J. Gromoll, M. Simoni, Absence of exon 10 of the human luteinizing hormone (LH) receptor impairs LH, but not human chorionic gonadotropin action, J Clin Endocrinol Metab 88 (5) (2003) 2242–2249.

[268] G. Meduri, A. Bachelot, M.P. Cocca, C. Vasseur, P. Rodien, F. Kuttenn, et al., Molecular pathology of the FSH receptor: new insights into FSH physiology, Mol Cell Endocrinol 282 (1–2) (2008) 130–142.

[269] K. Aittomaki, J.L. Lucena, P. Pakarinen, P. Sistonen, J. Tapanainen, J. Gromoll, et al., Mutation in the follicle-stimulating hormone receptor gene causes hereditary hypergonadotropic ovarian failure, Cell 82 (6) (1995) 959–968.

[270] G. Meduri, P. Touraine, I. Beau, O. Lahuna, A. Desroches, M.C. Vacher-Lavenu, et al., Delayed puberty and primary amenorrhea associated with a novel mutation of the human follicle-stimulating hormone receptor: Clinical, histological, and molecular studies, J Clin Endocrinol Metab 88 (8) (2003) 3491–3498.

[271] E. Kousta, C.G. Hadjiathanasiou, G. Tolis, A. Papathanasiou, Pleiotropic genetic syndromes with developmental abnormalities associated with obesity, J Pediatr Endocrinol Metab 22 (7) (2009) 581–592.

[272] L.J. Andrade, R. Andrade, C.S. Franca, A.V. Bittencourt, Pigmentary retinopathy due to Bardet-Biedl syndrome: Case report and literature review, Arq Bras Oftalmol 72 (5) (2009) 694–696.

[273] F. Muscatelli, T.M. Strom, A.P. Walker, E. Zanaria, D. Recan, A. Meindl, et al., Mutations in the DAX-1 gene give rise to both X-linked adrenal hypoplasia congenita and hypogonadotropic hypogonadism, Nature 372 (6507) (1994) 672–676.

[274] A.K. Iyer, E.R. McCabe, Molecular mechanisms of DAX1 action, Mol Genet Metab 83 (1–2) (2004) 60–73.

[275] J.H. Liu, A.H. Bill, Stress-associated or functional hypothalamic amenorrhea in the adolescent, Ann NY Acad Sci 1135 (2008) 179–184.

[276] B. Meczekalski, A. Podfigurna-Stopa, A. Warenik-Szymankiewicz, A.R. Genazzani, Functional hypothalamic amenorrhea: Current view on neuroendocrine aberrations, Gynecol Endocrinol 24 (1) (2008) 4–11.

[277] R.B. Perkins, J.E. Hall, K.A. Martin, Neuroendocrine abnormalities in hypothalamic amenorrhea: Spectrum, stability, and response to neurotransmitter modulation, J Clin Endocrinol Metab 84 (6) (1999) 1905–1911.

[278] A.B. Loucks, J.F. Mortola, L. Girton, S.S. Yen, Alterations in the hypothalamic–pituitary–ovarian and the hypothalamic–pituitary–adrenal axes in athletic women, J Clin Endocrinol Metab 68 (2) (1989) 402–411.

[279] J.D. Veldhuis, W.S. Evans, L.M. Demers, M.O. Thorner, D. Wakat, A.D. Rogol, Altered neuroendocrine regulation of gonadotropin secretion in women distance runners, J Clin Endocrinol Metab 61 (3) (1985) 557–563.

[280] D.I. Spratt, P. Cox, J. Orav, J. Moloney, T. Bigos, Reproductive axis suppression in acute illness is related to disease severity, J Clin Endocrinol Metab 76 (6) (1993) 1548–1554.

[281] R.R. Kalyani, S. Gavini, A.S. Dobs, Male hypogonadism in systemic disease, Endocrinol Metab Clin North Am 36 (2) (2007) 333–348.

[282] T. Kelesidis, I. Kelesidis, S. Chou, C.S. Mantzoros, Narrative review: The role of leptin in human physiology: Emerging clinical applications, Ann Intern Med 152 (2) (2010) 93–100.

[283] J.M. Castellano, V.M. Navarro, R. Fernandez-Fernandez, R. Nogueiras, S. Tovar, J. Roa, et al., Changes in hypothalamic KiSS-1 system and restoration of pubertal activation of the reproductive axis by kisspeptin in undernutrition, Endocrinology 146 (9) (2005) 3917–3925.

[284] J.M. Castellano, J. Roa, R.M. Luque, C. Dieguez, E. Aguilar, L. Pinilla, et al., KiSS-1/kisspeptins and the metabolic control of reproduction: physiologic roles and putative physiopathological implications, Peptides 30 (1) (2009) 139–145.

[285] A. Crown, D.K. Clifton, R.A. Steiner, Neuropeptide signaling in the integration of metabolism and reproduction, Neuroendocrinology 86 (3) (2007) 175–182.

[286] J.W. Hill, J.K. Elmquist, C.F. Elias, Hypothalamic pathways linking energy balance and reproduction, Am J Physiol Endocrinol Metab 294 (5) (2008) E827–E832.

[287] S.T. Skarda, M.R. Burge, Prospective evaluation of risk factors for exercise-induced hypogonadism in male runners, West J Med 169 (1) (1998) 9–12.

[288] D.J. Handelsman, Hypothalamic–pituitary gonadal dysfunction in renal failure, dialysis and renal transplantation, Endocr Rev 6 (2) (1985) 151–182.

[289] A.S. Lewis, C.H. Courtney, A.B. Atkinson, All patients with "idiopathic" hypopituitarism should be screened for hemochromatosis, Pituitary 12 (3) (2009) 273–275.

[290] J. Chahal, J. Schlechte, Hyperprolactinemia, Pituitary 11 (2) (2008) 141–146.

[291] J.A. Schlechte, Clinical practice, Prolactinoma, N Engl J Med 349 (21) (2003) 2035–2041.

[292] G. Page-Wilson, P.C. Smith, C.K. Welt, Prolactin suppresses GnRH but not TSH secretion, Horm Res 65 (1) (2006) 31–38.

[293] J. Burgos, P. Cobos, N. Vidaurrazaga, B. Prieto, I. Ocerin, R. Matorras, Ovarian hyperstimulation secondary to ectopic secretion of follicle-stimulating hormone. Literature review prompted by a case, Fertil Steril 92 (3) (2009) 1168 e5–e8.

[294] R.K. Iles, Ectopic hCGbeta expression by epithelial cancer: Malignant behaviour, metastasis and inhibition of tumor cell apoptosis, Mol Cell Endocrinol 260–262 (2007) 264–270.

[295] E. Brignardello, R. Manti, M. Papotti, E. Allia, D. Campra, G. Isolato, et al., Ectopic secretion of LH by an endocrine pancreatic tumor, J Endocrinol Invest 27 (4) (2004) 361–365.

[296] G. Piaditis, A. Angellou, G. Kontogeorgos, N. Mazarakis, T. Kounadi, G. Kaltsas, et al., Ectopic bioactive luteinizing hormone secretion by a pancreatic endocrine tumor, manifested as luteinized granulosa-thecal cell tumor of the ovaries, J Clin Endocrinol Metab 90 (4) (2005) 2097–2103.

[297] J.C. Carel, E.A. Eugster, A. Rogol, L. Ghizzoni, M.R. Palmert, F. Antoniazzi, et al., Consensus statement on the use of gonadotropin-releasing hormone analogs in children, Pediatrics 123 (4) (2009) e752–e762.

[298] G. Teilmann, C.B. Pedersen, T.K. Jensen, N.E. Skakkebaek, A. Juul, Prevalence and incidence of precocious pubertal development in Denmark: An epidemiologic study based on national registries, Pediatrics 116 (6) (2005) 1323–1328.

[299] M.R. Palmert, P.A. Boepple, Variation in the timing of puberty: Clinical spectrum and genetic investigation, J Clin Endocrinol Metab 86 (6) (2001) 2364–2368.

[300] L. de Vries, A. Kauschansky, M. Shohat, M. Phillip, Familial central precocious puberty suggests autosomal dominant inheritance, J Clin Endocrinol Metab 89 (4) (2004) 1794–1800.

[301] Y.M. Chan, K.A. Fenoglio-Simeone, S. Paraschos, L. Muhammad, M.M. Troester, Y.T. Ng, et al., Central precocious puberty due to hypothalamic hamartomas correlates with anatomic features but not with expression of GnRH, TGFalpha, or KISS1, Horm Res Paediatr 73 (5) (2010) 312–319.

[302] S. Nimkarn, M.I. New, Prenatal diagnosis and treatment of congenital adrenal hyperplasia, Pediatr Endocrinol Rev 4 (2) (2006) 99–105.

[303] A.P. Themmen, J.W. Martens, H.G. Brunner, Gonadotropin receptor mutations, J Endocrinol 153 (2) (1997) 179–183.

[304] V.N. Brito, A.C. Latronico, I.J. Arnhold, B.B. Mendonca, Update on the etiology, diagnosis and therapeutic management of sexual precocity, Arq Bras Endocrinol Metabol 52 (1) (2008) 18–31.

[305] C. Lussiana, B. Guani, C. Mari, G. Restagno, M. Massobrio, A. Revelli, Mutations and polymorphisms of the FSH receptor (FSHR) gene: Clinical implications in female fecundity and molecular biology of FSHR protein and gene, Obstet Gynecol Surv 63 (12) (2008) 785–795.

[306] M. Haywood, N. Tymchenko, J. Spaliviero, A. Koch, M. Jimenez, J. Gromoll, et al., An activated human follicle-stimulating hormone (FSH) receptor stimulates FSH-like activity in gonadotropin-deficient transgenic mice, Mol Endocrinol 16 (11) (2002) 2582–2591.

[307] U.B. Kaiser, The pathogenesis of the ovarian hyperstimulation syndrome, N Engl J Med 349 (8) (2003) 729–732.

[308] G. Smits, O. Olatunbosun, A. Delbaere, R. Pierson, G. Vassart, S. Costagliola, Ovarian hyperstimulation syndrome due to a mutation in the follicle-stimulating hormone receptor, N Engl J Med 349 (8) (2003) 760–766.

[309] C. Vasseur, P. Rodien, I. Beau, A. Desroches, C. Gerard, L. de Poncheville, et al., A chorionic gonadotropin-sensitive mutation in the follicle-stimulating hormone receptor as a cause of familial gestational spontaneous ovarian hyperstimulation syndrome, N Engl J Med 349 (8) (2003) 753–759.

[310] D.A. Ehrmann, Polycystic ovary syndrome, N Engl J Med 352 (12) (2005) 1223–1236.

[311] R.J. Chang, The reproductive phenotype in polycystic ovary syndrome, Nat Clin Pract Endocrinol Metab 3 (10) (2007) 688–695.

[312] S.K. Blank, C.R. McCartney, J.C. Marshall, The origins and sequelae of abnormal neuroendocrine function in polycystic ovary syndrome, Hum Reprod Update 12 (4) (2006) 351–361.

[313] C.R. McCartney, K.A. Prendergast, S.K. Blank, K.D. Helm, S. Chhabra, J.C. Marshall, Maturation of luteinizing hormone (gonadotropin-releasing hormone) secretion across puberty: Evidence for altered regulation in obese peripubertal girls, J Clin Endocrinol Metab 94 (1) (2009) 56–66.

[314] K.G. Ewens, D.R. Stewart, W. Ankener, M. Urbanek, J.M. McAllister, C. Chen, et al., Family-based analysis of candidate genes for polycystic ovary syndrome, J Clin Endocrinol Metab 95 (5) (2010) 2306–2315.

[315] M. Zitzmann, Testosterone deficiency, insulin resistance and the metabolic syndrome, Nat Rev Endocrinol 5 (12) (2009) 673–681.

[316] M. Ludwig, K.J. Doody, K.M. Doody, Use of recombinant human chorionic gonadotropin in ovulation induction, Fertil Steril 79 (5) (2003) 1051–1059.

[317] S. Bhasin, Approach to the infertile man, J Clin Endocrinol Metab 92 (6) (2007) 1995–2004.

[318] D. Buchter, H.M. Behre, S. Kliesch, E. Nieschlag, Pulsatile GnRH or human chorionic gonadotropin/human menopausal gonadotropin as effective treatment for men with hypogonadotropic hypogonadism: A review of 42 cases, Eur J Endocrinol 139 (3) (1998) 298–303.

[319] K.A. Martin, J.E. Hall, J.M. Adams, W.F. Crowley Jr., Comparison of exogenous gonadotropins and pulsatile gonadotropin-releasing hormone for induction of ovulation in hypogonadotropic amenorrhea, J Clin Endocrinol Metab 77 (1) (1993) 125–129.

[320] B.H. Vickery, Comparison of the potential for therapeutic utilities with gonadotropin-releasing hormone agonists and antagonists, Endocr Rev 7 (1) (1986) 115–124.

[321] A.R. Hoffman, W.F. Crowley Jr., Induction of puberty in men by long-term pulsatile administration of low-dose gonadotropin-releasing hormone, N Engl J Med 307 (20) (1982) 1237–1241.

[322] R.W. Whitcomb, W.F. Crowley Jr., Clinical review 4: Diagnosis and treatment of isolated gonadotropin-releasing hormone deficiency in men, J Clin Endocrinol Metab 70 (1) (1990) 3–7.

[323] R.P. Millar, Z.L. Lu, A.J. Pawson, C.A. Flanagan, K. Morgan, S.R. Maudsley, Gonadotropin-releasing hormone receptors, Endocr Rev 25 (2) (2004) 235–275.

[324] M.J. Karten, J.E. Rivier, Gonadotropin-releasing hormone analog design. Structure-function studies toward the development of agonists and antagonists: Rationale and perspective, Endocr Rev 7 (1) (1986) 44–66.

[325] C. Hayden, GnRH analogues: Applications in assisted reproductive techniques, Eur J Endocrinol 159 (Suppl. 1) (2008) S17–S25.

[326] I. Huhtaniemi, R. White, C.A. McArdle, B.E. Persson, Will GnRH antagonists improve prostate cancer treatment? Trends Endocrinol Metab 20 (1) (2009) 43–50.

[327] L.C. Layman, Genetics of human hypogonadotropic hypogonadism, Am J Med Genet 89 (4) (1999) 240–248.

[328] I. Huhtaniemi, M. Alevizaki, Mutations along the hypothalamic–pituitary–gonadal axis affecting male reproduction, Reprod Biomed Online 15 (6) (2007) 622–632.

CHAPTER

8

The Posterior Pituitary

Daniel G. Bichet

Université de Montréal, Hôpital du Sacré-Coeur de Montréal, Montréal (Québec), Canada

STRUCTURE OF THE NEUROHYPOPHYSIS: ANATOMY AND ELECTROPHYSIOLOGY OF VASOPRESSIN-PRODUCING CELLS

The hypothalamus, which is located at the anterior end of the diencephalon (Figure 8.1A), embodies a group of nuclei that form the floor and ventrolateral walls of the triangular-shaped third ventricle. A thin membrane called the lamina terminalis forms the anterior wall of this compartment and is believed to contain osmoreceptor cells in a structure known as the organum vasculosum. The subfornical organ (SFO) is also believed to contain these cells. The organum vasculosum of the lamina terminalis (OVLT), the SFO and the pituitary gland lack a blood–brain barrier. The supraoptic nucleus (SON) lies just dorsal to the optic chiasm and approximately 2 mm from the third ventricle. The paraventricular nucleus (PVN) lies closer to the thalamus in the suprachiasmatic portion of the hypothalamus, but it borders on the third ventricular space. These well-defined nuclei contain the majority of the large neuroendocrine cell bodies, known as the magnocellular or neurosecretory cells, that manufacture arginine-vasopressin and oxytocin [1].

The neurohypophysis consists of: (1) a set of hypothalamic nuclei, namely the SON and PVN which house the perikarya of the magnocellular neurons; (2) the axonal processes of the magnocellular neurons form the supraoptical hypophyseal tract; and (3) the neurosecretory material of these neurons which is carried on to the posterior pituitary gland (see Figure 8.1B). Immunocytochemical and radioimmunological studies have demonstrated that oxytocin and vasopressin are synthesized in separate populations of the supraoptic nuclei and the PVN neurons whose central and vascular projections have been described in great detail [2]. Some cells express the *AVP* gene and other cells express the *OXT* gene (see below). Immunohistochemical studies have revealed a second vasopressin neurosecretory pathway that transports high concentrations of the hormone to the anterior pituitary gland from parvocellular neurons to the hypophyseal portal system. In the portal system, the high concentration of AVP acts synergistically with corticotropin-releasing hormone (CRH) to stimulate adrenocorticotropin (ACTH) release from the anterior pituitary. More than half of the parvocellular neurons co-express both *CRH* and *AVP.* In addition, while passing through the median eminence and the hypophyseal stalk, magnocellular axons can also release arginine-vasopressin into the long portal system. Furthermore, a number of neuroanatomical studies have shown the existence of short portal vessels that allow communication between the posterior and anterior pituitary. Thus, in addition to parvocellular vasopressin, magnocellular vasopressin is able to influence ACTH secretion [3,4]. Other parvocellular neurons have been described, but their function is unknown or insufficiently characterized.

Oxytocin- and vasopressin-secreting cells can also be differentiated by their specific electrophysiological properties [5,6]. For example, in anesthetized lactating rats with suckling pups, oxytocin-secreting neurons are recognized by a slow irregular or continuous background firing which is interrupted every few minutes by a synchronous brief (1–2 seconds) high-frequency (50–80 Hz) burst of activity that causes oxytocin release and milk ejection. Vasopressin-secreting neurons are characterized by a unique phasic discharge pattern during activation by both osmotic stimuli and hemorrhage. In terms of their osmosensitivity, an elevation in the osmotic plasma pressure causes an increase in firing in both oxytocin- and vasopressin-secreting cells, but the firing is characteristically phasic in the vasopressin-secreting cells [5].

The Pituitary, Third Edition, DOI: 10.1016/B978-0-12-380926-1.10008-2

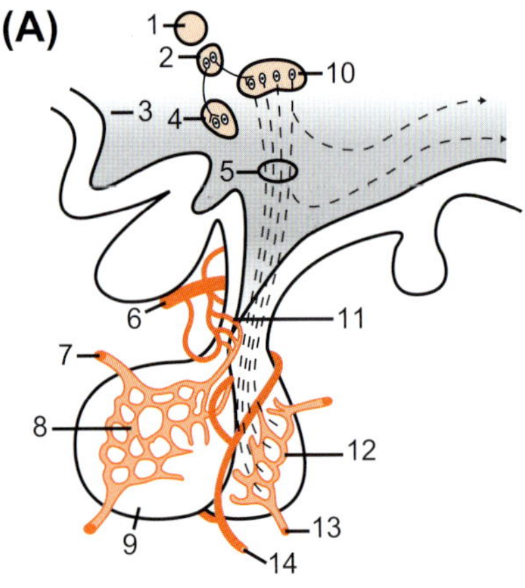

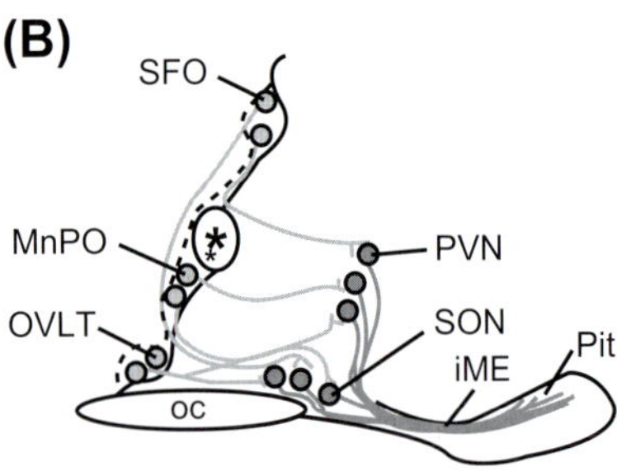

FIGURE 8.1 **A** Schematic representation of hypothalamus, posterior pituitary and surrounding structures. (1) Thirst center; (2) osmoreceptor; (3) lamina terminalis; (4) supraoptic nuclei; (5) supraopticohypophyseal tract; (6) superior hypophyseal artery; (7) vein to dural sinuses; (8) secondary capillary plexus; (9) anterior lobe hypophysis; (10) paraventricular nucleus; (11) sinusoids; (12) neurohypophysis; (13) vein to dural sinuses; (14) inferior hypophyseal artery **B** Schematic representation of the osmoregulatory pathway of the hypothalamus (sagittal section of midline of ventral brain around the third ventricle in mice). Neurons (lightly filled circles) in the lamina terminalis (OVLT), median preoptic nucleus (MnPO) and subfornical organ (SFO) – that are responsive to plasma hyptertonicity send efferent axonal projections (gray lines) to magnocellular neurons of the paraventricular (PVN) and supraoptic nuclei (SON). The OVLT is one of the brain circumventricular organs and is a key osmosensing site in the mammalian brain (see above). The processes (dark lines) of these magnocellular neurons form the hypothalamo–neurohypophyseal pathway that courses in the median eminence to reach the posterior pituitary, where neurosecretion of vasopressin and oxytocin occurs. *Modified from Wilson et al., 2002 [1] with permission, copyright (2002), National Academy of Sciences USA.*

THE VASOPRESSIN AND OXYTOCIN GENES

Homologues of vasopressin and oxytocin have evolved over 700 million years and have been identified in insects to vertebrates [7,8]. The *cis* and *trans* components important for vasopressin and oxytocin expression in magnocellular neurons have been conserved over 450 million years in the pufferfish isotocin and rat oxytocin genes [9,10]. Among these distant taxa (hydra, worms, insects and vertebrates), oxytocin and vasopressin-related peptides also play a general role in the modulation of social and reproductive behavior [7]. In contrast to this apparent conservation of function, the specific behaviors affected by these neuropeptides are notably species-specific [7].

Gene Structure

AVP and its corresponding carrier protein, neurophysin II, are synthesized as a composite precursor by the magnocellular and parvocellular neurons described previously. The precursor is packaged into neurosecretory granules and transported axonally in the stalk of the posterior pituitary (Figure 8.2) [11]. On route to the neurohypophysis, the precursor is processed into the active hormone (Figure 8.3). Prepro-vasopressin has 164 amino acids and is encoded by the 2.5 kb *AVP* gene located in chromosome region 20p13 [12]. The *AVP* gene (coding for AVP and neurophysin II) and the *OXT* gene (coding for oxytocin and neurophysin I) are located in the same chromosome region, at a very short distance from each other (12 kb in humans) in head-to-head orientation. Data from transgenic mouse studies indicate that the intergenic region between the *OXT* and the *AVP* genes contains the critical enhancer sites for cell-specific expression in the magnocellular neurons [11]. It is phylogenetically interesting to note that *cis* and *trans* components of this specific cellular expression have been conserved between the *Fugu* isotocin (the homologue of mammalian oxytocin) and rat oxytocin genes [9]. Exon 1 of the *AVP* gene encodes the signal peptide, AVP, and the NH_2-terminal region of NPII. Exon 2 encodes the central region of NPII, and exon 3 encodes the COOH-terminal region of NPII and the glycopeptide. Provasopressin is generated by the removal of the signal peptide from prepro-vasopressin and the addition of a carbohydrate chain to the glycopeptide. Additional post-translation processing occurs within neurosecretory vesicles during transport of the precursor protein to axon terminals in the posterior pituitary, yielding AVP, NPII and glycopeptide. The AVP–NPII complex forms tetramers that can self-associate to form higher oligomers [13].

In the posterior pituitary, AVP is stored in vesicles. Exocytotic release is stimulated by minute increases in serum osmolality (hypernatremia, osmotic regulation) and by more pronounced decreases in extracellular fluid (hypovolemia, nonosmotic regulation). Oxytocin and neurophysin I are released from the posterior pituitary by the suckling response in lactating females. The neuropeptides oxytocin and vasopressin are involved in new fascinating studies of the neurobiology of attachment [14], and central vasopressin and oxytocin receptors may regulate the autonomic expression of fear [15].

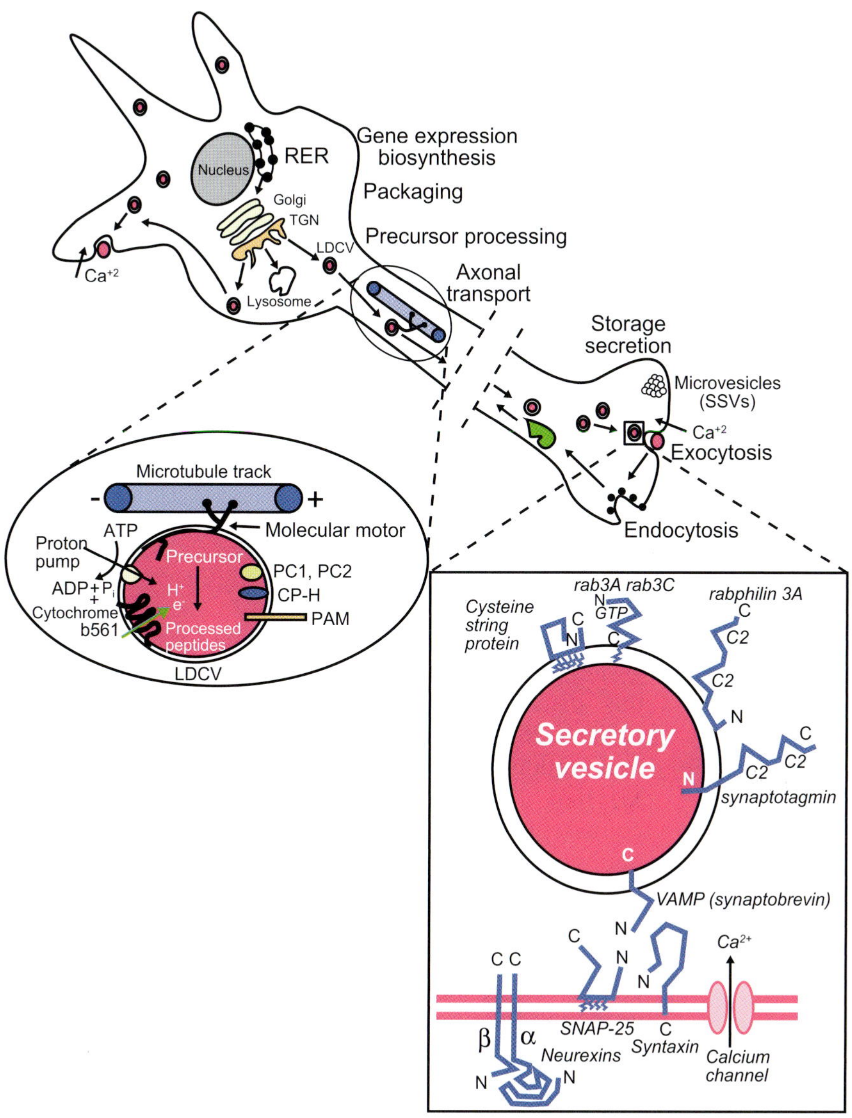

FIGURE 8.2 Peptidergic neuron. Cellular and molecular properties of a peptidergic neuron (neurosecretory cell) are shown. The structure of the neurosecretory cell is depicted schematically with notations of the various cell biological processes that occur in each topographic domain. Gene expression, protein biosynthesis and packaging of the protein into large dense core vesicles (LDCVs) in the cell body, where the nucleus, rough endoplasmic reticulum (RER) and Golgi apparatus are located. Enzymatic processing of the precursor proteins into the biologically active peptides occurs primarily in the LDCVS (see inset), often during the process of anterograde axonal transport of the LDCVS to the nerve terminals on microtubule tracks in the axon. Upon reaching the nerve terminal, the LDCVS are usually stored in preparation for secretion. Conduction of a nerve impulse (action potential) down the axon and its arrival in the nerve terminal causes an influx of calcium ions through calcium channels. The increased calcium ion concentration causes a cascade of molecular events that leads to neurosecretion (exocytosis). Recovery of the excess LDCV membrane after exocytosis is performed by endocytosis, but this membrane is not recycled locally and instead is retrogradely transported to the cell body for reuse or degradation in lysosomes. TGN, trans-Golgi network; SSV, small secretory vesicles; PC1 or PC2, prohormone convertase 1 or 2, respectively; CP-H, carboxypeptidase H; PAM, peptiylglycine-amidating monooxygenase. *From Gainer & Chin [305], Springer; and as adapted in Burbach et al [11], The American Physiological Society, used with permission.*

Expression of the Vasopressin Gene in Diabetes Insipidus Rats (Brattleboro Rats)

The animal model of diabetes insipidus that has been most extensively studied is the Brattleboro rat. Discovered in 1961, the rat lacks vasopressin and its neurophysin, whereas the synthesis of the structurally related hormone oxytocin is not affected by the mutation [16]. Its inability to synthesize vasopressin is inherited as an autosomal semirecessive trait. Schmale and Richter [17] isolated and sequenced the vasopressin gene from homozygous Brattleboro rats, and found that the defect is due to a single nucleotide deletion of a G residue within the second exon encoding the carrier protein neurophysin. The shift in the reading frame caused by this deletion predicts a precursor with an entirely different C terminus (Figure 8.4). The messenger RNA (mRNA) produced by the mutated gene encodes a normal AVP but an abnormal NPII moiety [17] which impairs transport and processing of the AVP-NPII precursor and its retention in the endoplasmic reticulum of the magnocellular neurons where it is produced [18,19]. Homozygous Brattleboro rats may still demonstrate some V2 (see below) antidiuretic effects since the administration of a selective nonpeptide V2 antagonist (SR 121463A, 10 mg/kg i.p.) induced a further increase in urine flow rate (200–354 ± 42 ml/24 h) and a decline in urinary osmolality (170 to 92 ± 8 mmol/kg) [20]. This decline in urine osmolality following the administration of a nonpeptide V2r antagonist could also be secondary to the "inverse agonist" properties of SR121463A: the intrinsic activity, or "tone," of the V2R would be deactivated by the SR121463A compound (for the inverse agonist properties of SR121463A see [21]). There is also

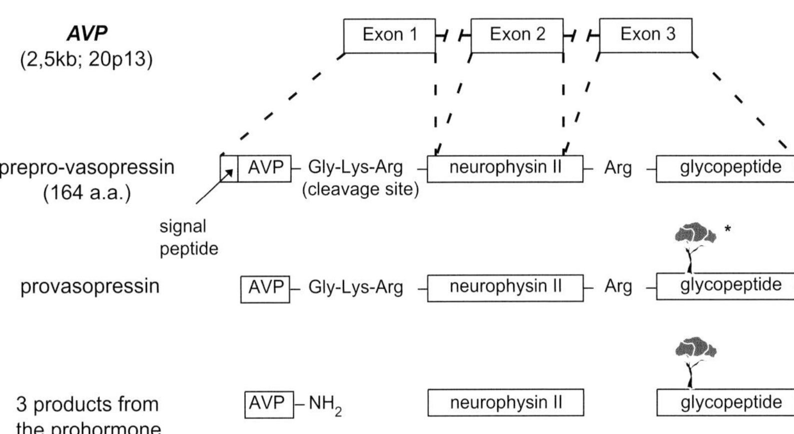

FIGURE 8.3 Cascade of vasopressin biosynthesis. SP, signal peptide; AVP, arginine-vasopressin; NP, neurophysin; GP, glycoprotein. *From Richter and Schmale [300]. See also [300].*

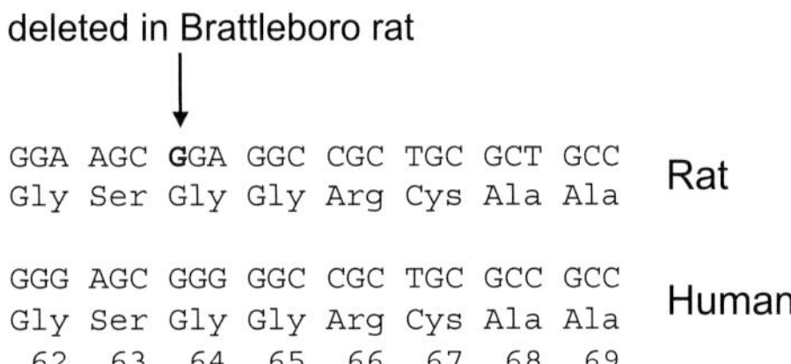

FIGURE 8.4 Neurophysin II genomic and amino acid sequence showing the 1 bp (G) deleted in the Brattleboro rat. The human sequence (GenBank entry M11166) is also shown. It is almost identical to the rat prepro sequence. In the Brattleboro rat, G1880 is deleted with a resultant frameshift after 63 amino acids (amino acid 1 is the first amino acid of neurophysin II).

an alternative explanation to this relatively high urine osmolality of 170 since, in Brattleboro rats, low levels of hormonally active AVP are produced from alternate forms of AVP pre-prohormone. Due to a process called molecular misreading, one transcript contains a 2 bp deletion downstream from the single nucleotide deletion that restores the reading frame and produces a variant AVP pre-prohormone that is smaller in length by one amino acid and differs from the normal product by only 13 amino acids in the neurophysin II moiety [22]. Oxytocin, which is present at enhanced plasma concentrations in Brattleboro rats, may be responsible for the antidiuretic activity observed [23,24]. Oxytocin is not stimulated by increased plasma osmolality in humans.

Expression of the Vasopressin Gene in Autosomal Dominant and Autosomal Recessive Diabetes Insipidus in Humans

Repaske et al. reported in 1990 [25] that the genetic locus for autosomal dominant central diabetes insipidus was within or near the gene encoding for AVP and suggested that a defective *AVP* gene might be the basis for this disease. Neurogenic diabetes insipidus (OMIM 125700) [26] is a now well characterized entity, secondary to mutations in the *AVP* gene (OMIM 192340; GenBank: M11166). This disorder is also referred to as central, cranial, pituitary, or more commonly, familial neurohypophyseal diabetes insipidus (FNDI). Patients with autosomal dominant FNDI retain some limited capacity to secrete AVP, and the polyuro–polydipsic symptoms usually appear after the first year of life, but there is considerable variation in age-of-onset. Over 50 *AVP* mutations segregating with autosomal neurogenic diabetes insipidus have been described [27,28]. The majority are dominant, but one recessive and one sequence variation have been reported to date [27,29,30]. The majority of mutations are located in the neurophysin (NP) II domain (codons 32–124), a region important for protein folding and sorting (see Figure 8.3) [31]. Transfection studies in mouse neuroblastoma Neuro 2A cells support that the mechanism(s) by which a dominant mutant allele causes neurogenic diabetes insipidus is a result of the accumulation of arginine-vasopressin fibrillar aggregates within the endoplasmic reticulum, a so-called toxic gain-of-function [28,30,32–35]. This process is mechanistically similar to that seen in other neurodegenerative diseases such as Huntington's and Parkinson's diseases [35]. Although the handling of misfolded AVP mutants could account for the delayed onset and progressive nature of dominant FNDI, the precise mechanism of magnocellular toxicity is still unknown [28]. An extremely rare form of FNDI is recessively inherited where the symptoms appear in infancy. Here, one mutation in the AVP gene has been reported to date in four families [29,36,37]. Comparative expression studies in

Neuro2A cells show that whereas dominant forms accumulate in the cytoplasm, recessive forms localize to the secretory granules at the tips of the cellular projections [32]. Moreover, in contrast to the dominant AVP mutants, it appears that recessive mutants do not exert progressive neurocytotoxicity.

Diabetes insipidus of nephrogenic origin (NDI) while rare, occurs more frequently than FNDI. Here, the disease results from the kidney's inability to use available AVP, and is associated with mutations in AVPR2 or in AQP2. In contrast to FNDI, the polyuro–polydipsic symptoms are present during the first week of life. Although errors in protein folding also represent the underlying basis for *AVPR2* and *AQP2* mutants responsible for NDI, the pathogenic mechanism is clearly different from FNDI. *AVPR2* missense mutations lead to the rapid degradation of the affected polypeptide but not to the accumulation of toxic aggregates, since the other important functions of the principal cells of the collecting ducts (where AVPR2 is expressed) are unaffected.

CHEMISTRY, PROCESSING AND METABOLISM OF AVP

AVP is a nonapeptide with a molecular weight of 1084 Da. The chemical structure of AVP and related peptides is given in Table 8.1 and Figure 8.5. It is a strongly basic molecule (isoelectric point pH 10.9) due to the amidation of three carboxyl groups. Lysine-vasopressin, the antidiuretic hormone of the pig family, has the less basic amino acid lysine at position 8, resulting in a lower isoelectric point (pH 10.0). Biological activity of these hormones is destroyed by oxidation or reduction of the disulfide bond [38,39].

Members of the vasopressin hormone family have been detected throughout the animal kingdom [40], comprising more than half a dozen variants including peptides such as vasotocin of nonmammalian vertebrates, the diuretic hormone of insects and the conopressins of mollusks. In vertebrates, their endocrine hormonal activity – controlling mainly water retention – is well documented, whereas in invertebrates, they may function primarily as neurotransmitters, although a hormonal diuretic activity has been demonstrated in the locust [41]. Acher and Chauvet [40] postulated the existence of a single ancestral peptide that developed along two evolutionary lines, one vasotocin-vasopressin and the other isotocin-mesotocin-oxytocin. However, recent evidence suggests that multiple genes, which code for numerous vasopressin-like hormones, are present in Australian macropods.

Neurophysins were first thought to be carrier-proteins for vasopressin and oxytocin. It is now recognized that NPI (for oxytocin) and NPII (for vasopressin) belong to the precursor of the respective hormone (see above section on the vasopressin and the oxytocin gene). After synthesis in the hypothalamic neurons, the vasopressin precursor migrates along the neuronal axons, many of which terminate in the posterior pituitary. The time from synthesis to release of the hormone into the systemic circulation is about 1.5 hours [42]. Pulse chase experiments indicate that cleavage occurs continuously during axonal transport [43], but both cleaved and uncleaved precursors [44] are present in the neurosecretory granules of the posterior pituitary. Only a small percentage of the synthetic peptide is released; some of the vasopressin-containing neurosecretory granules move away from the nerve endings and are unavailable for release. Once secreted into the circulation, vasopressin is accompanied, but not bound,

TABLE 8.1 Amino Acid Sequence of Arginine-vasopressin and Related Neurohypophyseal Nonapeptides*

	1 2 3 4 5		6 7 8 9	Distribution
Arginine-vasopressin	**Cys-Tyr-Phe-Glu(NH_2)-Asp(NH_2)-Cys-Pro-Arg-Gly(NH_2)**			**Most Mammals**
Lysine vasopressin	Phe	Glu(NH_2)	Lys	Pig family
Arginine vasotocin	lle	Glu(NH_2)	Arg	Nonmammalian vertebrates
Oxytocin	lle	Glu(NH_2)	Leu	Mammals, birds
Mesotocin	lle	Glu(NH_2)	lle	Reptiles
Isotocin	lle	Ser	lle	Fish
Glumitocin	lle	Ser	Glu(NH_2)	Fish
Valitocin	lle	Glu(NH_2)	Val	Fish
Aspartocin	lle	Asp(NH_2)	Leu	Fish

* *From Baylis [308], with permission.*

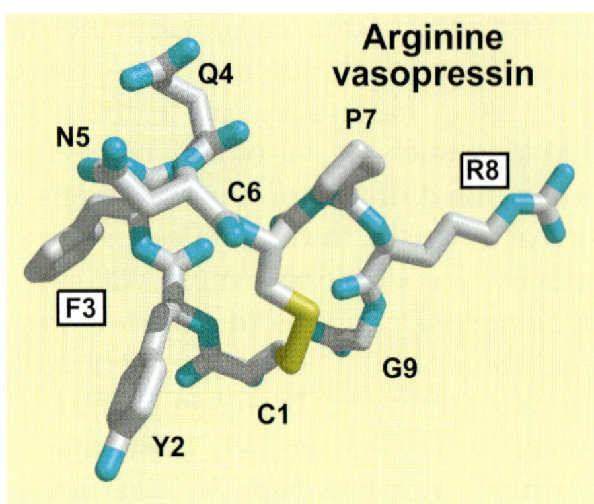

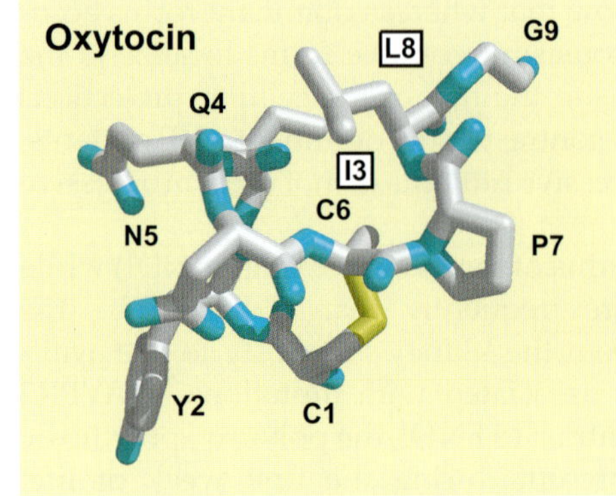

FIGURE 8.5 Contrasting structure of arginine-vasopressin (AVP) and oxytocin (OT). The peptides differ only by two amino acids F3 → I3 and R8 → L8 in AVP and OT, respectively. The conformation of AVP was obtained from [172] and the conformation of OT was obtained from the Protein Data Bank (PDB Id 1XY1). Note, for both hormones the formation of a disulfide bond between Cys residues at the 1 and 6 positions result in a peptide constituted of a 6-amino acid cyclic part and a 3-amino acid C-terminal part.

by its specific neurophysin. Neurophysins themselves do not appear to have any biological activity, but since they are synthesized and released with vasopressin and oxytocin, their concentrations in the plasma reflect any changes in the release of the active hormones (see below). The plasma half life of vasopressin is short, being about 5–15 minutes. Clearance is independent of plasma vasopressin concentration as it involves a liver- and kidney-dependent process. Vasopressin is not protein-bound, but large quantities of vasopressin are associated with the platelets in man [45] and dogs [46]. Platelet-rich plasma AVP concentrations are approximately five- to six-fold higher than those of platelet-depleted plasma. Furthermore, irreversible platelet aggregation could bring about intraplatelet AVP release [47]. However, osmotic stimulation of AVP release does not influence platelet-associated AVP concentrations [45].

CENTRAL NERVOUS SYSTEM MEDIATORS OF VASOPRESSIN AND OXYTOCIN RELEASE

Neurohypophyseal neurons receive an abundance of afferent connections and it is not surprising that a number of putative chemical mediators within the central nervous system have been shown to influence vasopressin and oxytocin release (for review, see [6]) (Table 8.2). The magnocellular neurons of the SON and PVN receive a dense noradrenergic innervation from the A_1 neurons in the ventrolateral medulla [48]. It has been shown that micromolar concentrations of norepinephrine and α agonists induce a dose-dependent release of vasopressin from perfused rat hypothalamic explants in vivo [49]. In particular, micromolar concentrations of norepinephrine and α agonists have been shown to evoke excitations, whereas norepinephrine and β agonists applied in millimolar concentrations evoke a reduction in the excitability of SON neurons [50]. Dopaminergic fibers innervate SON and PVN from the diencephalic A_{11}–A_{14} cell groups and may increase the activity of oxytocinergic neurons. Furthermore, endogenous cholinergic input to neurosecretory neurons may arise from cells located in the lateral hypothalamus [51]. In addition, the liaison between the subfornical organ (an osmoreceptor-sensing mechanism) and the SON and PVN may involve endogenous angiotensin II-immunoreactive pathways [52]. Finally, the presence of endogenous opioid peptides [53] and opioid receptors [54] in the neural lobe has led to the suggestion

TABLE 8.2 Putative Mediators of Arginine Vasopressin (AVP) Secretion*

Biogenic monoamines	Norepinephrine
	Dopamine
	Acetylcholine
	Serotonine
	γ-Aminobutyric acid (GABA)
	Glycine
	Histamine
Peptides	Angiotensin II
	Endogenous opioids
	Cholecystokinin (CCK)
	Substance P
	AVP
Others	NO
	Prostaglandins
	Electrolytes (potassium, calcium)

* *Adapted from Sklar and Schrier [309].*

that opioid peptides play a role in the release of neurohypophyseal hormones (see below, inhibition of vasopressin release by kappa agonists).

CONTROL OF AVP SECRETION

Osmotic Stimulation

Central mechanisms of osmosensation and systemic osmoregulation have recently been reviewed by Bourque [6]. Vasopressin release can be regulated by changes in either osmolality or cerebrospinal fluid (CSF) Na concentration. Mammals are osmoregulators; they have evolved mechanisms that maintain ECF osmolality near a stable value. Yet, although mammals strive to maintain a constant ECF osmolality, values measured in an individual can fluctuate around the set-point owing to intermittent changes in the rates of water intake and water loss (through evaporation or diuresis), and to variations in the rates of Na intake and excretion (natriuresis). In humans, for example, 40 minutes of strenuous exercise in the heat [55,56], or 24 hours of water deprivation [57], causes plasma osmolality to rise by more than 10 mosmol kg^{-1}. In a dehydrated individual, drinking the equivalent of two large glasses of water (~850 ml) lowers osmolality by approximately 6 mosmol kg^{-1} within 30 minutes [58]. Similarly, ingestion of 13 g of salt increases plasma osmolality by approximately 5 mosmol kg^{-1} within 30 minutes [59]. Although osmotic perturbations larger than these can be deleterious to health, changes in the 1–3% range play an integral part in the control of body-fluid homeostasis. Differences between the ECF osmolality and the desired set-point induce proportional homeostatic responses according to the principle of negative feedback [6]. ECF hyperosmolality stimulates the sensation of thirst, to promote water intake and the release of vasopressin to enhance water reabsorption in the kidney. By contrast, ECF hypo-osmolality suppresses basal VP secretion in rats and humans [60].

Osmoreceptors in the Brain and the Periphery

As summarized elegantly by Bourque [6] early studies provided clear evidence that "cellular dehydration" (that is, cell shrinking) was required for thirst and VP release to be stimulated during ECF hyperosmolality; these responses could be induced by infusions of concentrated solutions containing membrane-impermeable solutes, which extract water from cells, but not by infusions of solutes that readily equilibrate across the cell membrane (such as urea). Verney coined the term osmoreceptor to designate the specialized sensory elements. He further showed that these were present in the brain and postulated that they might comprise "tiny osmometers" and "stretch receptors" that would allow osmotic stimuli to be "transmuted into electrical" signals [61]. Osmoreceptors are therefore defined functionally as neurons that are endowed with an intrinsic ability to detect changes in ECF osmolality, and it is now known that both cerebral and peripheral osmoreceptors contribute to the body-fluid balance.

Peripheral Osmoreceptors

Experiments in animals and humans have indicated that there are peripheral osmoreceptors along the upper regions of the alimentary tract and in the blood vessels that collect solutes absorbed from the intestines. Specifically, such receptors are located in the oropharyngeal cavity [62], the gastrointestinal tract [59], the splanchnic mesentery [63], the hepatic portal vein and the liver. Osmoreceptors in these areas can therefore detect the osmotic strength of ingested materials and, through afferent connections to the CNS, induce anticipatory responses that might buffer the potential impact of ingestion-related osmotic perturbations. Indeed, water intake causes satiety in thirsty humans and animals before ECF hyperosmolality is fully corrected [64,65]. Similarly, gastric water loading has been shown to lower osmotically stimulated VP release long before any detectable reduction in ECF osmolality is observed [66]. The molecular and cellular structure of peripheral osmoreceptors is unknown. However, the information that they collect has been shown to reach the CNS through fibers that ascend in the vagus nerve [66,67].

Central Osmoreceptors

The primary cerebral osmoreceptors that modulate thirst and VP release are located in regions of the brain that are devoid of a blood–brain barrier such as the circumventricular organs [68]. The anterior ventral region of the third ventricle encloses the organum vasculosum laminae terminalis (OVLT), one of the brain's circumventricular organs [68]. The OVLT has therefore been proposed to serve as one of the key osmosensing sites in the mammalian brain [69]. In agreement with this hypothesis, functional MRI studies have shown that the anterior region of the third ventricle becomes activated during the onset of ECF hypertonicity in animals [70] and humans [64,71]. Neurons in the OVLT [72] and in the subfornical organ [73], as well as magnocellular neurosecretory cells (MNCs), i.e., the neuroendocrine cells manufacturing vasopressin itself, in the supraoptic nucleus (SON) [74,75] can operate as intrinsic osmoreceptors. Recordings in hypothalamic slices or explants have shown that hyperosmotic stimuli increase the firing rate in MNCs by depolarizing the membrane potential [76], and that this effect is caused by the activation of a nonselective cation current [77,78]. Conversely, hypo-osmotic stimuli inhibit firing by hyperpolarizing the membrane potential, an effect that is caused by the inhibition of a cation conductance that is active under resting conditions (Figure 8.6) [75,79]. MNCs encode dynamic changes in ECF osmolality through proportional changes in the probability of opening of nonselective cation channels [75,79].

This nonselective cation channel is likely a transient receptor potential vannilloid channel (TRPV) type 1 splice variant since magnocellular neurons in Trpv1$^{-/-}$ mice were not depolarized by hyperosmolality and showed blunted vasopressin release in response to hyperosmotic stimulation (Figure 8.7A) [80]. Bourque's group also demonstrated that this Trpv1 variant was also necessary to the anticipated vasopressin secretion associated with hyperthermia (Figure 8.7B) [81]. In summary, magnocellular neurons and thirst neurons express a variant of TRPV1 involved in tonicity, mainly hypertonicity, and thermic perception. Systemic hypotonicity is perceived by cells of the blood–brain barrier-deficient nuclei of the lamina terminalis, including those of the subfornical organ, organum vasculosum of the lamina terminalis and median preoptic nucleus, and the cation channel TRPV4 mediates this response [82,83].

Osmotic Threshold: Sensitivity or Gain of the Osmoreceptor/arginine-vasopressin Releasing Unit

The level of plasma osmolality at which hydrated subjects first responded to an intravenous infusion of 5% saline with a statistically significant fall in free water clearance (without a fall in osmolal clearance or creatinine excretion) was termed the osmotic threshold for vasopressin release [84]. This osmotic threshold, which was determined to be 288.5 mosm/kg [85], was raised by the administration of hydrocortisone [84] and plasma volume expansion [86] and lowered by plasma volume contraction [87].

With the development of sensitive radioimmunoassays, it was later demonstrated that, in healthy adults, the infusion of concentrated saline (850 mmol/L) caused a progressive rise in plasma osmolality and in plasma AVP concentrations [88–91]. A direct correlation between the two variables was established, defined by the function: pAVP = 0.30 (Posm − 280) (Figure 8.8). The abscissal intercept, 280 mmol/kg, is the osmotic threshold. Because this intercept falls below the limit of detection of the assay methods, this "set" of the osmoreceptor mechanism should be referred to as the theoretical threshold for vasopressin release. Whether AVP secretion can be completely suppressed or whether a linear versus an exponential model should be used remains unclear [91,92]. A close relationship has also been demonstrated between urine osmolality and AVP concentrations except in patients with nephrogenic diabetes insipidus (Figure 8.8). The exquisite sensitivity and gain of the osmoreceptor–AVP–renal reflex is given by the following example (Figure 8.9). A normally hydrated man may have a plasma osmolality of 287 mmol/kg, a plasma vasopressin concentration of 2 pg/ml and a urinary osmolality of 500 mmol/kg. With an increase of 1% in total body water, plasma osmolality will fall by 1% (2.8 mmol/kg), plasma AVP will decrease to 1 pg/ml and urinary osmolality will diminish to 250 mmol/kg. Similarly, it is only necessary to increase total body water by 2% to suppress the plasma AVP maximally (<0.25 pg/ml) and to maximally dilute the urine (<100 mmol/kg). In the opposite direction, a 2% decrease in total body water will increase plasma osmolality by 2% (5.6 mmol/kg), plasma AVP will rise from 2 to 4 pg/ml and urine will be maximally concentrated (>1000 mmol/kg). Thus, in the context of these sensitivity changes, a 1 mmol rise in plasma osmolality would be expected to increase plasma AVP by

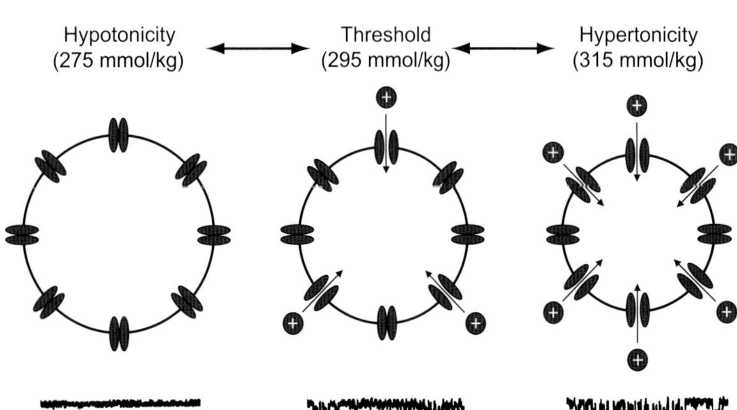

FIGURE 8.6 Stretch inactivated (SI) cationic channels transduce osmoreception. Under resting osmotic conditions (middle panel) a portion of the SI cationic channels is active and allows the influx of positive charge (diagram). Hypotonic stimulation (left) provokes cell swelling and inhibits channel activity, thereby hyperpolarizing the cell. In contrast, hypertonic stimulation (right) causes cell shrinkage. Activation of an increased number of channels under this condition augments charge influx and results in membrane depolarization. Traces representing changes in the activity of a single SI channel are shown below. *From Bourque and Oliet [301] with permission, Annual Reviews, Inc.*

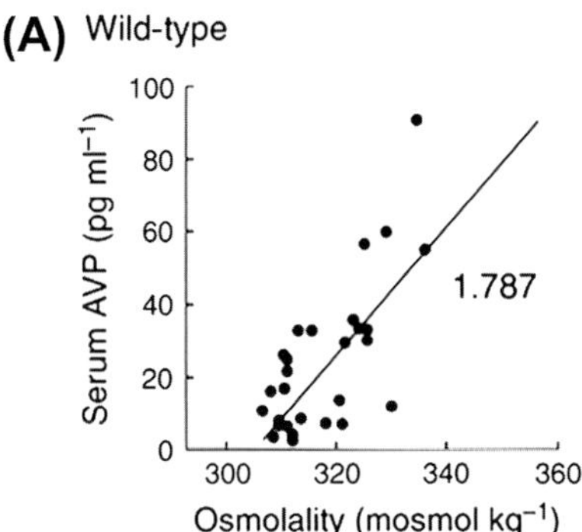

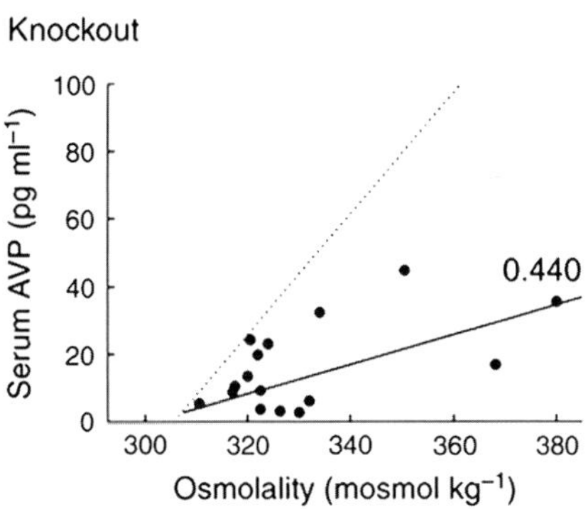

FIGURE 8.7A Trpv1$^{-/-}$ mice show defects in systemic osmoregulation. Linear regression analysis of the relation between serum AVP concentration and serum osmolality in wild-type and Trpv1$^{-/-}$ mice. In each case, mice were allowed to drink either water or 2% NaCl for 0–48 h and then were sampled in order to examine the effects of a systemic osmotic stimulus. Numbers on each graph show the slope of the best linear fit. The dotted line in the right graph repeats the regression observed in wild-type mice. *From Sharif-Naeini et al [80] with permission, Nature Publishing Group.*

0.38 pg/ml and urinary osmolality by 100 mmol/kg. Such a small change in plasma osmolality (measured by freezing point depression) or plasma AVP (by radioimmunoassay) may be undetectable yet of extreme physiological importance. For example, a patient with a 24-hour urinary solute load of 600 mmol must excrete 6 liters of urine with an osmolality of 100 mmol/kg to eliminate the solute; however, if the urine osmolality increases from 100 to 200 mmol/kg (due to an undetectable rise of 1 mmol in plasma osmolality and 0.38 pg/ml in plasma AVP), the obligatory 24-hour urine volume to excrete the 600 mmol solute load decreases substantially from 6 to 3 liters. Examination of Figure 8.9 demonstrates that a maximal antidiuresis is obtained when the plasma AVP concentration reaches 5 pg/ml. Greater hyperosmolality, although releasing more AVP, fails to conserve any more renal water, thus exposing the body to the potential of severe dehydration. This can be avoided by the stimulation of the thirst osmoreceptor at a plasma osmolality of 298 mmol/kg. However, recent studies, using a visual analogue scale, have demonstrated that the onset of thirst occurs at a considerably lower plasma osmolality than was previously recognized; the values were similar to those of the threshold for vasopressin release [93,94]. It has been shown in both animals [95] and humans [96–98] that the act of drinking ameliorates thirst and inhibits the secretion of vasopressin before changes occur in the extracellular fluid volume or osmolality. In humans, it has been shown that AVP secretion is inhibited independently of osmotic or gastric factors by the activation of the cold-sensitive oropharyngeal receptors [98]. The presence of such cold-sensitive oropharyngeal receptors may explain the desire of severely dehydrated patients, i.e., patients with diabetes insipidus (neurogenic or nephrogenic), for cold liquids.

There are considerable variations between individuals in osmoreceptor sensitivity and in the threshold for vasopressin release; however, these individual values remain constant for a relatively short period of time [99]. To determine if these interindividual differences are genetically influenced, Zerbe [99] compared the vasopressin osmolality relationships within monozygotic and dizygotic twin pairs. The threshold and sensitivity values correlated significantly within monozygotes but not within dizygotes, suggesting a genetic determinant for the set of the osmoregulatory system.

Pregnancy causes a lowering of the threshold for vasopressin secretion without altering the gain of the osmoreceptors in both rats [100] and humans [101], thus accounting for the hypo-osmolality of pregnancy. A role for human chorionic gonadotrophin in lowering this osmotic threshold has been postulated [102].

Vokes and coworkers [103] have demonstrated that osmoreceptor cells are insulin-sensitive, so that during insulin depletion they become impermeable to glucose and thus acquire an osmosensitivity to glucose. Durr et al. [104] pointed out that although glucose impermeability may account for the leftward shift in the AVP/plasma sodium relationship in insulin depletion, it cannot explain the simultaneous rightward shift observed in the AVP/plasma osmolality relationship [103]. Durr et al. [104] examined the respective roles of plasma osmolality and plasma tonicity (corrected or not for their relative cell permeability) in seven patients with diabetic ketoacidosis. They reasoned that decreasing permeability to glucose ($\sigma \rightarrow 1$) results in cell fasting and ketosis ($HCO_3^- \rightarrow 0$). Conversely, improved permeability ($\sigma \rightarrow 0$) corrects the metabolic acidosis ($HCO_3^- \rightarrow 26$). An empirical formula for the relative osmoreceptor cell permeability (σ) to glucose was derived from the plasma HCO_3^- as $\sigma = [26 - HCO_3^-]/26$. By using this concept of tonicity instead of osmolality, a three-dimensional plot was constructed ($Z = AX + BY + C$) in which the plasma AVP/sodium and AVP/plasma tonicity curves did not appear displaced. Thus, the increased osmotic and decreased sodium thresholds observed in diabetical ketoacidosis represent analytical artifacts, since they are unaltered when properly analyzed using the tonicity concept [104].

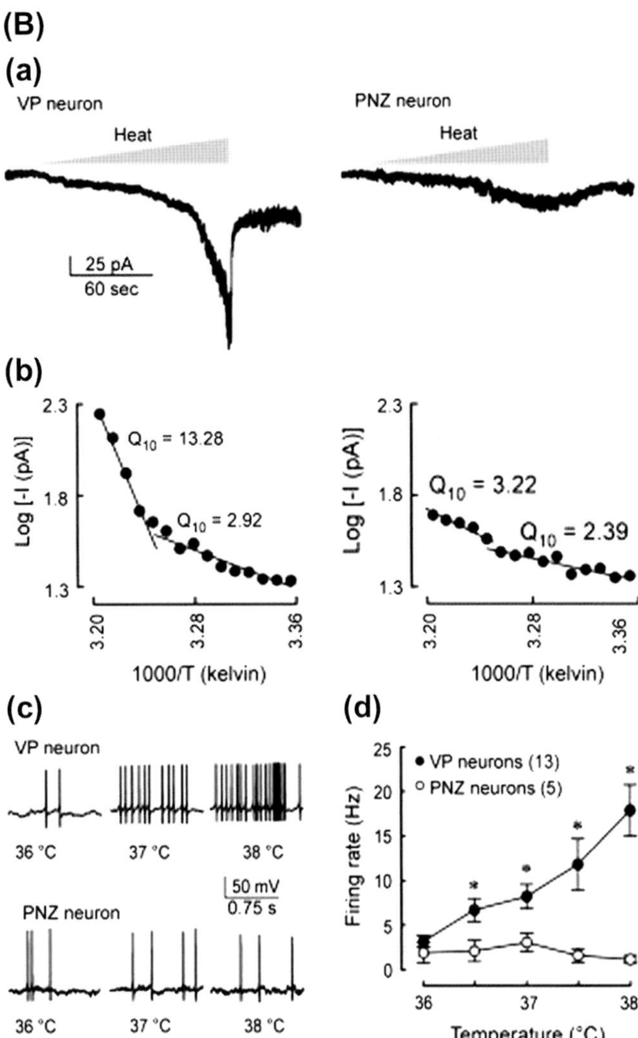

FIGURE 8.7B Vasopressin neurons are thermosensitive: (a) sample traces showing the effects of raising temperature (T) from 25°C to 39°C (heat, gray ramps) on holding current (VH −60mV) in single VP and PNZ neurons. VP neurons express but PNZ neurons do not express TRPV1. (b) Arrhenius plots of the data in (a). The log of the average absolute current at each temperature point was plotted against 1000/T (in °Kelvin). Separate linear regressions were fit through data taken between 25–35°C and between 35–39°C. The absolute value of the slope is the thermal coefficient, Q10. Note the greater thermosensitivity of the VP neuron above 35°C. (c) Sample traces demonstrate the effects of temperature on electrical activity in single VP and PNZ neurons recorded in current clamp. (d) Mean (± SEM) effect of temperature on action potential firing rate in VP (filled circles) and PNZ (empty circles) neurons (*$p<0.05$). *From ref [81] with permission.*

Baroregulation

It is now well established that afferent neural impulses arising from stretch receptors in the left atrium, carotid sinus and aortic arch inhibit the secretion of vasopressin. Conversely, when the discharge rate of these receptors is reduced, vasopressin secretion is enhanced (for review, see Norsk [105]). Moreover, the

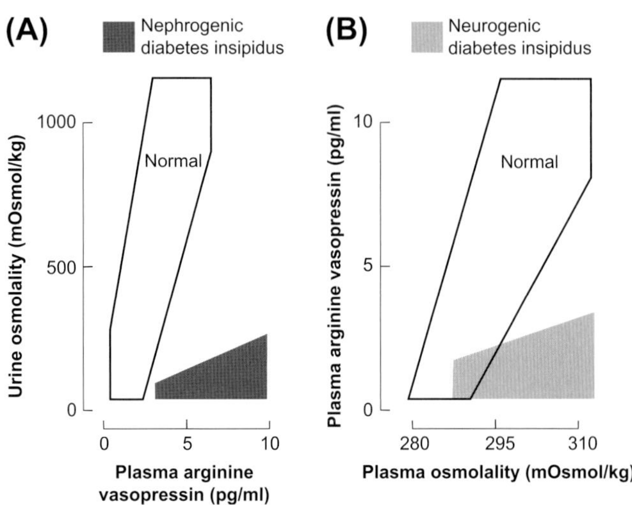

FIGURE 8.8 The relationship between plasma AVP and plasma osmolality during the infusion of hypertonic saline solution (left side). Patients with primary polydipsia and nephrogenic diabetes insipidus have values within the normal range (open area) in contrast to patients with neurogenic diabetes insipidus, who show subnormal plasma ADH responses (dark gray area). Relationship between urine osmolality and plasma ADH during dehydration and water loading (right side). Patients with neurogenic diabetes insipidus and primary polydipsia have values within the normal range (open area) in contrast to patients with nephrogenic diabetes insipidus, who have hypotonic urine despite high plasma ADH (light gray area). *Modified from Zerbe and Robertson [302].*

relative potency of the cardiac and sino-aortic reflexes in the release of vasopressin appears to vary among species. For example, the increase in plasma vasopressin that occurs during moderate hemorrhage in the dog is attributable primarily to reflex effects from cardiac receptors; sino-aortic receptors appear to exert only minor influences on vasopressin release in this situation. In contrast, sino-aortic receptors appear to play the dominant role in eliciting vasopressin secretion during blood loss in non-human primates and humans [105]. In humans, blood pressure reductions of as little as 5%, induced by the ganglion-blocking agent trimetaphan, significantly altered plasma AVP concentration [106]. Furthermore, an exponential relationship between plasma vasopressin and the percentage decline in mean arterial blood pressure has been observed with large decreases in blood pressure (Figure 8.10). Since an interdependence exists between osmoregulated and baroregulated AVP secretion (Figure 8.11) [107], under conditions of moderate hypovolemia, renal water excretion can be maintained around a lower set-point of plasma osmolality, thus preserving osmoregulation. As hypovolemia becomes more severe, plasma AVP concentrations attain extremely high values and baroregulation overrides the osmoregulatory system. An enhanced osmoreceptor sensitivity, but blunted baroregulation, has been described in elderly subjects [108].

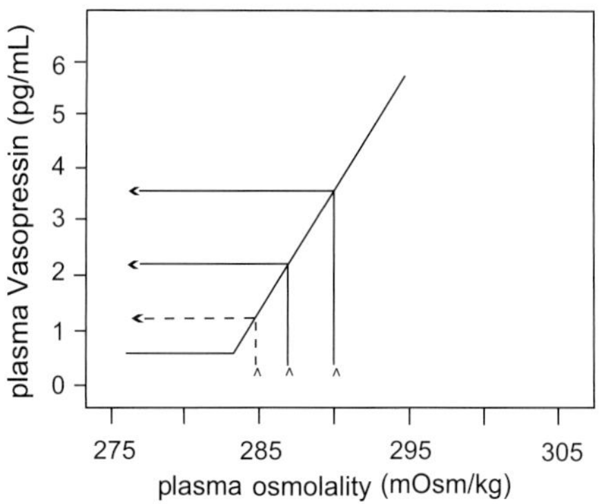

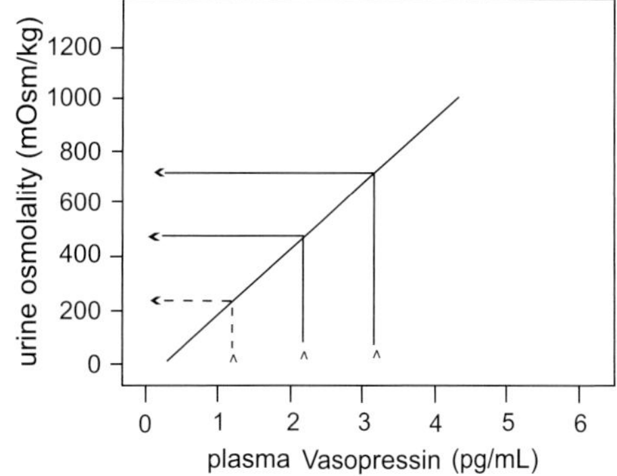

FIGURE 8.9 Schematic representation of the effect of small alterations in the basal plasma osmolality on (left) plasma vasopressin and (right) urinary osmolality in healthy adults. *Modified from Robertson et al. [90].*

Hormonal Influences on the Secretion of Vasopressin

Studies on the direct effects of various peptides and other biological substances on the release of vasopressin may be confounded by the hemodynamic effects of these substances, which indirectly modulate vasopressin release via the cardiovascular reflexes. For example, the infusion of pressor doses of norepinephrine increases both arterial blood pressure and left atrial pressure. Each of these changes is capable of eliciting a reflex inhibition of vasopressin release which should reduce plasma vasopressin. However, the inhibitory effects of the sino-aortic and cardiac reflexes on vasopressin release seem to be offset by the direct stimulatory effect of circulating norepinephrine. A similar situation may exist with the possible stimulation of vasopressin release by angiotensin. The direct stimulatory effect of angiotensin may be offset by inhibitory influences elicited from the cardiovascular reflexes. Angiotensin is a well-known dipsogen and has been shown to cause drinking in all the species tested [109]. Angiotensin II receptors have been described in the SFO and OVLT (for review see [110]). Brooks et al. [111] found that the infusion of exogenous angiotensin II increased vasopressin secretion and altered the baroreflex function in conscious dogs. Philips et al. [112] found that thirst and vasopressin secretion were stimulated in four out of ten healthy subjects infused with angiotensin II. Furthermore, the AVP concentrations were higher in the responders than in the nonresponders. These effects occurred at plasma angiotensin concentrations that were well above those measured under physiological conditions associated with thirst and vasopressin secretion, such as water deprivation.

To further assess the potential importance of angiotensin II in the regulation of vasopressin secretion in man, Morton et al. [113] submitted six normal subjects to a 3-day diet containing 10 mmol of sodium and 60 mmol of potassium per day. The mean cumulative sodium loss ($\pm$ SD) for the six subjects was 208 $\pm$ 94 mmol. Sodium restriction had no effect on serum sodium concentrations. Sodium depletion increased

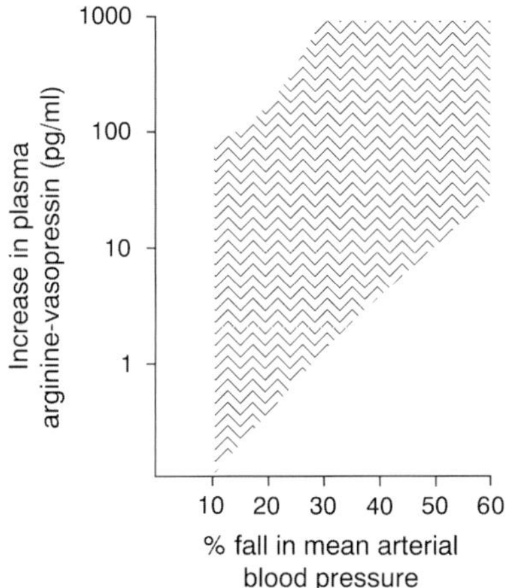

FIGURE 8.10 Increase in plasma arginine vasopressin AVP during hypotension (vertical lines). Note that a large diminution in blood pressure in normal humans induces large increments in AVP. *From Zerbe et al. [303], with permission.*

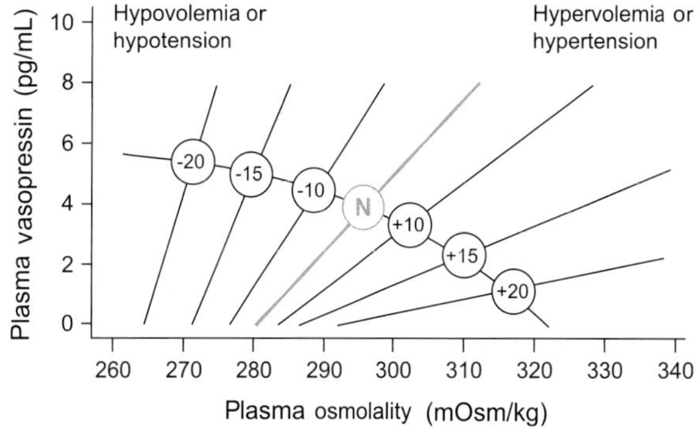

FIGURE 8.11 Schematic representation of the relationship between plasma vasopressin and plasma osmolality in the presence of differing states of blood volume and/or pressure. The line labeled N represents normovolemic normotensive conditions. Minus numbers to the left indicate percent fall, and positive numbers to the right, percent rise in blood volume or pressure. *Data from Vokes and Robertson [304].*

the circulating concentrations of angiotensin II more than five-fold ($p < 0.001$), but had no effect on plasma AVP concentrations. In short, physiologic concentrations of angiotensin II do not cause an increase in plasma vasopressin concentration in normal subjects. However, the complex interaction between the direct stimulatory and cardiovascular inhibitory influences has not been studied. Of interest, knockout models for angiotensinogen [114] or for AT1A receptor [115,116] did not alter thirst or water balance. Disruption of the AT2 receptor only induced mild abnormalities of thirst post dehydration [117].

The presence of endogenous opioid peptides and opioid receptors [118] in the neural lobe has led to the suggestion that opioid peptides play a role in the release of neurohypophyseal hormones. It is now recognized that opioid drugs exert their pharmacologic effects through an interaction with specific receptors. These receptors are classified into several types: μ, δ, σ and κ. μ Agonists such as morphine and methadone are responsible for the classical opiate effects of analgesia, respiratory depression and physical dependence. They typically cause an antidiuresis in hydrated animals and humans [119]. In contrast, κ agonists have analgesic properties, but do not cause respiratory depression or physical dependence at the dose required for analgesia. They have been shown to cause a water diuresis in experimental animals and in humans, probably by the inhibition of vasopressin secretion [120]. *κ* opioid agonists could have potential therapeutic benefits in the treatment of hyponatremia secondary to increased AVP secretion.

A very rapid and robust release of AVP is seen in humans after cholecystokinin (CCK) injection [121].

Nitric oxide is an inhibitory modulator of the hypothalamo–neurohypophyseal system in response to osmotic stimuli [122].

Vasopressin secretion is under the influence of a glucocorticoid-negative feedback system [123] and the vasopressin responses to a variety of stimuli (hemorrhage, hypoxia, hypertonic saline) in normal humans and animals appear to be attenuated or eliminated by pretreatment with glucocorticoids. Finally, nausea and emesis are potent stimuli of AVP release in humans and seem to involve dopaminergic neurotransmission [124].

The osmotic stimulation of AVP release by dehydration or hypertonic saline infusion, or both, is regularly used to test the AVP secretory capacity of the posterior pituitary. This secretory capacity can be assessed directly by comparing the plasma AVP concentration measured sequentially during a dehydration procedure with the normal values and then correlating the plasma AVP with the urinary osmolality measurements obtained simultaneously [125].

The AVP release can also be assessed indirectly by measuring plasma and urine osmolalities at regular intervals during the dehydration test [126]. The maximum urinary osmolality obtained during dehydration is compared with the maximum urinary osmolality obtained after the administration of vasopressin or dDAVP (Pitressin: 5 U SQ in adults; 1 U SQ in children) or 1-desamino[8-D-arginine]vasopressin [desmopressin (dDAVP)] (1–4 μg intravenously during 5–10 minutes).

The nonosmotic stimulation of AVP release can be used to assess the vasopressin secretory capacity of the posterior pituitary in a rare group of patients with essential hyponatremia and hypodipsia syndrome. Although some of these patients may have partial central diabetes insipidus, they respond normally to nonosmolar AVP release signals such as hypotension, emesis and hypoglycemia. In all other cases of suspected central diabetes insipidus, these nonosmotic stimulation tests will not give additional clinical information.

VASOPRESSIN RECEPTORS AND ANTAGONISTS

The four different receptor subtypes, respectively V_{1a}, V_{1b}, V_2 and oxytocin, have been cloned in mammals, lower vertebrates and invertebrates. These are four of 701 members of the rhodopsin family within the superfamily of guanine-nucleotide (G)-protein-coupled receptors [127] (see also the perspective by Perez [128] and recent comments on X-ray structure breakthroughs in the transmembrane-spanning region [129]). The V_{1a}, V_{1b}, V_2 and OT receptors are strikingly similar in both size and amino acid sequence. However, the V_{1a}, V_{1b} and OT receptors are selectively coupled to G-proteins of the $G_{q/11}$ family which mediate the activation of distinct isoforms of phospholipase C_β resulting in the breakdown of phosphoinositide lipids. The V_2 receptor, on the other hand, preferentially activates the G-protein, G_s, resulting in the activation of adenylyl cyclase.

The classical vascular smooth muscle contraction, platelet aggregation and hepatic glycogenolysis actions of AVP are mediated by the V_{1a} receptor that increases cytosolic calcium. In situ hybridization histochemistry using ^{35}S-labeled cRNA probes specific for the V_{1a} receptor mRNA showed high levels of V_{1a} receptor transcripts in the liver among hepatocytes surrounding central veins and in the renal medulla among the vascular bundles, the arcuate and interlobular arteries [130]. V_{1a} receptor mRNA was found to be extensively distributed throughout the brain where AVP may act as a neurotransmitter or a neuromodulator in addition to its classical role on vascular tone [14]. Brain AVP receptors have been proposed to mediate the effect of AVP on memory and learning, antipyresis, brain development, selective aggression and partner preference in rodents, cardiovascular responsivity, blood flow to the choroid plexus and cerebrospinal fluid production, regulation of smooth muscle tone in superficial brain vasculature and analgesia. It is, however, not known whether V_{1a} brain receptors respond to AVP released within the brain proper or whether the receptors also respond to AVP from the peripheral circulation [131].

V_{1b} receptors are not only expressed in the anterior pituitary [132] and kidney [133] as originally reported, but also in brain, uterus, thymus, heart, breast and lung [134]. The physiologic role of these extrapituitary V_{1b} receptors remains unknown, but some functions of AVP attributed in the past to V_{1a} receptors or OT receptors may be due to the activation of V_{1b} receptors [134,135]. In the rat adrenal medulla, AVP may regulate the adrenal functions by paracrine/autocrine mechanisms involving distinct AVP receptor subtypes: V_{1a} in the adrenal cortex and V_{1b} in the adrenal medulla [136].

V_2 transcripts are heavily expressed in cells of the renal collecting ducts (in humans and rodents) and in cells of the thick ascending limbs of the loops of Henle (in rodents only) [137].

Species specificity and partial agonist activity have frustrated the search to discover antidiuretic hormone receptor antagonists that are effective aquaretic agents in vivo. The compound SKF101926 (desGlyd$(CH_2)_5$D-Tyr(Et)VAVP) was shown to be a potent V_2 receptor antagonist having aquaretic activity in several animal species, including a primate species. However, SKF101926 lacked aquaretic activity and was a vasopressin agonist in humans [138]. The orally effective nonpeptide V_2 antagonists are aquaretic drugs potentially useful to treat various clinical syndromes with abnormal water retention [139–141].

CELLULAR ACTIONS OF VASOPRESSIN

The neurohypophyseal hormone AVP has multiple actions, including the inhibition of diuresis, contraction of smooth muscle, aggregation of platelets, stimulation of liver glycogenolysis, modulation of adrenocorticotropic hormone release from the pituitary, and central regulation of somatic functions (thermoregulation and blood pressure) and modulation of social and reproductive behavior. These multiple actions of AVP can be explained by the interaction of AVP with at least three types of G-protein-coupled receptors: the V_{1a} (vascular, hepatic and brain) and V_{1b} (anterior pituitary) receptors act through phosphatidylinositol hydrolysis to mobilize calcium, and the V_2 (kidney) receptor is coupled to adenylate cyclase [142–144].

The transfer of water across the principal cells of the collecting ducts is now known at such a detailed level that billions of molecules of water traversing the membrane can be represented; see useful teaching tools at http://www.mpibpc.gwdg.de/abteilungen/073/gallery.html and http://www.ks.uiuc.edu/research/aquaporins. The 2003 Nobel Prize in chemistry was awarded to Peter Agre and Roderick MacKinnon, who solved two complementary problems presented by the cell membrane: how does a cell let one type of ion through the lipid membrane to the exclusion of other ions? And how does it permeate water without ions? This contributed to a momentum and renewed interest in basic discoveries related to the transport of water and indirectly to diabetes insipidus. The first step in the action of AVP on water excretion is its binding to arginine vasopressin type 2 receptors (hereafter referred to as V_2 receptors) on the basolateral membrane of the collecting duct cells (Figure 8.12). The human *AVPR2* gene that codes for the V_2 receptor is located in chromosome region Xq28 and has three exons and two small introns [145,146]. The sequence of the cDNA predicts a polypeptide of 371 amino acids with seven transmembrane, four extracellular and four cytoplasmic domains (Figure 8.13). The activation of the V_2 receptor on renal collecting tubules stimulates adenylyl cyclase via the stimulatory G-protein (Gs) and promotes the cyclic adenosine monophosphate (cAMP)-mediated incorporation of water channels into the luminal surface of these cells. There are two ubiquitously expressed intracellular cAMP receptors: (1) the classical protein kinase A (PKA) that is a cAMP-dependent protein kinase, and (2) the recently discovered exchange protein directly activated by cAMP that is a cAMP-regulated guanine nucleotide exchange factor. Both of these receptors contain an evolutionally conserved cAMP-binding domain that acts as a molecular switch for sensing intracellular cAMP levels to control diverse biological functions [147]. Several proteins participating in the control of cAMP-dependent AQP2 trafficking have been identified; for example, A-kinase-anchoring proteins tethering PKA to cellular compartments; phosphodiesterases regulating the local cAMP level; cytoskeletal components such as F-actin and microtubules; small GTPases of the Rho family controlling cytoskeletal dynamics; motor proteins transporting AQP2-bearing vesicles to and from the plasma membrane for exocytic insertion and endocytic retrieval; and SNAREs inducing membrane fusions, hsc70, a chaperone important for endocytic retrieval. These processes are the molecular basis of the vasopressin-induced increase in the osmotic water permeability of the apical membrane of the collecting tubule [148–150].

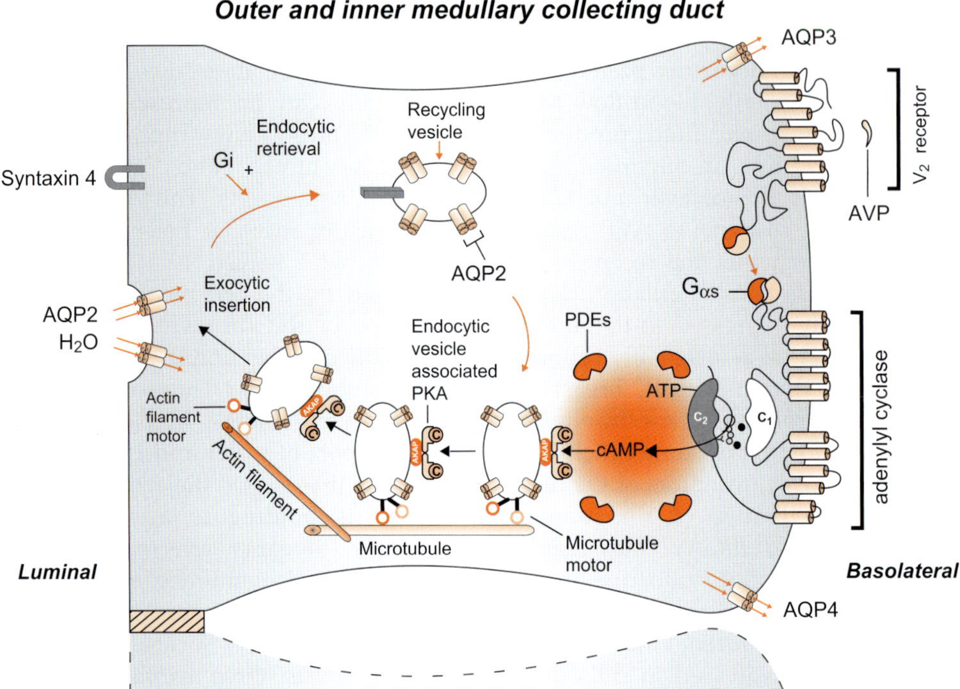

FIGURE 8.12 Schematic representation of the effect of vasopressin (AVP) to increase water permeability in the principal cells of the collecting duct. AVP is bound to the V_2 receptor (a G-protein-linked receptor) on the basolateral membrane. The basic process of G-protein-coupled receptor signaling consists of three steps: a hepta-helical receptor that detects a ligand (in this case, AVP) in the extracellular milieu, a G-protein ($G_{\alpha s}$) that dissociates into α-subunits bound to GTP and β-subunits after interaction with the ligand-bound receptor, and an effector (in this case, adenylyl cyclase) that interacts with dissociated G-protein subunits to generate small-molecule second messengers. AVP activates adenylyl cyclase, increasing the intracellular concentration of cAMP. The topology of adenylyl cyclase is characterized by two tandem repeats of six hydrophobic transmembrane domains separated by a large cytoplasmic loop and terminates in a large intracellular tail. The dimeric structure (C_1 and C_2) of the catalytic domains is represented. Conversion of ATP to cAMP takes place at the dimer interface. Two aspartate residues (in C_1) coordinate two metal cofactors (Mg^{2+} or Mn^{2+} represented here as two small black circles), which enable the catalytic function of the enzyme [305]. Adenosine is shown as an open circle and the three phosphate groups (ATP) are shown as smaller open circles. Protein kinase A (PKA) is the target of the generated cAMP. The binding of cAMP to the regulatory subunits of PKA induces a conformational change, causing these subunits to dissociate from the catalytic subunits. These activated subunits (C) as shown here are anchored to an aquaporin-2 (AQP2)-containing endocytic vesicle via an A-kinase anchoring protein. The local concentration and distribution of the cAMP gradient is limited by phosphodiesterases (PDEs). Cytoplasmic vesicles carrying the water channels (represented as homotetrameric complexes) are fused to the luminal membrane in response to AVP, thereby increasing the water permeability of this membrane. The dissociation of the A-kinase anchoring protein from the endocytic vesicle is not represented. Microtubules and actin filaments are necessary for vesicle movement toward the membrane. When AVP is not available, AQP2 water channels are retrieved by an endocytic process and water permeability returns to its original low rate. Aquaporin-3 (AQP3) and aquaporin-4 (AQP4) water channels are expressed constitutively at the basolateral membrane.

AVP also increases the water reabsorptive capacity of the kidney by regulating the urea transporter UT-A1 that is present in the inner medullary collecting duct, predominantly in its terminal part [151,152]. AVP also increases the permeability of principal collecting duct cells to sodium [153].

In summary, in the absence of AVP stimulation, collecting duct epithelia exhibit very low permeabilities to sodium urea and water. These specialized permeability properties permit the excretion of large volumes of hypotonic urine formed during intervals of water diuresis. By contrast, AVP stimulation of the principal cells of the collecting ducts leads to selective increases in the permeability of the apical membrane to water, urea and sodium.

These actions of vasopressin in the distal nephron are possibly modulated by prostaglandin E2, nitric oxide [154] and by luminal calcium concentration. High levels of E-prostanoid-3 receptors are expressed in the kidney [155]. However, mice lacking E-prostanoid-3 receptors for prostaglandin E2 were found to have quasi-normal regulation of urine volume and osmolality in response to various physiological stimuli [155]. An apical calcium/polycation receptor protein expressed in the terminal portion of the inner medullary collecting duct of the rat has been shown to reduce AVP-elicited osmotic water permeability when luminal calcium concentration rises [156]. This possible link between calcium and water metabolism may play a role in the pathogenesis of renal stone formation [156].

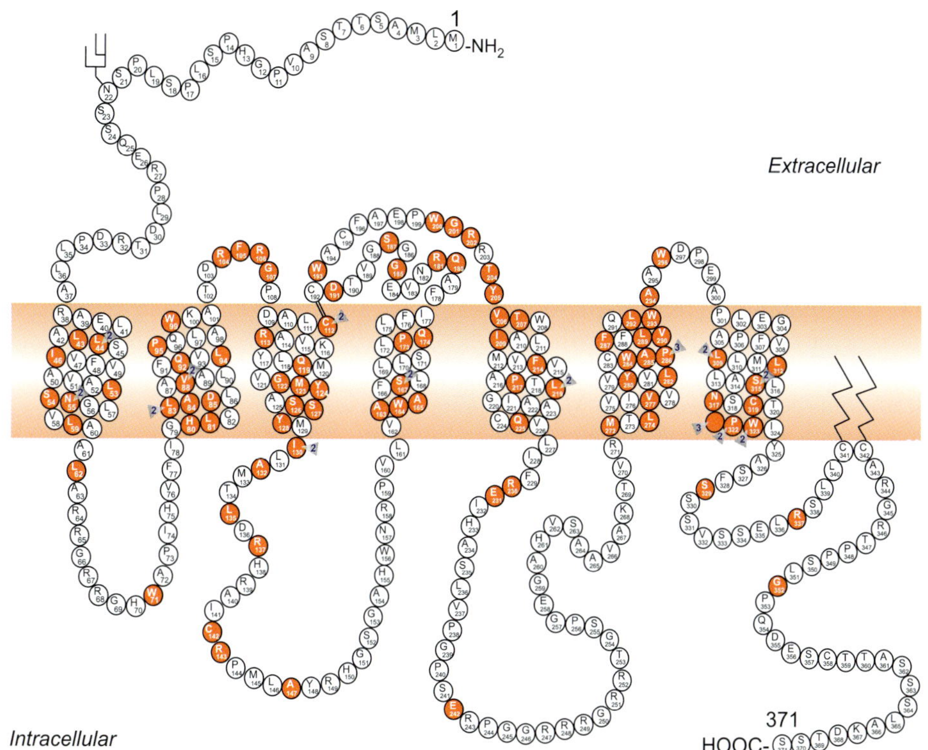

FIGURE 8.13 Schematic representation of the V_2 receptor and identification of 193 putative disease-causing AVPR2 mutations. Predicted amino acids are shown as the one-letter amino acid code. A solid symbol indicates a codon with a missense or nonsense mutation; a number indicates more than one mutation in the same codon; other types of mutations are not indicated on the figure. There are 95 missense, 18 nonsense, 46 frameshift deletion or insertion, seven inframe deletion or insertion, four splice-site and 22 large deletion mutations, and one complex mutation.

QUANTITATING RENAL WATER EXCRETION

Diabetes insipidus is characterized by the excretion of abnormally large volumes of hypo-osmotic urine (<250 mmol/kg). This definition excludes osmotic diuresis, which occurs when excess solute is being excreted, as with glucose in the polyuria of diabetes mellitus. Other agents that produce osmotic diuresis are mannitol, urea, glycerol, contrast media and loop diuretics. Osmotic diuresis should be considered when solute excretion exceeds 60 mmol/hour.

CLINICAL CHARACTERISTICS OF DIABETES INSIPIDUS DISORDERS

Neurogenic Diabetes Insipidus

Common Forms

Failure to synthesize or secrete vasopressin normally limits maximal urinary concentration and, depending on the severity of the disease, causes varying degrees of polyuria and polydipsia. Experimental destruction of the vasopressin-synthesizing areas of the hypothalamus (supraoptic and paraventricular nuclei) causes a permanent form of the disease. Similar results are obtained by sectioning the hypophyseal hypothalamic tract above the median eminence. Sections below the median eminence, however, produce only transient diabetes insipidus. Lesions to the hypothalamic–pituitary tract are frequently associated with a three-stage response both in experimental animals and in humans [157]: (1) an initial diuretic phase lasting from a few hours to 5–6 days; (2) a period of antidiuresis unresponsive to fluid administration. This antidiuresis is probably due to vasopressin release from injured axons and may last from a few hours to several days (because urinary dilution is impaired during this phase, continued water administration can cause severe hyponatremia); and (3) a final period of diabetes insipidus. The extent of the injury determines the completeness of the diabetes insipidus and, as already discussed, the site of the lesion determines whether the disease will be permanent.

Twenty-five percent of patients studied after transsphenoidal surgery developed spontaneous isolated hyponatremia, 20% developed diabetes insipidus and 46% remained normonatremic. Normonatremia, hyponatremia and diabetes insipidus were associated with increasing degrees of surgical manipulation of the posterior lobe and pituitary stalk during surgery [158]. Central diabetes insipidus observed after trans-sphenoidal surgery is often transient and only 2% of patients need long-term treatment with dDAVP [159].

The etiologies of central diabetes insipidus in adults and in children are listed in Table 8.3 [160–163].

Rare causes of central diabetes insipidus include leukemia, thrombotic thrombocytopenic purpura, pituitary apoplexy, sarcoidosis [164] and Wegener's granulomatosis, xanthoma disseminatum [165], septo-optico dysplasia and agenesis of the corpus callosum [166], metabolic (anorexia nervosa), lymphocytic hypophysitis [167], necrotizing infundibulo-hypophysitis [168]. Maghnie et al. [162] studied 79 patients with central diabetes insipidus. Additional deficits in anterior pituitary hormones were documented in 61% of patients, a median of 0.6 years (range: 0.1 to 18.0) after the onset of diabetes insipidus. The most frequent abnormality was growth hormone deficiency (59%), followed by hypothyroidism (28%), hypogonadism (24%) and adrenal insufficiency (22%). Seventy-five per cent of the patients with Langerhans cell histiocytosis had an anterior pituitary hormone deficiency that was first detected a median of 3.5 years after the onset of diabetes insipidus [162]. None of the patients with central diabetes insipidus secondary to *AVP* mutations developed anterior pituitary hormone deficiencies.

TABLE 8.3 Etiology of Hypothalamic Diabetes Insipidus in Children and Adults

	Children (%)	Children and Young Adults (%)	Adults (%)
Primary brain tumor[1]	49.5	22	30
before surgery	33.5		13
after surgery	16		17
Idiopathic (isolated or familial)	29	58	25
Histiocytosis	16	12	-
Metastatic cancer[2]	-		8
Trauma[3]	2.2	2.0	17
Postinfectious disease	2.2	6.0	-

[1]*Primary malignancy: craniopharyngioma, dysgerminoma, meningioma, adenoma, glioma, astrocytoma.*
[2]*Secondary: metastatic from lung or breast, lymphoma, leukemia, dysplastic pancytopenia.*
[3]*Trauma could be severe or mild.*
Data from Czernichow et al. [160], Greger et al. [161], Moses et al. [163], and Maghnie et al. [162].

Rare Forms

Autosomal Dominant and Recessive Neurogenic Diabetes Insipidus

Lacombe [169] and Weil [170] described a familial non-X-linked form of diabetes insipidus without any associated mental retardation. The descendants of the family described by Weil were later found to have autosomal dominant neurogenic diabetes insipidus [171–173]. Neurogenic diabetes insipidus (OMIM 125700) [26] is a well characterized entity, secondary to mutations in *AVP* (OMIM 192340). Patients with autosomal dominant neurogenic diabetes insipidus retain some limited capacity to secrete AVP during severe dehydration, and the polyuropolydipsic symptoms usually appear after the first year of life [174] when the infant's demand for water is more likely to be understood by adults. The expression of the vasopressin gene in autosomal dominant and autosomal recessive diabetes insipidus in humans has been described earlier in this chapter.

Wolfram Syndrome

Wolfram syndrome, also known as DIDMOAD, is an autosomal recessive neurodegenerative disorder accompanied by insulin-dependent diabetes mellitus and progressive optic atrophy. The acronym DIDMOAD describes the following clinical features of the syndrome: diabetes insipidus, diabetes mellitus, optic atrophy and sensorineural deafness. An unusual incidence of psychiatric symptoms has also been described in patients with this syndrome. These included paranoid delusions, auditory or visual hallucinations, psychotic behavior, violent behavior, organic brain syndrome typically in the late or preterminal stages of their illness, progressive dementia and severe learning disabilities or mental retardation, or both. Wolfram syndrome patients develop diabetes mellitus and bilateral optical atrophy mainly in the first decade of life, the diabetes insipidus is usually partial and of gradual onset, and the polyuria can be wrongly attributed to poor glycemic control. Furthermore, a severe hyperosmolar state can occur if untreated diabetes mellitus is associated with an unrecognized posterior pituitary deficiency. The dilatation of the urinary tract observed in DIDMOAD syndrome may be secondary to chronic high urine flow rates and, perhaps, to some degenerative aspects of the innervation of the urinary tract. The gene responsible for Wolfram syndrome, located in chromosome region 4p16.1, encodes a putative 890-amino acid transmembrane protein referred as wolframin. Wolframin is an endoglycosidase H-sensitive glycoprotein, which localizes primarily in the endoplasmic reticulum of a variety of neurons including neurons in the supraoptic nucleus and neurons in the lateral magnocellular division of the paraventricular nucleus [175,176]. Disruption of the *Wfs1* gene in mice causes progressive beta-cell loss and impaired stimulus-secretion coupling in insulin secretion, but central diabetes insipidus is not observed in $Wfs^{-/-}$ mice [177]. Miner1, another endoplasmic reticulum protein is causative in Wolfram syndrome 2 [178].

Syndrome of Hypernatremia and Hypodipsia

Some patients with the hypernatremia and hypodipsia syndrome may have partial central diabetes insipidus. These patients also have persistent hypernatremia that is not due to any apparent extracellular volume loss, absence or attenuation of thirst, and a normal renal response to AVP. In almost all the patients studied to date, the hypodipsia has been associated with cerebral lesions in the vicinity of the hypothalamus. It has been proposed that in these patients there is a "resetting" of the osmoreceptor because their urine tends to become concentrated or diluted at inappropriately high levels of plasma osmolality. However, using the regression analysis of plasma AVP concentration versus plasma osmolality, it has been shown that in some of these patients the tendency to concentrate and dilute urine at inappropriately high levels of plasma osmolality is due solely to a marked reduction in sensitivity or a gain in the osmoregulatory mechanism [179,180]. This finding is compatible with the diagnosis of partial central diabetes insipidus. In other patients, however, plasma AVP concentrations fluctuate in a random manner, bearing no apparent relationship to changes in plasma osmolality. Such patients frequently display large swings in serum sodium concentration and frequently exhibit hypodipsia. It appears that most patients with "essential hypernatremia" fit one of these two patterns (Figure 8.14). Both of these groups of patients consistently respond normally to nonosmolar AVP release signals, such as hypotension, emesis, or hypoglycemia, or all three. These observations suggest that: (1) the osmoreceptor may be anatomically as well as functionally separate from the nonosmotic efferent pathways and neurosecretory neurons for vasopressin and a hypothalamic lesion may impair the osmotic release of AVP while the nonosmotic release of AVP remains intact; and (2) the osmoreceptor neurons that regulate vasopressin secretion are not totally synonymous with those that regulate thirst, although they appear to be anatomically close if not overlapping.

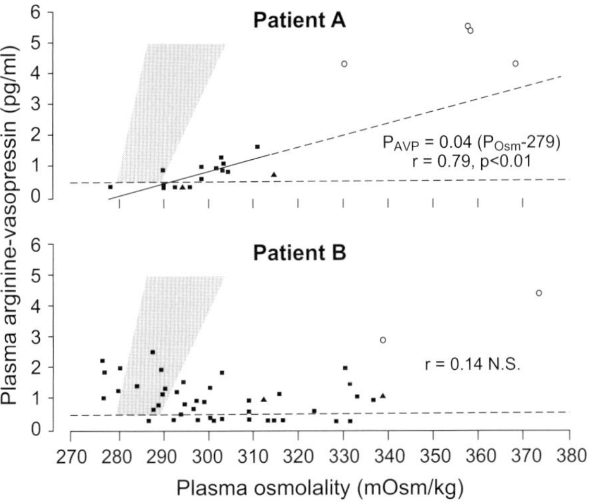

FIGURE 8.14 Plasma vasopressin as a function of "effective" plasma osmolality in two patients with adipsic hypernatremia. Unfilled circles indicate values obtained on admission; filled squares indicate those obtained during forced hydration; filled triangles indicate those obtained after 1–2 weeks of ad libitum water intake. Shaded areas indicate range of normal values. *From Robertson [306], with permission, Wolters Kluwer.*

Nephrogenic Diabetes Insipidus

In NDI, the kidney is unable to concentrate urine despite normal or elevated concentrations of the antidiuretic hormone arginine-vasopressin (AVP). In congenital NDI, the obvious clinical manifestations of the disease, that is polyuria and polydipsia, are present at birth and need to be immediately recognized to avoid severe episodes of dehydration. It is clinically useful to distinguish two types of hereditary NDI: a "pure" type characterized by loss of water only and a complex type characterized by loss of water and ions. Patients who have congenital NDI and bear mutations in the *AVPR2* or *AQP2* genes have a "pure" NDI phenotype with loss of water but normal conservation of sodium, potassium, chloride and calcium. Patients who bear inactivating mutations in genes (*SLC12A1, KCNJ1, CLCNKB, CLCNKA* and *CLCNKB* in combination, or *BSND*) that encode the membrane proteins of the thick ascending limb of the loop of Henle have a complex polyuropolydipsic syndrome with loss of water, sodium, chloride, calcium, magnesium and potassium. Most (>90%) of "pure" congenital NDI patients have mutations in the *AVPR2* gene, the Xq28 gene coding for the vasopressin V_2 (antidiuretic) receptor. In less than 10% of the families studied, congenital NDI has an autosomal recessive inheritance and mutations have been identified in the *AQP2* gene located in chromosome region 12q13, that is, the vasopressin-sensitive water channel. When studied in vitro, most *AVPR2* mutations lead to receptors that are trapped intracellularly and are unable to reach the plasma membrane. A minority of the mutant receptors reach the cell surface but are unable to bind AVP or to trigger an intracellular cAMP signal. Similarly, *AQP2* mutant proteins are trapped intracellularly and cannot be expressed at the luminal membrane. AVPR2 and AQP2-trafficking defects are correctable by chemical chaperones.

Loss-of-Function Mutations of the AVPR2

X-linked NDI (OMIM 304800) is secondary to *AVPR2* mutations, which result in a loss-of-function or dysregulation of the V_2 receptor [181].

Rareness and Diversity of AVPR2 Mutations

X-linked NDI is generally a rare disease in which the affected male patients do not concentrate their urine after administration of AVP [182]. Because this form is a rare, recessive X-linked disease, females are unlikely to be affected, but heterozygous females can exhibit variable degrees of polyuria and polydipsia because of skewed X chromosome inactivation. In Quebec, the incidence of this disease among males was estimated to be approximately 8.8 in 1,000,000 male live births [183]. A founder effect of two particular *AVPR2* mutations [184], one in Ulster Scot immigrants (the Hopewell mutation, W71X) and one in a large Utah kindred (the Cannon pedigree), results in an elevated prevalence of X-linked NDI in their descendants in certain communities in Nova Scotia, Canada and in Utah, USA [184]. These founder mutations have now spread all over the North American continent. To date, we have identified the W71X mutation in 42 affected males who reside predominantly in the Maritime Provinces of Nova Scotia and New Brunswick, and the L312X mutation has been identified in eight affected males who reside in central USA. We know of 98 living affected males of the Hopewell kindred and 18 living affected males of the Cannon pedigree. We also determined that the historical case report by Perry et al. [185] was related to the Hopewell pedigree and had the W71X mutation.

To date, about 200 putative disease-causing *AVPR2* mutations have been published in over 300 NDI families [186,187]. Approximately half of the mutations are missense mutations. Frameshift mutations owing to nucleotide deletions or insertions (24%), nonsense mutations (9%), large deletions (11%), in-frame deletions or insertions (4%), splice-site mutations (2%) and one complex mutation account for the remainder of the mutations [187–189]. Mutations have been identified in every domain, but on a per nucleotide basis about twice as many mutations occur in transmembrane domains compared with extracellular or intracellular domains. We previously identified private mutations, recurrent mutations and mechanisms of mutagenesis [190,191]. Ten recurrent mutations (D85N, V88M, R113W, Y128S, R137H, S167L, R181C, R202C, A294P and S315R) were found in 35 ancestrally independent families. The occurrence of the same mutation on different haplotypes was considered evidence for recurrent mutation. In addition, the most frequent mutations (D85N, V88N, R113W, R137H, S167L, R181C and R202C) occurred at potential mutational hot spots (a C-to-T or G-to-A nucleotide substitution at a CpG dinucleotide).

Most Mutant V2 Receptors are not Transported to the Cell Membrane and are Retained in the Intracellular Compartments

Classification of the defects of naturally occurring mutant human V_2 receptors can be based on a similar scheme to that used for the low-density lipoprotein receptor. Mutations have been grouped according to the function and subcellular localization of the mutant protein whose cDNA has been transiently transfected in a heterologous expression system [192]. Using this classification, type 1 mutant V_2 receptors reach the cell surface but display impaired ligand binding and are consequently unable to induce normal cAMP production. The dose-dependent AVP-stimulated cAMP production could be compared with the cAMP production obtained with the wild-type receptor using a protein-based bioluminescence resonance energy transfer cAMP biosensor that allows the measurement of cAMP in living cells [193]. The presence of mutant V_2 receptors on the surface of transfected cells can be determined pharmacologically. By carrying out saturation binding experiments using tritiated AVP, the number of cell surface mutant V_2 receptors and their apparent binding affinity can be compared with that of the wild-type receptor. In addition, the presence of cell surface receptors can be assessed directly by using immunodetection strategies to visualize epitope-tagged receptors in whole-cell immunofluorescence assays.

Type 2 mutant receptors have defective intracellular transport. This phenotype is confirmed by carrying out, in parallel, immunofluorescence experiments on cells that are intact (to demonstrate the absence of cell surface receptors) or permeabilized (to confirm the presence of intracellular receptor pools). In addition, protein expression is confirmed by western blot analysis of membrane preparations from transfected cells. It is likely that these mutant type 2 receptors accumulate in a pre-Golgi compartment because they are initially glycosylated but fail to undergo glycosyl-trimming maturation.

Type 3 mutant receptors are ineffectively transcribed and lead to unstable mRNAs which are rapidly degraded. This subgroup seems to be rare since northern blot analysis of cells expressing mutant AVPR2 receptors showed mRNAs of normal quantity and molecular size.

Most of the *AVPR2* mutants that we and other investigators have tested are type 2 mutant receptors. They did not reach the cell membrane and were trapped in the interior of the cell [194–198]. Other mutant G-protein-coupled receptors [199] and gene products causing genetic disorders are also characterized by protein misfolding. Mutations that affect the folding of secretory proteins, integral plasma membrane proteins, or enzymes destined to the endoplasmic reticulum, Golgi complex and lysosomes result in loss-of-function phenotypes irrespective of their direct impact on protein function because these mutant proteins are prevented from reaching their final destination [200,201]. Folding in the endoplasmic reticulum is the limiting step: mutant proteins that fail to fold correctly are initially retained in the endoplasmic reticulum and subsequently often degrade. Key proteins involved in the urine countercurrent mechanisms are good examples of this basic mechanism of misfolding. *AQP2* mutations responsible for autosomal recessive NDI are characterized by misrouting of the misfolded mutant proteins and are trapped in the endoplasmic reticulum [202]. Other mutant renal membrane proteins that are responsible for Gitelman syndrome [203], Bartter syndrome [204,205] and cystinuria [206] are also retained in the endoplasmic reticulum.

The *AVPR2* missense mutations are likely to impair folding and to lead to rapid degradation of the misfolded polypeptide and not to the accumulation of toxic aggregates (as is the case for AVP mutants that cause neurohypophyseal diabetes insipidus), because the other important functions of the principal cells of the collecting duct (where *AVPR2* is expressed) are entirely normal. These cells express the epithelial sodium channel (ENac). Decreased function of this channel results in a sodium-losing state [207]. This has not been observed in patients with *AVPR2* mutations. However, recent data showed that dDAVP could not stimulate sodium reabsorption in male patients with NDI bearing *AVPR2* mutations [153], but this is a V2R-specific effect [208]. By contrast, another type of conformational disease is characterized by the toxic retention of the misfolded protein. The relatively common Z mutation in α_1-antitrypsin deficiency not only causes retention of the mutant protein in the endoplasmic reticulum but also affects the secondary structure by insertion of the reactive center loop of one molecule into a destabilized β sheet of a second molecule [209]. These polymers clog up the endoplasmic reticulum of hepatocytes and lead to cell death and juvenile hepatitis, cirrhosis and hepatocarcinomas in these patients [210].

Nonpeptide Vasopressin Receptor Antagonists Act as Pharmacological Chaperones to Functionally Rescue Misfolded Mutant V_2 Receptors Responsible for X-linked NDI

If the misfolded protein/traffic problem responsible for so many human genetic diseases can be overcome and the mutant protein can be transported out of the endoplasmic reticulum to its final destination, these mutant proteins might be sufficiently functional [211]. Therefore, using pharmacological chaperones to promote escape from the endoplasmic reticulum is a possible therapeutic approach [195,198,200,212]. We used selective nonpeptide V_2 and V_1 receptor antagonists to rescue the cell surface expression and function of naturally occurring misfolded human V_2 receptors [194]. Since the beneficial effect of nonpeptide V_2 antagonists could be secondary to prevention or interference with endocytosis, we studied the R137H mutant previously reported to lead to constitutive endocytosis [213]. We found that the antagonist did not prevent the constitutive β-arrestin-mediated endocytosis [195]. These results indicate that as for other *AVPR2* mutants, the beneficial effects of the treatment result from the action of the pharmacological chaperones. In clinical studies, we administered a nonpeptide vasopressin antagonist SR49059 to five adult NDI patients bearing the del62-64, R137H, or W164S mutation. SR49059 significantly decreased urine volume and water intake and increased urine osmolality while sodium, potassium and creatinine excretions and plasma sodium were constant throughout the study [214]. This new therapeutic approach could be applied to the treatment of several hereditary diseases resulting from errors in protein folding and kinesis [211,212].

Since most human gene therapy experiments using viruses to deliver and integrate DNA into host cells are potentially dangerous [215], other treatments are being actively pursued. Torsten Schöneberg and colleagues [216] used aminoglycoside antibiotics because of their ability to suppress premature termination codons [217]. They demonstrated that geneticin, a potent aminoglycoside antibiotic, increased AVP-stimulated cAMP in cultured collecting duct cells prepared from E242X mutant mice. The urine-concentrating ability of heterozygous mutant mice was also improved.

Gain-of-Function of the Vasopressin V2 Receptor: Nephrogenic Syndrome of Inappropriate Antidiuresis

The clinical phenotype here is opposite to NDI. Rare cases of infants or adults with hyponatremia, concentrated urine and suppressed AVP plasma concentrations have been described bearing the mutations R137C or R137L in their *AVPR2* gene [218–221]. It is interesting to note that another mutation in the same codon (R137H) is a relatively frequent mutation causing classical NDI, albeit the phenotype may be milder in some patients [222]. With cell-based assays both R137C and R137L were found to have elevated basal signaling through the cAMP pathway and to interact with β-arrestins in an agonist-independent manner [223]. It is my opinion that *AVPR2* mutations with gain-of-function are extremely rare. We have sequenced the *AVPR2* gene in many patients with hyponatremia and never found a mutation. By contrast, we continue to identify new and recurrent loss-of-function *AVPR2* mutations in patients with classical NDI.

Loss-of-Function Mutations of AQP2

On the basis of desmopressin infusion studies and phenotypic characteristics of both male and female individuals who are affected with NDI, a non-X-linked form of NDI with a post-receptor (post cAMP) defect was suggested [224–226]. A patient who presented shortly after birth with typical features of NDI but who exhibited normal coagulation and normal fibrinolytic and vasodilatory responses to desmopressin was shown to be a compound heterozygote for two missense mutations (R187C and S217P) in the *AQP2* gene [227]. To date, 42 putative disease-causing *AQP2* mutations have been identified in 40 NDI families (Figure 8.15). The oocytes of the African clawed frog (*Xenopus laevis*) have provided a most useful experimental system for studying the function of many channel proteins. This convenient expression system was key to the discovery of AQP1 by Agre [228] because frog oocytes have very low permeability and survive even in freshwater ponds. Control oocytes are injected with water alone; test oocytes are injected with various quantities of synthetic transcripts from AQP1 or AQP2 DNA (cRNA). When subjected to a 20-mOsm osmotic shock, control oocytes have exceedingly low water permeability but test oocytes become highly permeable to water. These osmotic water-permeability assays demonstrated an absence or very low water transport for all of the cRNA with *AQP2* mutations. Immunofluorescence and immunoblot studies demonstrated that these recessive mutants were retained in the endoplasmic reticulum.

AQP2 mutations in autosomal recessive NDI, which are located throughout the gene, result in misfolded proteins that are retained in the endoplasmic reticulum. In contrast, the dominant mutations reported to date are located in the region that codes for the carboxyl terminus of AQP2. Dominant AQP2 mutants form heterotetramers with wt-AQP2 and are misrouted.

Complex Polyuropolydipsic Syndrome

In contrast to a "pure" NDI phenotype, with loss of water but normal conservation of sodium, potassium, chloride and calcium, in Bartter syndrome, patients' renal wasting starts prenatally and polyhydramnios often leads to prematurity. Bartter syndrome (OMIM 601678, 241200, 607364 and 602522) refers to a group of autosomal recessive disorders caused by inactivating mutations in genes (*SLC12A1*, *KCNJ1*, *CLCNKB*,

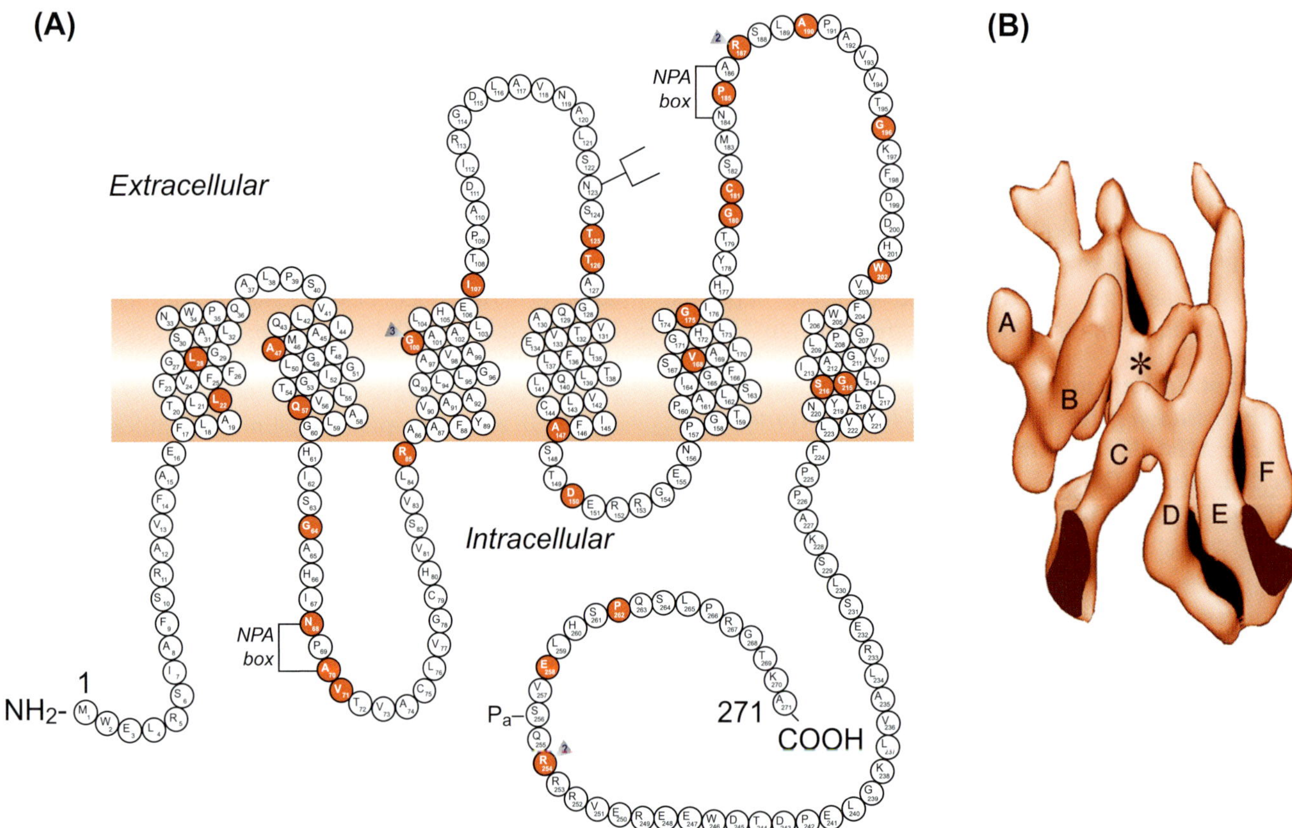

FIGURE 8.15 (A) Schematic representation of the aquaporin-2 protein and identification of 42 AQP2 mutations. A monomer is represented with six stretches of hydrophobic sequences that are suggestive of six transmembrane helices. The MIP proteins (see text) share an NPA (Asn-Pro-Ala) motif in each of the two prominent loops. AQP1 (and by analogy AQP2) is a homotetramer containing four independent aqueous channels. The location of the protein kinase A phosphorylation site is indicated. This site is possibly involved in the vasopressin-induced trafficking of AQP2 from intracellular vesicles to the plasma membrane and in the subsequent stimulation of endocytosis. (B) A surface-shaded representation of the six-helix barrel of the AQP1 protein viewed parallel to the bilayer. *Modified from [307].*

CLCNKA and *CLCNKB* in combination, or *BSND*) that encode membrane proteins of the thick ascending limb of the loop of Henle (for review see [229,230]). Although Bartter syndrome and Bartter's mutations are commonly used as a diagnosis, it is likely, as explained by Jeck et al. [231], that the two patients with a mild phenotype originally described by Dr. Bartter had Gitelman syndrome, a thiazide-like salt-losing tubulopathy with a defect in the distal convoluted tubule [231]. As a consequence, salt-losing tubulopathy of the furosemide type is a more physiologically appropriate definition.

Thirty percent of the filtered sodium chloride is reabsorbed in the thick ascending limb of the loop of Henle through the apically expressed sodium–potassium–chloride cotransporter NKCC2 (encoded by the *SLC12A1* gene), which uses the sodium gradient across the membrane to transport chloride and potassium into the cell. The potassium ions must be recycled through the apical membrane by the potassium channel ROMK (encoded by the *KCNJ1* gene). In the large experience of Seyberth and colleagues [232], who studied 85 patients with a hypokaliemic salt-losing tubulopathy, all 20 patients with *KCNJ1* mutations (except one) and all 12 patients with *SLC12A1* mutations were born as preterm infants after severe polyhydramnios. Of note, polyhydramnios was never seen during the pregnancies that led to infants bearing *AVPR2* or *AQP2* mutations. The most common causes of increased amniotic fluid include maternal diabetes mellitus, fetal malformations and chromosomal aberrations, twin-to-twin transfusion syndrome, rhesus incompatibility and congenital infections [233]. Postnatally, polyuria was the leading symptom in 19 of the 32 patients. Renal ultrasound revealed nephrocalcinosis in 31 of these patients. These patients with complex polyuropolydipsic disorders are often poorly recognized and may be confused with "pure" NDI. As a consequence, congenital polyuria does not suggest automatically *AVPR2* or *AQP2* mutations, and polyhydramnios, salt wasting, hypokaliemia and nephrocalcinosis are important clinical and laboratory characteristics that should be assessed. In patients with Bartter syndrome (salt-losing tubulopathy/furosemide type), the dDAVP test will only indicate a partial type of NDI. The algorithm proposed by Peters et al. [232] is useful since most mutations in *SLC12A1* and *KCNJ1* are found in the carboxyl terminus or in the last exon and, as a consequence, are amenable to rapid DNA sequencing. Nephropathic cystinosis, nephronophisis and apparent mineralocorticoid excess are also characterized by polyuria, polydipsia and poor urinary osmolality response to AVP [234].

Acquired NDI (Table 8.4)

Acquired NDI is much more common than congenital NDI but it is rarely as severe. The ability to produce hypertonic urine is usually preserved even though there is inadequate concentrating ability of the nephron. Polyuria and polydipsia are therefore moderate (3–4 L/day).

Among the more common causes of acquired NDI, lithium administration has become the most frequent cause; 54% of 1105 unselected patients on chronic lithium therapy developed NDI [235]. Nineteen percent of these patients had polyuria, as defined by a 24-hour urine output exceeding 3 L. The dysregulation of aquaporin-2 expression is the result of cytotoxic accumulation of lithium which enters via the epithelial sodium channel (ENaC) on the apical membrane and leads to the inhibition of signaling pathways that involve glycogen synthase kinase type 3 beta [236]. The concentration of lithium in urine of patients on well-controlled lithium therapy (i.e., 10–40 mOsmol/L) is sufficient to exert this effect. For patients on long-term lithium therapy, amiloride has been proposed to prevent the uptake of lithium in the collecting ducts, thus preventing the inhibitory effect of intracellular lithium on water transport [237].

Primary Polydipsia

Primary polydipsia is a state of hypotonic polyuria secondary to excessive fluid intake. Primary polydipsia was extensively studied by Barlow and de Wardener in 1959 [238]; however, the understanding of the pathophysiology of this disease has made little progress. Barlow and de Wardener [238] described seven women and two men who were compulsive water drinkers; their ages ranged from 48 to 59 years except for one patient who was 24 years old. Eight of these patients had histories of previous psychological disorders, which ranged from delusions, depression and agitation, to frank hysterical behavior. The other patient appeared normal. The consumption of water fluctuated irregularly from hour to hour or from day to day; in some patients, there were remissions and relapses lasting several months or longer. In eight of the patients, the mean plasma osmolality was significantly lower than normal. Vasopressin tannate in oil made most of these patients feel ill; in one, it caused overhydration. In four patients, the fluid intake returned to normal after electroconvulsive therapy or a period of continuous narcosis; the improvement in three was transient, but in the fourth it lasted 2 years. Polyuric female subjects might be heterozygous for de novo or previously unrecognized *AVPR2* mutations, may bear *AQP2* mutations and may be classified as compulsive water drinkers [239]. Therefore, the diagnosis of compulsive water drinking must be made with care and may represent our ignorance of yet undescribed pathophysiological mechanisms. G. Robertson [239] has described under the name "dipsogenic diabetes insipidus" a selective

TABLE 8.4 Acquired Causes of Nephrogenic Diabetes Insipidus

Chronic renal disease	Polycystic disease
	Medullary cystic disease
	Pyelonephritis
	Ureteral obstruction
	Far-advanced renal failure
Electrolyte disorders	Hypokalemia
	Hypercalcemia
Drugs	Alcohol
	Phenytoin
	Lithium
	Demeclocycline
	Acetohexamide
	Tolazamide
	Glyburide
	Propoxyphene
	Amphotericin
	Methoxyflurane
	Norepinephrine
	Vinblastine
	Colchicine
	Gentamicin
	Methicillin
	Isophosphamide
	Angiographic dyes
	Osmotic diuretics
	Furosemide and ethacrynic acid
Sickle cell disease	
Dietary abnormalities	Excessive water intake
	Decreased sodium chloride intake
	Decreased protein intake
Miscellaneous	Multiple myeloma
	Amyloidosis
	Sjogren's disease
	Sarcoidosis

defect in the osmoregulation of thirst. Three studied patients had, under basal conditions of ad libitum water intake, thirst, polydipsia, polyuria and high-normal plasma osmolality. They had a normal secretion of AVP, but osmotic threshold for thirst was abnormally low. These dipsogenic diabetes insipidus cases might represent up to 10% of all patients with diabetes insipidus [239].

Diabetes Insipidus and Pregnancy

PREGNANCY IN A PATIENT KNOWN TO HAVE DIABETES INSIPIDUS

An isolated deficiency of vasopressin without a concomitant loss of hormones in the anterior pituitary does not result in altered fertility, and with the exception of polyuria and polydipsia, gestation, delivery and lactation are uncomplicated [240]. Patients may require increasing dosages of dDAVP. The increased thirst may be due to a resetting of the thirst osmostat [102].

Increased polyuria also occurs during pregnancy in patients with partial NDI [241]. These patients may be obligatory carriers of the NDI gene [242] or may be homozygotes, compound heterozygotes or may have dominant AQP2 mutations.

SYNDROMES OF DIABETES INSIPIDUS THAT BEGIN DURING GESTATION AND REMIT AFTER DELIVERY

Barron et al. [243] described three pregnant women in whom transient diabetes insipidus developed late in gestation and subsequently remitted postpartum. In one of these patients, dilute urine was present despite high plasma concentrations of AVP. Hyposthenuria in all three patients was resistant to administered aqueous vasopressin. Because excessive vasopressinase activity was not excluded as a cause of this disorder, Barron et al. labeled the disease vasopressin resistant rather than NDI.

A well documented case of enhanced activity of vasopressinase has been described in a woman in the third trimester of a previously uncomplicated pregnancy [244]. She had massive polyuria and markedly elevated plasma vasopressinase activity. The polyuria did not respond to large intravenous doses of AVP but responded promptly to dDAVP, a vasopressinase-resistant analogue of AVP. The polyuria disappeared with the disappearance of the vasopressinase. It is suggested that pregnancy may be associated with several different forms of diabetes insipidus, including central, nephrogenic and vasopressinase-mediated [241,245–247].

INVESTIGATION OF A PATIENT WITH POLYURIA

Plasma sodium and osmolality are maintained within normal limits (136–143 mOsmol/L for plasma sodium; 275–290 mOsmol/kg for plasma osmolality) by a thirst–AVP–renal axis. Thirst and AVP release, both stimulated by increased osmolality, is a "double negative" feedback system [248]. Even when the AVP component of this "double negative" regulatory feedback system is lost, the thirst mechanism still preserves the plasma sodium and osmolality within the normal range, but at the expense of pronounced polydipsia and polyuria. Thus, the plasma sodium concentration or osmolality of an untreated patient with diabetes insipidus may be slightly greater than the mean normal value, but these small increases have no diagnostic significance.

Theoretically, it should be relatively easy to differentiate between neurogenic diabetes insipidus, NDI and primary polydipsia by comparing the osmolality of urine obtained during dehydration with that of urine obtained after the administration of dAVP. Patients with neurogenic diabetes insipidus should reveal a rapid increase in urinary osmolality, whereas it should increase normally in response to moderate dehydration in patients with primary polydipsia. However, for several reasons, these distinctions may not be as clear as one might expect [249]. First, chronic polyuria resulting from any cause interferes with the maintenance of the medullary concentration gradient and this "washout" effect diminishes the maximum concentrating ability of the nephron. The extent of the blunting varies in direct proportion to the severity of the polyuria. Hence, for any given basal urine output, the maximum urine osmolality achieved in the presence of saturating concentrations of AVP is depressed to the same extent in patients with primary polydipsia, neurogenic diabetes insipidus, or NDI (Figure 8.16). Second, most patients with neurogenic diabetes insipidus maintain a small, but detectable, capacity to secrete AVP during severe dehydration, and urinary osmolality may then increase to greater than the plasma osmolality. Third, patients referred to as partial diabetes insipidus (either neurogenic or nephrogenic) and patients with acquired NDI have an incomplete response to AVP and are able to concentrate their urine to varying degrees in a dehydration test. Finally, all polyuric states (whether neurogenic, nephrogenic, or psychogenic) can induce large dilatations of the urinary tract and bladder [250,251]. As a consequence, the urinary bladder of these patients has an increased residual capacity and changes in urinary osmolality induced by diagnostic maneuvers might be difficult to demonstrate.

Indirect Tests for Diabetes Insipidus

The measurement of urinary osmolality after dehydration and dDAVP administration is usually referred to as "indirect testing" because AVP secretion is indirectly assessed through changes in urinary osmolalities [126]. The patient is maintained on a complete fluid-restriction regimen until urinary osmolality reaches a plateau, as indicated by an hourly increase of less than 30 mOsmol/kg for at least three successive hours. After measuring the plasma osmolality, 2 μg dDAVP are administered subcutaneously. Urinary osmolality is measured 30 and 60 minutes later. The last urinary osmolality value obtained before the dDAVP injection and the highest value obtained after the injection are compared. In patients with severe neurogenic diabetes insipidus, urinary osmolality after dehydration is usually low (<200 mOsmol/kg) and increases more than 50% after dDAVP administration. In patients with

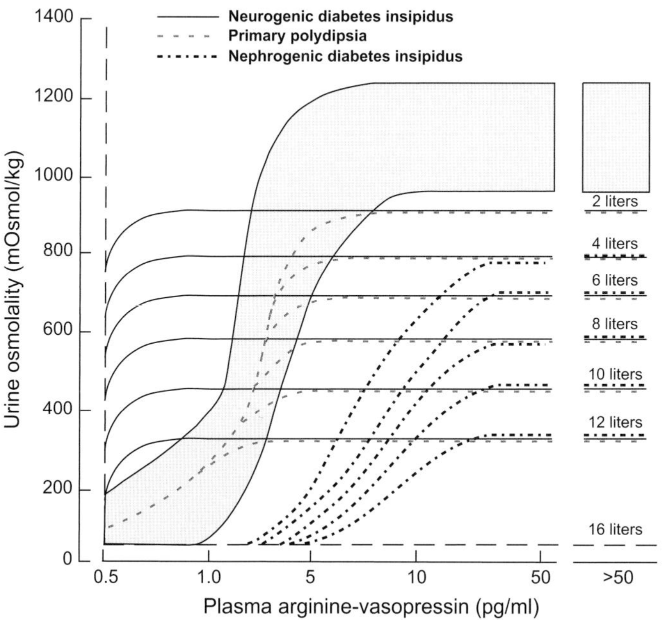

FIGURE 8.16 The relationship between urine osmolality and plasma vasopressin in patients with polyuria of diverse etiology and severity. Note that for each of the three categories of polyuria – neurogenic diabetes insipidus, nephrogenic diabetes insipidus and primary polydipsia – the relationship is described by a family of sigmoid curves that differ in height. These differences in height reflect differences in maximal concentrating capacity owing to "washout" of the medullary concentration gradient. They are proportional to the severity of the underlying polyuria (indicated in liters per day at the right end of each plateau) and are largely independent of the etiology. Thus, the three catagories of diabetes insipidus differ principally in the submaximal or ascending portion of the dose–response curve. In patients with partial neurogenic diabetes insipidus, this part of the curve lies to the left of normal, reflecting increased sensitivity to the antidiuretic effects of very low concentrations of plasma arginine-vasopressin (AVP). In contrast, in patients with partial nephrogenic diabetes insipidus, this part of the curve lies to the right of normal, reflecting decreased sensitivity to the antidiuretic effects of normal concentrations of plasma AVP. In primary polydipsia, this relationship is relatively normal. *From Robertson [249], with permission, Karger AG Basel.*

severe NDI, urinary osmolality after dehydration is also low (<200 mOsmol/kg) but does not increase after dDAVP administration (<20%). Urinary osmolality increases to variable degrees (10–50%) after dDAVP administration to patients with partial neurogenic or partial nephrogenic diabetes insipidus. In patients with primary polydipsia, maximum urinary osmolality will be obtained after dehydration (>295 mOsmol/kg) and does not increase after dDAVP administration (<10%).

Alternatively, plasma sodium and plasma and urinary osmolalities can be measured at the beginning of the dehydration procedure and at regular intervals (usually hourly) thereafter depending on the severity of the polyuria [252]. For example, an 8-year-old patient (body weight 31 kg) with a clinical diagnosis of congenital NDI (later found to bear an *AVPR2* mutation) continued to excrete large volumes of urine (300 ml/hour) during a short 4-hour dehydration test. During this time, the patient suffered from severe thirst, his plasma sodium was 155 mOsmol/L, plasma osmolality was 310 mOsmol/kg and urinary osmolality was 85 mOsmol/kg. The patient received 1 μg of dDAVP intravenously and was allowed to drink water. Repeated urinary osmolality measurements demonstrated a complete urinary resistance to dDAVP. It would have been dangerous and unnecessary to prolong the dehydration further in this young patient. Thus, the usual prescription of overnight dehydration should not be used in patients, and especially children, with severe polyuria and polydipsia (more than 30 ml/kg body weight per day). Great care should be taken to avoid any severe hypertonic state, arbitrarily defined as plasma sodium greater than 155 mOsmol/L.

Direct Tests of Diabetes Insipidus

The two approaches of Zerbe and Robertson are used [125], although they are expensive, time-consuming and difficult to carry out on young patients. In the first approach, during the dehydration test, plasma is collected hourly and assayed for AVP. The results are plotted on a nomogram depicting the normal relationship between plasma sodium or osmolality and plasma AVP in normal individuals (Figure 8.8). If the relationship goes below the normal range, the disorder is diagnosed as neurogenic diabetes insipidus.

In the second approach NDI can be differentiated from primary polydipsia by analyzing the relationship between plasma AVP and urinary osmolality at the end of the dehydration period (Figure 8.8). However, definitive differentiation might be impossible because a normal or even supranormal AVP response to increased plasma osmolality occurs in polydipsic patients. None of the patients with psychogenic or other forms of severe polydipsia studied by Robertson showed any evidence of pituitary suppression [249].

In a comparison of diagnoses based on indirect versus direct tests of AVP function in 54 patients with polyuria of diverse cause, Robertson [249] found that the indirect test was reliable only for patients with severe defects. Three severe NDI patients and 16 of 17 patients with severe neurogenic diabetes insipidus were accurately diagnosed. However, the error rate of the indirect test was about 50% in diagnosing partial neurogenic diabetes insipidus, partial NDI or primary polydipsia in patients who were able to concentrate their urine to varying degrees when water deprived. The benefits of combined direct and indirect testing of AVP function have been discussed by Stern and Valtin [253]. The diagnosis of primary polydipsia remains one of exclusion and the cause could be psychogenic [238] or inappropriate thirst [239,254]. Psychiatric patients with polydipsia and hyponatremia have unexplained defects in urinary dilution, the osmoregulation of water intake or the secretion of vasopressin [255].

Therapeutic Trial of dDAVP

In selected patients with an uncertain diagnosis, a closely monitored therapeutic trial of dDAVP (10 μg intranasally twice a day for 2–3 days) may be used to distinguish partial NDI from partial neurogenic diabetes insipidus or primary polydipsia. If dDAVP at this dosage causes a significant antidiuretic effect, NDI is effectively excluded. If polydipsia as well as polyuria is abolished and plasma sodium does not go below the normal range, the patient probably has neurogenic diabetes insipidus. Conversely, if dDAVP causes a reduction in urine output without reduction in water intake and hyponatremia appears, the patient probably has primary polydipsia. Since fatal water intoxication is a remote possibility, the dDAVP trial should be closely monitored.

The methods of differential diagnosis of diabetes insipidus are described in Tables 8.5 and 8.6.

Carrier Detection, Perinatal Testing and Early Treatment

The identification of mutations in the genes that cause hereditary diabetes insipidus allows the early diagnosis and management of at-risk members of families with identified mutations. We encourage physicians who follow families with autosomal neurogenic, X-linked and autosomal NDI to recommend mutation analysis before the birth of an infant because early diagnosis and treatment can avert the physical and mental retardation associated with episodes of dehydration. Diagnosis of X-linked NDI was accomplished by mutation testing of cultured amniotic cells ($n = 6$), chorionic villus samples ($n = 7$), or cord blood obtained at birth ($n = 31$) in 44 of

TABLE 8.5 Urinary Responses to Fluid Deprivation and Exogenous Vasopressin in Recognition of Partial Defects in Antidiuretic Hormone Secretion[a]

	Number of Cases	Maximum U_{osm}[b]	U_{osm} After Vasopressin	Percent Change (U_{osm})	U_{osm} Incrase After Vasopressin
Normal subjects	9	1068 ± 69	979 ± 79	− 9 ± 3	<9%
Complete central diabetes insipidus	8	168 ± 13	445 ± 52	183 ± 41	>50%
Partial central diabetes insipidus	11	438 ± 34	549 ± 28	28 ± 5	>9% <50%
Nephrogenic diabetes insipidus	2	123.5	174.5	42	<50%
Compulsive water drinking	7	738 ± 73	780 ± 73	5.0 ± 2.2	<9%

[a] *Data from Miller et al. [126].*
[b] *Urinary osmolality (U_{osm}) in mmol/kg.*

TABLE 8.6 Differential Diagnosis of Diabetes Insipidus*

1. Measure plasma osmolality and/or sodium concentration under conditions of ad libitum fluid intake. If they are above 295 mmol/kg and 143 mmol/L, the diagnosis of primary polydipsia is excluded and the work-up should proceed directly to step 5 and/or 6 to distinguish between neurogenic and nephrogenic diabetes insipidus. Otherwise:

2. Perform a dehydration test. If urinary concentration does not occur before plasma osmolality and/or sodium reach 295 mmol/kg or 143 mmol/L, the diagnosis of primary polydipsia is again excluded and the work-up should proceed to step 5 and/or 6. Otherwise:

3. Determine the ratio of urine to plasma osmolality at the end of the dehydration test. If it is less than 1.5, the diagnosis of primary polydipsia is again excluded and the work-up should proceed to step 5 and/or 6. Otherwise:

4. Perform a hypertonic saline infusion with measurements of plasma vasopressin and osmolality at intervals during the procedure. If the relationship between these two variables is subnormal, the diagnosis of diabetes insipidus is established. Otherwise:

5. Perform a vasopressin infusion test. If urine osmolality rises by more than 150 mosmol/kg above the value obtained at the end of the dehydration test, nephrogenic diabetes insipidus is excluded. Alternately:

6. Measure urine osmolality and plasma vasopressin at the end of the dehydration test. If the relationship is normal, the diagnosis of nephrogenic diabetes insipidus is excluded.

* *Data from Robertson [310].*

our patients. Twenty-one males were found to bear mutant sequences, 16 males were not affected and five females were not carriers. These affected patients were immediately given abundant water intake, a low-sodium diet and hydrochlorothiazide. They never experienced episodes of dehydration, and their physical and mental development is normal. Gene analysis is also important for the identification of nonobligatory female carriers in families with X-linked NDI. Most females heterozygous for a mutation in the V_2 receptor do not have clinical symptoms; few are severely affected [191,256,257]. Mutation detection in families with inherited neurogenic diabetes insipidus provides a powerful clinical tool for early diagnosis and management of subsequent cases, especially in early childhood, when diagnosis is difficult and the clinical risks are the greatest [258].

Neurogenic diabetes insipidus (central or Wolfram) is easily treated with dDAVP [259]. All complications of congenital NDI are prevented by an adequate water intake. Thus, patients should be provided with unrestricted amounts of water from birth to ensure normal development. In addition to a low-sodium diet, the use of diuretics (thiazides) or indometacin may reduce urinary output. This advantageous effect has to be weighed against the side effects of these drugs (thiazides: electrolyte disturbances; indometacin: reduction of the glomerular filtration rate and gastrointestinal symptoms).

RADIOIMMUNOASSAY OF AVP AND OTHER LABORATORY DETERMINATIONS

Radioimmunoassay of AVP

Three developments were basic to the elaboration of a clinically useful radioimmunoassay for plasma AVP [260,261]: (1) the extraction of AVP from plasma with petrol-ether and acetone and the subsequent elimination of nonspecific immunoreactivity; (2) the use of highly specific and sensitive rabbit antiserum; and (3) the use of a tracer (^{125}I-AVP) with high specific activity. These same extraction procedures are still widely used [88,89,101,103], and commercial tracers (^{125}I-AVP) and antibodies are available. AVP can also be extracted from plasma by using Sep-Pak C18 cartridges [262–264].

Blood samples collected in chilled 7 ml lavender-stoppered tubes containing EDTA are centrifuged at 4°C, 1000 g (3000 rpm in a usual laboratory centrifuge), for 20 minutes. This 20-minute centrifugation is mandatory for obtaining platelet-poor plasma samples because a large fraction of the circulating vasopressin is associated with the platelets in humans [89,265]. The tubes may be kept for 2 hours on slushed ice prior to centrifugation. Plasma is then separated, frozen at −20°C and extracted within 6 weeks of sampling. Details for sample preparation and assay procedure can be found in writings by Bichet and colleagues [88,89]. An AVP radioimmunoassay should be validated by demonstrating; (1) a good correlation between plasma sodium or osmolality and plasma AVP during dehydration and infusion of hypertonic saline solution (Figure 8.8); and (2) the inability to obtain detectable values of AVP in patients with severe central diabetes insipidus. Plasma AVP-immunoreactivity may be elevated in patients with diabetes insipidus following hypothalamic surgery [266].

In pregnant patients, the blood contains high concentrations of cystine aminopeptidase which can (in vitro) inactivate enormous quantities (ng $\times$ ml^{-1} $\times$ min^{-1}) of AVP. However, phenanthrolene effectively inhibits these cystine aminopeptidases. Measurements of copeptin by ELISA could, in the future, replace the difficult radioimmunological measure of AVP [267,268].

AQP2 Measurements

Urinary AQP2 excretion could be measured by radioimmunoassay or quantitative western analysis and could provide an additional indication of the responsiveness of the collecting duct to AVP.

Plasma Sodium, Plasma and Urine Osmolality

Measurements of plasma sodium, plasma and urinary osmolality should be immediately available at various intervals during dehydration procedures. Plasma sodium is easily measured by flame photometry or with a sodium-specific electrode [269]. Plasma and urinary osmolalities are also reliably measured by freezing point depression instruments with a coefficient of variation at 290 mmol/kg of less than 1%.

At variance with published data [89,125], we have found that plasma and serum osmolalities are equivalent (i.e., similar values are obtained). Blood taken in heparinized tubes is easier to handle because the plasma can be more readily removed after centrifugation. The tube used (green-stoppered tube) contains a minuscule concentration of lithium and sodium, which does not interfere with plasma sodium or osmolality measurements. Frozen plasma or urinary samples can be kept for further analysis of their osmolalities because the results obtained are similar to those obtained immediately after blood sampling, except in patients with severe renal failure. In the latter patients, plasma osmolality measurements are increased after freezing and thawing but the plasma sodium values remain unchanged.

Plasma osmolality measurements can be used to demonstrate the absence of unusual osmotically active substances (e.g., glucose and urea in high concentrations, mannitol, ethanol). With this information, plasma or serum sodium measurements are sufficient to assess the degree of dehydration and its relationship to plasma AVP. Nomograms describing the normal plasma sodium/plasma AVP relationship (Figure 8.8) are equally as valuable as classic nomograms describing the relationship between plasma osmolality and effective osmolality (i.e., plasma osmolality minus the contribution of "ineffective" solutes: glucose and urea).

Magnetic Resonance Imaging in Patients With Diabetes Insipidus

Magnetic resonance imaging (MRI) permits visualization of the anterior and posterior pituitary glands and the pituitary stalk. The pituitary stalk is permeated by numerous capillary loops of the hypophyseal–portal blood system. This vascular structure also provides the principal blood supply to the anterior pituitary lobe, because there is no direct arterial supply to this organ. In contrast, the posterior pituitary lobe has a direct vascular supply. Therefore, the posterior lobe can be more rapidly visualized in a dynamic mode after administration of a gadolinium (gadopentate dimeglumine) as contrast material during MRI. The posterior pituitary lobe is easily distinguished by a round, high-intensity signal (the posterior pituitary "bright spot") in the posterior part of the sella turcica on T_1-weighted images. Loss of the pituitary hyperintense spot or bright spot on a T_1-weighted MRI image reflects loss of functional integrity of the neurohypophysis and is a nonspecific indicator of neurohypophyseal diabetes insipidus regardless of the underlying cause [162,270]. It is now considered that the bright spot represents normal AVP storage in the posterior lobe of the pituitary, that the intensity is correlated with the amount of AVP and that after 60 years of age the signal is often less intense with irregularities in the normally smooth convex edge [271,272]. MRI is reported to be the best technique with which to evaluate the pituitary stalk and infundibulum in patients with idiopathic polyuria. A thickening or enlargement of the pituitary stalk may suggest an infiltrative process destroying the neurohypophyseal tract [273].

Treatment

In most patients with complete hypothalamic diabetes insipidus, the thirst mechanism remains intact. Thus, hypernatremia does not develop in these patients and they suffer only from the inconvenience associated with marked polyuria and polydipsia. If hypodipsia develops or access to water is limited, then severe hypernatremia can supervene. The treatment of choice for patients with severe hypothalamic diabetes insipidus is dDAVP, a synthetic, long-acting vasopressin analogue, with minimal vasopressor activity but a large antidiuretic potency. The usual intranasal daily dose is between 5 and 20 μg. To avoid the potential complication of dilutional hyponatremia, which is exceptional in these patients as a result of an intact thirst mechanism, dDAVP can be withdrawn at regular intervals to allow the patients to become polyuric. Aqueous vasopressin (Pitressin) or dDAVP (4.0 μg/1-mL ampule) can be used intravenously in acute situations such as after hypophysectomy or for the treatment of diabetes insipidus in the brain-dead organ donor. Pitressin tannate in oil and nonhormonal antidiuretic drugs are somewhat obsolete and now rarely used. For example, chlorpropamide (250–500 mg daily) appears to potentiate the antidiuretic action of circulating AVP, but troublesome side effects of hypoglycemia and hyponatremia do occur.

In the treatment of congenital NDI, an abundant unrestricted water intake should always be provided, and affected patients should be carefully followed during their first years of life. Water should be offered every 2 hours day and night, and temperature, appetite and growth should be monitored. The parents of these children easily accept setting their alarm clock every 2 hours during the night. Hospital admission may be necessary to allow continuous gastric feeding. A low-osmolar and low-sodium diet, hydrochlorothiazide (1–2 mg/kg/day) alone or with amiloride, and indometacin (0.75–1.5 mg/kg) substantially reduce water excretion and are helpful in the treatment of children. Many adult patients receive no treatment.

SYNDROME OF INAPPROPRIATE SECRETION OF THE ANTIDIURETIC HORMONE (SIADH)

Hyponatremia (defined as a plasma sodium below 130 mmol/L) is the most common disorder of body fluid and electrolyte balance encountered in the clinical practice of medicine, with incidences ranging from 1–2% in both acutely and chronically hospitalized patients [274,275]. Because a defect in renal water excretion, as reflected by hypo-osmolality, may occur in the presence of an excess or deficit of total body sodium or nearly normal total body sodium, it is useful to classify the hyponatremic states accordingly [276,277]. Moreover, since total body sodium is the primary determinant of the extracellular fluid (ECF) volume, bedside evaluation of the ECF volume allows for a convenient means of classifying hyponatremic patients [277,276] (Figure 8.17).

Patients with hyponatremia who show no evidence of either hypovolemia or edema constitute a select group. Although many of these patients may have SIADH (this syndrome is so named because the secretion of AVP cannot be accounted for by recognized osmotic or nonosmotic stimuli), endocrine disorders such as hypoparathyroidism, hypopituitarism with glucocorticoid deficiency, various pharmacological agents and emotional and physical stress may also cause euvolemic hyponatremia [277]. Psychotic patients with polydipsia and hyponatremia are also classified in this group of hyponatremic patients with normal total body sodium [255,278]. The diagnosis of SIADH is made primarily by excluding other causes of hyponatremia. It should be considered in the absence of hypovolemia, edematous disorders, endocrine dysfunction (including primary and secondary adrenal insufficiency and hypothyroidism), renal failure and drugs, all of which impair water excretion. Psychotic patients with polydipsia and hyponatremia have multiple disturbances in water regulation including alteration in osmoreceptor function, inappropriate thirst response, renal hypersensitivity to vasopressin and vasopressin-independent perturbation of urinary dilution. Thus, we recommend that these patients should not be classified as presenting with SIADH.

An animal model of antidiuretic-induced hyponatremia closely resembling clinical SIADH developed by Verbalis and coworkers using a continuous subcutaneous infusion of dDAVP in combination with dextrose drinking or the self-ingestion of a concentrated, nutritionally balanced liquid diet. A chronic, severe hyponatremia accompanied by an antidiuretic effect was obtained. Multiple hemodynamic and hormonal adaptive responses were also observed [279].

Since 1957 when Schwartz et al. [280] first described SIADH in two patients with bronchogenic carcinoma who were hyponatremic, clinically euvolemic with normal renal and adrenal function, and who had less than maximally dilute urine with appreciable urinary sodium concentrations (greater than 20 mmol/L), SIADH has been recognized in a variety of pathological

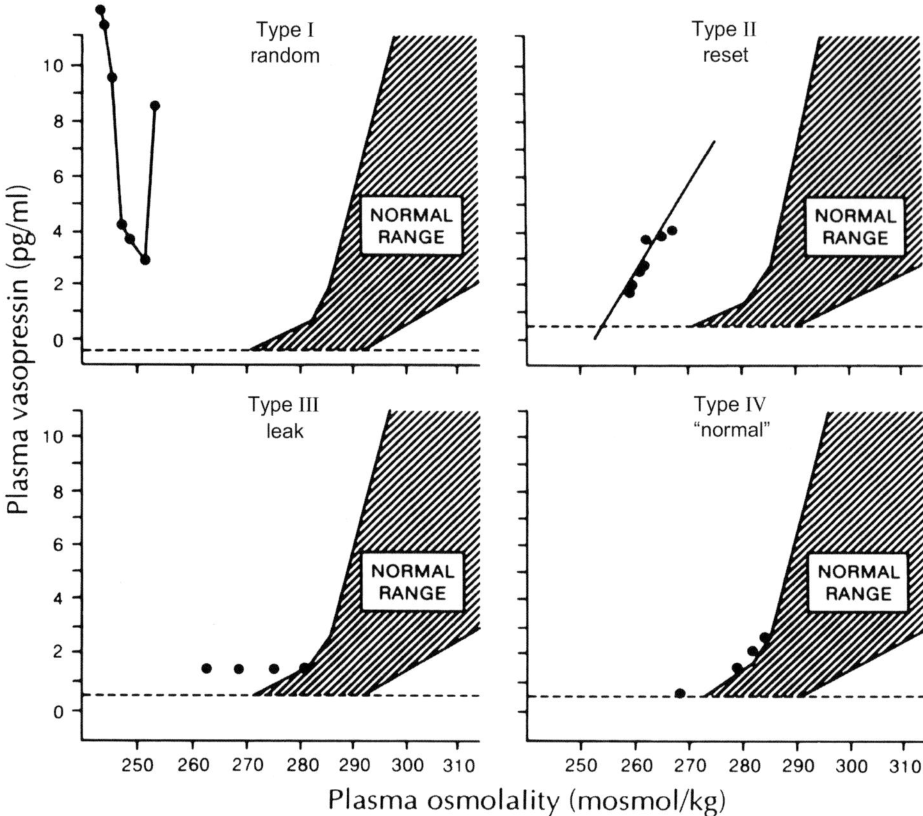

FIGURE 8.17 Plasma vasopressin as a function of plasma osmolality during the infusion of hypertonic saline in patients with syndrome of inappropriate secretion of antidiuretic hormone (SIADH). *From Robertson [306] with permission, Wolters Kluwer.*

processes. Various diseases, which may be accompanied by SIADH, are listed in Table 8.7. These diseases generally fall into three categories: (1) malignancies; (2) pulmonary disorders; and (3) central nervous system disorders. Human immunodeficiency virus (HIV) infection forms a new category of patients with SIADH, with as many as 35% of hospitalized patients affected. In these patients, *Pneumocystis carinii* pneumonia, CNS infections and malignancies play a role in the development of SIADH [281].

Tumors can synthesize and secrete AVP. Many tumors contain typical secretory granules and cultured tumor tissue has been shown to synthesize not only AVP but also the entire AVP precursor peptide, propressophysin [282,283]. Furthermore, tumor extracts have been found to contain AVP bioactivity and immunologically recognizable AVP [284]. Numerous reports have called attention to a rare tumor, olfactory neuroblastoma, which is frequently associated with chronic, occasionally symptomatic, hyponatremia [285].

In spite of the hyponatremia, patients with SIADH have a concentrated urine in which the urinary sodium concentration closely parallels the sodium intake, i.e., it is usually above 20 mmol/L. However, in the presence of sodium restriction or volume depletion these patients can conserve sodium normally and decrease their urinary sodium concentration to less than 10 mmol/L [286]. Serum uric acid has been found to be reduced in SIADH patients, whereas patients with other causes of hyponatremia have normal concentrations of serum uric acid [287]. Uric acid and phosphate clearances were found to be increased in patients with SIADH as a consequence of volume expansion and decreased tubular reabsorption [288]. Similarly, low serum blood urea nitrogen concentrations have been found in SIADH [289]. This is probably due to an increase in total body water, where urea is normally distributed, but a decrease in protein intake could also contribute. Plasma atrial natriuretic factor concentration has been found to be increased in patients with SIADH and to correlate with urinary sodium excretion [290,291]. Dillingham and Anderson [292] observed a direct inhibition of the renal epithelial water transport in rabbit collecting tubules perfused in vitro with 2 nmol of atriopeptin III. Nonoguchi et al. [293] found that physiological concentrations of atrial natriuretic factor caused an inhibition of vasopressin-stimulated osmotic water permeability in the rat terminal inner medullary collecting duct. Thus, although atrial natriuretic factor may antagonize the hydrosmotic effect of vasopressin, SIADH may

TABLE 8.7 Disorders Associated With Syndrome of Inappropriate Secretion of the Antidiuretic Hormone (SIADH)

Carcinomas	Small-cell carcinoma of the lung
	Carcinoma of the duodenum
	Carcinoma of the pancreas
	Thymoma
	Carcinoma of the ureter
	Lymphoma
	Ewing's sarcoma
	Mesothelioma
	Carcinoma of the bladder
	Prostatic carcinoma
	Olfactory neuroblastoma
Central nervous system disorders	Encephalitis (viral or bacterial)
	Meningitis (viral, bacterial, tuberculous, fungal)
	Head trauma
	Brain abscess
	Brain tumors
	Guillain-Barré syndrome
	Acute intermittent porphyria
	Subarachnoid hemorrhage of subdural hematoma
	Cerebellar and cerebral atrophy
	Cavernous sinus thrombosis
	Neonatal hypoxia
	Hydrocephalus
	Shy-Drager syndrome
	Rocky Mountain spotted fever
	Delirium tremens
	Cerebrovascular accident (cerebral thrombosis or hemorrhage)
	Acute psychosis
	Peripheral neuropathy
	Multiple sclerosis
Pulmonary disorders	Viral pneumonia
	Bacterial pneumonia
	Pulmonary abscess
	Tuberculosis
	Aspergillosis
	Positive-pressure breathing
	Asthma
	Pneumothorax
	Cystic fibrosis

nevertheless occur in the presence of increased plasma atrial natriuretic hormone concentrations.

Abnormal osmoregulation of vasopressin has been studied in 79 patients with SIADH [294]. These patients underwent either hypertonic saline or water loading or both and four patterns of responses were identified. The type I pattern, observed in 37% of the patients studied, consisted of large, erratic changes in plasma vasopressin concentrations with no relationship to the plasma osmolality. In type II (33% of the patients), the release of vasopressin was found, as in normal subjects, to correlate closely with the plasma osmolality; however, the osmotic threshold for vasopressin release was abnormally low. Theoretically, this group could correspond to the previously described patients with a "reset osmostat" which enabled the urine of these patients to become maximally dilute if they were sufficiently hyponatremic. Unfortunately, Zerbe et al. [294] did not publish any water load studies for these patients. Thus the ability of this group of SIADH patients to excrete a water load normally at a reduced osmotic threshold remains to be documented. In the type III patients, a constant, nonsuppressible basal "leak" of vasopressin with an otherwise normal osmotic release of vasopressin was observed. In type IV patients (14%), no detectable abnormalities in vasopressin secretion were observed. This suggested either a nonvasopressin-mediated mechanism or an increased sensitivity to normal amounts of vasopressin. These four types of SIADH did not correlate with the underlying clinical problems (Table 8.8). For example, bronchogenic carcinoma, a disorder that might be expected to feature ectopic production of vasopressin, was associated with all four categories of SIADH. The clinical relevance of this categorization of SIADH therefore remains to be elucidated.

SIGNS, SYMPTOMS AND TREATMENT OF HYPONATREMIA

The majority of the manifestations of hyponatremia are of a neuropsychiatric nature and include lethargy, psychosis, seizures and coma [295]. Elderly and young children with hyponatremia are most likely to become symptomatic. The degree of the clinical impairment is not strictly related to the absolute value of the lowered serum sodium concentration, but, rather, it relates to both the rate and the extent of the fall of ECF osmolality [295]. The mortality rate from acute symptomatic hyponatremia is difficult to determine. Arieff quotes a mortality rate of approximately 50% [296]. On the other hand, none of the ten acutely hyponatremic patients reported by Sterns had permanent neurologic sequelae [297]. As Berl [298] commented, the 50% mortality rate might be an exaggeration, but estimates

TABLE 8.8 Principal Clinical Diagnoses in Each of the Four Types of Syndrome of Inappropriate Secretion of the Antidiuretic Hormone (SIADH) Identified by Saline Infusion in 25 Patients*

Type	Number of Patients	Diagnoses
I	2	Acute respiratory failure
	1	Bronchogenic carcinoma
	1	Pulmonary tuberculosis
	1	Schizophrenia
	1	Rheumatoid arthritis
II	4	Bronchogenic carcinoma
	2	Cerebrovascular disease
	1	Tuberculous meningitis
	1	Acute respiratory disease
	1	Carcinoma of pharynx
III	3	Central nervous system disease
	2	Bronchogenic carcinoma
	1	Pulmonary tuberculosis
	1	Schizophrenia
IV	1	Bronchogenic carcinoma
	1	Diabetes mellitus, arteriosclerosis

* *From Robertson [306], with permission, Wolters Kluwer.*

suggesting that acute hyponatremia is a benign condition greatly underevaluate this potentially catastrophic electrolyte disturbance. Most patients who have seizures and coma have plasma sodium concentrations less than 120 mmol/L. The signs and symptoms are most likely related to the cellular swelling and cerebral edema that are associated with hyponatremia. Patients with SIADH whose plasma sodium concentrations are usually greater than 125 mmol/L rarely have significant symptoms related to hyponatremia itself and may not require specific treatment to raise their plasma sodium.

The treatment of symptomatic hyponatremic patients has been the subject of a large-scale debate in the literature [299]. This debate has been prompted by the description of both pontine (central pontine myelinolysis [CPM]) and extrapontine demyelinating lesions in patients whose hyponatremia has been treated. Numerous experiments (reviewed by Berl [298]) have demonstrated that hyponatremia per se is not the underlying cause of CPM, but that the corrections of hyponatremia of greater than 24-hour duration may play a central role in the development of CPM. The critical rate and the magnitude of the correction have been addressed and a "prudent" approach to the treatment has been published [281,298,299]. Virtually all investigators now agree that self-induced water intoxication, symptomatic hospital-acquired hyponatremia and hyponatremia-associated with intracranial pathology are true emergencies that demand prompt and definitive intervention with hypertonic saline. A 4–6 mmol/L increase in serum sodium concentration is adequate in the most seriously ill patients and this is best acheived with bolus infusions of 3% saline. Virtually all investigators now agree that overcorrection of chronic hyponatremia (which we define as 10 mmol/L in 24 hours, 18 mmol/L in 48 hours and 20 mmol/L in 72 hours) risks iatrogenic brain damage. Appropriate therapy should keep the patient safe from serious complications of hyponatremia while staying well clear of correction rates that risk iatrogenic injury. Accordingly, we suggest therapeutic goals of 6–8 mmol/L in 24 hours, 12–14 mmol/L in 48 hours and 14–16 mmol/L in 72 hours. Inadvertent overcorrection owing to a water diuresis may complicate any form of therapy, including the newly available vasopressin antagonists. Frequent monitoring of the serum sodium concentration and urine output are mandatory. Administration of desmopressin to terminate an unwanted water diuresis is an effective strategy to avoid or reverse overcorrection [299].

Acknowledgments

The author work cited in this chapter was supported by the Canadian Institutes of Health Research, the Kidney Foundation of Canada and the Fonds de la Recherche en Santé du Québec. DGB holds a Canada Research Chair in Genetics of Renal Diseases. We thank our coworkers, Marie-Françoise Arthus, Ellen Buschman, Mary Fujiwara, Michèle Lonergan and Kenneth Morgan; and many colleagues who contributed to our work.

References

[1] Y. Wilson, N. Nag, P. Davern, B.J. Oldfield, M.J. McKinley, U. Greferath, et al., Visualization of functionally activated circuitry in the brain, Proc Nat Acad Sci USA 99 (2002) 3252–3257.

[2] M.V. Sofroniew, Morphology of vasopressin and oxytocin neurones and their central and vascular projections, in: L. Cross (Ed.), The Neurohypophysis: Structure, Function, and Control, Elsevier, New York, 1983, pp. 101–114.

[3] K.T. Kalogeras, L.N. Nieman, T.C. Friedman, J.L. Doppman, G.B.J. Cutler, G.P. Chrousos, et al., Inferior petrosal sinus sampling in healthy human subjects reveals a unilateral corticotropin-releasing hormone-induced arginine vasopressin release associated with ipsilateral adrenocorticotropin secretion, J Clin Invest 97 (1996) 2045–2050.

[4] J.A. Yanovski, T.C. Friedman, L.K. Nieman, G.P. Chrousos, G.B. Cutler Jr., J.L. Doppman, et al., Inferior petrosal sinus AVP in patients with Cushing's syndrome, Clin Endocrinol (Oxf) 47 (1997) 199–206.

[5] L.P. Renaud, C.W. Bourque, T.A. Day, A.V. Ferguson, J.C.R. Randle, Electrophysiology of mammalian hypothalamic supraoptic and paraventricular neurosecretory cells, in: A.M. Poisner, J.M. Trifaro (Eds.), The Electrophysiology of the Secretory Cell, Elsevier, New York, 1985, pp. 165–194.

[6] C.W. Bourque, Central mechanisms of osmosensation and systemic osmoregulation, Nat Rev Neurosci 9 (2008) 519–531.

[7] Z.R. Donaldson, L.J. Young, Oxytocin, vasopressin, and the neurogenetics of sociality, Science 322 (2008) 900–904.

[8] P.C. Gwee, C.T. Amemiya, S. Brenner, B. Venkatesh, Sequence and organization of coelacanth neurohypophysial hormone genes: Evolutionary history of the vertebrate neurohypophysial hormone gene locus, BMC Evol Biol 8 (2008) 93.

[9] B. Venkatesh, S.L. Si-Hoe, D. Murphy, S. Brenner, Transgenic rats reveal functional conservation of regulatory controls between the Fugu isotocin and rat oxytocin genes, Proc Nat Acad Sci USA 94 (1997) 12462–12466.

[10] K. Tessmar-Raible, F. Raible, F. Christodoulou, K. Guy, M. Rembold, H. Hausen, et al., Conserved sensory-neurosecretory cell types in annelid and fish forebrain: Insights into hypothalamus evolution, Cell 129 (2007) 1389–1400.

[11] J.P. Burbach, S.M. Luckman, D. Murphy, H. Gainer, Gene regulation in the magnocellular hypothalamo–neurohypophysial system, Physiol Rev 81 (2001) 1197–1267.

[12] V.V. Rao, C. Loffler, J. Battey, I. Hansmann, The human gene for oxytocin-neurophysin I (OXT) is physically mapped to chromosome 20p13 by in situ hybridization, Cytogenet Cell Genet 61 (1992) 271–273.

[13] L. Chen, J.P. Rose, E. Breslow, D. Yang, W.R. Chang, W.F.J. Furey, et al., Crystal structure of a bovine neurophysin II dipeptide complex at 2.8 Angström determined from the single-wave length anomalous scattering signal of an incorporated iodine atom, Proc Nat Acad Sci USA 88 (1991) 4240–4244.

[14] T.R. Insel, The challenge of translation in social neuroscience: A review of oxytocin, vasopressin, and affiliative behavior, Neuron 65 (2010) 768–779.

[15] D. Huber, P. Veinante, R. Stoop, Vasopressin and oxytocin excite distinct neuronal populations in the central amygdala, Science 308 (2005) 245–248.

[16] H. Valtin, W.G. North, B.R. Edwards, M. Gellai, Animal models of diabetes insipidus, Front Horm Res 13 (1985) 105–126.

[17] H. Schmale, D. Richter, Single base deletion in the vasopressin gene is the cause of diabetes insipidus in Brattleboro rats, Nature 308 (1984) 705–709.

[18] H. Schmale, U. Bahnsen, S. Fehr, P. Nahke, D. Richter, Hereditary diabetes insipidus in man and rat, in: S. Jard, R. Jamison (Eds.), Vasopressin, Colloques INSERM/John Libbey Eurotext, Paris, 1991, pp. 57–62.

[19] D. Richter, Reflections on central diabetes insipidus: Retrospective and perspectives, in: P. Gross, D. Richter, G.L. Robertson (Eds.), Vasopressin, John Libbey Eurotext, Paris, 1993, pp. 3–14.

[20] C. Serradeil-Le Gal, C. Lacour, G. Valette, G. Garcia, L. Foulon, G. Galindo, et al., Characterization of SR 121463A, a highly potent and selective, orally active vasopressin V2 receptor antagonist, J Clin Invest 98 (1996) 2729–2738.

[21] F. Jean-Alphonse, S. Perkovska, M.C. Frantz, T. Durroux, C. Mejean, D. Morin, et al., Biased agonist pharmacochaperones of the AVP V2 receptor may treat congenital nephrogenic diabetes insipidus, J Am Soc Nephrol 20 (2009) 2190–2203.

[22] D.A. Evans, F.M. De Bree, M. Nijenhuis, A.A. Van Der Kleij, R. Zalm, N. Korteweg, et al., Processing of frameshifted vasopressin precursors, J Neuroendocrinol 12 (2000) 685–693.

[23] R.J. Balment, M.J. Brimble, M.L. Forsling, Oxytocin release and renal actions in normal and Brattleboro rats, Ann NY Acad Sci US 394 (1982) 241–253.

[24] C.L. Chou, S.R. DiGiovanni, A. Luther, S.J. Lolait, M.A. Knepper, Oxytocin as an antidiuretic hormone II. Role of V2 vasopressin receptor, Am J Physiol 269 (Renal Fluid Electrolyte Physiol 38) (1995) F78–F85.

[25] D.R. Repaske, J.A. Phillips, L.T. Kirby, W.J. Tze, A.J. D'Ercole, J. Battey, Molecular analysis of autosomal dominant neurohypophyseal diabetes insipidus, J Clin Endocrinol Metab 70 (1990) 752–757.

[26] V.A. McKusick, Online Mendelian Inheritance in Man OMIM, (TM), McKusick-Nathans Institute for Genetic Medicine, Johns Hopkins University (Baltimore, MD) and National Center for Biotechnology Information, National Library of Medicine, Bethesda, MD, 2000. World Wide Web URL: http://www.ncbi.nlm.nih.gov/omim/. 2000.

[27] J.H. Christensen, S. Rittig, Familial neurohypophyseal diabetes insipidus – an update, Semin Nephrol 26 (2006) 209–223.

[28] J. Birk, M.A. Friberg, C. Prescianotto-Baschong, M. Spiess, J. Rutishauser, Dominant pro-vasopressin mutants that cause diabetes insipidus form disulfide-linked fibrillar aggregates in the endoplasmic reticulum, J Cell Sci 122 (2009) 3994–4002.

[29] A. Abu Libdeh, F. Levy-Khademi, M. Abdulhadi-Atwan, E. Bosin, M. Korner, et al., Autosomal recessive familial neurohypophyseal diabetes insipidus: Onset in early infancy, Eur J Endocrinol 162 (2009) 221–226.

[30] C.M. Hedrich, A. Zachurzok-Buczynska, A. Gawlik, S. Russ, G. Hahn, et al., Autosomal dominant neurohypophyseal diabetes insipidus in two families. Molecular analysis of the vasopressin-neurophysin II gene and functional studies of three missense mutations, Horm Res 71 (2009) 111–119.

[31] D.R. Cool, S.B. Jackson, K.S. Waddell, Structural requirements for sorting pro-vasopressin to the regulated secretory pathway in a neuronal cell line, Open Neuroendocrinol J 1 (2008) 1–8.

[32] J.H. Christensen, C. Siggaard, T.J. Corydon, G.L. Robertson, N. Gregersen, L. Bolund, et al., Differential cellular handling of defective arginine vasopressin (AVP) prohormones in cells expressing mutations of the AVP gene associated with autosomal dominant and recessive familial neurohypophyseal diabetes insipidus, J Clin Endocrinol Metab 89 (2004) 4521–4531.

[33] M. Ito, J.L. Jameson, M. Ito, Molecular basis of autosomal dominant neurohypophyseal diabetes insipidus. Cellular toxicity caused by the accumulation of mutant vasopressin precursors within the endoplasmic reticulum, J Clin Invest 99 (1997) 1897–1905.

[34] R. Castino, C. Isidoro, D. Murphy, Autophagy-dependent cell survival and cell death in an autosomal dominant familial neurohypophyseal diabetes insipidus in vitro model, FASEB J 19 (2005) 1024–1026.

[35] N. Gregersen, P. Bross, S. Vang, J.H. Christensen, Protein misfolding and human disease, Annu Rev Genomics Hum Genet 7 (2006) 103–124.

[36] D.G. Bichet, M.-F. Arthus, M. Lonergan, K. Morgan, T.M. Fujiwara, Hereditary central diabetes insipidus: Autosomal dominant and autosomal recessive phenotypes due to mutations in the prepro-AVP-NPII gene, J Am Soc Nephrol 9 (1998) 386A.

[37] M.D. Willcutts, E. Felner, P.C. White, Autosomal recessive familial neurohypophyseal diabetes insipidus with continued secretion of mutant weakly active vasopressin, Hum Mol Genet 8 (1999) 1303–1307.

[38] A.V. Schally, Hormones of the neurohypophysis, in: W. Lock, A.V. Schally (Eds.), The Hypothalamus and Pituitary in Health and Disease, Charles C Thomas, Springfield, 1972, pp. 154–171.

[39] A.V. Schally, C.Y. Bowers, A. Kuroshima, Y. Ishida, W.H. Carter, T.W. Redding, Effect of lysine vasopressin dimers on blood pressure and some endocrine functions, Am J Physiol 207 (1964) 378–384.

[40] R. Acher, J. Chauvet, Structure, processing and evolution of the neurohypophysial hormone-neurophysin precursors, Biochimie 70 (1988) 1197–1207.

[41] J.P. Proux, The arginine vasopressin-like insect diurectic hormone, in: S. Jard, R. Jamison (Eds.), Vasopressin, Colloques INSERM/John Libbey Eurotext, Paris, 1991, pp. 367–373.

[42] H. Sachs, P. Fawcett, Y. Takabatake, R. Portanova, Biosynthesis and release of vasopressin and neurophysin, Recent Prog Horm Res 25 (1969) 447–491.

[43] H. Gainer, Y. Sarne, M.J. Brownstein, Biosynthesis and axonal transport of rat neurohypophysial proteins and peptides, J Cell Biol 73 (1977) 366–381.

[44] J.T. Russell, M.J. Brownstein, H. Gainer, Biosynthesis of vasopressin, oxytocin, and neurophysins: Isolation and characterization of two common precursors (propressophysin and prooxyphysin), Endocrinology 107 (1980) 1880–1891.

[45] D.G. Bichet, M.F. Arthus, M. Lonergan, Platelet vasopressin receptors in patients with congenital nephrogenic diabetes insipidus, Kidney Int 39 (1991) 693–699.

[46] L. Share, J.T. Crofton, D.P. Brooks, C.M. Chesney, Platelet and plasma vasopressin in dog during hydration and vasopressin infusion, Am J Physiol 249 (1985) R313–R316.

[47] G. Anfossi, E. Mularoni, M. Trovati, P. Massucco, L. Mattiello, G. Emanuelli, Arginine vasopressin release from human platelets after irreversible aggregation, Clin Sci (Colch) 78 (1990) 113–116.

[48] P.E. Sawchenko, L.W. Swanson, The organization of noradrenergic pathways from the brainstem to the paraventricular and supraoptic nuclei in the rat, Brain Res 257 (1982) 275–325.

[49] J.C. Randle, M. Mazurek, D. Kneifel, J. Dufresne, L.P. Renaud, Alpha 1-adrenergic receptor activation releases vasopressin and oxytocin from perfused rat hypothalamic explants, Neurosci Lett 65 (1986) 219–223.

[50] T.A. Day, J.C. Randle, L.P. Renaud, Opposing alpha- and beta-adrenergic mechanisms mediate dose-dependent actions of noradrenaline on supraoptic vasopressin neurones in vivo, Brain Res 358 (1985) 171–179.

[51] W.T. Mason, Y.W. Ho, F. Eckenstein, G.I. Hatton, Mapping of cholinergic neurons associated with rat supraoptic nucleus: Combined immunocytochemical and histochemical identification, Brain Res Bull 11 (1983) 617–626.

[52] A.V. Ferguson, L.P. Renaud, Systemic angiotensin acts at subfornical organ to facilitate activity of neurohypophysial neurons, Am J Physiol 251 (1986) R712–R717.

[53] S.J. Watson, H. Akil, W. Fischli, A. Goldstein, E. Zimmerman, G. Nilaver, et al., Dynorphin and vasopressin: Common localization in magnocellular neurons, Science 216 (1982) 85–87.

[54] R. Simantov, S.H. Snyder, Opiate receptor binding in the pituitary gland, Brain Res 124 (1977) 178–184.

[55] A.M. Edwards, M.E. Mann, M.J. Marfell-Jones, D.M. Rankin, T.D. Noakes, D.P. Shillington, Influence of moderate dehydration on soccer performance: Physiological responses to 45 min of outdoor match-play and the immediate subsequent performance of sport-specific and mental concentration tests, Br J Sports Med 41 (2007) 385–391.

[56] M. Saat, R.G. Sirisinghe, R. Singh, Y. Tochihara, Effects of short-term exercise in the heat on thermoregulation, blood parameters, sweat secretion and sweat composition of tropic-dwelling subjects, J Physiol Anthropol Appl Human Sci 24 (2005) 541–549.

[57] S.M. Shirreffs, S.J. Merson, S.M. Fraser, D.T. Archer, The effects of fluid restriction on hydration status and subjective feelings in man, Br J Nutr 91 (2004) 951–958.

[58] G. Geelen, J.E. Greenleaf, L.C. Keil, Drinking-induced plasma vasopressin and norepinephrine changes in dehydrated humans, J Clin Endocrinol Metab 81 (1996) 2131–2135.

[59] L.J. Andersen, T.U. Jensen, M.H. Bestle, P. Bie, Gastrointestinal osmoreceptors and renal sodium excretion in humans, Am J Physiol Regul Integr Comp Physiol 278 (2000) R287–R294.

[60] J.R. Claybaugh, A.K. Sato, L.K. Crosswhite, L.H. Hassell, Effects of time of day, gender, and menstrual cycle phase on the human response to a water load, Am J Physiol Regul Integr Comp Physiol 279 (2000) R966–R973.

[61] E. Verney, The antidiuretic hormone and the factors which determine its release, Proc R Soc London Ser B 135 (1947) 25–26.

[62] G. Kuramochi, I. Kobayashi, Regulation of the urine concentration mechanism by the oropharyngeal afferent pathway in man, Am J Nephrol 20 (2000) 42–47.

[63] S. Choi-Kwon, A.J. Baertschi, Splanchnic osmosensation and vasopressin: Mechanisms and neural pathways, Am J Physiol 261 (1991) E18–E25.

[64] G. Egan, T. Silk, F. Zamarripa, J. Williams, P. Federico, R. Cunnington, et al., Neural correlates of the emergence of consciousness of thirst, Proc Nat Acad Sci USA 100 (2003) 15241–15246.

[65] E.M. Stricker, M.L. Hoffmann, Presystemic signals in the control of thirst, salt appetite, and vasopressin secretion, Physiol Behav 91 (2007) 404–412.

[66] W. Huang, A.F. Sved, E.M. Stricker, Water ingestion provides an early signal inhibiting osmotically stimulated vasopressin secretion in rats, Am J Physiol Regul Integr Comp Physiol 279 (2000) R756–R760.

[67] T. Osaka, A. Kobayashi, S. Inoue, Vago-sympathoadrenal reflex in thermogenesis induced by osmotic stimulation of the intestines in the rat, J Physiol 540 (2002) 665–671.

[68] M.J. McKinley, R.M. McAllen, P. Davern, M.E. Giles, J. Penschow, N. Sunn, et al., The sensory circumventricular organs of the mammalian brain, Adv Anat Embryol Cell Biol 172 (III–XII) (2003) 1–122.

[69] T.N. Thrasher, L.C. Keil, D.J. Ramsay, Lesions of the organum vasculosum of the lamina terminalis (OVLT) attenuate osmotically-induced drinking and vasopressin secretion in the dog, Endocrinology 110 (1982) 1837–1839.

[70] H. Morita, T. Ogino, N. Fujiki, K. Tanaka, T.M. Gotoh, Y. Seo, et al., Sequence of forebrain activation induced by intraventricular injection of hypertonic NaCl detected by Mn^{2+} contrasted T1-weighted MRI, Auton Neurosci 113 (2004) 43–54.

[71] M.J. McKinley, D.A. Denton, B.J. Oldfield, L.B. De Oliveira, M.L. Mathai, Water intake and the neural correlates of the consciousness of thirst, Semin Nephrol 26 (2006) 249–257.

[72] S. Ciura, C.W. Bourque, Transient receptor potential vanilloid 1 is required for intrinsic osmoreception in organum vasculosum lamina terminalis neurons and for normal thirst responses to systemic hyperosmolality, J Neurosci 26 (2006) 9069–9075.

[73] J.W. Anderson, D.L. Washburn, A.V. Ferguson, Intrinsic osmosensitivity of subfornical organ neurons, Neuroscience 100 (2000) 539–547.

[74] S.H. Oliet, C.W. Bourque, Properties of supraoptic magnocellular neurones isolated from the adult rat, J Physiol 455 (1992) 291–306.

[75] S.H. Oliet, C.W. Bourque, Mechanosensitive channels transduce osmosensitivity in supraoptic neurons, Nature 364 (1993) 341–343.

[76] W.T. Mason, Supraoptic neurones of rat hypothalamus are osmosensitive, Nature 287 (1980) 154–157.

[77] C.W. Bourque, Ionic basis for the intrinsic activation of rat supraoptic neurones by hyperosmotic stimuli, J Physiol 417 (1989) 263–277.

[78] D.L. Qiu, T. Shirasaka, C.P. Chu, S. Watanabe, N.S. Yu, T. Katoh, et al., Effect of hypertonic saline on rat hypothalamic paraventricular nucleus magnocellular neurons in vitro, Neurosci Lett 355 (2004) 117–120.
[79] S.H. Oliet, C.W. Bourque, Steady-state osmotic modulation of cationic conductance in neurons of rat supraoptic nucleus, Am J Physiol 265 (1993) R1475–R1479.
[80] R. Sharif Naeini, M.F. Witty, P. Seguela, C.W. Bourque, An N-terminal variant of Trpv1 channel is required for osmosensory transduction, Nat Neurosci 9 (2006) 93–98.
[81] R. Sharif-Naeini, S. Ciura, C.W. Bourque, TRPV1 gene required for thermosensory transduction and anticipatory secretion from vasopressin neurons during hyperthermia, Neuron 58 (2008) 179–185.
[82] D.M. Cohen, The transient receptor potential vanilloid-responsive 1 and 4 cation channels: Role in neuronal osmosensing and renal physiology, Curr Opin Nephrol Hypertens 16 (2007) 451–458.
[83] W. Tian, Y. Fu, A. Garcia-Elias, J.M. Fernandez-Fernandez, R. Vicente, P.L. Kramer, et al., A loss-of-function nonsynonymous polymorphism in the osmoregulatory TRPV4 gene is associated with human hyponatremia, Proc Nat Acad Sci USA 106 (2009) 14034–14039.
[84] R.H. Aubry, H.R. Nankin, A.M. Moses, D.H. Streeten, Measurement of the osmotic threshold for vasopressin release in human subjects, and its modification by cortisol, J Clin Endocrinol Metab 25 (1965) 1481–1492.
[85] A.M. Moses, D.H. Streeten, Differentiation of polyuric states by measurement of responses to changes in plasma osmolality induced by hypertonic saline infusions, Am J Med 42 (1967) 368–377.
[86] A.M. Moses, M. Miller, D.H. Streeten, Quantitative influence of blood volume expansion on the osmotic threshold for vasopressin release, J Clin Endocrinol Metab 27 (1967) 655–662.
[87] A.M. Moses, M. Miller, Osmotic threshold for vasopressin release as determined by saline infusion and by dehydration, Neuroendocrinology 7 (1971) 219–226.
[88] D.G. Bichet, C. Kortas, B. Mettauer, C. Manzini, J. Marc-Aurele, J.L. Rouleau, et al., Modulation of plasma and platelet vasopressin by cardiac function in patients with heart failure, Kidney Int 29 (1986) 1188–1196.
[89] D.G. Bichet, M.-F. Arthus, J.N. Barjon, M. Lonergan, C. Kortas, Human platelet fraction arginine-vasopressin, J Clin Invest 79 (1987) 881–887.
[90] G.L. Robertson, R.L. Shelton, S. Athar, The osmoregulation of vasopressin, Kidney Int 10 (1976) 25–37.
[91] M. Hammer, J. Ladefoged, K. Olgaard, Relationship between plasma osmolality and plasma vasopressin in human subjects, Am J Physiol 238 (1980) E313–E317.
[92] P. Bie, Osmoreceptors, vasopressin, and control of renal water excretion, Physiol Rev 60 (1980) 961–1048.
[93] C.J. Thompson, J. Bland, J. Burd, P.H. Baylis, The osmotic thresholds for thirst and vasopressin release are similar in healthy man, Clin Sci 71 (1986) 651–656.
[94] G.L. Robertson, Abnormalities of thirst regulation, Kidney Int 25 (1984) 460–469.
[95] T.N. Thrasher, J.F. Nistal-Herrera, L.C. Keil, D.J. Ramsay, Satiety and inhibition of vasopressin secretion after drinking in dehydrated dogs, Am J Physiol 240 (1981) E394–E401.
[96] G. Geelen, L.C. Keil, S.E. Kravik, C.E. Wade, T.N. Thrasher, P.R. Barnes, et al., Inhibition of plasma vasopressin after drinking in dehydrated humans, Am J Physiol 247 (1984) R968–R971.
[97] J.M. Davison, E.A. Shiells, P.R. Philips, M.D. Lindheimer, Suppression of AVP release by drinking despite hypertonicity during and after gestation, Am J Physiol 254 (1988) F588–F592.
[98] R.A. Salata, J.G. Verbalis, A.G. Robinson, Cold water stimulation of oropharyngeal receptors in man inhibits release of vasopressin, J Clin Endocrinol Metab 65 (1987) 561–567.
[99] R.L. Zerbe, Genetic factors in normal and abnormal regulation of vasopressin secretion, in: R.W. Schrier (Ed.), Vasopressin, Raven Press, New York, 1985, pp. 213–220.
[100] J.A. Durr, B. Stamoutsos, M.D. Lindheimer, Osmoregulation during pregnancy in the rat. Evidence for resetting of the threshold for vasopressin secretion during gestation, J Clin Invest 68 (1981) 337–346.
[101] J.M. Davison, E.A. Gilmore, J. Durr, G.L. Robertson, M.D. Lindheimer, Altered osmotic thresholds for vasopressin secretion and thirst in human pregnancy, Am J Physiol 246 (1984) F105–F109.
[102] J.M. Davison, E.A. Shiells, P.R. Philips, M.D. Lindheimer, Serial evaluation of vasopressin release and thirst in human pregnancy. Role of human chorionic gonadotrophin in the osmoregulatory changes of gestation, J Clin Invest 81 (1988) 798–806.
[103] T.P. Vokes, P.R. Aycinena, G.L. Robertson, Effect of insulin on osmoregulation of vasopressin, Am J Physiol 252 (1987) E538–E548.
[104] J.A. Durr, W.H. Hoffman, J. Hensen, A.H. Sklar, T. el Gammal, C.M. Steinhart, Osmoregulation of vasopressin in diabetic ketoacidosis, Am J Physiol 259 (1990) E723–E728.
[105] P. Norsk, Influence of low- and high-pressure baroreflexes on vasopressin release in humans, Acta Endocrinol (Copenh) 121 (1989) 3–27.
[106] P.H. Baylis, Posterior pituitary function in health and disease, Clin Endocrinol Metab 12 (1983) 747–770.
[107] G.L. Robertson, Thirst and vasopressin function in normal and disordered states of water balance, J Lab Clin Med 101 (1983) 351–371.
[108] J.W. Rowe, K.L. Minaker, D. Sparrow, G.L. Robertson, Age-related failure of volume-pressure-mediated vasopressin release, J Clin Endocrinol Metab 54 (1982) 661–664.
[109] B. Rolls, E. Rolls, Thirst (Problems in the behavioural sciences), Cambridge University Press, Cambridge, UK, 1982.
[110] J.T. Fitzsimons, Angiotensin, thirst, and sodium appetite, Physiol Rev 78 (1998) 583–686.
[111] V.L. Brooks, L.C. Keil, I.A. Reid, Role of the renin–angiotensin system in the control of vasopressin secretion in conscious dogs, Circ Res 58 (1986) 829–838.
[112] P. Phillips, B. Rolls, J. Ledingham, J. Morton, M. Forsling, Angiotensin II-induced thirst and vasopressin release in man, Clin Science 68 (1985) 669–674.
[113] J. Morton, J. Connell, M. Hughes, G. Inglis, E. Wallace, The role of plasma osmolality, angiotensin II and dopamine in vasopressin release in man, Clin Endocrinol 23 (1985) 129–138.
[114] F. Nimura, P. Labosky, J. Kakuchi, S. Okubo, H. Yoshida, T. Oikawa, et al., Gene targeting in mice reveals a requirement for angiotensin in the development and maintenance of kidney morphology and growth factor regulation, J Clin Invest 96 (1995) 2947–2954.
[115] M. Ito, M.I. Oliverio, P.J. Mannon, C.F. Best, N. Maeda, O. Smithies, et al., Regulation of blood pressure by the type 1A angiotensin II receptor gene, Proc Nat Acad Sci USA 92 (1995) 3521–3525.
[116] T. Sugaya, S. Nishimatsu, K. Tanimoto, E. Takimoto, T. Yamagishi, K. Imamura, et al., Angiotensin II type 1a receptor-deficient mice with hypotension and hyperreninemia, J Biol Chem 270 (1995) 18719–18722.
[117] L. Hein, G.S. Barsh, R.E. Pratt, V.J. Dzau, B.K. Kobilka, Behavioural and cardiovascular effects of disrupting the angiotensin II type-2 receptor gene in mice, Nature 377 (1995) 744–747.

[118] R. Martin, K.H. Voigt, Enkephalins co-exist with oxytocin and vasopressin in nerve terminals of rat neurohypophysis, Nature 289 (1981) 502–504.

[119] R. DeBodo, The antidiuretic action of morphine and its mechanism, J Pharmacol Exp Ther 82 (1944) 74–85.

[120] K. Yamada, M. Nakano, S. Yoshida, Inhibition of elevated arginine vasopressin secretion in response to osmotic stimulation and acute haemorrhage by U-62066E, a kappa-opioid receptor agonist, Br J Pharmacol 99 (1990) 384–388.

[121] J.L. Abelson, J. Le Melledo, D.G. Bichet, Dose response of arginine vasopressin to the CCK-B agonist pentagastrin, Neuropsychopharmacology 24 (2001) 161–169.

[122] H. Wang, J.F. Morris, Constitutive nitric oxide synthase in hypothalami of normal and hereditary diabetes insipidus rats and mice: Role of nitric oxide in osmotic regulation and its mechanism, Endocrinology 137 (1996) 1745–1751.

[123] H. Raff, Glucocorticoid inhibition of neurohypophysial vasopressin secretion, Am J Physiol 252 (1987) R635–R644.

[124] J.W. Rowe, R.L. Shelton, J.H. Helderman, R.E. Vestal, G.L. Robertson, Influence of the emetic reflex on vasopressin release in man, Kidney Int 16 (1979) 729–735.

[125] R.L. Zerbe, G.L. Robertson, A comparison of plasma vasopressin measurements with a standard indirect test in the differential diagnosis of polyuria, N Engl J Med 305 (1981) 1539–1546.

[126] M. Miller, T. Dalakos, A.M. Moses, H. Fellerman, D.H. Streeten, Recognition of partial defects in antidiuretic hormone secretion, Ann Intern Med 73 (1970) 721–729.

[127] R. Fredriksson, M.C. Lagerstrom, L.G. Lundin, H.B. Schioth, The G-protein-coupled receptors in the human genome form five main families. Phylogenetic analysis, paralogon groups, and fingerprints, Mol Pharmacol 63 (2003) 1256–1272.

[128] D.M. Perez, The evolutionarily triumphant G-protein-coupled receptor, Mol Pharmacol 63 (2003) 1202–1205.

[129] S. Topiol, M. Sabio, X-ray structure breakthroughs in the GPCR transmembrane region, Biochem Pharmacol 78 (2009) 11–20.

[130] N.L. Ostrowski, W.S. Young II, M.A. Knepper, S.T. Lolait, Expression of vasopressin V1a and V2 receptor messenger ribonucleic acid in the liver and kidney of embryonic, developing, and adult rats, Endocrinol 133 (1993) 1849–1859.

[131] N.L. Ostrowski, S.J. Lolait, W.S. Young III, Cellular localization of vasopressin V1a receptor messenger ribonucleic acid in adult male rat brain, pineal, and brain vasculature, Endocrinol 135 (1994) 1511–1528.

[132] T. Sugimoto, M. Saito, S. Mochizuki, Y. Watanabe, S. Hashimoto, H. Kawashima, Molecular cloning and functional expression of a cDNA encoding the human V1b vasopressin receptor, J Biol Chem 269 (1994) 27088–27092.

[133] Y. de Keyzer, C. Auzan, F. Lenne, C. Beldjord, M. Thibonnier, X. Bertagna, et al., Cloning and characterization of the human V3 pituitary vasopressin receptor, FEBS Letts 356 (1994) 215–220.

[134] S.J. Lolait, A.-M. O'Carroll, L.C. Mahan, C.C. Felder, D.C. Button, W.S. Young III, et al., Extrapituitary expression of the rat V1b vasopressin receptor gene, Proc Nat Acad Sci USA 92 (1995) 6783–6787.

[135] C. Serradeil-Le Gal, D. Raufaste, S. Derick, J. Blankenstein, J. Allen, B. Pouzet, et al., Biological characterization of rodent and human vasopressin V1b receptors using SSR-149415, a nonpeptide V1b receptor ligand, Am J Physiol Regul Integr Comp Physiol 293 (2007) R938–R949.

[136] E. Grazzini, A.M. Lodboerer, A. Perez-Martin, D. Joubert, G. Guillon, Molecular and functional characterization of V1b vasopressin receptor in rat adrenal medulla, Endocrinology 137 (1996) 3906–3914.

[137] R.A. Fenton, M.A. Knepper, Mouse models and the urinary concentrating mechanism in the new millennium, Physiol Rev 87 (2007) 1083–1112.

[138] N.L. Allison, C.R. Albrightson-Winslow, D.P. Brooks, F.L. Stassen, W.F. Huffman, R.M. Stote, et al., Species heterogeneity and antidiuretic hormone antagonists: What are the predictors? in: A.W.J. Cowley, J.F. Liard, D.A. Ausiello (Eds.), Vasopressin: Cellular and Integrative Functions Raven Press, New York, 1988, pp. 207–214.

[139] M. Manning, S. Stoev, B. Chini, T. Durroux, B. Mouillac, G. Guillon, Peptide and non-peptide agonists and antagonists for the vasopressin and oxytocin V1a, V1b, V2 and OT receptors: research tools and potential therapeutic agents, Prog Brain Res 170 (2008) 473–512.

[140] G. Decaux, A. Soupart, G. Vassart, Non-peptide arginine-vasopressin antagonists: The vaptans, Lancet 371 (2008) 1624–1632.

[141] Berl, T. Quittnat-Pelletier, F. Verbalis, J. G. Schrier, R. W. Bichet, D. G. Ouyang, J. et al., Oral tolvaptan is safe and effective in chronic hyponatremia. J Am Soc Nephrol 21 705–712.

[142] M. Thibonnier, P. Coles, A. Thibonnier, M. Shoham, The basic and clinical pharmacology of nonpeptide vasopressin receptor antagonists, Annu Rev Pharmacol Toxicol 41 (2001) 175–202.

[143] C. Serradeil-Le Gal, J. Wagnon, J. Simiand, G. Griebel, C. Lacour, G. Guillon, et al., Characterization of (2S,4R)-1-[5-chloro-1-[(2,4-dimethoxyphenyl)sulfonyl]-3-(2-methoxy-phenyl)-2-oxo-2,3-dihydro-1H-indol-3-yl]-4-hydroxy-N,N-dimethyl-2-pyrrolidine carboxamide (SSR149415), a selective and orally active vasopressin V1b receptor antagonist, J Pharmacol Exp Ther 300 (2002) 1122–1130.

[144] H. Walum, L. Westberg, S. Henningsson, J.M. Neiderhiser, D. Reiss, W. Igl, et al., Genetic variation in the vasopressin receptor 1a gene (AVPR1A) associates with pair-bonding behavior in humans, Proc Nat Acad Sci USA 105 (2008) 14153–14156.

[145] M. Birnbaumer, A. Seibold, S. Gilbert, M. Ishido, C. Barberis, A. Antaramian, et al., Molecular cloning of the receptor for human antidiuretic hormone, Nature 357 (1992) 333–335.

[146] A. Seibold, P. Brabet, W. Rosenthal, M. Birnbaumer, Structure and chromosomal localization of the human antidiuretic hormone receptor gene, Am J Hum Genet 51 (1992) 1078–1083.

[147] H. Rehmann, A. Wittinghofer, J.L. Bos, Capturing cyclic nucleotides in action: Snapshots from crystallographic studies, Nat Rev Mol Cell Biol 8 (2007) 63–73.

[148] S. Nielsen, J. Frokiaer, D. Marples, T.H. Kwon, P. Agre, M.A. Knepper, Aquaporins in the kidney: From molecules to medicine, Physiol Rev 82 (2002) 205–244.

[149] M. Boone, P.M. Deen, Physiology and pathophysiology of the vasopressin-regulated renal water reabsorption, Pflugers Arch 456 (2008) 1005–1024.

[150] P.I. Nedvetsky, G. Tamma, S. Beulshausen, G. Valenti, W. Rosenthal, E. Klussmann, Regulation of aquaporin-2 trafficking, Handb Exp Pharmacol (2009) 133–157.

[151] B. Yang, L. Bankir, A. Gillespie, C.J. Epstein, A.S. Verkman, Urea-selective concentrating defect in transgenic mice lacking urea transporter UT-B, J Biol Chem 277 (2002) 10633–10637.

[152] C.P. Smith, Mammalian urea transporters, Exp Physiol 94 (2009) 180–185.

[153] L. Bankir, S. Fernandes, P. Bardoux, N. Bouby, D.G. Bichet, Vasopressin-V2 receptor stimulation reduces sodium excretion in healthy humans, J Am Soc Nephrol 16 (2005) 1920–1928.

[154] T. Morishita, M. Tsutsui, H. Shimokawa, K. Sabanai, H. Tasaki, O. Suda, et al., Nephrogenic diabetes insipidus in mice lacking all nitric oxide synthase isoforms, Proc Nat Acad Sci USA 102 (2005) 10616–10621.

[155] E.F. Fleming, K. Athirakul, M.I. Oliverio, M. Key, J. Goulet, B.H. Koller, et al., Urinary concentrating function in mice lacking EP3 receptors for prostaglandin E2, Am J Physiol 275 (1998) F955–F961.

[156] J.M. Sands, M. Naruse, M. Baum, I. Jo, S.C. Hebert, E.M. Brown, et al., Apical extracellular calcium/polyvalent cation-sensing receptor regulates vasopressin-elicited water permeability in rat kidney inner medullary collecting duct, J Clin Invest 99 (1997) 1399–1405.

[157] J.G. Verbalis, A.G. Robinson, A.M. Moses, Postoperative and post-traumatic diabetes insipidus, in: P. Czernichow, A.G. Robinson (Eds.), Frontiers of Hormone Research, S. Karger, Basel, Switzerland, 1985, pp. 247–265.

[158] B.R. Olson, J. Gumowski, D. Rubino, E.H. Oldfield, Pathophysiology of hyponatremia after transsphenoidal pituitary surgery, J Neurosurg 87 (1997) 499–507.

[159] E.C. Nemergut, Z. Zuo, J.A. Jane Jr., E.R. Laws Jr., Predictors of diabetes insipidus after transsphenoidal surgery: A review of 881 patients, J Neurosurg 103 (2005) 448–454.

[160] P. Czernichow, R. Pomarede, R. Brauner, R. Rappaport, Neurogenic diabetes insipidus in children, in: P. Czernichow, A.G. Robinson (Eds.), Frontiers of Hormone Research, S. Karger, Basel, Switzerland, 1985, pp. 190–209.

[161] N.G. Greger, R.T. Kirkland, G.W. Clayton, J.L. Kirkland, Central diabetes insipidus. 22 years' experience, Am J Dis Child 140 (1986) 551–554.

[162] M. Maghnie, G. Cosi, E. Genovese, M.L. Manca-Bitti, A. Cohen, S. Zecca, et al., Central diabetes insipidus in children and young adults, N Engl J Med 343 (2000) 998–1007.

[163] A.M. Moses, S.A. Blumenthal, D.H.P. Streeten, Acid-base and electrolyte disorders associated with endocrine disease: Pituitary and thyroid, in: A.I. Arieff, R.A. De Fronzo (Eds.), Fluid, Electrolyte and Acid-Base Disorders, Churchill Livingstone, New York, 1985, pp. 851–892.

[164] F. Fery, L. Plat, P. van de Borne, E. Cogan, J. Mockel, Impaired counterregulation of glucose in a patient with hypothalamic sarcoidosis, N Engl J Med 340 (1999) 852–856.

[165] W.D. Odell, R.S. Doggett, Xanthoma disseminatum, a rare cause of diabetes insipidus, J Clin Endocrinol Metab 76 (1993) 777–780.

[166] N. Masera, D.B. Grant, R. Stanhope, M.A. Preece, Diabetes insipidus with impaired osmotic regulation in septo-optic dysplasia and agenesis of the corpus callosum, Arch Dis Child 70 (1994) 51–53.

[167] H. Imura, K. Nakao, A. Shimatsu, Y. Ogawa, T. Sando, I. Fujisawa, et al., Lymphocytic infundibuloneurohypophysitis as a cause of central diabetes insipidus, N Engl J Med 329 (1993) 683–689.

[168] S.R. Ahmed, D.P. Aiello, R. Page, K. Hopper, J. Towfighi, R.J. Santen, Necrotizing infundibulo-hypophysitis: A unique syndrome of diabetes insipidus and hypopituitarism, J Clin Endocrinol Metab 76 (1993) 1499–1504.

[169] U.L. Lacombe, Imprimerie et Fonderie de Rignoux, De la polydipsie, Paris, 1841, pp 87.

[170] A. Weil, Ueber die hereditare form des diabetes insipidus, Archives fur Pathologische Anatomie und Physiologie and fur Klinische Medicine (Virchow's Archives) 95 (1884) 70–95.

[171] J.W. Camerer, Eine ergänzung des Weilschen diabetes-insipidus-stammbaumes, Archiv für Rassen-und Gesellschaftshygiene Biologie 28 (1935) 382–385.

[172] W. Dölle, Eine weitere ergänzung des Weilschen diabetes-insipidus-stammbaumes, Zeitschrift für Menschliche Vererbungs-und Konstitutionslehre 30 (1951) 372–374.

[173] A. Weil, Ueber die hereditare form des diabetes insipidus, Deutches Archiv fur Klinische Medizin 93 (1908) 180–290.

[174] R. Rittig, G.L. Robertson, C. Siggaard, L. Kovacs, N. Gregersen, J. Nyborg, et al., Identification of 13 new mutations in the vasopressin-neurophysin II gene in 17 kindreds with familial autosomal dominant neurohypophyseal diabetes insipidus, Am J Hum Genet 58 (1996) 107–117.

[175] E. Domenech, M. Gomez-Zaera, V. Nunes, Study of the WFS1 gene and mitochondrial DNA in Spanish Wolfram syndrome families, Clin Genet 65 (2004) 463–469.

[176] K. Takeda, H. Inoue, Y. Tanizawa, Y. Matsuzaki, J. Oba, Y. Watanabe, et al., WFS1 (Wolfram syndrome 1) gene product: predominant subcellular localization to endoplasmic reticulum in cultured cells and neuronal expression in rat brain, Hum Mol Genet 10 (2001) 477–484.

[177] H. Ishihara, S. Takeda, A. Tamura, R. Takahashi, S. Yamaguchi, D. Takei, et al., Disruption of the WFS1 gene in mice causes progressive beta-cell loss and impaired stimulus-secretion coupling in insulin secretion, Hum Mol Genet 13 (2004) 1159–1170.

[178] A.R. Conlan, H.L. Axelrod, A.E. Cohen, E.C. Abresch, J. Zuris, D. Yee, et al., Crystal structure of Miner1: The redox-active 2Fe-2S protein causative in Wolfram Syndrome 2, J Mol Biol 392 (2009) 143–153.

[179] R.L. Howard, D.G. Bichet, R.W. Schrier, Hypernatremic and polyuric states, in: D.W. Seldin, G. Giebisch (Eds.), The Kidney: Physiology and Pathophysiology, second ed., Raven Press, Ltd, New York, 1992, pp. 1753–1778.

[180] R.K. Crowley, M. Sherlock, A. Agha, D. Smith, C.J. Thompson, Clinical insights into adipsic diabetes insipidus: A large case series, Clin Endocrinol (Oxf) 66 (2007) 475–482.

[181] T.M. Fujiwara, D.G. Bichet, Molecular biology of hereditary diabetes insipidus, J Am Soc Nephrol 16 (2005) 2836–2846.

[182] D.G. Bichet, T.M. Fujiwara, et al., Nephrogenic diabetes insipidus, in: C.R. Scriver, A.L. Beaudet, W.S. Sly, D. Vallee, B. Childs, K.W. Kinzler (Eds.), The Metabolic and Molecular Bases of Inherited Disease, eighth ed., McGraw-Hill, New York, 2001, pp. 4181–4204.

[183] M.-F. Arthus, M. Lonergan, M.J. Crumley, A.K. Naumova, D. Morin, L. De Marco, et al., Report of 33 novel AVPR2 mutations and analysis of 117 families with X-linked nephrogenic diabetes insipidus, J Am Soc Nephrol 11 (2000) 1044–1054.

[184] D.G. Bichet, M.-F. Arthus, M. Lonergan, G.N. Hendy, A.J. Paradis, T.M. Fujiwara, et al., X-linked nephrogenic diabetes insipidus mutations in North America and the Hopewell hypothesis, J Clin Invest 92 (1993) 1262–1268.

[185] T.L. Perry, G.C. Robinson, J.M. Teasdale, S. Hansen, Concurrence of cystathioninuria, nephrogenic diabetes insipidus and severe anemia, N Engl J Med 276 (1967) 721–725.

[186] M.F. Arthus, M. Lonergan, T.M. Fujiwara, D.G. Bichet, Clinical and genetic approaches to the diagnosis of congenital polyuro-polydipsic syndromes, The NDI Foundation 2004 Global Conference, Phoenix, Arizona, 2004, pp 55.

[187] E. Spanakis, E. Milord, C. Gragnoli, AVPR2 variants and mutations in nephrogenic diabetes insipidus: Review and missense mutation significance, J Cell Physiol 217 (2008) 605–617.

[188] N.B. Knops, K.K. Bos, M. Kerstjens, K. van Dael, Y.J. Vos, Nephrogenic diabetes insipidus in a patient with L1 syndrome: A new report of a contiguous gene deletion syndrome including L1CAM and AVPR2, Am J Med Genet A 146A (2008) 1853–1858.

[189] M. Fujimoto, K. Imai, K. Hirata, R. Kashiwagi, Y. Morinishi, K. Kitazawa, et al., Immunological profile in a family with nephrogenic diabetes insipidus with a novel 11 kb deletion in AVPR2 and ARHGAP4 genes, BMC Med Genet 9 (2008) 42.

[190] D.G. Bichet, M. Birnbaumer, M. Lonergan, M.-F. Arthus, W. Rosenthal, P. Goodyer, et al., Nature and recurrence of AVPR2 mutations in X-linked nephrogenic diabetes insipidus, Am J Hum Genet 55 (1994) 278–286.
[191] M.F. Arthus, M. Lonergan, M.J. Crumley, A.K. Naumova, D. Morin, L.A. De Marco, et al., Report of 33 novel AVPR2 mutations and analysis of 117 families with X-linked nephrogenic diabetes insipidus, J Am Soc Nephrol 11 (2000) 1044–1054.
[192] H.H. Hobbs, D.W. Russell, M.S. Brown, J.L. Goldstein, The LDL receptor locus in familial hypercholesterolemia: Mutational analysis of a membrane protein, Annu Rev Genet 24 (1990) 133–170.
[193] L.S. Barak, A. Salahpour, X. Zhang, B. Masri, T.D. Sotnikova, A.J. Ramsey, et al., Pharmacological characterization of membrane-expressed human trace amine-associated receptor 1 (TAAR1) by a bioluminescence resonance energy transfer cAMP biosensor, Mol Pharmacol 74 (2008) 585–594.
[194] J.P. Morello, A. Salahpour, A. Laperrière, V. Bernier, M.-F. Arthus, M. Lonergan, et al., Pharmacological chaperones rescue cell-surface expression and function of misfolded V2 vasopressin receptor mutants, J Clin Invest 105 (2000) 887–895.
[195] V. Bernier, M. Lagace, M. Lonergan, M.F. Arthus, D.G. Bichet, M. Bouvier, Functional rescue of the constitutively internalized V2 vasopressin receptor mutant R137H by the pharmacological chaperone action of SR49059, Mol Endocrinol 18 (2004) 2074–2084.
[196] R. Hermosilla, M. Oueslati, U. Donalies, E. Schonenberger, E. Krause, A. Oksche, et al., Disease-causing V(2) vasopressin receptors are retained in different compartments of the early secretory pathway, Traffic 5 (2004) 993–1005.
[197] S. Wuller, B. Wiesner, A. Loffler, J. Furkert, G. Krause, R. Hermosilla, et al., Pharmacochaperones post-translationally enhance cell surface expression by increasing conformational stability of wild-type and mutant vasopressin V2 receptors, J Biol Chem 279 (2004) 47254–47263.
[198] J.H. Robben, M. Sze, N.V. Knoers, P.M. Deen, Functional rescue of vasopressin V2 receptor mutants in MDCK cells by pharmacochaperones: Relevance to therapy of nephrogenic diabetes insipidus, Am J Physiol Renal Physiol 292 (2007) F253–F260.
[199] T. Schoneberg, A. Schulz, H. Biebermann, T. Hermsdorf, H. Rompler, K. Sangkuhl, Mutant G-protein-coupled receptors as a cause of human diseases, Pharmacol Ther 104 (2004) 173–206.
[200] K. Romisch, A cure for traffic jams: Small molecule chaperones in the endoplasmic reticulum, Traffic 5 (2004) 815–820.
[201] P.M. Conn, J.A. Janovick, Trafficking and quality control of the gonadotropin releasing hormone receptor in health and disease, Mol Cell Endocrinol 299 (2009) 137–145.
[202] B.K. Tamarappoo, A.S. Verkman, Defective aquaporin-2 trafficking in nephrogenic diabetes insipidus and correction by chemical chaperones, J Clin Invest 101 (1998) 2257–2267.
[203] S. Kunchaparty, M. Palcso, J. Berkman, H. Velazquez, G.V. Desir, P. Bernstein, et al., Defective processing and expression of thiazide-sensitive Na-Cl cotransporter as a cause of Gitelman's syndrome, Am J Physiol 277 (1999) F643–F649.
[204] M. Peters, S. Ermert, N. Jeck, C. Derst, U. Pechmann, S. Weber, et al., Classification and rescue of ROMK mutations underlying hyperprostaglandin E syndrome/antenatal Bartter syndrome, Kidney Int 64 (2003) 923–932.
[205] A. Hayama, T. Rai, S. Sasaki, S. Uchida, Molecular mechanisms of Bartter syndrome caused by mutations in the BSND gene, Histochem Cell Biol 119 (2003) 485–493.
[206] J. Chillaron, R. Estevez, I. Samarzija, S. Waldegger, X. Testar, F. Lang, et al., An intracellular trafficking defect in type I cystinuria rBAT mutants M467T and M467K, J Biol Chem 272 (1997) 9543–9549.
[207] A. Bonnardeaux, D.G. Bichet, Inherited disorders of the renal tubule, in: B.M. Brenner (Ed.), Brenner & Rector's The Kidney, seventh ed., Saunders, Philadelphia, 2004, pp. 1697–1741.
[208] J. Perucca, D.G. Bichet, P. Bardoux, N. Bouby, L. Bankir, Sodium excretion in response to vasopressin and selective vasopressin receptor antagonists, J Am Soc Nephrol 19 (2008) 1721–1731.
[209] D.A. Lomas, D.L. Evans, J.T. Finch, R.W. Carrell, The mechanism of Z alpha 1-antitrypsin accumulation in the liver, Nature 357 (1992) 605–607.
[210] M.W. Lawless, C.M. Greene, A. Mulgrew, C.C. Taggart, S.J. O'Neill, N.G. McElvaney, Activation of endoplasmic reticulum-specific stress responses associated with the conformational disease Z alpha 1-antitrypsin deficiency, J Immunol 172 (2004) 5722–5726.
[211] F.E. Cohen, J.W. Kelly, Therapeutic approaches to protein-misfolding diseases, Nature 426 (2003) 905–909.
[212] A. Ulloa-Aguirre, J.A. Janovick, S.P. Brothers, P.M. Conn, Pharmacologic rescue of conformationally-defective proteins: Implications for the treatment of human disease, Traffic 5 (2004) 821–837.
[213] L.S. Barak, R.H. Oakley, S.A. Laporte, M.G. Caron, Constitutive arrestin-mediated desensitization of a human vasopressin receptor mutant associated with nephrogenic diabetes insipidus, Proc Nat Acad Sci USA 98 (2001) 93–98.
[214] V. Bernier, J.P. Morello, A. Zarruk, N. Debrand, A. Salahpour, M. Lonergan, et al., Pharmacologic chaperones as a potential treatment for X-linked nephrogenic diabetes insipidus, J Am Soc Nephrol 17 (2006) 232–243.
[215] D.J. Glover, H.J. Lipps, D.A. Jans, Towards safe, non-viral therapeutic gene expression in humans, Nat Rev Genet (2005) 299–310.
[216] K. Sangkuhl, A. Schulz, H. Rompler, J. Yun, J. Wess, T. Schoneberg, Aminoglycoside-mediated rescue of a disease-causing nonsense mutation in the V2 vasopressin receptor gene in vitro and in vivo, Hum Mol Genet 13 (2004) 893–903.
[217] A.S. Mankin, S.W. Liebman, Baby, don't stop! Nat Genet 23 (1999) 8–10.
[218] B.J. Feldman, S.M. Rosenthal, G.A. Vargas, R.G. Fenwick, E.A. Huang, M. Matsuda-Abedini, et al., Nephrogenic syndrome of inappropriate antidiuresis, N Engl J Med 352 (2005) 1884–1890.
[219] G. Decaux, F. Vandergheynst, Y. Bouko, J. Parma, G. Vassart, C. Vilain, Nephrogenic syndrome of inappropriate antidiuresis in adults: High phenotypic variability in men and women from a large pedigree, J Am Soc Nephrol 18 (2007) 606–612.
[220] S. Soule, C. Florkowski, H. Potter, D. Pattison, M. Swan, P. Hunt, et al., Intermittent severe, symptomatic hyponatraemia due to the nephrogenic syndrome of inappropriate antidiuresis, Ann Clin Biochem 45 (2008) 520–523.
[221] M.A. Marcialis, V. Faa, V. Fanos, M. Puddu, M.C. Pintus, A. Cao, et al., Neonatal onset of nephrogenic syndrome of inappropriate antidiuresis, Pediatr Nephrol 23 (2008) 2267–2271.
[222] K. Kalenga, A. Persu, E. Goffin, E. Lavenne-Pardonge, P.J. van Cangh, D.G. Bichet, et al., Intrafamilial phenotype variability in nephrogenic diabetes insipidus, Am J Kidney Dis 39 (2002) 737–743.
[223] M. Kocan, H.B. See, N.G. Sampaio, K.A. Eidne, B.J. Feldman, K.D. Pfleger, Agonist-independent interactions between beta-arrestins and mutant vasopressin type II receptors associated with nephrogenic syndrome of inappropriate antidiuresis, Mol Endocrinol 23 (2009) 559–571.
[224] B. Brenner, U. Seligsohn, Z. Hochberg, Normal response of factor VIII and von Willebrand factor to 1-deamino-8D-

arginine vasopressin in nephrogenic diabetes insipidus, J Clin Endocrinol Metab 67 (1988) 191–193.
[225] N. Knoers, L.A. Monnens, A variant of nephrogenic diabetes insipidus: V2 receptor abnormality restricted to the kidney, Eur J Pediatr 150 (1991) 370–373.
[226] J.M. Langley, J.W. Balfe, T. Selander, P.N. Ray, J.T. Clarke, Autosomal recessive inheritance of vasopressin-resistant diabetes insipidus, Am J Med Genet 38 (1991) 90–94.
[227] P.M.T. Deen, M.A.J. Verdijk, N.V.A.M. Knoers, B. Wieringa, L.A.H. Monnens, C.H. van Os, et al., Requirement of human renal water channel aquaporin-2 for vasopressin-dependent concentration of urine, Science 264 (1994) 92–95.
[228] P. Agre, Aquaporin water channels (Nobel Lecture), Angew Chem Int Ed Engl 43 (2004) 4278–4290.
[229] D.G. Bichet, Nephrogenic diabetes insipidus: New developments, Nephrology Self-Assessment Program 3 (2004) 187–191.
[230] D.G. Bichet, T.M. Fujiwara, Reabsorption of sodium chloride – lessons from the chloride channels, N Engl J Med 350 (2004) 1281–1283.
[231] N. Jeck, K.P. Schlingmann, S.C. Reinalter, M. Komhoff, M. Peters, S. Waldegger, et al., Salt handling in the distal nephron: Lessons learned from inherited human disorders, Am J Physiol Regul Integr Comp Physiol 288 (2005) R782–R795.
[232] M. Peters, N. Jeck, S. Reinalter, A. Leonhardt, B. Tonshoff, G.G. Klaus, et al., Clinical presentation of genetically defined patients with hypokalemic salt-losing tubulopathies, Am J Med 112 (2002) 183–190.
[233] S. Marek, I. Tekesin, L. Hellmeyer, M. Komhoff, H.W. Seyberth, R.F. Maier, et al., [Differential diagnosis of a polyhydramnion in hyperprostaglandin E syndrome: A case report], Z Geburtshilfe Neonatol 208 (2004) 232–235.
[234] D. Bockenhauer, W. van't Hoff, A. Lehnhardt, M. Subtirelu, F. Hildebrandt, D.G. Bichet, Secondary nephrogenic diabetes insipidus as a complication of inherited renal diseases, submitted (2010).
[235] R. Boton, M. Gaviria, D.C. Batlle, Prevalence, pathogenesis, and treatment of renal dysfunction associated with chronic lithium therapy, Am J Kidney Dis 10 (1987) 329–345.
[236] J.P. Grunfeld, B.C. Rossier, Lithium nephrotoxicity revisited, Nat Rev Nephrol 5 (2009) 270–276.
[237] D.C. Batlle, A.B. von Riotte, M. Gaviria, M. Grupp, Amelioration of polyuria by amiloride in patients receiving long-term lithium therapy, N Engl J Med 312 (1985) 408–414.
[238] E.D. Barlow, H.E. de Wardener, Compulsive water drinking, Q J Med New Series 28 (1959) 235–258.
[239] G.L. Robertson, Dipsogenic diabetes insipidus: A newly recognized syndrome caused by a selective defect in the osmoregulation of thirst, Trans Assoc Am Physicians 100 (1987) 241–249.
[240] J.A. Amico, Diabetes insipidus and pregnancy, in: P. Czernichow, A.G. Robinson (Eds.), Frontiers of Hormone Research, Karger, Basel, Switzerland, 1985, pp. 266–277.
[241] Y. Iwasaki, Y. Oiso, K. Kondo, S. Takagi, K. Takatsuki, H. Hasegawa, et al., Aggravation of subclinical diabetes insipidus during pregnancy, N Engl J Med 324 (1991) 522–526.
[242] H. Forssman, On hereditary diabetes insipidus, with special regard to a sex-linked form, Acta Med Scand 159 (1945) 1–196.
[243] W.M. Barron, L.H. Cohen, L.A. Ulland, W.E. Lassiter, E.M. Fulghum, D. Emmanouel, et al., Transient vasopressin-resistant diabetes insipidus of pregnancy, N Engl J Med 310 (1984) 442–444.
[244] J.A. Durr, J.G. Hoggard, J.M. Hunt, R.W. Schrier, Diabetes insipidus in pregnancy associated with abnormally high circulating vasopressinase activity, N Engl J Med 316 (1987) 1070–1074.
[245] U.C. Brewster, J.P. Hayslett, Diabetes insipidus in the third trimester of pregnancy, Obstet Gynecol 105 (2005) 1173–1176.
[246] A.K. Hiett, J.R. Barton, Diabetes insipidus associated with craniopharyngioma in pregnancy, Obstet Gynecol 76 (1990) 982–984.
[247] M.D. Lindheimer, Polyuria and pregnancy: Its cause, its danger, Obstet Gynecol 105 (2005) 1171–1172.
[248] A. Leaf, Neurogenic diabetes insipidus, Kidney Int 15 (1979) 572–580.
[249] G.L. Robertson, Diagnosis of diabetes insipidus, in: P. Czernichow, A.G. Robinson (Eds.), Frontiers of Hormone Research, Karger, Basel, 1985, pp. 176–189.
[250] S.D. Boyd, S. Raz, R.M. Ehrlich, Diabetes insipidus and nonobstructive dilatation of urinary tract, Urology 16 (1980) 266–269.
[251] B. Gautier, P. Thieblot, A. Steg, Mégauretère, mégavessie et diabète insipide familial, Sem Hop 57 (1981) 60–61.
[252] D. Bichet, Nephrogenic diabetes insipidus, in: A. Davison, J. Cameron, J. Grunfeld, D. Kerr, E. Ritz, C. Winearls (Eds.), Oxford Textbook of Clinical Nephrology, second ed., Oxford University Press, New York, 1998, pp. 1095–1109.
[253] P. Stern, H. Valtin, Verney was right, but. [editorial], N Engl J Med 305 (1981) 1581–1582.
[254] G.L. Robertson, Differential diagnosis of polyuria, Annu Rev Med 39 (1988) 425–442.
[255] M.B. Goldman, D.J. Luchins, G.L. Robertson, Mechanisms of altered water metabolism in psychotic patients with polydipsia and hyponatremia, N Engl J Med 318 (1988) 397–403.
[256] A. Oksche, J. Dickson, R. Schülein, H.W. Seyberth, M. Müller, W. Rascher, et al., Two novel mutations in the vasopressin V2 receptor gene in patients with congenital nephrogenic diabetes insipidus, Biophys Biochem Res Com 205 (1994) 552–557.
[257] A.F. van Lieburg, M.A.J. Verdijk, F. Schoute, M.J.L. Ligtenberg, B.A. van Oost, F. Waldhauser, et al., Clinical phenotype of nephrogenic diabetes insipidus in females heterozygous for a vasopressin type 2 receptor mutation, Hum Genet 96 (1995) 70–78.
[258] W.L. Miller, Molecular genetics of familial central diabetes insipidus, J Clin Endocrinol Metab 77 (1993) 592–595.
[259] D.G. Bichet, Nephrogenic and central diabetes insipidus, in: R.W. Schrier, C.W. Gottschalk (Eds.), Diseases of the Kidney, sixth ed., Little, Brown and Company, New York, 1997, pp 2429–2449.
[260] G.L. Robertson, L.A. Klein, J. Roth, P. Gorden, Immunoassay of plasma vasopressin in man, Proc Nat Acad Sci USA 66 (1970) 1298–1305.
[261] G.L. Robertson, E.A. Mahr, S. Athar, T. Sinha, Development and clinical application of a new method for the radioimmunoassay of arginine vasopressin in human plasma, J Clin Invest 52 (1973) 2340–2352.
[262] E. Hartter, W. Woloszczuk, Radioimmunological determination of arginine vasopressin and human atrial natriuretic peptide after simultaneous extraction from plasma, J Clin Chem Clin Biochem 24 (1986) 559–563.
[263] F.T. LaRochelle Jr., W.G. North, P. Stern, A new extraction of arginine vasopressin from blood: The use of octadecasilylsilica, Pflugers Arch 387 (1980) 79–81.
[264] K.A. Ysewijn-Van Brussel, A.P. De Leenheer, Development and evaluation of a radioimmunoassay for Arg8-vasopressin, after extraction with Sep-Pak C18, Clin Chem 31 (1985) 861–863.

[265] J.J. Preibisz, J.E. Sealey, J.H. Laragh, R.J. Cody, B.B. Weksler, Plasma and platelet vasopressin in essential hypertension and congestive heart failure, Hypertension 5 (1983) I129–I138.
[266] J.R. Seckl, D.B. Dunger, J.S. Bevan, Y. Nakasu, C. Chowdrey, C.W. Burke, et al., Vasopressin antagonist in early postoperative diabetes insipidus, Lancet 355 (1990) 1353–1356.
[267] N.G. Morgenthaler, J. Struck, C. Alonso, A. Bergmann, Assay for the measurement of copeptin, a stable peptide derived from the precursor of vasopressin, Clin Chem 52 (2006) 112–119.
[268] S. Jochberger, C. Velik-Salchner, V.D. Mayr, G. Luckner, V. Wenzel, G. Falkensammer, et al., The vasopressin and copeptin response in patients with vasodilatory shock after cardiac surgery: A prospective, controlled study, Intensive Care Med 35 (2009) 489–497.
[269] A.H. Maas, O. Siggaard-Andersen, H.F. Weisberg, W.G. Zijlstra, Ion-selective electrodes for sodium and potassium: A new problem of what is measured and what should be reported, Clin Chem 31 (1985) 482–485.
[270] J. De Buyst, G. Massa, C. Christophe, S. Tenoutasse, C. Heinrichs, Clinical, hormonal and imaging findings in 27 children with central diabetes insipidus, Eur J Pediatr 166 (2007) 43–49.
[271] I. Fujisawa, Magnetic resonance imaging of the hypothalamic–neurohypophyseal system, J Neuroendocrinol 16 (2004) 297–302.
[272] F. Cattin, F. Bonneville, C. Chayep, et al., Imagerie par resonnance magnetique du diabete insipide, Feuill Radiol 45 (2005) 425–434.
[273] R. Rappaport, Magnetic resonance imaging in pituitary disease, Growth Genetics & Hormones 11 (1995) 1–5.
[274] A. Upadhyay, B.L. Jaber, N.E. Madias, Epidemiology of hyponatremia, Semin Nephrol 29 (2009) 227–238.
[275] G. Decaux, The syndrome of inappropriate secretion of antidiuretic hormone (SIADH), Semin Nephrol 29 (2009) 239–256.
[276] T. Berl, R.J. Anderson, K.M. McDonald, R.W. Schrier, Clinical disorders of water metabolism, Kidney Int 10 (1976) 117–132.
[277] D.G. Bichet, R. Kluge, R.L. Howard, R.W. Schrier, Hyponatremic states, in: D.W. Seldin, G. Giebisch (Eds.), The Kidney: Physiology and Pathophysiology, second ed., Raven Press, New York, 1992, pp. 1727–1751.
[278] T. Berl, Psychosis and water balance [editorial], N Engl J Med 318 (1988) 441–442.
[279] J.G. Verbalis, The syndrome of inappropriate antidiuretic hormone secretion and other hypoosmolar disorders, in: R.W. Schrier, C.W. Gottschalk (Eds.), Diseases of the Kidney, sixth ed., Little, Brown and Company, Boston, 1997, pp. 2393–2427.
[280] W.B. Schwartz, W. Bennett, S. Curelop, F.C. Bartter, A syndrome of renal sodium loss and hyponatremia probably resulting from inappropriate secretion of antidiuretic hormone, Am J Med 23 (1957) 529–542.
[281] T. Berl, S. Kumar, Disorders of water metabolism, in: R.J. Johnson, J. Feehally (Eds.), Comprehensive Clinical Nephrology, Mosby, London, 2000, pp. 9.1–9.20.
[282] E. Sausville, D. Carney, J. Battey, The human vasopressin gene is linked to the oxytocin gene and is selectively expressed in a cultured lung cancer cell line, J Biol Chem 260 (1985) 10236–10241.
[283] S. Smitz, J.J. Legros, P. Franchimont, M. le Maire, Identification of vasopressin-like peptides in the plasma of a patient with the syndrome of inappropriate secretion of antidiuretic hormone and an oat cell carcinoma, Acta Endocrinol (Copenh) 119 (1988) 567–574.
[284] J.G. Verbalis, Tumoral hyponatremia [editorial], Arch Intern Med 146 (1986) 1686–1687.
[285] G. Schwaab, C. Micheau, C. Le Guillou, L. Pacheco, P. Marandas, C. Domenge, et al., Olfactory esthesioneuroma: A report of 40 cases, Laryngoscope 98 (1988) 872–876.
[286] K.D. Nolph, R.W. Schrier, Sodium, potassium and water metabolism in the syndrome of inappropriate antidiuretic hormone secretion, Am J Med 49 (1970) 534–545.
[287] L.H. Beck, Hypouricemia in the syndrome of inappropriate secretion of antidiuretic hormone, N Engl J Med 301 (1979) 528–530.
[288] P. Falardeau, J. Proulx, T. Nawar, C. Caron, P. Montambault, G.E. Plante, Clinical and biochemical profiles of inappropriate secretion of antidiuretic hormone, Proceedings of the Seventh International Congress of Nephrology D-32 (1978).
[289] G. Decaux, F. Genette, J. Mockel, Hypouremia in the syndrome of inappropriate secretion of antidiuretic hormone, Ann Intern Med 93 (1980) 716–717.
[290] C. Manoogian, M. Pandian, L. Ehrlich, D. Fisher, R. Horton, Plasma atrial natriuretic hormone levels in patients with the syndrome of inappropriate antidiuretic hormone secretion, J Clin Endocrinol Metab 67 (1988) 571–575.
[291] K. Kamoi, T. Ebe, O. Kobayashi, M. Ishida, F. Sato, O. Arai, et al., Atrial natriuretic peptide in patients with the syndrome of inappropriate antidiuretic hormone secretion and with diabetes insipidus, J Clin Endocrinol Metab 70 (1990) 1385–1390.
[292] M.A. Dillingham, R.J. Anderson, Inhibition of vasopressin action by atrial natriuretic factor, Science 231 (1986) 1572–1573.
[293] H. Nonoguchi, J.M. Sands, M.A. Knepper, Atrial natriuretic factor inhibits vasopressin-stimulated osmotic water permeability in rat inner medullary collecting duct, J Clin Invest 82 (1988) 1383–1390.
[294] R. Zerbe, L. Stropes, G. Robertson, Vasopressin function in the syndrome of inappropriate antidiuresis, Annu Rev Med 31 (1980) 315–327.
[295] A.I. Arieff, Effects on the central nervous system of hypernatremic and hyponatremic states, Kidney Int 10 (1976) 104–116.
[296] A.I. Arieff, Osmotic failure: Physiology and strategies for treatment, Hosp Pract (Off Ed) 23 (1988) 173–178. 183-184, 187-189 passim.
[297] R.H. Sterns, Severe symptomatic hyponatremia: Treatment and outcome. A study of 64 cases, Ann Intern Med 107 (1987) 656–664.
[298] T. Berl, Treating hyponatremia: Damned if we do and damned if we don't [clinical conference], Kidney Int 37 (1990) 1006–1018.
[299] R.H. Sterns, S.U. Nigwekar, J.K. Hix, The treatment of hyponatremia, Semin Nephrol 29 (2009) 282–299.
[300] D. Richter, H. Schmale, Molecular aspects of the expression of the vasopressin gene, in: P. Czernichow, A.G. Robinson (Eds.), Frontiers of Hormone Research, S. Karger, Basel, 1985, pp. 37–41.
[301] C.W. Bourque, S.H.R. Oliet, Osmoreceptors in the central nervous system, Annu Rev Physiol 59 (1997) 601–619.
[302] R.L. Zerbe, G.L. Robertson, Disorders of ADH, Med North America 13 (1984) 1570–1574.
[303] R.L. Zerbe, D.P. Henry, G.L. Robertson, Vasopressin response to orthostatic hypotension, Am J Med 74 (1983) 265–271.
[304] T.P. Vokes, G.L. Robertson, Physiology of secretion of vasopressin, in: P. Czernichow, A.G. Robinson (Eds.), Front Horm Res: Diabetes Insipidus in Man, Karger, 13 (1985) 127–155.
[305] H. Gainer, H. Chin, Molecular diversity in neurosecretion: reflections on the hypothalamo-neurohypophysial system. Cell Mol Neurobiol 18 (1998) 211–230.

[306] G.L. Robertson, The physiopathology of ADH secretion, in: G. Tolis, F. Labrie, J.B. Martin, F. Naftolin (Eds.), Clinical Neuroendocrinology: A Pathophysiological Approach, Raven Press, New York, 1979, pp. 247–260.

[307] A. Cheng, A.N. van Hoek, M. Yeager, A.S. Verkman, A.K. Mitra, Three-dimensional organization of a human water channel, Nature 387 (1997) 627–630.

[308] P.H. Baylis, Vasopressin and its neurophysin, in: L.J. Degroot, J.M. Besser, G.F.J. Cahill, J.C. Marshall, D.H. Nelson, W.D. Odell, et al. (Eds.), Endocrinology, second ed., W. B Saunders, Philadelphia, 1989, pp. 213–229.

[309] A.H. Sklar, R.W. Schrier, Central nervous system mediators of vasopressin release, Physiol Rev 63 (1983) 1243–1280.

[310] G.L. Robertson, Diseases of the posterior pituitary, in: D. Felig, J.D. Baxter, A.E. Broadus, L.A. Frohman (Eds.), Endocrinology and Metabolism, McGraw-Hill, New York, 1981, pp. 251–277.

SECTION II

HYPOTHALAMIC–PITUITARY DISORDERS

CHAPTER

9

The Hypothalamus

Glenn D. Braunstein

Cedars-Sinai Medical Center, Los Angeles, USA

ANATOMY

The hypothalamus is one of the major portions of the diencephalon, and is situated at the base of the brain below the thalamus and above the pituitary (Figures 9.1 and 9.2). The anterior margin of the optic chiasm forms the anterior boundary of the hypothalamus, while the posterior margins of the mamillary bodies delineate the posterior boundary. The lateral borders are less well defined and vary at different levels. They are composed of the optic tracts, internal capsule, pes pedunculi, globus pallidus and ansa lenticularis [1]. Between the chiasm and the mamillary bodies on the ventral surface is the tuber cinereum from which the pituitary stalk arises. The third ventricle lies in the center of the hypothalamus and is connected to the lateral ventricles through the foramen of Monro, and to the fourth ventricle by the aqueduct of Sylvius. The overall dimensions of the hypothalamus are approximately 1.5 (top-to-bottom) × 1.5 (front-to-back) × 1.3 (side-to-side) cm, and the weight is about 2.5 g [2].

This relatively small structure is packed with groups of nerve cell bodies which form distinct nuclei (see Figures 9.1 and 9.2). These nuclei can be divided into three zones (periventricular, medial, lateral) or four regions moving anterior to posterior (preoptic, supraoptic, tuberal and mamillary) (Table 9.1) [3–5]. In addition to the nuclei, numerous afferent and efferent fibers connect the hypothalamus to the cerebral cortex and the brain stem.

HYPOTHALAMIC FUNCTIONS

A number of functions have been ascribed to the hypothalamus based upon animal studies, clinical observations of disease states involving the hypothalamus, and electrical stimulation or destruction of hypothalamic regions in humans. Because of the close association of hypothalamic nuclei to afferent and efferent tracts from cortical, thalamic, limbic, midbrain and spinal regions, it has been difficult to localize

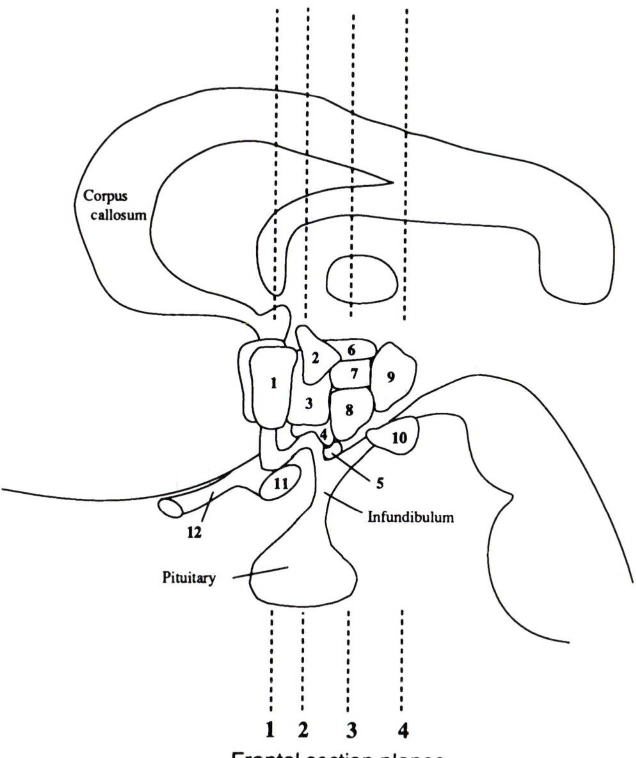

FIGURE 9.1 Schematic representation of lateral brain section demonstrating hypothalamic nuclei. Dashed lines represent the frontal (coronal) section planes illustrated in Figures 9.2 and 9.3. Key to numbers: 1, preoptic nucleus; 2, paraventricular nucleus; 3, anterior hypothalamic area; 4, supraoptic nucleus; 5, arcuate nucleus; 6, dorsal hypothalamic area; 7, dorsomedial nucleus; 8, ventromedial nucleus; 9, posterior hypothalamic area; 10, mamillary body; 11, optic chiasm; 12, optic nerve.

The Pituitary, Third Edition, DOI: 10.1016/B978-0-12-380926-1.10009-4

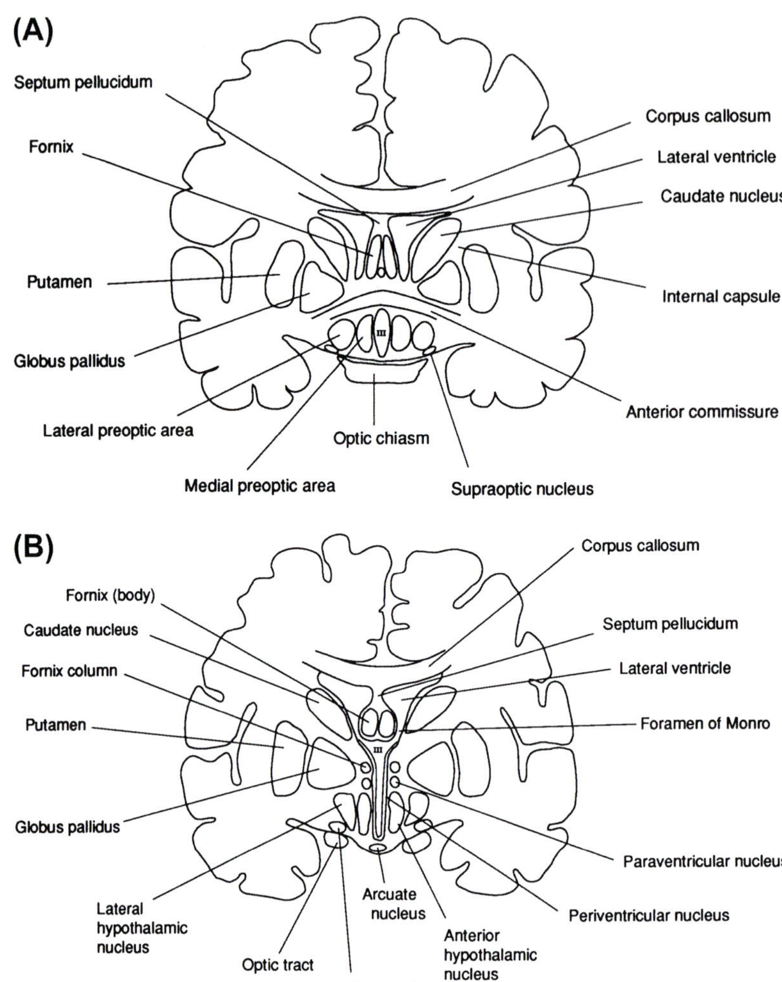

FIGURE 9.2 Frontal (coronal) sections of the hypothalamic regions. (A) Represents the preoptic region (frontal section plane 1 in Figure 9.1); (B) represents the supraoptic region (frontal section plane 2 in Figure 9.1);

(*continued*)

precisely specific functions to specific nuclei in the hypothalamus. A lesion in a nucleus may also damage or interrupt transmissions from adjacent nerve fibers. Indeed, the nucleus may only serve as a synaptic junction for neural transmissions that begin and terminate elsewhere. In addition, many nuclei appear to subserve multiple functions, and more than one pair of nuclei may be involved with the same function. For example, the ventromedial nucleus is involved in appetite control, emotional expression and short-term memory retention. The following sections summarize the current concepts regarding the normal functions of the hypothalamus. The reader is referred to several publications which review the clinical and experimental evidence upon which these summaries are based [3,6–9].

Water Metabolism

Arginine-vasopressin (AVP; antidiuretic hormone [ADH]) is synthesized in the nerve cell bodies of the magnocellular neurons of the supraoptic and paraventricular nuclei. The hormone is packaged in secretory granules with a specific neurophysin and transported through axoplasmic streaming down long axons that terminate in the pituitary stalk and posterior pituitary. AVP is released into the blood when serum osmolarity increases or vascular volume decreases. Blood volume status is monitored by stretch receptors present in the left atrium and large pulmonary veins, while serum osmolarity changes are detected by peripheral and hypothalamic osmoreceptors. Increased serum osmolarity is the dominant stimulus for AVP release, and this is mediated primarily through the hypothalamic osmoreceptors located in the medial preoptic anterior hypothalamic region.

Osmoreceptors located in the lateral preoptic anterior hypothalamic region stimulate thirst in response to increased serum osmolarity [6]. Hypovolemia and hypotension also stimulate thirst. AVP acts on the V_2 receptors of the distal tubules and collecting ducts of the kidneys and increases their water permeability

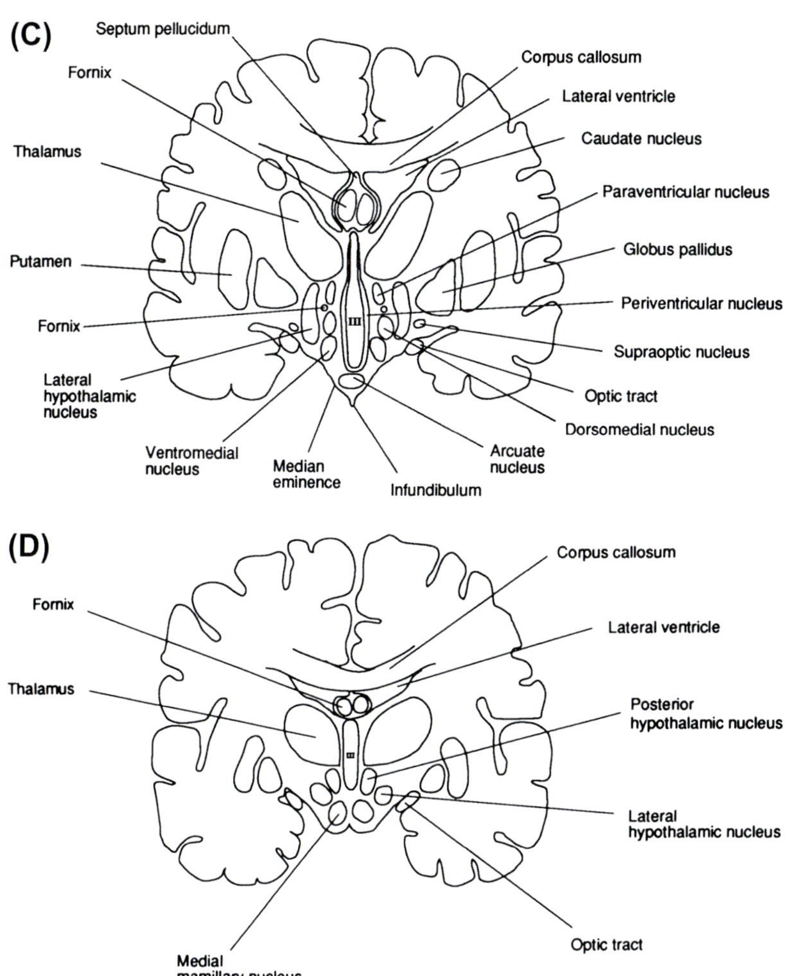

FIGURE 9.2 (C) represents the tuberal region (frontal section plane 3 in Figure 9.1); (D) represents the mamillary region (frontal section plane 4 in Figure 9.1).

through the aquaporin-II water channels, allowing water to be reabsorbed from the urine into the hypertonic renal medullary interstitial region, from which it re-enters the bloodstream. This reabsorbed water along with the water ingested in response to activation of the thirst mechanism re-establishes volume and decreases osmolarity, closing the feedback loop [10].

Other factors that stimulate the release of AVP include hypotension, nausea, vomiting, nicotine, hypoglycemia, hypoxia, barbiturates, β-adrenergic drugs, morphine, tricyclic antidepressants, cholinergic drugs and angiotensin II infusions. AVP release is inhibited by ethanol, atropine, α-adrenergic drugs, diphenylhydantoin and chlorpromazine [10].

Temperature Regulation

The preoptic anterior hypothalamus harbors receptors for warmth ("warm receptors"), as well as "cold receptors" that respond to cold. When peripheral warm receptors are stimulated by a rise in ambient temperature, and the hypothalamic adrenergic warm receptors are activated by an increase in the temperature of the blood, efferent signals are transmitted to the lateral portion of the posterior hypothalamus via the median forebrain bundle. This leads to activation of the heat-dissipating responses of vasodilatation and sweating. In contrast, activation of peripheral cold receptors through a decrease in environmental temperature, or activation of the serotonergic hypothalamic cold receptors, leads to medially placed neurons in the posterior hypothalamus activating the heat production and conservation mechanisms of shivering and vasoconstriction [6,7,11].

Appetite Control

The physiology of caloric homeostasis is incompletely understood. Feeding behavior involves cerebral, cortical, limbic and hypothalamic input. Animal studies have defined the ventromedial medial nucleus as the "satiety center," which inhibits feeding when stimulated and leads to hyperphagia when destroyed. In addition, a "feeding center" is present in the lateral hypothalamus,

TABLE 9.1 Major Hypothalamic Nuclei

	Zone		
Region	**Periventricular**	**Medial**	**Lateral**
Preoptic	Preoptic periventricular nucleus	Medial preoptic nucleus	Lateral preoptic nucleus
	Anterior periventricular nucleus		
Supraoptic	Suprachiasmatic nucleus	Anterior hypothalamic nucleus	Lateral portion of supraoptic nucleus
	Paraventricular nucleus	Medial portion of supraoptic nucleus	
Tuberal	Arcuate (infundibular) nucleus	Dorsomedial hypothalamic nucleus	Lateral hypothalamic nucleus
		Ventromedial hypothalamic nucleus	
Mamillary	Posterior hypothalamic nucleus	Premamillary nucleus	Lateral mamillary nucleus
		Medial mamillary nucleus	Intercalatus nucleus

Modified from [3–5].

whereby stimulation leads to hyperphagia and destruction to hypophagia [11,12]. The mechanisms by which the body monitors caloric balance are unknown. Peripheral lipid sensors, intestinal mechanoreceptors, hepatic glucoreceptors and hypothalamic glucoreceptors have been proposed [7]. The hypothalamus does contain glucoreceptors, and hypoglycemia can stimulate them to increase feeding behavior, but these receptors do not appear to be of physiologic importance [7].

There are a number of humeral factors that are involved in appetite. These include leptin, derived from adipocytes, which interacts with leptin receptors present on neurons in the arcuate nucleus [13]. One set of leptin-sensitive neurons express orexigenic peptides, neuropeptide Y and agouti-related peptide, while another group of neurons expresses cocaine and amphetamine-related transcript and proopiomelanocortin. These neurons in turn interact with hypothalamic melanocortin-4 receptor-expressing neurons. Additional hypothalamic factors that affect appetite experimentally include melanin-concentrating hormone, orexins, endocannabinoids, brain-derived neutrotrophic factor and nesfatin-1 [13–15]. Other peripherally produced factors that affect appetite include cholecystokinin, peptide YY, ghrelin, obestatin, glucagons-like peptide-1 and oxyntomodulin [16,17].

Sleep–Wake Cycle and Circadian Rhythm Control

The most important area governing wakefulness is the reticular activating system of the brain stem. Lesions in this area result in coma, a state in which the individual cannot be aroused, even with noxious stimuli. The anterior hypothalamus contains a "sleep center," stimulation of which leads to inhibition of the reticular activating system and sleep, from which, in contrast to coma, the animal or individual can be aroused. Stimulation of the posterior hypothalamus ("wakefulness center") leads to wakefulness and arousal. The normal sleep–wake cycle is regulated in part by the suprachiasmatic nucleus which integrates retinal stimuli during the day and pineal gland melatonin secretion at night [18]. The suprachiasmatic nuclei also control the circadian rhythms in anterior pituitary hormone release, as well as other physiologic rhythms [19]. Many of these rhythms are entrained through the visual system via the retinohypothalamic tract [20].

Regulation of Visceral (Autonomic) Functions

Integration of sympathetic and parasympathetic autonomic nervous system activity is an important function of the hypothalamus. Stimulation of the "sympathetic region" in the posteromedial hypothalamus results in activation of the thoracolumbar autonomic response and a "fight-or-flight" reaction with pupillary dilatation, a rise in blood pressure, tachycardia, increased cardiac output, tachypnea, piloerection, vasoconstriction of the α-adrenergic receptor visceral vascular beds and vasodilatation of the β-adrenergic responsive blood vessels in skeletal muscle [8]. Stimulation of the "parasympathetic region" in the preoptic anterior hypothalamus leads to increased vagal and sacral autonomic response with pupillary constriction, bradycardia, hypotension, increased blood flow in the visceral vascular bed and decreased flow in the muscle blood vessels [7,8]. Because of the multitude of autonomic fibers running through the hypothalamus, stimulation of one area may result in a sympathetic response, while a parasympathetic type of response may be found with stimulation of an adjacent area.

Other types of autonomic function that have been described in non-human animal studies include stimulation of micturition and defecation with electrical stimulation of the medial tuberal region [3], increased motility activity of the gastrointestinal tract with stimulation of the preoptic anterior hypothalamus and posterior dorsolateral regions and reduced bowel motility with ventromedial hypothalamic stimulation [3,7]. Gastric juice volume, acidity and pepsin content are increased with stimulation of the anteromedial hypothalamus, as well as the tegmentum of the brain stem [6].

Emotional Expression and Behavior

Through the use of electrode stimulation or production of lesions in various hypothalamic regions of animals, as well as clinical observations on humans with hypothalamic diseases, the ventromedial nucleus has been found to play an important role in integrating cortical input with regard to behavior. Lesions in this area lead to rage with aggressive, often violent, behavior associated with activation of the sympathetic nervous system [7]. This behavior is referred to as "sham rage" to distinguish it from voluntary or cortical rage. The autonomic response is probably mediated through activation of the posterior hypothalamic sympathetic area. In man, electrical stimulation of the medial or posterior hypothalamus results in the sensations of fear or horror, while apathy and reduced activity are found with destructive lesions in these areas [8,21,22]. Lesions in the limbic system in the region of the caudal hypothalamus have been associated with aggressive, hypersexual behavior [23]. A "pleasure center" located in the medial forebrain bundle in the lateral hypothalamus of rats has been described [6], this has a "nourishing region" around the septal area, stimulation of which leads to lapping, licking and chewing [3].

Memory

Memory is a complex process that requires an intact brain stem reticular formation, limbic system and hypothalamus. Short-term or recent memory requires intact ventromedial nuclei and hippocampus [6,7]. The role of the mamillary nuclei and dorsal medial nucleus in short-term memory is presently unclear.

Control of Anterior Pituitary Function

The hypothalamus synthesizes and secretes several hypophysiotropic releasing and inhibitory hormones that regulate anterior pituitary function. The physiologic and pharmacologic factors that control the hypothalamic–pituitary–target organ axes are described in detail elsewhere in this volume. Several immunohistochemical studies have localized the various factors in the hypothalamus. Although the nerve cell bodies in which the factors are synthesized are widely distributed throughout the hypothalamus, the axons converge at the median eminence (neurovascular zone) as part of the tuberoinfundibular system and terminate on or near the hypothalamohypophyseal portal vessels in which they discharge hypophysiotropic substances under appropriate stimulation.

The highest concentrations of nerve cell bodies for gonadotropin-releasing hormone (GnRH) are located in the medial basal hypothalamus and preoptic areas [25]. Thyrotropin-releasing hormone (TRH) neurons are found in the suprachiasmatic, preoptic medial and paraventricular nuclei [26], while corticotropin-releasing hormone (CRH) has been localized to the paraventricular nucleus [27]. Growth-hormone-releasing hormone (GHRH)-containing neurons are found in the arcuate nucleus [28], as are neurons synthesizing somatostatin [29]. Dopaminergic neurons, which presumably inhibit prolactin secretion through dopamine release into the hypothalamohypophyseal portal vessels, are found primarily in the arcuate nucleus, with smaller amounts found in the dorsomedial, ventromedial, periventricular, paraventricular nuclei and median forebrain bundle [30]. In addition to the peptides and amines with established physiologic pituitary regulatory functions, the hypothalamus is replete with a large number of biologically active substances, many of which are located in the same neurons that harbor the hypophysiotropic factors (Table 9.2).

PATHOPHYSIOLOGICAL PRINCIPLES

Considering the large number of important physiologic functions that depend upon the integrity of the hypothalamus, the close proximity of the nuclei and tracts, and the small overall size of the structure, one would anticipate that diseases involving the hypothalamus would give rise to a plethora of clinical syndromes. Indeed, this is the case, but despite the diversity of findings from patient to patient, several general principles regarding the pathophysiology of signs and symptoms of hypothalamic dysfunction have been established through careful clinical observation [7,31–35].

1. The spectrum of diseases that can affect the hypothalamus is large, and different lesions may produce identical signs and symptoms of hypothalamic damage. Multiple pathologic processes in each of the major disease categories can involve the hypothalamus (Table 9.3). Bauer reviewed 60 patients with hypothalamic involvement by a variety of diseases documented by

TABLE 9.2 Biologically Active Substances Present in Paraventricular and Arcuate Nucleus Neurons

PARAVENTRICULAR NUCLEUS
Magnocellular division
Angiotensin II
Cholecystokinin
Glucagon
Oxytocin
Peptide 7B2
Proenkephalin B (dynorphin, rimorphin, α-neoendorphin)
Vasopressin
Parvocellular division
Angiotensin II
Atrial natriuretic factor
Cholecystokinin
Corticotropin-releasing hormone
Dopamine
Follicle-stimulating hormone-releasing factor
γ-Aminobutyric acid
Galanin
Glucagon
Neuropeptide Y
Neurotensin
Peptide 7B2
Proenkephalin A (methionine enkephalin, leucine enkephalin, BAM 22P, metorphamide, [Met]enkephalin-Arg^6-Phe^7 -Leu^8, [Met]enkephalin-Arg^6 -Gly^7-Leu^8)
Somatostatin
Thyrotropin-releasing hormone
Vasopressin
Vasoactive intestinal polypeptide/Peptide histidine isoleucine
ARCUATE NUCLEUS
Acetylcholine
Dopamine
Galanin
γ-Aminobutyric acid
Growth hormone-releasing hormone
Neuropeptide Y
Neurotensin
Pancreatic polypeptide
Proenkephalin A
Prolactin
Proopiomelanocortin (adrenocorticotropic hormone, β-lipotropin, γ-melanocyte-stimulating hormone, β-endorphin)
Somatostatin
Substance P

From Lechan [24].

autopsy [31,32]. Despite the diversity of pathologic abnormalities, 78% had neuro-ophthalmologic abnormalities (in 13% these were the first manifestations), 75% developed pyramidal tract or sensory nerve involvement, 65% had headaches, 62% showed extrapyramidal cerebellar signs and 40% exhibited recurrent vomiting. Findings more specific to the hypothalamus included precocious puberty in 40% (undoubtedly reflecting a selection bias due to the types of case reports in which autopsies were performed), diabetes insipidus in 35%, hypogonadism in 32%, somnolence in 30%, dysthermia in 28% and obesity or emaciation in 25%. Although most of the different hypothalamic syndromes can result from a large proportion of the diseases listed in Table 9.3, some pathologic processes result in a restricted number of syndromes. For instance, the gliosis of the supraoptic and paraventricular nuclei that occurs in familial or idiopathic diabetes insipidus has diabetes insipidus as its only hypothalamic manifestation. Similarly, hamartomas have precocious puberty and galastic seizures as their primary manifestations, due to their endocrine activity and/or their specific location in the tuber cinereum. Many of the pathologic processes have characteristic appearances on magnetic resonance imaging that are helpful diagnostically [36].

2. As a general rule, patients with systemic illnesses such as sarcoidosis, histiocytosis and infections that involve the hypothalamus usually, but not uniformly, have nonhypothalamic manifestations of the disease process. Isolated sarcoid lesions may be found in the hypothalamus, but more commonly ophthalmologic and extracranial disease coexists. Unifocal eosinophilic granulomas have been described in the hypothalamus, but usually such involvement reflects disseminated histiocytosis and bony lesions generally are also present. Tuberculous meningitis, neurosyphilis and viral illnesses are rarely confined to the hypothalamus, although hypothalamic symptoms may be early manifestations of the disease.
3. The site of a lesion causing a dysfunction does not necessarily correspond to the site from which the function emanates. As noted above, the hypothalamic nuclei are closely packed and interspersed among various fiber tracts whose origins or destinations may be the cerebral cortex, midbrain, thalamus, limbic system, spinal cord, or even other nuclei within the hypothalamus. Since disease processes involving the hypothalamus tend to be rather large in relation to the size of the hypothalamus, it is rare to find a lesion involving only one nucleus or a single tract. Therefore, it is not

TABLE 9.3 Etiologies of Hypothalamic Dysfunction

Congenital	Nutritional/Metabolic
Acquired	Anorexia nervosa
Developmental malformations	Kernicterus
Anencephaly	Wernicke-Korsakoff syndrome
Porencephaly	Weight loss
Agenesis of the corpus callosum	
Septooptic dysplasia	**Degenerative**
Suprasellar arachnoid cyst	Glial scarring
Colloid cyst of the third ventricle	Parkinson's
Hamartoma	
Aqueductal stenosis	**Infectious**
Trauma	Bacterial
Intraventricular hemorrhage	Meningitis
Genetic (familial or sporadic cases)	Mycobacterial
Hypothalamic hypopituitarism	Tuberculosis
Familial diabetes insipidus	Spirochetal
Prader-Willi syndrome	Syphilis
Bardet-Biedl syndrome	
Wolfram's syndrome	**Viral**
Pallister-Hall syndrome	Cytomegalovirus
	Encephalitis
Tumors	Jakob-Creutzfeldt
Primary intracranial tumors	Kuru
Angioma of the third ventricle	Poliomyelitis
Craniopharyngioma	Varicella
Ependymoma	
Ganglioneuroma	**Vascular**
Germ cell tumors	Aneurysm
Glioblastoma multiforme	Arteriovenous malformation
Glioma	Pituitary apoplexy
Hamartoma	Subarachnoid hemorrhage
Hemangioma	Vasculitis
Lipoma	
Lymphoma	**Trauma**
Medulloblastoma	Birth injury
Meningioma	Head injury
Neuroblastoma	Postneurosurgical
Pinealomas	
Pituitary tumors	**Functional**
Plasmacytoma	Diencephalic epilepsy
Sarcoma	Drugs
Metastatic tumors	Hayek-Peake syndrome
	Idiopathic SIADH
Infiltrative	Kleine-Levin syndrome
Histiocytosis	Periodic syndrome of Wolff
Leukemia	Psychosocial deprivation syndrome
Sarcoidosis	
	Other
Immunologic	Radiation
Idiopathic diabetes insipidus	Porphyria
Paraneoplastic syndrome	Toluene exposure

surprising that in Bauer's series most patients had mixtures of neurologic or neuro-ophthalmologic signs and symptoms in addition to endocrine abnormalities [31,32].

4. The clinical manifestations depend in part upon the rate of progression of the disease process. Patients with small, rapidly progressive lesions often develop symptoms early, while slowly progressive lesions may remain asymptomatic for long periods, allowing some to obtain relatively immense size before clinical evidence of the disease becomes apparent. Presumably in the latter instance, the slow growth allows for the other areas of the hypothalamus or extrahypothalamic regions to compensate for the deficits induced by the lesion. Acute insults, such as vascular accidents or trauma, tend to result in decreased consciousness, hyperthermia and diabetes insipidus, which may be transient if the patient survives the initial injury. Chronic lesions tend to alter cognitive ability and endocrine function, and are not reversible.
5. Although lesions that involve a single, unilateral area of the hypothalamus may result in symptoms, most lesions resulting in chronic hypothalamic syndromes are bilateral, though not necessarily symmetrical. Since most of the hypothalamic functions are controlled by one or more pairs of nuclei, destruction of a single nucleus usually is not sufficient to result in a clinical syndrome. From a pathophysiologic standpoint, this implies that pathologic processes that are multiple (i.e., metastatic tumors, granulomatous diseases), arise in or around the third ventricle (colloid cysts), cause enlargement of the third ventricle (pinealomas, germ cell tumors, midbrain gliomas, aqueductal stenosis), or impinge upon or invade the floor of the hypothalamus (craniopharyngiomas, optic gliomas, pituitary adenomas) will be more likely to result in clinical signs and symptoms of hypothalamic disease than will diseases that affect the lateral portions of the hypothalamus.
6. Lesions involving hypothalamic nuclei may give different syndromes depending upon whether the lesion results in stimulation or destruction of the nuclei. Thus, stimulatory lesions in the tuberal area may result in precocious puberty, while destructive lesions may lead to hypogonadism. Hyperthermia is associated with stimulation of the preoptic region, while hypothermia is the clinical consequence of destruction of the same area.
7. The clinical manifestations of hypothalamic disease depend upon the age of onset. As a rule, the hypothalamus of neonates is quite immature, and diseases afflicting the neonatal or infant hypothalamus present different symptoms than the

same disease affecting the same region in an older child or an adult. The diencephalic syndrome of infancy due to a glioma involving the anterior hypothalamus is an example of this phenomenon. The affected infants eat seemingly adequate quantities of food, yet lose weight. They tend to be hyperactive and euphoric. After the age of 2 years, the surviving infants undergo a dramatic change by gaining weight, becoming obese and displaying irritable behavior [7]. Another type of age-related disease manifestation is the effect of hypopituitarism due to hypothalamic abnormalities. Gonadotropin deficiency that occurs before puberty will result in a lack of pubertal changes with maintenance of the sexually infantile state. Acquired hypothalamic hypogonadism that has its onset in an adult may lead to some regression of secondary sexual characteristics, but such individuals do not appear sexually infantile. GH deficiency due to hypothalamic disease in a prepubertal individual is associated with short stature, while a similar deficiency in an adult is clinically inapparent.

MANIFESTATIONS OF HYPOTHALAMIC DISEASE

Keeping the above general principles in mind, and based upon careful pathologic studies of patients with hypothalamic diseases, a topographic map of the hypothalamus which correlates clinical findings with anatomic sites of lesions can be constructed (Figure 9.3) [37–47].

Disorders of Water Metabolism

Central Diabetes Insipidus

This condition results from a partial or complete absence of AVP. Without sufficient AVP, the distal tubules and collecting ducts of the kidneys are unable to adequately reabsorb water, leaving the urine inappropriately hypotonic relative to the plasma osmolarity. The persistent diuresis leads to polyuria (up to 10–12 L/day) and nocturia, which in turn stimulates the thirst mechanism to bring about water-seeking behavior and polydipsia. If the osmoreceptor mechanism is intact and the patient is conscious and has access to fluids, the plasma osmolarity may be maintained within the normal range. However, if the osmoreceptors of the thirst center are damaged, or if the patient is unable to ingest adequate quantities of water, hypernatremic dehydration may occur and result in rapid deterioration of the sensorium from lethargy to stupor to coma. Patients with lesser deficiencies of AVP may release enough of the hormone to maintain adequate water balance under basal conditions. In contrast to patients with complete diabetes insipidus, patients with partial diabetes insipidus may increase their urine osmolarity to a level above their plasma osmolarity during dehydration. However, in both conditions, the administration of exogenous vasopressin to a dehydrated patient will result in a further increase in urine osmolarity, while dehydrated normal individuals will show little or no further increase in urine osmolarity after a standard dehydration test.

Diabetes insipidus results from lesions involving the magnocellular neurons of the supraoptic and paraventricular nuclei or that interrupt the supraopticohypophyseal tracts that terminate in the pituitary stalk or posterior pituitary. Such lesions are commonly found in patients with hypothalamic disorders. Transient diabetes insipidus may be found in individuals with posterior pituitary or low pituitary stalk lesions, manipulation of the pituitary stalk during resection of a pituitary adenoma, or in patients with acute, reversible hypothalamic lesions. In Bauer's series of anatomically proven chronic hypothalamic lesions, 21 (35%) of the patients had diabetes insipidus at some time during the course of their illness [31,32]. Although it was the second most frequent manifestation of hypothalamic disease, in only 3% of cases was diabetes insipidus the initial manifestation. Diabetes insipidus is often associated with hypogonadism and obesity, reflecting the anterior, medial hypothalamic localization of lesions affecting the supraoptic and paraventricular nuclei.

The spectrum of pathologic lesions accounting for diabetes insipidus from two large series is shown in Table 9.4 [48–51]. Idiopathic diabetes insipidus comprises the largest single category of causes and over a third of these patients have circulating vasopressin cell antibodies suggesting an autoimmune etiology [52]. In this condition, loss of magnocellular nerve cell bodies and gliosis is found in the supraoptic and paraventricular nuclei [53]. The same pathologic findings are present in patients with familial central diabetes insipidus but these patients do not have anti-AVP antibodies. Rather, mutations in the vasopressin precursor molecule gene have been found in some families [54]. Both sex-linked recessive and autosomal dominant forms of this latter condition have been described. An autosomal recessive form (Wolfram's syndrome) exists, composed of central diabetes insipidus, insulin-dependent diabetes mellitus, primary optic atrophy, bilateral sensorineural deafness, and in some families, autonomic neurogenic bladder and ataxia [55]. Degeneration of the paraventricular and, to a lesser extent, the supraoptic nuclei have been noted in this syndrome, as has atrophy of the posterior pituitary [55].

Deficiency of ADH is frequently seen with hypothalamic involvement by suprasellar germinomas (93%) [56,57], pineal germinomas (40%) [56,58], the chronic disseminated form of histiocytosis (50%) [59] and sarcoidosis (58%) [60–63]. Diabetes insipidus may also be found in patients with septo-optic dysplasia (22%) [64–67], pinealomas (18%) [58], hypothalamic gliomas (15%) [68,69] and craniopharyngiomas (22%) [56].

Adipsic or Essential Hypernatremia (Cerebral Salt Retention Syndrome)

Damage to the osmoreceptors in the anterior medial and anterior lateral preoptic regions of the hypothalamus may bring about essential hypernatremia which is characterized by chronic, fluctuating elevations of serum sodium (and chloride), often to dangerously high levels, despite the spontaneous ingestion of amounts of fluid (1–2 L/day) that are capable of maintaining appropriate plasma osmolarity in otherwise normal adults. Affected individuals have an impaired thirst mechanism, demonstrating hypodipsia or adipsia despite the marked elevations in serum sodium. Nevertheless, these patients have a normal volume of extracellular fluid and are not dehydrated, and, therefore, maintain a normal blood pressure, pulse rate, blood–urea nitrogen, serum creatinine and creatinine clearance. Since vascular volume status also regulates AVP release, these patients can release AVP and concentrate their urine with volume depletion. However, even while hypernatremic, an oral or intravenous intake of a large volume of water only results in inhibition of AVP release due to increased volume, culminating in the excretion of a dilute urine. Most of these patients do have partial diabetes insipidus, as their urine osmolarity does increase with exogenous administration of AVP [7,31,32,34,70,71].

Clinically, few symptoms reflecting hypernatremia are found with serum sodium concentrations below 160 mmol/L. Above this level, patients develop fatigue, lethargy, weakness, muscle tenderness and cramps, anorexia, depression and irritability. Stupor and frank coma may be found with sodium concentrations greater than 180 mmol/L. Although the pituitary gland at autopsy is normal, anterior pituitary hormone deficiencies are found in 71% of patients, reflecting the hypothalamic etiology of the hypopituitarism [70]. Obesity has been noted also in 43% of the patients. Additionally, hypertriglyceridemia has been found in five of six subjects (83%) in whom this measurement has been reported [70].

The pathologic processes that have been associated with essential hypernatremia include suprasellar germinomas, histiocytosis, sarcoidosis, craniopharyngiomas, ruptured aneurysms, optic nerve gliomas, pineal tumors, trauma, hydrocephalus, cysts, inflammatory conditions and toluene exposure [72]. Recently a few children have been described with essential hypernatremia but without a structural hypothalamic defect being found (Hayek–Peake syndrome). They demonstrate recurrent hypernatremia, hypodipsia, obesity, hyperprolactinemia, hypothyroidism, hyperlipidemia, lethargy, increased perspiration and in some cases, central hypoventilation [73,74]. The findings suggest a functional derangement in the anterior medial hypothalamic region with involvement of the osmoreceptors and the ventral medial nucleus.

Syndrome of Inappropriate Secretion of ADH (SIADH)

This condition is characterized by serum hypo-osmolarity (Posm <275 mOsm/kg) and hyponatremia, an inappropriately concentrated urine (Uosm >100 mOsm/kg) for the low serum osmolarity, continued urinary excretion of sodium despite the low serum sodium, and hypouricemia in a patient with normal renal, adrenal and thyroid function, and who does not exhibit findings of extracellular fluid volume expansion (i.e., no evidence of congestive heart failure, cirrhosis, or other edematous states) [75]. This condition may be due to drugs, activation of peripheral volume receptors, peripheral neuropathies, ectopic production of AVP from neoplasms, or intracranial processes. In some individuals the syndrome is due to a decrease in the set-point for the serum osmolarity release of AVP. Indeed, SIADH may occur, usually transiently, following head trauma, intracranial bleeds, meningitis, encephalitis, transsphenoidal pituitary surgery and other neurosurgical procedures. It has also been noted in some patients with hydrocephalus, craniopharyngiomas, germinomas, pinealomas, central pontine myelinolysis and acute intermittent porphyria [56,75]. In the latter situation it is not clear whether this is a reflection of a hypothalamic lesion or the result of a peripheral neuropathy [7,34]. An idiopathic, cyclic form of the syndrome has been found in young women with menstrual irregularities and enlarged lateral ventricles. No hypothalamic pathology has been identified in patients with the idiopathic variety [10].

Besides symptoms from the underlying disease, these patients demonstrate the clinical findings of water intoxication. Mild decrements in serum sodium, between 130 and 120 mmol/L, generally result in weight gain without edema, anorexia, nausea, vomiting, headache, weakness, withdrawal and lethargy. Mental confusion is common at concentrations below 120 mmol/L, and seizures and coma may also develop, especially if the decrease in sodium occurs rapidly.

Cerebral salt wasting due to central nervous system disease or post-neurosurgical procedures may also

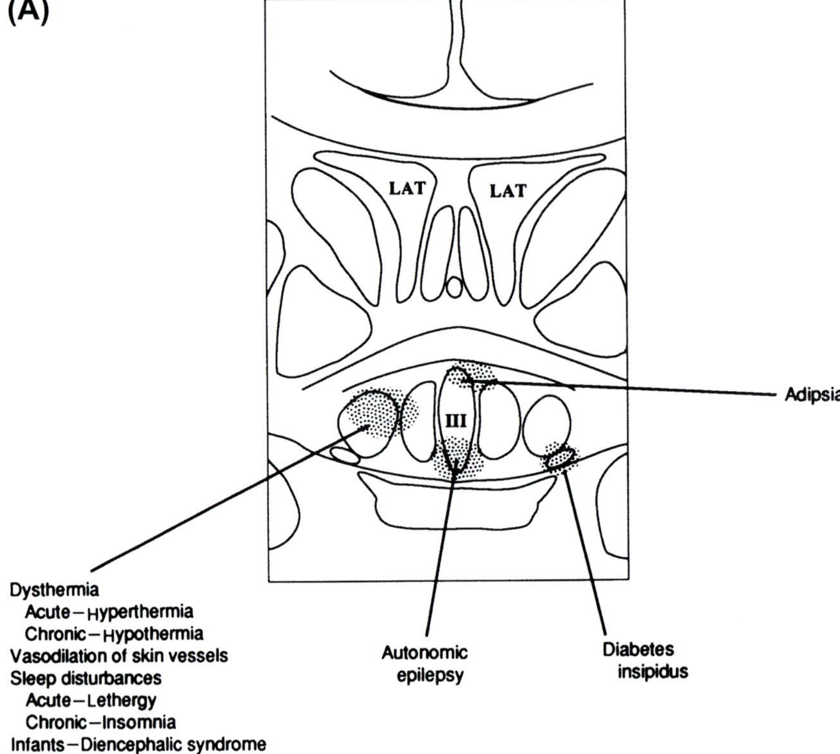

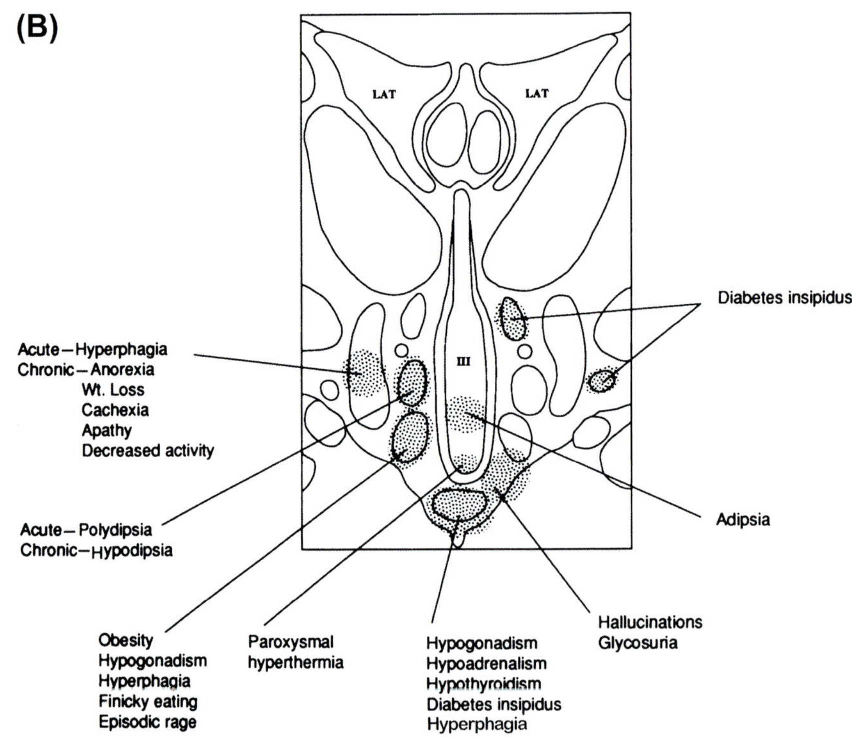

FIGURE 9.3 Clinical findings associated with hypothalamic lesions located at various anatomical sites. Clinicopathologic correlation based upon multiple studies [33–42]. (A) Corresponds to the region depicted in Figure 9.2A; (B) corresponds to the region depicted in Figure 9.2C;

(continued)

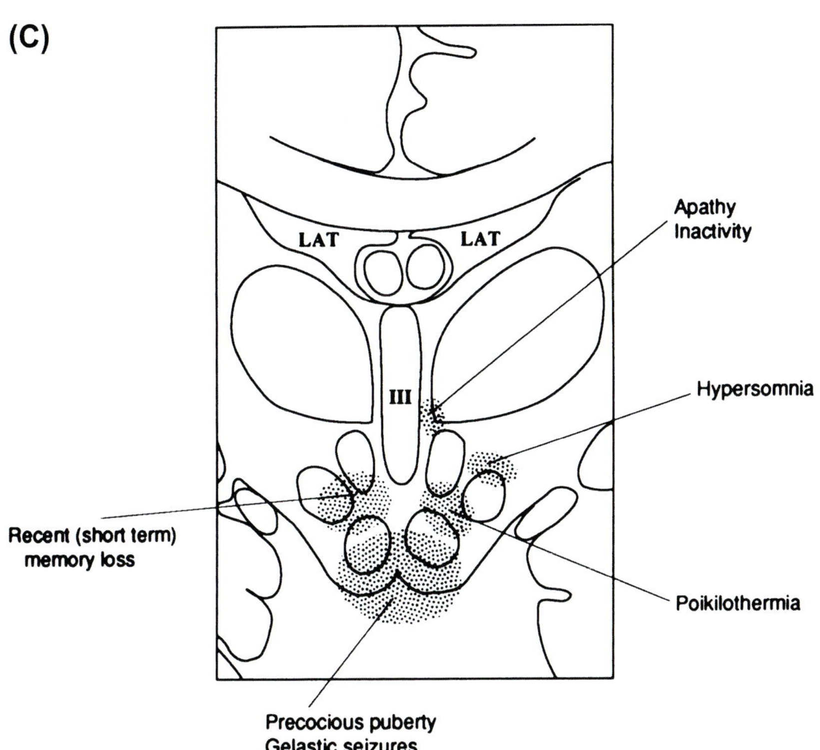

FIGURE 9.3 (C) corresponds to the section depicted in Figure 9.2D.

cause hyponatremia. Unlike SIADH, these patients are hypovolemic rather than eu- or hypervolemic as in SIADH. Disruption of the renal sympathetic nervous system input and increased production of a central naturetic factor are the mechanisms proposed for this syndrome [76].

Dysthermia

Hyperthermia

Acute injury to the anterior hypothalamic and preoptic areas from intracranial bleeds, neurosurgical procedures in the region of the floor of the third ventricle, or trauma may result in temperature elevations up to 41°C, tachycardia and unconsciousness that generally lasts for less than 2 weeks if the patient survives. With such lesions, heat production continues, while the heat-dissipating mechanisms fail to respond appropriately. The pulse rate in patients with hyperthermia due to hypothalamic lesions is not increased to the same extent for a given elevation in temperature as is the pulse rate in patients with fever from infections or inflammatory processes [3,6,7,31,32].

Acute hyperthermia to 41°C or greater is a characteristic of the neuroleptic malignant syndrome. This syndrome develops in susceptible individuals over 24–72 hours following exposure to phenothiazines, butyrophenones, thioxanthenes, or ioxapine. The potential for development of the syndrome roughly parallels

TABLE 9.4 Etiologies of Diabetes Insipidus

Etiology	Number of Patients	Percentage
Idiopathic/familial	179	44
Neoplasm		
Primary intracranial	89	22
Metastatic	15	4
Lymphoma	3	1
Leukemia	3	1
Trauma	20	5
Histiocytosis	35	8
Infectious		
Neurosyphilis	9	2
Meningitis	3	1
Postencephalitic	5	1
Sarcoidosis	4	1
Other*	46	11
Total	411	100

* *Cerebral atherosclerosis, birth injury, postvaccinal, giant cell granuloma, systemic illness, postirradiation, congenital malformation and postoperative.*
Adapted from [48–51].

the antidopaminergic D_2 receptor potency of the neuroleptic drug. It has been hypothesized that the syndrome results from basal ganglia dopamine D_2 receptor blockade which activates heat generation through muscle contraction, impairment of heat dissipation through hypothalamic injury, and inhibition of diaphoresis through a peripheral anticholinergic effect of the neuroleptics [77]. Autopsy studies have shown injury in the preoptic medial and tuberal nuclei [77]. Other clinical characteristics of the syndrome include hypertonicity of the skeletal muscles with "lead-pipe" type of rigidity, fluctuating consciousness varying from agitation to stupor to coma, and instability of the autonomic nervous system reflected by pallor, diaphoresis, wide swings in blood pressure, tachycardia and arrhythmias, tremors and akinesis. Leukocytosis, elevations of serum creatine phosphokinase and nonspecific encephalopathic findings on electroencephalography (EEG) are also found [78]. The syndrome lasts 5–10 days and currently carries a 20–30% mortality rate [78].

Altered mental status, autonomic nervous system instability, abnormal neuromuscular activity and hyperthermia also occur with the serotonin syndrome caused by methamphetamine and cocaine intoxication or use of stimulants and antidepressants [78]. Malignant hyperthermia occurs in susceptible individuals during and following anesthesia and is characterized by hyperthermia, hypotension and muscle rigidity, and is due to increased calcium release in skeletal muscles [78].

Sustained or chronic hyperthermia is found with lesions in the tuberoinfundibular region. Ten percent of the patients in Bauer's series exhibited chronic hyperthermia [31,32], which may result from loss of heat-dissipating mechanisms, stimulation of the heat-conservation mechanisms, or elevation of the set-point for activation of the heat dissipation [7]. Patients with chronic hypothalamic hyperthermia do not exhibit the generalized malaise that accompanies elevated temperatures due to infections, and also have paradoxical peripheral vasoconstriction with cold, clammy extremities. The hyperthermia may respond to sedatives or anticonvulsant medications, but not to salicylates [31,32].

Spontaneous paroxysmal hyperthermia of probable hypothalamic origin but without pathologic lesions in the hypothalamus has been described in a few patients. In most individuals, the episodes occur sporadically and are characterized by shaking chills, fever, hypertension, vomiting and peripheral vasoconstriction. Resolution over minutes to hours is accompanied by vasodilatation and diaphoresis. A similar syndrome occurring at regular 3-week intervals was described by Wolff, and may represent a form of diencephalic epilepsy [7,79,80].

Hypothermia

Chronic hypothermia with temperatures below 32°C was present in 12% of the patients described by Bauer [31,32], and this finding was usually associated with large lesions involving the anterior and/or posterior hypothalamus. Destruction of the thermoregulatory mechanisms by such lesions results in an inability to generate heat through shivering and vasoconstriction. Hypothermia has been noted in third-ventricular and large hypothalamic neoplasms, poliomyelitis, neurosyphilis, sarcoidosis, multiple sclerosis, gliosis of the anterior hypothalamus, posterior hypothalamic neuronal pyknosis in Parkinson's disease, and with the periventricular and mamillary body destruction seen with Wernicke's encephalopathy [60,80–83].

Episodic or paroxysmal hypothermia, also known as diencephalic autonomic epilepsy, is a distinct syndrome in which body temperatures abruptly decrease, often to 32°C or lower, over a period of minutes to days, associated with a variety of signs and symptoms of autonomic nervous system dysfunction [7,37,84–90]. The frequency of attacks varies from daily to decades apart. Patients experience flushing, diaphoresis, fatigue, hypotension, bradycardia, salivation, lacrimation, pupillary dilatation, Cheyne-Stokes respirations, nausea, vomiting, asterixis, ataxia and obtundation. Thus, during the episodes heat generation is impaired and heat loss is increased due to the vasodilatation and sweating. EEG slowing occurs during the episodes. Recovery occurs spontaneously over hours to days, and is associated with heat generation through shivering and vasoconstriction. Attacks often begin in the teenage years and the frequency and duration of attacks may increase as the patient ages. Some degree of thermal regulation is maintained during the episodes, since experimentally lowering the temperature further results in shivering and vasoconstriction, suggesting that there is a resetting of the thermostat during the episodes [89]. This syndrome has been found in some patients with tumors involving the floor and lower walls of the third ventricle [37,84]. In others, gliosis and loss of the arcuate nucleus and the premamillary area have been noted at autopsy. In addition, approximately half of the patients with episodic hypothermia have an agenesis of the corpus callosum, a combination given the eponym "Shapiro's syndrome" [85,86]. Such patients may also have hypogonadism, precocious puberty, diabetes insipidus, reset osmostat and GH deficiency [85,88–90].

Poikilothermia

This condition – the tendency of the individual to assume the ambient temperature – results from loss of both heat conservation and heat-loss homeostatic mechanisms. Wide fluctuations of temperature are seen, and affected patients do not experience thermal discomfort, or attempt to alter their environment to maintain their core body temperature [91]. This condition, noted in 1.7% of the patients in Bauer's series, is found with large lesions involving the posterior hypothalamus and rostral mesencephalon, as well as in patients with both anterior and posterior hypothalamic destruction [7,31,32]. Poikilothermia may also be found in Wernicke's encephalopathy and multiple sclerosis [7].

Disorders of Caloric Balance

Hypothalamic Obesity

Obesity is a common finding in patients with hypothalamic diseases, occurring in approximately 25% of individuals with anatomically proven lesions, although rarely is it the initial manifestation of hypothalamic dysfunction [31,32]. Most patients with hypothalamic obesity have large lesions or extensive involvement of multiple areas of the hypothalamus. Nevertheless, based upon careful study of the few patients with well-described, discrete lesions, it is clear that bilateral destruction of the ventromedial nucleus results in obesity in man, as it does in experimental studies in animals [3,12,31,32,39,40,44]. In patients with documented structural involvement, close to 90% have a neoplasm, most often a craniopharyngioma (approximately 60%) [12,92]. Approximately 6% are the result of inflammatory or granulomatous processes including sarcoidosis, tuberculosis, arachnoiditis and encephalitis, 5% are post-traumatic and 2% are due to leukemic infiltration [12].

As would be anticipated from the location of the lesions that lead to obesity, other clinical findings are commonly present. In a series of 69 patients analyzed by Bray and Gallagher, 72% had headaches, 72% had decreased vision or visual field abnormalities, 56% exhibited reproductive dysfunction such as amenorrhea, impotence, or diminished libido, 35% had disordered water metabolism with diabetes insipidus, polyuria, and/or polydipsia, 40% were somnolent, 20% had behavioral abnormalities and 7% had seizures [12]. The association between obesity and hypogonadism has long been noted since Froehlich described his patient, who was subsequently found to have a craniopharyngioma, with "dystrophic adiposogenitalis." The affective disorders that coexist with hypothalamic obesity vary from antisocial behavior to sham rage [40].

The obesity is clearly the result of hyperphagia. In many instances the abnormality appears to reflect a resetting of the satiety set-point. This is best seen in patients with obesity that develops following trauma. Most affected individuals gain weight for approximately 6 months following the trauma, followed by a period of stabilization as the energy expenditure equals the caloric content of the ingested food, with a subsequent gradual decrease in food intake and a loss of weight [12]. Similarly, patients with tumor destruction of the ventromedial nuclei may develop hyperphagia and a rapid gain in weight, followed by a plateau and then a further weight gain as the neoplasm grows [7]. Some patients display an indiscriminate food intake and will even ingest left-over scraps destined for the garbage, while others will show a finickiness that closely resembles that seen in rats with bilateral lesions in the ventromedial nuclei [12]. These patients have hyperinsulinemia to a greater extent than patients with essential obesity, and it has been proposed that this is due to enhanced insulin secretion through stimulation of the vagus nerve, as increased vagal firing rate has been noted in animals with ventromedial nucleus lesions [92]. In addition to hyperphagia and hyperinsulinemia, lowered basal metabolic rate and deficient GH, TSH and gonadotropins may contribute to the weight gain [92]. Hypothalamic obesity occurs in the Prader-Willi syndrome, in patients with leptin and leptin receptor deficiency, proopiomelanocortin mutations and mutations of the melanocortin-4 receptor [92].

Hypothalamic Cachexia in Adults

In Bauer's series, 18% of the patients exhibited substantial weight loss, 7% had anorexia and 8% were bulimic [31,32]. Destruction of both the ventromedial nuclei and the lateral hypothalamus leads to anorexia and emaciation, as do lesions isolated to the lateral hypothalamus [39,40,42]. The features of the lateral hypothalamic syndrome include rapid weight loss, muscle wasting, decreased activity, and hypophagia leading to cachexia and death. The most common lesions accounting for this syndrome are neoplasms, although cysts and malignant multiple sclerosis also have been described as causes [39,42].

Diencephalic Syndrome of Infancy

In 1951, Russell described an unusual syndrome in infants with hypothalamic tumors of severe emaciation despite an apparently good food intake, associated with an alert appearance and euphoric affect, and nystagmoid eye movements [93]. The majority (80%) of these infants have been found to have low-grade hypothalamic or optic nerve gliomas that destroy the ventromedial nuclei [6,7,94]. Rarely ependymomas, gangliogliomas and dysgerminomas give rise to the syndrome [94]. The infants appear normal at birth and demonstrate normal feeding and developmental parameters during the first 3–12 months. Towards the end of the first year of life, the infants begin to lose weight and subcutaneous fat, show signs of hyperactivity and a cheerful, happy affect, but continue to grow normally. They exhibit an alert appearance secondary to eyelid retraction (Collier sign) [94]. Other findings including nystagmus, pallor, vomiting, tremor and optic atrophy may be present (Table 9.5). Endocrine evaluation is generally normal, although absent diurnal variation in plasma cortisol concentrations, low insulin-like growth factor-I levels and elevated basal serum GH levels with a paradoxical rise following a glucose load, have been found [34,95]. The elevated GH levels are not specific to these patients, since other illnesses associated with weight loss, such as anorexia nervosa, are also accompanied by such elevations. Usually the infants succumb to the tumor and emaciation by the age of 2 years. Paradoxically, infants who survive beyond age 2, either due to spontaneous stabilization or therapy, often maintain their good appetite, gain weight and become obese. In addition, their pleasant personality is replaced by irritability and rage, and they may develop somnolence and precocious puberty [6,94]. This syndrome nicely illustrates the fact that the manifestations of hypothalamic disease are related in part to the age of patient and maturity of the hypothalamus.

Anorexia Nervosa

The typical patient with anorexia nervosa is a young, white female from a middle to upper socioeconomic background who inappropriately views herself as obese, and, therefore, severely restricts her food intake, exercises excessively and may engage in bulimic binges with self-induced vomiting, and diuretic and cathartic abuse. The typical age of onset is less than 25 years, the patients lose more than 15% of their weight, and are usually 25% below their ideal body weight. Amenorrhea is a characteristic finding and often precedes the weight loss, and may persist even after the patient regains her weight [94]. A number of endocrine abnormalities have been noted. A prepubertal pattern of gonadotropin release is characteristically present with low basal serum luteinizing hormone (LH) and follicle-stimulating hormone (FSH) concentrations, a prepubertal, apulsitile 24-hour LH-secretory pattern, a diminished LH response to GnRH, and a loss of the positive feedback effect of estrogen on LH secretion [96]. With weight gain, the patients enter a "second puberty," developing nocturnal secretory pulses of LH, and eventually an adult pattern of pulsatile LH release throughout the day and night [96]. The GnRH response also returns to normal.

Basal serum GH levels are normal or elevated, and rise paradoxically following a glucose load. The GH response to GHRH is normal, but the response to L-dopa and apomorphine is impaired [96]. A rise in serum GH levels may also occur following an injection of TRH, a response also found in patients with acromegaly, depression, chronic renal failure and cirrhosis [96]. The major mediator of GH action, insulin-like growth factor-I (IGF-I, somatomedin-C), is low, suggesting that the elevations in serum GH are due to decreased feedback inhibition by IGF-I. A reduction in tonic inhibition of GH secretion through a lowering of somatostatin has been suggested following the finding of decreased somatostatin levels in the cerebrospinal fluid [96]. The GH abnormalities revert to normal with weight gain.

Patients with anorexia nervosa also exhibit abnormalities in the hypothalamic–pituitary–adrenal axis. Plasma adrenocorticotropic hormone (ACTH) concentrations are diminished, while plasma cortisol levels are elevated, reflecting a decrease in the clearance of cortisol, since the cortisol production rate remains normal [96]. As is found in patients with Cushing's syndrome, depression and obesity, the reduction in plasma or serum cortisol is inadequate following the administration of dexamethasone. An attenuated response to a bolus injection of CRH has also been found. The abnormalities return to normal following weight gain.

These individuals share many clinical features with hypothyroid patients, including dry skin with a yellowish hue due to hypercarotemia, scalp hair loss, bradycardia and hypothermia. Their thyroid function tests are similar to those seen in patients with the "sick euthyroid syndrome." Thus, serum thyroxine levels

TABLE 9.5 Clinical Findings in 78 Patients with Diencephalic Syndrome of Infancy

Feature	Percentage
Emaciation	100
Alert appearance	87
Increased vigor and/or hyperkinesis	63
Vomiting	63
Euphoria	60
Pallor	55
Hydrocephalus	36
Nystagmus	51
Irritability	32
Optic atrophy	22
Tremor	23
Sweating	15
Large hands/feet	<5
Large genitalia	<5
Polyuria	<5
Papilledema	<5
Endocrine abnormalties	89

From [94] and [95].

are in the low-normal or frankly low range, the triiodothyronine concentrations are low, the reverse triiodothyronine levels are elevated, and the thyroid-stimulating hormone (TSH) concentrations are in the low-normal range. The serum TSH response to TRH is either normal or shows a delayed rise with a peak at 45 or 60 minutes, characteristic of hypothalamic hypothyroidism. As with the other hormonal abnormalities, the thyroid dysfunction resolves with weight gain.

Although most patients with classical anorexia nervosa do not have hypothalamic anatomic abnormalities, there is convincing evidence that this disorder has a component of hypothalamic dysfunction. In addition to the neuroendocrine abnormalities noted above, these patients may have hyperprolactinemia with galactorrhea, a poikilothermic type of thermal dysregulation and a partial diabetes insipidus [97]. It is unknown whether the hypothalamic abnormalities reflect a primary hypothalamic etiology of pathophysiologic importance to the genesis of anorexia nervosa, or whether the dysfunction is an epiphenomenon of a major psychiatric derangement and the associated weight loss.

Diencephalic Glycosuria

Transient hyperglycemia and glycosuria may occur following hypothalamic injury that results in lesion of the tuberoinfundibular region [3,98]. This has been most commonly noted after basal skull fractures, intracranial hemorrhage, or surgery near the floor of the third ventricle. Although each of these entities is associated with elevated concentrations of ACTH, glucocorticoids, GH and catecholamines, which have insulin-contraregulatory effects, the occurrence of hyperglycemia with injuries to the tuberoinfundibular region and not with injuries to other areas of the hypothalamus which may also be associated with elevations of the same hormones, suggests that other factors are involved. This may be analogous to pique hyperglycemia found with brain stem lesions.

Sleep—Wake Cycle And Circadian Abnormalities

Alterations in consciousness and the sleep—wake cycle rhythm are relatively common in patients with hypothalamic disease. Somnolence is most often seen, is found in 30% of patients, and is the presenting symptom in about 10% of individuals with proven hypothalamic disease [31,32]. Acute injury to the hypothalamus may result in coma, as can lesions involving the periaqueductal gray matter, mamillary bodies, or the mid-brain reticular activating system [6,7]. Drowsiness, hypersomnolence and emotional lethargy frequently accompany posterior hypothalamic lesions, often in association with hypothermia [3,7]. Historically, hypothalamic hypersomnia was commonly seen in the 1918 pandemic of Von Economo's encephalitis and as a manifestation of thiamine deficiency as part of Wernicke's encephalopathy [3,6,7]. Neoplasms account for the majority of documented cases at present. Hypersomnia, drowsiness, or stupor is found in approximately 18% of patients with craniopharyngiomas [98], 15% of patients with suprasellar germinomas and 26% of patients with nongerminomatous pineal tumors [58]. Approximately 40% of patients with hypersomnolence also have hypothalamic obesity [12].

Insomnia is an infrequent manifestation of hypothalamic disease. Hyperactivity and diminished duration of sleep have been noted in patients with anterior and preoptic hypothalamic lesions [99]. More commonly, anterior hypothalamic or anterior tuberal lesions result in alterations of the sleep—wake cycle, with daytime somnolence and nocturnal hyperactivity [7,45,99]. This is especially common with cystic craniopharyngiomas, and may resolve with drainage of the cyst fluid. Lesions in the tuberal region also have been associated with a syndrome resembling akinetic mutism in which the patient is mute, shows little spontaneous movement, is not responsive to verbal stimuli and yet appears awake [99].

A hypothalamic etiology for narcolepsy has been suggested because the syndrome has been found following encephalitis, third ventricular tumors, multiple sclerosis and head injuries, although the majority are idiopathic without a demonstratable pathologic basis [3]. Narcolepsy most commonly occurs in obese males with an onset in the teenage years, and is characterized by sudden attacks of falling asleep for minutes to hours [3]. Unlike normal sleep, these patients enter the stage of rapid eye movement sleep immediately and do not pass through the nonrapid eye movement stage [3,100]. Low levels of hypocretin-1, a key modulator of sleep—wake cycle stability, have been found in patients with narcolepsy [100].

Lesions that damage the suprachiasmatic region are associated with disordered circadian rhythms of the sleep—wake cycle, and body temperature and cognitive functioning [101].

Behavioral Abnormalities

Lesions involving the ventromedial nuclei are associated with rage reactions with emotional lability, agitation, and aggressive and destructive behavior that occur spontaneously [7,45]. During the episodes, there is usually activation of the autonomic nervous system with tachycardia, a rise in blood pressure, diaphoresis and pupillary dilatation. Similar sham rage reactions are found with lesions of the medial temporal lobes or orbitofrontal cortex [7].

Medial posterior hypothalamic lesions or destruction of the mamillary bodies is characteristically associated with apathy, somnolence, hypoactivity and general indifference. Vocal and auditory unresponsiveness and akinetic mutism have also been noted with lesions in this region [3,7].

Confabulation and short-term memory deficits are characteristic of Korsakoff's psychosis due to Wernicke's encephalopathy, which is associated with widespread lesions involving the mamillary bodies, periaqueductal gray matter and thalamus. These abnormalities appear to be the result of damage to the medial dorsal thalamus rather than the hypothalamus, although ependymal cysts and gliomas involving the third ventricle may be associated with similar findings, possibly through compression of the thalamus [3,6,7].

Sexual dysfunction occurs commonly with hypothalamic disorders. Hypogonadism was present in 32% of the patients analyzed by Bauer, with the majority of the lesions located around the floor of the third ventricle and involving the anterior hypothalamus, ventromedial nuclei and the tuberoinfundibular regions [31,32]. Symptoms include decreased libido and impotence in men, and amenorrhea in women. The pathogenesis most likely is due to abnormalities in GnRH secretion.

Hypersexual behavior may accompany lesions in the limbic system, medial temporal lobe and the caudal hypothalamus [102]. The Kline-Levin syndrome appears to have a genetic predisposition with an environmental trigger, which may result in reduced dopaminergic tone in the hypothalamus [103]. The syndrome usually involves adolescent boys who exhibit recurrent episodes of somnolence, with periodic arousal associated with irritability, incoherent speech, hallucinations, forgetfulness, compulsive gorging of food (megaphagia), masturbation and other sexual activity. The symptoms generally develop over a 2–4-day period with a vague sensation of malaise and headache. The episodes occur at 3–6-month intervals, and usually last 5–7 days, although they may last for several weeks. Spontaneous resolution is the rule in late adolescence or early adulthood. The syndrome also occurs in adolescent girls linked to their menstrual cycles [3,103].

Diencephalic Epilepsy

Diencephalic epilepsy broadly encompasses any seizure activity arising from the hypothalamus, although the term was originally used by Penfield in his description of a patient with a third ventricular cholesteatoma and periodic hypothermia and associated autonomic discharge [84]. Periodic hypothermia with absence of the corpus callosum (Shapiro's syndrome) and periodic hyperthermia (Wolff's syndrome) are also forms of diencephalic epilepsy.

Gelastic or laughing seizures are seen primarily in children with hamartomas of the tuber cinereum (50%) and other lesions near the floor of the third ventricle and extending to the mamillary region [104]. During a typical seizure the child stops his activity, makes laughing, giggling, or bubbling noises and develops a grimacing appearance from unilateral or bilateral clonic movements of the ocular, palpebral and/or buccal muscles [104,105]. There also may be dacrystic seizures, characterized by a crying quality with grimacing. During the episode the child does not lose consciousness, although the gelastic seizure may be followed by a grand mal or petit mal seizure [105]. The diagnosis is established by stereotyped recurrences, absence of precipitating factors, concomitance of other ictal manifestations, epileptiform abnormalities on EEG and no other obvious cause for pathologic laughter [104,105]. It is unclear whether the seizure is the consequence of compression of the mamillary region, interference with the neural connections with the limbic system, or reflects associated cerebral malformations [104,105].

NEUROGENIC (CUSHING'S) ULCERS

Since stimulation of the preoptic and anterior medial hypothalamic areas in animals results in enhanced secretion of gastric acid and pepsin, it has been proposed that the neurogenic ulcers found with acute hypothalamic lesions may be a consequence of irritation of the diencephalic parasympathetic center and subsequent vagus nerve activation [106]. Indeed, vagotomy abolishes the occurrence of experimental neurogenic ulcers [7]. However, neurogenic ulcers, which can occur anywhere in the gastrointestinal tract, and gastric hemorrhages from superficial erosive gastritis, are found with a wide variety of central nervous system (CNS) problems including trauma, infections, vascular accidents, multiple sclerosis and intracranial surgery. In addition to vagal activation which may occur at levels other than in the hypothalamus, the lesions may also activate the sympathetic nervous system with enhanced catecholamine secretion, and the hypothalamic–pituitary–adrenal axis with resulting hypercortisolemia. These factors, along with drugs used to treat CNS diseases (e.g., glucocorticoids), may increase the likelihood of nonspecific gastrointestinal tract ulceration.

DISORDERED CONTROL OF ANTERIOR–PITUITARY FUNCTION

Hyperfunction Syndromes

Precocious Puberty

Sexual precocity is considered to be present when secondary sexual development begins below the age of 8 years in girls and 9 years in boys. Isosexual precocious puberty due to CNS mechanisms is called true or complete precocious puberty, while that due to primary gonadal or adrenal abnormalities, or tumors that produce human chorionic gonadotropin (hCG) ectopically is referred to as incomplete precocious puberty. In Bauer's series of patients with pathologically proven hypothalamic lesions, true precocious puberty was noted in 24 of the 60 cases (40%), most often due to neoplasms (60%), especially those located in the posterior hypothalamus at or near the mamillary bodies, or hamartomas in the region of the tuber cinereum (20%) [31,32]. However, Bauer's series overrepresents the true frequency of hypothalamic neoplasms and hamartomas, since 80% of the affected individuals with central precocious puberty are girls, and idiopathic precocious puberty is the diagnosis in close to 70% [106–109]. There is a marked gender difference in the underlying etiologies accounting for central precocious puberty. While the majority of girls have idiopathic early activation of the hypothalamic–pituitary–ovarian axis, idiopathic precocious puberty accounts for only 10% of the cases in boys [107–109]. Approximately half of the boys and only 16% of the girls have hypothalamic hamartomas, while 35% of the boys and 7% of the girls have benign or malignant neoplasms [107]. The spectrum of etiologies responsible for central precocious puberty is shown in Table 9.6.

At the onset of normal puberty the hypothalamus appears to become less sensitive to the inhibitory influences of the gonadal steroids on the arcuate nucleus, which controls the pulsatile release of GnRH. This leads to enhanced secretion of pituitary gonadotropins which in turn leads to enhanced gonadal steroid secretion and the appearance of secondary sexual characteristics. The process continues until adult levels of gonadotropins and sex steroid hormones are achieved. Patients with idiopathic precocious puberty go through the same sequence, and this condition presumably represents a premature activation of the normal gonadotropin regulatory system. The finding that some patients without structural lesions in the central nervous system have a family history of early puberty or even precocious puberty supports this hypothesis. Patients with neoplasms, inflammatory conditions, or conditions associated with increased intracranial pressure also may have premature activation of the normal pubertal maturation process due to the mass, pressure, or irritative effects on the basal hypothalamus. In addition, germinomas may secrete hCG which may directly stimulate the gonads to secrete sex steroid hormones. Premature activation of the normal process is seen in some patients who initially have incomplete precocious puberty due to congenital adrenal hyperplasia or the McCune-Albright polyostotic fibrous dysplasia syndrome in which the hypothalamus is bathed with sex steroid hormone concentrations that are elevated for the patient's chronological age. In susceptible individuals lowering of the sex hormone levels through adrenal or gonadal suppression may be followed by the appearance of central precocious puberty, presumably due to functional hypothalamic alterations from the previously elevated sex steroid hormone levels. The precocious puberty found in patients with hypothalamic hamartomas may be the result of premature activation of the

TABLE 9.6 Causes of Central Precocious Puberty

Idiopathic	**Inflammatory conditions**
Congenital abnormalities	Tuberculosis
Hypothalamic hamartoma	Sarcoidosis
Arachnoid cyst	Meningoencephalitis
Myelomeningocele	
Aqueductal stenosis with hydrocephalus	**Subdural hematoma**
Tuberous sclerosis	**Primary hypothyroidism**
Congenital optic nerve hypoplasia	
Congenital adrenal hyperplasia	
McCune-Albright syndrome	
Neoplasms	
Optic nerve glioma	
Hypothalamic glioma	
Neurofibroma	
Astrocytoma	
Ependymoma	
Infundibuloma	
Medulloblastoma	
Meningoma	
Pinealoma	
Neuroblastoma	
Germinoma	
Craniopharyngioma	

Data compiled from [66,67,107–110].

normal pubertal mechanisms or secondary to direct secretion of GnRH from the hamartoma, since GnRH is present in neurons that comprise the hamartoma [111]. The cause of the precocious puberty in children with primary hypothyroidism and galactorrhea with elevated levels of TSH and prolactin (the Van Wyk-Grumbach syndrome) is unknown, but is probably not due to premature activation of the normal hypothalamic–pituitary–gonadal axis, since treatment of such patients with thyroxine results in cessation of further progression of precocious puberty [112].

Acromegaly

As discussed elsewhere in this book, over 98% of patients with acromegaly have a pituitary adenoma. Rarely, GH itself is secreted ectopically [113,114]. A small number of acromegalics have ectopic production of GHRH from benign or malignant carcinoid or pancreatic islet cell tumors, adrenal adenoma, pheochromocytoma, or lung carcinoma [115]. Acromegaly has also been found in patients with hypothalamic hamartomas, gangliocytomas, gliomas and choristomas which contain and presumably secrete excessive quantities of GHRH [115–120]. Most of these tumors have extended into or been located within the sella turcica in close proximity to the anterior pituitary. Of interest, the predominant anterior pituitary lesion is a pituitary adenoma, and not pituitary hyperplasia [119,120]. Since the hypothalamus is the physiologic source of GHRH, it is reasonable to speculate that GH-producing pituitary adenomas actually represent neoplastic transformation secondary to excessive stimulation of the somatotropes to high concentrations of hypothalamic GHRH. Support for this hypothesis includes the unconfirmed finding of nonsuppressed plasma GHRH concentrations in a series of patients with GH-secreting pituitary adenomas [121]; the paradoxical increase in serum GH following a bolus injection of TRH in acromegalics with typical pituitary adenomas, similar to the response that is found in patients with GHRH-secreting neoplasms [115]; the recurrence of GH hypersecretion and acromegaly following apparently successful transsphenoidal removal of an adenoma, presumably reflecting the development of a second adenoma; and the finding that some patients have a favorable therapeutic response to progestogens or chlorpromazine which probably have a hypothalamic locus of action [122]. The finding that pituitary adenomas are of monoclonal origin is a strong argument against this hypothesis [123].

Cushing's Disease

This refers to the pituitary-dependent form of Cushing's syndrome associated with bilateral adrenal cortical hyperplasia, excessive secretion of ACTH and cortisol, and the presence of a pituitary adenoma. This form must be differentiated from the pituitary-dependent variety that is secondary to excessive ectopic production of CRH, and the pituitary-independent ectopic ACTH syndrome, adrenal neoplasms and bilateral micronodular adrenal hyperplasia. A hypothalamic etiology for Cushing's disease has long been suggested, and the hypersecretion of ACTH may reflect an altered set-point for feedback inhibition at the hypothalamus by circulating glucocorticoids [124]. Patients with Cushing's disease demonstrate a loss of the circadian periodicity of GH, PRI and ACTH, as well as sleep abnormalities that remain following correction at the hypercortisolism [124]. Historically, many patients with Cushing's disease recount a severe emotional stress, such as a death in the family or a separation, that immediately precedes the onset of the disease [125]. In addition, although over 80% of patients with Cushing's disease are found to have a pituitary adenoma at the time of surgery, cortisol hypersecretion may persist after apparently successful removal of the neoplasm or an adenoma may recur after transsphenoidal adenomectomy, despite initial post-operative re-establishment of normal hypothalamic–pituitary–adrenal dynamics [126,127]. A number of the pituitary adenomas have been found to secrete ACTH in vitro in response to CRH [124]. Cyproheptadine, a serotonin antagonist, bromocriptine, a dopamine receptor agonist, and sodium valproate, which increases gamma aminobutyric acid concentrations, lower ACTH and cortisol concentrations and reverse the clinical manifestations in some patients with Cushing's disease, possibly through a hypothalamic rather than direct pituitary action [128–131]. Finally, Cushing's disease has been associated with an intrasellar gangliocytoma which produced CRH, indicating that these neural neoplasms have the capacity to directly stimulate the corticotropes [132]. However, the clonal origin of corticotrope adenomas, the presence of a discrete adenoma rather than hyperplasia at surgery, the high cure rate following transsphenoidal removal of the adenoma and the low concentration of CRH in the CSF of patients with Cushing's disease strongly suggest a somatic mutation is responsible for corticotrope adenoma formation, although hypothalamic factors may be needed for promoting clonal expansion of the abnormal corticotrope cell [124,133,134].

Hyperprolactinemia

Since the lactotropes in the anterior pituitary are normally under tonic inhibition by dopamine synthesized and secreted by the hypothalamus, it is common for hyperprolactinemia to be present in patients with structural abnormalities of the hypothalamus. Amenorrhea and galactorrhea in women, and erectile dysfunction in men, are present to a variable extent. The menstrual abnormalities, libido and potency problems are difficult to assess because of the high frequency of concomitant gonadotropin deficiency. Most patients have serum prolactin concentrations below 70 ng/ml although an occasional patient will have a level up to 150 ng/ml. Hyperprolactinemia was present in 55% of adults with craniopharyngioma [135]. In a series of patients with hypothalamic tumors, Imura and coworkers found hyperprolactinemia in 36% of patients with craniopharyngiomas, in 79% of patients with suprasellar germinomas and in 14% of patients harboring a pineal germinoma [58]. Galactorrhea was less frequently seen, being found in 4, 3 and 0% of patients with the three types of tumor, respectively [58].

Prolactin-secreting microadenomas of the pituitary may be caused by a hypothalamic dopamine deficiency with resultant disinhibition of the lactotropes leading to lactotrope hyperplasia and neoplasia. In support of this hypothesis is the finding of such hyperplasia of the lactotropes in some patients with prolactin-secreting adenomas, and the recurrence of adenomas following successful removal of microadenomas as assessed by a return to normal prolactin dynamics in response to provocative tests [136,137]. However, the monoclonal origin of prolactinomas argues against this hypothesis [136]. A large group of patients with hyperprolactinemia do not have obvious structural abnormalities in the hypothalamus or pituitary microadenomas visualized by computed tomography (CT) or magnetic resonance imaging (MRI) scans. The serum prolactin in response to provocative and inhibitory agents in patients with idiopathic hyperprolactinemia is qualitatively indistinguishable from that in patients with prolactin-secreting microadenomas. Indeed, some patients with idiopathic hyperprolactinemia when followed over time will develop a microadenoma, adding support to the concept that idiopathic hyperprolactinemia and prolactin-secreting pituitary tumors are on a continuum, with hypothalamic dopamine deficiency being the etiology of both conditions.

Hypofunction Syndromes

Acquired Hypogonadotropic Hypogonadism

This condition is commonly found in patients with organic lesions in the hypothalamus. Almost one-third of the patients in Bauer's series had hypogonadism, with 84% of the lesions located in the floor of the third ventricle involving the tuberoinfundibular and more anterior regions of the hypothalamus [31,32]. The etiology is probably multifactorial in most instances. The mechanisms include destruction of GnRH-secreting neurons, disruption of the median eminence where the GnRH peptidergeric axons converge, interference with the "pulse generator" that is responsible for the normal pulsatile release of LH and FSH, damage to the hypothalamohypophyseal portal system and/or hyperprolactinemia.

Patients with neoplasms and inflammatory conditions have a high frequency of neuro-ophthalmologic abnormalities (52%), diabetes insipidus (47%) and obesity (42%) [31,32]. Hypothalamic hypogonadism with prepubertal onset results in a lack of pubertal development. Thus, both sexes will have diminished growth of axillary and pubic hair, unless ACTH deficiency coexists, in which case pubic and axillary hair will be absent because of the lack of adrenal androgens. Males will not develop chin, sideburn, moustache, chest, abdominal, or back terminal hair growth; nor will the voice deepen or muscles develop into the adult pattern. The testicles will remain small and the penis does not enlarge. Females will not experience breast development, uterine enlargement, vaginal cornification and adult mucus production, or menstruation. If GH secretion remains normal, affected individuals may continue to grow and acquire eunuchoidal proportions in which the upper segment (crown to pubis) to lower segment (pubis to floor) ratio is less than 1, and the arm span exceeds total height by 5 cm or more. This occurs because the cartilaginous epiphyseal growth plates of the long bones grow under the influence of GH and do not fuse, as this requires pubertal levels of androgens and estrogens. Acquired hypogonadism developing postpubertally results in amenorrhea, vaginal dryness and some regression of breast glandular tissue in women. Men experience gradual loss of body and pubic hair, decreased muscular development, testicular atrophy, decreased libido and erectile dysfunction. With long-standing hypogonadism, both sexes may develop fine wrinkling around the corners of the eyes and lips and osteopenia. The characteristic hormonal findings are low levels of LH and FSH in association with low concentrations of gonadal steroids. The gonadotropin response to a single bolus injection of GnRH may be normal or low, but characteristically increases if the patient receives multiple priming doses given every 90 minutes. Males have a low seminal plasma volume and oligo- or azoospermia.

Congenital (Idiopathic) Gonadotropin Deficiency

Deficiency of LH may occur alone or together with FSH resulting in hypogonadotropic hypogonadism, and gonadotropin deficiency may be present as part of the multiple tropic hormone deficiencies that are seen in idiopathic panhypopituitarism. The most common form of isolated gonadotropin deficiency is Kallmann's syndrome, also known as olfactory–genital dysplasia. This syndrome, which occurs sporadically or as an X-linked dominant or autosomal dominant trait with incomplete penetrance, is due to a defect in hypothalamic GnRH synthesis or secretion. The X chromosome linked syndrome is due to defects in the *KAL1* gene resulting in altered expression of anosmin, a neural cell adhesion molecule. This leads to failure of the GnRH neurons to migrate to the hypothalamus from the olfactory placode [138]. Males are affected more frequently than females. Cryptorchidism and microphallus may be present at birth owing to the lack of normal fetal testicular testosterone production in late gestation as a result of deficient fetal gonadotropin secretion. Puberty fails to occur at all in the severe, complete form of the syndrome, or may be markedly delayed and incomplete in the partial form [138]. In addition to the gonadal abnormalities, other defects are present. The most common associated problem is hyposmia or anosmia due to agenesis or hypoplasia of the olfactory bulbs. Color blindness, nerve deafness, cleft palate, exostosis and renal abnormalities may also be present. In addition to the prepubertal levels of LH, FSH and sex steroids, these patients exhibit a deficient release of LH or FSH following a bolus injection of GnRH. After several weeks of priming the pituitary gonadotropes with pulsatile boluses of GnRH given at 90-minute intervals, the gonadotropin response to a bolus injection of GnRH approaches normal, indicating that the initial inadequate gonadotrope response represented secondary atrophy of the gonadotrope due to the lack of endogenous GnRH secretion. Full fertility in these patients may be achieved with small doses of GnRH given by infusion pump every 90 minutes [138].

Mutations of fibroblast growth factor-1 receptor gene occurs in 7–10% of patients with autosomal dominant congenital hypogonadotropic hypogonadism and is associated with both anosmia and normosmia. Approximately 5% of patients with idiopathic hypogonadotropic hypogonadism will have a loss-of-function mutation in the GnRH-receptor gene [138]. LH deficiency, with normal levels of FSH, has been termed the "fertile eunuch syndrome" since these patients have hypogonadism with prepubertal levels of testosterone, deficient secondary sexual development and large testes with evidence of spermatogenesis. Unlike the small, prepubertal testes seen in patients with combined gonadotropin deficiency, these patients experience testicular growth because of normal serum concentrations of FSH which stimulate the growth of the seminiferous tubules that normally account for 85% of the adult testicular volume.

Gonadotropin deficiency is also present in patients with mutations in the genes for leptin, the leptin receptor, G-protein-coupled receptor-54, and dosage-sensitive sex-reversal-adrenal hypoplasia congenital critical region on the X chromosome, gene 1, as well as in patients with complex, presumably hypothalamic, syndromes including the Prader-Willi, Laurence-Moon and Bardet-Biedl syndromes [138].

Acquired Hypothalamic GH Deficiency

Growth failure due to structural abnormalities in the hypothalamus is common, and may be multifactorial in origin including deficiency of GH, thyrotropin and gonadotropins, as well as nutritional abnormalities. Growth retardation is present in about one-third of children with craniopharyngiomas [56,98,135], 40% of patients with the chronic disseminated form of histiocytosis [59] and 10–40% of individuals with suprasellar germinomas [56,58]. Formal testing for GH secretory response in patients with hypothalamic disease yields an even higher frequency of abnormalities. For instance, 85–95% of patients with craniopharyngioma have an inadequate rise in serum GH following provocative stimuli [98]. In these patients, the GH deficiency is presumed due to inadequate synthesis, release, or transmission of GHRH to the somatotropes. Indeed, many patients with hypothalamic structural abnormalities demonstrate a rise in serum GH following a bolus injection of GHRH, indicating the presence of functional somatotropes [139].

Congenital GH Deficiency

Congenital absence of GH due to hypothalamic structural or functional abnormalities is seen in several midline developmental abnormalities including anencephaly, holoprosencephaly, transsphenoidal encephalocele, septooptic dysplasia, and some patients with simple cleft lip and palate [140]. In most affected patients GH deficiency coexists with deficiencies of one or more of the other tropic hormones. Studies have suggested that approximately one-third of these patients develop their hormone abnormalities due to a traumatic transection of the pituitary stalk during delivery, while the remainder have a defective induction of the mediobasal brain structures, which results in a failure of the pituitary lobes to fuse and an absence or hypoplasia of the pituitary stalk [140,141].

GH deficiency occurs on a familial basis, either as part of familial panhypopituitarism or as an isolated defect. In panhypopituitarism, GH deficiency is the most common abnormality, followed by gonadotropin, then ACTH and finally TSH deficiency or deficiencies. Both autosomal recessive and X-linked recessive transmission have been described, although most cases appear to be sporadic [140]. Most of these patients exhibit a rise in anterior pituitary hormones following bolus injections of the releasing hormones, but not in response to provocative stimuli that work through the release of endogenous hypothalamic releasing hormones. Congenital GH deficiency is also due to defects in a variety of genes involved in pituicyte differentiation [140]. Monotropic growth hormone deficiency may be found in patients with abnormalities in the GH gene family found on chromosome 17, in which case the pituitary is unable to produce GH or secretes a biologically inactive form. However, the majority of patients with monotropic GH deficiency actually have a hypothalamic etiology, with an absence of appropriate secretion of GHRH. These patients have GH-containing somatotropes in their anterior pituitary, but are unable to secrete adequate quantities because of inadequate stimulation from the hypothalamus. Most are capable of releasing GH following the exogenous administration of GHRH.

Clinically, patients with congenital GH deficiency have normal birth length and weight. Males may exhibit micropenis, especially if gonadotropin deficiency coexists. Growth retardation generally becomes apparent during the latter part of the first year, and both height age and bone age are delayed. Untreated patients develop proportional short stature, an increase in subcutaneous fat, a "pinched facies" with a high forehead, and fine wrinkling of the skin around the corners of the mouth and eyes. Hypoglycemia may occur during infancy, since GH is an insulin antagonist, but later insulin deficiency may develop resulting in abnormal glucose tolerance. Puberty may be delayed even in the absence of gonadotropin deficiency. Exogenous GH replacement therapy stimulates linear growth, restores normal glucose tolerance and allows puberty to progress normally [140].

Hypothalamic Hypoadrenalism

Abnormalities of the hypothalamic–pituitary–adrenal cortex axis, as revealed by blood or urine steroid measurements or provocative tests, are relatively common in patients with congenital or acquired structural disorders of the hypothalamus. Even with normal baseline corticosteroids, abnormalities in the normal circadian variation of these steroids are frequently seen [142]. Over half of patients with craniopharyngiomas, suprasellar germinomas and septo-optic dysplasia demonstrate deficient glucocorticoid levels or ACTH responses to stimuli that function via the hypothalamus [13,57,64–67,98,135,143]. CRH administration to patients with hypothalamic structural abnormalities does result in the release of ACTH from the pituitary. Congenital monotropic ACTH deficiency is rare, and theoretically could result from either an abnormality in CRH production or secretion or a defect in the corticotrope cells in the pituitary [144]. There is at present insufficient information available to localize the locus of abnormality in these patients. A hypothalamic etiology of the ACTH deficiency found in some patients with congenital panhypopituitarism is implied by the finding that these patients can release other "deficient" anterior pituitary hormones with hypothalamic-releasing factors.

The clinical manifestations of tertiary adrenal insufficiency include hypoglycemia in childhood, especially if GH deficiency coexists, and occasionally hypotension. Acute adrenocortical insufficiency rarely occurs spontaneously, but may be precipitated with stresses such as surgery, infections, or trauma. In this situation nausea, vomiting and hypotension may be found. Unlike patients with primary adrenocortical insufficiency, hyperpigmentation and the electrolyte abnormalities that reflect aldosterone deficiency (hyponatremia and hyperkalemia) are not seen.

Hypothalamic Hypothyroidism

Tertiary hypothyroidism is found in one-third to one-half of patients with craniopharyngiomas, suprasellar germinomas and septo-optic dysplasia [56,57,66–67,98,134]. Characteristically these patients have low serum concentrations of free thyroxine; normal, low and occasionally slightly elevated levels of serum TSH (the latter possibly representing a TSH molecule with reduced biologic activity) [145]; and a quantitatively normal or exaggerated, but delayed peak in serum TSH concentrations following a bolus injection of TRH [56,57,66,67]. Normally, the highest concentrations of TSH are found between 15 and 30 minutes after TRH, while in patients with hypothalamic hypothyroidism, peak levels are found between 90 and 120 minutes. Similar delayed responses can be seen in patients with hypothyroidism due to primary pituitary disease [146].

The clinical manifestations of hypothalamic hypothyroidism are similar, but less severe than those found with primary hypothyroidism and include thyroid gland atrophy, lethargy, cold intolerance, dry skin with a pasty, yellow hue, hypothermia, bradycardia, constipation and weight gain.

SPECIFIC HYPOTHALAMIC DISORDERS

A number of syndromes have been described in which affected patients exhibit abnormalities in hypothalamic function, but do not have obvious structural defects in the hypothalamus (Table 9.7). Some, like the Prader-Willi, Bardet-Bidl and Laurence-Moon syndromes, may be congenital with fixed defects, while others, such as anorexia nervosa (discussed above) or the emotional deprivation syndrome, are acquired and reversible.

Prader-Willi Syndrome

In 1956, Prader, Labhart and Willi described a syndrome whose major features were fetal hypotonia, hyperphagia, obesity, short stature, mental retardation

TABLE 9.7 Complex Syndromes of Presumed Hypothalamic Origin or with Hypothalamic Involvement

Syndrome	Major manifestations
Congenital Prader-Willi	Hypotonia
	Hyperphagia
	Obesity
	Short stature
	Mental retardation
	Hypogonadism
Bardet-Biedl	Pigmentary retinopathy
	Obesity
	Mental retardation
	Polydactyly
	Hypogonadism
Wolfram	Central diabetes insipidus
	Insulin-dependent diabetes mellitus
	Optic atrophy
	Sensorineural deafness
Hayek-Peake	Adipsia or hypodipsia
	Recurrent hypernatremia
	Obesity
	Hyperprolactinemia
	Hypothyroidism
	Hypertriglyceridemia
	Central hypoventilation
Septooptic-pituitary dysplasia	Absent septum pellucidum
	Optic nerve hypoplasia
	Agenesis of corpus callosum
	Visual defects
	Mental retardation
	Short stature
	Hypothalamic hypopituitarism
Acquired Anorexia nervosa	Anorexia
	Weight loss
	Behavioral abnormalities
	Bradycardia
	Hypogonadism
	Thermal dysregulation
	Partial diabetes insipidus
	Hyperprolactinemia
Environmental deprivation	Short stature
	Polydipsia
	Polyphagia
	Bizarre behavior
	Emotional/mental retardation
Pseudocyesis	Amenorrhea
	Symptoms of pregnancy
	Abdominal distension
	Hyperprolactinemia
	Persistent corpus luteum

and hypogonadism [147]. The prevalence of the syndrome has been estimated to be approximately 1 per 10–16,000 live births [148,149]. The major clinical features derived from several series of studied patients are tabulated in Table 9.8. The clinical manifestations begin before birth with reduced fetal movement, an increased incidence of breech presentation and prematurity, and low birth weight. Profound muscle hypotonia may be present at birth resulting in a poor sucking response, often necessitating gavage feeding. The affected infants may exhibit multiple somatic anomalies including a narrow bitemporal diameter of the cranium, strabismus, hypertelorism, almond-shaped eyes, upslanting palpebral fissure, low-set ears, micrognathism, an ogival palate, clinodactyly, and small hands and feet [148–151]. During late infancy or early childhood, hyperphagia develops, with often indiscriminate food-seeking behavior, resulting in obesity, which reaches morbid proportions in many individuals. These patients also have short stature, which during childhood and adolescence is associated with a delayed bone age. In the series of patients studied by Bray and associates, the mean height was 149 cm and the mean weight 114 kg [148]. Mental and developmental retardation is almost always present, and personality problems, such as stubbornness, temper tantrums and inadequate peer interactions have been noted in over two-thirds of such individuals [148–151]. Hypogonadism is a prominent feature, especially in males. Cryptorchidism and scrotal hypoplasia are generally present at birth, undoubtedly due to inadequate fetal testicular androgen production; the penis is small and the testes immature [148]. Labial hypoplasia has been noted in affected females [149]. There is a variable degree of sexual maturation that occurs during adolescence or adulthood, and even precocious puberty has been noted in a few patients [148–151].

Endocrine studies have demonstrated normal thyroid function tests, including normal responses to TRH, normal ACTH and cortisol dynamics in response to provocative stimuli, and normal prolactin concentrations [148,150]. GH responses to various secretagogues have been blunted, but resemble the response seen in patients with simple obesity, although unlike obesity, IGF-I levels are reduced [150]. Although early reports suggested that type II diabetes mellitus was frequently present in these patients, more recent studies have shown that the glucose intolerance and insulin resistance are similar to that found in weight-matched subjects with simple obesity [148,150]. The hypogonadism is associated with low testosterone in males and low estradiol in females, and low basal serum LH and FSH concentrations [148,150]. GnRH tests are abnormal in most of the patients, with a marked blunting of the

TABLE 9.8 Clinical Features of 163 Patients with Prader-Willi Syndrome

Criteria	Abnormality	Percentage Affected
Major	Neonatal hypotonia	93
	Feeding problems in infancy	87
	Excessive weight gain	82
	Typical facial features	88
	HypogonadismHHy	70
	Developmental delay	98
	Hyperphagia	91
Minor	Decreased fetal activity	71
	Behavior problems	78
	Sleep disturbances	76
	Short stature	76
	Hypopigmentation	73
	Small hands and/or feet	89
	Eye abnormalities	66
	Thick saliva	89
	Articulation defects	80
	Skin-picking	83
	Cryptorchidism	85
	Delayed bone age	66

Adapted from [148,149].

gonadotropin response, reflecting a longstanding GnRH deficiency. Indeed, chronic treatment with GnRH will increase the LH and FSH response to a bolus injection of GnRH. Treatment of patients with clomiphene citrate, a competitive inhibitor of estradiol, has been found to increase basal LH, FSH and sex steroid hormones, and to restore the gonadotropin response to GnRH to normal [148]. Collectively, these results indicate that the hypogonadotropism is hypothalamic in origin. There is little information available about nonendocrine hypothalamic function. Some patients have been noted to have abnormalities in temperature control and heat generation, also pointing to a hypothalamic abnormality [148].

Most patients with Prader-Willi syndrome develop it sporadically, although a few familial cases have been reported [152]. The syndrome is due to an abnormality in genomic imprinting. Most affected patients have a deletion of the paternally contributed chromosome 15q11-q13, which is normally the active gene at this site [151]. The few autopsy studies that have been carried out have failed to demonstrate any histopathologic abnormalities in the hypothalamus [148].

TABLE 9.9 Clinical Features of Bardet-Biedl Syndrome

	Percentage Affected	
Abnormality	Men (n = 188)	Women (n = 133)
Pigmentary retinopathy and other ocular manifestations	93.6	92.5
Obesity	89.4	94.7
Developmental delay	86.7	85.0
Polydactyly	76.1	73.7
Hypogonadism	76.1	51.9

Adapted from Klein and Ammann [153].

Bardet-Biedl Syndrome

The cardinal features of this syndrome are tapetoretinal degeneration, obesity, mental retardation, polydactyly and hypogonadotropic hypogonadism (Table 9.9). In over two-thirds of the patients, an extra digit is found in one or more of the extremities (hexadactyly), while other digital abnormalities such as syndactyly and/or brachydactyly are seen in 10–15% of individuals [153]. The retinopathy, which in the early stages may not be pigmentary, begins in early childhood and is associated with night blindness, decreased visual acuity and an abnormal electroretinogram response. By age 20, almost three-fourths of the patients are blind or near blind, and this figure rises to 86% by age 30 [153]. Obesity and associated glucose intolerance begin in early childhood. Variable degrees of mental retardation are present, with 36% being classified as mild, 12% moderate and 9% severe [153]. In addition, a variety of behavioral abnormalities have been noted including emotional lability and short attention span. The hypogonadism affects males more frequently than females (see Table 9.9). Other associated abnormalities noted include nerve deafness (9%), renal abnormalities (glomerulosclerosis, mesangial proliferation, renal cysts; 13%), brachycephaly (50%), and rarely diabetes insipidus and hyperlipidemia [153,154].

The disorder is transmitted in an autosomal recessive fashion, with a prevalence of 1 per 160,000 births [153]. Although the hypothalamic hypogonadism, obesity and occasional coexistence of central diabetes insipidus strongly suggest hypothalamic involvement, the few pathologic studies performed to date have not demonstrated a histopathologic abnormality in the hypothalamus [155]. The pathogenesis of the presumed hypothalamic dysfunction may involve a transient internal hydrocephalus during the eighth to ninth embryonic weeks, resulting in an enlargement of the third ventricle causing a diencephalic lesion [153]. Linkage studies and positional cloning techniques have identified a group of genes involved with cilium, and it has been proposed that Bardet-Biedl syndrome is due to defects in the immotile sensory cilia function [154].

Several other syndromes that resemble Bardet-Biedl syndrome have been described. The Laurence-Moon syndrome includes retinal pigmentary degeneration, mental retardation, hypogonadism, progressive spastic paraparesis and distal muscle weakness, but no polydactyly [156]. The Biemond syndrome, also inherited as an autosomal recessive condition, consists of hypogonadotropic hypogonadism, mental retardation, polydactyly or brachydactyly, obesity, and iris coloboma, rather than retinitis pigmentosa [153,157]. The Alstrom-Hallgren syndrome, transmitted as an autosomal recessive defect, is associated with atypical tapetoretinal degeneration, obesity, diabetes mellitus, nerve deafness, acanthosis nigricans and hypogonadism. In contrast to Bardet-Biedl syndrome, the hypogonadism is due to primary gonadal failure, rather than to hypothalamic dysfunction [153,157]. At least three other syndromes with overlapping features with the above disorders have been described by other authors [157]. It is likely that they represent heterogeneous expression of the same or a closely related genetic abnormality.

Septo-optic–Pituitary Dysplasia

The cardinal features of the septo-optic–pituitary dysplasia syndrome (De Morsier syndrome) are anterior midline prosencephalic developmental defects including an absent septum pellucidum and/or agenesis of the corpus callosum, bilateral or unilateral optic nerve hypoplasia, and hypothalamic hypopituitarism (Table 9.10) [64–67,158–160]. In addition to the above anatomic defects, other defects and dysmorphic features may be present. These include cleft palate, syndactyly, low-set ears, misshapen pinnae, hypertelorism, mongoloid slants of the palpebral fissures, micropenis and agenesis of the olfactory nerves. The optic nerve atrophy is manifest by a small optic disc, one-third to one-half the normal size, and variable degrees of visual impairment [64–67,160].

The syndrome occurs sporadically, with an estimated incidence of 1 in 10,000 live births [161]. The etiology is unknown and is probably multifactorial, although rare cases have been described in patients with mutations of the homeobox gene, *HESX1* [159,161]. The affected individuals are usually the first-born of a young woman whose pregnancy may have been complicated by toxemia [66]. Birth weight is normal, but the infants demonstrate poor feeding, vomiting, prolonged neonatal hyperbilirubinemia and hypoglycemia. Cerebral palsy with hemiplegia, diplegia, or quadriplegia is relatively common, as are developmental delay and seizures [66].

The most common endocrine abnormality is short stature associated with GH deficiency. Clinically this is followed by ACTH deficiency, diabetes insipidus, and hypothyroidism, although abnormalities in the hypothalamic–pituitary–thyroid axis can be demonstrated in over 60% of patients by TRH testing [64–67,158,159]. The relatively low frequency of hypogonadism reported in these patients undoubtedly reflects the fact that the mean age of diagnosis

TABLE 9.10 Clinical, Anatomic and Biochemical Features of Septo-optic–Pituitary Dysplasia

Feature	Number Abnormal/ Number Studied	Percentage Abnormal
ANATOMIC		
Hypoplastic optic nerves	230/230	100
Absent septum pellucidum	99/162	61
Agenesis of corpus callosum	9/117	8
CLINICAL: NONENDOCRINE		
Visual problems	112/195	52
Developmental delay	92/206	45
Cerebral palsy	42/151	28
Nystagmus	101/230	44
Seizures	22/59	37
Neonatal jaundice	10/44	23
Neonatal hypoglycemia	19/115	16
CLINICAL: ENDOCRINE		
Short stature	41/61	67
Decreased growth rate	41/67	61
Diabetes insipidus	43/193	22
Precocious puberty	7/106	7
ENDOCRINE TESTING		
Human growth hormone deficiency	140/189	74
Adrenocorticotropic hormone deficiency	69/183	38
Thyroid stimulating hormone deficiency	45/187	24
Abnormal thyrotropin-releasing hormone test	11/18	61.1
Gonadotropin deficiency	7/74	9
Hyperprolactinemia	7/32	22
Multiple hormone deficiencies	75/174	43

Compiled from [64–67,158-160].

of the disorder is 4.9 years [64–67], which is too young to detect hypogonadotropic hypogonadism. However, some children have been noted to have micropenis, which may be a reflection of prenatal fetal hypogonadotropism [65,158]. Examination of the hypothalamus at autopsy has demonstrated absence of the supraoptic and paraventricular nuclei, hypoplasia of the posterior pituitary, ependymal scars around the third ventricle and a normal anterior pituitary, supporting the hypothalamic locus of the hypopituitarism [162].

Environmental Deprivation Syndrome (Psychosocial Short Stature)

Children presenting with this unusual, reversible syndrome have a constellation of signs and symptoms that suggest hypothalamic dysfunction. These include short stature, polydipsia, polyphagia, emotional or mental retardation, and bizarre behavior (Table 9.11) [163,164]. The majority of children have onset of the syndrome before the age of 2, and over half have a social history of divorced or separated parents, or significant marital strife at home resulting in a disturbed parent–child relationship. Males are more frequently affected than females. Short stature is generally the presenting complaint and is associated with a retarded bone age and inadequate GH response to insulin hypoglycemia. The upper-to-lower body size ratio is normal for age, as is tooth eruption. Body weight is low for the chronological age and in most instances for the height age. Polydipsia and polyphagia are uniformly present. Indeed, these children have been noted to eat two to three times the amount of food compared to their siblings. Bulky, foul-smelling stools have been noted in many of the subjects, which together with the polyphagia, low weight and short stature, often leads to an evaluation for malabsorption, which is not present in these children. Bizarre behavior is a common concomitant of the syndrome. The patients often steal food and hide it around their houses, and most have been discovered to have eaten food retrieved from garbage cans. They also drink water from toilet bowls and stagnant pools, and tend to wander at night in search of food or water. Emotional retardation is clearly present manifest by shyness and a tendency to play alone, temper tantrums, delayed toilet training and retarded speech [163–165].

Endocrine testing reveals normal urine concentrating ability, normal thyroid function in most patients, inadequate adrenocortical response to provocative testing, along with the poor GH responses to stimuli. Thus, these patients appear to have a form of idiopathic hypopituitarism. However, when they are removed from their home environment, their polydipsia, polyphagia and food-stealing rapidly cease. They gain weight, and some even become obese. In addition, they exhibit rapid linear growth, showing a "catch-up" growth phenomenon, and return of the GH abnormalities to normal [165]. If they are once again placed in their home environment, growth rapidly ceases. The pathogenesis of this complex syndrome is unclear, but it is likely that it represents a psychophysiologic reaction to the adverse environment.

TABLE 9.11 Clinical Features of 13 Patients with Environmental Deprivation Syndrome

Feature	Percentage
Short stature	100
Retarded bone age	77
Low weight for height	85
Abnormal human growth hormone dynamics	75*
Polydipsia	100
Polyphagia	100
Gorging and vomiting	69
Foul-smelling stools	62
Bizarre behavior	100
Food-stealing	92
Eating from garbage cans	85
Nocturnal wandering	54
Drinking from toilet bowl	46
Emotional/mental retardation	100
Low IQ	100†
Retarded speech	85
Playing alone	69
Shy	69
Temper tantrums	69
Protuberant abdomen	100
Depressed (infantile) nasal bridge	100

** Based on eight patients.*
†Based on IQ testing of eight children "who were easily distracted during the test period."
From Powell et al. [163,164].

Pseudocyesis

Pseudocyesis or false pregnancy represents a hysterical conversion reaction in a woman who either desperately wishes to conceive, or is extremely fearful of becoming pregnant. The woman develops amenorrhea, progressive abdominal distension, morning sickness, sensations of fetal activity, breast engorgement with a prominent venous pattern, and, at times, galactorrhea [166–169]. Hyperprolactinemia is present in the majority of women, and may be of pathophysiologic significance, in that its luteotropic activity may be the cause of the persistent corpus luteum found in these individuals. In addition, LH levels may be elevated which may also account for maintenance of the corpus luteum [166]. When confronted with the diagnosis, some women experience a rapid decrease in abdominal girth, which was due to gaseous distension of the intestine, cessation of galactorrhea and resumption of menses. This syndrome, along with anorexia nervosa and the environmental deprivation syndrome, illustrate the profound influence that the cerebral cortex has on the hypothalamus.

Hypothalamic Hamartoma

Hamartomas are benign heterotrophic hyperplastic malformations composed of a fibrous glial matrix with mature ganglion cells and occasional myelinated nerve fibers [111,170]. They range in size between a few millimeters and 3.5 cm, with the majority being less than 1.5 cm, and usually are located in the posterior hypothalamus between the tuber cinereum and the mamillary bodies [111,170]. They are felt to represent a midline dysraphic syndrome with displacement of cells from the mamillary region as the infundibulum moves behind the notochord [170].

As indicated in Table 9.12 [171–177], a little more than half of the affected individuals are males, and most patients present before the age of 4 years [171–178]. Close to 90% of the patients develop precocious puberty with pubertal or adult concentrations of sex steroid hormones and gonadotropins [111,172,175]. Over half have neurodevelopmental delay with low intelligence quotient and seizures. Often the seizures are gelastic or laughing seizures with brief lapses without loss of consciousness [111,171–173,178]. Emotional lability and sham rage may also be present. Gross neurologic abnormalities are usually absent, although large hamartomas may be associated with ataxia and nystagmus due to pontine compression [179]. There is also a tendency for the patients to become obese in late childhood and adolescence [179].

Three hypotheses have been proposed to explain the precocious puberty in these patients. First, the hamartoma may mechanically stimulate the median eminence to secrete GnRH. Support for this explanation is the finding that some hamartomas associated with precocious puberty are devoid of nerve cell bodies, and that precocious puberty is also found in some patients with suprasellar arachnoid cysts and craniopharyngiomas located in the same region, suggesting that pressure on the median eminence is of etiologic significance. Alternatively, these lesions may interrupt interneuronal pathways that tonically inhibit the GnRH-secreting neurons in the median eminence, allowing these neurons to be disinhibited and begin secreting GnRH [111,170].

TABLE 9.12 Clinical Features of Patients with Hypothalamic Hamartomas

Feature	Number Abnormal/ Number Studied	Percentage
SEX		
Male	56/105	53
Female	49/105	47
AGE OF ONSET		
Birth	10/76	13
<2 years (including at birth)	47/76	62
2–4 years	17/105	22
5–8 years	5/76	6
AGE AT DIAGNOSIS		
<2 years	26/58	45
2–4 years	20/58	34
5–8 years	8/58	14
ASSESSMENT OF SEXUAL PRECOCITY		
Precocious puberty present	46/57	81
Tanner stage 3 or more (males)	17/21	81
Tanner stage 3 or more (females)	9/9	100
Menses	7/9	78
Bone age > chronological age by 3 + years	23/27	85
Height age > chronological age by 3 + years	14/29	48
DEVELOPMENT AND NEUROLOGIC ASSESSMENT		
Neurodevelopmental delay	24/4026/47	55
Seizures	44/81	54
Hyperactivity/tremors/ laughing spells	31/81	38
Signs of increased intracranial pressure	5/24	20.8

Data are combined from [171–178].

The finding that an occasional patient with precocious puberty may actually have a hamartoma that is not attached to the hypothalamus, argues against precocious puberty being the direct result of hypothalamic pressure [119,180]. The third suggestion is that the hamartoma acts as an "accessory hypothalamus" directly secreting GnRH, which in turn stimulates the gonadotropes to secrete gonadotropins [111,173]. Indeed, several of these hamartomas have been found to contain GnRH, and cerebrospinal fluid GnRH concentrations in patients with hypothalamic hamartoma-associated precocious puberty have been found to be elevated [173,181].

That GnRH is involved in the pathogenesis of the precocious puberty is evidenced by the pubertal or adult gonadotropin response to a bolus injection of GnRH [175,182], and the response to the therapeutic administration of long-acting analogues of GnRH, which act directly on the gonadotropes to down-regulate the GnRH receptors. This results in a lowering of basal levels of sex steroid hormones and gonadotropins, inhibition of the gonadotropin response to a bolus injection of GnRH, a cessation of menses, and a deceleration of the advancing bone age and growth rate [109,175]. Indeed, treatment of the precocious puberty with GnRH analogues is the therapy of choice for this disorder, since in most instances, the hamartoma does not appear to progress, and attempts at total neurosurgical removal in the past have been associated with high operative or postoperative mortalities and neurologic disabilities [173,183]. Although more recent data suggest that 60% of the patients undergoing gamma-knife surgery have some degree of improvement [183], surgery should be restricted to those patients who have signs of increased intracranial pressure or neurologic deterioration from progressive growth of the hamartoma.

The Pallister-Hall syndrome is a complex autosomal dominant disorder associated with a frameshift mutation of the GLI-Kruppel family member 3 gene located on chromosome 7p13 [184]. It includes hypothalamic hamartoma, which often occupies the space between the optic chiasm and interpeduncular fossa, and pituitary dysplasia with hypopituitarism [185–188]. The hypopituitarism is manifest by micropenis and cryptorchidism in affected males and the presence of hypoadrenalism. Associated craniofacial malformations include large fontanelles, a shortened midface, short nose with long philtrum, posteriorly rotated ears, cleft uvula and palate, microglossia, cleft larynx, hypoplasia of the epiglottis and occasional natal teeth or buccal frenula. Limb abnormalities such as postaxial polydactyly, syndactyly, nail dysplasia, clinodactyly of the fifth fingers, shortened fourth metacarpals and/or metatarsals, and pes cavus are commonly found. Other anomalies noted with this syndrome are congenital heart disease, hypoplastic renal dysplasia, abnormal lung segmentation and imperforate anus. The genetic basis of this disorder is unknown, but it is linked to 7p13 [184].

Germ Cell Tumors

Germ cell tumors are broadly classified into germinomas (seminomas; 65% of intracranial germ cell neoplasms) and nongerminomatous germ cell tumors. The latter group includes teratomas, embryonal carcinomas, endodermal sinus tumors and choriocarcinomas, which account for 18, 5, 7 and 5%, respectively, of the germ cell tumors [58]. The incidence of these neoplasms in Western countries is between 0.4 and 3.4% of primary intracranial neoplasms, while the incidence in the Far East is several-fold higher [58,189]. Germinomas and nongerminomatous germ cell tumors differ with regard to their age of onset, sex ratio, site of primary neoplasm and prognosis. The peak age of diagnosis is 10–12 years, with patients with nongerminomatous tumors generally presenting earlier than individuals with germinomas. The male/female sex ratio is 1.88:1 for patients with germinoma, and 3.25:1 for those with nongerminomatous germ cell tumor [58]. Ninety-five percent of patients with intracranial germ cell neoplasms have the primary lesion located in the region of the third ventricle, between the suprasellar cistern and the pineal gland, with the majority of the germinomas being found in the suprasellar region and most of the nongerminomatous tumors located in the pineal area [58].

The cardinal clinical features of suprasellar germ cell tumors are listed in Table 9.13 [56,57,189–193]. The triad of diabetes insipidus, visual field abnormalities, and clinical and/or biochemical evidence of anterior pituitary hormone deficiency is present in many patients, reflecting the anatomic involvement of the optic chiasm, median eminence and region of the third ventricle. Some patients with occult intracranial germinomas present with diabetes insipidus and pituitary stalk thickening [194]. Other manifestations of hypothalamic dysfunction include abnormalities in appetite control with both emaciation and obesity being found, and the adipsia/hypernatremia syndrome characterized by severe proximal muscle weakness: polyuria, adipsia or hypodipsia, hypernatremia and hypertriglyceridemia [56,190]. In an exhaustive review of a large number of patients with germ cell tumors, Jennings and colleagues noted that patients with germinomas, most of whom had primary lesions in the suprasellar region, exhibited a variety of neurologic abnormalities including hydrocephalus (21%), obtundation (15%), Parinaud's sign (paralysis of the upward gaze, 14%), pyramidal tract signs (11%), ataxia (9%), diplopia (10%), seizures (3%), choreoathetosis (2%), dementia (2%) and psychosis (1%) [58]. In contrast, patients with nongerminomatous germ cell tumors, usually involving the pineal gland, tended to demonstrate more neurologic abnormalities due to obstruction of the third ventricle and aqueduct of Sylvius and less endocrine disturbances [195]. Thus, 47% had hydrocephalus, 34% Parinaud's sign, 26% obtundation, 21% pyramidal tract signs, 19% ataxia, 18% diabetes insipidus, and only 19% had evidence of hypothalamic–anterior pituitary failure [58]. Of interest, approximately 5% of patients with intracranial germ cell tumors develop precocious puberty [56–58,190,191].

TABLE 9.13 Clinical Features and Pituitary Function Evaluation in Patients with Suprasellar Germ Cell Tumors

Feature	Number Abnormal/ Number Studied	Percentage
Diabetes insipidus	104/112	93
Clinical hypopituitarism	34/43	79
Chiasmal visual field defect	48/81	59
Headache	13/28	46
Emaciation	17/50	34
Growth failure	24/81	30
Adipsia/hypenatremia	9/42	21
Delayed or regression of sexual development	6/44	14
Nausea/vomiting	4/28	14
Obesity	7/60	12
Precocious puberty	2/41	5
Hormonal evaluation	40/41	98
Abnormal growth hormone dynamics		
Abnormal response to gonadotropin-releasing hormone	30/34	88
Hyperprolactinemia	47/62	76
Abnormal adrenocorticotropic hormone dynamics	20/30	67
Low thyroxine or abnormal thyrotropin-releasing hormone response	34/42	81

Data are restricted to tumors involving the suprasellar region and do not include germ cell tumors of the pineal.
Data are compiled from [56,57,189–193].

This may occur as a pressure effect of the neoplasm on the median eminence, or, alternatively, as a result of the production of hCG by the neoplasm [196]. Choriocarcinomas or the syncytiotrophoblastic giant cells present in the other types of germ cell neoplasms secrete hCG, which directly stimulates the Leydig cells of the testes to produce androgens, resulting in sexual precocity. The testes of affected individuals show Leydig cell hyperplasia with no spermatogenesis since FSH levels are suppressed [196]. Precocious puberty is extremely rare in girls with germ cell tumors, probably because of the requirement of FSH for ovarian estradiol production [197].

Intracranial germ cell neoplasms spread by direct invasion of the hypothalamus or through seeding into the ventricles or subarachnoid pathways [58]. Poor prognostic features include neoplastic involvement of the hypothalamus, third ventricle, or spinal cord, and histologic tumor type, with germinomas having the best prognosis, choriocarcinomas the worst, and the other varieties falling in between [58,198].

The mainstay of therapy for these neoplasms has been radiation therapy, with the best results being seen in patients with germinomas who receive 4000–6000 rads to the tumor. Extirpative surgery and chemotherapy are generally reserved for patients with aggressive, radioresistant tumors [58,198].

Optic Chiasm and Hypothalamic Gliomas

Gliomas of the optic pathways tend to be low-grade pilocytic astrocytomas, occurring primarily in children, with close to 40% being found in those under 2 years of age and 80% under 10 [68,69,199–203]. These tumors account for 4–6% of brain tumors in children and adolescents [204]. Approximately one-fourth of optic pathway gliomas are intraorbital, while three-fourths arise in the optic chiasm, optic tract, or hypothalamus. Tumors of the chiasm and hypothalamus are grouped together because they tend to infiltrate and involve both structures, and it is often impossible to differentiate between tumors originating in one structure or the other. Von Recklinghausen's neurofibromatosis (Type 1) is a major predisposing factor for the development of these tumors and is present in 20–25% of patients with gliomas of the optic pathways [69,200].

Intraorbital optic nerve gliomas rarely involve the hypothalamus or pituitary. The major clinical manifestations are unilateral visual loss, proptosis of the ipsilateral eye, papilledema, strabismus and nystagmus [69,176,205,206]. In contrast, optic chiasm/hypothalamic gliomas are associated with endocrine disturbances, visual field abnormalities, diabetes insipidus, hydrocephalus and the diencephalic syndrome of infancy, in addition to decreased visual acuity, optic atrophy and papilledema (Table 9.14) [68,69,199–202].

Therapy of these tumors has been controversial. Some authorities have argued that these tumors are indolent and behave more like hamartomatous lesions than neoplasms, and, therefore, do not require therapy unless they continue to grow and cause neurologic dysfunction [205]. Others have advocated radiation therapy, citing improvement or stabilization of the visual abnormalities and inhibition of tumor growth, or a delayed time to recurrence [68,199,202,206]. From a prognostic standpoint, patients with intraorbital gliomas have a considerably better prognosis than do patients with chiasmatic/hypothalamic gliomas. In one long-term study, 85% of patients with optic nerve gliomas survived 17 years, while only 44% of patients with chiasmatic/hypothalamic lesions lived 19 years [200]. There is also evidence that optic pathway gliomas in patients with neurofibromatosis

TABLE 9.14 Clinical Features of Patients with Optic Chiasm/ Hypothalamic Glioma

Feature	Number Abnormal/ Number Studied	Percentage
Sex		
Male	95/164	58
Female	69/164	42
Age of onset <2 years of age	28/73	38
Associated neurofibromatosis	20/112	18
Decreased visual acuity	83/125	66
Optic atrophy	54/101	54
Anterior pituitary dysfunction	23/48	48
Growth retardation	7/32	22
Precocious puberty	11/76	14
Delayed puberty	8/56	14
Hypothyroidism	2/33	6
Panhypopituitarism	2/33	6
Hypothalamic involvement	23/68	34
Papilledema/increased intracranial pressure	23/69	33
Hydrocephalus	29/92	32
Visual field abnormalities	24/80	30
Microcephaly	5/24	21
Diencephalic syndrome	11/53	21
Headache	23/116	20
Ataxia/hemiparesis	9/57	16
Nausea/vomiting	5/33	15
Diabetes insipidus	9/61	15
Seizures	4/52	8
Exophthalmos	4/68	6
Behavioral abnormalities	1/24	4

Data are compiled from [68,69,199–202].

behave in a more benign fashion than do gliomas in patients without neurofibromatosis [200,205].

Craniopharyngioma

Craniopharyngiomas are benign neoplasms derived from cell rests of Rathke's pouch origin, that often behave in a malignant fashion due to local growth and infiltration of surrounding tissue [98]. They account for approximately 2.5% of brain tumors and 5–10% of brain neoplasms in children [98,207]. The male/female sex ratio is 1.2–1.4:1 [208,209]. Almost half the patients present before the age of 20, with the median age of 22 years [98,209]. Most of the tumors are cystic or partially cystic, while 15% are solid [98]. The clinical presentation and prognosis depend upon the age of the patient, the location of the neoplasm and its size [98,208].

Children generally present with signs and symptoms of increased intracranial pressure including headache (often occurring intermittently in the morning), vomiting (occasionally in a projectile fashion), papilledema (31%) and hydrocephalus [98,203,207,210]. Decreased visual acuity and visual field abnormalities are also common. Short stature due to GH deficiency is the most prevalent hormonal abnormality, being found in close to 43% of the children, with diabetes insipidus being the second most common clinical endocrinologic disorder (22%) although endocrine abnormalities are the presenting complaint in less than 15% of the patients [211]. Abnormalities of the sleep–wake cycle and excessive somnolence occur more frequently in children than in adults [98,208,209,212]. In contrast, visual abnormalities, especially a progressive diminution of vision and an asymmetric bitemporal hemianopsia, are the most common presenting symptoms in adults [98,209,212]. Other prominent symptoms in this group are headache, deterioration of cognitive abilities, personality change, vomiting, weight gain and hypogonadism [98,209,212]. In addition to the signs and symptoms of raised intracranial pressure, visual abnormalities, hypothalamic dysfunction and deficiencies of the anterior pituitary tropic hormones, a variety of additional neurologic findings may be present in both children and adults. Lateral extension of the neoplasm into the cavernous sinus may damage cranial nerves III, IV and VI, which results in diplopia and abnormalities of the extraocular muscles, and a portion of cranial nerve V, which leads to facial pain. Temporal lobe involvement is associated with temporal lobe seizures, while posterior extension to the midbrain may give rise to cerebellar ataxia and pyramidal tract findings [98,203,209]. The clinical and biochemical features of craniopharyngiomas derived from several series of patients are summarized in Table 9.15 [56,98,140,143,207–210].

Children with craniopharyngiomas differ from adults in several other respects. They are more likely to have an enlarged sella turcica on skull roentgenography (64% vs. 27%) [209], calcification of the tumor on skull X-ray (76% vs. 21%) [209], larger tumors (91% $\geq$ 3 cm in children vs. 60% in adults) [208] and a better prognosis [208].

The therapy of these neoplasms has been a matter of controversy for decades. In the past, radical excision carried unacceptably high mortality and morbidity rates [207,209]. However, recent studies using modern microsurgical techniques, including approaching the tumors through the transsphenoidal route, have claimed

TABLE 9.15 Clinical and Biochemical Features of Patients with Craniopharyngioma

Feature	Number Abnormal/ Number Studied	Percentage
Anterior pituitary dysfunction	269/296	91
Gonadotropin deficiency*	218/304	72
Clinical hypogonadism	182/506	36
Growth hormone deficiency*	189/268	70
Short stature/delayed bone age	418/1294	32
Adrenocorticotropic hormone deficiency*	185/480	38
Thyroid-stimulating hormone deficiency	169/522	32
Multiple hormone deficiency	246/296	83
Hyperprolactinemia*	224/567	40
Galactorrhea	12/296	4
Precocious puberty	21/363	6
Decreased visual acuity/visual field defect	945/1390	68
Headache	836/1200	70
Obesity	228/685	33
Vomiting	312/922	34
Mental deterioration	221/866	26
Diabetes insipidus	316/1439	22
Papilledema	197/826	24
Hydrocephalus	16/102	15.7
Somnolence	69/383	18
Ataxia	48/280	17
Pyramidal tract signs	4/67	6
Cranial nerve palsy	29/379	8

** Results from biochemical testing.*
Data are compiled from [56,98,140,143,207–210].

excellent results although there remains a 25% recurrence rate [207,210,212,213]. The most conservative approach balancing the associated risks with radical, total resection, and the need for local control of tumor growth is to partially resect the tumor and deliver 5000–6000 rads of postoperative radiation to the residual neoplasm [208,214]. This carries a 21% recurrence rate [210]. Following surgery, one-half or more of the patients develop hyperphagia, obesity, hyperinsulinemia and normal growth despite growth hormone deficiency, possibly reflecting damage to the ventromedial hypothalamus [98,215].

Suprasellar Meningiomas

Meningiomas arising from the tuberculum sellae, diaphragma sellae and planum sphenoidale may encroach upon, but not invade, the hypothalamus. These benign neoplasms have a male/female sex ratio of 1:2–3, and become symptomatic in adults. The peak incidence is between the ages of 40–55 years [216,217]. Over 80% of the patients present with a complaint of slow loss of vision in one eye, and over 90% have objective evidence of diminished visual acuity. Other neuro-ophthalmologic signs and symptoms include poor color perception, an afferent pupillary light defect, abnormal visual fields (80%), pallor of the optic discs (83%), the Foster-Kennedy syndrome (7.2%) and abnormal extraocular movements (3.6%) [216]. Headache is also common, being found in 35–55% of the patients. It generally is of poor localizing value, although some patients will have ipsilateral orbital pain. Deterioration of cognitive function, confusion and memory loss may be found in approximately 20% of patients [204]. Endocrine abnormalities have been found in 22% of patients, most commonly hypogonadism (13%), hypothyroidism (14%) and diabetes insipidus (4.8%). Close to 40% of the patients are obese [216].

These tumors contain estrogen receptors and may increase in size during pregnancy or even during the menstrual cycle [218]. The latter feature may account for some of the fluctuation in the signs and symptoms noted in patients with these tumors. Surgical resection is the treatment of choice for these lesions, and results in improved vision in about 50–60% of patients, and stabilization of the visual defect in an additional 30–40% [216,217].

Suprasellar Arachnoid Cyst

Developmental defects in the arachnoid membrane in the suprasellar region may allow for the development of a large, fluid-filled closed cyst that causes symptoms through a mass effect. The majority (70%) of patients with this congenital anomaly present before 5 years of age [219,220]. The major findings are related to hydrocephalus with increased intracranial pressure from obstruction to cerebrospinal fluid flow through the foramen of Monro (Table 9.16 [219,221]). Symptoms and signs related to compression of the brain stem, thalamus and the optic tracts are also common. GH and ACTH deficiency, and precocious puberty are the primary endocrinologic problems encountered in children affected with this rare abnormality.

The treatment is surgical decompression. Although a number of procedures have been developed, percutaneous ventriculocystostomy appears to be an effective technique with low morbidity [219]. Following the procedure, the elevated intracranial pressure returns to

TABLE 9.16 Clinical Features of Patients with Suprasellar Arachnoid Cysts

Feature	Number Abnormal/ Number Studied	Percentage
Hydrocephalus	21/25	84
Increased head size	17/25	68
Headache/papilledema	5/25	20
Drowsiness/vomiting	2/25	8
Brain stem/thalamic compression	14/20	70
Spasticity	11/20	55
Ataxia	6/20	30
Tremor	4/20	20
Head bobbing	12/106	11
Hypothalamic–pituitary dysfunction	9/18	50
Growth hormone deficiency	4/18	22
Adrenocorticotropic hormone deficiency	4/18	22
Precocious puberty	4/18	22
Optic nerve/chiasm compression	9/25	36
Optic pallor	7/25	28
Visual acuity/field defect	6/25	24

Adapted from [219,221].

normal and there is an increase in the IQ of the child [219]. Endoscopic fenestration of the cysts also appears to have excellent results with low morbidity [222].

Colloid Cyst of the Third Ventricle

Colloid cysts are usually located in the roof of the third ventricle or rarely in the area of the septum pellucidum [223]. They generally present clinically between the ages of 30 and 60 years, and there is a male/female sex ratio of 2–3:1 [224–226]. There are three major clinical presentations that these patients exhibit [225]. A little over one-third will have symptoms and signs of increased intracranial pressure, complaining of a nonspecific headache and vomiting, and exhibiting papilledema. Approximately 10–20% will develop a fluctuating or progressive dementia, often with gait disturbance and urinary incontinence, a combination that closely resembles normal pressure hydrocephalus. Another 20% will present with a history of intermittent attacks of headache, vomiting and visual disturbances, followed by loss of consciousness for a variable period, and then recovery. The headache is often of sudden onset with a frontal localization, usually precipitated by head movement such as lying down. The pain intensity rises rapidly, and the patient develops nausea and vomiting until he or she loses consciousness [225,226]. This "classical" presentation is due to the cyst acting as a ball-valve obstructing the foramen of Monro or the aqueduct of Sylvius. A similar mechanism is probably responsible for the drop attacks that can occur abruptly in these patients. Approximately 10–20% of patients in several series suffer sudden death, presumably from acute obstruction to the flow of cerebrospinal fluid [224,225]. Both microsurgical and endoscopic techniques are effective in treating these cysts [226].

Infiltrative Disorders

Hypothalamic–Pituitary Sarcoidosis

Sarcoidosis involves the intracranial central nervous system in 5–15% of patients with the disease, and affects the hypothalamic–pituitary region in about 0.5% of cases [68,227]. The sarcoid granulomas have a predilection for the basal hypothalamus and floor of the third ventricle, as well as the posterior, but not the anterior, pituitary [62,63,228]. Both sexes are equally involved, and over 80% of patients have evidence of systemic involvement with sarcoidosis, especially hilar adenopathy, which is present on chest X-rays in two-thirds of cases [60,61]. The common clinical manifestations in these patients are diabetes insipidus (37.5%), visual acuity and/or visual field abnormalities (53%), other dysfunction of other cranial nerves (especially VII, I, V and VIII; 44%) and evidence of other central nervous system involvement (71%) [60,61,63,229–231]. In addition to the diabetes insipidus, hypothalamic involvement is manifest by thermal dysregulation (hypothermia, hyperthermia, and poikilothermia), somnolence, personality changes, abnormalities of thirst with resetting of the osmostat and obesity [60,61,63,228–230,232]. Hypothalamic hypopituitarism is also present in virtually all of the patients with hypothalamic involvement. GH deficiency is the most common abnormality (92%), followed by gonadotropin deficiency (79%), ACTH deficiency (58%), hyperprolactinemia (20%) and hypothyroidism (6%) [61,63,233]. Following a bolus injection of TRH the patients who have hypothyroidism associated with a low basal TSH have a rise in TSH. Similarly, the hypogonadal patients show a rise in gonadotropins following GnRH infusion [61]. Most patients with sarcoidosis involving the CNS, including the hypothalamus, receive therapeutic doses of glucocorticoids. Several authors have described improvement in some of the clinical manifestations of hypothalamic–pituitary sarcoidosis, especially the visual dysfunction, following such therapy, although it is uncommon for longstanding abnormalities, especially diabetes insipidus, to improve [61–63,233].

Langerhans Cell Histiocytosis

Langerhans cell histiocytosis represents a clonal proliferation of dendritic cells that resemble normal epidermal Langerhans cells derived from CD34+ stem cells from the bone marrow [234]. Hypothalamic involvement with Langerhans' cell histiocytosis occurs primarily in the chronic, disseminated form, Hand-Schuller-Christian disease, and occasionally by a unifocal eosinophilic granuloma [59,234,235]. The classical triad of Hand-Schuller-Christian disease consists of exophthalmos, lytic lesions of the membranous bones and diabetes insipidus. Diabetes insipidus is found in close to one-half of the patients with this multisystem form of the disease and about a quarter of all patients with histiocytosis [59,234]. The other common clinical manifestation of hypothalamic involvement is growth retardation, found in 40% of patients with prepubertal onset of disease, due to abnormalities in the formation and/or release of GHRH by the hypothalamus [59,139,236]. Hyperprolactinemia, hypothalamic hypogonadism and disorders of thirst are also seen in some patients [234]. Obesity from hyperphagia may also occur from the hypothalamic involvement [235]. Low-dose radiation therapy and chemotherapy have been utilized to treat the disease, but have not been successful in reversing the diabetes insipidus or growth retardation [59,234].

Leukemia

Diabetes insipidus due to leukemic infiltration or thrombosis of the small vessels of the hypothalamus or posterior pituitary is a rare manifestation of acute leukemia. Close to three-quarters of the patients have acute nonlymphoblastic leukemia, 14% have acute lymphoblastic leukemia, 10% chronic myelocytic leukemia and 3% have chronic lymphocytic leukemia [237]. Antileukemic therapy generally fails to resolve the diabetes insipidus. The relatively low frequency of acute lymphoblastic leukemia associated with diabetes insipidus may reflect the prophylactic central nervous system radiation and intrathecal chemotherapy these patients receive [237].

Paraneoplastic Syndrome

Lymphocytic and histiocytic infiltration of the hypothalamus in patients with nonmetastatic neural crest tumors can result in a syndrome of hypersomnia. hyperphagia, obesity, polyuria, respiratory irregularity, temperature fluctuations and aggressive behavior, presumably as a paraneoplastic phenomenon [238,239].

Effect of Brain Irradiation on Hypothalamic Function

It has been known for decades that patients who receive therapeutic irradiation to the pituitary–hypothalamic region for the treatment of pituitary adenomas or primary suprasellar neoplasms may develop hypopituitarism, either as a direct result of the radiation or as a consequence of the mass effects of the neoplasm. Nevertheless, it commonly was felt that the normal hypothalamus and pituitary are relatively radioresistant. However, histologic studies have shown areas of necrosis in the hypothalamus following cranial irradiation and it is now being increasingly recognized that pituitary and especially hypothalamic dysfunction may be a long-term, adverse consequence of irradiation to the head and neck for disease outside of the sellar region. Thus, whole-brain irradiation for acute lymphoblastic leukemia or primary brain tumors, or more localized radiation for the treatment of nasopharyngeal cancer, paranasal sinus tumors, and other head and neck neoplasms have been found to be associated with hypothalamic and pituitary dysfunction and decreased pituitary gland height on magnetic resonance imaging [240–247]. The risk factors that have been identified include the dose of irradiation, with higher doses being associated with a higher risk, the interval over which the radiotherapy is delivered, the age of the patient, with children and adolescents being more susceptible than adults, and the interval following completion of the radiation therapy and the time that the patient is specifically tested for damage [246,248]. Many of the early series of patients studied were referred for evaluation of short stature or hypothalamic dysfunction; objective endocrine abnormalities were quite common in these cases [242,244,246]. One of the most important studies that examined the topic is the investigation by Samaan and colleagues [243]. They studied 166 patients who received a median of 5000 rads to the hypothalamus and 5700 rads to the pituitary during treatment of nasopharyngeal carcinoma and paranasal sinus tumors [243]. These patients were not selected because of signs or symptoms of hypothalamic or pituitary disease, and studies in 65 of the patients were performed prospectively. They found that 66.8% of the patients had one or more hormonal abnormalities that suggested a hypothalamic lesion, while 40% had evidence of primary pituitary dysfunction. The prevalence of the various anterior pituitary hormone abnormalities was directly related to the number of years between completion of the therapy and the evaluation, as shown in Figure 9.4. The earliest abnormality was found with GH secretion, with onset of the dysfunction being documented a mean of 2.6 years following therapy, and the last abnormality to be detected involved ACTH secretion,

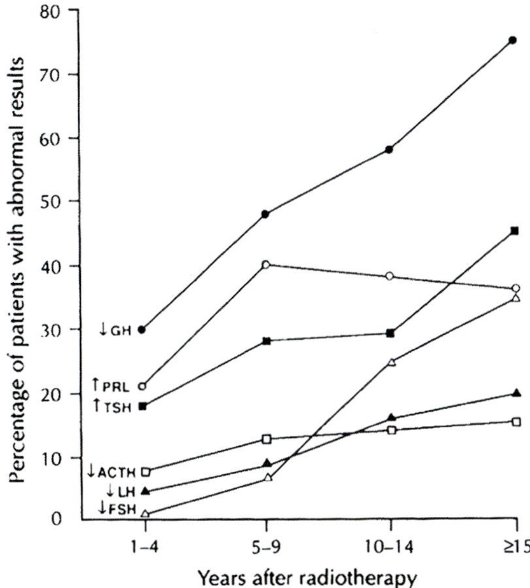

FIGURE 9.4 Percentages of 166 patients with head and neck irradiation who have abnormal hormonal levels following radiotherapy. *Data from Samaan et al. [243].* In this group of patients the thyroid-stimulating hormone (TSH) tended to be elevated, reflecting primary hypothyroidism secondary to the head and neck radiation. ACTH, adrenocorticotropic hormone; FSH, follicle-stimulating hormone; GH, growth hormone; LH, luteinizing hormone; PRL, prolactin.

which was found a mean of 6 years following the therapy [243]. Younger patients tended to have more GH deficiency than adults, while adults tended to have a greater frequency of ACTH and LH deficiency than did younger individuals. Serial serum prolactin levels appear to be a relatively sensitive and easy means to detect hypothalamic–pituitary dysfunction in patients who receive head and neck irradiation [243,244]. Other manifestations of hypothalamic dysfunction that have been noted in patients who received whole-brain irradiation include alterations in personality, appetite, thirst and sleep–wake cycle [246,249].

References

[1] P.M. Daniel, M.M.L. Prichard, Studies of the hypothalamus and the pituitary gland, Acta Endocrinol 80 (suppl 201) (1975) 1–216.

[2] P.M. Daniel, C.S. Treip, The pathology of the hypothalamus, Clin Endocrinol Metab 3 (1977) 3–19.

[3] B. Boshes, Syndromes of the diencephalon. The hypothalamus and the hypophysis, in: P.J. Vinken, G.W. Bruyn (Eds.), Localization in clinical neurology. Handbook of clinical neurology, vol. 2, North-Holland Publishing Cop, Amsterdam, 1969, pp. 432–468.

[4] H.D. Kirgis, W. Locke, Anatomy and embryology, in: W. Locke, A.V. Schally (Eds.), The hypothalamus and pituitary in health and disease, Charles C. Thomas, Springfield, 1972, pp. 3–21.

[5] S.R. Bruesch, Anatomy of the human hypothalamus, in: J.R. Givens, A.E. Kitabchi, J.T. Robertson (Eds.), The hypothalamus, Year Book Medical Publishers Inc, Chicago, 1984, pp. 1–16.

[6] P.W. Carmel, Surgical syndromes of the hypothalamus, Clin Neurosurg 27 (1980) 133–159.

[7] F. Plum, R. Van Uitert, Nonendocrine diseases and disorders of the hypothalamus, in: S. Reichlin, R.J. Baldessarini, J.B. Martin (Eds.), The hypothalamus, Raven Press, New York, 1978, pp. 415–473.

[8] K. Sano, Y. Mayanagi, H. Sekino, M. Ogashiwa, B. Ishijima, Results of stimulation and destruction of the posterior hypothalamus in man, J Neurosurg 33 (1970) 689–707.

[9] A.D. Garnica, M.L. Netzloff, A.L. Rosenbloom, Clinical manifestations of hypothalamic tumors, Ann Clin Lab Sci 10 (1980) 474–485.

[10] J.G.H. Verbalis, Disorders of body water homeostasis, Best Practice & Res Clin Endocrinol Metab 17 (2003) 471–503.

[11] A.A. Romanovsky, Thermoregulation: Some concepts have changed. Functional architecture of the thermoregulatory system, Am J Physiol Regul Integr Comp Physiol 292 (2007) R37–R46.

[12] G.A. Bray, T.F. Gallagher Jr., Manifestations of hypothalamic obesity in man: A comprehensive investigation of eight patients and a review of the literature, Medicine 54 (1975) 301–330.

[13] M.W. Schwartz, S.C. Woods, D. Porte Jr., R.J. Seeley, D.G. Baskin, Central nervous system control of food intake, Nature 404 (2000) 661–671.

[14] R.D. Cone, Anatomy and regulation of the central melanocortin system, Nature Neurosci 8 (2005) 571–578.

[15] W.S. Dhillo, Appetite regulation: An overview, Thyroid 17 (2007) 433–445.

[16] A.P. Coll, I.S. Farooqi, S. O'Rahilly, The hormonal control of food intake, Cell 129 (2007) 251–262.

[17] S.C. Higgins, M. Gueorguiev, M. Korbonits, Ghrelin, the peripheral hunger hormone, Ann Med 39 (2007) 116–136.

[18] C.B. Saper, T.E. Scammell, J. Lu, Hypothalamic regulation of sleep and circadian rhythms, Nature 437 (2005) 1257–1263.

[19] J. Aschoff, Circadian rhythms: General features and endocrinological aspects, in: D.T. Krieger (Ed.), Endocrine rhythms, Raven Press, New York, 1979, pp. 1–61.

[20] R.Y. Moore, The anatomy of central neural mechanisms regulating endocrine rhythms, in: D.T. Krieger (Ed.), Endocrine rhythms, Raven Press, New York, 1979, pp. 63–87.

[21] J.R. Schvarcz, R. Driollet, E. Rios, O. Betti, Stereotactic hypothalamotomy for behavior disorders, J Neurol Neurosurg Psych 35 (1972) 356–359.

[22] E.A. Spiegel, H.T. Wycis, Multiplicity of subcortical localization of various functions, J Nerv Ment Dis 147 (1968) 45–48.

[23] K. Poeck, G. Pilleri, Release of hypersexual behavior due to a lesion in the limbic system, Acta Neurol Scand 41 (1965) 233–244.

[24] R.M. Lechan, Neuroendocrinology of pituitary hormone regulation, Endocrinol Metab Clin 16 (1987) 475–501.

[25] G. Pelletier, Localization of active peptides in brain, in: M. Motta (Ed.), Endocrine functions of the brain, Raven Press, New York, 1980, pp. 155–169.

[26] T. Hokfelt, K. Fuxe, O. Johansson, S.J. Jeffocate, N. White, Thyrotropin-releasing hormone (TRH) in the central nervous system as revealed with immunohistochemistry, Eur J Pharmacol 34 (1975) 389–392.

[27] G. Pelletier, L. Desy, J. Cote, H. Vaudry, Immunocytochemical localization of corticotropin-releasing factor-like immunoreactivity in the human hypothalamus, Neurosci Lett 41 (1983) 259–263.

[28] G. Pelletier, L. Desy, J. Cote, G. Lefevre, H. Vaudry, Light microscope immunohistochemical localization of growth hormone-releasing factor (GRF) in the human hypothalamus, Cell Tissue Res 245 (1986) 461–464.
[29] L. Desy, G. Pelletier, Immunohistochemical localization of somatostatin in the human hypothalamus, Cell Tissue Res 184 (1977) 491–497.
[30] M. Palkovits, M. Brownstein, J.M. Saavedra, J. Axelrod, Norepinephrine and dopamine content of hypothalamic nuclei of the rat, Brain Res 77 (1974) 137–149.
[31] H.G. Bauer, Endocrine and other clinical manifestations of hypothalamic disease. A survey of 60 cases, with autopsies, J Clin Endocrinol Metab 14 (1954) 13–31.
[32] H.G. Bauer, Endocrine and metabolic conditions related to pathology in the hypothalamus: A review, J Nerv Ment Dis 128 (1959) 323–338.
[33] N.M. Dott, Surgical aspects of the hypothalamus, in: W.E. Le Gros Clark, J. Beattie, G. Riddoch, N.M. Dott (Eds.), The hypothalamus. Morphological, functional, clinical and surgical aspects, Oliver and Boyd, London, 1938, pp. 131–185.
[34] L.A. Frohman, Clinical aspects of hypothalamic disease, in: M. Motta (Ed.), The endocrine functions of the brain, Raven Press, New York, 1980, pp. 419–446.
[35] G. Riddoch, Clinical aspects of hypothalamic derangement, in: W.E. Le Gros Clark, J. Beattie, G. Riddoch, N.M. Dott (Eds.), The hypothalamus. Morphological, functional, clinical and surgical aspects, Oliver and Boyd, London, 1938, pp. 101–130.
[36] S.N. Saleem, A.-H.M. Said, D.H. Lee, Lesions of the hypothalamus: MR imaging diagnostic features, RadioGraphics 27 (2007) 1087–1108.
[37] A.J. McLean, Autonomic epilepsy, Arch Neurol 32 (1934) 189–197.
[38] A.B. Rothballer, G.S. Dugger, Hypothalamic tumor. Correlation between symptomatology, regional anatomy, and neurosecretion, Neurology 5 (1955) 160–177.
[39] L.E. White, R.F. Hain, Anorexia in association with a destructive lesion of the hypothalamus, AMA Arch Pathol 68 (1959) 275–281.
[40] A.G. Reeves, F. Plum, Hyperphagia, rage, and dementia accompanying a ventromedial hypothalamic neoplasm, Arch Neurol 20 (1969) 616–624.
[41] R.H. Fox, T.W. Davies, F.P. Marsh, H. Urich, Hypothermia in a young man with an anterior hypothalamic lesion, Lancet (1970) 185–188.
[42] K. Lewin, D. Mattingly, R.R. Millis, Anorexia nervosa associated with hypothalamic tumour, Br Med J 2 (1972) 629–630.
[43] N. Kamalian, R.E. Keesey, G.M. Zurhein, Lateral hypothalamic demyelination and cachexia in a case of "malignant" multiple sclerosis, Neurology 25 (1975) 25–30.
[44] G.G. Celesia, C.R. Archer, H.D. Chung, Hyperphagia and obesity: Relationship to medial hypothalamic lesions, JAMA 246 (1981) 151–153.
[45] R.M. Haugh, W.R. Markesbery, Hypothalamic astrocytoma. Syndrome of hyperphagia, obesity, and disturbances of behavior and endocrine and autonomic function, Arch Neurol 40 (1983) 560–563.
[46] W.J. Schwartz, N.A. Busis, E.T. Hedley-Whyte, A discrete lesion of ventral hypothalamus and optic chiasm that disturbed the daily temperature rhythm, J Neurol 233 (1986) 1–4.
[47] J. Pinkney, J. Wilding, G. Williams, I. MacFarlane, Hypothalamic obesity in humans: What do we know and what can be done? Obesity Reviews 3 (2002) 27–34.
[48] H. Blotner, Primary or idiopathic diabetes insipidus: A system disease, Metabolism 7 (1958) 191–200.
[49] W.A. Scherbaum, J.A.H. Wass, G.M. Besser, G.F. Bottazzo, D. Doniach, Autoimmune cranial diabetes insipidus: Its association with other endocrine diseases and with histiocytosis X, Clin Endocrinol 25 (1986) 411–420.
[50] R.V. Randall, E.C. Clark, H.W. Dodge Jr., et al., Scientific exhibit: Diabetes insipidus. Current concepts in the production of antidiuretic hormone. Clinical and experimental observations, Postgrad Med 29 (1961) 97–107.
[51] M. Maghnie, G. Cosi, E. Genovese, et al., Central diabetes insipidus in children and young adults, N Engl J Med 343 (2000) 998–1007.
[52] M. Maghnie, S. Ghirardello, A. De Bellis, et al., Idiopathic central diabetes insipidus in children and young adults is commonly associated with vasopressin-cell antibodies and markers of autoimmunity, Clin Endocrinol 65 (2006) 470–478.
[53] C. Bergeron, K. Kovacs, C. Ezrin, C. Mizzen, Hereditary diabetes insipidus: An immunohistochemical study of the hypothalamus and pituitary gland, Acta Neuropathol 81 (1991) 345–348.
[54] J.F. McLeod, L. Kouvacs, M.B. Gaskill, et al., Familial neurohypophyseal diabetes insipidus associated with a signal peptide mutation, J Clin Endocrinol Metab 77 (1997). 599A–599G.
[55] J.A.L. Minton, L.A. Rainbow, C. Ricketts, T.G. Barrett, Wolfram syndrome, Rev Endocrine Metab Dis 4 (2003) 53–59.
[56] H. Imura, Y. Kato, Y. Nakai, Endocrine aspects of tumors arising from suprasellar, third ventricular regions, Prog Exp Tumor Res 30 (1987) 313–324.
[57] M. Buchfelder, R. Fahlbusch, M. Walther, K. Mann, Endocrine disturbances in suprasellar germinomas, Acta Endocrinol 120 (1989) 337–342.
[58] M.T. Jennings, R. Gelman, F. Hochberg, Intracranial germ-cell tumors: Natural history and pathogenesis, J Neurosurg 63 (1985) 155–167.
[59] H. Stosel, G.D. Braunstein, Endocrine abnormalities associated with Langerhans cell histiocytosis, Endocrinologist 1 (1991) 393–397.
[60] P. Delaney, Neurologic manifestations in sarcoidosis. Review of the literature, with a report of 23 cases, Ann Int Med 87 (1977) 336–345.
[61] C.A. Stuart, F.A. Neelon, H.F. Lebovitz, Hypothalamic insufficiency: The cause of hypopituitarism in sarcoidosis, Ann Int Med 88 (1978) 589–594.
[62] H. Bihan, V. Christozova, J.-L. Dumas, et al., Sarcoidosis. Clinical, hormonal, and magnetic resonance imaging (MRI) manifestations of hypothalamic–pituitary disease in 9 patients and review of the literature, Medicine 86 (2007) 259–268.
[63] D.L. Vesely, A. Maldonado, G.S. Levey, Partial hypopituitarism and possible hypothalamic involvement in sarcoidosis, Am J Med 62 (1977) 425–431.
[64] S.A. Arslanian, W.E. Rothfus, T.P. Foley Jr., D.J. Becker, Hormonal metabolic, and neuroradiologic abnormalities associated with septo-optic dysplasia, Acta Endocrinol 107 (1984) 282–288.
[65] N. Isenberg, M. Rosenblum, J.S. Parks, The endocrine spectrum of septo-optic dysplasia, Clin Pediatr 23 (1984) 632–636.
[66] D. Margalith, J.E. Jan, A.Q. McCormick, W.J. Tze, J. Lapointe, Clinical spectrum of congenital optic nerve hypoplasia: Review of 51 patients, Develop Med Child Neurol 26 (1984) 311–322.
[67] D. Margalith, W.J. Tze, J.E. Jan, Congenital optic nerve hypoplasia with hypothalamic–pituitary dysplasia, Amer J Dis Child 139 (1985) 361–366.
[68] C. Roberson, K. Till, Hypothalamic gliomas in children, J Neurol Neurosurg Psych 37 (1974) 1047–1052.

[69] A. Borit, E.P. Richardson Jr., The biological and clinical behaviour of pilocytic astrocytomas of the optic pathways, Brain 105 (1982) 161–187.
[70] F.R. De Rubertis, M.F. Michelis, B.B. Davis, "Essential" hypernatremia. Report of three cases and review of the literature, Arch Intern Med 134 (1974) 889–895.
[71] S.G. Ball, B. Vaidja, P.H. Baylis, Hypothalamic adipsic syndrome: Diagnosis and management, Clin Endocrinol 47 (1997) 405–409.
[72] S. Teelucksingh, C.R. Steer, C.J. Thompson, et al., Hypothalamic syndrome and central sleep apnoea associated with toluene exposure, Quart J Med 78 (1991) 185–190.
[73] A. Hayek, G.T. Peake, Hypothalamic adipsia without demonstrable structural lesion, Pediatrics 70 (1982) 275–278.
[74] S.K. Du Rivage, R.J. Winter, R.T. Brouillette, C.E. Hung, Z. Noah, Idiopathic hypothalamic dysfunction and impaired control of breathing, Pediatrics 75 (1985) 896–898.
[75] D.H. Ellison, T. Berl, The syndrome of inappropriate antidiuresis, N Engl J Med 356 (2007) 2064–2072.
[76] B.F. Palmer, Hyponatremia in patients with central nervous system disease: SIADH versus CSW, Trends Endocrinol Metab 14 (2003) 182–187.
[77] E. Horn, B. Lach, Y. Lapierre, P. Hrdina, Hypothalamic pathology in the neuroleptic malignant syndrome, Am J Psych 145 (1988) 617–620.
[78] D.E. Rusyniak, J.E. Sprague, Hyperthermic syndromes induced by toxins, Clin Lab Med 26 (2006) 165–184.
[79] J.B. Martin, S. Reichlin, Clinical Neuroendocrinology, FA Davis Co, Philadelphia, 1987.
[80] S.M. Wolff, R.C. Adler, E.R. Buskirk, R.H. Thompson, A syndrome of periodic hypothalamic discharge, Am J Med 36 (1964) 956–967.
[81] R. Sandyk, R.P. Iacono, C.R. Bamford, The hypothalamus in Parkinson disease, Ital J Neurol Sci 8 (1987) 227–234.
[82] N. Weiss, D. Hasboun, S. Demeret, et al., Paroxysmal hypothermia as a clinical feature of multiple sclerosis, Neurology 72 (2009) 193–195.
[83] H.R. Haak, J.J. van Hilten, R.A.C. Roos, A.E. Meinders, Functional hypothalamic derangement in a case of Wernicke's encephalopathy, Netherlands J Med 36 (1990) 291–296.
[84] W. Penfield, Diencephalic autonomic epilepsy, Arch Neurol Psychiat 22 (1929) 358–369.
[85] W.R. Shapiro, G.H. Williams, F. Plum, Spontaneous recurrent hypothermia accompanying agenesis of the corpus callosum, Brain 92 (1969) 423–436.
[86] R.H. Fox, D.C. Wilkins, J.A. Bell, et al., Spontaneous periodic hypothermia: Diencephalic epilepsy, Br Med J 2 (1973) 693–695.
[87] A.D. Mooradian, G.K. Morley, R. McGeachie, S. Lundgren, J.E. Morley, Spontaneous periodic hypothermia, Neurology 34 (1984) 79–82.
[88] P. Bannister, P. Sheridan, M.D. Penney, Chronic reset osmoreceptor response, agenesis of the corpus callosum, and hypothalamic cyst, J Pediatr 104 (1984) 97–99.
[89] S.R. Page, S.S. Nussey, J.S. Jenkins, S.G. Wilson, D.A. Johnson, Hypothalamic disease in association with dysgenesis of the corpus callosum, Postgrad Med J 65 (1989) 163–167.
[90] R.T. Kloos, Spontaneous periodic hypothermia, Medicine 74 (1995) 268–280.
[91] M.A. MacKenzie, Pathophysiology and clinical implications of human poikilothermia, Ann NY Acad Sci 813 (1997) 738–740.
[92] J. Pinkney, J. Wilding, G. Williams, I. MacFarlane, Hypothalamic obesity in humans: What do we know and what can be done? Obesity Rev 3 (2002) 27–34.
[93] A. Russell, A diencephalic syndrome of emaciation in infancy and childhood, Arch Dis Child 26 (1951) 274.
[94] I.M. Burr, A.E. Slonim, R.K. Danish, N. Gadoth, I.J. Butler, Diencephalic syndrome revisited, J Pediatr 88 (1976) 439–444.
[95] A. Fleischman, C. Brue, T.Y. Poussaint, et al., Diencephalic syndrome: A cause of failure to thrive and a model of partial growth hormone resistance, Pediatrics 115 (2005) e742–e748.
[96] M.T. Munoz, J. Argente, Anorexia nervosa in female adolescents: Endocrine and bone mineral density disturbances, Eur J Endocrinol 147 (2002) 275–286.
[97] R.S. Mecklenberg, D.L. Loriaux, R.H. Thompson, A.E. Anderson, M.B. Lipsett, Hypothalamic dysfunction in patients with anorexia, Medicine 53 (1974) 147–159.
[98] N. Karavitaki, S. Cudlip, C.B.T. Adams, J.A.H. Wass, Craniopharyngiomas, Endo Rev 27 (2006) 371–397.
[99] J.B. Martin, S. Reichlin, Clinical Neuroendocrinology, FA Davis Co, Philadelphia, 1987. 411.
[100] S. Nishino, Clinical and neurobiological aspects of narcolepsy, Sleep Med 8 (2007) 373–399.
[101] R.A. Cohen, H.E. Albers, Disruption of human circadian and cognitive regulation following a discrete hypothalamic lesion: A case study, Neurology 41 (1991) 726–729.
[102] F. Fenzi, A. Simonati, F. Crosato, et al., Clinical features of Kleine-Levin syndrome with localized encephalitis, Neuropediatrics 24 (1993) 292–295.
[103] I. Arnulf, J.M. Zeitzer, J. File, N. Farber, E. Mignot, Kleine-Levin syndrome: A systemic review of 186 cases in the literature, Brain 128 (2005) 2763–2776.
[104] S. Striano, P. Striano, C. Sarappa, P. Boccella, The clinical spectrum and natural history of gelastic epilepsy–hypothalamic hamartoma syndrome, Seizure 14 (2005) 232–239.
[105] A.S. Harvey, J.L. Freeman, Epilepsy in hypothalamic hamartoma: Clinical and EEG features, Semin Pediatr Neurol 14 (2007) 60–64.
[106] P.W. Carmel, Vegetative dysfunctions of the hypothalamus, Acta Neurochir 75 (1985) 113–121.
[107] R.R. Shankar, O.H. Pescovitz, Precocious puberty, Adv Endocrin Metab 6 (1995) 55–89.
[108] W. Chemaitilly, C. Trivin, L. Adan, V. Gall, C. Sainte-Rose, R. Brauner, Central precocious puberty: Clinical and laboratory features, Clin Endocrinol 54 (2001) 289–294.
[109] A. Muir, Precocious puberty, Pediatrics in Review 27 (2006) 373–380.
[110] L.M. Weinberger, F.C. Grant, Precocious puberty and tumors of the hypothalamus, Arch Int Med 67 (1941) 762–792.
[111] K. Arita, K. Kurisu, Y. Kiura, K. Iida, H. Otsubo, Hypothalamic hamartoma, Neurol Med Chir Tokyo 45 (2005) 221–231.
[112] A. Chattopadhyay, V. Kumar, M. Marulaiah, Polycystic ovaries, precocious puberty and acquired hypothyroidism: The Van Wyk and Grumbach syndrome, J Pediatr Surg 38 (2003) 1390–1392.
[113] S. Melmed, C. Ezrin, K. Kovacs, R.S. Goodman, L.A. Frohman, Acromegaly due to secretion of growth hormone by an ectopic pancreatic islet-cell tumor, N Engl J Med 312 (1985) 9–17.
[114] F. Beuschlein, C.J. Strasburger, V. Siegerstetter, et al., Acromegaly caused by secretion of growth hormone by a non-Hodgkin's lymphoma, N Engl J Med 342 (2000) 1871–1876.
[115] M. Losa, K. von Werder, Pathophysiology and clinical aspects of the ectopic GH-releasing hormone syndrome, Clin Endocrinol 47 (1997) 123–135.
[116] S.L. Asa, J.M. Bilbao, K. Kovacks, J.A. Linfoot, Hypothalamic neuronal hamartoma associated with pituitary growth hormone cell adenoma and acromegaly, Acta Neuropathol 52 (1980) 231–234.

[117] S.L. Asa, B.W. Scheithauer, J.M. Bilbao, et al., A case for hypothalamic acromegaly: A clinicopathological study of six patients with hypothalamic gangliocytomas producing growth hormone releasing factor, J Clin Endocrinol Metab 58 (1984) 796–803.

[118] W. Saeger, M.J.A. Puchner, D.K. Ludecke, Combined sellar gangliocytomas and pituitary adenoma in acromegaly or Cushing's disease, Virchows Archiv A Path Anat Histopath 425 (1994) 93–99.

[119] W. Muller, Uber das gemeinsame Vorkommen eines Hypophysenadenome mit einem Gangliocytoma in zwein faillen. Ein Beitrag zur Frage der Neurosekretion, Acta Neurochir 7 (1956) 13.

[120] R.H. Rhodes, J.J. Dusseau, A.S. Boyd Jr., K.M. Knigg, Intrasellar neuraladenophypopophyseal choristoma. A morphological and immunocytochemical study, J Neuropathol Exp Neurol 41 (1982) 267–271.

[121] I. Shimon, S. Melmed, Growth hormone- and growth-hormone-releasing hormone-producing tumors, Cancer Treatment Res 89 (1997) 1–24.

[122] S. Melmed, I. Jackson, D. Kleinberg, A. Klibanski, Current treatment guidelines for acromegaly, J Clin Endocrinol Metab 83 (1998) 2646–2652.

[123] S. Melmed, Acromegaly pathogenesis and treatment, J Clin Invest 119 (2009) 3189–3202.

[124] B.M.K. Biller, Pathogenesis of pituitary Cushing's syndrome. Pituitary versus hypothalamic, Endocrinol Clin N Amer 23 (1994) 547–554.

[125] S. Gifford, J.G. Gunderson, Cushing's disease as a psychosomatic disorder: A selective review of the clinical and experimental literature and a report of ten cases, Perspect Biol Med 13 (1970) 169–221.

[126] S.W. Lamberts, S.Z. Stefanko, S.A. DeLang, et al., Failure of clinical remission after transsphenoidal removal of a microadenoma in a patient with Cushing's disease: Multiple hyperplastic and adenomatous cell nests in surrounding pituitary tissues, J Clin Endocrinol Metab 50 (1980) 793–795.

[127] B.M.K. Biller, A.B. Grossman, P.M. Steward, et al., Treatment of adrenocorticotropin-dependent Cushing's syndrome: A consensus statement, J Clin Endocrin Metab 93 (2008) 2454–2462.

[128] D.T. Krieger, L. Amorosa, F. Linick, Cyproheptadine-induced remission of Cushing's disease, N Engl J Med 293 (1975) 893–896.

[129] H.U. Lankford, H.S. Tucker, W.G. Blackard, A cyproheptadine-reversible defect in ACTH control persisting after removal of the pituitary tumor in Cushing's disease, N Engl J Med 305 (1981) 1244–1248.

[130] F. Cavagnini, C. Invitti, E.E. Polli, Sodium valproate in Cushing's disease, Lancet (1984) 162–163.

[131] S.W.J. Lamberts, J.G. Klijn, M. deQuijada, et al., The mechanism of the suppressive action of bromocriptine on adrenocorticotropin secretion in patients with Cushing's disease and Nelson's syndrome, J Clin Endocrinol Metab 51 (1980) 307–311.

[132] S.L. Asa, K. Kovacs, G.T. Tindall, D.L. Barrow, E. Horvath, P. Vecsei, Cushing's disease associated with an intrasellar gangliocytoma producing corticotrophin-releasing factor, Ann Int Med 101 (1984) 789–793.

[133] B.M.K. Biller, J.M. Alexander, N.T. Zervas, et al., Clonal origins of adrenocorticotropin-secreting pituitary tissue in Cushing's disease, J Clin Endocrinol Metab 75 (1992) 1303–1309.

[134] G. Faglia, A. Spada, The role of hypothalamus in pituitary neoplasia, Clin Endocrinol 9 (1995) 225–242.

[135] N. Karavitaki, C. Brufani, J.T. Warner, et al., Craniopharyngiomas in children and adults: Systemic analysis of 121 cases with long-term follow-up, Clin Endocrinol 62 (2005) 397–409.

[136] A. Spada, G. Mantovani, A. Lania, Pathogenesis of prolactinomas, Pituitary 8 (2005) 7–15.

[137] S.L. Feigenbaum, D.E. Downey, C.B. Wilson, R.B. Jaffe, Transsphenoidal pituitary resection for preoperative diagnosis of prolactin-secreting pituitary adenoma in women: Long term follow-up, J Clin Endocrinol Metab 81 (1996) 1711–1719.

[138] L.C. Layman, Hypogonadotropic hypogonadism, Endocrinol Metab Clin N Am 36 (2007) 283–296.

[139] J.L.C. Borges, R.M. Blizzard, M.C. Gelato, et al., Effects of human pancreatic tumour growth hormone releasing factor on growth hormone and somatomedin C levels in patients with idiopathic growth hormone deficiency, Lancet (1983) 119–124.

[140] M. Dattani, M. Preece, Growth hormone deficiency and related disorders: Insights into causation, diagnosis, and treatment, Lancet 363 (2004) 1977–1987.

[141] F. Triulzi, G. Scotti, B. di Natale, et al., Evidence of a congenital midline brain anomaly in pituitary dwarfs: A magnetic resonance imaging study in 101 patients, Pediatrics 93 (1994) 409–416.

[142] D.T. Krieger, H.P. Krieger, Circadian variation of the plasma 17-hydroxycorticosteroids in central nervous system disease, J Clin Endocrinol Metab 26 (1966) 929–940.

[143] O. Korsgaard, J. Lindholm, P. Rasmussen, Endocrine function in patients with suprasellar and hypothalamic tumours, Acta Endocrinol 83 (1976) 1–8.

[144] M. Andrioli, F.P. Giraldi, F. Cavagnini, Isolated corticotrophin deficiency, Pituitary 9 (2006) 289–295.

[145] L. Persani, E. Ferretti, S. Borgato, G. Faglia, P. Beck-Peccoz, Circulating thyrotropin bioactivity in sporadic central hypothyroidism, J Clin Endocrinol Metab 85 (2000) 3631–3635.

[146] A. Mehta, P.C. Hindmarsh, R.G. Stanhope, C.E. Brain, M.A. Preece, M.T. Dattani, Is the thyrotropin-releasing hormone test necessary in the diagnosis of central hypothyroidism in children? J Clin Endocrinol Metab 88 (2003) 5696–5703.

[147] A. Prader, A. Labhart, H. Willi, Ein syndrome von adipositas, Kleinwuchs, Kryptorchismus, und Oligophrenie nach myotonieartigen Zustand im Neugeborenenalter, Schweiz Med Wochenschr 86 (1956) 1260–1261.

[148] G.A. Bray, W.T. Dahms, R.S. Swerdloff, R.H. Fiser, R.L. Atkinson, R.E. Carrel, The Prader-Willi syndrome: A study of 40 patients and a review of the literature, Medicine 62 (1983) 59–80.

[149] M. Gunay-Aygun, S. Schwartz, S. Heeger, M.A. O'Riordan, S.B. Cassidy, The changing purpose of Prader-Willi syndrome clinical diagnostic criteria and proposed revised criteria, Pediatrics 108 (2001) 1–5.

[150] P. Burman, E.M. Ritzen, A.C. Lindgren, Endocrine dysfunction in Prader-Willi syndrome: A review with special reference to GH, Endocrine Rev 22 (2001) 787–799.

[151] A.P. Goldstone, Prader-Willi syndrome: Advances in genetics, pathophysiology and treatment, Trends in Endocrinol Metab 15 (2004) 12–20.

[152] C. Sapienza, J.G. Hall, Genetic imprinting in human disease, in: C.R. Scriver, A.R. Beaudet, W.S. Sly (Eds.), The metabolic and molecular basis of inherited disease, vol. 1, McGraw-Hill Inc., New York, 1995, pp. 437–458.

[153] D. Klein, F. Ammann, The syndrome of Laurence-Moon-Bardet-Biedl and allied diseases in Switzerland. Clinical, genetic and epidemiological studies, J Neuro Sci 9 (1969) 479–513.

[154] J.L. Tobin, P.L. Beales, Bardet-Biedl syndrome: Beyond the cilium, Pediatr Nephrol 22 (2007) 926–936.

[155] W. Stiggelbout, The Bardet-Biedl syndrome. Including Hutchinson-Laurence-Moon syndrome, in: P.J. Vinken, G.W. Bruyn (Eds.), Handbook of clinical neurology, vol. 13, North-Holland, Amsterdam, 1972, pp. 380–413.

[156] P.L. Beales, A.M. Warner, G.A. Hitman, et al., Bardet-Biedl syndrome: A molecular and phenotypic study of 18 families, J Med Genet 34 (1997) 922–928.
[157] J.A. Edwards, P.K. Sethi, A.J. Scoma, R.M. Bannerman, L.A. Frohman, A new familial syndrome characterized by pigmentary retinopathy, hypogonadism, mental retardation, nerve deafness and glucose intolerance, Amer J Med 60 (1976) 23–32.
[158] N.H. Birkebaek, L. Patel, N.B. Wright, et al., Endocrine status in patients with optic nerve hypoplasia: Relationship to midline central nervous system abnormalities and appearance of the hypothalamic–pituitary axis on magnetic resonance imaging, J Clin Endocrinol Metab 88 (2003) 5281–5286.
[159] A. Polizzi, P. Pavone, P. Iannetti, L. Manfre, M. Ruggieri, Septo-optic dysplasia complex: A heterogeneous malformation syndrome, Pediatr Neurol 34 (2006) 66–71.
[160] M.L. Garcia, E.B. Ty, M. Taban, A.D. Rothner, D. Rogers, E.I. Traboulsi, Systemic and ocular findings in 100 patients with optic nerve hypoplasia, J Child Neurol 21 (2006) 949–956.
[161] L. Patel, R.J.Q. McNally, E. Harrison, I.C. Lloyd, P.E. Clayton, Geographical distribution of optic nerve hypoplasia and septo-optic dysplasia in northwest Endgland, J Pediatr 148 (2006) 85–88.
[162] U. Roessmann, M.E. Velasco, E.J. Small, A. Hori, Neuropathology of "septo-optic dysplasia" (de Morsier syndrome) with immunohistochemical studies of the hypothalamus and pituitary gland, J Neuropath Exp Neurol 46 (1987) 597–608.
[163] G.F. Powell, J.A. Brasel, R.M. Blizzard, Emotional deprivation and growth retardation simulating idiopathic hypopituitarism. I. Clinical evaluation of the syndrome, N Engl J Med 276 (1967) 1271–1278.
[164] G.F. Powell, J.A. Brasel, S. Raiti, R.M. Blizzard, Emotional deprivation and growth retardation simulating idiopathic hypopituitarism. II. Endocrinologic evaluation of the syndrome, N Engl J Med 276 (1967) 1279–1283.
[165] B.C. Gohlke, F.L. Frazer, R. Stanhope, Body mass index and segmental proportion in children with different subtypes of psychosocial short stature, Eur J Pediatr 161 (2002) 250–254.
[166] S.S.C. Yen, R.W. Rebar, W. Quesenberry, Pituitary function in pseudocyesis, J Clin Endocrinol Metab 43 (1976) 132–136.
[167] T. Zuber, J. Kelly, Pseudocyesis, Am Fam Phys 30 (1984) 131–134.
[168] G.W. Small, Pseudocyesis: An overview, Canadian J Psych 31 (1986) 452–457.
[169] M.A. Bray, A. Muneyyirci-Delale, G.D. Kofinas, F.I. Reyes, Circadian, ultradian, and episodic gonadotropin and prolactin secretion in human pseudocyesis, Acta Endocrinol 124 (1991) 501–509.
[170] P.R. Sharma, Hamartoma of the hypothalamus and tuber cincereum: A brief review of the literature, J Postgrad Med 33 (1987) 1–13.
[171] G.N. Breningstall, Gelastic seizures, precocious puberty, and hypothalamic hamartoma, Neurology 35 (1985) 1180–1183.
[172] J. Takeuchi, H. Handa, Pubertas praecox and hypothalamic hamartoma, Neurosurg Rev 8 (1985) 225–231.
[173] H.I. Hochman, D.M. Judge, S. Reichlin, Precocious puberty and hypothalamic hamartoma, Pediatrics 67 (1981) 236–244.
[174] C. Diebler, G. Ponsot, Hamartomas of the tuber cinereum, Neuroradiology 25 (1983) 93–101.
[175] F. Comite, O.H. Pescovitz, K.G. Rieth, Luteinizing hormone-releasing hormone analog treatment of boys with hypothalamic hamartoma and true precocious puberty, J Clin Endocrinol Metab 59 (1984) 888–892.
[176] M. Sato, Y. Ushio, N. Arita, H. Mogami, Hypothalamic hamartoma: Report of two cases, Neurosurgery 16 (1985) 198–206.
[177] J.M. Valdueza, L. Cristante, O. Dammann, et al., Hypothalamic hamartomas: With special reference to gelastic epilepsy and surgery, Neurosurgery 34 (1994) 949–958.
[178] D. Nguyen, S. Singh, M. Zaatreh, et al., Hypothalamic hamartomas: Seven cases and review of the literature, Epilepsy Behavior 4 (2003) 246–258.
[179] C.F. List, C.E. Dowman, B.S. Bagehi, J. Bebin, Posterior hypothalamic hamartomas and gangliogliomas causing precocious puberty, Neurology 8 (1958) 164–174.
[180] E. Ilgren, M. Briggs, A. Anysly-Green, Precocious puberty in a 3-year-old girl associated with parasellar ganglionic hamartoma, Clin Neuropathol 2 (1983) 95–98.
[181] D.M. Judge, H.E. Kulin, R. Page, R. Santen, S. Trapukd, Hypothalamic hamartoma: A source of luteinizing-hormone-releasing factor in precocious puberty, N Engl J Med 296 (1977) 7–10.
[182] J. Takeuchi, H. Handa, Pubertas praecox and hypothalamic hamartoma, Neurosurg Rev 8 (1985) 225–231.
[183] J. Regis, D. Scavarda, M. Tamura, et al., Epilepsy related to hypothalamic hamartomas: Surgical management with special reference to gamma knife surgery, Childs Nerv Syst 22 (2006) 881–895.
[184] E.A. Boudreau, K. Liow, C.M. Frattali, et al., Hypothalamic hamartomas and seizures: Distinct natural history of isolated and Pallister-Hall syndrome cases, Epilepsia 46 (2005) 42–47.
[185] J.G. Hall, P.D. Pallister, S.K. Clarren, et al., Congenital hypothalamic hamartoblastoma, hypopituitarism, imperforate anus, and postaxial polydactyly – a new syndrome? Part I: Clinical, causal, and pathogenetic considerations, Am J Med Gen 7 (1980) 47–74.
[186] S.K. Clarren, E.C. Alvord Jr., J.G. Hall, Congenital hypothalamic hamartoblastoma, hypopituitarism, imperforate anus, and postaxial polydactyly – a new syndrome? Part II: Neuropathological considerations, Am J Med Gen 7 (1980) 75–83.
[187] L.G. Biesecker, M. Abbott, J. Allen, et al., Report from the workshop on Pallister-Hall syndrome and related phenotypes, Am J Med Gen 65 (1996) 76–81.
[188] L.G. Biesecker, J.M. Graham Jr., Pallister-Hall syndrome, J Med Genet 33 (1996) 585–589.
[189] J. Takeuchi, H. Handa, I. Nagata, Suprasellar germinoma, J Neurosurg 49 (1978) 41–48.
[190] C.A. Sklar, M.M. Grumbach, S.L. Kaplan, F.A. Conte, Hormonal and metabolic abnormalities associated with central nervous system germinoma in children and adolescents and the effect of therapy: Report of 10 patients, J Clin Endocrinol Metab 52 (1981) 9–16.
[191] L.R. Simson, I. Lampe, M.R. Abell, Suprasellar germinomas, Cancer 22 (1968) 533–544.
[192] T. Aida, H. Abe, K. Fujieda, N. Matsuura, Endocrine functions in children with suprasellar germinoma, Neurol Med Chir 33 (1993) 152–157.
[193] S. Nishio, T. Inamura, I. Takeshita, et al., Germ cell tumor in the hypothalamo–neurohypophysial region: Clinical features and treatment, Neurosurg Rev 16 (1993) 221–227.
[194] S.L. Mootha, A.J. Barkovich, M.M. Grumbach, et al., Idiopathic hypothalamic diabetes insipidus, pituitary stalk thickening, and the occult intracranial germinoma in children and adolescents, J Clin Endocrinol Metab 82 (1997) 1362–1367.
[195] C.R. Nichols, E.P. Fox, Extragonadal and pediatric germ cell tumors, Hemat/Oncol Clinics N Amer 5 (1991) 1189–1209.
[196] C. Navarro, J.M. Corretger, A. Sancho, J. Rovira, I. Morales, Paraneoplastic precocious puberty. Report of a new case with hepatoblastoma and review of the literature, Cancer 56 (1985) 1725–1729.

[197] O. Kubo, N. Yamasaki, Y. Kamijo, K. Amano, K. Kitamura, R. Demura, Human chorionic gonadotropin produced by ectopic pinealoma in a girl with precocious puberty, J Neurosurg 47 (1977) 101–105.
[198] R.J. Packer, B.H. Cohen, K. Coney, Intracranial germ cell tumors, The Oncologist 5 (2000) 312–320.
[199] R.J. Packer, I.N. Sutton, L.T. Bilaniuk, et al., Treatment of chiasmatic hypothalamic gliomas of childhood and chemotherapy: An update, Ann Neurol 23 (1988) 79–85.
[200] J.A. Rush, B.R. Younge, R.J. Campbell, C.S. MacCarty, Optic glioma. Long-term follow up of 85 histopathologically verified cases, Ophthalmology 89 (1982) 1213–1219.
[201] F. Helcl, H. Petraskova, Gliomas of visual pathways and hypothalamus in children – a preliminary report, Acta Neurochir 35 (suppl) (1985) 106–110.
[202] L.A. Rodriguez, M.S.B. Edwards, V.A. Levin, Management of hypothalamic gliomas in children: An analysis of 33 cases, Neurosurgery 26 (1990) 242–247.
[203] A.D. Rogol, Pituitary and parapituitary tumors of childhood and adolescence, in: J.R. Givens, A.E. Kitabchi, J.T. Robertson (Eds.), Hormone-secreting pituitary tumors, Year Book Medical Publishers, Inc, Chicago, 1981, pp. 349–375.
[204] G.E. Keles, A. Banerjee, D. Puri, M.S. Bergen, Supratentorial gliomas, in: N. Gupta, A. Banerjee, D. Hass-Kogan (Eds.), Pediatric CNS Tumors, Springer, New York, 2004, pp. 1–26.
[205] E. Alshail, J.J. Rutka, L.E. Becker, H.J. Hoffman, Optic chiasmatic-hypothalamic glioma, Brain Pathol 7 (1997) 799–806.
[206] C.S. MacCarty, A.S. Boyd Jr., D.S. Childs Jr., Tumors of the optic nerve and optic chiasm, J Neurosurg 33 (1970) 439–444.
[207] R.N. Kjellberg, Craniopharyngiomas, in: G.T. Tindall, W.F. Collins (Eds.), Clinical management of pituitary disorders, Raven Press, New York, 1979, pp. 373–388.
[208] B.-C. Wen, D.H. Hussey, J. Staples, et al., A comparison of the roles of surgery and radiation therapy in the management of craniopharyngiomas, Int J Rad Oncol Bio Phys 16 (1989) 17–24.
[209] R.V. Randall, E.R. Laws Jr., C.F. Abboud, Clinical presentation of craniopharyngiomas. A brief review of 300 cases, in: J.R. Givens, A.E. Kitabchi, J.T. Robertson (Eds.), The hypothalamus, Year Book Medical Publishers Inc., Chicago, 1984, pp. 312–333.
[210] R.A. Sanford, M.S. Muhlbauer, Craniopharyngioma in children, Neurologic Clinics 9 (1991) 453–465.
[211] C.A. Sklar, Craniopharyngioma: Endocrine abnormalities at presentation, Pediatr Neurosurg 21 (suppl 1) (1994) 18–20.
[212] M.G. Yasargil, M. Curcic, M. Kis, G. Stegenthaler, P.J. Teddy, P. Roth, Total removal of craniopharyngiomas. Approaches and long-term results in 144 patients, J Neurosurg 73 (1990) 3–11.
[213] M. Samn, M. Tatagiba, Surgical management of craniopharyngiomas: A review, Neurol Med Chir 37 (1997) 141–149.
[214] E.G. Fischer, K. Welch, J. Shillito Jr., K.R. Winston, N.J. Tarbell, Craniopharyngiomas in children. Long-term effects of conservative surgical procedures combined with radiation therapy, J Neurosurg 73 (1990) 534–540.
[215] C.A. Sklar, Craniopharyngioma: Endocrine sequelae of treatment, Pediatr Neurosurg 21 (1994) 120–123.
[216] J.E. Finn, L.A. Mount, Meningiomas of the tuberculum sellae and planum sphenoidale. A review of 83 cases, Arch Ophthalmol 92 (1974) 23–97.
[217] J.H. Chi, M.W. McDermott, Tuberculum sellae meningiomas, Neurosurg Focus 14 (2003) 1–6.
[218] M. Banna, Pathology and clinical manifestations, in: J. Hankinson, M. Banna (Eds.), Pituitary and parapituitary tumours, WB Saunders, London, 1976, pp. 13–58.
[219] A. Pierre-Kahn, L. Capelle, R. Brauner, et al., Presentation and management of suprasellar arachnoid cysts. Review of 20 cases, J Neurosurg 73 (1990) 355–359.
[220] G.R.I.V. Harsh, M.S.P. Edwards, C.B. Wilson, Intracranial arachnoid cysts in children, J Neurosurg 69 (1986) 835–842.
[221] Z.H. Rappaport, Suprasellar arachnoid cysts: Options in operative management, Acta Neurochir 122 (1993) 71–75.
[222] G. Pradilla, G. Jallo, Arachnoid cysts: Case series and review of the literature, Neurosurg Focus 22 (2007) 1–4.
[223] J.B. Martin, S. Reichlin, Clinical Neuroendocrinology, FA Davis Co, Philadelphia, 1987, 534.
[224] J.R. Little, C.S. MacCarty, Colloid cysts of the third ventricle, J Neurosurg 39 (1974) 230–235.
[225] R. Kelly, Colloid cysts of the third ventricle. Analysis of twenty-nine cases, Brain 74 (1951) 23–65.
[226] D. Hellwig, B.L. Bauer, M. Schulte, S. Gatscher, T. Riegel, H. Bertalanffy, Neuroendoscopic treatment for colloid cysts of the third ventricle: the experience of a decade, Neurosurgery 52 (2003) 525–533.
[227] A. Silverstein, M.M. Feuer, L.E. Siltzbach, Neurologic sarcoidosis, Arch Neurol 12 (1965) 1–11.
[228] C.A. Stuart, F.A. Neelon, H.E. Lebovitz, Disordered control of thirst in hypothalamic–pituitary sarcoidosis, N Engl J Med 303 (1980) 1078–1082.
[229] J.L. Winnacker, K.L. Becker, S. Katz, Endocrine aspects of sarcoidosis, N Engl J Med 278 (1968) 427–434.
[230] J.L. Winnacker, K.L. Becker, S. Katz, Endocrine aspects of sarcoidosis (concluded), N Engl J Med 278 (1968) 483–492.
[231] N.H. Bell, Endocrine complications of sarcoidosis, Endocrinol Metab Clin N Am 20 (1991) 645–654.
[232] D.L. Vesely, Hypothalamic sarcoidosis: A new cause of morbid obesity, South Med J 82 (1989) 758–761.
[233] K. Nakao, K. Noma, B. Sato, S. Yano, Y. Yamamura, T. Tachibana, Serum prolactin levels in eighty patients with sarcoidosis, Europ J Clin Invest 8 (1978) 37–40.
[234] P. Makras, K.I. Alexandraki, G.P. Chrousos, A.B. Grossman, G.A. Kaltsas, Endocrine manifestations in Langerhans cell histiocytosis, Trends in Endocrinol Metab 18 (2007) 252–257.
[235] M.C.M. Amato, L.L.K. Elias, J. Elias, et al., Endocrine disorders in pediatric-onset Langerhans cell histiocytosis, Horm Met Res 38 (2006) 746–751.
[236] G.D. Braunstein, P.O. Kohler, Pituitary function in Hand-Schuller-Christian disease. Evidence for deficient growth-hormone release in patients with short stature, N Engl J Med 286 (1972) 1225–1229.
[237] P. Ra'anani, O. Shpilberg, M. Berezin, I. Ben-Bassat, Acute leukemia relapse presenting as central diabetes insipidus, Cancer 73 (1994) 2312–2316.
[238] K. Nunn, R. Ouvrier, T. Sprague, S. Arbuckle, M. Docker, Idiopathic hypothalamic dysfunction: A paraneoplastic syndrome, J Child Neurol 12 (1997) 276–281.
[239] N. Sirvent, E. Berard, P. Chastagner, F. Feillet, K. Wagner, D. Sommelet, Hypothalamic dysfunction associated with neuroblastoma: Evidence for a new paraneoplastic syndrome? Med Pediatr Oncology 40 (2003) 326–328.
[240] M.D. Littley, S.M. Shalet, C.G. Beardwell, Radiation and hypothalamic–pituitary function, Bailliere's Clin Endocrinol Metab 4 (1990) 147–175.
[241] L.S. Constine, P.D. Woolf, D. Cann, et al., Hypothalamic–pituitary dysfunction after radiation for brain tumors, N Engl J Med 328 (1993) 87–94.

[242] G.E. Richards, W.M. Wara, M.M. Grumbach, S.L. Kaplan, G.E. Sheline, F.A. Conte, Delayed onset of hypopituitarism: Sequelae of therapeutic irradiation of central nervous system, eye, and middle ear tumors, J Pediatr 89 (1976) 553–559.
[243] N.A. Samaan, P.N. Schultz, K.-P.P. Yang, et al., Endocrine complications after radiotherapy for tumors of the head and neck, J Lab Clin Med 109 (1987) 364–372.
[244] J.I. Mechanick, F.H. Hochberg, A. LaRocque, Hypothalamic dysfunction following whole-brain irradiation, J Neurosurg 65 (1986) 490–494.
[245] K.S.L. Lam, V.K.C. Tse, C. Wang, R.T.T. Yeung, J.T.C. Ma, J.H.C. Ho, Early effects of cranial irradiation on hypothalamic–pituitary function, J Clin Endocrinol Metab 64 (1987) 418–424.
[246] G. Costin, Effects of low-dose cranial radiation on growth hormone seretory dynamics and hypothalamic–pituitary function, Amer J Dis Child 142 (1988) 847–852.
[247] E. Pääkkö, K. Talvensaari, J. Pyhtinen, M. Lanning, Decreased pituitary gland height after radiation treatment to the hypothalamic–pituitary axis evaluated by MR, Am J Neuroradiol 15 (1994) 537–541.
[248] S.M. Shalet, Radiation and pituitary dysfunction, N Engl J Med 328 (1993) 131–133.
[249] C.R. Kelsey, L.B. Marks, Somnolence syndrome after focal radiation therapy to the pineal region: Case report and review of the literature, J Neuro-Oncology 78 (2006) 153–156.

CHAPTER

10

Anterior Pituitary Failure

John D. Carmichael

Pituitary Center, Cedars-Sinai Medical Center, Los Angeles, CA, USA

INTRODUCTION

Hypopituitarism results from the failure of one or more pituitary hormones to be produced or secreted from the anterior pituitary. The anterior lobe of the pituitary is responsible for the production and secretion of hormones that affect specific peripheral glandular tissues. The anterior pituitary is under control of the hypothalamus via hypophysiotropic neurohormonal regulation, which integrates feedback mechanisms that govern secretion of hypothalamic factors, pituitary hormones and peripheral hormones.

Peripheral stimuli from a wide array of sources prompt modulation of the neurohormonal control of anterior pituitary function, including production and secretion of pituitary hormones. These hormones are released into the circulation, resulting in specific systemic effects. Anterior pituitary failure can result from the disruption of any step in the production, stimulation, secretion and regulation of these hormones.

ETIOLOGY

The causes of anterior pituitary failure are varied (Table 10.1). The etiology of pituitary failure can be broadly divided into structural causes and functional causes. Normal physiologic secretion of pituitary hormones relies on intact hypothalamic control of pituitary function, transport of hypophysiotropic hormones from the hypothalamus to the pituitary via the portal blood supply, and normal functioning of the anterior pituitary hormone-secreting cells. Mass lesions arising from the pituitary or hypothalamus can affect normal pituitary or hypothalamic function and cause deficiency of one or more pituitary hormones. Structural abnormalities rooted in the embryologic development of the adenohypophysis can lead to deficiencies in one or more pituitary hormones. These and other structural causes are generally not reversible without invasive intervention. Functional causes of pituitary deficiency are present without extrinsic or intrinsic mass, and are generally reversible, once the underlying etiology is discovered and treated. In contrast, genetic or congenital causes may not have structural manifestations, cause failure of one or more pituitary hormones and are not reversible.

MORTALITY

Hypopituitarism is associated with an increased mortality compared to the normal population. Epidemiologic studies of patients with hypopituitarism have demonstrated an excess standardized mortality ratio of 1.2–2.2 years [1–3], often ascribed to a higher incidence of cardiovascular and cerebrovascular events. Despite numerous studies, risk attributable to hormonal replacement remains a controversial issue. Deficiency in growth hormone has been implicated as a cause for increased mortality in subjects with hypopituitarism, but long-term controlled studies are not available to adequately point toward this deficiency as the sole mediator of increased mortality. Imprecise and excessive glucocorticoid replacement carries with it an increased morbidity, but this too has not been adequately studied to determine its role in excess mortality in patients with hypopituitarism.

STRUCTURAL CAUSES OF PITUITARY FAILURE

Mass Lesions

Pituitary Tumors

Pituitary adenomas are the most common cause of hypopituitarism. Lesions arising from monoclonal cells

The Pituitary, Third Edition, DOI: 10.1016/B978-0-12-380926-1.10010-0

TABLE 10.1 Causes of Anterior Pituitary Failure

Neoplastic
Pituitary adenoma
Pituitary carcinoma
Craniopharyngioma
Pituicytoma
Fibroma
Glioma
Meningioma
Paraganglioma
Teratoma
Chordoma
Angioma
Sarcoma
Ependymoma
Germinoma
Cysts
Rathke's cleft, arachnoid, epidermoid, dermoid
Ganglioneuroma
Astrocytoma
Metastatic
Breast, lung, colon, prostate
TREATMENT OF SELLAR, PARASELLAR AND HYPOTHALAMIC DISEASE
Surgery
Radiotherapy
Radiosurgery
INFILTRATIVE DISEASE
Autoimmune
Lymphocytic hypophysitis
Granulomatous
Sarcoidosis
Langerhans cell histiocytosis
Giant cell granuloma
Granulomatous hypophysitis
Xanthomatous hypophysitis
Wegener's granulomatosis
Hemochromatosis

TABLE 10.1 Causes of Anterior Pituitary Failure—cont'd

EMPTY SELLA
IDIOPATHIC
VASCULAR
Pituitary tumor apoplexy
Sheehan's syndrome
Intrasellar carotid artery aneurysm
Subarachnoid hemorrhage
GENETIC (SEE TABLE 10.2)
Combined pituitary hormone deficiencies
Isolated pituitary hormone deficiencies
DEVELOPMENTAL
Midline cerebral and cranial malformations
Pituitary hypoplasia or aplasia
Ectopic pituitary
Basal encephalocele
TRAUMATIC
Head injury
Perinatal trauma
INFECTIOUS
Bacterial
Viral
Fungal
Tuberculosis
Syphilis
MEDICATIONS
Opiates
Glucocorticoid therapy
Megestrol acetate
Suppressive thyroxine treatment
Dopamine
Sex steroid treatment
GnRH agonists
SYSTEMIC DISEASE
Obesity
Anorexia nervosa
Chronic illness

of pituitary origin are the most common sellar lesions, account for approximately 15% of all intracranial lesions, and are classified by cell type and size. Microadenomas are tumors with a greatest diameter of less than 10 mm. These masses are common, with an estimated incidence ranging from 1.5–27% based on autopsy series [4]. Nonsecretory microadenomas are rarely associated with hypopituitarism, and have a benign natural course [5]. Macroadenomas are less common but are frequently associated with hypopituitarism. The mechanism responsible for diminished pituitary function appears to be increased intrasellar pressure causing compression of the portal vessel blood supply to the normal pituitary, or compression of the pituitary stalk, interrupting hypothalamic control over pituitary secretion [6]. Hyperprolactinemia is commonly seen in patients with nonprolactinoma tumors due to interruption of the normal suppressive effects of dopaminergic tone from the hypothalamus. The resultant compression can lead to decreased secretion of one or many pituitary hormones. Hyperprolactinemia alone can cause hypopituitarism, specifically isolated hypogonadotropic hypogonadism, via a short feedback loop interrupting GnRH pulse regulation in the hypothalamus, with resultant decreases in LH and FSH secretion. Since the mechanism of pituitary dysfunction appears to be related to pressure-mediated effects, it is not surprising that pituitary recovery is anticipated in some, but not all, cases of pituitary mass lesions after surgical or medical decompression.

PITUITARY SURGERY

Hypopituitarism is a known risk of pituitary surgery. A number of factors contribute to the risk of hypopituitarism following surgery on a sellar mass including the size of tumor, degree of invasiveness and the level of experience of the surgeon. New hypopituitarism is found in less than 5% of patients undergoing pituitary surgery [7–9]. Further details regarding the outcomes of surgery are found in Chapter 21.

Nonpituitary Neoplasms

A number of nonpituitary neoplastic lesions can cause hypopituitarism due to their proximity to the pituitary gland and hypothalamus. Craniopharyngiomas arise from the remnants of Rathke's pouch and may be cystic, solid, or mixed tumors. Due to the involvement of the pituitary stalk and hypothalamus, craniopharyngiomas frequently present with diabetes insipidus (up to 38%), in addition to some degree of anterior pituitary failure (up to 95%) [10].

Metastatic lesions from breast, lung, colon and prostate primary tumors have been described in the sella. These tumors generally spread to the hypothalamus or posterior pituitary prior to invasion of the anterior pituitary. Diabetes insipidus may result from metastatic lesions; however, other manifestations of pituitary failure are rare, especially since the time to develop symptomatic hypopituitarism is lengthy and patients may not live long enough for symptoms to be apparent.

Other rare solid tumors in the parasellar area can cause hypopituitarism. These include pituiticytomas, fibromas, parasellar meningiomas, paragangliomas, teratomas and germ cell tumors, chordomas and angiomas [11–13]. Sarcomas are a rare cause of hypopituitarism which arise from structures adjacent to the pituitary and cause compression of the adenohypophysis. These include fibrosarcomas, osteosarcomas and undifferentiated sarcomas [14–16].

Cystic Lesions

Cystic lesions found in the region of the sella may cause pituitary dysfunction and include cystic adenomas, Rathke's cleft cysts, arachnoid cysts, epidermoid cysts and dermoid cysts [17]. Rathke's cleft cysts arise from cystic remnants during the formation of Rathke's pouch. They are thin-walled cysts lined by cuboidal or columnar ciliated epithelium. The size and growth rate of these lesions is variable. They may be intrasellar, intrasellar with extrasellar extension, or rarely entirely suprasellar. Arachnoid cysts are derived from the arachnoid membrane and are usually located in the suprasellar subarachnoid space. Epidermoid cysts are rare causes of hypopituitarism. These unilocular cysts are slow-growing and lined by laminated squamous epithelium, and rarely become malignant. Dermoid cysts have a firm fibrous capsule, lined by keratinized squamous epithelium. Other tissue types may be present in the cyst wall [18].

Aneurysms

Aneurysms of the cavernous portion of the carotid artery or branches from the circle of Willis may compress the hypothalamic/pituitary unit resulting in hypopituitarism [19]. The appearance of an aneurysm in the parasellar area may resemble a pituitary adenoma, and careful consideration of this entity is required prior to invasive interventions.

Infiltrative Lesions

Lymphocytic Hypophysitis

Lymphocytic hypophysitis is characterized by lymphocytic infiltration and destruction of the pituitary resulting in various degrees of hypopituitarism. It is commonly seen in the postpartum period and during pregnancy, and is most likely due to an autoimmune process, although subtle variations in histopathology may indicate two separate underlying immune processes [20]. It is predominately seen in women; however, a growing number of reports in children and men have been described.

Infiltration may affect the anterior pituitary (hypophysitis), the infundibulum and posterior pituitary (infundibulohypophysitis), or both. The anterior pituitary is most commonly affected resulting in pituitary hormone deficits, without diabetes insipidus. Infiltration of the posterior pituitary and infundibulum may present with diabetes insipidus and hyperprolactinemia, and infiltration of the entire hypophysis is rarely seen but presents with both anterior and posterior pituitary dysfunction. There are three forms of hypophysitis: lymphocytic, granulomatous and xanthogranulomatous. Lymphocytic infiltration has been shown to be mostly cytotoxic T-lymphocyte cells that cause anterior pituicyte destruction and replacement with fibrosis. The presence of giant cells and granulomatous formation suggests the more rare entity, granulomatous hypophysitis. Granulomatous hypophysitis occurs in equal frequency in men and women and has a reported incidence of 1:1,000,000 [21]. Xanthomatous hypophysitis is exceedingly rare and is characterized by the presence of foamy macrophages, lymphocytes and plasma cells [22,23]. Hypophysitis is generally a primary disease of the pituitary; however, it has been associated with infectious etiologies, Langerhans cell histiocytosis, sarcoidosis, Wegener's granulomatosis, Crohn's disease, Takayasu arteritis, and ruptured cysts [21].

Patients generally present with symptoms of a pituitary mass, either with headaches or visual disturbances, and symptoms of pituitary insufficiency. Since it is commonly associated with pregnancy and the postpartum period, failure of lactation and lack of menses may be one of the first signs of disease. Symptoms of multiple pituitary deficiencies occur in 75% of cases [24–27]. Thyrotroph and corticotroph cells appear to be affected more frequently in lymphocytic hypophysitis with sparing of the gonadal axis. Prolactin levels may range from undetectable to elevated, with low levels of prolactin attributable to destruction of lactotrophs, an uncommon finding in other pituitary masses. Elevated levels of prolactin may be expected during pregnancy and the postpartum period, but have been reported in men and nonpregnant women [21,28].

Characteristically, MRI shows an enlarged pituitary gland, and suprasellar extension is common [22,24,26]. The findings are usually distinguishable from pituitary adenomas [29]. With hypophysitis, the gland is symmetrically enlarged with uniform enhancement with gadolinium. The gland is usually low signal on T_1-weighted images and high signal on T_2-weighted images. Images obtained later in the disease process may demonstrate shrinkage, fibrosis and an empty sella [21].

The diagnosis of hypophysitis should be strongly considered in female patients who are pregnant or who have recently delivered, and have symptoms of pituitary insufficiency. A heightened index of suspicion should be present in patients with other autoimmune disease processes. Biopsy of the mass is necessary to definitively make the diagnosis; however, a presumptive diagnosis can be made in the proper clinical setting with typical imaging characteristics, rapid development of symptoms, and hypopituitarism affecting ACTH secretion and TSH secretion with a serum prolactin level below the normal range.

The natural course of history of lymphocytic hypophysitis is variable. The disease is marked by initial inflammation, infiltration and enlargement of the gland, accompanied by mass effects. Destruction of the gland follows with resultant hypopituitarism of varying degrees. Cases of spontaneous partial and complete recovery have been documented, with complete resolution of the pituitary mass [30–32]. Management of lymphocytic hypophysitis ranges from conservative management to more aggressive resection of the mass. Corticosteroid therapy has been advocated, but the effects are variable [21]. All patients require appropriate replacement of deficient pituitary hormones, with attempts to withdraw replacement after the acute phase to assess for recovery of pituitary function.

Sarcoidosis and Other Granulomatous Diseases

Central nervous system involvement occurs in approximately 5–15% of patients with sarcoidosis. These granulomatous lesions of the hypothalamus commonly result in hypopituitarism and diabetes insipidus [33]. Sarcoidosis is generally not seen in the hypothalamic region without evidence of systemic involvement. Infiltration can be visualized on MRI in the hypothalamus, infundibulum, or pituitary. Corticosteroid therapy often improves the appearance of the lesion, but deficits in pituitary function usually remain [33]. Giant cell granuloma is a rare cause of pituitary failure, affecting primarily the anterior pituitary [34]. Langerhans cell histiocytosis is a rare proliferative disease characterized by infiltration of organs by abnormal dendritic cells [34,35]. Hypopituitarism generally is caused by infiltration of the hypothalamus and is found in 20% of cases. Wegener's granulomatosis is a rare cause of pituitary insufficiency, with partial or panhypopituitarism [36]. Other forms of granulomatous disease have been associated with failing pituitary function including idiopathic giant cell hypophysitis, Takayasu's disease, Cogan's syndrome and Crohn's disease [34].

Hemochromatosis

Hereditary hemochromatosis is an autosomal recessive disorder and is a rare cause of hypopituitarism [37]. Excessive absorption of dietary iron leads to iron overload. Hypopituitarism is the result of iron infiltration of the anterior pituitary. Hypogonadism is the most common pituitary manifestation, with preferred uptake of iron by gonadotroph cells [38]. Secondary hypogonadism is also reported, and infiltration at multiple areas may be seen in more severe disease. TSH and ACTH deficiencies have been described but are less common.

Pituitary Irradiation

Hypopituitarism is a well-known complication of radiation treatment of pituitary tumors and other masses and malignancies, and has been extensively documented and reviewed [39]. Advances in stereotactic techniques and delivery systems providing focused beams of various types of radiation have the theoretical benefit of precise treatment of the disease without adverse effects on normal surrounding tissue. Despite these advances, the pituitary tissue often receives significant doses of radiation during therapy, with the propensity to develop hypopituitarism over the years following treatment [40–43]. As an example, 76 patients with secretory adenomas were treated with stereotactic radiosurgery and observed for a mean of 96 months. Remission of secretory function was achieved in 45% of these patients with 23% experiencing new hypopituitarism [40]. In comparison, prior long-term evaluation of hypopituitarism following radiation therapy demonstrates up to 80% prevalence of new deficits in gonadotroph, thyrotroph, or adrenocorticotroph function [44–46]. Whether newer modalities utilizing stereotactic gamma knife radiosurgery are less prone to complications of hypopituitarism is yet to be determined, as few studies have been published with large numbers of treated patients.

Pituitary adenomas are the most common sellar masses treated with radiation therapy. Residual secretory tumors and nonfunctioning adenomas are treated for control of hormonal activity and tumor growth. Multiple adverse effects of radiation therapy include optic neuropathy, second brain tumors, vascular injury, as well as hypopituitarism, necessitating lifelong monitoring [47]. Radiotherapy is commonly delivered in fractionated doses of 1.8 Gy over 25 fractions, for a total dose of 45 Gy. Radiosurgery, utilizing doses of 15–30 Gy during a single session, has been used more frequently in the past decade. The incidence of radiation-induced hypopituitarism varies from study to study and reaches 100% in some series [39].

A number of effects of radiation on normal and neoplastic tissue may be responsible for hypopituitarism seen after treatment. DNA damage induced by ionizing radiation may have acute or delayed effects on cell replication, possibly explaining the delayed onset of hypopituitarism. Degenerative changes in glial cells may lead to damage to the hypothalamic supportive structures causing chronic and subacute neural damage. Vascular damage leads to long-term damage to pituitary and parasellar tissues [39].

Hypothalamic damage is likely responsible for early radiation-induced hypopituitarism, whereas pituitary damage is more associated with late-onset hypopituitarism. Typically, growth hormone and gonadotropin secretion are more susceptible to effects of radiation than TSH or ACTH secretion. The mechanism underlying this expected progression of deficiencies is unknown. Most patients present with a typical progression of deficiencies starting with GH deficiency, gonadotropin deficiency, ACTH deficiency, progressing to TSH deficiency [48]. However, any deficiency can arise at any time, even years after the radiation treatment.

Infectious Etiologies

A wide array of infectious agents has been described as etiologies of pituitary insufficiency. These are, however, all rare causes of pituitary failure. Most infectious etiologies spread via hematogenous spread or by direct extension. Bacterial infections with abscess formation have been described, with a variety of pathogens as a bacterial source: *Staphylococcus aureus, Streptococcus pyogenes, Pseudomonas, Klebsiella ozaenae, Bacteroides*, Gram-positive *Coryneform* rods, have all been associated with abscess formation [49]. Fungal infections caused by *Aspergillosis, Coccidiomycosis, Candida albicans* and *Histoplasmosis* have been described [34]. Granulomatous infections from *Mycobacterium tuberculosis* have been described. Syphilitic gummatous lesions have been described. Hypopituitarism in the setting of HIV infection has been described, as well as other viral pathogens [50].

Pituitary Hemorrhage

Apoplexy

Pituitary tumor apoplexy is a rare event resulting in spontaneous hemorrhage or infarction of a pituitary adenoma [51]. Sudden hemorrhage increases the intrasellar volume and pressure compressing surrounding structures, portal vessels and normal pituitary tissue. The increase in pressure results in sudden onset of headache, visual disturbance and acute pituitary insufficiency [52]. Subclinical hemorrhage may be present in existing pituitary adenomas; however, this entity is distinctly separate from the syndrome of acutely deteriorating pituitary function in the setting of hemorrhage into the pituitary adenoma [53]. Spontaneous hemorrhage may be present without clinically significant symptoms in up to 25% of patients [51,53].

The true incidence of pituitary tumor apoplexy or subclinical hemorrhage is difficult to establish. It is a rare event, with reported incidences ranging from 0.6–27.7%, but these estimates may include subclinical cases [54]. Nearly 50% of cases occur in patients without prior knowledge of a pituitary adenoma. All types of pituitary tumors are susceptible to apoplectic events, and men appear to be affected more commonly than women. Most cases present in the fifth or sixth decade of life, but cases have spanned the first through eighth decades.

Patients present with acute onset of headache and visual disturbance, including cranial nerve palsies resulting in extraocular muscle defects. Neurological signs may be present, including an altered level of consciousness and meningismus. Generalized symptoms are not uncommon with nausea and vomiting, malaise and lethargy frequently reported. Endocrine dysfunction contributes to the morbidity and mortality associated with pituitary tumor apoplexy with acute ACTH deficiency having a central role. The extent of pituitary dysfunction varies with adrenal insufficiency occurring in 50–100% of cases, thyroid dysfunction present in 25–75% of cases and gonadal function impaired in 60–100% of cases [51]. Noncontrast CT scan of the sella turcica reveals acute hemorrhage, and MRI of the sella may be helpful to elucidate the extent of parasellar involvement. Hemorrhage is more evident on MRI in the subacute phase than during the acute phase.

Sheehan's Syndrome

The pituitary gland normally enlarges during pregnancy. Postpartum pituitary necrosis occurs in women who suffer large-volume hemorrhage during delivery, resulting in hypovolemic shock and ischemia. Usual causes of hypovolemia include placenta previa or retained placenta, leading to blood loss, hypovolemia and necrosis of the enlarged pituitary due to the limited blood supply. Loss of pituitary function may be partial or complete. Due to advances in obstetrical care, and peripartum supportive measures, Sheehan's syndrome is not commonly encountered.

Congenital and Inheritable Pituitary Insufficiency

Developmental Pituitary Dysfunction

Pituitary development occurs after midline cell migration from Rathke's pouch. Structural pituitary abnormalities are seen with midline anomalies such as corpus callosum and anterior commissure defects. Congenital absence of the pituitary and ectopic pituitary tissue is rarely encountered, although functional ectopic posterior pituitary tissue is sometimes incidentally noted on brain or pituitary imaging. Craniofacial anomalies such as cleft lip and palate, septo-optic dysplasia and basal encephalocele often present with varying degrees of pituitary dysfunction and hypoplasia. Children with congenital malformations and structural defects impairing pituitary function require lifelong replacement of pituitary deficiencies. Improvements in imaging techniques over the years have led to improved detection of structural abnormalities accompanying pituitary and hypothalamic deficits. Patients may present with a small pituitary, complete or partial empty sella, ectopic posterior pituitary, or pituitary stalk abnormalities.

Genetic Factors

Mutations of several genes including those responsible for pituitary hormone production, hormone receptors and pituitary development can cause hypopituitarism (Table 10.2) [55]. Several transcription factors involved in pituitary development and function have been identified in recent years and mutations in any of these factors may lead to multiple or isolated pituitary deficiencies [56]. Mutations in genes specific for single pituitary hormones and receptors give rise to isolated hormonal deficiencies. Morphological changes, often but not always limited to the pituitary and parasellar region, may be evident. The roles of these transcriptional factors are complex and interdependent upon each other in many circumstances. The embryogenesis and development of the pituitary and the roles that each of these factors play in development of the adenohypophysis is addressed elsewhere in this text (see Chapter 1).

Prop-1 (OMIM601538) is the most common factor associated with multiple pituitary deficiencies occurring in as many as 50% of patients with combined pituitary deficits. The gene, located on chromosome 5q, is required for subsequent Pit-1 activation. Several human mutations have been described associated with deficiencies in GH, TSH, PRL and gonadotropins. Human Prop-1 mutations are associated with deficiencies in Pit-1-dependent cell lines (GH, PRL, TSH) and impaired gonadotroph and corticotroph reserve, despite these latter cell lines not being Pit-1-dependent. Several mutations have been associated with the phenotype of multiple pituitary deficiencies. The inheritance mode is autosomal recessive, thus patients are homozygous for either deletion or missense frameshift mutations. The resulting protein product is truncated and nonfunctional. GA or AG deletions in a Prop-1 hotspot on exon 2 result in a coding frameshift and termination at codon 109. Siblings that are unaffected are either heterozygous or homozygous for a normal Prop-1 sequence on both alleles. Prop-1 gene mutations are frequently found in patients with combined pituitary hormone deficiencies occurring in as many as 30–50% of affected subjects [57]. Clinical features most often include a presentation of hypogonadism, with delayed or absent puberty. Some patients will enter puberty spontaneously and present with late-onset hypogonadotropic hypogonadism, similar to patients with acquired disease [58]. Patients may develop or present with adrenal

TABLE 10.2 Genetic Disorders of Hypothalamo–Pituitary Development in Humans

Gene	Phenotype	Inheritance
Isolated hormone abnormalities		
GH1	Isolated GH deficiency	AR, AD
GHRHR	Isolated GH deficiency	AR
TSH-ß	Isolated TSH deficiency	AR
TRHR	Isolated TSH deficiency	AR
TPIT	Isolated ACTH deficiency	AR
GnRHR	HH	AR
PCI	ACTH deficiency, hypoglycemia, HH, obesity	AR
POMC	ACTH deficiency, obesity, red hair	AR
DAX1	Adrenal hypoplasia congenital and HH	XL
CRH	CRH deficiency	AR
KAL1	Kallman syndrome, renal angenesis, synkinesia	XL
FGFR1	Kallman syndrome, cleft lip and palate, facial dysmorphism	AD, AR
Leptin	HH, obesity	AR
Leptin-R	HH, obesity	AR
GPR54	HH	AR
Kisspeptin	HH	AR
FSH-ß	Primary amenorrhea, defective spermatogenesis	AR
LH-ß	Delayed puberty	AR
PROK2	Kallman syndrome, severe sleep disorder, obesity	AD
PROKR2	Kallman syndrome	AD, AR
AVP-NP11	Diabetes insipidus	AR, AD
Combined pituitary hormone deficiency		
POU1F1	GH, TSH and prolactin deficiencies	AR, AD
PROP1	GH, TSH, LH, FSH, prolactin and evolving ACTH deficiencies	AR
Specific syndrome		
HESX1	Septo-optic dysplasia	AR, AD
LHX3	GH, TSH, LH, FSH, prolactin deficiencies, limited neck rotation	AR
LHX4	GH, TSH, ACTH deficiencies with cerebellar abnormalities	AD
SOX3	Hypopituitarism and mental retardation	XL
GLI2	Holoprosencephaly and multiple midline defects	AD
SOX2	Anophthalmia, hypopituitarism, esophageal atresia	AD
GLI3	Pallister-Hall syndrome	AD
PITX2	Rieger syndrome	AD

R, receptor; GH, growth hormone; AR, autosomal recessive; AD, autosomal dominant; TSH, thyroid-stimulating hormone; ACTH, adrenocorticotrophic hormone; HH, hypogonadotrophic hypogonadism; XL, X-linked; CRH, corticotrophin-releasing hormone; LH, luteinizing hormone; FSH, follicle-stimulating hormone.

Reproduced with permission from [54].

insufficiency or panhypopituitarism [59]. The appearance of the pituitary on MRI may be hypoplastic or normal. Cystic changes may be present with the appearance of empty sella. Linear growth arrest becomes evident after the age of 3, with height severely lower than expected. Eunicoid habitus and reduced upper to lower body proportions may be seen. Affected adults usually have short stature and lack secondary sexual characteristics [60].

The Pou1F1 gene (formerly known as Pit-1) (OMIM173110) is located on chromosome 3p11 and contains two protein domains, the POU-specific and the POU-homeo [56]. Both of these domains are necessary for DNA binding, transcription of the GH and PRL genes and regulating PRL, TSH-ß and Pit-1 genes. The Pit-1 nuclear protein activates the transcription of the PRL, GH, TSH and GHRH receptor genes. Pit-1 acts with coactivator proteins such as cyclic AMP response element-binding (CREB) protein, P-Lim, Ptx-1, HESX-1 and Zn-15. Pit-1 expression is autoregulated, and is restricted to the anterior pituitary. Its expression is necessary for development of lactotrophs, somatotrophs, and thyrotrophs. Most mutations in Pou1F1 are recessive, but five autosomal dominant mutations have been described. The most common dominant mutation is the R271W mutation [61]. Inactivating mutations of the gene result in varied pituitary hormone deficiencies [62]. However, several Pou1F1 mutations have characteristic clinical phenotypes [57]. In general, GH and prolactin deficiencies are the first to become apparent clinically, with TSH deficiency presenting later in childhood [63]. The anterior pituitary may be small or normal on MRI, with normal posterior pituitary.

HESX1 (Rpx) is the earliest known transcriptional marker of the developing pituitary and is limited to

Rathke's pouch. The expression of HESX1 is essential for normal forebrain and pituitary formation. HESX1 expression declines as specific pituitary cell types develop and is longer expressed in the mature pituitary. The gene is located on chromosome 3p212 and encodes a 185-amino acid protein that competes with Prop-1 protein for DNA binding. Septo-optic dysplasia is associated with a homozygous Arg53Cys homeodomain mutation, but only accounts for approximately 1% of subjects affected by septo-optic dysplasia. Affected patients have panhypopituitarism, possibly related to the anatomical and structural anomalies associated with the syndrome.

Lhx4 and Lhx3 are members of the LIM homeodomain protein family and mutations of each have been described with combined pituitary hormone deficiencies. LHX3 is expressed in the anterior and intermediate lobes of the pituitary, spinal cord and medulla. Three LHX3 isoforms have been identified in humans, including hLHX3a, hLHX3b and hM2-LHX3. Patients with mutations in LHX3 have deficiencies in GH, PRL, TSH and gonadotropins [64]. They also demonstrate abnormal pituitary morphology and a rigid cervical spine limiting rotation [65]. LHX3 homozygous mutations are a rare form of hypopituitarism accounting for 2.2% of patients with panhypopituitarism. Mutations in the LHX4 gene result in the arrest of the formation of Rathke's pouch and a hypoplastic pituitary. Mutations in the LHX4 gene prohibit activation of both Prop-1 and Pou1F1, resulting in pituitary failure [66]. In addition to pituitary deficiencies, findings of ectopic posterior pituitary, cerebellar abnormalities, Chiari malformation and poorly developed sella turcica have been described [63].

OTX2 is a transcription factor required for formation of forebrain structures. Mutations have been implicated in syndromes of anophthalmia and microphthalmia in humans. Heterozygous mutations have been associated with eye abnormalities and variable pituitary defects [67,68]. MRI appearance of the pituitary is small or normal with an ectopic posterior pituitary. OTX2 mutations have also rarely been reported in patients with pituitary deficits without ocular anomalies [69].

Isolated hormone deficiencies also occur due to genetic mutations in genes encoding hormones and receptors. Congenital isolated GH deficiency is mostly sporadic, with an incidence of approximately 1:4000 to 1:10,000 live births. Four familial forms comprise 5–30% of cases [70,71]. Isolated GHD may be autosomal dominant, autosomal recessive or X-linked. Autosomal recessive forms are associated with mutations in GH1 and GHRHR genes. Autosomal dominant forms have been described due to mutations in GH1 gene. An X-linked form is associated with agammaglobulinemia or hypogammaglobulinemia, but no gene has been found associated with this syndrome [63].

Autosomal recessive mutations in TBX19 (TPIT) are the primary cause of congenital isolated ACTH deficiency [72]. Mutations result in profound hypoglycemia, seizures and cholestatic jaundice, and may be an under-appreciated cause of neonatal mortality. Basal plasma levels of ACTH and cortisol are very low with lack of ACTH stimulation after CRH administration. POMC mutations are also associated with isolated ACTH deficiency [73].

Septo-optic dysplasia (de Morsier syndrome) is a heterogeneous syndrome. Diagnosis relies upon the presence of two of the three following features: optic nerve hypoplasia, midline forebrain defects (agenesis of the corpus callosum and absent septum pellucidum) and pituitary hypoplasia. Pituitary insufficiency is variable in this condition [74]. Approximately 30% of patients have all three features, with hypopituitarism evident in approximately 60%, and 60% with absent septum pellucidum. Optic nerve abnormalities may be unilateral or bilateral, and this may be the initial presenting feature. Neurological symptoms are common, ranging from focal deficits to developmental delay. Hypopituitarism ranges from isolated GH deficiency to panhypopituitarism. Gonadotropin secretion may be retained. Pituitary deficiencies may develop over time, and usually do not include posterior pituitary deficits. The etiology is multifactorial, with cases usually being sporadic, and multiple factors including genetic and environmental exposures being implicated. Mutations in HESX1, SOX2 and SOX3 have been implicated, but the majority of cases do not have an identifiable mutation [75].

Prader-Willi syndrome is a genetic disease characterized by hypotonia, short stature, hyperphagia, mild mental retardation, obesity and hypogonadotropic hypogonadism. The defects indicate a hypothalamic source for dysfunction in growth, sexual development, hunger and satiety. Details regarding Prader-Willi syndrome are addressed in Chapter 9.

Kallman's syndrome is an X-linked recessive syndrome caused by mutations in the KAL1 gene on the Xp22.3 region of the X chromosome coding for anosmin-1. The syndrome consists of hypogonadotropic hypogonadism accompanied by one or more congenital abnormalities including anosmia, midline facial anomalies, renal agenesis, neurologic abnormalities, deafness and color blindness.

Traumatic Brain Injury

It has long been known that traumatic brain injury can cause hypopituitarism. The incidence of post-traumatic hypopituitarism was thought to be rare until recent studies demonstrated the high prevalence after head trauma [76,77]. In 2000, a retrospective review characterized 367 patients with hypopituitarism following traumatic brain injury [77]. Patients in this retrospective study suffered from deficiencies in all pituitary axes. Since then, a number of studies have examined the effects of traumatic brain injury on pituitary function. Disparate methods of assessment of pituitary function, degrees of traumatic brain injury, and varying definitions of post-traumatic hypopituitarism have contributed to a wide variation in incidence and prevalence of hypopituitarism following traumatic brain injury [78]. However, it seems evident that hypopituitarism is a common consequence of traumatic brain injury with a prevalence of at least 25% [76].

Hypopituitarism results from local trauma to the vasculature supplying the anterior pituitary. The major blood supply is from the hypophyseal portal circulation. The inferior hypophyseal artery branches off from the internal carotid artery, supplying a small portion of the adenohypophysis and posterior pituitary. Edema, hemorrhage, increased cranial pressure and skull fracture can compress the normal pituitary and vasculature, causing damage. Mechanical injury to the stalk and infundibulum also may contribute to insufficient pituitary function. Hypopituitarism may manifest in the acute setting following head trauma, including secondary hypogonadism, TSH deficiency and hyperprolactinemia [79]. After recovery, patients may have persistent deficiencies, or may develop late onset of pituitary deficiencies during the first year after trauma.

A systematic review of hypopituitarism following traumatic brain injury demonstrated a prevalence of 15–50% in patients with a history of head trauma, and a prevalence of 38–55% in patients with subarachnoid hemorrhage [80]. A total of 809 patients with traumatic brain injury were studied, with GH deficiency seen in 6–33%, gonadotropin deficiency in 2–20%, ACTH deficiency in 0–19%, TSH deficiency in 1–10% and multiple deficiencies seen in 4–12% [80]. With the number of hospitalizations and deaths from traumatic brain injuries occurring each year totaling approximately 180–250 persons per 100,000 population, it is clear that a large segment of the population has been overlooked in the diagnosis and treatment of hypopituitarism [81,82]. Increased awareness is necessary at the primary care level and in subspecialty practice to fully address this cause of hypopituitarism. Additionally, further prospective studies are needed to elaborate the optimal timing of assessment and benefit of replacement in these patients.

Empty Sella Syndrome

Replacement of sellar contents with cerebrospinal fluid can impact pituitary function. Empty sella syndrome can occur as a primary event, theoretically due to weakness of the diaphragma sella and herniation of the arachnoid space into the sella, or can be secondary to surgery, radiation, or infarction of a pre-existing adenoma or other mass. Primary empty sella may be associated with increased intracranial pressure [83]. The appearance of an empty sella on MRI usually consists of either a complete or partial filling of the sellar space with CSF. Pituitary tissue may be visibly compressed against the floor of the sella. In most circumstances, an empty sella is an incidental finding with normal pituitary function. However, one large case series reported endocrine abnormalities in approximately 20% of patients with partial or complete empty sella [83]. The most common endocrine abnormality reported was hyperprolactinemia (10%) and panhypopituitarism was present in 4%. Isolated GH deficiency was also noted in 4% of patients.

FUNCTIONAL CAUSES OF PITUITARY FAILURE

Multiple disorders associated with functional disruption of pituitary hormone secretion are usually limited to an isolated pituitary hormone, and are generally reversible when the underlying cause is corrected. Critical illness can have a profound impact on pituitary function and can lead to low levels of multiple pituitary hormones and target hormones. These abnormalities, as well as other functional causes of pituitary failure, are covered in detail in other chapters (see Chapters 9 and 11).

Functional Central Adrenal Insufficiency

Central adrenal insufficiency due to suppression of the hypothalamic–pituitary–adrenal (HPA) axis after glucocorticoid administration is the most common cause of adrenal insufficiency. The dose, duration of therapy and frequency of administration all put patients at risk for adrenal insufficiency once the treatment is stopped. Glucocorticoid administration suppresses both ACTH and CRH secretion. This results in eventual adrenal cortex atrophy and failure to maintain normal cortisol levels. Multiple sources of exogenous glucocorticoids have been implicated in causing adrenal insufficiency, including oral, inhaled [84,85], topical [86] and injections [87]. Concomitant retroviral therapy for HIV infection may exacerbate the suppression [87,88]. Recovery from adrenal insufficiency during glucocorticoid withdrawal can be prolonged, with some cases extending as long as 18 months after the therapeutic regimen. During this period, replacement doses are given to avoid symptomatic adrenal insufficiency, stress doses are advised during illness or physiologic stress, and medic alert bracelets should be worn.

During the recovery period of the HPA axis, corticotroph activity recovers prior to adequate adrenal cortex recovery. Periodic assessment of adrenal activity with synthetic ACTH stimulation, coordinated with appropriate temporary holding of replacement glucocorticoids, will assist in the management of adrenal insufficiency and establish HPA axis recovery.

In addition to exogenous glucocorticoid therapy, longstanding endogenous glucocorticoid excess has a suppressive effect on the normal secretion of CRH, pituitary corticotroph activity and ACTH secretion. Cure of Cushing's syndrome from an adrenal source or an ACTH-dependent source can render the patient adrenally insufficient. Similar to assessment and treatment of patients with adrenal insufficiency due to exogenous steroid excess, patients recovering from endogenous glucocorticoid excess should be treated with replacement glucocorticoids, given stress doses when appropriate and advised to wear a medic alert bracelet. Recovery of normal adrenal function can be months after successful treatment of endogenous Cushing's syndrome.

Treatment with megestrol acetate, a medication used primarily to increase appetite in patients with wasting and failure to maintain normal weight, can cause adrenal insufficiency when withdrawn. Megestrol acetate is a progestin with glucocorticoid activity, and while symptoms of adrenal insufficiency are rare during therapy, treatment with stress doses of glucocorticoids is necessary in times of physiologic stress to avoid adrenal crisis.

Functional Central Hypothyroidism

Central hypothyroidism occurs in a few settings due to functional causes that are reversible with time. Recovery of thyrotroph activity after longstanding hyperthyroidism occurs in both exogenous administration of thyroid hormone and after cure of endogenous hyperthyroidism. Treatment of hyperthyroid states with antithyroid drugs, radioactive iodine and surgery may render the patient hypothyroid for a number of weeks. Prolonged exogenous thyroid hormone treatment of thyroid nodules, goiter, or thyroid cancer, with the intent to suppress TSH, can lead to central hypothyroidism for a short duration after discontinuation of therapy.

In addition to suppression by thyroid hormone, other medications and hormones can have suppressive effects on TSH secretion. Dopamine, glucocorticoids and somatostatin analogues have all been reported to suppress TSH secretion. These medications rarely lead to clinically significant or prolonged hypothyroidism. Nonthyroidal illness may also have a transient, nonclinically significant phase of hypothyroidism, which recovers during the recovery phase of the nonthyroidal illness.

Functional Hypogonadotropic Hypogonadism

Failure of the gonadal axis can result from functional defects that occur in the absence of structural or genetic causes. In females, a common cause of amenorrhea is commonly referred to as hypothalamic amenorrhea or functional amenorrhea. Functional amenorrhea may result from weight loss, hypocaloric diet, exercise, or stress. Similarly in some, but not all, men dietary restriction or extreme exercise may cause a hypogonadotropic hypogonadism. Endocrine abnormalities associated with anorexia nervosa are discussed in Chapter 9.

Hyperprolactinemia causes impairment of the gonadal axis in both men and women. Any cause of hyperprolactinemia can interfere with GnRH pulse generation in the hypothalamus via a short feedback loop causing decreased gonadotropin secretion and a reduction in sex steroid secretion. Treatment of hyperprolactinemia results in normalization of the gonadal axis in most cases, with resolution of the hypogonadotropic hypogonadism.

Prolonged use of testosterone can result in suppression of the gonadal axis with variable time to recover after cessation of therapy. Testosterone can also have a suppressive effect on residual spermatogenesis during treatment. Similarly, GnRH analogues, commonly used in treatment of prostate cancer, result in suppression of gonadotroph secretion and hypogonadism.

Obesity is associated with lower levels of testosterone in men. Hypogonadism in obesity is predominately primary; however, in cases of morbid obesity the etiology can be central in origin, with laboratory findings consistent with hypogonadotropic hypogonadism [89].

Functional Growth Hormone Deficiency

There are multiple factors that negatively impact GH secretion, with obesity and visceral adiposity being one of the most common causes of low levels of GH, both during 24-hour sampling and after stimulation with various secretagogues [90]. Low levels of growth hormone present in obese individuals improve with weight loss, either from diet and exercise or from bariatric surgery.

Children can have transient growth failure due to nongrowth-hormone endocrine abnormalities, psychosocial causes and idiopathic isolated GH deficiencies. GH secretion is impaired in the setting of hypothyroidism, Cushing's syndrome, delayed puberty and isolated ACTH deficiency. Approximately 40% of children diagnosed with idiopathic GH deficiency in childhood are found to be GH sufficient when retested as adults. Psychosocial dwarfism is covered in Chapter 9.

CLINICAL MANIFESTATIONS

The clinical manifestations of anterior pituitary failure are variable depending upon the age and gender of onset, the pituitary axes affected and the underlying disease. The presentation and findings associated with each individual pituitary hormone will be described here, with the associated manifestations specific to gender and age.

Manifestations of Secondary Adrenal Insufficiency

Symptoms of secondary adrenal insufficiency can present insidiously with a gradual onset or abruptly with symptoms of adrenal crisis [91]. Chronic symptoms are largely nonspecific and consist of weakness, lethargy, malaise, nausea or abdominal pain, loss of appetite, arthralgias and myalgias. Presenting features are often associated with hypoglycemia, hypotension, or hyponatremia. Hypoglycemia stems from impaired gluconeogenesis and hyponatremia from SIADH associated with low levels of cortisol and the impaired excretion of free water with adrenal insufficiency. Adrenal crisis usually presents with hypotension in the setting of concomitant illness, and can be fatal if untreated.

Presentation of secondary insufficiency is similar to that of primary adrenal insufficiency with a few exceptions that are characteristic of ACTH deficiency with intact mineralocorticoid secretion. Unique to secondary adrenal insufficiency is the sparing of aldosterone secretion due to the preservation of renin and angiotensin control of aldosterone production and secretion by the adrenal cortex. With mineralocorticoid activity, severe hypotension is rare unless acute stress is present. Hyperkalemia, volume depletion and dehydration are not usually part of the clinical presentation. Second, the characteristic pigmentation of primary adrenal insufficiency is absent in ACTH deficiency due to absence of the increase in proopiomelanocortin (POMC)-derived peptides. In fact, due to a deficiency of melanocyte-stimulating hormone, patients with prolonged secondary adrenal insufficiency may be pale and experience diminished capacity to tan after exposure to sunlight.

Secondary adrenal insufficiency can be partial in its impairment, and symptoms may only manifest in times of physiologic stress. Symptomatic manifestations may be slow and insidious, especially if the impairment is not noticeably progressive. Patients presenting with acute ACTH deficiency may become symptomatic from either acute loss of ACTH, as in pituitary apoplexy, or from a failure to increase exogenous steroid dosing in the face of acute physiologic stress. Cardiovascular collapse can be fatal but can be responsive to steroid administration, if administered promptly.

Patients who present with secondary adrenal insufficiency usually have signs and symptoms of the underlying cause or concomitant findings suggestive of central ACTH deficiency. They may have a history of glucocorticoid use, and may appear cushingoid. Loss of other pituitary function may be present, especially the presence of central hypothyroidism. Patients presenting with endocrine active pituitary tumors, nonfunctioning pituitary tumors, other sellar masses, or signs of congenital malformations and midline defects should be evaluated for adrenal insufficiency. Laboratory evaluation may reveal mild anemia, neutropenia, hypoglycemia, or hyponatremia.

Adrenal Androgen Insufficiency

Hypopituitarism and secondary adrenal insufficiency may result in low serum levels of adrenal androgens, including androstenedione, DHEA, DHEA-S and testosterone [92]. Absence of adrenal androgens is of minimal consequence to males who retain testosterone secretion or are treated with testosterone replacement. Women who lack adrenal androgens may exhibit hair loss, unexplained fatigue, depressed mood, reduced sense of well-being, reduced stamina and loss of libido [93,94].

Manifestations of Thyrotropin Deficiency

Clinical features of central hypothyroidism are virtually indistinguishable from that of primary hypothyroidism [95]. Fatigue, lethargy, cold intolerance, constipation, dry skin, brittle hair, bradycardia, facial edema and normocytic anemia are common findings in patients with hypothyroidism. Physical exam findings may include thinning of the lateral portion of the eyebrows, a sallow appearance to the skin and a delayed relaxation phase of deep tendon reflexes. In addition to characteristic thyroid function studies, laboratory evaluation may reveal lipid abnormalities with a high total cholesterol and low HDL cholesterol. The presentation is variable with some patients being asymptomatic or unaware of symptoms and some patients having symptoms of profound hypothyroidism. Goiter is not a feature of secondary hypothyroidism.

Manifestations of Hypogonadotropic Hypogonadism

Adult Males

The presenting features of men with hypogonadotropic hypogonadism are variable and do not necessarily correlate to levels of circulating testosterone [96]. Adult males presenting with new-onset hypogonadotropic hypogonadism may present with impaired libido, impotence, decreased body and facial hair, decreased muscle mass, osteopenia or osteoporosis and atrophy of the testes. Laboratory findings may include hypercholesterolemia and decreased sperm count.

Prepubertal Males

Manifestations of hypogonadism prior to puberty may go unnoticed until puberty is delayed, defined as the absence of secondary sexual characteristics at an age more than two standard deviations above the population mean for the onset of puberty. The clinical staging of puberty has been established by James Tanner and is widely used (Figures 10.1–10.4) [97,98]. The average age for the first signs of puberty in boys is 14 with increase in testicular size being the first sign. Boys with prepubertal hypogonadism have a small penis, small testes and prostate, and scant pubic and axillary hair. They may exhibit long arms and legs with a eunicoid habitus if epiphyseal closure has been delayed. Their voices may remain high in pitch and they may have gynecomastia.

Males with pubertal delay due to congenital loss of GnRH, LH, or FSH secretion may exhibit congenital abnormalities consistent with abnormal development of the hypothalamic–pituitary axis. Patients may have midline defects, cryptorchidism, cleft lip or palate. Headaches, visual disturbance, anosmia, or mental retardation suggest a congenital gonadotropin deficiency.

Hypogonadotropic hypogonadism must be differentiated from constitutional pubertal delay, and a family history may help in making this diagnosis. However, other than expectant observation there is no method to accurately differentiate between these two entities [99]. Serial measurements of height, weight, arm span, testicular size may help clarify the diagnosis over a few years.

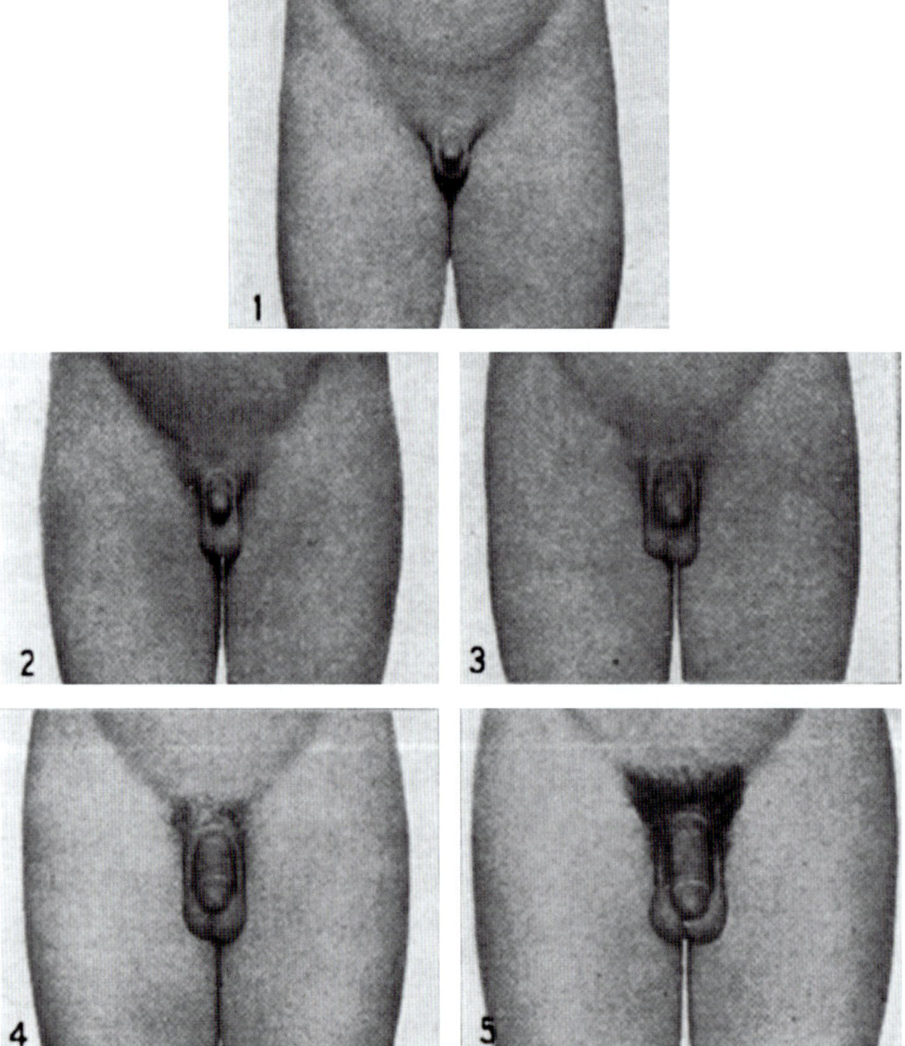

FIGURE 10.1 Clinical staging of male genital development. Tanner stages 1–5 depicted. *Used with permission from [97].*

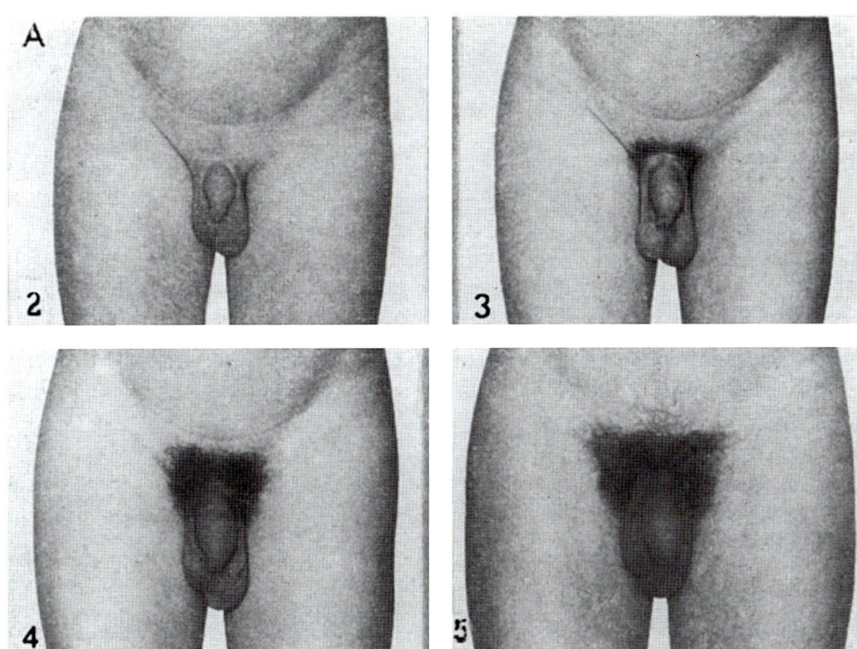

FIGURE 10.2 Clinical staging of male pubic hair development. Tanner stages 2–5 depicted. *Used with permission from [97].*

Stimulation testing can be performed but often does not clearly distinguish between these two diagnoses.

Neonatal Males

Infants presenting with hypogonadotropic hypogonadism may have the presence of a micropenis and cryptorchidism [100]. It is critical to assess the patient for concomitant pituitary deficiencies, as GH deficiency and ACTH deficiency are associated with a high risk of death due to hypoglycemia or cortisol deficiency [101].

Female Hypogonadotropic Hypogonadism

Adult Females (Secondary Amenorrhea)

The hallmark of hypogonadotropic hypogonadism occurring after puberty in premenopausal females is amenorrhea occurring for at least 3 consecutive months. Common causes of secondary amenorrhea in women are pregnancy, functional hypothalamic amenorrhea, hyperprolactinemia and polycystic ovarian syndrome. Women with hypogonadotropic hypogonadism are infertile, since

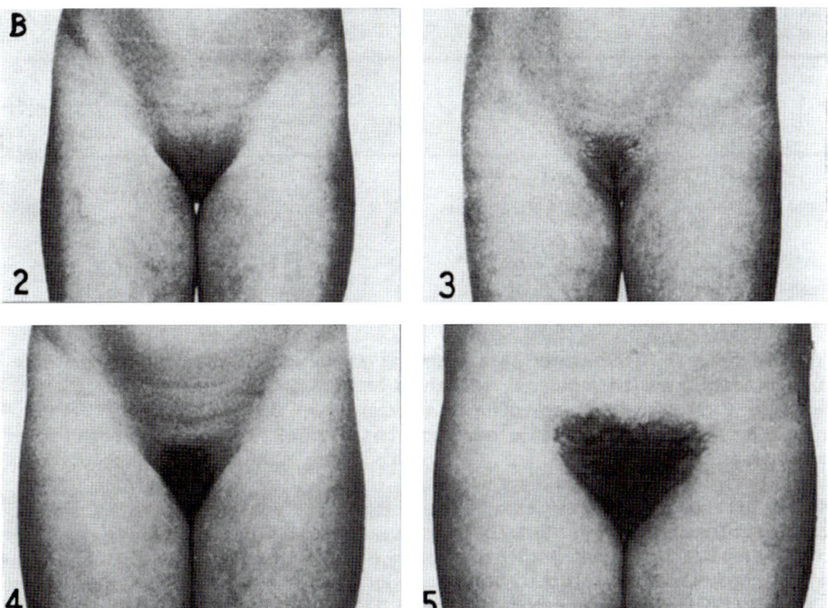

FIGURE 10.3 Clinical staging of female pubic hair development. Tanner stages 2–5 depicted. *Used with permission from [98].*

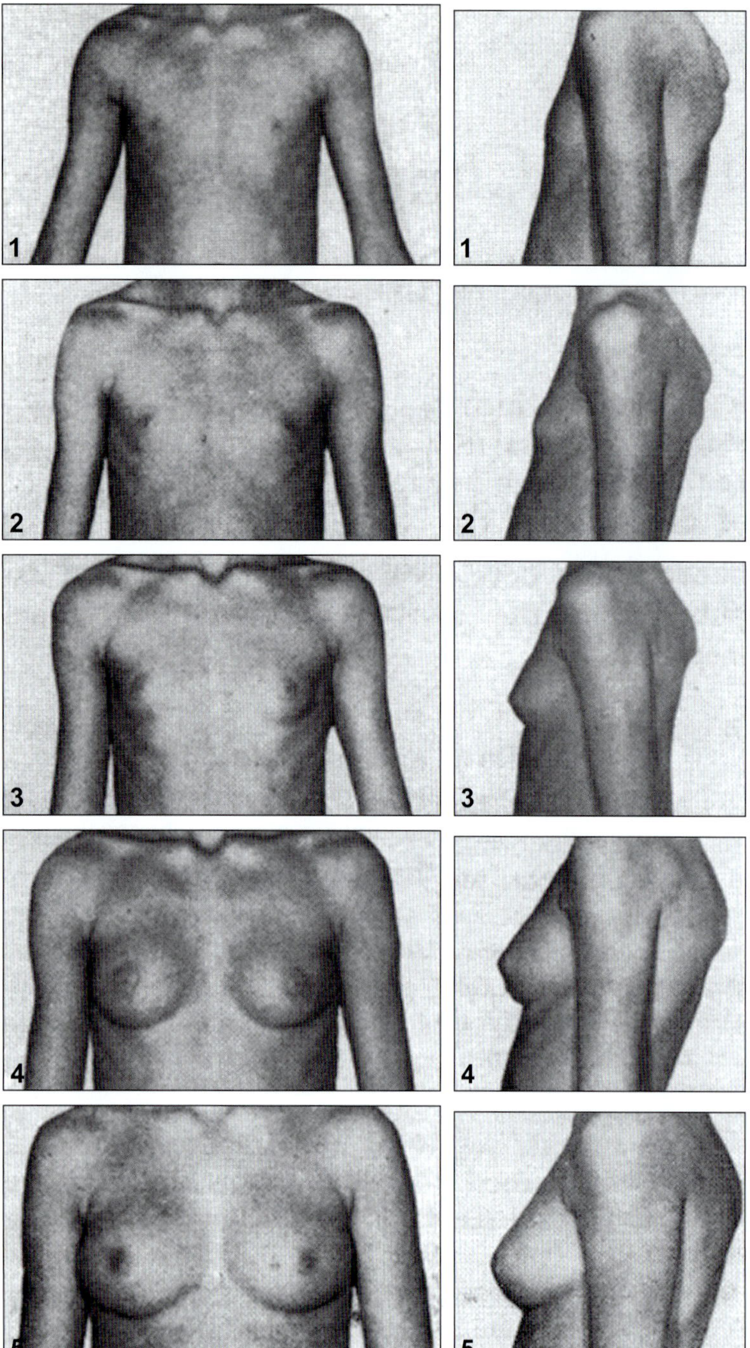

FIGURE 10.4 Clinical staging of female pubertal breast development. Tanner stages 1–5 depicted. *Used with permission from [98].*

they lack the hormones responsible for the usual regulation of follicle stimulation and ovulation. Decreased estrogen production results in symptoms similar to menopause: hypoestrogenic symptoms such as osteoporosis, decreased vaginal secretion, dyspareunia, decreased libido and atrophy of breast tissue. Postmenopausal women with hypogonadotropic hypogonadism do not manifest clinical symptoms due to deficiencies of gonadotropins, but may manifest symptoms due to other pituitary hormone deficiencies.

Primary Amenorrhea/Pubertal Delay

Hypogonadotropic hypogonadism in young females may manifest itself as an absence of menses and a complete lack of development of secondary sexual characteristics, with or without normal growth. Staging of pubertal development in girls has been established by Tanner (Figures 10.3 and 10.4) [98]. Occasionally patients may have partial pubertal development with pubertal arrest; however, complete absence of pubertal development is more common.

Growth Hormone Deficiency

Adult Onset

Clinical features of growth hormone deficiency in the adult are covered in detail in Chapter 4. The features of GH deficiency in the adult include abnormal body composition with increased visceral adiposity and decreased lean muscle mass. Patients may exhibit psychological impairment with reduced energy, social isolation, emotional lability, anxiety and depressed mood. They are typically overweight with increased central adiposity. Their skin may be cool to the touch, dry and thin. Patients have reduced muscle strength, reduction in exercise performance and may exhibit a depressed affect [102].

CARDIOVASCULAR RISK

Retrospective studies have demonstrated that patients with hypopituitarism who have not been treated for GHD have a higher mortality than patients on conventional replacement therapy [3]. This increase in mortality is largely due to cerebrovascular and cardiovascular disease [103]. Lipid profiles of GHD subjects have been variable in retrospective studies and database reviews. Subjects with GHD have higher total cholesterol levels and higher LDL levels than normal subjects [104]. Triglyceride levels have been found to be elevated [105]. Measurements of HDL levels in GHD subjects have varied. It appears that the severity and duration of GHD may be associated with the severity of the cardiovascular risk, as IGF-I levels are inversely associated with LDL levels [106,107]. Prevalence of hypertension in GHD adults is unclear. Some studies have reported higher prevalence compared to normal populations [108], while others have not found elevated blood pressures in GHD subjects [109]. The KIMS database has a prevalence of 15% of GHD adults with hypertension [104]. Other cardiovascular risk factors have been studied and found to be elevated in patients with GHD. Carotid intima media thickness is increased in subjects with GHD [110]. Higher levels of fibrinogen, PAI-1 and tPA have been found in GHD subjects [110]. Inflammatory markers such as CRP, IL-6 and homocysteine, which are associated with increased cardiovascular risk, are elevated in subjects with GHD [111,112]. Finally, left ventricular function appears to be diminished in subjects with GHD [109].

Childhood-onset GHD

Patients with congenital or childhood-onset GHD have short stature and fail to grow at a normal rate. Children with congenital GHD are born with normal height and weight, but serial measurements of height and weight demonstrate a failure to progress normally. The growth curve of acquired growth hormone deficiency is characteristic of growth failure with normal growth for a period of time and progressive fall in height away from the mean. Height tends to be affected more than weight and they appear overweight for their height, with a propensity for central weight gain in the abdomen and chest. Arm span is normal and they are normally proportioned in regard to upper and lower segment ratios. Dentition may be delayed and the voice high-pitched. When GHD is concomitant with ACTH deficiency, children may present with hypoglycemia. This is most commonly seen in abnormal development of the anterior pituitary or with idiopathic hypopituitarism. Midline developmental abnormalities such as cleft lip or palate, septo-optic dysplasia, a single incisor and congenital roaming nystagmus are associated with congenital GHD.

Prolactin Deficiency

Prolactin deficiency manifests itself solely with the inability to lactate in the postpartum time period. Absence of lactation may portend deficiencies in other pituitary hormones, warranting investigation.

DIAGNOSTIC TESTING

The diagnosis of anterior pituitary failure requires the assessment of the integrity of the various stimulatory hormones secreted by the pituitary (Table 10.3). For the assessment of certain axes, dynamic testing is required due to the pulsatility of the pituitary hormones, and in others, dual assessment of the trophic hormone and target gland hormone is sufficient. The selection of the appropriate test can differ depending upon the age of the patient. Over the years, various tests have been developed and have either fallen out of favor due to advances in other testing methodologies, convenience of other methods of testing, or the discontinuation of key components of the tests themselves.

Assay Variability

In general, assessment of pituitary function is reliant on the measurement of hormones in serum. Distinguishing normal responses to stimulation testing, or normal basal serum levels from those of patients with pituitary insufficiency is also dependent upon establishing generalizable cutoff points that can be applied to clinical practice. It is well understood that as the field of clinical biochemistry advances, the methodology for assays will evolve. Techniques change and require validation, and therefore, cutoff points established under prior conditions require re-evaluation. A great deal of variability is inherent in the various methodologies employed by laboratories to measure hormones and

TABLE 10.3 Pituitary Hormone Diagnostic Testing

Pituitary Axis	Test	Method	Expected Results
Corticotroph assessment	Serum cortisol	Basal testing (morning, 07:00–09:00 h)	Normal: Serum cortisol level ≥18 μg/dl Insufficient: <3 μg/dl Indeterminate: 3–18 μg/dl
	Insulin tolerance test	Insulin (0.05–0.15 U/kg intravenously) Serum measurements of cortisol at 0, 30, 60 minutes	Symptomatic hypoglycemia, blood glucose <40 mg/dl required for interpretation Normal: Peak cortisol ≥18 μg/dl Insufficient: Serum cortisol level <18 μg/dl
	Overnight metyrapone test	Metyrapone 30 mg/kg administered at midnight Serum measurements of cortisol and 11-deoxycortisol at 08:00 the following morning	Serum cortisol <7 μg/dl confirms enzymatic blockade Normal: Serum 11-deoxycortisol >7 μg/dl Insufficient: Serum 11-deoxycortisol <7 μg/dl Caveat: Adrenal crisis possible is basal cortisol ≤ μg/kg
	ACTH stimulation test	Synthetic 1–24 ACTH (250 μg IV or IM or 1 μg IV) Serum measurements of cortisol at 0, 30, 60 minutes	Normal: Serum cortisol level ≥18 μg/dl Insufficient: Serum cortisol level <8 μg/dl Caveat: False-negative results possible in acute or subacute timeframe
Thyrotroph assessment	Thyroid-stimulating hormone (TSH), free thyroxine index (FTI) or free thyroxine (fT4)	Basal testing	Normal: Normal serum levels of fT4 or FTI, combined with normal serum TSH Central hypothyroidism: Low levels of fT4 or FTI; low, normal, or high serum level of TSH
Gonadotroph assessment (males)	Serum testosterone, luteinizing hormone (LH) and follicle-stimulating hormone (FSH)	Basal testing (morning, 07:00–09:00 h)	Normal: Serum testosterone level within the normal range, normal LH, FSH Hypogonadotropic hypogonadism: Serum testosterone level below lower limits of normal, LH and FSH low or normal
Gonadotroph assessment (females)	Serum estradiol, LH, FSH	Basal testing	Normal: Results are variable in menstruating women Normal postmenopausal women: Elevated LH, FSH; low serum estradiol Normal prepubertal females: Low LH, FSH, estradiol Gonadotroph failure: Low levels of LH, FSH, estradiol (primary amenorrhea, secondary central amenorrhea, postmenopausal gonadotroph deficiency)
Somatotroph assessment	Serum IGF-I, IGFBP-3 (children)	Basal testing	Normal: Serum IGF-I within the age- and gender-adjusted normal range Serum IGFBP-3 within the age- and gender-adjusted normal range Growth hormone (GH) deficient: Serum IGF-I levels below 84 μg/dl (assay specific) with three or more additional pituitary deficits Serum IGFBP-3 below lower limits of normal
	Insulin tolerance test	Insulin (0.05–0.15 U/kg intravenously) Serum measurements of GH at 0, 30, 60 minutes	Symptomatic hypoglycemia, blood glucose <40 mg/dl required for interpretation. Normal: Peak GH response >5.1 μg/L Severe GH deficiency: Peak GH <3 μg/L GH deficient: Peak GH ≤5.1 μg/L
	GHRH–arginine stimulation test	GHRH (1 μg/kg IV bolus) arginine 30 g IV infusion over 30 minutes Serum measurement of GH at 0, 30, 60, 90, 120, 150, 180 minutes	Responses variable Normal: Peak GH ≥9 μg/L (ideal body weight ± 15%) GH deficiency: BMI <25: Peak GH ≤11.5 μg/L BMI 25–30: Peak GH ≤8.0 μg/L BMI ≥30: Peak GH ≤4.2 μg/L
	Glucagon stimulation test	Glucagon 1 mg IM; 1.5 mg IM if weight >90 kg Serum measurement of GH and glucose at 0, 30, 60, 90, 120, 150, 180, 210 and 240 minutes	Normal: Peak GH >3 μg/L GH deficiency: Peak GH ≤3 μg/L

establish normative data. It should therefore be recognized that cutoff points established with one technique might not apply to other techniques. The interassay and intra-assay variation of laboratory measurement is largely unrecognized, but various quality assessment studies have demonstrated certain vulnerabilities in our generalized use of cutoff points established with one technique [113–116].

The focus of this section is testing of anterior pituitary function. However, diagnostic testing of genetic causes of combined pituitary hormonal deficits is commercially available for testing POU1F1 and PROP1 genetic defects. Specific recommendations for testing other pituitary deficiencies in certain circumstances (i.e., traumatic brain injury) are addressed at the end of this section.

Assessment of Pituitary Function

Corticotroph Assessment

An intact hypothalamic–pituitary–adrenal axis is reflected by normal secretion of cortisol by the adrenal cortex. Cortisol secretion is pulsatile and follows a diurnal pattern with serum levels highest in the early morning and lowest at midnight. Due to the pulsatile secretion pattern, there is a great deal of overlap in serum cortisol levels between patients with adrenal insufficiency and intact HPA function. It is for this reason that dynamic testing, either with direct stimulation of the adrenal cortex or corticotrophs or through an integrated stimulus such as hypoglycemia, is usually necessary to assess corticotroph function.

BASAL TESTING

Laboratory measurement of serum cortisol reflects total cortisol levels, and as such is subject to fluctuations in cortisol-binding globulin. Measurement of random basal serum cortisol or ACTH is generally not helpful in the assessment of adrenal insufficiency due to the pulsatile nature of secretion and the extensive overlap of values obtained from healthy control subjects. When performed, they are most helpful when obtained in the morning (07:00–09:00 h). An intact HPA axis can be inferred by a serum cortisol level >18 ng/ml [114,117–119]. Serum cortisol levels below 3 ng/ml are highly suggestive of adrenal insufficiency in morning samples, but can be found in normal subjects during other times of day. Values between these levels require dynamic testing for diagnosis.

DYNAMIC TESTING

INSULIN TOLERANCE TESTING The insulin tolerance test (ITT) is widely regarded as the gold standard test for testing for adrenal insufficiency. It is particularly useful for detecting secondary adrenal insufficiency. Intravenous insulin is administered (0.1 units/kg) with the intention of inducing hypoglycemia. Symptomatic hypoglycemia, with blood glucose values below 40 mg/dl, is required to evoke a reliable central stress response with activation of the HPA axis. Higher doses may be required in patients with insulin resistance or acromegaly [120]. The test is contraindicated in patients older than 60 years, with a risk of seizures, or suspicion or history of cardiovascular disease. The test should be performed in specialized centers and with precautions to avoid consequences of potential adrenal crisis. Measurements are obtained at 0, 30 and 60 minutes with serum cortisol levels greater than 18 ng/ml indicating a normal response [120–122]. The ITT will elicit few false-negatives and some false-positives [123]. The test is not frequently performed, but remains a valuable tool in the assessment of adrenal insufficiency especially following recent pituitary surgery [114,118,124–126].

OVERNIGHT METYRAPONE TEST Metyrapone inhibits the enzyme 11ß-hydroxylase, preventing the conversion of 11-deoxycortisol to cortisol in the adrenal cortex. For the overnight metyrapone test 30 mg/kg of metyrapone is administered at midnight with measurement of cortisol and 11-deoxycortisol at 08:00 the following morning. Serum cortisol levels below 7 μg/dl confirm adequate enzyme inhibition [114,126]. After metyrapone, the normal response is a significant rise in serum 11-deoxycortisol. Serum levels below 7 μg/dl are consistent with adrenal insufficiency [114,118,119,126]. The metyrapone test does not induce hypoglycemia as the ITT does, but relies on an intact HPA axis to elicit the response to abrupt lowering of cortisol levels. The test can be administered on an outpatient basis. However, there is a risk for adrenal crisis, and metyrapone should not be administered to subjects with baseline morning cortisol values less than 7 μg/dl. The metyrapone test is not frequently performed due to the limited availability of the drug, but is an effective method for testing the integrity of the entire HPA axis.

ACTH STIMULATION TESTING The most common test to assess adrenal insufficiency is the administration of synthetic adrenocorticotropic hormone (1–24 ACTH 250 μg). Synthetic preparations maintain the full potency of endogenous ACTH. The injection can be administered intravenously or intramuscularly, and both methods give equivalent results [114,124]. Injection of 250 μg of synthetic ACTH leads to supraphysiological levels approximately 1000-fold higher than the normal physiological peak, which provides ample stimulation of the adrenal cortex [114,127]. Baseline serum cortisol levels are obtained, and measurements of the serum cortisol response at 30 and 60 minutes are subsequently obtained. The test can be performed at any time of day and need not be done in the fasting state. This short test has largely replaced an 8-hour infusion test, due to its ease of use and similar cortisol responses. Peak serum cortisol levels above 18 ng/dl are regarded as a sufficient response to stimulation, indicating normal adrenal reserve.

The ACTH stimulation is especially useful for diagnosing cases of chronic adrenal insufficiency or primary adrenal insufficiency. The ACTH stimulation test is also helpful in the diagnosis of secondary adrenal insufficiency because of adrenal atrophy caused by long-term deficiency of ACTH. The duration and extent of ACTH deficiency are directly related to the degree of adrenal atrophy and the utility of the ACTH stimulation test in making the diagnosis of secondary adrenal insufficiency. Patients with partial ACTH deficiency or complete ACTH deficiency due to recent trauma or surgery may have false-negative test results with the use of ACTH stimulation. Time necessary to develop adrenal atrophy in the absence of ACTH is variable, and the ACTH stimulation test is not recommended within 2 weeks of a known insult to the pituitary or hypothalamus.

A low-dose ACTH stimulation test (1–24 ACTH 1 μg) has been developed to address the issue of poor sensitivity in the standard ACTH stimulation test. A 1-μg dose is not commercially prepared and must be diluted by injecting a 250 μg dose into 249 ml of normal saline. One milliliter is withdrawn from the mixture and administered intravenously. Initial studies demonstrated improved sensitivity for the diagnosis of secondary adrenal insufficiency [114,128,129]. Performance of the test may be inaccurate due to techniques involving dilution and administration of the low-dose test. Although the dose is reduced from the standard 250 μg dose, the 1 μg dose still delivers a supraphysiologic concentration to the adrenal cortex and similar results of the two concentrations have been demonstrated by multiple investigators [124].

CRH STIMULATION The CRH stimulation test is performed by administration of ovine or human corticotrophin-releasing hormone (100 μg IV) with subsequent measurement of cortisol and ACTH at time 0, 15, 30, 45, 60, 90 and 120 minutes. Normal response is a two- to four-fold increase in ACTH from baseline, peaking at 15–30 minutes. Peak cortisol levels follow at 60 minutes post CRH injection.

COMPARISON OF TESTS

The ITT has generally been regarded as the gold standard test for the diagnosis of adrenal insufficiency and it has been validated against the cortisol response to surgical stress [114,130]. When comparing the ITT to ACTH stimulation tests performance is excellent for the diagnosis of primary adrenal insufficiency [124]. Discrepancies have been found, however, when comparing the ITT to the ACTH stimulation test in secondary insufficiency. Results are often concordant, but investigators have found a number of subjects who have normal ACTH-stimulated responses who later fail the ITT [114,124,131–136]. While the ITT is considered the gold standard, it is not infallible and the majority of conflicting results often are in subjects whose results are near established cutoff points for diagnosis [114].

A metaanalysis explored the utility of the 250 μg ACTH stimulation test for the diagnosis of primary adrenal insufficiency and secondary adrenal insufficiency and the 1 μg ACTH stimulation test for secondary adrenal insufficiency [124]. Using receiver operator characteristics (ROC) analysis, the standard ACTH stimulation test performed well in the diagnosis of primary adrenal insufficiency with a sensitivity of 97% at a specificity of 95%. Sensitivities for the 250 μg test and the 1 μg test in the diagnosis of secondary adrenal insufficiency were 57% and 61% for summary ROC curves, set at a specificity of 95%. The standard ACTH and low-dose ACTH tests performed similar to each other in the diagnosis of secondary insufficiency [124].

The CRH test has been compared to basal cortisol and ITT for assessment of adrenal function in patients with suspected HPA insufficiency [137]. One study determined that a serum cortisol level of ≤13 μg/dl had a 96% specificity and a 76% sensitivity [137]. Basal cortisol levels in this study had 100% sensitivity and 61% specificity for a cutoff point of 10.3 μg/dl.

TESTING AFTER PITUITARY SURGERY

The ITT is also regarded as the gold standard for assessing adrenal reserve after recent pituitary surgery. The ACTH stimulation test is being used in some centers due to its ease of performance [114,125]. A false-negative rate of 3% in postsurgical patients has been demonstrated with a predictive value of 97% [114,138]. However, others have found higher false-negative rates, especially when performed within 1 week of surgery [114,139]. During the first 4–6 weeks of the postoperative period, ACTH testing has been found to be more unreliable and should be utilized after the immediate postoperative period has passed [114].

Diagnosis of Adrenal Androgen Deficiency in Women

Making the diagnosis of androgen insufficiency in women rests on three essential criteria [94]. First, the woman must present with clear evidence of clinical symptoms compatible with androgen deficiency: diminished sense of well-being, persistent fatigue and changes in sexual function. Second, effects of estrogen deficiency should be isolated from effects of androgen deficiency by only considering the diagnosis in the setting of adequate serum estrogen levels. This can be accomplished by endogenous production or replacement. Third, free testosterone values should be at or below the lowest quartile of the normal range for women in their reproductive years, bearing in mind that there is not a sufficiently sensitive assay or threshold for women with androgen insensitivity [94].

Thyrotroph Assessment

The assessment of thyrotroph function is measured with basal sampling of thyroid-stimulating hormone (TSH) and concomitant measurement of free thyroxine (fT4). The diagnosis is made when TSH levels are inappropriately low or normal in conjunction with low levels of fT4, and the appropriate clinical findings suggestive of central hypothyroidism are present. TSH testing is widely accepted as the test of choice for the initial evaluation of hypothyroidism in the general population, and it is useful in the diagnosis of primary hypothyroidism. However, one cannot make the diagnosis of central hypothyroidism with TSH alone, and therefore clinical suspicion must prompt the evaluation of the peripheral hormone (fT4). TSH values are reportedly normal in 84% of subjects with central hypothyroidism, elevated in 8% and low in only 8% of patients [95]. Serum levels of fT4 provide the highest accuracy for the diagnosis of central hypothyroidism, whereas other hormonal measurements are neither sensitive nor specific enough for diagnosis [140–142]. Combined pituitary hormone deficiencies may affect the diagnostic work-up of central hypothyroidism, with GH deficiency altering thyroid hormone metabolism [143].

TRH TESTING

Dynamic testing of thyrotroph reserve may be helpful in differentiating hypothalamic causes of central hypothyroidism from pituitary causes. TRH is no longer commercially available in the US and its diagnostic utility in thyroid disease has largely been supplanted by the current sensitive TSH assay. The test is performed by measuring TSH, fT4 and free triiodothyronine (fT3) after an intravenous injection of TRH. The responses provide information regarding the integrity of the thyrotroph cells and the biologic activity of the TSH secreted by the pituitary. Dynamic testing is rarely indicated as it does not improve the diagnostic reliability above standard nondynamic testing in patients with pituitary adenomas [144]. It may be helpful in the evaluation of patients with low-normal serum TSH and low-normal serum fT4 levels in the setting of known hypothalamic–pituitary disease, but the limited availability of TRH limits the practical application of such testing [145].

Gonadotroph Assessment

ADULT MALES

The initial biochemical assessment of central or hypogonadotropic hypogonadism in adult males is performed by the measurement of morning levels of testosterone in conjunction with measurement of the gonadotropins: luteinizing hormone (LH) and follicle-stimulating hormone (FSH). Testosterone levels vary widely due to circadian rhythms, seasonal variation and episodic secretion. Results may be altered by concurrent illness, medications and changes in sex-hormone-binding globulin levels. Repeating the measurement of testosterone after initial low testosterone values are found is recommended [146]. LH and FSH have short half lives in serum and FSH may yield more accurate results in a single serum sample due to its longer half life. Pooling of LH in 2–3 samples taken 20–30 minutes apart may improve the accuracy of the specimen [147]. Dynamic testing is usually not necessary in adults, and imaging studies are more practical for the assessment of hypothalamic and pituitary disease in adults [147].

ADOLESCENT MALES

In addition to the assessment of gonadotropins and testosterone, the assessment of hypogonadism in adolescent males may require stimulation testing. GnRH is not currently available in the United States, yet its use and the use of other dynamic tests remain as diagnostic tools in distinguishing constitutional delay of puberty (CDP) from hypogonadotropic hypogonadism. Basal total testosterone levels of >1.7 nmol/L may suggest CDP [148–150], but further dynamic testing may be necessary. As previously discussed, the diagnosis of hypogonadotropic hypogonadism versus CDP is often not resolved with stimulation testing, and the diagnosis is most reliably made with expectant observation [99]. However, the following stimulation tests are discussed for reference.

GNRH STIMULATION TESTING GnRH 100 μg is administered intravenously with measurement of LH and FSH taken at 0, 15, 30, 45, 60 and 90 min [147]. Priming with GnRH may be necessary with GnRH delivered via infusion pump every 90 min for 36 hours prior to the GnRH stimulation test. Testing can be performed with GnRH analogues with measurement of gonadotropins at 0 and 4 hours after a single subcutaneous injection [147]. Analogues provide the benefit of longer duration of action and a priming effect with the one injection. Normal response for the classic GnRH test is a rise of LH and FSH with a peak between 15 and 60 minutes. When performed with GnRH priming, the LH peak is lower than the standard GnRH test.

Normal response with GnRH analogues is an LH peak 3–4 hours after injection and an FSH peak 3–6 hours after injection. A blunted rise in gonadotropins is usually seen in pituitary disease or longstanding hypothalamic disease.

CLOMIPHENE STIMULATION TEST The administration of clomiphene inhibits estrogen feedback centrally, interrupting the negative feedback of estrogen GnRH release, and causing a rise in LH and FSH [147]. The test is cumbersome with 100 mg of clomiphene citrate administered for 5–7 days with sampling of LH and FSH at days 0, 4, 7 and 10. A doubling of LH and a 20–50% rise in FSH indicate a normal hypothalamic–pituitary response. The test does not distinguish between hypothalamic and pituitary disease, nor does it assist in the differentiation of constitutional pubertal delay and hypogonadotropic hypogonadism. The test is therefore not recommended for differential diagnosis of delayed puberty.

hCG STIMULATION TEST The hCG stimulation test is utilized to distinguish between testicular agenesis and cryptorchidism in infants, and can be used to diagnose hypogonadism versus delayed puberty in peripubertal males. Two different protocols are in use. In pubertal boys a single dose of hCG (5000 IU intramuscularly) is administered. Serum testosterone is measured at baseline and every 24 h for 5 days. Other protocols suggest repeated hCG injections, 1000 IU daily for 3 days or 2000 IU daily on days 0 and 2. Testosterone is sampled at 0, 48 and 72 hours. In infants, a flat response to hCG is consistent with testicular agenesis. Increased levels of testosterone suggest undescended testes, which should be localized. In peripubertal males, a 2–3-fold increase in testosterone is seen more commonly in constitutional delay in puberty, whereas patients with hypogonadotropic hypogonadism do not have a dramatic rise in testosterone. Studies have shown that testosterone levels above 8 nmol/L are consistent with constitutional delay in puberty, whereas values less than three are seen in hypogonadotropic hypogonadism [150,151]. These criteria result in a positive predictive value of 100% and negative predictive value of 80%. Intermediate values are inconclusive and 29% of these patients remain unclassified after further testing [147].

ADULT FEMALES

The evaluation of gonadotroph function in postmenopausal females entails basal measurement of LH and FSH. As gonadotroph function in postmenopausal females does not involve stimulation of ovarian secretion of estrogen, menstruation, or ovulation, the levels of LH and FSH may be used indirectly to assess the overall functioning of the pituitary when damage is suspected. Normal postmenopausal elevations imply normal pituitary function, and lower levels may indicate pituitary dysfunction. Postmenopausal elevation of gonadotropins may decline with advancing age and may not be a specific indicator of pituitary dysfunction.

The evaluation of premenopausal females who have gone through puberty relies initially on the assessment of regular menses. Regular menstrual cycles imply, but do not guarantee, normal function of the gonadotropic axis. If secondary amenorrhea is present, a work-up of underlying causes is initiated (including measurement of hCG, TSH, FSH and prolactin). Elevated serum FSH levels indicate primary ovarian failure, while normal serum levels of LH or FSH indicate a central cause. Low or normal FSH or LH levels indicate a central cause, which may be genetic, structural, or functional, and a thorough evaluation of underlying causes should be pursued.

PRIMARY AMENORRHEA As with adolescent males with a delay in onset of puberty, females with delayed puberty should undergo an evaluation of the underlying cause. No test will reliably differentiate between constitutional delay of puberty and hypogonadotropic hypogonadism. Expectant observation is the only reliable way to distinguish between these two entities. Once a careful history and physical have been performed, imaging studies and biochemical testing are performed. Testing of pituitary function in females with suspected hypothalamic or pituitary function usually begins with baseline measurement of LH, FSH and estradiol. Levels of estradiol, LH and FSH are typically low in patients with constitutional delay of puberty and hypogonadotropic hypogonadism. GnRH testing is not recommended since it may not reliably distinguish between constitutional delay of puberty and GnRH deficiency.

Somatotroph Assessment

ADULTS

The diagnosis of GH deficiency in adults relies on biochemical testing, due to the absence of specific signs and symptoms. Further, there are no auxological criteria associated with GHD in adults as there are in children who display a lack of growth. Diagnostic testing should be performed in the appropriate clinical context. Patients who should be considered for testing include those with known hypothalamic–pituitary disease or dysfunction, a history of cranial irradiation, or patients with a history of childhood-onset growth hormone deficiency. Recent consensus guidelines have emphasized the importance of including patients with a history of traumatic brain injury or subarachnoid hemorrhage [152,153].

In most circumstances, making the diagnosis of GHD in adults requires dynamic stimulation testing. Individuals with known genetic causes of GHD, childhood-onset GHD due to irreversible structural causes of GHD, or GHD due to embryological developmental causes need not be retested if they were found to be GH-deficient in childhood. Patients who have childhood-onset GHD should be retested as adults if they do not have one of these genetic or structural afflictions, since approximately 40% of children with GHD are found to be GH sufficient when retested as adults [154,155].

Other patients with adult-onset GH deficiency do not require stimulation testing to make a diagnosis. Patients with multiple pituitary hormone deficits and low serum IGF-I levels have a high likelihood of having GHD. A review of data from the U.S. Hypopituitary Control and Complications Study (HypoCCS) revealed that of the 817 subjects included in the study at that time, a variety of stimulation tests had been performed on these subjects [156]. The percentage of subjects with severe GH deficiency defined by peak response to stimulation testing was 41%, 67%, 83%, 96% and 99% for subjects with zero, one, two, three and four other pituitary hormone deficits, respectively. The positive predictive value of having three or four pituitary hormone deficits (TSH deficiency, ACTH deficiency, gonadotropin deficiency with LH and FSH considered together, or central diabetes insipidus) was 96% and 99%, respectively. Serum IGF-I levels, measured by Esoterix Endocrinology laboratories, had a positive predictive value of 96% for the diagnosis of adult GHD when serum levels were less than 84 μg/L. The presence of either a serum IGF-I level below 84 μg/L or three or more pituitary hormone deficiencies provided a positive predictive value of 95% for adult GHD, with a specificity of 89% and sensitivity of 69%. When combined, the PPV and specificity increased to 100% when three or more pituitary hormone deficiencies and a low serum IGF-I level were present. The combination of two or more pituitary hormone deficiencies and a low IGF-I yields a PPV and specificity of 99% [156]. Many practitioners and insurers have accepted these criteria as being sufficient evidence for the diagnosis of GHD, without the need for stimulation testing.

Stimulation testing is required for all adults not meeting the above criteria. There are multiple stimulation tests available for use in the diagnosis of GHD. While the ITT had widely been regarded as the test of choice for the diagnosis of GHD in adults [157], the test was rarely performed in the US due to the intensive nature of the test, contraindications for use in some patients, and the potential risks of performing the test. Alternative tests have been used, such as the combined use of GHRH and arginine with great success in separating GHD subjects from healthy controls [158].

Cutoff points for the diagnosis of GHD vary depending upon the test performed, the assay employed and multiple physiologic factors influencing the GH response to secretagogues. Known physiologic factors affecting the dynamic testing of GH secretion include gender, BMI, visceral adiposity, sex steroid status and age [159]. Responses to some secretagogues do not appear to attenuate with age [160].

A multicenter study evaluated the sensitivity and specificity of six tests for the diagnosis of GH deficiency in adults [161]. The ITT, combined GHRH–arginine test, combined arginine and L-dopa, arginine alone, L-dopa alone and serum IGF-I were compared. Subjects were determined to be GHD based on multiple pituitary hormone deficits and controls were matched for BMI, gender, age and estrogen status. Of the six tests performed, the ITT and combination of GHRH and arginine performed with the greatest accuracy.

With GHRH in limited supply, alternate tests to the GHRH–arginine and insulin tolerance tests are needed. Injection of glucagon results in GH secretion from the pituitary and stimulation testing has been validated against the insulin tolerance test [162,163]. Comparison of the glucagon stimulation test to the ITT has demonstrated that a cutoff of 3 μg/L provides 100% sensitivity and 100% specificity in diagnosing adults with GH deficiency [163]. Other investigators have found 97% and 88% sensitivity and specificity, respectively, using ROC curve analysis [164]. The test is safe and well tolerated. Studies are required to develop the same level of validation established for the GHRH–arginine test, as there are no studies establishing appropriate cutoff points for potential physiologic confounders of testing such as BMI.

Alternate tests have been used in the past including arginine alone, L-dopa, clonidine, and the combination of L-dopa and arginine. These tests do not attain adequate accuracy and are not recommended as alternate tests to the ITT or GHRH–arginine stimulation test [153,161]. Promising alternatives include investigational compounds such as synthetic GH secretagogues, GHRP-2 and GHRP-6; however, these secretagogues have been utilized in combination with GHRH, which currently limits their use.

THE INSULIN TOLERANCE TEST Hypoglycemia is a potent stimulus for GH secretion. Growth hormone levels generally peak 40–90 minutes after insulin administration, and only after a sufficient stimulus of hypoglycemia is attained. The test is performed in the fasting state and baseline measurements of glucose and GH are obtained. If desired, assessment of the HPA axis can be performed simultaneously, with measurement of cortisol after hypoglycemia is attained. Bedside glucose monitoring is required. Regular insulin is injected at a dose of 0.1 units/kg intravenously. Higher doses of 0.15–0.2 units/kg may be necessary in patients with insulin resistant states such as obesity, Cushing's syndrome, or acromegaly. Lower doses (0.05 units/kg) are advisable if panhypopituitarism is suspected. The ITT is contraindicated in patients with ischemic cardiovascular disease, seizure disorders, patients with traumatic brain injury and the elderly. Severe GH deficiency has been defined as a peak response to the ITT of 3 μg/L and more recent data demonstrate that this cutoff represents the first percentile of responses in normal lean individuals [157,165]. A cutoff of 5.1 μg/L provides the best sensitivity and specificity by ROC curve analysis [161].

GHRH–ARGININE STIMULATION TEST The combination of GHRH and arginine has been touted as the most appealing alternative to the ITT in the diagnosis of adults with suspected GH deficiency [152,153]. The GHRH–arginine test has become a well-validated test for the diagnosis of GH deficiency; however, GHRH is in limited supply, and is currently not available in the US, making its widespread use challenging. The peak response to the test is clearly higher than those of other provocative tests with normal lean subjects having peaks greater than 9 μg/L [166]. The test is performed by infusing GHRH, 1 μg/kg by IV bolus, followed by a 30 g infusion of arginine over 30 minutes. GH is measured every half hour for 3 hours. Based on ROC curve analysis a cutoff point of 4.1 μg/L provides a 95% sensitivity and 91% specificity [161]. One study provided weight-based cutoff points in three BMI categories: lean (BMI <25; ≤ 11.5 μg/L; 99% sensitivity, 84% specificity), overweight (BMI ≥ 25 and <30; ≤ 8.0 μg/L 97% sensitivity, 76% specificity) and obese (BMI ≥ 30; ≤ 4.2 μg/L; 94% sensitivity, 78% specificity) [167].

GLUCAGON STIMULATION TEST With the limited availability of GHRH and the contraindications and safety issues related to hypoglycemia with the ITT, the glucagon stimulation test has emerged as a viable alternate test for GH deficiency in the adult. GH peaks approximately 120–180 minutes after glucagon stimulation [168,169]. The glucagon stimulation test is performed in the fasting state, with baseline values for glucose and GH obtained prior to administration of 1 mg intramuscularly of glucagon. The dose is increased to 1.5 mg for patients weighing greater than 90 kg. Glucose and GH are measured serially every 30 minutes for 4 hours. A normal GH response is greater than 3 μg/L. Glucose measurements are not necessary for interpretation, but are obtained for safety. Hypoglycemia during the test is uncommon; however, late hypoglycemia may occur and patients are instructed to eat small, frequent meals after completion of the test. Patients may feel nausea during and after the test. Antiemetics may be considered during the test.

RECOMMENDATIONS

Current recommendations for the diagnosis of GH deficiency include the consideration of the diagnosis in the appropriate clinical context. Evaluation proceeds with investigation of other pituitary hormone deficits and IGF-I secretion. If three or more pituitary deficiencies are present, and the serum IGF-I level is low compared to age- and gender-matched populations, the diagnosis of GHD is almost certain, and stimulation testing may not be necessary. If suspicion remains and there are two or fewer pituitary deficits or a normal IGF-I, stimulation testing should be performed after replacement of other pituitary hormone deficits is completed. Recommended stimulation tests include the ITT (if no contraindications are present), the GHRH–arginine stimulation test, or the glucagon stimulation test. Cutoff points specific to the test, and to the BMI for GHRH–arginine test, should be employed to diagnose GH deficiency in the adult.

SOMATOTROPH ASSESSMENT IN CHILDREN

The diagnosis of GHD in children is based on auxological signs of growth failure. In contrast to the diagnosis of GHD in adults, auxological signs are regarded as the most important tool in the diagnostic work-up [99]. Serial length or height data are plotted on growth charts, along with weight measurements (Figure 10.5A–D) [170]. Height velocity can be determined with serial measurements using velocity charts.

Diagnostic testing begins by ruling out other causes of growth failure, such as hypothyroidism, chronic disease and skeletal disorders. Again in contrast to adults, the measurement of serum IGF-I levels is an excellent screening tool for the investigation of GHD. Measured with IGFBP-3, and bone age, these tests provide an initial step in the diagnosis of GH deficiency in children. IGF-I and IGFBP-3 reflect an integrated assessment of GH secretion. Unlike the pulsatile secretion of GH, IGF-I and IGFBP-3 have long half lives in serum of 12 h and 16 h, respectively. While IGF-I and IGFBP-3 are excellent screening tests, there are caveats that prevent their exclusive use. Serum IGF-I values are low in early life, with overlap between GHD patients and normal children. IGF-I production is affected by nutritional status in adults and children, and may not accurately reflect GH secretion. IGF-I levels are also affected by comorbidities such as renal failure, hepatic failure, diabetes and hypothyroidism, limiting its usefulness in these settings. IGF-I levels do not distinguish between GH insensitivity and GH deficiency.

IGF-I and IGFBP-3 measurement should be interpreted in relation to gender- and age-related normative data. IGFBP-3 is the major carrier protein of the IGF-

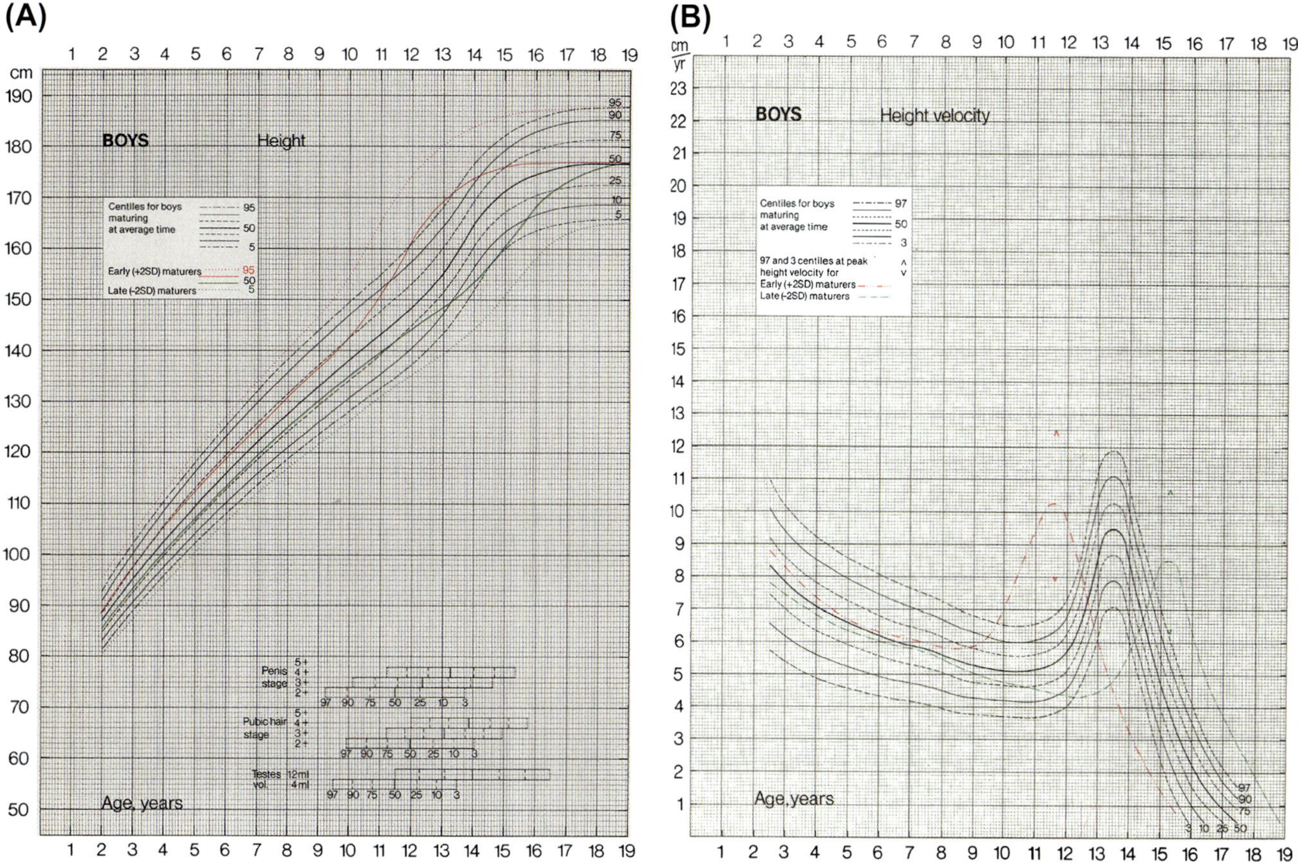

FIGURE 10 5 Height and growth velocity curves for American boys and girls. Figure 10.5A Height, American boys. Height depicted for the 50th percentile (solid black line) with 95th and 5th percentiles depicted (dashed lines). Early maturers (+2 SD) depicted in red (50th percentile, solid; 95th percentile, dotted) and late maturers (−2 SD) depicted in green (50th percentile, solid; 5th percentile, dotted). Figure 10.5B Height velocity, American boys. Height velocity depicted for average males (black). 50th percentile, solid; 3rd percentile and 97th percentile, dashed. Early maturers depicted in red. Late maturers depicted in green. (*continued*).

binding protein family. Normative data for IGFBP-3 are less related to age, and are therefore a good test for young children and infants.

GH STIMULATION TESTING IN CHILDREN

As in adults, GH stimulation testing is an important part of the diagnostic work-up of children with suspected GH deficiency. Also, as in adults, there are a number of limitations to their use. GH stimulation testing is not physiological, in that the secretagogues used do not reflect normal GH secretion in an individual. The cutoff points determined for each test are arbitrary, as there is no one true gold standard stimulation test for GH deficiency in children.

Measurement of GH secretion relies upon the use of pharmacological secretagogues and physiological stimuli. Physiologic causes of GH secretion include exercise, sleep and fasting. There are a number of pharmacologic secretagogues used in the testing of GH secretion including L-dopa, clonidine, propranolol, glucagon, arginine and the insulin tolerance test. The diagnosis of GHD in children requires subnormal responses to two secretagogues, unless there is a known genetic defect or multiple pituitary deficits.

GH stimulation testing is performed in the fasting state. Serial measurements of GH are obtained after the administration of one or a combination of secretagogues. The following tests are utilized in the diagnosis of children. Details regarding tests that are used in the diagnosis of both adults and children are provided in the above section on testing adults.

AGENTS USED FOR GH STIMULATION TESTING IN CHILDREN Arginine is infused at a dose of 0.5 g/kg body weight (up to a maximum of 40 g) over 30 minutes. Serum GH is measured at baseline and at 30-minute intervals for 2 hours [171]. Clonidine is administered at a dose of 5 μg/kg (maximum dose of 250 μg), and peaks approximately 1 hour after baseline. Clonidine may cause hypotension and hypoglycemia, and monitoring is performed during the test. GHRH is not commonly recommended for use in children because it may yield a false-negative result, since the defect in children is usually in the hypothalamic regulation of GH release.

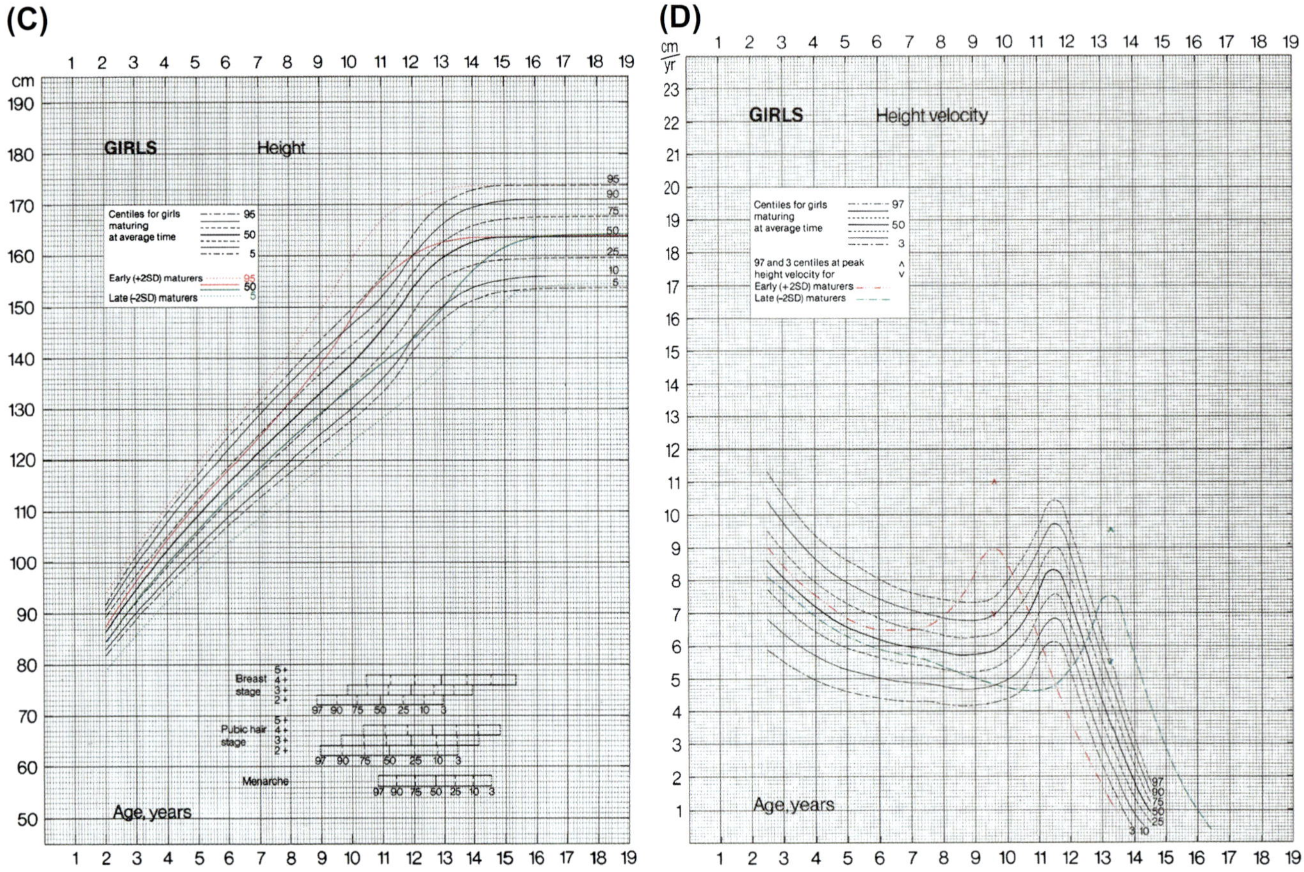

FIGURE 10 5 Figure 10.5C Height, American girls. Height depicted for the 50th percentile (solid black line) with 95th and 5th percentiles depicted (dashed lines). Early maturers (+2 SD) depicted in red (50th percentile, solid; 95th percentile, dotted) and late maturers (−2 SD) depicted in green (50th percentile, solid; 5th percentile, dotted) Figure 10.5D Height velocity, American girls. Height velocity depicted for average females (black). 50th percentile, solid; 3rd percentile and 97th percentile, dashed. Early maturers depicted in red. Late maturers depicted in green. *Used with permission from [170].*

The combination of arginine and GHRH is commonly used in adults and adolescents transitioning to adult care. Insulin-induced hypoglycemia is a potent stimulant of GH reserve, however it is not commonly used in children due to the safety concerns of inducing hypoglycemia. Glucagon causes transient hyperglycemia and consequent insulin secretion and GH secretion. It is safer than the insulin tolerance test. Glucagon is administered at a dose of 0.03 mg/kg subcutaneously in children (maximum 1 mg) and serum samples are obtained at 30-minute intervals for 3 hours after the stimulus. More details regarding the use of GH stimulation testing are provided in the section regarding diagnosis of adults with GH deficiency.

Lactotroph Assessment

The measurement of prolactin is performed more commonly for assessment of hypersecretion than in the work-up of pituitary failure. Prolactin is the most resilient anterior pituitary hormone to local damage, and usually remains normal or slightly elevated in the setting of other anterior pituitary hormone deficiencies. Basal measurement of prolactin with a current two-site immunometric sandwich assay is adequate to assess for deficiency; however, dynamic testing with TRH stimulation has been performed in the past to assess pituitary reserve. This approach has been supplanted by more specific assessments of individual pituitary axes. TRH would be injected intravenously with an expected increase in prolactin of 2.5-fold from baseline 15–30 minutes after injection. Response times are variable, and many normal subjects have been found to have blunted responses [172].

Special Consideration

Evaluation of Patients After Traumatic Brain Injury

Due to the high prevalence of hypopituitarism after traumatic brain injury and the high incidence of traumatic brain injury, a systematic approach toward the evaluation of hypopituitarism in subjects at risk after TBI is required. Despite the high prevalence of hypopituitarism due to TBI, and a consensus statement regarding the testing of hypopituitarism in this setting, there remains controversy regarding the appropriate work-up of hypopituitarism in these patients [80]. Patients who have suffered traumatic brain injury or subarachnoid hemorrhage should be evaluated immediately to assess for any acute loss of anterior or posterior pituitary function. Deficiencies of vasopressin and ACTH can be life-threatening and should be immediately addressed. Deficiencies in gonadal steroids, thyroid hormone and growth hormone are not necessary in the acute phase. Patients who have a history of TBI should be assessed periodically within the first 12 months after the initial insult, as hypopituitarism can be transient, or develop late after recovery. Testing of the HPA axis requires stimulation testing, but may be uncovered with assessment of a morning serum cortisol. Basal testing of thyroid function and the gonadal axis is sufficient for appraisal of these hormones. GH deficiency should be assessed with stimulation testing in most circumstances, unless multiple pituitary deficiencies are present with a low IGF-I, and not before 12 months after the inciting event [152].

Evaluation of Pituitary Function in Critical Illness

The effects of critical illness on pituitary function are addressed in Chapter 11. The evaluation of pituitary function is challenging in the acute care setting. Changes in hypothalamic and pituitary function are evident in acute illness, and may be adaptive responses to critical illness. Diagnosing adrenal insufficiency in the ICU setting is challenging due to multiple factors including a lack of uniform criteria for the diagnosis, physiological factors affecting free and total serum cortisol levels, the lack of an appropriate test, and the lack of reliable methods to measure free cortisol levels in serum [173]. Basal levels of total serum cortisol may indicate adrenal insufficiency, but cutoff levels vary widely in the literature. A cutoff of 15 μg/dl has been proposed as a level that best identifies patients who would benefit from glucocorticoid therapy during critical illness [174]. However, concomitant hypoalbuminemia may indicate lower levels of cortisol-binding globulin, and therefore lower levels of total serum cortisol. Patients with albumin levels less than 2.5 g/dl may be best identified as adrenally insufficient with a cutoff level of 10 μg/dl [174–176]. Measurements of serum-free cortisol, either directly or through the use of a calculated index, are appealing but not widely available or rapidly performed [173,177]. Dynamic testing carries undue risk to critically ill patients (ITT, metyrapone), are not validated in this setting (CRH stimulation, glucagon, low-dose ACTH stimulation), or do not reflect pituitary insufficiency (all ACTH stimulation tests). The 250 μg ACTH stimulation test may have prognostic value with a rise in serum cortisol levels of <9 μg/dl portending an increased risk of mortality in critically ill patients. Changes in other pituitary axes in critical illness are discussed in Chapter 11.

TREATMENT OF HYPOPITUITARISM

The treatment of hypopituitarism is directed toward removal of the underlying cause if possible, with a potential for recovery of normal pituitary function and replacement of deficient hormones. Hormone replacement for pituitary insufficiency can be implemented in three ways depending upon the hormonal axis involved and the desired outcome: (1) replacement of the hormone secreted by the target gland; (2) replacement of an analogue of the deficient pituitary hormone; and (3) administration of an analogue of a hypothalamic-releasing factor.

Recovery of Pituitary Function After Neurosurgical Treatment

Recovery of pituitary function in subjects with some degree of preoperative hypopituitarism has been reported by a number of investigators [7,178–181]. Improvement in pituitary function can occur in the immediate postoperative period [182]. Transsphenoidal resection of pituitary tumors was accompanied by improvement in pituitary function in 36–65% [7]. Deterioration of pituitary function after surgery appears to be low with reported values of 1.4–32% and no change in pituitary function noted in 24–54% [7]. Smaller preoperative tumor size and higher prolactin levels were found to be positively related to pituitary hormone recovery, whereas patient age did not correlate to recovery of pituitary function, in one study [7]. Other investigators have demonstrated higher chances of pituitary recovery in younger, nonhypertensive patients and in patients without the complication of CSF leak [178].

Hormonal Replacement

Glucocorticoid Replacement

ACTH deficiency is potentially life-threatening and its replacement is the highest priority when considering hormonal replacement for hypopituitary patients. Initiation of other hormonal replacement, especially thyroid hormone or growth hormone, can lead to an adrenal crisis. It is crucial to either ensure an intact HPA axis, or treat ACTH deficiency prior to initiating other hormonal therapies. Treatment of ACTH deficiency is accomplished by replacing endogenous adrenal cortisol secretion with a glucocorticoid equivalent. Optimal therapy would closely mimic the normal diurnal variation of cortisol, although this goal is often met with difficulty due to the complexity of administration required to replicate normal human physiology. In contrast to primary adrenal failure, wherein glucocorticoid and mineralocorticoid replacement are necessary, secondary adrenal insufficiency requires only glucocorticoid replacement. Mineralocorticoid secretion is preserved, since it is under the control of the renin–angiotensin system.

There is no consensus on the best method for adrenal glucocorticoid replacement, nor is there an accepted method to test for optimal dosing or long-term monitoring of replacement therapy. Dosing has shifted away from the 12–15 mg/m^2 dosing that was previously believed to be necessary to 10–12 mg/m^2 based on isotope studies that demonstrated a lower daily cortisol production rate than was previously determined.

Replacement of glucocorticoids can be accomplished using multiple dosing regimens, but administration of hydrocortisone of 15–20 mg per day in divided doses, has been the standard approach toward replacement. Twice daily dosing (with 10–15 mg of hydrocortisone in the morning and 5 mg in the early afternoon) is one method of replacing glucocorticoids. Early afternoon doses provide the patient with less sleep interference compared to doses given later in the day. Thrice daily dosing (10 mg in the morning, 5 mg at lunchtime and 5 mg in the afternoon) has also been advocated and has been shown to more closely mimic the normal diurnal variation in cortisol production during the day than conventional twice daily dosing [183].

Monitoring of glucocorticoid replacement is done solely on clinical grounds, as there has not been an accurate method to determine the appropriate dose, and interindividual variation is common. Some practitioners rely on weight-based dosing, surface-area-based dosing, or fixed dosages, yet there have not been adequate randomized, powered studies to establish a best method to determine appropriate dosing. Biochemical markers of appropriate dosing are not helpful. ACTH is not helpful in either primary or secondary adrenal insufficiency [184]. Measurement of 24-hour urinary free cortisol is not helpful as there is a great degree of interindividual variation in cortisol excretion after glucocorticoid absorption, renal excretion is transiently elevated immediately after absorption and saturation of cortisol binding globulin, and normative data from patients with intact HPA activity is not applicable to patients on replacement dosing [184]. Cortisol day curves have been used, but are not validated by controlled studies. In the absence of biochemical markers, clinical judgment must be used to avoid symptoms associated with under- or overreplacement. Underreplacement may be associated with weight loss, fatigue, afternoon headaches, nausea, abdominal pain and myalgias. Overreplacement may be associated with weight gain, obesity, hypertension, hyperglycemia, osteoporosis and possibly cushingoid features. Osteoporosis has been reported in patients taking doses of 30 mg of hydrocortisone daily or greater, but lower doses have not been associated with osteoporosis [185–188].

Instructions regarding dosing for sick days and other times of physiologic stress need to be given to patients receiving glucocorticoid replacement. Patients dependent upon glucocorticoid medication do not respond to physiologic stress with increased levels of corticosteroids, and therefore require increased dosing. Doubling or tripling an oral dose of glucocorticoid therapy for febrile illnesses or administration of 100–150 mg per day of hydrocortisone for other serious physiologic stressors for 2–3 days, with a tapering dose if indicated, is required depending upon the severity of the illness or surgical intervention. Patients should be instructed to wear a bracelet or other form of identification to alert others to their steroid dependence in the case of emergencies.

ANDROGEN REPLACEMENT IN WOMEN

Adult women with hypopituitarism affecting adrenal androgen production have a deficiency in androgen production, with decreased levels of DHEA, DHEA-S, androstenedione and testosterone [189]. DHEA replacement has been shown in controlled studies to improve symptoms of androgen deficiency in women with primary and secondary adrenal insufficiency [190–194]. DHEA is not available in an FDA-approved form, but is available as a dietary supplement. These supplements are not controlled and the quality and content of DHEAS preparations that are available over-the-counter demonstrate a high degree of variability and unreliable amounts of drug provided in each dose [195]. Large prospective randomized studies of DHEA supplementation in women are lacking but studies using 50 mg daily of DHEA have demonstrated increased levels of DHEA, DHEA-S and testosterone. Side effects, such as hirsutism, increased sweating, facial acne and alopecia, are infrequent and are reversible with discontinuation of DHEA.

Transdermal testosterone replacement in women has been studied in several placebo-controlled phase III clinical trials. A 300 μg daily patch was investigated in women who were surgically postmenopausal and in female patients with hypopituitarism. Improvements in mood, sexual function and testosterone levels were seen in the treatment group [196–199]. Long-term safety data are lacking, however, and therefore there is no FDA-approved formulation providing this dose.

Thyroid Hormone Replacement

Replacement of the thyroid axis in secondary, tertiary, or central hypothyroidism is usually done with synthetic

L-thyroxine (LT4). Nonsynthetic preparations of thyroid hormone replacement are available, but synthetic formulations are preferred due to their uniform potency. As stated above, it is necessary to exclude adrenal insufficiency prior to the initiation of thyroxine replacement due to the potential to precipitate an adrenal crisis. Thyroxine increases the metabolism of cortisol and an unmet demand for glucocorticoid secretion may result in an Addisonian crisis. LT4 circulates bound to thyroid-binding globulin and is converted in peripheral tissues by T4-5′-deiodonase to the more biologically potent thyroid hormone triiodothyronine (T3). Synthetic T3 is available as a thyroid hormone replacement, but should not be used as monotherapy in the long-term treatment of hypothyroidism. Combined therapy with T4 and T3 analogues has been explored and there are conflicting reports in the literature. Despite early positive findings [200], combined therapy has been shown in multiple randomized, double-blind controlled trials not to be more advantageous in improving mood, quality of life and neuropsychological function [201–207]. Combined therapy often is associated with multiple side effects of the T3 component including palpitations, anxiety and diaphoresis. Proponents of combined therapy suggest there is a benefit to those who remain symptomatic despite adequate T4 replacement, but the benefit is not clearly demonstrated by changes in biological endpoints, psychometric testing, or psychological assessments [208].

Oral L-thyroxine is available from multiple manufacturers and the mean replacement dose is 1.5 ± 0.3 μg/kg/day [142]. There is considerable interindividual variation, however, and the dosing for hypothyroid replacement may vary widely. LT4 should be given consistently, and patients are instructed to take the medication on an empty stomach, separately from other medications to avoid effects on absorption. The mean bioavailability of LT4 is approximately 80% but reduced absorption has been demonstrated with concurrent intake of medication, inflammatory bowel disease and short bowel syndrome.

The half life of LT4 is approximately 7 days, with daily administration providing a steady level of drug in the circulation. Hence, dose adjustments should be followed by a reassessment of the steady-state level 6 weeks after the dosing change. Additionally, holding a dose when required to do so for surgery or other reasons does not significantly affect drug levels and can be reinitiated as soon as possible without harm. If necessary, intravenous replacement can be done with LT4 (at a ratio of 1:2 for IV:PO dosing) during prolonged periods of time when a patient cannot take the medication by mouth. Concomitant medications may alter the metabolism of LT4 and higher doses may be required if medications such as rifampin, phenobarbital, carbemazepine, or phenytoin are being administered [209,210].

Monitoring replacement of levothyroxine for central hypothyroidism differs from that of primary hypothyroidism in that TSH measurement is not helpful in determining appropriate dosing. As in diagnosis, the TSH does not appropriately or reliably respond to changes in circulating T4 or T3 levels. Free thyroxine or free thyroxine index measurements are used to adjust dosing in central hypothyroidism. Free T3 levels have been advocated as well [95,142]. However, T3 levels are preserved in hypothyroid states and may not accurately guide replacement dosing [201]. Measurement of total T4 and T3 levels is not helpful in dosing changes [95,142]. The target for dosing LT4 replacement is to attain levels of free thyroxine in the upper half of the normal range.

Dosing adjustments are necessary during pregnancy or after initiating estrogen replacement therapy due to the changes in levels of thyroid-binding globulin. Free thyroxine levels (preferably utilizing the free thyroxine index) are useful in reaching the appropriate dose. As with nonhypopituitary patients, adequate thyroxine levels are necessary for good fetal health, and increases of approximately 30% are expected during pregnancy [210]. After the initiation of estrogen therapy, dosing adjustments should be made every 6–8 weeks to ensure proper serum levels of thyroxine.

The treatment of neonates and children requires higher doses of thyroxine compared to adults, and treatment should begin with the estimated full dose to prevent adverse effects of hypothyroidism on neurological development [211]. Treatment of neonatal central hypothyroidism should start with 12–17 μg/kg of LT4, with adjustment every 2–3 weeks as needed based on free T4 and T3 measurements. The goal of therapy is to achieve levels within the age-adjusted normal range. Progressively lower doses will be required as the child ages.

Gonadal Steroid Replacement

Deficiencies in LH and FSH manifest in various ways depending upon the age of onset and the degree of deficiency. The method of treatment of hypogonadism also depends upon the desired outcome of therapy. Treatment of hypogonadism varies dramatically depending upon whether puberty has occurred, fertility is desired, or menopause has occurred in females. Similar considerations are made for males who have not undergone puberty or desire fertility.

FEMALE HYPOGONADOTROPIC HYPOGONADISM

ESTROGEN REPLACEMENT IN ADULT WOMEN

Large epidemiological studies evaluating the impact of hormone replacement therapy (HRT) for long-term preventative therapy during postmenopausal years have drastically altered the approach toward standard therapy during menopause [212–216]. The long-term use of HRT during menopause for cardiovascular risk reduction and prevention of osteoporosis is no longer recommended due to the risks associated with breast cancer and cardiovascular outcomes. In concordance with these findings, the treatment of women with HRT in the setting of hypopituitarism has been re-evaluated. Women who have reached an age commensurate with the postmenopausal state are no longer treated with HRT for long-term preventative reasons. In younger women, it is recommended to take HRT until the average age of menopause (approximately 50 years of age) [216]. Studies in young women have demonstrated cardiovascular benefits to treatment of estrogen deficiency [1], and the risk for osteoporosis increases with early menopause from either secondary or primary causes [212,213].

Transdermal preparations of estradiol are preferred over oral preparations [217,218]. Oral estrogen replacement is subject to hepatic first-pass metabolism. Avoiding this first-pass metabolism has many beneficial effects including reduced synthesis of clotting factors and inflammatory proteins associated with increased cardiovascular risk [217], reduced synthesis of sex-hormone-binding globulin, and absence of the growth-hormone-resistant effect of estrogen on IGF-I production in the liver [218,219]. As with other cases of estrogen replacement, women with an intact uterus taking estrogen due to pituitary insufficiency should take concomitant progesterone therapy. Multiple treatment options are available for progestin therapy, but daily or monthly administration is preferred.

TESTOSTERONE REPLACEMENT IN MEN Treatment of hypogonadism in males consists of replacement of deficiencies in testosterone and sperm production, if fertility is desired. Testosterone therapy is aimed at restoring serum testosterone levels to within the normal range. There are multiple testosterone preparations available to use for treatment of hypogonadism. Administration of testosterone is hampered by first-pass hepatic metabolism, rendering oral administration of testosterone ineffective. Testosterone enanthate and testosterone cypionate are injectable forms of testosterone that have been used for many years in the treatment of hypogonadism. Injection of these lipophilic preparations results in a slow release of testosterone into the circulation. Dosing averages approximately 100 mg per week, with less frequent dosing resulting in higher excursions above the normal range immediately after injection. A standard approach toward treatment is initiating injections of 200 mg every 2 weeks with dose titration based on mid-cycle values. More frequent dosing may be more acceptable to some men who prefer not to have the fluctuation in serum levels of testosterone seen with less frequent injections. The advantage of testosterone injections is the ability to not apply medication on a daily basis. The disadvantage is that an intramuscular injection requires a large-bore needle and specialized training to administer.

Transdermal preparations are supplied in patch and gel form. Each must be applied daily. The patch is applied to the arm or torso, and delivers a stable amount of testosterone over a 24-hour period. One disadvantage of the patch delivery system is the frequent occurrence of rash. Gel preparations are well-tolerated forms of administration that are applied daily. As with the patch, serum levels of testosterone remain stable over a 24-hour period. Care must be taken to limit the potential for transfer to another individual by contact, and instructions are given to patients for strict hand washing and placement of the gel in an area less likely to contact others.

Successful replacement should lead to achieving normal serum testosterone levels and initiation of virilization or maintenance of virilization in adults. Libido and energy levels should improve with therapy, and if persistent may indicate another cause for these symptoms. Replacement therapy also leads to improved muscle strength and fat-free mass, as well as improvements in bone mineral density [146]. Improvements in bone health are most dramatic in those subjects with lower baseline evaluations and in previously untreated patients [220].

INDUCING FERTILITY IN MALES Spermatogenesis can be achieved with treatment of secondary hypogonadism due to pituitary disease through the use of gonadotropins, or gonadotropin-releasing hormone (GnRH), in men with hypothalamic disease. Human chorionic gonadotropin (hCG) is an LH analogue that has a longer half life and stimulates Leydig cells in the testes to produce and secrete testosterone. Recombinant LH is available but is less effective due to its shorter half life. Local production of testosterone produces levels of testosterone in the testes much greater than replacement of testosterone alone. This higher level of testosterone is necessary for spermatogenesis. In most cases hCG treatment is sufficient to induce spermatogenesis [221].

INDUCING PUBERTY IN MALES When hypogonadism precedes puberty and secondary sexual characteristics have not developed, the induction of puberty is required to achieve normal adulthood. Administration of testosterone is the treatment of choice for the induction of puberty when fertility is not immediately desired and development of secondary sex characteristics is the goal. Testosterone is administered at low doses and gradually increased in dose and frequency to achieve stimulation of a pubertal growth spurt and secondary sexual characteristics.

In cases where puberty is constitutionally delayed, treatment is required only temporarily until spontaneous gonadotropin secretion occurs. However, in cases of anterior pituitary failure as the underlying etiology, spontaneous gonadotropin secretion is not expected and treatment modalities should not rely on normal pituitary function. Treatment of delayed puberty with GnRH treatment will result in release of both LH and FSH from the gonadotroph cells. Treatment will result in complete development with testicular growth, spermatogenesis and virilization.

For the majority of patients with hypogonadotropic hypogonadism, GnRH therapy is ineffective in replacing the gonadal axis due to destruction of gonadotroph cells and an inability to secrete LH and FSH. LH, FSH, hCG and TSH are glycoproteins with similar α-subunit structure and individualized β-subunits. hCG has been utilized as monotherapy to induce puberty in males, and is necessary for testicular development and spermatogenesis [222,223].

Growth Hormone Replacement

Treatment of GHD should be addressed after all other pituitary deficiencies have been addressed and sufficiently treated. The treatment of GHD is performed by daily subcutaneous injection of a recombinant form of human growth hormone. Recombinant preparations of GH have replaced preparations made from cadaveric tissue since 1985. Cadaveric GH preparations were associated with cases of Creutzfeldt-Jakob disease, halting its use worldwide.

ADULT-ONSET GHD

The FDA approved the treatment of GH-deficient adults with GH in 1996. The treatment of GH deficiency in adults is directed at improving symptoms of body composition (increased abdominal adiposity and loss of muscle mass and bone mineral density), increasing strength and exercise performance, improving the cardiovascular risk profile, correcting abnormalities in cardiac structure and intima media thickness of the carotid artery, and improving mood and sense of well being [224]. Discontinuation of GH therapy results in reversal of the beneficial effects. While it is suggested that GH replacement therapy improves overall mortality it has not been proven to restore the higher mortality rates associated with GH deficiency back to normal.

There are several preparations of GH commercially available and each is supplied at a potency of 3 IU/mg, using the WHO reference preparation 88/624. Initiation of therapy should begin after careful exclusion of absolute contraindications for therapy, including active malignancy, benign intracranial hypertension and preproliferative or proliferative diabetic retinopathy. Initiation of GH therapy in adults should be at low doses of 0.15–0.3 mg given subcutaneously prior to bedtime. A general principle to follow is to initiate dosing in younger subjects with a dose of 0.3 mg and titrate the dose every 1–2 months based on the IGF-I response. For older adults doses of 0.15 mg daily should be started with monthly titration as tolerated.

Initial trials of GH therapy used weight-based dosing regimens that resulted in an unacceptable level of adverse effects that were directly related to dose. Dosages have been reduced and the method of initiation and titration changed to reflect an individualized dose based on IGF-I levels [225]. Trials comparing weight-based strategies to IGF-I-based titration demonstrated 50% fewer adverse events in the individualized, IGF-I-based regimens compared to weight-based dosing. Final doses were lower in the individualized titration groups [226,227].

In general women require higher doses of GH to achieve normal IGF-I levels compared to men. Additionally, women with matched IGF-I responses may reap fewer expected benefits of GH therapy than men [228,229]. Changes in estrogen therapy, either discontinuation of estrogen or switching from oral to transdermal estrogen may be accompanied by a lowering of GH dose.

GH secretion diminishes with age, and dosing in older adults may need to be lower to avoid side effects and to maintain a serum IGF-I level within the age- and gender-matched normative range.

Clinical Benefits of GH Replacement

BODY COMPOSITION

GH replacement imparts a reliable change in body composition through increased lipolysis. Subjects with GHD are found to have an increased amount of visceral adiposity [230–232], and GH treatment diminishes this visceral fat deposit over months of therapy [233–236]. Effects are also seen in subcutaneous fat, with an overall treatment response of improvements in total body fat. Untreated subjects with GHD also have decreased lean muscle mass, and treatment of GHD has been shown to increase lean muscle mass [233,235,237,238]. Some studies have demonstrated an increase in strength, although this result has not been universally seen [234,235,239,240]. Some studies have shown an increase in exercise capacity and physical performance, but again, not all studies have demonstrated this improvement [241–243].

BONE DENSITY

Multiple studies have demonstrated decreased bone mineral density by DEXA or quantitative CT scan, independent of glucocorticoid replacement and hypogonadism. The prevalence of osteoporosis is increased in subjects with childhood-onset GHD compared to adult-onset GHD, with rates of 35% and 20%, respectively [153]. The severity of GHD also correlates with the extent of osteopenia [106]. Histological examination of bone marrow biopsies reveals an increase in trabecular bone, increased reabsorption and increased osteoid thickness in GHD individuals [244]. Fracture rates in GHD subjects are increased compared to control groups [245–247]. Replacement of GH in GH-deficient adults has an anabolic effect on bone, with effects on both bone formation and reabsorption. Long-term therapy exerts a beneficial effect on bone mineral density, as determined by DXA, with subjects having the greatest incremental improvement when initial Z-score values were lowest [248]. Improvement in bone mineral density appears to be more dramatic in men compared with women [249,250].

CARDIOVASCULAR MARKERS

GH treatment has multiple beneficial effects on cardiovascular health to improve risk factors associated with cardiovascular-related morbidity and mortality. Studies have demonstrated improved flow-mediated dilatation and a reduction in arterial stiffness [251]. Several studies have demonstrated a small reduction in blood pressure [252]. C-reactive protein and homocysteine concentrations decrease with GH replacement [111,112]. Some studies have demonstrated increases in HDL and decreases in LDL and total cholesterol with replacement [233,237,252–256]. GH therapy may worsen insulin resistance and cause a small increase in fasting plasma glucose levels. The effect of GH on insulin metabolism is variable however, and it is unclear what the long-term, individual effects on insulin resistance are in subjects treated with GH. Initial increases in free fatty acids may worsen insulin resistance. Longer-term effects on decreased adipose tissue and increased lean muscle mass may impart an improvement in glucose metabolism. Increased intima medial thickness has been shown to improve with GH replacement [237,257,258] and cardiac function measured by echocardiography improves with GH therapy. Notable improvements are seen in left ventricle (LV) mass, LV end diastolic volume and stroke volume [259]. Despite the improvements in cardiovascular risk factors, replacement of GH has not been clearly shown to improve the increased cardiovascular and cerebrovascular mortality associated with hypopituitarism.

QUALITY OF LIFE

The effects of GH replacement on quality of life have been varied in studies. Some studies have shown a benefit, others have shown little or no change. Improvement in quality of life appears to be more likely when initial scores are low; however, this improvement does not correlate to improvements in IGF-I levels [260–262].

Monitoring Therapy

After dose titration is complete, monitoring should be implemented with careful periodic review of side effects, and biannual assessment of serum IGF-I levels and clinical outcomes. A lipid panel and fasting blood glucose should be measured annually. Bone mineral density should be monitored with DEXA if the baseline assessment is found to be low at 1–2-year intervals, and consideration should be made for additional therapies directed at bone density loss. Measurement of thyroxine should also be performed, and adjustments made in replacement, if indicated [153].

Children and Adolescents

Once the diagnosis of GH deficiency is made in children, treatment should begin to improve linear growth. There is wide variability in responses to GH therapy and dosing should be adjusted based on the growth response and the serum levels of IGF-I. Unlike adults, dosing is weight based, and initial dosing depends upon the preparation used but ranges from approximately 0.18–0.3 mg/kg/week subcutaneously divided into equal daily doses. The treatment goal is to achieve levels above mid-normal range of IGF-I adjusted for age and Tanner stage.

GH therapy is effective at increasing final height and improving growth velocity. If administered at an early age, patients can reach a height within the mid-parenteral target range [263]. Predictors of response to GH therapy have been established based on large databases: gender, gap between target height and height at beginning of puberty, dose of GH at beginning of puberty, age at onset of puberty, and age at end of growth. Other factors such as diet, dosing schedule, response to testing stimuli, exercise and psychological well being may also contribute to the response to therapy.

Special considerations should be made when treatment of adolescents with GH is continued into adulthood. While final height is achieved once the epiphyses are closed, GH replacement has ongoing benefits through the transition period into adulthood. Complete development of muscle mass and peak bone mass are GH-dependent and continue after final height is reached. It has been recommended that treatment be continued through the transition period, rather than interrupt GH therapy and resume treatment in adulthood [264]. Controlled clinical trials have demonstrated a detrimental effect on interruption of GH replacement on fat distribution, muscle mass, cardiac performance and bone mass [254,265–269]. During the transition phase, dosing of GH should be closely monitored and reduced to conform to the normal decline in GH secretion that occurs in late puberty. During puberty dosing of GH varies widely. But during the transition phase the dosing should restart using a nonweight-based dosing method at 0.2–0.5 mg daily, and adjustments made based on the age- and gender-matched serum IGF-I level [264]. Serum IGF-I levels should be monitored every 6 months and adjusted if necessary. Long-term follow-up should include body composition measurements (BMI, hip and waist measurement, height and weight), cardiovascular measurements (heart rate, blood pressure) and assessment of quality of life. Bone mineral density and lipid profiles should be assessed at baseline and proceed according to adult guidelines during the transition period. Thyroxine and glucocorticoid replacement should be reassessed with dose changes in GH therapy adjusted if necessary [264].

References

[1] J.W. Tomlinson, N. Holden, R.K. Hills, K. Wheatley, R.N. Clayton, A.S. Bates, et al., Association between premature mortality and hypopituitarism. West Midlands Prospective Hypopituitary Study Group, Lancet 357 (9254) (2001) 425–431.

[2] A.S. Bates, W. Van't Hoff, P.J. Jones, R.N. Clayton, The effect of hypopituitarism on life expectancy, J Clin Endocrinol Metab 81 (3) (1996) 1169–1172.

[3] T. Rosen, B.A. Bengtsson, Premature mortality due to cardiovascular disease in hypopituitarism, Lancet 336 (8710) (1990) 285–288.

[4] M.E. Molitch, E.J. Russell, The pituitary "incidentaloma," Ann Intern Med 112 (12) (1990) 925–931.

[5] N. Karavitaki, K. Collison, J. Halliday, J.V. Byrne, P. Price, S. Cudlip, et al., What is the natural history of nonoperated nonfunctioning pituitary adenomas? Clin Endocrinol (Oxf) 67 (6) (2007) 938–943.

[6] B.M. Arafah, D. Prunty, J. Ybarra, M.L. Hlavin, W.R. Selman, The dominant role of increased intrasellar pressure in the pathogenesis of hypopituitarism, hyperprolactinemia, and headaches in patients with pituitary adenomas, J Clin Endocrinol Metab 85 (5) (2000) 1789–1793.

[7] P. Nomikos, C. Ladar, R. Fahlbusch, M. Buchfelder, Impact of primary surgery on pituitary function in patients with non-functioning pituitary adenomas – a study on 721 patients, Acta Neurochir (Wien) 146 (1) (2004) 27–35.

[8] A. Tabaee, V.K. Anand, Y. Barron, D.H. Hiltzik, S.M. Brown, A. Kacker, et al., Endoscopic pituitary surgery: A systematic review and meta-analysis, J Neurosurg 111 (3) (2009) 545–554.

[9] N. Fatemi, J.R. Dusick, M.A. de Paiva Neto, D.F. Kelly, The endonasal microscopic approach for pituitary adenomas and other parasellar tumors: A 10-year experience, Neurosurgery 63 (4 Suppl 2) (2008) 244–256, discussion 56.

[10] N. Karavitaki, S. Cudlip, C.B. Adams, J.A. Wass, Craniopharyngiomas, Endocr Rev 27 (4) (2006) 371–397.

[11] R. Valdez, P. McKeever, W.G. Finn, S. Gebarski, B. Schnitzer, Composite germ cell tumor and B-cell non-Hodgkin's lymphoma arising in the sella turcica, Hum Pathol 33 (10) (2002) 1044–1047.

[12] T. Beems, J.A. Grotenhuis, P. Wesseling, Meningioma of the pituitary stalk without dural attachment: Case report and review of the literature, Neurosurgery 45 (6) (1999) 1474–1477.

[13] S.Q. Wolfe, J. Bruce, J.J. Morcos, Pituicytoma: Case report, Neurosurgery 63 (1) (2008) E173–E174, discussion E4.

[14] A. Massier, B.W. Scheithauer, H.C. Taylor, C. Clark, L. Llerena, Sclerosing epithelioid fibrosarcoma of the pituitary, Endocr Pathol 18 (4) (2007) 233–238.

[15] J. Zhong, S.T. Li, X.H. Yao, B. Jin, L. Wan, An intrasellar rhabdomyosarcoma misdiagnosed as pituitary adenoma, Surg Neurol 68 (Suppl 2) (2007) S29–S33, discussion S.

[16] K.K. Gnanalingham, A. Chakraborty, M. Galloway, T. Revesz, M. Powell, Osteosarcoma and fibrosarcoma caused by post-operative radiotherapy for a pituitary adenoma. Case report, J Neurosurg 96 (5) (2002) 960–963.

[17] J. Iqbal, I. Kanaan, M. Al Homsi, Non-neoplastic cystic lesions of the sellar region presentation, diagnosis and management of eight cases and review of the literature, Acta Neurochir (Wien) 141 (4) (1999) 389–397, discussion 97-8.

[18] M.J. Harrison, S. Morgello, K.D. Post, Epithelial cystic lesions of the sellar and parasellar region: A continuum of ectodermal derivatives? J Neurosurg 80 (6) (1994) 1018–1025.

[19] H.M. Heshmati, V. Fatourechi, S.A. Dagam, D.G. Piepgras, Hypopituitarism caused by intrasellar aneurysms, Mayo Clin Proc 76 (8) (2001) 789–793.

[20] S. Mirocha, R.B. Elagin, S. Salamat, J.C. Jaume, T regulatory cells distinguish two types of primary hypophysitis, Clin Exp Immunol 155 (3) (2009) 403–411.

[21] M.E. Molitch, M.P. Gillam, Lymphocytic hypophysitis, Horm Res 68 (Suppl 5) (2007) 145–150.

[22] P. Caturegli, C. Newschaffer, A. Olivi, M.G. Pomper, P.C. Burger, N.R. Rose, Autoimmune hypophysitis, Endocr Rev 26 (5) (2005) 599–614.

[23] A. Gutenberg, R. Buslei, R. Fahlbusch, M. Buchfelder, W. Bruck, Immunopathology of primary hypophysitis: Implications for pathogenesis, Am J Surg Pathol 29 (3) (2005) 329–338.

[24] A. Bellastella, A. Bizzarro, C. Coronella, G. Bellastella, A.A. Sinisi, A. De Bellis, Lymphocytic hypophysitis: A rare or under-estimated disease? Eur J Endocrinol 149 (5) (2003) 363–376.

[25] K.M. Lury, Inflammatory and infectious processes involving the pituitary gland, Top Magn Reson Imaging 16 (4) (2005) 301–306.

[26] J.A. Rivera, Lymphocytic hypophysitis: Disease spectrum and approach to diagnosis and therapy, Pituitary 9 (1) (2006) 35–45.

[27] N. Beressi, J.P. Beressi, R. Cohen, E. Modigliani, Lymphocytic hypophysitis. A review of 145 cases, Ann Med Interne (Paris) 150 (4) (1999) 327–341.

[28] E. Thodou, S.L. Asa, G. Kontogeorgos, K. Kovacs, E. Horvath, S. Ezzat, Clinical case seminar: Lymphocytic hypophysitis: Clinicopathological findings, J Clin Endocrinol Metab 80 (8) (1995) 2302–2311.

[29] E.K. Pressman, S.M. Zeidman, U.M. Reddy, J.I. Epstein, H. Brem, Differentiating lymphocytic adenohypophysitis from pituitary adenoma in the peripartum patient, J Reprod Med 40 (4) (1995) 251–259.

[30] T. Ishihara, M. Hino, H. Kurahachi, H. Kobayashi, M. Kajikawa, K. Moridera, et al., Long-term clinical course of two cases of lymphocytic adenohypophysitis, Endocr J 43 (4) (1996) 433–440.

[31] D. Castle, J.C. de Villiers, R. Melvill, Lymphocytic adenohypophysitis. Report of a case with demonstration of spontaneous tumour regression and a review of the literature, Br J Neurosurg 2 (3) (1988) 401–405.

[32] S. Leiba, B. Schindel, R. Weinstein, I. Lidor, S. Friedman, S. Matz, Spontaneous postpartum regression of pituitary mass with return of function, JAMA 255 (2) (1986) 230–232.

[33] H. Bihan, V. Christozova, J.L. Dumas, R. Jomaa, D. Valeyre, A. Tazi, et al., Sarcoidosis: Clinical, hormonal, and magnetic resonance imaging (MRI) manifestations of hypothalamic–pituitary disease in 9 patients and review of the literature, Medicine (Baltimore) 86 (5) (2007) 259–268.

[34] R. Carpinteri, I. Patelli, F.F. Casanueva, A. Giustina, Pituitary tumours: Inflammatory and granulomatous expansive lesions of the pituitary, Best Pract Res Clin Endocrinol Metab 23 (5) (2009) 639–650.

[35] P. Makras, K.I. Alexandraki, G.P. Chrousos, A.B. Grossman, G.A. Kaltsas, Endocrine manifestations in Langerhans cell histiocytosis, Trends Endocrinol Metab 18 (6) (2007) 252–257.

[36] T.Y. Yong, J.Y. Li, L. Amato, K. Mahadevan, P.J. Phillips, P.S. Coates, et al., Pituitary involvement in Wegener's granulomatosis, Pituitary 11 (1) (2008) 77–84.

[37] A.S. Lewis, C.H. Courtney, A.B. Atkinson, All patients with "idiopathic" hypopituitarism should be screened for hemochromatosis, Pituitary 12 (3) (2009) 273–275.

[38] J.H. McDermott, C.H. Walsh, Hypogonadism in hereditary hemochromatosis, J Clin Endocrinol Metab 90 (4) (2005) 2451–2455.

[39] A. Fernandez, M. Brada, L. Zabuliene, N. Karavitaki, J.A. Wass, Radiation-induced hypopituitarism, Endocr Relat Cancer 16 (3) (2009) 733–772.

[40] F. Castinetti, M. Nagai, I. Morange, H. Dufour, P. Caron, P. Chanson, et al., Long-term results of stereotactic radiosurgery in secretory pituitary adenomas, J Clin Endocrinol Metab 94 (9) (2009) 3400–3407.

[41] G. Minniti, D.C. Gilbert, M. Brada, Modern techniques for pituitary radiotherapy, Reviews in Endocrine & Metabolic Disorders 10 (2) (2009) 135–144.

[42] C. Hoybye, T. Rahn, Adjuvant gamma knife radiosurgery in non-functioning pituitary adenomas; low risk of long-term complications in selected patients, Pituitary 12 (3) (2009) 211–216.

[43] F.E. Snead, R.J. Amdur, C.G. Morris, W.M. Mendenhall, Long-term outcomes of radiotherapy for pituitary adenomas, Int J Radiat Oncol Biol Phys 71 (4) (2008) 994–998.

[44] G. Barrande, M. Pittino-Lungo, J. Coste, D. Ponvert, X. Bertagna, J.P. Luton, et al., Hormonal and metabolic effects of radiotherapy in acromegaly: Long-term results in 128 patients followed in a single center, J Clin Endocrinol Metab 85 (10) (2000) 3779–3785.

[45] M.W. McCord, J.M. Buatti, E.M. Fennell, W.M. Mendenhall, R.B. Marcus Jr., A.L. Rhoton, et al., Radiotherapy for pituitary adenoma: Long-term outcome and sequelae, Int J Radiat Oncol Biol Phys 39 (2) (1997) 437–444.

[46] N.R. Biermasz, H. van Dulken, F. Roelfsema, Long-term follow-up results of postoperative radiotherapy in 36 patients with acromegaly, J Clin Endocrinol Metab 85 (7) (2000) 2476–2482.

[47] G. Minniti, M.L. Jaffrain-Rea, M. Osti, V. Esposito, A. Santoro, F. Solda, et al., The long-term efficacy of conventional radiotherapy in patients with GH-secreting pituitary adenomas, Clin Endocrinol (Oxf) 62 (2) (2005) 210–216.

[48] M.D. Littley, S.M. Shalet, C.G. Beardwell, S.R. Ahmed, G. Applegate, M.L. Sutton, Hypopituitarism following external radiotherapy for pituitary tumours in adults, Q J Med 70 (262) (1989) 145–160.

[49] P. Dutta, A. Bhansali, P. Singh, N. Kotwal, A. Pathak, Y. Kumar, Pituitary abscess: Report of four cases and review of literature, Pituitary 9 (3) (2006) 267–273.

[50] S. Bhasin, A.B. Singh, M. Javanbakht, Neuroendocrine abnormalities associated with HIV infection, Endocrinol Metab Clin North Am 30 (3) (2001) 749–764.

[51] R.N. Nawar, D. AbdelMannan, W.R. Selman, B.M. Arafah, Pituitary tumor apoplexy: A review, J Intensive Care Med 23 (2) (2008) 75–90.

[52] D.H. Zayour, W.R. Selman, B.M. Arafah, Extreme elevation of intrasellar pressure in patients with pituitary tumor apoplexy: Relation to pituitary function, J Clin Endocrinol Metab 89 (11) (2004) 5649–5654.

[53] F. Zhang, J. Chen, Y. Lu, X. Ding, Manifestation, management and outcome of subclinical pituitary adenoma apoplexy, J Clin Neurosci 16 (10) (2009) 1273–1275.

[54] M. Verrees, B. Arafah, W. Selman, Pituitary tumor apoplexy: Characteristics, treatment, and outcomes, Neurosurg Focus 16 (4) (2004) E6.

[55] A. Mehta, M.T. Dattani, Developmental disorders of the hypothalamus and pituitary gland associated with congenital hypopituitarism, Best Pract Res Clin Endocrinol Metab 22 (1) (2008) 191–206.

[56] C. Romero, S. Nesi-França, S. Radovick, The molecular basis of hypopituitarism, Trends Endocrinol Metab 20 (2009) 506–516.

[57] J.P. Turton, R. Reynaud, A. Mehta, J. Torpiano, A. Saveanu, K.S. Woods, et al., Novel mutations within the POU1F1 gene associated with variable combined pituitary hormone deficiency, J Clin Endocrinol Metab 90 (8) (2005) 4762–4770.

[58] J. Deladoey, C. Fluck, A. Buyukgebiz, B.V. Kuhlmann, A. Eble, P.C. Hindmarsh, et al., "Hot spot" in the PROP1 gene responsible for combined pituitary hormone deficiency, J Clin Endocrinol Metab 84 (5) (1999) 1645–1650.

[59] G. Agarwal, V. Bhatia, S. Cook, P.Q. Thomas, Adrenocorticotropin deficiency in combined pituitary hormone deficiency patients homozygous for a novel PROP1 deletion, J Clin Endocrinol Metab 85 (12) (2000) 4556–4561.

[60] A.L. Rosenbloom, A.S. Almonte, M.R. Brown, D.A. Fisher, L. Baumbach, J.S. Parks, Clinical and biochemical phenotype of familial anterior hypopituitarism from mutation of the PROP1 gene, J Clin Endocrinol Metab 84 (1) (1999) 50–57.

[61] L.E. Cohen, F.E. Wondisford, A. Salvatoni, M. Maghnie, F. Brucker-Davis, B.D. Weintraub, et al., A "hot spot" in the Pit-1 gene responsible for combined pituitary hormone deficiency: Clinical and molecular correlates, J Clin Endocrinol Metab 80 (2) (1995) 679–684.

[62] B. Andersen, M.G. Rosenfeld, POU domain factors in the neuroendocrine system: Lessons from developmental biology provide insights into human disease, Endocr Rev 22 (1) (2001) 2–35.

[63] K.S. Alatzoglou, M.T. Dattani, Genetic forms of hypopituitarism and their manifestation in the neonatal period, Early Hum Dev 85 (2009) 705–712.

[64] B. Kristrom, A.M. Zdunek, A. Rydh, H. Jonsson, P. Sehlin, S.A. Escher, A novel mutation in the LIM homeobox 3 gene is responsible for combined pituitary hormone deficiency, hearing impairment, and vertebral malformations, J Clin Endocrinol Metab 94 (4) (2009) 1154–1161.

[65] I. Netchine, M.L. Sobrier, H. Krude, D. Schnabel, M. Maghnie, E. Marcos, et al., Mutations in LHX3 result in a new syndrome revealed by combined pituitary hormone deficiency, Nat Genet 25 (2) (2000) 182–186.

[66] K. Machinis, S. Amselem, Functional relationship between LHX4 and POU1F1 in light of the LHX4 mutation identified in patients with pituitary defects, J Clin Endocrinol Metab 90 (9) (2005) 5456–5462.

[67] N.K. Ragge, A.G. Brown, C.M. Poloschek, B. Lorenz, R.A. Henderson, M.P. Clarke, et al., Heterozygous mutations of OTX2 cause severe ocular malformations, Am J Hum Genet 76 (6) (2005) 1008–1022.

[68] A. Wyatt, P. Bakrania, D.J. Bunyan, R.J. Osborne, J.A. Crolla, A. Salt, et al., Novel heterozygous OTX2 mutations and whole gene deletions in anophthalmia, microphthalmia and coloboma, Hum Mutat 29 (11) (2008) E278–E283.

[69] D. Diaczok, C. Romero, J. Zunich, I. Marshall, S. Radovick, A novel dominant negative mutation of OTX2 associated with combined pituitary hormone deficiency, J Clin Endocrinol Metab 93 (11) (2008) 4351–4359.

[70] P.E. Mullis, Genetic control of growth, Eur J Endocrinol 152 (1) (2005) 11–31.

[71] L.M. Hernandez, P.D. Lee, C. Camacho-Hubner, Isolated growth hormone deficiency, Pituitary 10 (4) (2007) 351–357.

[72] B. Lamolet, A.M. Pulichino, T. Lamonerie, Y. Gauthier, T. Brue, A. Enjalbert, et al., A pituitary cell-restricted T box factor, Tpit, activates POMC transcription in cooperation with Pitx homeoproteins, Cell 104 (6) (2001) 849–859.

[73] K. Clement, B. Dubern, M. Mencarelli, P. Czernichow, S. Ito, K. Wakamatsu, et al., Unexpected endocrine features and normal pigmentation in a young adult patient carrying a novel homozygous mutation in the POMC gene, J Clin Endocrinol Metab 93 (12) (2008) 4955–4962.

[74] E.A. Webb, M.T. Dattani, Septo-optic dysplasia, Eur J Hum Genet 18 (2010) 393–397.

[75] D. Kelberman, M.T. Dattani, Genetics of septo-optic dysplasia, Pituitary 10 (4) (2007) 393–407.

[76] A. Agha, C.J. Thompson, Anterior pituitary dysfunction following traumatic brain injury (TBI), Clin Endocrinol (Oxf) 64 (5) (2006) 481–488.

[77] S. Benvenga, A. Campenni, R.M. Ruggeri, F. Trimarchi, Clinical review 113: Hypopituitarism secondary to head trauma, J Clin Endocrinol Metab 85 (4) (2000) 1353–1361.

[78] N.E. Kokshoorn, M.J. Wassenaar, N.R. Biermasz, F. Roelfsema, J.W. Smit, J.A. Romijn, et al., Hypopituitarism following traumatic brain injury: Prevalence is affected by the use of different dynamic tests and different normal values, Eur J Endocrinol 162 (1) (2010) 11–18.

[79] A. Agha, B. Rogers, M. Sherlock, P. O'Kelly, W. Tormey, J. Phillips, et al., Anterior pituitary dysfunction in survivors of traumatic brain injury, J Clin Endocrinol Metab 89 (10) (2004) 4929–4936.

[80] H.J. Schneider, I. Kreitschmann-Andermahr, E. Ghigo, G.K. Stalla, A. Agha, Hypothalamopituitary dysfunction following traumatic brain injury and aneurysmal subarachnoid hemorrhage: A systematic review, JAMA 298 (12) (2007) 1429–1438.

[81] M. Bondanelli, M.R. Ambrosio, M.C. Zatelli, L. De Marinis, E.C. degli Uberti, Hypopituitarism after traumatic brain injury, Eur J Endocrinol 152 (5) (2005) 679–691.

[82] H.J. Schneider, G. Aimaretti, I. Kreitschmann-Andermahr, G.-K. Stalla, E. Ghigo, Hypopituitarism, Lancet 369 (9571) (2007) 1461–1470.

[83] L. De Marinis, S. Bonadonna, A. Bianchi, G. Maira, A. Giustina, Primary empty sella, J Clin Endocrinol Metab 90 (9) (2005) 5471–5477.

[84] E.W. Zollner, Hypothalamic–pituitary–adrenal axis suppression in asthmatic children on inhaled corticosteroids (Part 2) – the risk as determined by gold standard adrenal function tests: A systematic review, Pediatr Allergy Immunol 18 (6) (2007) 469–474.

[85] E.W. Zollner, Hypothalamic–pituitary–adrenal axis suppression in asthmatic children on inhaled corticosteroids: Part 1. Which test should be used? Pediatr Allergy Immunol 18 (5) (2007) 401–409.

[86] S.P. Durmazlar, B. Oktay, C. Eren, F. Eskioglu, Cushing's syndrome caused by short-term topical glucocorticoid use for erythrodermic psoriasis and development of adrenal insufficiency after glucocorticoid withdrawal, Eur J Dermatol 19 (2) (2009) 169–170.

[87] P.J. Danaher, T.L. Salsbury, J.A. Delmar, Metabolic derangement after injection of triamcinolone into the hip of an HIV-infected patient receiving ritonavir, Orthopedics 32 (6) (2009) 450.

[88] R.M. St Germain, S. Yigit, L. Wells, J.E. Girotto, J.C. Salazar, Cushing syndrome and severe adrenal suppression caused by fluticasone and protease inhibitor combination in an HIV-infected adolescent, AIDS Patient Care STDS 21 (6) (2007) 373–377.

[89] R.D. Stanworth, T.H. Jones, Testosterone in obesity, metabolic syndrome and type 2 diabetes, Front Horm Res 37 (2009) 74–90.

[90] M.H. Rasmussen, Obesity, growth hormone and weight loss, Mol Cell Endocrinol 316 (2) (2010) 147–153.

[91] G. Reimondo, S. Bovio, B. Allasino, M. Terzolo, A. Angeli, Secondary hypoadrenalism, Pituitary 11 (2) (2008) 147–154.

[92] K.K. Miller, G. Sesmilo, A. Schiller, D. Schoenfeld, S. Burton, A. Klibanski, Androgen deficiency in women with hypopituitarism, J Clin Endocrinol Metab 86 (2) (2001) 561–567.

[93] M.E. Wierman, R. Basson, S.R. Davis, S. Khosla, K.K. Miller, W. Rosner, et al., Androgen therapy in women: An Endocrine Society Clinical Practice guideline, J Clin Endocrinol Metab 91 (10) (2006) 3697–3710.

[94] G. Bachmann, J. Bancroft, G. Braunstein, H. Burger, S. Davis, L. Dennerstein, et al., Female androgen insufficiency: The Princeton consensus statement on definition, classification, and assessment, Fertil Steril 77 (4) (2002) 660–665.

[95] O. Alexopoulou, C. Beguin, P. De Nayer, D. Maiter, Clinical and hormonal characteristics of central hypothyroidism at diagnosis and during follow-up in adult patients, Eur J Endocrinol 150 (1) (2004) 1–8.

[96] L.C. Layman, Hypogonadotropic hypogonadism, Endocrinol Metab Clin North Am 36 (2) (2007) 283–296.

[97] W.A. Marshall, J.M. Tanner, Variations in the pattern of pubertal changes in boys, Arch Dis Child 45 (239) (1970) 13–23.

[98] W.A. Marshall, J.M. Tanner, Variations in pattern of pubertal changes in girls, Arch Dis Child 44 (235) (1969) 291–303.

[99] R.G. Rosenfeld, K. Albertsson-Wikland, F. Cassorla, S.D. Frasier, Y. Hasegawa, R.L. Hintz, et al., Diagnostic controversy: The diagnosis of childhood growth hormone deficiency revisited, J Clin Endocrinol Metab 80 (5) (1995) 1532–1540.

[100] B. Bin-Abbas, F.A. Conte, M.M. Grumbach, S.L. Kaplan, Congenital hypogonadotropic hypogonadism and micropenis: Effect of testosterone treatment on adult penile size why sex reversal is not indicated, J Pediatr 134 (5) (1999) 579–583.

[101] M.M. Grumbach, A window of opportunity: The diagnosis of gonadotropin deficiency in the male infant, J Clin Endocrinol Metab 90 (5) (2005) 3122–3127.

[102] P.V. Carroll, E.R. Christ, B.A. Bengtsson, L. Carlsson, J.S. Christiansen, D. Clemmons, et al., Growth hormone deficiency in adulthood and the effects of growth hormone replacement: A review. Growth Hormone Research Society Scientific Committee, J Clin Endocrinol Metab 83 (2) (1998) 382–395.

[103] J. Svensson, B.A. Bengtsson, T. Rosen, A. Oden, G. Johannsson, Malignant disease and cardiovascular morbidity in hypopituitary adults with or without growth hormone replacement therapy, J Clin Endocrinol Metab 89 (7) (2004) 3306–3312.

[104] J. Verhelst, R. Abs, Cardiovascular risk factors in hypopituitary GH-deficient adults, Eur J Endocrinol 161 (Suppl 1) (2009) S41–S49.

[105] S.A. Beshyah, D.G. Johnston, Cardiovascular disease and risk factors in adults with hypopituitarism, Clin Endocrinol (Oxf) 50 (1) (1999) 1–15.

[106] A. Colao, C. Di Somma, R. Pivonello, S. Loche, G. Aimaretti, G. Cerbone, et al., Bone loss is correlated to the severity of growth hormone deficiency in adult patients with hypopituitarism, J Clin Endocrinol Metab 84 (6) (1999) 1919–1924.

[107] H. de Boer, G.J. Blok, H.J. Voerman, M. Phillips, J.A. Schouten, Serum lipid levels in growth hormone-deficient men, Metabolism: Clinical Experimental 43 (2) (1994) 199–203.

[108] A. Sanmartí, A. Lucas, F. Hawkins, S. Webb, A. Ulied, Observational study in adult hypopituitary patients with untreated growth hormone deficiency (ODA study). Socio-economic impact and health status. Collaborative ODA (Observational GH Deficiency in Adults) Group, Eur J Endocrinol 141 (5) (1999) 481–489.

[109] A. Colao, C. Di Somma, A. Cuocolo, M. Filippella, F. Rota, W. Acampa, et al., The severity of growth hormone deficiency correlates with the severity of cardiac impairment in 100 adult patients with hypopituitarism: An observational, case-control study, J Clin Endocrinol Metab 89 (12) (2004) 5998–6004.

[110] A. Colao, C. Di Somma, M. Savanelli, M. De Leo, G. Lombardi, Beginning to end: Cardiovascular implications of growth hormone (GH) deficiency and GH therapy, Growth Horm IGF Res 16 (Suppl A) (2006) S41–S48.

[111] G. Sesmilo, B.M. Biller, J. Llevadot, D. Hayden, G. Hanson, N. Rifai, et al., Effects of growth hormone administration on inflammatory and other cardiovascular risk markers in men with growth hormone deficiency. A randomized, controlled clinical trial, Ann Intern Med 133 (2) (2000) 111–122.

[112] G. Sesmilo, B.M. Biller, J. Llevadot, D. Hayden, G. Hanson, N. Rifai, et al., Effects of growth hormone (GH) administration on homocyst(e)ine levels in men with GH deficiency: A randomized controlled trial, J Clin Endocrinol Metab 86 (4) (2001) 1518–1524.

[113] L. Wood, D.H. Ducroq, H.L. Fraser, S. Gillingwater, C. Evans, A.J. Pickett, et al., Measurement of urinary free cortisol by tandem mass spectrometry and comparison with results obtained by gas chromatography-mass spectrometry and two commercial immunoassays, Ann Clin Biochem 45 (Pt 4) (2008) 380–388.

[114] I. Wallace, S. Cunningham, J. Lindsay, The diagnosis and investigation of adrenal insufficiency in adults, Ann Clin Biochem 46 (Pt 5) (2009) 351–367.

[115] J. Cohen, G. Ward, J. Prins, M. Jones, B. Venkatesh, Variability of cortisol assays can confound the diagnosis of adrenal insufficiency in the critically ill population, Intensive Care Med 32 (11) (2006) 1901–1905.

[116] A. Pokrajac, G. Wark, A.R. Ellis, J. Wear, G.E. Wieringa, P.J. Trainer, Variation in GH and IGF-I assays limits the applicability of international consensus criteria to local practice, Clin Endocrinol (Oxf) 67 (1) (2007) 65–70.

[117] S. Grinspoon, B. Biller, Clinical review 62: Laboratory assessment of adrenal insufficiency, J Clin Endocrinol Metab 79 (4) (1994) 923–931.

[118] W. Oelkers, Adrenal insufficiency, N Engl J Med 335 (16) (1996) 1206–1212.

[119] W. Arlt, B. Allolio, Adrenal insufficiency, Lancet 361 (9372) (2003) 1881–1893.

[120] R. Salvatori, Adrenal insufficiency, JAMA 294 (19) (2005) 2481–2488.

[121] L.K. Nieman, Dynamic evaluation of adrenal hypofunction, J Endocrinol Invest 26 (7 Suppl) (2003) 74–82.

[122] M. Andrioli, F.P. Giraldi, F. Cavagnini, Isolated corticotrophin deficiency, Pituitary 9 (4) (2006) 289–295.

[123] C.H. Courtney, A.S. McAllister, D.R. McCance, P.M. Bell, D.R. Hadden, H. Leslie, et al., Comparison of one week 0900 h serum cortisol, low and standard dose synacthen tests with a 4 to 6 week insulin hypoglycaemia test after pituitary surgery in assessing HPA axis, Clin Endocrinol (Oxf) 53 (4) (2000) 431–436.

[124] R.I. Dorin, C.R. Qualls, L.M. Crapo, Diagnosis of adrenal insufficiency, Ann Intern Med 139 (3) (2003) 194–204.

[125] R.M. Reynolds, P.M. Stewart, J.R. Seckl, P.L. Padfield, Assessing the HPA axis in patients with pituitary disease: A UK survey, Clin Endocrinol (Oxf) 64 (1) (2006) 82–85.

[126] A.M. Suliman, T.P. Smith, M. Labib, T.M. Fiad, T.J. McKenna, The low-dose ACTH test does not provide a useful assessment of the hypothalamic–pituitary–adrenal axis in secondary adrenal insufficiency, Clin Endocrinol (Oxf) 56 (4) (2002) 533–539.

[127] J. Mayenknecht, S. Diederich, V. Bähr, U. Plöckinger, W. Oelkers, Comparison of low and high dose corticotropin stimulation tests in patients with pituitary disease, J Clin Endocrinol Metab 83 (5) (1998) 1558–1562.

[128] K. Tordjman, A. Jaffe, Y. Trostanetsky, Y. Greenman, R. Limor, N. Stern, Low-dose (1 microgram) adrenocorticotrophin (ACTH) stimulation as a screening test for impaired hypothalamo–pituitary–adrenal axis function: Sensitivity, specificity and accuracy in comparison with the high-dose (250 microgram) test, Clin Endocrinol (Oxf) 52 (5) (2000) 633–640.

[129] L.M. Thaler, L.S. Blevins Jr., The low dose (1-microg) adrenocorticotropin stimulation test in the evaluation of patients with suspected central adrenal insufficiency, J Clin Endocrinol Metab 83 (8) (1998) 2726–2729.

[130] F.S. Plumpton, G.M. Besser, The adrenocortical response to surgery and insulin-induced hypoglycemia in corticosteroid-treated and normal subjects, Br J Surg 55 (11) (1968 Nov) 857.

[131] S.J. Hurel, C.J. Thompson, M.J. Watson, M.M. Harris, P.H. Baylis, P. Kendall-Taylor, The short synacthen and insulin stress tests in the assessment of the hypothalamic–pituitary–adrenal axis, Clin Endocrinol (Oxf) 44 (2) (1996) 141–146.

[132] J. Lindholm, The insulin hypoglycaemia test for the assessment of the hypothalamic–pituitary–adrenal function, Clin Endocrinol (Oxf) 54 (3) (2001) 283–286.

[133] R.P. Dullaart, S.H. Pasterkamp, J.A. Beentjes, W.J. Sluiter, Evaluation of adrenal function in patients with hypothalamic and pituitary disorders: Comparison of serum cortisol, urinary free cortisol and the human-corticotrophin releasing hormone test with the insulin tolerance test, Clin Endocrinol (Oxf) 50 (4) (1999) 465–471.

[134] S.E. Borst, T. Mulligan, Testosterone replacement therapy for older men, Clin Interv Aging 2 (4) (2007) 561–566.

[135] F. Ammari, B. Issa, E. Millward, M. Scanion, A comparison between short ACTH and insulin stress tests for assessing hypothalamo–pituitary–adrenal function, Clin Endocrinol (Oxf) 44 (4) (1996) 473–476.

[136] M. Schmiegelow, U. Feldt-Rasmussen, A.K. Rasmussen, M. Lange, H.S. Poulsen, J. Muller, Assessment of the hypothalamo–pituitary–adrenal axis in patients treated with radiotherapy and chemotherapy for childhood brain tumor, J Clin Endocrinol Metab 88 (7) (2003) 3149–3154.

[137] I.L. Schmidt, H. Lahner, K. Mann, S. Petersenn, Diagnosis of adrenal insufficiency: Evaluation of the corticotropin-releasing hormone test and basal serum cortisol in comparison to the insulin tolerance test in patients with hypothalamic–pituitary–adrenal disease, J Clin Endocrinol Metab 88 (9) (2003) 4193–4198.
[138] H.K. Gleeson, B.R. Walker, J.R. Seckl, P.L. Padfield, Ten years on: Safety of short synacthen tests in assessing adrenocorticotropin deficiency in clinical practice, J Clin Endocrinol Metab 88 (5) (2003) 2106–2111.
[139] C.H. Courtney, A.S. McAllister, D.R. McCance, D.R. Hadden, H. Leslie, B. Sheridan, et al., The insulin hypoglycaemia and overnight metyrapone tests in the assessment of the hypothalamic–pituitary–adrenal axis following pituitary surgery, Clin Endocrinol (Oxf) 53 (3) (2000) 309–312.
[140] J.O. Jorgensen, J. Moller, T. Laursen, H. Orskov, J.S. Christiansen, J. Weeke, Growth hormone administration stimulates energy expenditure and extrathyroidal conversion of thyroxine to triiodothyronine in a dose-dependent manner and suppresses circadian thyrotrophin levels: Studies in GH-deficient adults, Clin Endocrinol (Oxf) 41 (5) (1994) 609–614.
[141] A. Lania, L. Persani, P. Beck-Peccoz, Central hypothyroidism, Pituitary 11 (2) (2008) 181–186.
[142] E. Ferretti, L. Persani, M.L. Jaffrain-Rea, S. Giambona, G. Tamburrano, P. Beck-Peccoz, Evaluation of the adequacy of levothyroxine replacement therapy in patients with central hypothyroidism, J Clin Endocrinol Metab 84 (3) (1999) 924–929.
[143] M.R. Martins, F.C. Doin, W.R. Komatsu, T.L. Barros-Neto, V.A. Moises, J. Abucham, Growth hormone replacement improves thyroxine biological effects: Implications for management of central hypothyroidism, J Clin Endocrinol Metab 92 (11) (2007) 4144–4153.
[144] M.L. Hartoft-Nielsen, M. Lange, A.K. Rasmussen, S. Scherer, T. Zimmermann-Belsing, U. Feldt-Rasmussen, Thyrotropin-releasing hormone stimulation test in patients with pituitary pathology, Horm Res 61 (2) (2004) 53–57.
[145] H. Atmaca, F. Tanriverdi, C. Gokce, K. Unluhizarci, F. Kelestimur, Do we still need the TRH stimulation test? Thyroid 17 (6) (2007) 529–533.
[146] S. Bhasin, G.R. Cunningham, F.J. Hayes, A.M. Matsumoto, P.J. Snyder, R.S. Swerdloff, et al., Testosterone therapy in adult men with androgen deficiency syndromes: An Endocrine Society Clinical Practice Guideline, J Clin Endocrinol Metab 91 (6) (2006) 1995–2010.
[147] A.M. Isidori, E. Giannetta, A. Lenzi, Male hypogonadism, Pituitary 11 (2) (2008) 171–180.
[148] F. Wu, D. Brown, G. Butler, H. Stirling, C. Kelnar, Early morning plasma testosterone is an accurate predictor of imminent pubertal development in prepubertal boys, J Clin Endocrinol Metab 76 (1) (1993) 26–31.
[149] M. Forest, Sexual maturation of the hypothalamus: Pathophysiological aspects and clinical implications, Acta Neurochir (Wien) 75 (1–4) (1985) 23–42.
[150] V. Degros, C. Cortet-Rudelli, B. Soudan, D. Dewailly, The human chorionic gonadotropin test is more powerful than the gonadotropin-releasing hormone agonist test to discriminate male isolated hypogonadotropic hypogonadism from constitutional delayed puberty, Eur J Endocrinol 149 (1) (2003) 23–29.
[151] L. Dunkel, J. Perheentupa, R. Sorva, Single versus repeated dose human chorionic gonadotropin stimulation in the differential diagnosis of hypogonadotropic hypogonadism, J Clin Endocrinol Metab 60 (2) (1985) 333–337.
[152] K.K. Ho, Consensus guidelines for the diagnosis and treatment of adults with GH deficiency II: A statement of the GH Research Society in association with the European Society for Pediatric Endocrinology, Lawson Wilkins Society, European Society of Endocrinology, Japan Endocrine Society, and Endocrine Society of Australia, Eur J Endocrinol 157 (6) (2007) 695–700.
[153] M.E. Molitch, D.R. Clemmons, S. Malozowski, G.R. Merriam, S.M. Shalet, M.L. Vance, et al., Evaluation and treatment of adult growth hormone deficiency: an Endocrine Society Clinical Practice Guideline, J Clin Endocrinol Metab 91 (5) (2006) 1621–1634.
[154] V. Gasco, G. Corneli, G. Beccuti, F. Prodam, S. Rovere, J. Bellone, et al., Retesting the childhood-onset GH-deficient patient, Eur J Endocrinol 159 (Suppl 1) (2008) S45–S52.
[155] J. Donaubauer, W. Kiess, J. Kratzsch, T. Nowak, H. Steinkamp, H. Willgerodt, et al., Re-assessment of growth hormone secretion in young adult patients with childhood-onset growth hormone deficiency, Clin Endocrinol (Oxf) 58 (4) (2003) 456–463.
[156] M.L. Hartman, B.J. Crowe, B.M. Biller, K.K. Ho, D.R. Clemmons, J.J. Chipman, Which patients do not require a GH stimulation test for the diagnosis of adult GH deficiency? J Clin Endocrinol Metab 87 (2) (2002) 477–485.
[157] Consensus guidelines for the diagnosis and treatment of adults with growth hormone deficiency, summary statement of the Growth Hormone Research Society Workshop on Adult Growth Hormone Deficiency, J Clin Endocrinol Metab 83 (2) (1998) 379–381.
[158] G. Aimaretti, G. Corneli, P. Razzore, S. Bellone, C. Baffoni, E. Arvat, et al., Comparison between insulin-induced hypoglycemia and growth hormone (GH)-releasing hormone + arginine as provocative tests for the diagnosis of GH deficiency in adults, J Clin Endocrinol Metab 83 (5) (1998) 1615–1618.
[159] G. Corneli, V. Gasco, F. Prodam, S. Grottoli, G. Aimaretti, E. Ghigo, Growth hormone levels in the diagnosis of growth hormone deficiency in adulthood, Pituitary 10 (2) (2007) 141–149.
[160] E. Ghigo, S. Goffi, M. Nicolosi, E. Arvat, F. Valente, E. Mazza, et al., Growth hormone (GH) responsiveness to combined administration of arginine and GH-releasing hormone does not vary with age in man, J Clin Endocrinol Metab 71 (6) (1990) 1481–1485.
[161] B.M. Biller, M.H. Samuels, A. Zagar, D.M. Cook, B.M. Arafah, V. Bonert, et al., Sensitivity and specificity of six tests for the diagnosis of adult GH deficiency, J Clin Endocrinol Metab 87 (5) (2002) 2067–2079.
[162] K. Yuen, B. Biller, M. Molitch, D. Cook, Clinical review: Is lack of recombinant growth hormone (GH)-releasing hormone in the United States a setback or time to consider glucagon testing for adult GH deficiency? J Clin Endocrinol Metab 94 (8) (2009) 2702–2707.
[163] J.M. Gomez, R.M. Espadero, F. Escobar-Jimenez, F. Hawkins, A. Pico, J.L. Herrera-Pombo, et al., Growth hormone release after glucagon as a reliable test of growth hormone assessment in adults, Clin Endocrinol (Oxf) 56 (3) (2002) 329–334.
[164] F. Conceição, A. da Costa e Silva, A. Leal Costa, M. Vaisman, Glucagon stimulation test for the diagnosis of GH deficiency in adults, J Endocrinol Invest 26 (11) (2003) 1065–1070.
[165] G. Aimaretti, C. Baffoni, L. DiVito, S. Bellone, S. Grottoli, M. Maccario, et al., Comparisons among old and new provocative tests of GH secretion in 178 normal adults, Eur J Endocrinol 142 (4) (2000) 347–352.

[166] E. Ghigo, G. Aimaretti, L. Gianotti, J. Bellone, E. Arvat, F. Camanni, New approach to the diagnosis of growth hormone deficiency in adults, Eur J Endocrinol 134 (3) (1996 Mar) 352–356.
[167] G. Corneli, C. Di Somma, R. Baldelli, S. Rovere, V. Gasco, C.G. Croce, et al., The cut-off limits of the GH response to GH-releasing hormone-arginine test related to body mass index, Eur J Endocrinol 153 (2) (2005) 257–264.
[168] K. Leong, A. Walker, I. Martin, D. Wile, J. Wilding, I. MacFarlane, An audit of 500 subcutaneous glucagon stimulation tests to assess growth hormone and ACTH secretion in patients with hypothalamic–pituitary disease, Clin Endocrinol (Oxf) 54 (4) (2001) 463–468.
[169] S. Orme, A. Price, A. Weetman, R. Ross, Comparison of the diagnostic utility of the simplified and standard i.m. glucagon stimulation test (IMGST), Clin Endocrinol (Oxf) 49 (6) (1998) 773–778.
[170] J.M. Tanner, P.S. Davies, Clinical longitudinal standards for height and height velocity for North American children, J Pediatr 107 (3) (1985) 317–329.
[171] E. Richmond, A. Rogol, Growth hormone deficiency in children, Pituitary 11 (2) (2008) 115–120.
[172] R. Le Moli, E. Endert, E. Fliers, T. Mulder, M. Prummel, J. Romijn, et al., Establishment of reference values for endocrine tests. II: Hyperprolactinemia, Neth J Med 55 (2) (1999) 71–75.
[173] M. Bondanelli, M.C. Zatelli, M.R. Ambrosio, E.C. degli Uberti, Systemic illness, Pituitary 11 (2) (2008) 187–207.
[174] B.M. Arafah, Hypothalamic pituitary adrenal function during critical illness: Limitations of current assessment methods, J Clin Endocrinol Metab 91 (10) (2006) 3725–3745.
[175] A. Beishuizen, L.G. Thijs, I. Vermes, Patterns of corticosteroid-binding globulin and the free cortisol index during septic shock and multitrauma, Intensive Care Med 27 (10) (2001) 1584–1591.
[176] P.E. Marik, G.P. Zaloga, Adrenal insufficiency in the critically ill: A new look at an old problem, Chest 122 (5) (2002) 1784–1796.
[177] A.H. Hamrahian, T.S. Oseni, B.M. Arafah, Measurements of serum free cortisol in critically ill patients, N Engl J Med 350 (16) (2004) 1629–1638.
[178] N. Fatemi, J. Dusick, M. de Paiva Neto, D. Kelly, The endonasal microscopic approach for pituitary adenomas and other parasellar tumors: A 10-year experience, Neurosurgery 63 (4 Suppl 2) (2008) 244–256, discussion 56.
[179] S.M. Webb, M. Rigla, A. Wagner, B. Oliver, F. Bartumeus, Recovery of hypopituitarism after neurosurgical treatment of pituitary adenomas, J Clin Endocrinol Metab 84 (10) (1999) 3696–3700.
[180] B. Arafah, J. Brodkey, A. Manni, M. Velasco, B. Kaufman, O. Pearson, Recovery of pituitary function following surgical removal of large nonfunctioning pituitary adenomas, Clin Endocrinol (Oxf) 17 (3) (1982) 213–222.
[181] B.M. Arafah, Reversible hypopituitarism in patients with large nonfunctioning pituitary adenomas, J Clin Endocrinol Metab 62 (6) (1986) 1173–1179.
[182] B. Arafah, S. Kailani, K. Nekl, R. Gold, W. Selman, Immediate recovery of pituitary function after transsphenoidal resection of pituitary macroadenomas, J Clin Endocrinol Metab 79 (2) (1994) 348–354.
[183] T.A. Howlett, An assessment of optimal hydrocortisone replacement therapy, Clin Endocrinol (Oxf) 46 (3) (1997) 263–268.
[184] W. Arlt, The approach to the adult with newly diagnosed adrenal insufficiency, J Clin Endocrinol Metab 94 (4) (2009) 1059–1067.
[185] W. Arlt, C. Rosenthal, S. Hahner, B. Allolio, Quality of glucocorticoid replacement in adrenal insufficiency: Clinical assessment vs. timed serum cortisol measurements, Clin Endocrinol (Oxf) 64 (4) (2006) 384–389.
[186] C. Florkowski, S. Holmes, J. Elliot, R. Donald, E. Espiner, Bone mineral density is reduced in female but not male subjects with Addison's disease, NZ Med J 107 (972) (1994) 52–53.
[187] P. Zelissen, R. Croughs, P. van Rijk, J. Raymakers, Effect of glucocorticoid replacement therapy on bone mineral density in patients with Addison disease, Ann Intern Med 120 (3) (1994) 207–210.
[188] E. Jodar, M.P. Valdepenas, G. Martinez, A. Jara, F. Hawkins, Long-term follow-up of bone mineral density in Addison's disease, Clin Endocrinol (Oxf) 58 (5) (2003) 617–620.
[189] K.K. Miller, Androgen deficiency in women, J Clin Endocrinol Metab 86 (6) (2001) 2395–2401.
[190] G. Johannsson, P. Burman, L. Wiren, B.E. Engstrom, A.G. Nilsson, M. Ottosson, et al., Low dose dehydroepiandrosterone affects behavior in hypopituitary androgen-deficient women: A placebo-controlled trial, J Clin Endocrinol Metab 87 (5) (2002) 2046–2052.
[191] P.J. Hunt, E.M. Gurnell, F.A. Huppert, C. Richards, A.T. Prevost, J.A. Wass, et al., Improvement in mood and fatigue after dehydroepiandrosterone replacement in Addison's disease in a randomized, double blind trial, J Clin Endocrinol Metab 85 (12) (2000) 4650–4656.
[192] E.M. Gurnell, V.K. Chatterjee, Dehydroepiandrosterone replacement therapy, Eur J Endocrinol 145 (2) (2001) 103–106.
[193] W. Arlt, F. Callies, J.C. van Vlijmen, I. Koehler, M. Reincke, M. Bidlingmaier, et al., Dehydroepiandrosterone replacement in women with adrenal insufficiency, N Engl J Med 341 (14) (1999) 1013–1020.
[194] A. Brooke, L. Kalingag, F. Miraki-Moud, C. Camacho-Hübner, K. Maher, D. Walker, et al., Dehydroepiandrosterone improves psychological well-being in male and female hypopituitary patients on maintenance growth hormone replacement, J Clin Endocrinol Metab 91 (10) (2006) 3773–3779.
[195] J. Parasrampuria, K. Schwartz, R. Petesch, Quality control of dehydroepiandrosterone dietary supplement products, JAMA 280 (18) (1998) 1565.
[196] K.K. Miller, B.M. Biller, C. Beauregard, J.G. Lipman, J. Jones, D. Schoenfeld, et al., Effects of testosterone replacement in androgen-deficient women with hypopituitarism: A randomized, double-blind, placebo-controlled study, J Clin Endocrinol Metab 91 (5) (2006) 1683–1690.
[197] J. Simon, G. Braunstein, L. Nachtigall, W. Utian, M. Katz, S. Miller, et al., Testosterone patch increases sexual activity and desire in surgically menopausal women with hypoactive sexual desire disorder, J Clin Endocrinol Metab 90 (9) (2005) 5226–5233.
[198] G.D. Braunstein, D.A. Sundwall, M. Katz, J.L. Shifren, J.E. Buster, J.A. Simon, et al., Safety and efficacy of a testosterone patch for the treatment of hypoactive sexual desire disorder in surgically menopausal women: A randomized, placebo-controlled trial, Arch Intern Med 165 (14) (2005) 1582–1589.
[199] J.E. Buster, S.A. Kingsberg, O. Aguirre, C. Brown, J.G. Breaux, A. Buch, et al., Testosterone patch for low sexual desire in surgically menopausal women: A randomized trial, Obstet Gynecol 105 (5 Pt 1) (2005) 944–952.
[200] R. Bunevicius, G. Kazanavicius, R. Zalinkevicius, A.J. Prange Jr., Effects of thyroxine as compared with thyroxine plus triiodothyronine in patients with hypothyroidism, N Engl J Med 340 (6) (1999) 424–429.
[201] J. Jonklaas, B. Davidson, S. Bhagat, S. Soldin, Triiodothyronine levels in athyreotic individuals during levothyroxine therapy, JAMA 299 (7) (2008) 769–777.

[202] B.C. Appelhof, E. Fliers, E.M. Wekking, A.H. Schene, J. Huyser, J.G. Tijssen, et al., Combined therapy with levothyroxine and liothyronine in two ratios, compared with levothyroxine monotherapy in primary hypothyroidism: A double-blind, randomized, controlled clinical trial, J Clin Endocrinol Metab 90 (5) (2005) 2666–2674.

[203] H.F. Escobar-Morreale, J.I. Botella-Carretero, M. Gomez-Bueno, J.M. Galan, V. Barrios, J. Sancho, Thyroid hormone replacement therapy in primary hypothyroidism: A randomized trial comparing L-thyroxine plus liothyronine with L-thyroxine alone, Ann Intern Med 142 (6) (2005) 412–424.

[204] W. Siegmund, K. Spieker, A.I. Weike, T. Giessmann, C. Modess, T. Dabers, et al., Replacement therapy with levothyroxine plus triiodothyronine (bioavailable molar ratio 14:1) is not superior to thyroxine alone to improve well-being and cognitive performance in hypothyroidism, Clin Endocrinol (Oxf) 60 (6) (2004) 750–757.

[205] P.W. Clyde, A.E. Harari, E.J. Getka, K.M. Shakir, Combined levothyroxine plus liothyronine compared with levothyroxine alone in primary hypothyroidism: A randomized controlled trial, JAMA 290 (22) (2003) 2952–2958.

[206] J.P. Walsh, L. Shiels, E.M. Lim, C.I. Bhagat, L.C. Ward, B.G. Stuckey, et al., Combined thyroxine/liothyronine treatment does not improve well-being, quality of life, or cognitive function compared to thyroxine alone: A randomized controlled trial in patients with primary hypothyroidism, J Clin Endocrinol Metab 88 (10) (2003) 4543–4550.

[207] A.M. Sawka, H.C. Gerstein, M.J. Marriott, G.M. MacQueen, R.T. Joffe, Does a combination regimen of thyroxine (T4) and 3,5,3'-triiodothyronine improve depressive symptoms better than T4 alone in patients with hypothyroidism? Results of a double-blind, randomized, controlled trial, J Clin Endocrinol Metab 88 (10) (2003) 4551–4555.

[208] H.F. Escobar-Morreale, J.I. Botella-Carretero, F. Escobar del Rey, G. Morreale de Escobar, Review: Treatment of hypothyroidism with combinations of levothyroxine plus liothyronine, J Clin Endocrinol Metab 90 (8) (2005) 4946–4954.

[209] W.M. Wiersinga, Thyroid hormone replacement therapy, Horm Res 56 (Suppl 1) (2001) 74–81.

[210] C.G. Roberts, P.W. Ladenson, Hypothyroidism. Lancet 363 (9411) (2004) 793–803.

[211] K. Selva, S. Mandel, L. Rien, D. Sesser, R. Miyahira, M. Skeels, et al., Initial treatment dose of L-thyroxine in congenital hypothyroidism, J Pediatr 141 (6) (2002) 786–792.

[212] S.O. Skouby, F. Al-Azzawi, D. Barlow, J. Calaf-Alsina Erdogan Ertungealp, A. Gompel, A. Graziottin, et al., Climacteric medicine: European Menopause and Andropause Society (EMAS) 2004/2005 position statements on peri- and post-menopausal hormone replacement therapy, Maturitas 51 (1) (2005) 8–14.

[213] M. Hickey, S.R. Davis, D.W. Sturdee, Treatment of menopausal symptoms: What shall we do now? Lancet 366 (9483) (2005) 409–421.

[214] C.M. Farquhar, J. Marjoribanks, A. Lethaby, Q. Lamberts, J.A. Suckling, Long term hormone therapy for perimenopausal and postmenopausal women, Cochrane Database Syst Rev (3) (2005) CD004143.

[215] Hormone therapy for the prevention of chronic conditions in postmenopausal women, recommendations from the U.S. Preventive Services Task Force, Ann Intern Med 142 (10) (2005) 855–860.

[216] National Institutes of Health State-of-the-Science Conference statement, management of menopause-related symptoms, Ann Intern Med 142 (12 Pt 1) (2005) 1003–1013.

[217] D.V. Menon, W. Vongpatanasin, Effects of transdermal estrogen replacement therapy on cardiovascular risk factors, Treat Endocrinol 5 (1) (2006) 37–51.

[218] P.M. Mah, J. Webster, P. Jonsson, U. Feldt-Rasmussen, M. Koltowska-Haggstrom, R.J. Ross, Estrogen replacement in women of fertile years with hypopituitarism, J Clin Endocrinol Metab 90 (11) (2005) 5964–5969.

[219] K.C. Leung, G. Johannsson, G.M. Leong, K.K. Ho, Estrogen regulation of growth hormone action, Endocr Rev 25 (5) (2004) 693–721.

[220] J.S. Finkelstein, A. Klibanski, R.M. Neer, S.H. Doppelt, D.I. Rosenthal, G.V. Segre, et al., Increases in bone density during treatment of men with idiopathic hypogonadotropic hypogonadism, J Clin Endocrinol Metab 69 (4) (1989) 776–783.

[221] D. Finkel, J. Phillips, P. Snyder, Stimulation of spermatogenesis by gonadotropins in men with hypogonadotropic hypogonadism, N Engl J Med 313 (11) (1985) 651–655.

[222] E. Delemarre, B. Felius, Delemarre-van de Waal H, Inducing puberty. Eur J Endocrinol 159 (Suppl 1) (2008) S9–S15.

[223] Y. Okada, T. Onishi, Pubertal growth spurt induced by human chorionic gonadotropin in hypogonadotropic growth hormone-deficient children, Endocrinol Jpn 36 (5) (1989) 695–703.

[224] H. de Boer, G.J. Blok, E.A. Van der Veen, Clinical aspects of growth hormone deficiency in adults, Endocr Rev 16 (1) (1995) 63–86.

[225] W.M. Drake, S.J. Howell, J.P. Monson, S.M. Shalet, Optimizing GH therapy in adults and children, Endocr Rev 22 (4) (2001) 425–450.

[226] A.R. Hoffman, C.J. Strasburger, A. Zagar, W.F. Blum, A. Kehely, M.L. Hartman, Efficacy and tolerability of an individualized dosing regimen for adult growth hormone replacement therapy in comparison with fixed body weight-based dosing, J Clin Endocrinol Metab 89 (7) (2004) 3224–3233.

[227] G. Johannsson, T. Rosen, B.A. Bengtsson, Individualized dose titration of growth hormone (GH) during GH replacement in hypopituitary adults, Clin Endocrinol (Oxf) 47 (5) (1997) 571–581.

[228] D.M. Cook, W.H. Ludlam, M.B. Cook, Route of estrogen administration helps to determine growth hormone (GH) replacement dose in GH-deficient adults, J Clin Endocrinol Metab 84 (11) (1999) 3956–3960.

[229] P. Burman, A.G. Johansson, A. Siegbahn, B. Vessby, F.A. Karlsson, Growth hormone (GH)-deficient men are more responsive to GH replacement therapy than women, J Clin Endocrinol Metab 82 (2) (1997) 550–555.

[230] G. Johannsson, P. Marin, L. Lonn, M. Ottosson, K. Stenlof, P. Bjorntorp, et al., Growth hormone treatment of abdominally obese men reduces abdominal fat mass, improves glucose and lipoprotein metabolism, and reduces diastolic blood pressure, J Clin Endocrinol Metab 82 (3) (1997) 727–734.

[231] S.A. Beshyah, A. Henderson, C. Baynes, D. Copping, W. Richmond, D.G. Johnston, Post-heparin plasma lipase activity in hypopituitary adults, Horm Res 44 (2) (1995) 69–74.

[232] D.M. Hoffman, A.J. O'Sullivan, J. Freund, K.K. Ho, Adults with growth hormone deficiency have abnormal body composition but normal energy metabolism, J Clin Endocrinol Metab 80 (1) (1995) 72–77.

[233] A.F. Attanasio, P.C. Bates, K.K. Ho, S.M. Webb, R.J. Ross, C.J. Strasburger, et al., Human growth hormone replacement in adult hypopituitary patients: Long-term effects on body composition and lipid status – 3-year results from the HypoCCS Database, J Clin Endocrinol Metab 87 (4) (2002) 1600–1606.

[234] A. Chrisoulidou, S.A. Beshyah, O. Rutherford, T.J. Spinks, J. Mayet, P. Kyd, et al., Effects of 7 years of growth hormone replacement therapy in hypopituitary adults, J Clin Endocrinol Metab 85 (10) (2000) 3762–3769.
[235] A.R. Hoffman, J.E. Kuntze, J. Baptista, H.B. Baum, G.P. Baumann, B.M. Biller, et al., Growth hormone (GH) replacement therapy in adult-onset GH deficiency: Effects on body composition in men and women in a double-blind, randomized, placebo-controlled trial, J Clin Endocrinol Metab 89 (5) (2004) 2048–2056.
[236] B.A. Bengtsson, S. Eden, L. Lonn, H. Kvist, A. Stokland, G. Lindstedt, et al., Treatment of adults with growth hormone (GH) deficiency with recombinant human GH, J Clin Endocrinol Metab 76 (2) (1993) 309–317.
[237] J. Gibney, J.D. Wallace, T. Spinks, L. Schnorr, A. Ranicar, R.C. Cuneo, et al., The effects of 10 years of recombinant human growth hormone (GH) in adult GH-deficient patients, J Clin Endocrinol Metab 84 (8) (1999) 2596–2602.
[238] K.A. Al-Shoumer, K. Ali, V. Anyaoku, R. Niththyananthan, D.G. Johnston, Overnight metabolic fuel deficiency in patients treated conventionally for hypopituitarism, Clin Endocrinol (Oxf) 45 (2) (1996) 171–178.
[239] G. Johannsson, G. Grimby, K.S. Sunnerhagen, B.A. Bengtsson, Two years of growth hormone (GH) treatment increase isometric and isokinetic muscle strength in GH-deficient adults, J Clin Endocrinol Metab 82 (9) (1997) 2877–2884.
[240] J. Svensson, K.S. Sunnerhagen, G. Johannsson, Five years of growth hormone replacement therapy in adults: Age- and gender-related changes in isometric and isokinetic muscle strength, J Clin Endocrinol Metab 88 (5) (2003) 2061–2069.
[241] R.C. Cuneo, F. Salomon, C.M. Wiles, R. Hesp, P.H. Sonksen, Growth hormone treatment in growth hormone-deficient adults. II. Effects on exercise performance, J Appl Physiol 70 (2) (1991) 695–700.
[242] L.J. Woodhouse, S.L. Asa, S.G. Thomas, S. Ezzat, Measures of submaximal aerobic performance evaluate and predict functional response to growth hormone (GH) treatment in GH-deficient adults, J Clin Endocrinol Metab 84 (12) (1999) 4570–4577.
[243] T. Elgzyri, J. Castenfors, E. Hagg, C. Backman, M. Thoren, M. Bramnert, The effects of GH replacement therapy on cardiac morphology and function, exercise capacity and serum lipids in elderly patients with GH deficiency, Clin Endocrinol (Oxf) 61 (1) (2004) 113–122.
[244] N. Bravenboer, P. Holzmann, H. de Boer, G.J. Blok, P. Lips, Histomorphometric analysis of bone mass and bone metabolism in growth hormone deficient adult men, Bone 18 (6) (1996) 551–557.
[245] P. Vestergaard, J.O. Jorgensen, C. Hagen, H.C. Hoeck, P. Laurberg, L. Rejnmark, et al., Fracture risk is increased in patients with GH deficiency or untreated prolactinomas – a case-control study, Clin Endocrinol (Oxf) 56 (2) (2002) 159–167.
[246] C. Wuster, R. Abs, B.A. Bengtsson, H. Bennmarker, U. Feldt-Rasmussen, E. Hernberg-Stahl, et al., The influence of growth hormone deficiency, growth hormone replacement therapy, and other aspects of hypopituitarism on fracture rate and bone mineral density, J Bone Miner Res 16 (2) (2001) 398–405.
[247] T. Rosen, L. Wilhelmsen, K. Landin-Wilhelmsen, G. Lappas, B.A. Bengtsson, Increased fracture frequency in adult patients with hypopituitarism and GH deficiency, Eur J Endocrinol 137 (3) (1997) 240–245.
[248] G. Johannsson, T. Rosen, I. Bosaeus, L. Sjostrom, B.A. Bengtsson, Two years of growth hormone (GH) treatment increases bone mineral content and density in hypopituitary patients with adult-onset GH deficiency, J Clin Endocrinol Metab 81 (8) (1996) 2865–2873.
[249] M. Bex, R. Abs, D. Maiter, A. Beckers, G. Lamberigts, R. Bouillon, The effects of growth hormone replacement therapy on bone metabolism in adult-onset growth hormone deficiency: A 2-year open randomized controlled multicenter trial, J Bone Miner Res 17 (6) (2002) 1081–1094.
[250] W.M. Drake, J. Rodriguez-Arnao, J.U. Weaver, I.T. James, D. Coyte, T.D. Spector, et al., The influence of gender on the short- and long-term effects of growth hormone replacement on bone metabolism and bone mineral density in hypopituitary adults: A 5-year study, Clin Endocrinol (Oxf) 54 (4) (2001) 525–532.
[251] J.C. Smith, L.M. Evans, I. Wilkinson, J. Goodfellow, J.R. Cockcroft, M.F. Scanlon, et al., Effects of GH replacement on endothelial function and large-artery stiffness in GH-deficient adults: A randomized, double-blind, placebo-controlled study, Clin Endocrinol (Oxf) 56 (4) (2002) 493–501.
[252] P. Maison, S. Griffin, M. Nicoue-Beglah, N. Haddad, B. Balkau, P. Chanson, Impact of growth hormone (GH) treatment on cardiovascular risk factors in GH-deficient adults: A meta-analysis of blinded, randomized, placebo-controlled trials, J Clin Endocrinol Metab 89 (5) (2004) 2192–2199.
[253] T. Kearney, C.N. de Gallegos, A. Proudler, K. Parker, V. Anayaoku, P. Bannister, et al., Effects of short- and long-term growth hormone replacement on lipoprotein composition and on very-low-density lipoprotein and low-density lipoprotein apolipoprotein B100 kinetics in growth hormone-deficient hypopituitary subjects, Metabolism: Clinical and Experimental 52 (1) (2003) 50–59.
[254] A. Colao, C. Di Somma, M. Salerno, L. Spinelli, F. Orio, G. Lombardi, The cardiovascular risk of GH-deficient adolescents, J Clin Endocrinol Metab 87 (8) (2002) 3650–3655.
[255] A.F. Attanasio, S.W. Lamberts, A.M. Matranga, M.A. Birkett, P.C. Bates, N.K. Valk, et al., Adult growth hormone (GH)-deficient patients demonstrate heterogeneity between childhood onset and adult onset before and during human GH treatment. Adult Growth Hormone Deficiency Study Group, J Clin Endocrinol Metab 82 (1) (1997) 82–88.
[256] N. Mauras, O.H. Pescovitz, V. Allada, M. Messig, M.P. Wajnrajch, B. Lippe, et al., Limited efficacy of growth hormone (GH) during transition of GH-deficient patients from adolescence to adulthood: A phase III multicenter, double-blind, randomized two-year trial, J Clin Endocrinol Metab 90 (7) (2005) 3946–3955.
[257] F. Borson-Chazot, A. Serusclat, Y. Kalfallah, X. Ducottet, G. Sassolas, S. Bernard, et al., Decrease in carotid intima-media thickness after one year growth hormone (GH) treatment in adults with GH deficiency, J Clin Endocrinol Metab 84 (4) (1999) 1329–1333.
[258] M. Pfeifer, R. Verhovec, B. Zizek, J. Prezelj, P. Poredos, R.N. Clayton, Growth hormone (GH) treatment reverses early atherosclerotic changes in GH-deficient adults, J Clin Endocrinol Metab 84 (2) (1999) 453–457.
[259] P. Maison, P. Chanson, Cardiac effects of growth hormone in adults with growth hormone deficiency: A meta-analysis, Circulation 108 (21) (2003) 2648–2652.
[260] M. Rosilio, W.F. Blum, D.J. Edwards, E.P. Shavrikova, D. Valle, S.W. Lamberts, et al., Long-term improvement of quality of life during growth hormone (GH) replacement therapy in adults with GH deficiency, as measured by questions on life satisfaction-hypopituitarism (QLS-H), J Clin Endocrinol Metab 89 (4) (2004) 1684–1693.
[261] R.D. Murray, C.J. Skillicorn, S.J. Howell, C.A. Lissett, A. Rahim, L.E. Smethurst, et al., Influences on quality of life in GH deficient adults and their effect on response to treatment, Clin Endocrinol (Oxf) 51 (5) (1999) 565–573.

[262] R.D. Murray, S.M. Shalet, Adult growth hormone replacement: Lessons learned and future direction, J Clin Endocrinol Metab 87 (10) (2002) 4427–4428.

[263] E.O. Reiter, D.A. Price, P. Wilton, K. Albertsson-Wikland, M.B. Ranke, Effect of growth hormone (GH) treatment on the near-final height of 1258 patients with idiopathic GH deficiency: Analysis of a large international database, J Clin Endocrinol Metab 91 (6) (2006) 2047–2054.

[264] P.E. Clayton, R.C. Cuneo, A. Juul, J.P. Monson, S.M. Shalet, M. Tauber, Consensus statement on the management of the GH-treated adolescent in the transition to adult care, Eur J Endocrinol 152 (2) (2005) 165–170.

[265] L.E. Underwood, K.M. Attie, J. Baptista, Growth hormone (GH) dose-response in young adults with childhood-onset GH deficiency: A two-year, multicenter, multiple-dose, placebo-controlled study, J Clin Endocrinol Metab 88 (11) (2003) 5273–5280.

[266] S.M. Shalet, E. Shavrikova, M. Cromer, C.J. Child, E. Keller, J. Zapletalova, et al., Effect of growth hormone (GH) treatment on bone in postpubertal GH-deficient patients: A 2-year randomized, controlled, dose-ranging study, J Clin Endocrinol Metab 88 (9) (2003) 4124–4129.

[267] W.M. Drake, P.V. Carroll, K.T. Maher, K.A. Metcalfe, C. Camacho-Hubner, N.J. Shaw, et al., The effect of cessation of growth hormone (GH) therapy on bone mineral accretion in GH-deficient adolescents at the completion of linear growth, J Clin Endocrinol Metab 88 (4) (2003) 1658–1663.

[268] N. Vahl, A. Juul, J.O. Jorgensen, H. Orskov, N.E. Skakkebaek, J.S. Christiansen, Continuation of growth hormone (GH) replacement in GH-deficient patients during transition from childhood to adulthood: A two-year placebo-controlled study, J Clin Endocrinol Metab 85 (5) (2000) 1874–1881.

[269] G. Johannsson, K. Albertsson-Wikland, B.A. Bengtsson, Discontinuation of growth hormone (GH) treatment: Metabolic effects in GH-deficient and GH-sufficient adolescent patients compared with control subjects. Swedish Study Group for Growth Hormone Treatment in Children, J Clin Endocrinol Metab 84 (12) (1999) 4516–4524.

CHAPTER

11

Pituitary Function in Systemic Disorders

Harold E. Carlson

Stony Brook University, Stony Brook, NY, USA

INTRODUCTION

The pituitary gland may be affected by a wide variety of systemic disorders (Table 11.1). In some instances, the pituitary is directly involved by the same processes that also afflict other organs, while in other disorders, the primary disease process has indirect, distant effects on pituitary function.

TABLE 11.1 Systemic Disorders Affecting the Pituitary

Direct Involvement	Indirect Involvement
Iron overload	Any severe systemic illness
Sarcoidosis	Aging
Wegener's granulomatosis	Obesity
Tuberculosis	Diabetes mellitus
HIV infection	Renal failure
Syphilis	Liver disease
Bacterial or fungal abscess	Primary hypothyroidism
Toxoplasmosis	Thyrotoxicosis
Hemorrhagic fever with renal syndrome	Hypoadrenalism
Snakebite (Russell's viper)	Malnutrition
Langerhans' cell histiocytosis	
Metastatic cancer	
Multiple endocrine neoplasia syndrome	
Polyglandular endocrine autoimmunity	
Amyloidosis	

DISORDERS DIRECTLY AFFECTING THE PITUITARY

Iron Overload

Patients with excessive tissue iron deposits, either from idiopathic hemochromatosis, multiple transfusions, or prolonged use of pharmaceutic iron supplements, often develop hypogonadism [1–9]. Female patients appear to suffer from this complication less frequently than males, perhaps because of the protective effects of monthly menstrual blood loss. Although occasional patients appear to have primary testicular failure or hypothalamic pathology as the cause of the hypogonadism [4,5,10,11], pituitary gonadotropic insufficiency is responsible for the hypogonadism in the vast majority of cases. This conclusion is supported by findings of low basal serum gonadotropin levels, impaired gonadotropin responses to gonadotropin-releasing hormone (GnRH) [1,3–7,9–12,14], even with prolonged, pulsatile GnRH administration [9,10,13] and generally intact testosterone responses to human chorionic gonadotropin (hCG) stimulation [1,5,7,9,13]. In nearly all patients, the secretion of growth hormone (GH), thyrotropin (thyroid-stimulating hormone; TSH) and adrenocorticotropic hormone (ACTH) is normal [1,3–6,9,12,14], although GH deficiency has been identified in some patients with transfusion iron overload [15]. A minority of patients have a modest impairment in prolactin (PRL) secretion, primarily revealed as diminished PRL responses in stimulation tests with thyrotropin-releasing hormone (TRH) or chlorpromazine [5,6,12,16]. These findings correlate well with histochemical observations localizing pituitary iron deposits primarily to the gonadotrophs and, less frequently, to the lactotrophs [17]. Pituitary iron deposition may also be visualized radiologically; in hemochromatosis, the anterior pituitary may have abnormally low signal

The Pituitary, *Third Edition*, DOI: 10.1016/B978-0-12-380926-1.10011-2

intensity on T_2-weighted magnetic resonance (MR) images [18]. In some cases, gonadotropin and thyrotropin secretion and end-organ function have improved following iron depletion therapy [10,19–21], but in other patients pituitary function is unchanged by these procedures [9,12]. In children who receive multiple transfusions for thalassemia major, early intensive iron chelation therapy may prevent pituitary damage, allowing normal pubertal development to take place [1].

Sarcoidosis

Sarcoid granulomas involve the central nervous system (CNS) in about 5% of cases, and there is evidence of hypothalamic or pituitary dysfunction in about one-third of these [22–24]. Anatomically, both the hypothalamus and pituitary may be affected; visual symptoms often result from involvement of the optic chiasm [22,24–26]. On computed tomography (CT) scanning, CNS sarcoid lesions usually show contrast enhancement, generally without surrounding edema or calcification [29]. The appearance of CNS sarcoid lesions on MR scanning is more variable; the majority of lesions enhance with gadolinium [24,29,30]. Recent reports suggest that sarcoid lesions in the CNS and elsewhere are often visualized on positron emission tomography using ^{18}F-fluorodeoxyglucose [31]. Patients with hypothalamic–pituitary involvement usually have extensive involvement of many organ systems with sarcoidosis, but occasional instances of isolated hypothalamic–pituitary disease have been reported [25].

Studies using provocative testing have demonstrated a high prevalence of hypothalamic dysfunction, with intact pituitary hormonal responses to releasing factors but impaired responses to clomiphene, metyrapone and insulin hypoglycemia [32–34]. Hyperprolactinemia occurs [23,24,32,35], but is not a universal finding in patients with hypothalamic–pituitary involvement [24,32,33]. Disturbances of water metabolism are common and include diabetes insipidus, primary polydipsia and the syndrome of inappropriate antidiuretic hormone secretion (SIADH) [24,32–34,36–39]. Other reported features of hypothalamic dysfunction have included polyphagia with morbid obesity [40] and disordered temperature regulation and vascular control [41].

Therapy with corticosteroids or other immunosuppressive agents usually does not improve hypothalamic–pituitary function, but occasional beneficial responses have been noted [24,32,39]. Hormone replacement therapy is given as indicated.

Wegener's Granulomatosis

A small number of patients have been reported with Wegener's granulomatosis involving the pituitary. Diabetes insipidus is the most common endocrine manifestation, but anterior pituitary hypofunction has also been described. Radiologic studies usually show pituitary enlargement and thickening of the stalk [42,43].

Infectious Diseases

Tuberculosis has a predilection for involvement of the basilar meninges and may therefore occasionally involve tissues in the sellar region, sometimes producing anterior or posterior pituitary insufficiency [44,45]. Tuberculous meningitis may also cause SIADH [46]. Radiologically, pituitary tuberculomas may resemble other sellar mass lesions; thickening of the stalk is seen in some cases [44,45]. Syphilitic infections of the hypothalamus or pituitary are rare; they usually take the form of a gumma which may be asymptomatic or may produce local mass effects or pituitary hypofunction [47,48]. Pyogenic and fungal infections of the pituitary, usually in the form of abscesses, are rare [49,50]. Whipple's disease and Chagas' disease may also occasionally involve the pituitary [51,52]. Although Lyme disease may affect the central nervous system (CNS), there have been no reports of pituitary dysfunction in this condition.

In the acquired immune deficiency syndrome (AIDS), the hypothalamus and pituitary may be infected with the human immunodeficiency virus (HIV) or any of a variety of opportunistic pathogens, including cytomegalovirus, *Pneumocystis carinii*, *Cryptococcus neoformans* and *Toxoplasma gondii* [53–56]; in some cases pituitary function was impaired [54,57,58]. CNS lymphomas may also involve the pituitary of AIDS patients [56]. Even in the absence of pituitary infection, functional abnormalities of the pituitary are common in AIDS, reflecting the changes accompanying any severe systemic illness (see below); these include the euthyroid sick syndrome and hypogonadotropic hypogonadism [59–63]. Occasional patients may have ACTH deficiency [64], GH deficiency [65], hypergonadotropic hypogonadism [66], increased gonadal function [67] and enhanced secretion of ACTH, TSH, LH, GH, or PRL [68,69]. Hyponatremia due to SIADH is common and usually secondary to pulmonary or CNS pathology [60,63]. It is clear that the spectrum of endocrine abnormalities in AIDS is broad, and that much more study is needed to define their pathogenesis.

Hemorrhagic fever with renal syndrome is a viral illness characterized by fever, hypotension, capillary leak and acute renal failure; several varieties of Asian and European hantaviruses cause the syndrome. Approximately 20% of the infected patients in one series developed pituitary hormone deficiencies. Pituitary atrophy and empty sella were seen radiologically. Autopsy studies have shown pituitary hemorrhage and necrosis [70]. A wide variety of viral infections causing encephalitis may occasionally result in hypothalamic–pituitary dysfunction, presumably from damage to neural structures [71].

Langerhans' Cell Histiocytosis

Langerhans' cell histiocytosis (also known as histiocytosis X or Hand-Schuller-Christian disease) is characterized by involvement of more than one site or system by lesions composed of lipid-laden histiocytes, eosinophils, lymphocytes and plasma cells. The hypothalamus and posterior pituitary are frequent sites of involvement, which may be demonstrated radiologically as enhancing mass lesions on CT or as bright, gadolinium-enhancing areas on MR scanning. Thickening of the pituitary stalk is common and the posterior pituitary bright spot is frequently absent in patients with diabetes insipidus [72–74]. Diabetes insipidus (DI) is the most common endocrine disturbance, occurring in about one-quarter of the patients, followed by growth retardation and other anterior pituitary hormone deficiencies in a minority of subjects [72,75–78]. Hypothalamic or stalk pathology appears to be responsible for the majority of cases of GH and gonadotropin deficiency, since these patients do respond to GH-releasing hormone (GHRH) and GnRH, especially when given in repeated pulsatile doses [79,80]. Hyperprolactinemia, seen in some patients, also points to a hypothalamic or stalk disturbance, and may contribute to the suppression of gonadotropins.

Although the mass effect of hypothalamic and stalk lesions may itself result in DI, there is also evidence that autoimmune factors may play a role in the condition's pathogenesis. Scherbaum et al. [81] have detected autoantibodies to vasopressin-secreting hypothalamic cells in 54% of patients with DI due to Langerhans' cell histiocytosis. Since the Langerhans' cell histiocyte may function as an antigen-presenting cell, infiltration of these cells into the hypothalamus could lead to immunologically mediated destruction of vasopressin neurons [81]. Such a mechanism could conceivably account for the occurrence of DI in patients who have no hypothalamic or posterior pituitary lesions at autopsy [82].

Hormone replacement is indicated in the treatment of endocrine deficiencies in histiocytosis; corticosteroids, cytotoxic chemotherapy and radiation therapy have rarely been effective in restoring endocrine function in patients with hypothalamic involvement [72,75–78].

Snakebite

In south Asia, bites and envenomation by Russell's viper are common. The venom contains powerful procoagulants whose action results in disseminated intravascular coagulation, while other toxins damage capillary endothelia, leading to spontaneous hemorrhage, edema and shock. Acute renal failure is the usual cause of death [83]. Autopsy studies frequently show fibrin thrombi in the anterior pituitary, along with hemorrhage and necrosis [83], and recent investigations have documented a high prevalence of hypopituitarism in long-term survivors [84,85]. It is likely that hypopituitarism may contribute to the morbidity and mortality of the acute stage of illness in the initial hours and days postenvenomation [84,85]. Pituitary necrosis and hypopituitarism appear to be uncommon following bites of other species of poisonous snakes, with only one other case being reported following a bite by the jararacucu of Brazil [86].

Metastatic Cancer

Cancer metastases have been found in the hypothalamus, pituitary or sella turcica in 1–27% of autopsied cancer cases [87–89]. Pituitary metastases are frequently located in the posterior lobe, which receives blood from the systemic circulation via the inferior hypophyseal artery. In contrast, the anterior lobe does not have a significant direct, systemic blood supply, being supplied principally by the hypothalamic–pituitary portal system. Breast and lung cancers are the most common types associated with pituitary metastases [90,91]. Most pituitary and hypothalamic metastases are asymptomatic, but about 7% result in DI and a smaller number show anterior pituitary insufficiency [90–93]. Occasionally, pituitary metastasis may be the presenting feature of an occult primary cancer [90,91,93], leading to confusion with a primary pituitary adenoma. The presence of headache, extraocular palsies and DI are features suggesting pituitary metastasis [90,92,93]. Stereotactic radiation therapy has improved neurological symptoms and diabetes insipidus in some cases [94].

Polyglandular Syndromes

Pituitary tumors occur commonly in the syndrome of multiple endocrine neoplasia (MEN) type 1, along with pancreatic islet cell tumors and hyperparathyroidism [95,96]. Pituitary neoplasms may also occasionally be found in patients with features of MEN type 2A (consisting of medullary carcinoma of the thyroid, pheochromocytoma and hyperparathyroidism); these cases have raised the concept of "overlap" syndromes [96–99]. Many of these "overlap" cases involve the co-occurrence of pheochromocytoma and acromegaly; detailed examination of three of these cases has shown that the pheochromocytoma was producing GHRH and the pituitary lesion was actually somatotroph hyperplasia rather than an adenoma [96,98,99]. Thus, at least some of these "overlap" cases may represent an isolated pheochromocytoma with secondary pituitary hyperfunction due to production of a hormonal stimulating factor by the adrenal tumor. Similarly, other presumed cases of MEN type 1 have been shown to actually represent an isolated pancreatic islet cell tumor which produced GHRH, resulting in somatotroph hyperplasia and acromegaly [100].

Another recently described syndrome, termed the "Carney complex," consists of myxomas, spotty mucocutaneous pigmentation and endocrine overactivity (testicular tumors, pigmented nodular adrenocortical hyperplasia and acromegaly). The syndrome is due to inactivating mutations in the gene coding for the 1α regulatory subunit of protein kinase A (PRKAR1A) and is inherited in an autosomal dominant fashion. No other pituitary lesions have been found in the cases described to date and clinical acromegaly has occurred in only about 10% of patients [101,102]. Cyclic AMP-mediated stimulation of GH secretion also appears to be responsible for the occasional cases of acromegaly occurring in the McCune-Albright syndrome, due to activating mutations of the $G_s\alpha$-subunit of the G-protein which activates adenylate cyclase [103].

In polyglandular autoimmune states, clinical involvement of the pituitary is rare [104]. Lymphocytic hypophysitis, an uncommon disorder of pregnant and postpartum women, is associated in some cases with other evidence of endocrine autoimmunity [105]. Antibodies to pituitary tissue have been found in some patients with lymphocytic hypophysitis and in a variety of other endocrine autoimmune disorders, as well as in some patients with the primary empty sella syndrome and Sheehan's syndrome, but, to date, the functional significance of these antibodies remains unclear [105,106].

Amyloidosis

Microscopic amyloid deposits are frequently seen in blood vessel walls and interstitial areas in normal human pituitaries from elderly subjects [107], and amyloid may be deposited in pituitary blood vessels in patients with systemic amyloidosis [108]. Pituitary function is usually intact; however, very few cases of hypopituitarism have been reported [109]. Spherical deposits of amyloid have occasionally been found in the lactotroph cells of prolactin-secreting pituitary adenomas. The amyloid is apparently composed of prolactin fragments and does not deposit in other tissues [110].

GENERAL EFFECTS OF SYSTEMIC ILLNESS ON PITUITARY FUNCTION

Illness, injury and stress, if sufficiently severe, produce a constellation of endocrine changes that are, in general, independent of the specific type of illness.

ACTH and Adrenal Function

With acute stress and illness, ACTH and cortisol secretion are increased [111–116]. Although this is, in part, due to increased release of corticotropin-releasing hormone (CRH), other factors (e.g., vasopressin, interleukin-1) may also play a role in stimulating ACTH secretion [111–114]. Adrenal androgen secretion is also acutely stimulated early in the course of illness but falls below normal when the illness continues for a week or more [111,115,116]. Additionally, adrenal aldosterone secretion is impaired in critical illness despite stimulation with angiotensin II [117]. Taken together, these observations suggest an adaptive adrenocortical shift in steroid production away from androgens and mineralocorticoids in order to maximize cortisol secretion.

In recent years, the concept of "relative adrenal insufficiency" has been proposed as a contributor to mortality in septic shock. At present, there is no clear consensus on the existence, diagnosis, or treatment of this condition. Current data suggest that there is no readily available laboratory test to diagnose sepsis-related adrenal insufficiency, and, in addition, there has been no survival benefit shown for glucocorticoid therapy [118–122].

TSH

Prolonged physical stress or illness (e.g., major surgery, severe infections) results in the so-called "non-thyroidal illness syndrome" or "euthyroid sick syndrome" [112,114,123,124]. In its milder form, there is an alteration in the peripheral metabolism of thyroxine (T_4) such that production of triiodothyronine (T_3) is decreased while the production of reverse T_3 is increased; deiodination of reverse T_3 is impaired, further contributing to a rise in its serum concentration. Serum T_4 and TSH levels are normal, and T_3 and reverse T_3 concentrations return to normal following recovery [114].

In severe, usually life-threatening, illness, the same changes in serum T_3 and reverse T_3 occur but, in addition, serum T_4 falls [112,114,123,124]. Although conflicting data have been published, free T_4 levels are generally normal, with the fall in total T_4 being produced by changes in concentration or affinity of serum carrier proteins for thyroid hormones [114,123]. Normal serum free T_4 levels would predict normal levels of TSH and, indeed, this seems to be the case in most patients [114,123]. During the recovery phase, serum TSH may be transiently mildly elevated, with a later return to normal as serum T_4 normalizes [114,123]. No clear benefit has been shown when patients with the nonthyroidal illness syndrome have been treated with either T_3 or T_4 [114,123,125–128].

PRL

Stress, injury and illness often raise serum PRL [112,114], though levels return to normal with recovery.

GH

GH secretion is frequently stimulated by stress, injury and illness, though serum insulin-like growth factor-I (IGF-I) is low [112,114]. Both GH and IGF-I return to normal after recovery [129].

Gonadotropins

In the initial hours of stress or surgery, there is a transient rise in serum luteinizing hormone (LH) which rapidly returns to normal [112,130]. When stress or illness continues for days to weeks, serum LH and follicle-stimulating hormone (FSH) remain normal or fall to low levels, associated with a fall in serum total testosterone and free testosterone in men [112,130,131]; similar decreases in serum gonadotropins have been observed in women [116,132]. GnRH administration stimulates LH and FSH secretion during severe illness, although these responses are sometimes blunted [112,131,133]. These observations may relate, in part, to the duration and severity of illness and to the need for repetitive GnRH stimulation to elicit normal gonadotropin responses in hypothalamic disorders [134].

The mechanisms producing hypogonadotropic hypogonadism during illness are unclear; possibilities include the suppressive effect of circulating cytokines, increased aromatization of androgens to estrogens and overproduction of endogenous opioids, all of which may suppress gonadotropin secretion [112,131,133].

Several authors have drawn parallels between the hypogonadism of severe illness and the nonthyroidal illness syndrome; indeed, the occurrence of hypogonadism seems to correlate with depressed serum thyroid hormone levels [112,131]. Although the mechanisms may be different, the changes in both cases may operate to conserve the body's resources during periods of extreme stress.

PITUITARY ALTERATIONS IN SPECIFIC SYSTEMIC DISORDERS

Aging

Though not strictly a disease, aging is associated with certain changes in the pituitary. Pituitary size, assessed radiologically, decreases mildly with age [135,136], although the weight of the gland is maintained [137]. This change in density suggests a qualitative change in the pituitary; indeed, there is a decrease in pituitary parenchymal cells with age [137] and an increase in fibrosis [138]. Most of the decrease in pituitary parenchymal cells is due to fewer and smaller somatotrophs [137]; lactotrophs change little [137,139] and gonadotrophs may be enlarged [140].

Functional changes also occur. The most dramatic, of course, is the loss of ovarian function at the menopause, with a consequent elevation of serum LH and FSH due to activation of normal feedback mechanisms [141]. Similar changes, albeit more gradual and of lesser magnitude, take place in many normal elderly men, in whom some degree of testicular failure develops. Total serum testosterone falls while serum sex-hormone-binding globulin (SHBG) increases, with more dramatic falls in free or bioavailable testosterone [142,143]. Serum LH and FSH are often normal, but may be elevated in some patients [142–144]. Although GnRH secretion appears to be diminished [145], testicular responsiveness to LH or hCG is also decreased [145,146]. Concurrent obesity and medical comorbidities appear to further modulate the effects of aging [142–144].

GH secretion also declines with age, and 24-hour integrated serum GH concentrations are reduced in elderly subjects. This is primarily due to a reduction in the amplitude and duration of GH secretory pulses, especially those occurring during sleep [145,146]. As a consequence, serum IGF-I and GH-dependent IGF-binding proteins are also decreased [146–148]. It is not clear whether the primary defect in GH secretion is at the hypothalamic or pituitary level, since GH responses in the elderly to insulin hypoglycemia and arginine have been reported to be normal [145] or reduced [190,191]. GH responses to GHRH have been shown to be reduced in the elderly [145,149]. Consistent with this finding, the number and size of somatotrophs in the pituitary has been shown to be reduced in aged subjects [137]. These findings could be explained either by a chronic decrease in endogenous GHRH, an increase in somatostatin tone, or a primary pituitary process, independent of hypothalamic regulatory factors; there are few data bearing on this point. IGF-I responses to either endogenous or exogenous GH are intact in the elderly [146,150].

It has been suggested that decreased GH secretion and decreased serum IGF-I are causally related to the decrease in lean body mass and increase in adiposity seen with aging or to decreased sex steroid production in the elderly [145,150]. In therapeutic trials, administration of recombinant biosynthetic human GH to elderly subjects normalized serum IGF-I levels, increased lean body mass and decreased adipose tissue mass [150,151]. Despite these apparent benefits, small but significant increases in blood pressure, serum insulin and blood glucose concentrations, along with the occurrence of edema, arthralgias and carpal tunnel syndrome in subjects given GH, do raise questions about the safety of its long-term administration to wide segments of the adult population [150]. There is also a theoretical concern that increased GH or IGF-I could promote the development or progression of neoplasia.

Basal serum PRL concentrations are probably changed little with aging, as are PRL responses to various secretagogues [152,153], although individual studies have reported decreased, increased, or unaltered responses. Major confounding effects of illness, drugs and decreased gonadal function may account for these discrepant results.

With aging, serum T_3 levels fall modestly, perhaps due to medical comorbidities and the nonthyroidal illness syndrome, while serum T_4 remains nearly stable; in most (though not all) studies, serum TSH increases slightly with advancing age [153–155]. The rise in average TSH levels is not due to a high prevalence of autoimmune thyroid failure, since it is observed even when subjects with positive antithyroid antibodies and any family history of thyroid disease are excluded from consideration [156,157]. Most studies agree that the TSH response to TRH is diminished in the elderly [153–155].

In the absence of disease, the pituitary–adrenal axis appears to be generally intact in the elderly, although several studies have reported modest increases in basal plasma cortisol and ACTH secretion, and less suppression of cortisol by dexamethasone, particularly in elderly women [158–160]. In contrast, both basal and stimulated plasma levels of dehydroepiandrosterone (DHEA) and DHEA-sulfate are markedly diminished in elderly subjects [142,159].

Obesity

Several aspects of pituitary function are altered in obesity. Most dramatic is the decrease in GH secretion. Both spontaneous and stimulated GH secretion are blunted, and are improved following weight loss [161–165]. Despite decreased GH secretion, serum total IGF-I levels are generally within the normal range, although perhaps somewhat lower than age-matched subjects of normal weight [161,165]. Serum free IGF-I has been reported to be increased, however, and may contribute to the suppression of GH secretion in obesity [166,167].

PRL secretion is minimally altered in obesity. Basal and 24-hour integrated PRL levels are normal in obese subjects, although PRL responses to a variety of pharmacologic agents (TRH, dopamine antagonists) may be blunted in some patients [161,168]. Although most of these responses improve after weight loss, the blunted PRL response to insulin-induced hypoglycemia may persist, suggesting an intrinsic hypothalamic abnormality [168].

In most obese men, testicular function is normal. Serum total testosterone may be low, however, due to reduced concentrations of its carrier protein, sex-hormone-binding globulin; free testosterone concentrations are usually normal, as are serum LH and FSH [161,169,170]. In some extremely obese men, however, even free testosterone is depressed; this appears to be due to suppression of LH by excessive estrogens produced by aromatization of androgens in adipose tissue [161].

Obese postmenopausal women also have increased aromatization of androgens to estrogens in adipose tissue. Obese premenopausal women, especially those with abdominal obesity, may suffer from hyperandrogenism, increased serum LH, and polycystic ovary syndrome [169].

Serum concentrations of thyroid hormones and TSH are normal in obesity, both basally and following stimulation by TRH [161]. Likewise, serum cortisol, urinary free cortisol and plasma ACTH are usually normal in obese subjects [161], though some patients with abdominal obesity may have modest increases in urinary free cortisol, salivary cortisol, and cortisol responses to stress, ACTH or administration of CRH-arginine vasopressin [171].

Diabetes Mellitus

A variety of pituitary abnormalities have been reported in diabetics. Infarction of the adenohypophysis may occur without antecedent hypotension, and may lead to hypopituitarism [172]. Functional abnormalities may also occur in the absence of anatomic changes; many of these reports have been contradictory, with normal, increased, or decreased responses to various stimulation tests recorded [173]. The most consistent abnormality has been an elevation of basal serum GH in poorly controlled diabetics; most, but not all, investigators have found that basal GH returns to normal when the diabetes is better controlled. Despite the chronic hyperglycemia, GH responses to provocative stimuli are generally intact in diabetes [173]. Serum IGF-I is decreased in poorly controlled diabetics and increases with improved diabetic control [173,174].

Renal Failure

A host of endocrine abnormalities occur in uremia; many affect the pituitary. Basal serum GH is normal or elevated in uremia and GH regulation is disturbed, with diminished responses to hypoglycemia, exaggerated responses to L-dopa and GHRH and paradoxical GH responses to TRH and hyperglycemia [175–177]. Serum IGF-I concentrations are normal or elevated in uremic plasma, but somatomedin bioactivity is decreased due to the presence of circulating inhibitors and changes in IGF-binding proteins [175–177].

Serum PRL is modestly increased in many uremic patients, due principally to increased hormone secretion rather than decreased PRL clearance [178,179]. It persists despite dialysis, but is reversed by successful renal transplantation [178]. The role of secondary hyperparathyroidism in the causation of uremic hyperprolactinemia is unclear [180,181].

Hypogonadism is common in uremia and probably multifactorial in origin; gonadal function is not improved by dialysis, but is usually normalized by renal transplantation [178,179]. There is evidence for both central and gonadal defects in the pathogenesis of uremic hypogonadism. In most patients, serum gonadotropins are normal or elevated, with a normal or blunted response to GnRH; testicular responsiveness to hCG is also blunted [178].

The pituitary–thyroid axis is mildly deranged in uremia. Thyroid hormone concentrations are normal or low, and serum TSH is normal. Conversion of T_4 to T_3 is decreased, although reverse T_3 levels are normal. The serum TSH response to TRH is depressed and delayed. In general, the changes seen in uremia resemble those seen in the "euthyroid sick" or "nonthyroidal illness" syndrome, with the exception of the normal serum reverse T_3 level. Dialysis has little effect on the disordered thyroid function, but renal transplantation may correct most of the defects; residual abnormalities persisting after transplantation may be due to the effects of immunosuppressive therapy [182,183].

The hypothalamic–pituitary–adrenal axis is probably basically intact in renal failure, with normal serum concentrations of cortisol and a normal diurnal rhythm [178]. Nevertheless, a prolonged half life of cortisol in the serum, coupled with accelerated degradation and poor oral absorption of dexamethasone, results in incomplete suppressibility of cortisol in uremia [184]; measurements of serum dexamethasone can ensure a valid test.

Liver Disease

Chronic liver disease produces a wide variety of endocrine disturbances. In patients with cirrhosis, basal serum GH is increased, and paradoxical increases in GH are observed following glucose ingestion or TRH administration [185,186]. These features appear to be independent of the etiology or structural changes seen in liver disease, as they may be observed with cirrhosis of any cause [185]. Serum levels of IGF-I are depressed in patients with chronic liver disease [185]; reduced negative feedback effects of IGF-I on GH secretion may contribute to the disordered GH regulation, as may changes in brain neurotransmitters that occur as a result of altered amino acid metabolism [187]. The abnormalities of GH secretion appear to return toward normal after successful liver transplantation, although the effects of immunosuppressive drugs and residual encephalopathy complicate interpretation of the data [188].

Thyroid hormone measurements are altered in patients with most chronic liver diseases, primarily as a consequence of changes in peripheral thyroid hormone metabolism. Thus, serum T_3 is usually reduced and serum reverse T_3 elevated in cirrhosis, while serum T_4 is generally normal and serum TSH normal or mildly elevated [185,189]. This picture of the "euthyroid sick" or "nonthyroidal illness" syndrome appears to be related to the degree of hepatocyte dysfunction and is not a feature of portosystemic shunting [190]. In contrast to advanced alcoholic cirrhosis, patients with infectious hepatitis, chronic active hepatitis and primary biliary cirrhosis may have elevated serum levels of thyroxine-binding globulin, thereby raising total serum T_4 and T_3, although free hormone levels and serum TSH are usually normal [189].

The pituitary–adrenal axis is altered minimally in cirrhosis. Serum concentrations of corticosteroid-binding globulin are often decreased, and the serum half lives of both cortisol and dexamethasone are prolonged in cirrhotics, apparently as a consequence of hepatic parenchymal damage [114].

Gonadal function and gonadotropin secretion are altered in patients with cirrhosis; many of the changes appear to correlate with the degree of liver dysfunction, although some may be specifically due to the toxic effects of ethanol on the testis. Men with advanced cirrhosis usually have decreased serum concentrations of total and free testosterone; estradiol is normal or mildly increased, and estrone considerably increased. The increased estrogen concentrations are primarily a consequence of increased peripheral aromatization of androgens (especially androstenedione) rather than decreased hepatic removal. Serum LH is normal or moderately elevated [179,185]. It has been argued that the failure of LH to rise substantially in the face of low free testosterone concentrations suggests concurrent hypothalamic–pituitary dysfunction; however, these findings may be due to the gonadotropin-suppressing effects of elevated serum estradiol, estrone and other estrogen metabolites (e.g., 16-hydroxy-estrone) [185,192]. Seminiferous tubule damage may be seen in cirrhotics and alcoholics, with a rise in serum FSH concentrations [185,193]. Gonadotropin responses to GnRH are intact or blunted [185,191,193].

Premenopausal women with alcoholic liver disease have lower serum estradiol but higher serum estrone levels than healthy women, again presumably due to alterations in peripheral steroid metabolism. Gonadotropin concentrations are normal or low, and respond normally to GnRH [179,194,195]. Thus, in summary, gonadal function is depressed in cirrhotics and further worsened by alcoholism [179]. There is partial reversal of these abnormalities following liver transplantation [179,191].

Serum PRL is sometimes mildly elevated in cirrhotic patients [179,185,193,195,196]; this may reflect the potentiating effects of estrogens on PRL release plus disordered hypothalamic neurotransmitter function [196].

Hypothyroidism

Besides elevating serum TSH concentrations, primary hypothyroidism may have other effects on the pituitary. Activation of the thyrotrophs by loss of thyroid hormone negative feedback may result in thyrotroph hyperplasia, sometimes sufficient to mimic a pituitary tumor [197–201]. Moderate hyperprolactinemia (usually less than 100 ng/ml) is occasionally seen, generally in patients with severe hypothyroidism [199–203]; the mechanism is unclear, but may involve an increase in TRH [204]. GH synthesis is decreased, and its secretion blunted, both basally and in response to provocative testing [205–207]. Although cortisol turnover is decreased, serum cortisol and ACTH concentrations are generally normal [207]. In hypothyroid men, total, free and bioavailable serum testosterone levels are low, as is serum sex-hormone-binding globulin; however, serum gonadotropin levels are in the normal range, suggesting a hypothalamic–pituitary defect; these changes are normalized when euthyroidism is restored [208–211]. Severely hypothyroid children may experience precocious puberty associated with mildly elevated serum FSH levels [212–214]; in addition, very high serum TSH concentrations may also stimulate the gonadal FSH receptor [215,216].

Hyperthyroidism

TSH secretion is suppressed by negative feedback in patients with thyroid hormone excess. In addition, PRL response to TRH or dopamine antagonists is usually blunted in hyperthyroidism, though the basal serum PRL level is normal [217,218]. Serum gonadotropin concentrations are normal or mildly elevated in hyperthyroid patients [209,210]. GH secretion is normal or blunted [206].

Adrenal Insufficiency

In addition to the expected feedback elevation of ACTH secretion, patients with primary adrenal insufficiency may have elevations in serum TSH and PRL levels. Although this is often due to coexistent primary hypothyroidism, in some patients the elevations in TSH and PRL appear to be related to glucocorticoid deficiency, and fall rapidly with cortisol replacement therapy [219–222].

Malnutrition

Malnutrition impairs production of IGF-I [114,223, 224], and is often associated with increased basal GH secretion, perhaps due to decreased negative feedback [114,207,224–226]; additionally, paradoxical increases in GH may be seen following glucose loading or TRH administration [114]. Basal serum PRL concentrations are usually not altered by fasting or malnutrition, but the PRL response to TRH may be diminished, modestly increased, or unchanged [227,228]. ACTH and cortisol secretion are increased [226,229–232].

Starvation or severe carbohydrate restriction induces the "euthyroid sick" or "nonthyroidal illness" syndrome, often accompanied by a slight decrease in basal and TRH-stimulated TSH secretion [112,114,123,124,228,230].

Changes in gonadotropin secretion induced by malnutrition have been more variable; hypogonadism is frequently seen in states of prolonged decreases in calorie intake. However, although most studies have reported normal or decreased serum gonadotropins [114,179,229–236], others report increased serum gonadotropin concentrations [237]. These differences may reflect varying prevalences of specific nutrient deficiencies, initial body weight and concurrent illness. The gonadotropin response to GnRH is, on balance, probably normal [114,179,233–235]. Taken together, these findings suggest a primary hypothalamic abnormality in malnutrition- or fasting-induced pituitary hormone changes.

References

[1] N. Bronspiegel-Weintrob, N.F. Olivieri, B. Tyler, et al., Effect of age at the start of iron chelation therapy on gonadal function in β-thalassemia major, N Engl J Med 323 (1990) 713–719.

[2] J.H. McDermott, C.H. Walsh, Hypogonadism in hereditary hemochromatosis, J Clin Endocrinol Metab 90 (2005) 2451–2455.

[3] Schafter AI, R.G. Cheron, R. Dluhy, et al., Clinical consequences of acquired transfusional iron overload in adults, N Engl J Med 304 (1981) 319–324.

[4] B. Charbonnel, M. Chupin, A. LeGrand, J. Guillon, Pituitary function in idiopathic haemochromatosis: Hormonal study in 36 male patients, Acta Endocrinol 98 (1981) 178–183.

[5] L.W. McNeil, L.C. McKee Jr., D. Lorber, D. Rabin, The endocrine manifestations of hemochromatosis, Am J Med Sci 285 (1983) 7–13.

[6] C. Walton, W.F. Kelly, I. Laing, D.E. Bullock, Endocrine abnormalities in idiopathic haemochromatosis, Q J Med 52 (1983) 99–110.

[7] H.K. Kley, W. Stremmel, C. Niederau, et al., Androgen and estrogen response to adrenal and gonadal stimulation in idiopathic hemochromatosis: Evidence for decreased estrogen formation, Hematology 5 (1985) 251–256.
[8] M.J. Cunningham, E.A. Macklin, E.J. Neufeld, A.R. Cohen, Complications of β-thalassemia major in North America, Blood 104 (2004) 34–39.
[9] C. Wang, S.C. Tso, D. Todd, Hypogonadotropic hypogonadism in severe β-thalassemia: Effect of chelation and pulsatile gonadotropin-releasing hormone therapy, J Clin Endocrinol Metab 68 (1989) 511–516.
[10] T.M. Kelly, C.Q. Edwards, A.W. Meikle, J.P. Kushner, Hypogonadism in hemochromatosis: Reversal with iron depletion, Ann Intern Med 101 (1984) 629–632.
[11] T.C. Williams, L.A. Frohman, Hypothalamic dysfunction associated with hemochromatosis, Ann Intern Med 103 (1985) 550–551.
[12] E.G. Lufkin, W.P. Baldus, E.J. Bergstralh, P.C. Kao, Influence of phlebotomy treatment on abnormal hypothalamic–pituitary function in genetic hemochromatosis, Mayo Clin Proc 62 (1987) 473–479.
[13] L. Duranteau, P. Chanson, J. Blumberg-Tick, et al., Non-responsiveness of serum gonadotropins and testosterone to pulsatile GnRH in hemochromatosis suggesting a pituitary defect, Acta Endocrinol 128 (1993) 351–354.
[14] C.H. Walsh, A.L. Murphy, S. Cunningham, T.J. McKenna, Mineralocorticoid and glucocorticoid status in idiopathic haemochromatosis, Clin Endocrinol 41 (1994) 439–443.
[15] K.E. Oerter, G.A. Kamp, P.J. Munson, et al., Multiple hormone deficiencies in children with hemochromatosis, J Clin Endocrinol Metab 76 (1993) 357–361.
[16] C.L. Levy, H.E. Carlson, Decreased prolactin reserve in hemochromatosis, J Clin Endocrinol Metab 47 (1978) 444–446.
[17] C. Bergeron, K. Kovascs, Pituitary siderosis: A histologic immunocytologic and ultrastructural study, Am J Pathol 93 (1978) 295–306.
[18] M.I. Argyropoulou, D.N. Kiortsis, L. Astrakas, et al., Liver, bone marrow, pancreas and pituitary gland iron overload in young and adult thalassemic patients: A T2 relaxometry study, Eur Radiol 17 (2007) 3025–3030.
[19] L.J. Siemons, C.H. Mahler, Hypogonadotropic hypogonadism in hemochromatosis: Recovery of reproductive function after iron depletion, J Clin Endocrinol Metab 65 (1987) 585–587.
[20] K. Farmaki, I. Tzoumari, C. Pappa, et al., Normalisation of total body iron load with very intensive combined chelation reverses cardiac and endocrine complications of thalassemia major, Br J Haematol 148 (2010) 466–475.
[21] M. Hudec, M. Grigerova, C.H. Walsh, Secondary hypothyroidism in hereditary hemochromatosis: Recovery after iron depletion, Thyroid 18 (2008) 255–257.
[22] F.G. Joseph, N.J. Scolding, Neurosarcoidosis: A study of 30 new cases, J Neurol Neurosurg Psychiatry 80 (2009) 297–304.
[23] N. Porter, H.L. Beynon, H.S. Randeva, Endocrine and reproductive manifestations of sarcoidosis, Q J Med 96 (2003) 553–561.
[24] H. Bihan, V. Christozova, J.-L. Dumas, et al., Sarcoidosis. Clinical, hormonal and magnetic resonance imaging (MRI) manifestations of hypothalamic–pituitary disease in 9 patients and review of the literature, Medicine 86 (2007) 259–268.
[25] F.G. Lawton, C.G. Beardwell, S.M. Shalet, R.A. Daws, Hypothalamic–pituitary disease as the sole manifestation of sarcoidosis, Postgrad Med J 58 (1982) 771–772.
[26] R.A. Tang, J.C. Grotta, K.F. Lee, Y.E. Lee, Chiasmal syndrome in sarcoidosis, Arch Ophthalmol 101 (1983) 1069–1073.
[27] W.H. Daughaday, R.M. Burde, R.G. Jost, F. Pikul, Visual impairment, pituitary dysfunction, and hilar adenopathy in a young man, Am J Med 80 (1986) 259–268.
[28] B.S. Brooks, T. El Gammal, G.D. Hungerford, et al., Radiologic evaluation of neurosarcoidosis: Role of computed tomography, AJNR 3 (1982) 513–521.
[29] W.S. Hayes, J.L. Sherman, B.J. Stern, et al., MR and CT evaluation of intracranial sarcoidosis, AJNR 8 (1987) 841–847.
[30] K.M. Lury, J.K. Smith, M.G. Matheus, M. Castillo, Neurosarcoidosis – review of imaging findings, Semin Roentgenol 39 (2004) 495–504.
[31] N. Aide, M. Benayoun, K. Kerrou, et al., Impact of (^{18}F)-fluorodeoxyglucose ((^{18}F)-FDG) imaging in sarcoidosis: Unsuspected neurosarcoidosis discovered by (^{18}F)-FDG PET and early metabolic response to corticosteroid therapy, Br J Radiol 80 (2007) e67–e71.
[32] C.A. Stuart, F.A. Neelon, H.E. Lebovitz, Hypothalamic insufficiency: The cause of hypopituitarism in sarcoidosis, Ann Intern Med 88 (1978) 589–593.
[33] M.H. Jawadi, T.J. Hanson, J.E. Schemmel, et al., Hypothalamic sarcoidosis and hypopituitarism, Horm Res 12 (1980) 1–9.
[34] F. Fery, L. Plat, P. Van de Borne, et al., Impaired counterregulation of glucose in a patient with hypothalamic sarcoidosis, N Engl J Med 340 (1990) 852–856.
[35] K. Nakao, K. Noma, B. Sato, et al., Serum prolactin levels in 80 patients with sarcoidosis, Eur J Clin Invest 8 (1978) 37–40.
[36] C.A. Stuart, F.A. Neelon, H.A. Lebovitz, Disordered control of thirst in hypothalamic–pituitary sarcoidosis, N Engl J Med 303 (1980) 1078–1082.
[37] J.L. Kirkland, D.J. Pearson, C. Goddard, I. Davies, Polyuria and inappropriate secretion of arginine vasopressin in hypothalamic sarcoidosis, J Clin Endocrinol Metab 56 (1983) 269–272.
[38] C. Bullmann, M. Faust, A. Hoffmann, et al., Five cases with central diabetes insipidus and hypogonadism at first presentation of neurosarcoidosis, Eur J Endocrinol 142 (2000) 365–372.
[39] R.P. Tabuena, S. Nagai, T. Handa, et al., Diabetes insipidus from neurosarcoidosis: Long-term follow-up for more than eight years, Intern Med 43 (2004) 960–966.
[40] D.L. Vesely, Hypothalamic sarcoidosis: A new cause of morbid obesity, South Med J 82 (1989) 758–761.
[41] C.G. Wathen, I. Campbell, A.C. Douglas, Hypothalamic malfunction in cerebral sarcoidosis with abnormalities in temperature regulation and vascular control, Sarcoidosis 5 (1988) 74–76.
[42] P. Dutta, M. Hayatbhat, A. Bhansali, et al., Wegener's granulomatosis presenting as diabetes insipidus, Exp Clin Endocrinol Diab 114 (2006) 533–536.
[43] T.Y. Yong, J.Y.Z. Li, L. Amato, et al., Pituitary involvement in Wegener's granulomatosis, Pituitary 11 (2008) 77–84.
[44] M.C. Sharma, R. Arora, A.K. Mahapatra, et al., Intrasellar tuberculoma – an enigmatic pituitary infection: A series of 18 cases, Clin Neurol Neurosurg 102 (2000) 72–77.
[45] P. Petrossians, P. Delvenne, P. Flandroy, et al., An unusual pituitary pathology, J Clin Endocrinol Metab 83 (1998) 3454–3458.
[46] J. Smith, R. Godwin-Austen, Hypersecretion of anti-diuretic hormone due to tuberculous meningitis, Postgrad Med J 56 (1980) 41–44.
[47] D. Nolt, R. Saad, A. Kouatli, et al., Survival with hypopituitarism from congenital syphilis, Pediatrics 109 (2002) e63.
[48] K.M. Fargen, J.E. Alvernia, C.S. Lin, M. Melgar, Cerebral syphilitic gummata: A case presentation and analysis of 156 reported cases, Neurosurgery 64 (2009) 568–576.

[49] G.E. Vates, M.S. Berger, C.B. Wilson, Diagnosis and management of pituitary abscess: A review of twenty-four cases, J Neurosurg 95 (2001) 233–241.
[50] P. Ciapetta, A. Calace, P.I. D'Urso, N. DeCandia, Endoscopic treatment of pituitary abscess: Two case reports and literature review, Neurosurg Rev 31 (2008) 237–246.
[51] M. Brändle, P. Ammann, G.A. Spinas, et al., Relapsing Whipple's disease presenting with hypopituitarism, Clin Endocrinol 50 (1999) 399–403.
[52] H.-J.H. Choi, M. Cornford, L. Wang, et al., Acute Chagas' disease presenting with a suprasellar mass and panhypopituitarism, Pituitary 7 (2004) 111–114.
[53] J. Ferreiro, H.V. Vinters, Pathology of the pituitary gland in patients with the acquired immune deficiency syndrome (AIDS), Pathology 20 (1988) 211–213.
[54] S.A. Milligan, M.S. Katz, P.C. Craven, et al., Toxoplasmosis presenting as panhypopituitarism in a patient with the acquired immune deficiency syndrome, Am J Med 77 (1984) 760–764.
[55] T. Sano, K. Kovacs, B.W. Scheithauer, et al., Pituitary pathology in acquired immunodeficiency syndrome, Arch Pathol Lab Med 113 (1989) 1066–1070.
[56] L. Mosca, G. Costanzi, C. Antonacci, et al., Hypophyseal pathology in AIDS, Histol Histopathol 7 (1992) 291–300.
[57] W.M. Sullivan, G.G. Kelley, P.G. O'Connor, et al., Hypopituitarism associated with hypothalamic CMV infection in a patient with AIDS, Am J Med 92 (1992) 221–223.
[58] A.M. Moses, D.G. Thomas, M.C. Canfield, G.H. Collins, Central diabetes insipidus due to cytomegalovirus infection of the hypothalamus in a patient with acquired immunodeficiency syndrome: A clinical, pathological, and immunohistochemical case study, J Clin Endocrinol Metab 88 (2003) 51–54.
[59] A.S. Dobs, M.A. Dempsey, P.W. Ladenson, B.E. Polk, Endocrine disorders in men infected with human immunodeficiency virus, Am J Med 84 (1987) 611–616.
[60] D.C. Aron, Endocrine complications of the acquired immunodeficiency syndrome, Arch Intern Med 149 (1989) 330–333.
[61] J.S. Lo Presti, J.C. Fried, C.A. Spencer, J.T. Nicoloff, Unique alternations of thyroid hormone indices in the acquired immunodeficiency syndrome (AIDS), Ann Intern Med 110 (1989) 970–975.
[62] F. Raffi, J.-M. Brisseau, B. Planchon, et al., Endocrine function in 98 HIV-infected patients: A prospective study, AIDS 5 (1991) 729–733.
[63] D.E. Sellmeyer, C. Grunfeld, Endocrine and metabolic disturbances in human immunodeficiency virus infection and the acquired immune deficiency syndrome, Endocr Rev 17 (1996) 518–532.
[64] L. Membreno, I. Irony, W. Dere, et al., Adrenocortical function in acquired immunodeficiency syndrome (AIDS), J Clin Endocrinol Metab 65 (1987) 482–487.
[65] T.T.C. Ng, I.P.M. O'Connel, E.G.L. Wilkins, Growth hormone deficiency coupled with hypogonadism in AIDS, Clin Endocrinol 41 (1994) 689–694.
[66] T.S. Croxson, W.E. Chapman, L.K. Miller, et al., Changes in the hypothalamic–pituitary–gonadal axis in human immunodeficiency virus infected homosexual men, J Clin Endocrinol Metab 68 (1989) 317–321.
[67] J.A. Merenich, M.T. McDermott, A.A. Asp, et al., Evidence of endocrine involvement early in the course of human immunodeficiency virus infection, J Clin Endocrinol Metab 70 (1990) 566–571.
[68] O. Lortholary, N. Christeff, P. Casassus, et al., Hypothalamo–pituitary–adrenal function in human immunodeficiency virus-infected men, J Clin Endocrinol Metab 81 (1996) 791–796.
[69] L.D. Wilson, M.P.M. Truong, A.R. Barber, T.T. Aoki, Anterior pituitary and pituitary-dependent target organ function in men infected with the human immunodeficiency virus, Metabolism 45 (1996) 738–746.
[70] M. Stojanovic, S. Pekic, G. Cvijovic, et al., High risk of hypopituitarism in patients who recovered from hemorrhagic fever with renal syndrome, J Clin Endocrinol Metab 93 (2008) 2722–2728.
[71] S. Schaefer, N. Boegershausen, S. Meyer, et al., Hypothalamic-pituitary insufficiency following infectious diseases of the central nervous system, Eur J Endocrinol 158 (2008) 3–9.
[72] P. Makras, K.I. Alexandraki, G.P. Chrousos, et al., Endocrine manifestations in Langerhans cell histiocytosis, Trends Endocrinol Metab 18 (2007) 252–257.
[73] P. Makras, C. Samara, M. Antoniou, et al., Evolving radiological features of hypothalamo–pituitary lesions in adult patients with Langerhans cell histiocytosis (LCH), Neuroradiol 48 (2006) 37–44.
[74] A. Varan, A. Cila, C. Akyüz, et al., Radiological evaluation of patients with pituitary Langerhans cell histiocytosis at diagnosis and at follow-up, Ped Hematol Oncol 25 (2008) 567–574.
[75] G.A. Kaltsas, T.B. Powles, J. Evanson, et al., Hypothalamo–pituitary abnormalities in adult patients with Langerhans cell histiocytosis: Clinical, endocrinological, and radiological features and response to treatment, J Clin Endocrinol Metab 85 (2000) 1370–1376.
[76] J. Donadieu, M.-A. Rolon, C. Thomas, et al., Endocrine involvement in pediatric-onset Langerhans cell histiocytosis: A population-based study, J Pediatr 144 (2004) 344–350.
[77] R. Haupt, V. Nanduri, M.G. Calevo, et al., Permanent consequences in Langerhans cell histiocytosis patients: A pilot study from the Histiocyte Society Late Effects Study Group, Pediatr Blood Cancer 42 (2004) 438–444.
[78] J. Donadieu, M.-A. Rolon, I. Pion, et al., Incidence of growth hormone deficiency in pediatric-onset Langerhans cell histiocytosis: Efficacy and safety of growth hormone treatment, J Clin Endocrinol Metab 89 (2004) 604–609.
[79] J.G. Rothman, P.J. Snyder, R.D. Utiger, Hypothalamic endocrinopathy in Hand-Schuller-Christian disease, Ann Intern Med 88 (1978) 512–513.
[80] M.C. Gelato, D.L. Loriaux, G.R. Merriam, Growth hormone responses to growth hormone-releasing hormone in Hand-Schuller-Christian disease, Neuroendocrinology 50 (1989) 259–264.
[81] W.A. Scherbaum, J.A.H. Wass, G.M. Besser, et al., Autoimmune cranial diabetes insipidus: Its association with other endocrine diseases and with histiocytosis X, Clin Endocrinol 25 (1986) 411–420.
[82] R. Gramatovici, G.J. D'Angio, Radiation in soft-tissue lesions in histiocytosis X (Langerhans' cell histiocytosis), Med Ped Oncol 16 (1988) 259–262.
[83] Than-Than, N. Francis, Tin-Nu-Swe, et al., Contribution of focal haemorrhage and microvascular fibrin deposition of fatal envenoming by Russell's viper (*Vipera russelli siamensis*) in Burma, Acta Trop 46 (1989) 23–38.
[84] Tun-Pe, D.A. Warrell, Tin-Nu-Swe, et al., Acute and chronic pituitary failure resembling Sheehan's syndrome following bites by Russell's viper in Burma, Lancet (1987) 763–767.
[85] C. Proby, Tha-Aung, Thet-Win, et al., Immediate and long-term effects on hormone levels following bites by the Burmese Russell's viper, Q J Med 75 (1989) 399–411.
[86] R. Milani, M.T. Jorge, F.P. Ferraz de Campos, et al., Snake bites by the jararacucu (*Bothrops jararacussu*): Clinico pathological studies of 29 proven cases in Sao Paulo state, Brazil, Q J Med 90 (1997) 323–334.

[87] K. Kovacs, Metastatic cancer of the pituitary gland, Oncology 27 (1973) 533–542.
[88] U. Roessmann, B. Kaufman, R.L. Friede, Metastatic lesions in the sella turcica and pituitary gland, Cancer 25 (1970) 478–480.
[89] M.B. Max, M.D.F. Deck, D.A. Rottenberg, Pituitary metastasis: Incidence in cancer patients and clinical differentiation from pituitary adenoma, Neurology 8 (1981) 998–1002.
[90] A. Morita, F.B. Meyer, E.R. Laws Jr., Symptomatic pituitary metastases, J Neurosurg 89 (1998) 69–73.
[91] H.M. Heshmati, B.W. Scheithauer, W.F. Young Jr., Metastases to the pituitary gland, Endocrinologist 12 (2002) 45–49.
[92] D.R. Fassett, W.T. Couldwell. Metastases to the pituitary gland, Neurosurg Focus 16 (4) :Article 8
[93] J. Komninos, V. Vlassopoulou, D. Protopapa, et al., Tumors metastatic to the pituitary gland: Case report and literature review, J Clin Endocrinol Metab 89 (2004) 574–580.
[94] H. Kano, A. Niranjan, D. Kondziolka, et al., Stereotactic radiosurgery for pituitary metastases, Surg Neurol 72 (2009) 248–256.
[95] G. Piecha, J. Chudek, A. Wiecek, Multiple endocrine neoplasia type 1, Eur J Intern Med 19 (2008) 99–103.
[96] B.W. Scheithauer, E.R. Laws Jr., K. Kovacs, et al., Pituitary adenomas of the multiple endocrine neoplasia type I syndrome, Sem Diag Pathol 4 (1987) 205–211.
[97] J. Baughan, C. DeGara, D. Morrish, A rare association between acromegaly and pheochromocytoma, Am J Surg 182 (2001) 185–187.
[98] L.V. Neto, G.F. Taboada, L.L. Correa, et al., Acromegaly secondary to growth hormone-releasing hormone secreted by an incidentally discovered pheochromocytoma, Endocr Pathol 18 (2007) 46–52.
[99] K.A. Roth, D.M. Wilson, J. Eberwine, et al., Acromegaly and pheochromocytoma: A multiple endocrine syndrome caused by a plurihormonal adrenal medullary tumor, J Clin Endocrinol Metab 63 (1986) 1421–1426.
[100] M.O. Thorner, R.L. Perryman, M.J. Cronin, et al., Somatotroph hyperplasia. Successful treatment of acromegaly by removal of a pancreatic islet cell tumor secreting a growth hormone-releasing factor, J Clin Invest 70 (1982) 965–977.
[101] D. Wilkes, D.A. McDermott, C.T. Basson, Clinical phenotypes and molecular genetic mechanisms of Carney complex, Lancet Oncol 6 (2005) 501–508.
[102] S.A. Boikos, C.A. Stratakis, Pituitary pathology in patients with Carney complex: Growth hormone producing hyperplasia or tumors and their association with other abnormalities, Pituitary 9 (2006) 203–209.
[103] A. Horvath, C.A. Stratakis, Clinical and molecular genetics of acromegaly: MEN 1, Carney complex, McCune-Albright syndrome, familial acromegaly and genetic defects in sporadic tumors, Rev Endocr Metab Disord 9 (2008) 1–11.
[104] C.J. Owen, T.D. Cheetham, Diagnosis and management of polyendocrinopathy syndromes, Endocrinol Metab Clin N Am 38 (2009) 419–436.
[105] P. Caturegli, C. Newschaffer, A. Olivi, et al., Autoimmune hypophysitis, Endocr Rev 26 (2005) 599–614.
[106] P. Caturegli, I. Lupi, M. Landek-Salgado, et al., Pituitary autoimmunity: 30 years later, Autoimmunity Rev 7 (2008) 631–637.
[107] S. Storkel, J. Bohl, H.-M. Schneider, Senile amyloidosis: Principles of localization in a heterogeneous form of amyloidosis, Virchows Arch (Pathol Anat) 44 (1983) 145–161.
[108] T. Ishihara, T. Nagasawa, T. Yokota, et al., Amyloid protein of vessels in leptomeninges, cortices, choroid plexuses, and pituitary glands from patients with systemic amyloidosis, Hum Pathol 20 (1989) 891–895.
[109] M.S. Las, M.I. Surks, Hypopituitarism associated with systemic amyloidosis, NY State J Med 83 (1983) 1183–1185.
[110] P. Wiesli, M. Brändle, S. Brandner, et al., Extensive spherical amyloid deposition presenting as a pituitary tumor, J Endocrinol Invest 26 (2003) 552–555.
[111] P. Schuetz, B. Müller, The hypothalamic–pituitary adrenal axis in critical illness, Endocrinol Metab Clin N Am 35 (2006) 823–838.
[112] L. Langouche, G. Van den Berghe, The dynamic neuroendocrine response to stress, Endocrinol Metab Clin N Am 35 (2006) 777–791.
[113] B.M. Arafah, Hypothalamic pituitary adrenal function during critical illness: Limitations of current assessment methods, J Clin Endocrinol Metab 91 (2006) 3725–3745.
[114] M. Bondanelli, M.C. Zatelli, M.R. Ambrosio, E.C. Degli Uberti, Systemic illness, Pituitary 11 (2008) 187–207.
[115] C.G. Semple, S.E. Gray, G.H. Beastall, Adrenal androgens and illness, Acta Endocrinol 116 (1987) 155–160.
[116] D.I. Spratt, C. Longcope, P.M. Cox, et al., Differential changes in serum concentrations of androgens and estrogens (in relation to cortisol) in postmenopausal women with acute illness, J Clin Endocrinol Metab 76 (1993) 1542–1547.
[117] R.D. Zipser, M.W. Davenport, K.L. Martin, et al., Hyperreninemic hypoaldosteronism in the critically ill: A new entity, J Clin Endocrinol Metab 53 (1981) 867–873.
[118] C.L. Sprung, D. Annane, D. Keh, et al., Hydrocortisone therapy for patients with septic shock, N Engl J Med 358 (2008) 111–124.
[119] L. Richardson, S. Hunter, Is steroid therapy ever of benefit to patients in the intensive care unit going into septic shock? Interactive Cardiovasc Ther Surg 7 (2008) 898–905.
[120] P.E. Marik, Critical illness-related corticosteroid insufficiency, Chest 135 (2009) 181–193.
[121] M.G. Annetta, R. Maviglia, R. Proietti, M. Antonelli, Use of corticosteroids in critically ill septic patients: A review of mechanisms of adrenal insufficiency in sepsis and treatment, Curr Drug Targets 10 (2009) 887–894.
[122] D.L. Loriaux, M. Fleseriu, Relative adrenal insufficiency, Curr Opin Endocrinol Diab Obes 16 (2009) 392–400.
[123] S.M. Adler, L. Wartofsky, The nonthyroidal illness syndrome, Endocrinol Metab Clin N Am 36 (2007) 657–672.
[124] L. Mebis, Y. Debaveye, T.J. Visser, G. Van den Berghe, Changes within the thyroid axis during the course of critical illness, Endocrinol Metab Clin N Am 35 (2006) 807–821.
[125] G.A. Brent, J.M. Hershman, Thyroxine therapy in patients with severe nonthyroidal illnesses and low serum thyroxine concentration, J Clin Endocrinol Metab 63 (1986) 1–8.
[126] R.A. Becker, G.M. Vaughan, M.G. Ziegler, et al., Hypermetabolic low triiodothyronine syndrome of burn injury, Crit Care Med 10 (1982) 870–875.
[127] E.L. Kaptein, E. Beale, L.S. Chan, Thyroid hormone therapy for obesity and nonthyroidal illness: A systematic review, J Clin Endocrinol Metab 94 (2009) 3663–3675.
[128] G. Bello, G. Paliani, M.G. Annetta, et al., Treating nonthyroidal illness syndrome in the critically ill patient: Still a matter of controversy, Curr Drug Targets 10 (2009) 778–787.
[129] D. Mesotten, G. Van den Berghe, Changes within the growth hormone/insulin-like growth factor I/IGF binding protein axis during critical illness, Endocrinol Metab Clin N Am 35 (2006) 793–805.
[130] D.I. Spratt, S.T. Bisas, I. Beitins, et al., Both hyper- and hypogonadotropic hypogonadism occur transiently in acute illness: Bio- and immunoreactive gonadotropins, J Clin Endocrinol Metab 75 (1992) 1562–1570.

[131] D.I. Spratt, R.S. Kramer, J.R. Morton, et al., Characterization of a prospective human model for study of the reproductive hormone responses to major illness, Am J Physiol Endocrinol Metab 295 (2008) E63–E69.
[132] D.I. Spratt, P. Cox, J. Orav, et al., Reproductive axis suppression in acute illness is related to disease severity, J Clin Endocrinol Metab 76 (1993) 1548–1554.
[133] G. Van den Berghe, F. Weekers, R.C. Baxter, et al., Five-day pulsatile gonadotropin-releasing hormone administration unveils combined hypothalamic–pituitary–gonadal defects underlying profound hypoandrogenism in men with prolonged critical illness, J Clin Endocrinol Metab 80 (2001) 3217–3226.
[134] T. Hashimoto, K. Miyai, T. Uozumi, et al., Effect of prolonged LH-releasing hormone administration on gonadotropin response in patients with hypothalamic and pituitary tumors, J Clin Endocrinol Metab 41 (1975) 712–716.
[135] K. Hayakawa, Y. Konishi, T. Matsuda, et al., Development and aging of brain midline structures: Assessment with MR imaging, Radiology 172 (1989) 172–177.
[136] S.N. Lurie, P.M. Doraiswamy, M.M. Husain, et al., In vivo assessment of pituitary gland volume with magnetic resonance imaging: The effect of age, J Clin Endocrinol Metab 71 (1990) 505–508.
[137] Y.-K. Sun, Y.-P. Xi, C.M. Fenoglio, et al., The effect of age on the number of pituitary cells immunoreactive to growth hormone and prolactin, Hum Pathol 15 (1984) 169–180.
[138] M.W. Shanklin, Age changes in the histology of the human pituitary, Acta Anat 19 (1953) 290–304.
[139] S.L. Asa, G. Penz, K. Kovacs, C. Ezrin, Prolactin cells in the human pituitary. A quantitative immunocytochemical analysis, Arch Pathol Lab Med 106 (1982) 360–363.
[140] K. Kovacs, E. Horvath, C. Ezrin, Anatomy and histology of the normal and abnormal pituitary gland, in: L.J. De Groot, G.M. Besser, G.F. Cahill Jr., et al. (Eds.), Endocrinology, second ed., WB Saunders Co, Philadelphia, 1989, pp. 264–283.
[141] J.E. Hall, Neuroendocrine changes with reproductive aging in women, Semin Reprod Med 25 (2007) 344–351.
[142] J.M. Kaufman, A. Vermeulen, The decline of androgen levels in elderly men and its clinical and therapeutic implications, Endocr Rev 26 (2005) 833–876.
[143] C.A. Allan, R.I. McLachlan, Age-related changes in testosterone and the role of replacement therapy in older men, Clin Endocrinol 60 (2004) 653–670.
[144] A. Tajar, G. Forti, T.W. O'Neill, et al., Characteristics of secondary, primary and compensated hypogonadism in aging men: Evidence from the European male aging study, J Clin Endocrinol Metab 95 (2010) 1810–1818.
[145] J.D. Veldhuis, Aging and hormones of the hypothalamic–pituitary axis: Gonadotropic axis in men and somatotropic axes in men and women, Ageing Res Rev 7 (2008) 189–208.
[146] E. Corpas, S.M. Harman, S.R. Blackman, Human growth hormone and human aging, Endocr Rev 14 (1993) 20–39.
[147] J.R. Florini, P.N. Prinz, N.W. Vitiello, R.L. Hintz, Somatomedin-C levels in healthy young and old men: Relationship to peak and 24-hour integrated levels of growth hormone, J Gerontol 40 (1985) 2–7.
[148] L.R. Donahue, S.J. Hunter, A.P. Sherblom, C. Rosen, Age-related changes in serum insulin-like growth factor-binding proteins in women, J Clin Endocrinol Metab 71 (1990) 575–579.
[149] R. Giordano, G. Aimaretti, F. Lanfranco, et al., Testing pituitary function in aging individuals, Endocrinol Metab Clin N Am 34 (2005) 895–906.
[150] M. Sherlock, A.A. Toogood, Aging and the growth hormone/insulin like growth factor-I axis, Pituitary 10 (2007) 189–203.
[151] D. Rudman, A.G. Feller, H.S. Najraj, et al., Effects of human growth hormone in men over 60 years old, N Engl J Med 323 (1990) 1–6.
[152] C.T. Sawin, H.E. Carlson, A. Geller, et al., Serum prolactin and aging: Basal values and changes with estrogen use and hypothyroidism, J Gerontol 44 (1989) M131–M135.
[153] M.R. Blackman, Pituitary hormones in aging men, Endocrinol Metab Clin N Am 16 (1987) 981–994.
[154] M. Stan, J.C. Morris, Thyrotropin-axis adaptation in aging and chronic disease, Endocrinol Metab Clin N Am 34 (2005) 973–992.
[155] M. Habra, N.J. Sarlis, Thyroid and aging, Rev Endocrinol Metab Disord 6 (2005) 145–154.
[156] M.I. Surks, J.G. Hollowell, Age-specific distribution of serum thyrotropin and antithyroid antibodies in the US population: Implications for the prevalence of subclinical hypothyroidism, J Clin Endocrinol Metab 92 (2007) 4575–4582.
[157] G. Atzmon, N. Barzilai, J.G. Hollowell, et al., Extreme longevity is associated with increased serum thyrotropin, J Clin Endocrinol Metab 94 (2009) 1251–1254.
[158] T.E. Seeman, R.J. Robbins, Aging and hypothalamic–pituitary–adrenal response to challenge in humans, Endocr Rev 15 (1994) 233–260.
[159] E. Ferrari, L. Cravella, B. Muzzoni, et al., Age-related changes of the hypothalamic–pituitary–adrenal axis: Pathophysiologic correlates, Eur J Endocrinol 144 (2001) 319–329.
[160] D.M. Keenan, F. Roelfsema, B.J. Carroll, et al., Sex defines the age dependence of endogenous ACTH-cortisol dose responsiveness, Am J Physiol Integr Comp Physiol 297 (2009) R515–R523.
[161] P. Kokkoris, F.X. Pi-Sunyer, Obesity and endocrine disease, Endocrinol Metab Clin N Am 32 (2003) 895–914.
[162] M.E.V. Mora, M. Manco, E. Capristo, et al., Growth hormone and ghrelin secretion in severely obese women before and after bariatric surgery, Obesity 15 (2007) 2012–2018.
[163] V. Gasco, G. Corneli, S. Rovere, et al., Diagnosis of adult GH deficiency, Pituitary 11 (2008) 121–128.
[164] S. Camastra, M. Manco, S. Frascerra, et al., Daylong pituitary hormones in morbid obesity: Effects of bariatric surgery, Int J Obesity 33 (2009) 166–172.
[165] M.H. Rasmussen, A. Hvidberg, A. Juul, et al., Massive weight loss restores 24-hour growth hormone release profiles and serum insulin-like growth factor-I levels in obese subjects, J Clin Endocrinol Metab 80 (1995) 1407–1415.
[166] J. Frystyk, E. Vestbo, C. Skjaerbaek, et al., Free insulin-like growth factors in human obesity, Metabolism 44 (Suppl 10) (1995) 37–44.
[167] J. Argente, N. Caballo, V. Barrios, et al., Multiple endocrine abnormalities of the growth hormone and insulin-like growth factor axis in prepubertal children with exogenous obesity: Effect of short- and long-term weight reduction, J Clin Endocrinol Metab 82 (1997) 2076–2083.
[168] P.G. Kopelman, Physiopathology of prolactin secretion in obesity, Int J Obes 24 (Suppl.2) (2000) S104–S108.
[169] R. Pasquali, Obesity and androgens: Facts and perspectives, Fertil Steril 85 (2006) 1319–1340.
[170] M. Diaz-Arjonilla, M. Schwarcz, R.S. Swerdloff, C. Wang, Obesity, low testosterone levels and erectile dysfunction, Int J Impot Res 21 (2009) 89–98.
[171] P. Anagnostis, V.G. Athyros, K. Tziomalos, et al., The pathogenetic role of cortisol in the metabolic syndrome: A hypothesis, J Clin Endocrinol Metab 94 (2009) 2692–2701.
[172] A.A. Tahrani, T.E.T. West, A.F. Macleod, An unusual case of severe hypoglycaemia in Type 1 diabets mellitus. Antepartum pituitary failure: A case report and literature review, Exp Clin Endocrinol Diab 115 (2007) 136–138.

[173] H. Alrefai, H. Allababidi, S. Levy, J. Levy, The endocrine system in diabetes mellitus, Endocrine 18 (2002) 105–119.

[174] K. Ekström, J. Salemyr, I. Zachrisson, et al., Normalization of the IGF-IGFBP axis by sustained nightly insulinization in type 1 diabetes, Diab Care 30 (2007) 1357–1360.

[175] G. Johannsson, J. Ahlmén, End-stage renal disease: Endocrine aspects of treatment, Growth Horm IGF Res 13 (2003) S94–S101.

[176] P. Iglesias, J.J. Diez, M.J. Fernández-Reyes, J. Méndez, et al., Growth hormone, IGF-1 and its binding proteins (IGFBP-1 and -3) in adult uraemic patients undergoing peritoneal dialysis and haemodialysis, Clin Endocrinol 60 (2004) 741–749.

[177] S. Mahesh, F. Kaskel, Growth hormone axis in chronic kidney disease, Pediatr Nephrol 23 (2008) 41–48.

[178] D.J. Handelsman, Hypothalamic–pituitary–gonadal dysfunction in renal failure, dialysis and renal transplantation, Endocr Rev 6 (1985) 151–182.

[179] A. Karagiannis, F. Harsoulis, Gonadal dysfunction in systemic diseases, Eur J Endocrinol 152 (2005) 501–513.

[180] I. Zovková, I. Sotornik, R.L. Kancheva, Adenohypophyseal–gonadal dysfunction in male hemodialyzed patients before and after subtotal parathyroidectomy, Nephron 74 (1996) 536–540.

[181] F.-F. Chou, C.-H. Lee, K. Shu, et al., Improvement in sexual function in male patients after parathyroidectomy for secondary hyperparathyroidism, J Am Coll Surg 193 (2001) 486–492.

[182] V.S. Lim, Thyroid function in patients with chronic renal failure, Am J Kidney Dis 38 (Suppl. 1) (2001) S80–S84.

[183] P. Iglesias, J.J. Diez, Thyroid dysfunction and kidney disease, Eur J Endocrinol 160 (2009) 503–515.

[184] R.J. Workman, W.K. Vaughn, W.J. Stone, Dexamethasone suppression testing in chronic renal failure: Pharmacokinetics of dexamethasone and demonstration of a normal hypothalamic–pituitary–adrenal axis, J Clin Endocrinol Metab 63 (1986) 741–746.

[185] B. Zietz, G. Lock, B. Plach, et al., Dysfunction of the hypothalamic–pituitary–glandular axes and relation to Child-Pugh classification in male patients with alcohol and virus-related cirrhosis, Eur J Gastroenterol Hepatol 15 (2003) 495–501.

[186] T. Agner, C. Hagen, B.N. Andersen, L. Hegedus, Pituitary–thyroid function and thyrotropin, prolactin and growth hormone responses to TRH in patients with chronic alcoholism, Acta Med Scand 220 (1986) 57–62.

[187] S. Naomi, J. Tajiri, J. Inoue, et al., Interrelation between plasma amino acid composition and growth hormone secretion in patients with liver cirrhosis, Endocrinol Jpn 31 (1984) 557–564.

[188] D.H. Van Thiel, J.S. Gavaler, A. Sanghvi, Pituitary and thyroid hormone levels before and after orthotopic hepatic transplantation and their responses to thyrotropin-releasing hormone, J Clin Endocrinol Metab 60 (1985) 569–574.

[189] R. Malik, H. Hodgson, The relationship between the thyroid gland and the liver, Q J Med 95 (2002) 559–569.

[190] W.J. Kalk, D. Russet, H.C. Seftel, L.A. Van der Walt, Pituitary and thyroid function before and after portocaval anastomosis in patients with normal liver, J Clin Endocrinol Metab 51 (1980) 1450–1453.

[191] D.J. Handelsman, S. Strasser, J.A. McDonald, et al., Hypothalamic–pituitary–testicular function in end-stage non-alcoholic liver disease before and after liver transplantation, Clin Endocrinol 43 (1995) 331–337.

[192] J. Fishman, C. Martucci, Biological properties of 16α-hydroxy estrone: Implications in estrogen physiology and pathophysiology, J Clin Endocrinol Metab 51 (1980) 611–615.

[193] M. Valimaki, M. Salaspuro, M. Harkonen, R. Ylikahri, Liver damage and sex hormones in chronic male alcoholics, Clin Endocrinol 17 (1982) 469–477.

[194] M. Valimaki, R. Pelkonen, M. Salaspuro, et al., Sex hormones in amenorrheic women with alcoholic liver disease, J Clin Endocrinol Metab 59 (1984) 133–138.

[195] H. Bell, N. Raknerud, J.A. Falch, et al., Inappropriately low levels of gonadotropins in amenorrheic women with alcoholic and non-alcoholic cirrhosis, Eur J Endocrinol 132 (1995) 444–449.

[196] M. Borzio, R. Caldara, C. Ferrari, et al., Growth hormone and prolactin secretion in liver cirrhosis: Evidence for dopaminergic dysfunction, Acta Endocrinol 97 (1981) 441–447.

[197] B.W. Scheithauer, K. Kovacs, R.Y. Randall, N. Ryan, Pituitary gland in hypothyroidism. Histologic and immunocytologic study, Arch Pathol Lab Med 109 (1985) 499–504.

[198] B.R.F. Lecky, S.L. Lightman, T.D.M. Williams, et al., Myxoedema presenting with chiasmal compression: Resolution after thyroxine replacement, Lancet i (1987) 1347–1350.

[199] N.J. Sarlis, F. Brucker-Davis, J.L. Doppman, M.C. Skarulis, MRI-demonstrable regression of a pituitary mass in a case of primary hypothyroidism after a week of acute thyroid hormone therapy, J Clin Endocrinol Metab 82 (1997) 808–811.

[200] T. Shimono, H. Hatabu, K. Kasagi, et al., Rapid progression of pituitary hyperplasia in humans with primary hypothyroidism: Demonstration with MR imaging, Radiology 213 (1999) 383–388.

[201] C. Alves, A.C. Alves, Primary hypothyroidism in a child simulating a prolactin-secreting adenoma, Childs Nerv Syst 24 (2008) 1505–1508.

[202] L.H. Fish, C.N. Mariash, Hyperprolactinemia, infertility, and hypothyroidism. A case report and literature review, Arch Intern Med 148 (1988) 709–711.

[203] W. Raber, A. Gessl, P. Nowotny, H. Vierhapper, Hyperprolactinemia in hypothyroidism: Clinical significance and impact of TSH normalization, Clin Endocrinol 58 (2003) 185–191.

[204] J.M.M. Rondeel, W.J. DeGreef, W. Klootwijk, T.J. Visser, Effects of hypothyroidism on hypothalamic release of thyrotropin-releasing hormone in rats, Endocrinology 130 (1992) 651–656.

[205] C.J. Mirell, M. Yanagisawa, R. Lau, et al., Influence of thyroidal status on pituitary content of thyrotropin β- and α-subunit, growth hormone, and prolactin messenger ribonucleic acids, Mol Endocrinol 1 (1987) 408–412.

[206] A. Giustina, J.D. Veldhuis, Pathophysiology of the neuroregulation of growth hormone secretion in experimental animals and the human, Endocr Rev 19 (1998) 717–797.

[207] K.L. Cohen, Metabolic, endocrine, and drug-induced interference with pituitary function tests: A review, Metabolism 26 (1977) 1165–1177.

[208] P. Donnelly, C. White, Testicular dysfunction in men with primary hypothyroidism; reversal of hypogonadotrophic hypogonadism with replacement thyroxine, Clin Endocrinol 52 (2000) 197–201.

[209] G.E. Krassas, N. Pontikides, Male reproductive function in relation to thyroid alterations, Best Practice Res Clin Endocrinol Metab 18 (2004) 183–195.

[210] A.W. Meikle, The interrelationships between thyroid dysfunction and hypogonadism in men and boys, Thyroid 14 (Suppl 1) (2004) S17–S25.

[211] A. Kumar, B.P. Mohanty, L. Rani, Secretion of testicular steroids and gonadotrophins in hypothyroidism, Andrologia 39 (2007) 253–260.

[212] J.M. Bruder, M.H. Samuels, W.J. Bremner, et al., Hypothyroidism-induced macroorchidism: Use of a gonadotropin-releasing hormone agonist to understand its mechanism and augment adult stature, J Clin Endocrinol Metab 80 (1995) 11–16.

[213] W. Chemaitilly, C. Thalassinos, S. Emond, E. Thibaud, Metrorrhagia and precocious puberty revealing hypothyroidism in a child with Down's syndrome, Arch Dis Child 88 (2003) 330–331.
[214] A. Karthikeyan, J.C. Agwu, Precocious puberty, Clin Ped 47 (2008) 718–719.
[215] J.N. Anasti, M.R. Flack, J. Froehlich, et al., A potential novel mechanism for precocious puberty in juvenile hypothyroidism, J Clin Endocrinol Metab 80 (1995) 276–279.
[216] G.L. Ryan, X. Feng, C. Brasil d'Alva, et al., Evaluating the roles of follicle-stimulating hormone receptor polymorphisms in gonadal hyperstimulation associated with severe juvenile primary hypothyroidism, J Clin Endocrinol Metab 92 (2007) 2312–2317.
[217] H.E. Carlson, C.T. Sawin, L.G. Krugman, et al., Effect of thyroid hormones on the prolactin response to thyrotropin-releasing hormone in normal persons and euthyroid goitrous patients, J Clin Endocrinol Metab 47 (1978) 275–279.
[218] E. Ciccarelli, M. Zini, S. Grottoli, et al., Impaired prolactin response to arginine in patients with hyperthyroidism, Clin Endocrinol 41 (1994) 371–374.
[219] E.G. Lever, C.G. McKerron, Auto-immune Addison's disease associated with hyperprolactinemia, Clin Endocrinol 21 (1984) 451–457.
[220] T.D. Stryker, M.E. Molitch, Reversible hyperthyrotropinemia, hyperthyroxinemia, and hyperprolactinemia due to adrenal insufficiency, Am J Med 79 (1985) 271–276.
[221] M.E. Kelver, M. Nagamani, Hyperprolactinemia in primary adrenocortical insufficiency, Fertil Steril 44 (1985) 423–425.
[222] A.A.A. Ismail, W.A. Burr, P.L. Walker, Acute changes in serum thyrotropin in treated Addison's disease, Clin Endocrinol 30 (1989) 225–230.
[223] J.E. Abdenur, M.T. Pugliese, C. Cervantes, et al., Alterations in spontaneous growth hormone (GH) secretion and the response to GH-releasing hormone in children with non-organic nutritional dwarfing, J Clin Endocrinol Metab 75 (1992) 930–934.
[224] A. Juul, Serum levels of insulin-like growth factor I and its binding proteins in health and disease, Growth Horm IGF Res 13 (2003) 113–170.
[225] K.Y. Ho, J.D. Veldhuis, M.L. Hohnson, et al., Fasting enhances growth hormone secretion and amplifies the complex rhythms of growth hormone secretion in man, J Clin Invest 81 (1988) 968–975.
[226] J. Palmblad, L. Levi, A. Burger, et al., Effects of total energy withdrawal (fasting) on the levels of growth hormone, thyrotropin, cortisol, adrenaline, noradrenaline, T_4, T_3, and rT_3 in healthy males, Acta Med Scand 201 (1977) 15–22.
[227] S. Rojdmark, A. Nygren, Thyrotropin and prolactin responses to thyrotropin-releasing hormone: Influence of fasting- and insulin-induced changes in glucose metabolism, Metabolism 32 (1983) 1013–1018.
[228] H.E. Carlson, E.J. Drenick, I.J. Chopra, J.M. Hershman, Alterations in basal and TRH-stimulated serum levels of thyrotropin, prolactin, and thyroid hormones in starved obese men, J Clin Endocrinol Metab 45 (1977) 707–713.
[229] D.J. Becker, The endocrine responses to protein calorie malnutrition, Ann Rev Nutr 3 (1983) 187–212.
[230] J.D. Veldhuis, A. Iranmanesh, W.S. Evans, et al., Amplitude suppression of the pulsatile mode of immunoradiometric luteinizing hormone release in fasting-induced hypoandrogenemia in normal men, J Clin Endocrinol Metab 76 (1993) 587–593.
[231] M.L. Vance, M.O. Thorner, Fasting alters pulsatile and rhythmic cortisol release in normal man, J Clin Endocrinol Metab 68 (1989) 1013–1018.
[232] M. Bergendahl, M.L. Vance, A. Iranmanesh, et al., Fasting as a metabolic stress paradigm selectively amplifies cortisol secretory burst mass and delays the time of maximal nyctohemeral cortisol concentrations in healthy men, J Clin Endocrinol Metab 81 (1996) 692–699.
[233] Y. Nakamura, Y. Yoshimura, T. Oda, et al., Clinical and endocrine studies on patients with amenorrhea associated with weight loss, Clin Endocrinol 23 (1985) 643–651.
[234] S. Rojdmark, Increased gonadotropin responsiveness to gonadrotropin-releasing hormone during fasting in normal subjects, Metabolism 36 (1987) 21–26.
[235] A. Klibanski, I.Z. Beitins, T. Badger, et al., Reproductive function during fasting in men, J Clin Endocrinol Metab 53 (1981) 258–263.
[236] L.J. Hoffer, I.Z. Beitins, N.-H. Kyung, B.R. Bistrian, Effects of severe dietary restriction on male reproductive hormones, J Clin Endocrinol Metab 62 (1986) 288–292.
[237] S.R. Smith, M.K. Chhetri, A.J. Johanson, et al., The pituitary—gonadal axis in men with protein-calorie malnutrition, J Clin Endocrinol Metab 41 (1975) 60–69.

CHAPTER

12

The Pituitary Gland in Pregnancy and the Puerperium

Harold E. Carlson

Stony Brook University, Stony Brook, NY, USA

NORMAL PREGNANCY

In response to a changing hormonal milieu, the human pituitary gland undergoes a remarkable transformation during pregnancy. Substances produced by the fetoplacental unit greatly modify maternal hypophyseal structure and function. In the case of some hormones, for example prolactin (PRL) or oxytocin, such changes clearly play an important functional role in pregnancy, labor and the puerperium. In the case of others, such as growth hormone (GH), the changes in the maternal pituitary seem to be a coincidental side effect of processes involved in stimulating fetal growth.

Anatomic Changes

During pregnancy, the anterior pituitary enlarges greatly; pituitary weight increases by about 33% [1], as does cross-sectional area (assessed histologically [2]) and gland volume (assessed radiologically by magnetic resonance imaging [MRI] techniques [3]). This enlargement results in an upward convexity of the superior surface of the gland when visualized radiologically [3]. The adenohypophysis also becomes hyperintense on T_1-weighted images during pregnancy [4]. The pituitary stalk remains in its normal midline position, but the posterior pituitary, normally seen as an intense T_1-weighted signal on MRI, is not visualized in the third trimester of gestation [3]. Postpartum, adenohypophyseal enlargement regresses, although perhaps not totally [1–3].

Microscopically, the anterior pituitary enlargement is due to an increased number of lactotrophs [2,5,6]. The percentage of lactotrophs in the pituitary gland rises from about 15–20% of total pituitary cells in men and nulliparous women to approximately 50% at the end of normal gestation [2,5]. Following delivery, the percentage of lactotrophs falls, especially if lactation is not continued [2,5]; regression may not be complete, however, as shown by the finding that about 25% of total pituitary cells in nonpregnant multiparous women are lactotrophs [5].

Other changes noted during pregnancy in immunohistochemical studies include a modest diminution in the relative number of somatotrophs [2,6], a major decrease in the proportion of stainable gonadotrophs [2], and no change in the proportions of thyrotrophs or corticotrophs [2]. Some of the somatotrophs may convert to mammosomatotrophs or lactotrophs during pregnancy [6].

In the human fetus, a distinct intermediate lobe of the pituitary exists. After birth, this structure gradually regresses, so that in the adult there is no recognizable intermediate lobe [7]. Based on limited evidence, this situation does not change during pregnancy.

HORMONE SECRETION

The changes that occur in circulating pituitary hormones during normal pregnancy are listed in Table 12.1.

PRL

To prepare the breast for lactation, the secretion of PRL increases greatly during pregnancy; serum levels rise to approximately 20–40 ng/ml at the end of the first trimester, 50–150 ng/ml by the end of the second trimester and 100–400 ng/ml at term (Figure 12.1) [8,10]. The massive hyperestrogenemia of pregnancy is generally deemed responsible for this increase in PRL

The Pituitary, *Third Edition*, DOI: 10.1016/B978-0-12-380926-1.10012-4

TABLE 12.1 Summary of Maternal Pituitary Function Changes During Normal Pregnancy and Postpartum Period

Hormone	Pregnancy	Postpartum
Prolactin	Increases progressively throughout gestation	Stimulated by suckling; falls rapidly in the absence of breastfeeding
Gonadotropins	Suppressed in first few weeks and remain low throughout gestation	In the absence of breastfeeding, return to normal within 1–2 months; suppressed by active lactation
Thyrotropin	No change except for a transient dip at 9–13 weeks' gestation	No change
Growth hormone	Suppressed during second half of gestation	Return to normal within a few weeks' postpartum
Corticotropin	Probable modest increase in plasma ACTH, remaining in normal range	Return to normal within 1 week
Vasopressin	No change in plasma levels, though production rate increased in third trimester	No change in plasma levels
Oxytocin	No change except for increase in plasma levels during labor	Stimulated acutely by nipple stimulation and maternal psychic factors

secretion, since estrogen is a known stimulus to both PRL synthesis and secretion, as well as lactotroph proliferation [10–12]. It is not clear, however, whether the effect of estrogen is predominantly a direct stimulatory effect on the lactotroph, an indirect effect mediated by decreased hypothalamic dopamine (DA) release into the portal circulation, or perhaps an indirect effect mediated by other potential trophic factors (e.g., vasoactive intestinal polypeptide, VIP [13]) acting on the lactotroph. Animal evidence has suggested that estrogen may induce changes in the pattern of pituitary blood supply, such that a greater fraction of adenohypophyseal blood flow is derived from the systemic circulation (with low DA concentration) and less from the hypothalamic–pituitary portal circulation (with high DA concentrations) [14]. It is likely that some combination of these factors is responsible for the hyperprolactinemia of pregnancy.

During pregnancy, PRL is also produced by uterine tissues, principally the decidua, and secreted into the amniotic fluid [15,16]. PRL is found in extremely high concentration in amniotic fluid, peaking at about 4000–6000 ng/ml near the end of the second trimester, and falling to about 200–800 ng/ml at term [17,18]. Very little of this decidual PRL enters the maternal circulation, however, as revealed by low serum PRL concentrations despite high amniotic fluid PRL in pregnant women with pre-existing PRL deficiency [19–21] and pregnant women in whom pituitary PRL secretion has been suppressed by bromocriptine [22–24]. Elevated

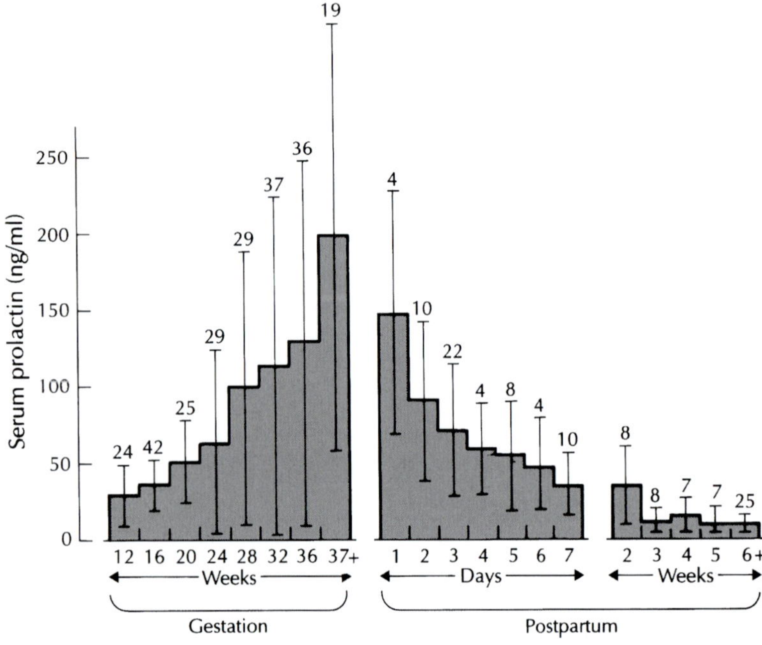

FIGURE 12.1 Mean (± SD) serum prolactin concentrations during normal pregnancy and the postpartum period. The number of subjects sampled at each time point is indicated. *From Hwang et al. [10].*

serum PRL levels in the fetus appear to be largely derived from fetal pituitary secretion and reach 80–500 ng/ml at term [8,17,24].

The dynamics of normal PRL regulation appear to be preserved in pregnancy. Although baseline serum PRL levels are elevated, responses to thyrotropin-releasing hormone (TRH), sleep, arginine infusion and meals are present [8,26–29]. In absolute terms, the observed increments in serum PRL in response to these stimuli are normal. Since baseline PRL levels are elevated, however, the proportional increase (expressed as multiples of baseline) is diminished during pregnancy.

Following delivery, serum PRL levels decline fairly quickly in nonnursing mothers, falling to approximately normal prepregnancy levels by 1–3 weeks postpartum (Figure 12.1) [8,30]. In nursing mothers, each episode of suckling activates a neural reflex arc to acutely stimulate PRL release, prolonging the decline in baseline levels; somewhat larger PRL responses occur with afternoon or evening suckling episodes compared to the morning [8,25,31]. Nevertheless, as nursing episodes become less frequent, baseline serum PRL values eventually return to near prepregnancy levels, despite continued intermittent bursts of PRL secretion coincident with episodes of suckling (Figure 12.2). As the suckling episodes become less frequent, the magnitude of the suckling-induced bursts of PRL secretion also diminishes [8,25,30,31]. The maintenance of hyperprolactinemia by frequent nursing episodes results in prolonged suppression of gonadotropins and extends the period of postpartum amenorrhea and infertility [32].

There is a permanent 50% decrease in basal and stimulated levels of serum PRL following the first pregnancy in normal women. This change occurs regardless of the maternal age at first pregnancy and is not influenced by breastfeeding or by subsequent pregnancies [33]. The authors of this report speculated that such changes in PRL secretion might bear some relationship to the known protective effects of an early first pregnancy against breast cancer.

In addition to the changes in total serum PRL concentrations during pregnancy, there are qualitative changes in the circulating molecular species of PRL as well. In nonpregnant women, gel filtration chromatography has revealed that most circulating PRL has an apparent molecular weight of about 22 kDa; small amounts appear at column elution positions corresponding to approximately 45 kDa and 100–150 kDa [34–36]. The relative abundance of the 22 kDa form may increase modestly during pregnancy [34,36,37]. In contrast, more dramatic changes appear to take place in the proportion of circulating PRL which is glycosylated. In nonpregnant women in the basal state, the majority of circulating PRL is glycosylated; during late pregnancy and lactation, most circulating PRL is nonglycosylated [38–40]. Since glycosylation may alter the biological activity of PRL [41], regulation of this step may be important in initiating and sustaining lactation.

Gonadotropins

Confirming the immunohistochemical observation that pituitary gonadotrophs are decreased in number during pregnancy [2], maternal pituitary content of luteinizing hormone (LH) is also gradually diminished through the course of gestation [42]; although pituitary follicle-stimulating hormone (FSH) content during pregnancy has not been specifically measured, it presumably also decreases, since immunologically stainable FSH is diminished [2].

Basal maternal serum levels of both LH and FSH are decreased as early as 6–7 weeks of gestation and are

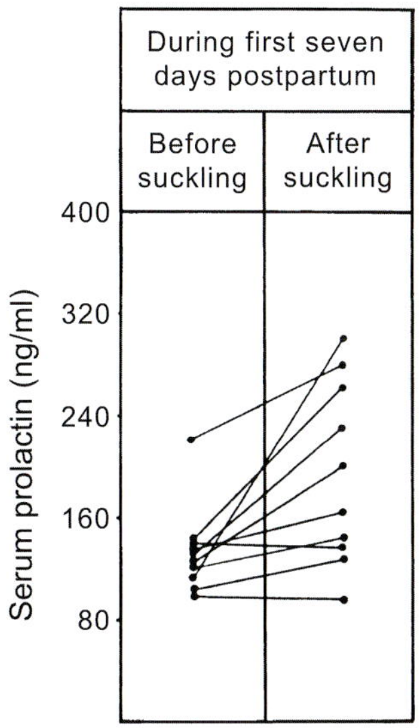

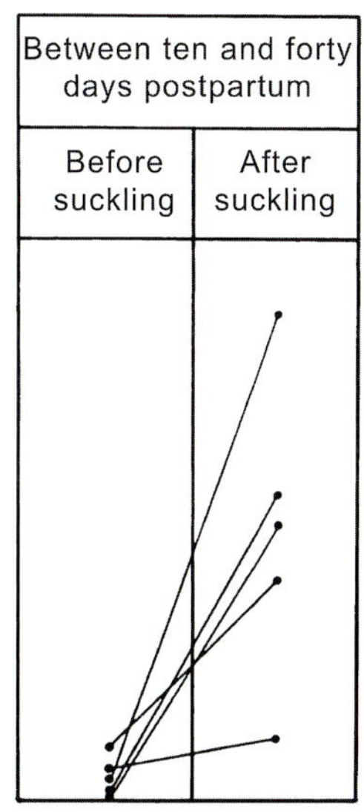

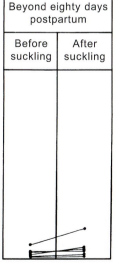

FIGURE 12.2 Serum prolactin responses to suckling in normal postpartum women. Note the diminished response beyond 80 days' postpartum. *From Tyson et al. [8].*

frequently undetectable thereafter. The LH and FSH response to gonadotropin-releasing hormone (GnRH) decreases in parallel with the decrease in basal serum levels of these hormones and remains suppressed into the puerperium [43–45].

The decreased pituitary content of gonadotropins, decreased serum levels of LH and FSH, and the decreased pituitary responsiveness to GnRH all appear to reflect a profound suppression of pituitary gonadotropin synthesis and secretion in response to marked increases in estrogen and progesterone [45,46] (initially from the corpus luteum and decidua, and later from the placenta), PRL (from the maternal pituitary) and inhibin (from the corpus luteum and placenta [47–49]). In addition to stimulating the corpus luteum, hCG may also have a direct suppressive effect on LH (but not FSH) secretion [50].

As the serum concentrations of these suppressive substances fall in the puerperium, maternal gonadotropin secretion resumes, along with responsiveness to GnRH [43,44,46,51]. LH and FSH responses to GnRH are actually exaggerated in the second postpartum month before settling back to normal [51,52].

Gonadotropin secretion by the human fetal pituitary is present by the end of the first trimester, and fetal serum LH and FSH levels peak at about 20 weeks' gestation at adult castrate values; serum levels of both LH and FSH are several times higher in female fetuses than males. In both sexes, serum gonadotropin concentrations then fall in the last trimester of pregnancy, reaching low prepubertal values at term [53–55]. Fetal gonadotropins are excreted into the amniotic fluid, but do not reach the maternal circulation in significant amounts [56].

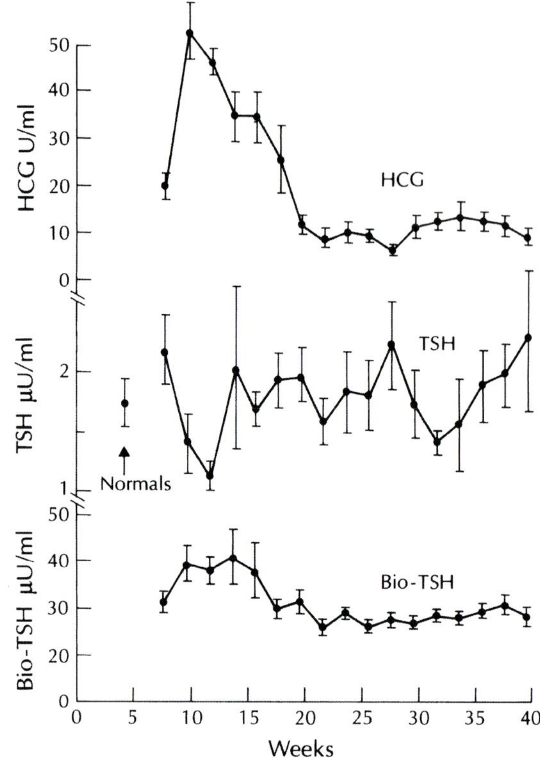

FIGURE 12.3 Mean (± SE) serum concentrations of hCG, TSH and bioassayable thyroid-stimulating activity (Bio-TSH) during normal pregnancy. Note the transient dip in immunoreactive TSH coincident with the peak of serum hCG at 9–12 weeks' gestation. *From Harada et al. [59].*

Thyrotropin

The well-known increase in serum thyroxine-binding globulin which occurs during pregnancy in response to hyperestrogenemia results in a progressive rise in maternal total serum thyroxine (T_4) and triiodothyronine (T_3) concentrations [57,58]. Serum concentrations of free T_4 and free T_3 are either normal throughout or slightly increased during early pregnancy [57,58]. Maternal serum thyrotropin (thyroid-stimulating hormone; TSH) concentrations are generally stable throughout pregnancy except for a small decrease around 9–13 weeks' gestation, coincident with peak maternal serum hCG concentrations (Figure 12.3) [57–60]. Since hCG has weak thyroid-stimulating activity [57,61], it has been postulated that the high concentrations of hCG near the end of the first trimester result in mild thyroid overactivity that, in turn, slightly suppresses maternal pituitary TSH secretion [57–63]. Although early research suggested there might be another placental thyroid stimulator (termed chorionic thyrotropin), most recent studies have concluded that no such hormone exists, and that the thyroid-stimulating properties of placental extracts can be completely accounted for by chorionic gonadotropin [57,59]. Maternal TSH responsiveness to TRH is usually normal in pregnancy [26,44,57,64].

In the fetus, serum T_4 and TSH are low until midgestation, at which point TSH begins to increase, rising to mildly elevated levels (10–15 μU/ml) by the end of the second trimester and declining slightly to about 10 μU/ml at term; the elevation in serum TSH in the second half of gestation is associated with (and presumably causes) a progressive rise in fetal serum T_4. Throughout pregnancy, fetal and maternal TSH secretion proceed independently, since the placenta is impermeable to TSH and only modestly permeable to thyroid hormones [57,65,66]. Within 30 minutes after delivery, there is an acute surge of fetal TSH secretion which may reach 60–80 μU/ml; decline from this peak is fairly rapid over the next several days of life [65].

Adrenocorticotropin (ACTH)

The maternal hypothalamic–pituitary–adrenal (HPA) axis undergoes significant changes during pregnancy.

The causes and consequences of these changes are still unclear, however.

There is general agreement that maternal total serum cortisol gradually increases throughout pregnancy, with a preservation of normal diurnal rhythmicity [67–77]. Part of the rise in total serum cortisol is attributed to an estrogen-induced increase in its principal serum carrier protein, corticosteroid-binding globulin (CBG) [71,75–82]. There is, in addition, a clear rise in serum free cortisol [68,71,75,76,83], salivary free cortisol [74,77] and urinary free cortisol [67,68,70,75,78,79, 84,85]; values for urinary free cortisol at term are above the usual normal range and are comparable to levels seen in nonpregnant patients with Cushing's syndrome.

Maternal plasma ACTH is generally within the normal range, although mean levels have been variously reported as higher [67,72–74,84] or lower [69,86] than those seen in nonpregnant women. Plasma ACTH levels rise gradually through pregnancy [69,72,79,84]. Complicating this picture is the observation that the placenta produces ACTH [67,79,84,86,87]; the relative contribution of placental ACTH to total maternal plasma ACTH is unknown.

Finally, plasma concentrations of corticotropin-releasing hormone (CRH), predominantly of placental origin [79,88–91], have been reported to be greatly elevated in late pregnancy [67,72,73,79,92–94]. Much of this CRH is bound to a specific serum carrier protein and is not biologically active in the maternal circulation [73,79,95,96], although it may have local paracrine effects in the placenta [88,90], and probably contributes to the activation of the maternal HPA axis during pregnancy [67,79].

In an effort to further define the regulation of the HPA axis during pregnancy, a variety of stimulation and suppression tests have been performed. Maternal adrenals are hyperresponsive to ACTH during pregnancy, after both acute and more prolonged (8-hour) stimulation [79,82,97]. Total serum cortisol, the serum free cortisol index and urine free cortisol all show incomplete suppression following dexamethasone administration, in both the overnight test [79,82] and after prolonged dexamethasone ingestion [79,84]. Finally, maternal ACTH responses to exogenous CRH are blunted during pregnancy, and larger CRH doses than usual are required to elicit a response [73,79].

The mechanisms underlying these changes are, at present, largely speculative; possibilities include the following:

1. An increase in CBG levels due to hyperestrogenemia, although simple elevation in CBG does not appear to raise free cortisol [77].
2. Antagonism of glucocorticoid action by progesterone [79,98], resulting in a state of relative cortisol resistance, with an elevation in the set-point for negative feedback by cortisol on ACTH secretion. One study has shown, however, that a relatively brief (days) elevation of serum progesterone to pregnancy levels is not sufficient to elevate free cortisol [77].
3. Autonomous secretion of ACTH by the placenta, leading to nonsuppressibility of maternal ACTH and cortisol. However, this would result in the loss of the normal diurnal rhythm.
4. Tonic hypersecretion of CRH by the placenta with resulting mild chronic ACTH and cortisol hypersecretion, along with down-regulation of the acute response to CRH.
5. An effect of estrogen, through undefined mechanisms, to raise the set-point for feedback of free cortisol on ACTH secretion [77,79].
6. A synergistic stimulatory effect of vasopressin and CRH on ACTH secretion, an effect which may not suppress readily with dexamethasone [99]. Vasopressin secretion is enhanced in late pregnancy in order to overcome the enhanced vasopressin degradation due to placental vasopressinase [100].

Whatever the mechanism, the changes in the maternal HPA axis rapidly return to normal within a few weeks postpartum [72,79,94,101].

GH

The secretion of GH (somatotropin) by the maternal pituitary is profoundly suppressed during the second half of pregnancy. When measured by the usual clinical radioimmunoassay (RIA) or immunoradiometric assay (IRMA) methodologies, both basal and stimulated serum GH levels are low in maternal plasma [25,102–107]. Despite this, maternal serum levels of insulin-like growth factor-I (IGF-I; somatomedin-C) are, if anything, slightly elevated in pregnancy [105–108], and are normalized in pregnant women with GH deficiency [109–113].

This apparent paradox is explained by the observation that the placenta secretes large amounts of a variant form of growth hormone (termed placental growth hormone [PGH]), which is apparently not produced by other tissues [104–108,114–117]. This variant form of GH is not measured in most commercial assays for pituitary hGH, although it may crossreact partially in some research RIAs [104,106]. Placental GH is secreted in a nonpulsatile fashion into the maternal circulation beginning in the late first trimester; its concentration rises progressively to term, and then falls rapidly after delivery [107,108]. When assayed by a human liver radioreceptor method, measurements of total serum "GH-like" activity in pregnancy yield values of about 65 ng/ml; only 3% of this is derived from maternal pituitary secretion of "normal" GH, and only 12% from the GH-like actions of chorionic somatomammotropin (placental lactogen) [105]. The elevated serum levels of PGH and IGF-I probably exert a negative feedback effect on the maternal hypothalamus and pituitary, resulting in a blunting of pituitary GH secretion [102–107]. High serum levels of estrogen present during pregnancy may limit the increase in maternal serum IGF-I levels, since estrogens block the normal stimulation of IGF-I production by GH [118,119].

The placenta also produces GH-releasing hormone (GHRH) [120]; its role in the regulation of placental or fetal GH production is unknown. Similarly, the human placenta has been shown to produce IGF-I [121], but it is not known whether this process is stimulated by GH-like hormones or whether placental IGF-I production plays any important role in the regulation of growth or metabolism during pregnancy.

The fetal pituitary secretes GH normally during gestation [122]; this may not be necessary for fetal IGF production, however, since serum IGF-I and IGF-II are normal in anencephalic fetuses [123].

Posterior Pituitary

During pregnancy, the plasma osmolality set-point for vasopressin release is lowered from the nonpregnant value of about 285 mOsm/kg to about 275–280 mOsm/kg. Peripheral plasma vasopressin levels and vasopressin responses to changes in plasma tonicity remain normal [124]. Vasopressin degradation is increased in pregnancy, however, due to placental vasopressinase, and vasopressin secretion rises in order to keep pace and maintain normal plasma vasopressin levels [100].

Plasma oxytocin concentrations do not appear to rise during pregnancy until the late stages of labor; then, stretching of the vaginal wall results in reflex release of oxytocin which stimulates myometrial contractions and thereby assists in expelling the fetus and placenta. In the postpartum period, oxytocin also assists with breastfeeding; nipple stimulation and/or maternal awareness of a hungry infant reflexively release oxytocin, which produces contraction of the myoepithelial cells of the mammary gland, resulting in milk ejection [125–127].

SHEEHAN'S SYNDROME

Postpartum necrosis of the pituitary (Sheehan's syndrome) may be the most common cause of hypopituitarism worldwide [128]. Hypotension, usually caused by severe hemorrhage at the time of delivery, is the major causal factor [129,130]. Antepartum hemorrhage due to nonobstetric causes may also result in pituitary infarction [131,132]. The hyperplastic pituitary of pregnancy may have a tenuous blood supply to begin with, and the enlarged gland may also compress its feeding blood vessels against the wall of the sella. Additionally, local or systemic vasoconstrictors released during shock may lead to vasospasm of pituitary arterioles [133], further contributing to tissue hypoperfusion.

In its complete form, Sheehan's syndrome typically presents the picture of gradually evolving postpartum panhypopituitarism [129,134–136]. Failure to lactate and rapid breast involution are usually the earliest signs, followed by a failure to resume menses and a lack of regrowth of shaved pubic and/or axillary hair. Signs and symptoms of hypothyroidism and hypoadrenalism gradually develop over a period of months to years. Skin pigmentation decreases, especially in the areolar and genital areas, and poor tanning is noted.

Posterior pituitary involvement may also occur. Overt diabetes insipidus (DI) has been reported but is unusual [136–139]; more subtle defects in vasopressin secretion and maximal urinary concentrating ability are common [140–143] and correspond to the high incidence of posterior pituitary infarcts and neuronal loss in the supraoptic and paraventricular nuclei seen in anatomic studies [144,145]. In some patients, latent DI becomes overt when glucocorticoid therapy is instituted, probably due to the suppressive effects of glucocorticoids on residual vasopressin secretion [146] and perhaps also to direct renal effects of glucocorticoids in facilitating free water excretion [147].

Mental disturbance is common in Sheehan's syndrome, and is usually manifest as an organic psychosis [148–150]; this frequently responds to hormone replacement therapy.

As in other forms of secondary adrenal insufficiency, basal mineralocorticoid production is not impaired, although there may be blunted responses of both renin and aldosterone to upright posture and volume depletion. This blunting is largely corrected by thyroid hormone and glucocorticoid replacement [151,152].

Other features of Sheehan's syndrome include hyperlipidemia, which is probably related to hypothyroidism [153,154]. Several cases of bone marrow aplasia which responded to hormone replacement have been reported [155], and one case of hypomagnesemia with cardiac arrhythmia was noted [156].

Pituitary infarction in Sheehan's syndrome is frequently not total, and partial hypopituitarism is common, with selective loss of one or more hormones [21,130,135,136,157–161]. Preservation of gonadotropin secretion may allow normal menses and even subsequent pregnancy [162–166].

Special mention should be made of the increased vulnerability of the pituitary to infarction in pregnant patients with diabetes mellitus [167,168], probably related to pre-existing vascular disease. In pregnant diabetics, pituitary infarction may be seen without antecedent hypotension and may occur antepartum [169,170].

Recently, antipituitary and antihypothalamus antibodies have been detected in the serum of 30–60% of patients with Sheehan's syndrome [171,172]. It is possible that these antibodies only represent a marker of prior antigen release from necrotic pituitary or hypothalamic tissue; alternatively, they could possibly play a role in the gradual emergence of pituitary hormone deficiencies following the initial infarction of part of the gland.

Diagnosis of Sheehan's Syndrome

To confirm the clinical diagnosis, pituitary function is tested in the usual fashion. The finding of low or normal serum levels of TSH, ACTH, LH and FSH in the presence of subnormal levels of T_4, cortisol and estradiol, respectively, supports the diagnosis of secondary end-organ failure. In most patients, a subnormal serum level of IGF-I (somatomedin-C) can be taken as prima facie evidence of GH deficiency.

Stimulation tests (insulin hypoglycemia, arginine infusion, GHRH infusion) may be used to establish a diagnosis of GH deficiency, and are usually necessary to diagnose PRL deficiency, since basal PRL levels are rarely so low as to be considered subnormal. Deficient PRL responses to TRH or dopamine antagonists are among the most consistent abnormalities seen in patients with Sheehan's syndrome [135,136,159,161,173].

Assessment of TSH, LH and FSH reserve with TRH and GnRH tests has yielded interesting results. Despite hypothyroidism, basal TSH levels are often within the normal range and frequently show a small or normal response to TRH, sometimes with a delayed peak [153,154,159,161,173,174]. Similarly, basal LH and FSH levels may be normal in hypogonadal patients, and often show some response to GnRH [159,161]. These findings suggest suprapituitary disease, and may be due either to anatomic damage to the hypothalamus [145] or, perhaps more likely, to the survival of islands of anterior pituitary tissue no longer supplied with hypothalamic releasing factors due to destruction of the portal circulation [133].

Radiologic studies of the pituitary are also generally performed to exclude the presence of a mass lesion. Acutely, MRI scanning reveals an enlarged, low-density sellar mass, often with rim enhancement following contrast administration [175,176]. Necrotic tissue is gradually reabsorbed, and in longstanding Sheehan's syndrome, the sella turcica is frequently "empty," filled only with CSF [157,160,174,177–179]. In a substantial minority of patients, small remnants of pituitary tissue may be seen on a CT scan [160,174,177]. Sellar volume is small in patients with Sheehan's syndrome, and shows no relation to the time elapsed since the postpartum hemorrhage [179]. This suggests that the sella in Sheehan's syndrome patients may have been small to begin with; in a small, rigid sella, the hyperplastic pituitary may be more likely to compress its blood supply, thus predisposing the gland to infarction if hypotension ensues [180].

Treatment of Sheehan's Syndrome

In most instances, end-organ replacement hormone therapy with L-thyroxine, glucocorticoid and sex hormones are given as indicated; growth hormone and vasopressin may be replaced as needed. Hormone replacement is particularly important in patients with Sheehan's syndrome who become pregnant, since both fetal and maternal mortality is increased in unreplaced patients [162].

LYMPHOCYTIC HYPOPHYSITIS

Lymphocytic hypophysitis is a rare disorder characterized by lymphocytic infiltration and destruction of the anterior pituitary. Several hundred cases have been reported in the literature to date. Most of the reported cases have been women in their reproductive years, and in nearly all of these the disorder presented in late pregnancy or up to about 1 year postpartum. Patients whose symptoms develop during pregnancy generally present with features of a sellar mass (headache, visual disturbance), while patients presenting postpartum may have signs and symptoms of hypopituitarism in addition to those due to pituitary enlargement [181–184]. Radiologically, the pituitary mass cannot always be distinguished from adenoma or other neoplasms on CT or MRI scans. MRI findings suggestive of lymphocytic hypophysitis include: low signal intensity on T_1- and high signal intensity on T_2-weighted imaging; marked, homogeneous contrast enhancement; symmetrical mass, often with suprasellar extension; contrast enhancement of adjacent dura ("dural tail"); thickened pituitary stalk; intact sellar floor [181–186].

Pituitary function testing may reveal complete or partial hypopituitarism; interestingly, when partial defects occur, ACTH deficiency is commonly present, while GH and gonadotropin secretion may be preserved, a contrast to the usual findings in patients with pituitary tumors [181–184]. This pattern of hormone loss presumably reflects specific immunologic damage to a target cell population. Approximately 25% of the patients have prolactin deficiency and 25% have hyperprolactinemia [182], probably due to stalk compression. Around 15–20% of patients have had DI in the absence of surgical intervention.

Some investigators have subdivided lymphocytic hypophysitis into three subtypes: lymphocytic adenohypophysitis, involving primarily the anterior pituitary, with a female, peripartum predominance; lymphocytic infundibulo-neurohypophysitis, involving primarily the posterior pituitary, with less of a female predominance and no association with pregnancy; and lymphocytic panhypophysitis, involving both the anterior and posterior pituitary lobes with a mild female predominance but no relationship to pregnancy [182]. It is not clear how these subtypes differ in their pathogenesis.

Pathogenesis

When sectioned, the pituitary is firm and sometimes gritty. It may be enlarged early in the course of the disease and later frequently becomes atrophic. Microscopically, the gland is infiltrated with lymphocytes and plasma cells, sometimes forming germinal centers. Fibrosis is often present, especially in the later stages, when pituicytes are scant [181,182].

Consistent with this picture of autoimmune hypophysitis, circulating antipituitary antibodies have been found in some cases; unfortunately, antipituitary antibodies are also found in healthy controls and in patients with other diseases [181,182,187,188], making their measurement of little use clinically. About 30% of patients with lymphocytic hypophysitis have had evidence of other endocrine autoimmunity, including thyroiditis, pernicious anemia, adrenalitis, diabetes mellitus and parathyroiditis; thyroid autoimmunity has been the most common associated abnormality [182].

Course and Treatment

About 8% of the patients have died of lymphocytic hypophysitis, probably from adrenal insufficiency [182]. In some patients, pituitary function spontaneously improves, whereas in others, partial defects worsen with time. Some patients are left with an empty sella turcica, prompting confusion with Sheehan's syndrome [181–184]. Treatment therefore consists of hormone replacement as needed, and surgery to relieve visual symptoms due to suprasellar extension. Surgical biopsy with partial debulking is also useful in establishing a definite diagnosis, which may guide further therapy. Glucocorticoids may have restored normal hormone secretion and decreased the size of the pituitary mass in some patients [181–184], but these cases are difficult to distinguish from spontaneous shrinkage. There has been no randomized, controlled trial of high-dose corticosteroids or other immunosuppressive therapy; nevertheless, many case reports have described temporary or long-term improvement following glucocorticoid therapy, and a therapeutic trial of such treatment is not unreasonable [181–184]. Stereotactic radiotherapy has been used successfully to treat two patients with recurrent lymphocytic hypophysitis [189]; further experience is needed with this modality.

PROLACTINOMA

The problem of prolactinoma during pregnancy is discussed in Chapter 15.

CUSHING'S SYNDROME

Pregnancy rarely occurs in patients with Cushing's syndrome. Gonadotropin secretion is suppressed by excess cortisol [190,191], resulting in oligomenorrhea or amenorrhea in 75% of patients [192,193]. The presence of physiologic hypercortisolism during normal pregnancy [67–85] and the frequent occurrence of weight gain, hypertension and hyperglycemia in pregnancy combine to obscure the diagnosis of Cushing's syndrome in pregnant women.

The most common cause (about 50%) of Cushing's syndrome in pregnancy is an adrenal tumor, most of which (80%) are benign [194,195]. This is in distinct contrast to the situation in nonpregnant adults, where pituitary-dependent bilateral adrenal hyperplasia (Cushing's disease) accounts for about two-thirds of all cases, and where adrenal adenomas and carcinomas occur with approximately equal frequency [192,193]. The reasons for this unusual occurrence of hyperfunctioning adrenal adenomas are unclear. The high frequency of benign adrenal adenomas could conceivably relate to excessive stimulation of adrenal growth during pregnancy by placental ACTH [67,79,87,88], placental GH [104,107], or other growth factors. Recently, patients have been described with ACTH-independent Cushing's syndrome during pregnancy associated with adrenal tumors or bilateral adrenal hyperplasia, either diffuse or macronodular; in some cases, the hypercortisolism resolved spontaneously following delivery, suggesting that an adrenal stimulator produced by the fetoplacental unit might be responsible for the Cushing's syndrome. The mechanism of tumor development and hypercortisolism may involve the expression of hormone receptors in the adrenal glands, which become activated only when normal pregnancy hormones (e.g., hCG) are present [196–199]. In one of these cases, cortisol production was, in fact, stimulated by hCG and LH [198].

As previously discussed, plasma total and free cortisol are increased during normal pregnancy, as is urinary free cortisol, and suppression of these parameters by exogenous dexamethasone is incomplete [78,79,82,84,195]. These measurements must therefore be compared to pregnancy norms in order to make the diagnosis of Cushing's syndrome during pregnancy (Table 12.2). Careful examination of diurnal rhythmicity of serum cortisol may be valuable, since this rhythm is preserved in normal pregnancy and is generally absent in Cushing's syndrome [68,70,79,195]. Additionally, urinary 17-hydroxycorticosteroids are not increased during normal pregnancy, so this parameter, rather than urinary free cortisol, may be a useful measurement [200]. Complete nonsuppressibility of plasma or urinary cortisol by high-dose dexamethasone would suggest autonomous production by an adrenal tumor or ectopic ACTH syndrome, but borderline suppressibility in low-dose or overnight testing may still be normal [79,195]. Short-term administration of dexamethasone for testing purposes poses little or no risk to either mother or fetus.

Measurements of plasma ACTH have been undetectable in most but not all cases of adrenal tumor causing Cushing's syndrome in pregnancy, and in the high-normal range in pregnant patients with pituitary-dependent Cushing's disease [79,195]. Thus, a detectable level of ACTH in plasma does not necessarily exclude adrenal tumor; this ACTH may originate from the placenta [67,78,79,84,87,88].

Radiologic studies to evaluate the pituitary and adrenal glands during pregnancy are necessarily limited; ultrasonography and MRI are the preferred techniques.

The major risks to the fetus of maternal Cushing's syndrome are premature labor, which occurs in about 50–60% of patients, and intrauterine growth retardation, seen in about 38%; perinatal death occurs in about 15% [79,194,195,201]. Although the fetal HPA axis may be suppressed by excess maternal cortisol crossing the placenta, neonatal adrenal insufficiency is unusual [195]. The major maternal complications are hypertension (68%) and gestational diabetes mellitus (25%) [195]. Cardiac failure occurs in 3% of patients [195]. Poor wound healing and postoperative infections often complicate cesarean section performed on patients with uncontrolled Cushing's syndrome. Maternal mortality was 2% in one report [195].

Very mild cases of Cushing's syndrome during pregnancy may be managed expectantly with careful monitoring, deferring definitive therapy until after delivery. More severe cases, including those in which adrenal carcinoma is suspected, need surgical intervention. A small number of patients with pituitary-dependent Cushing's disease have been subjected to transsphenoidal adenomectomy during pregnancy, with generally good results [79,195]. Adrenalectomy for adrenal tumors may be performed in the second trimester, often laparoscopically, with cure of hypercortisolism in most patients [195,202,203]. Drug treatment with metyrapone has been used in several cases, usually with no apparent harm to the fetus, although in one patient metyrapone therapy exacerbated maternal hypertension and may have contributed to pre-eclampsia [79].

ACROMEGALY

Patients with acromegaly frequently have menstrual disturbances, and many are amenorrheic, either from anatomic interference with normal pituitary function

TABLE 12.2 Pituitary-Adrenal Function Tests During Pregnancy

Test	Nonpregnant	Pregnant
Plasma cortisol (mean (SD) μg/dl)	a.m. 12.3 (6.6)	Second trimester: a.m. 26.9 (9.5)
	p.m. 1.4 (1.2)	p.m. 12.7 (3.7)
		Third trimester: a.m. 26.4 (11.3)
		p.m. 14.3 (3.4)
Urinary free cortisol (UFC) (μg/24 h)	<50	30–150
Urinary 17-hydroxysteroids (17-OHCS) (mg/24 h)	2–10	2–10
Overnight dexamethasone suppression test (plasma cortisol; μg/dl)	≤1.8 (mean 1.5 [1.2])	Mean 4.6 (0.8) (in third trimester)
Low-dose dexamethasone (0.5 mg q 6h x 2 days) suppression	Urinary 17-OHCS ≤4 mg	Urinary 17-OHCS ≤4 mg
test*	UFC ≤20 μg	UFC 40–80 μg
Response to cosyntropin, 0.25 mg (plasma cortisol; μg/dl)	Peak >18	Second trimester: peak >23
		Third trimester: peak >21

* *Urinary 17-OHCS or UFC excreted in 24 hours.*

All values, especially those for urinary free cortisol, are approximate, and are subject to considerable interlaboratory variability; patient values should be compared to local norms.

or concurrent hyperprolactinemia [204,205]. Nevertheless, patients with acromegaly occasionally become pregnant. In general, the presence of GH excess does not alter the pregnancy in any important way; theoretically, there could be a tendency toward more maternal hypertension and gestational diabetes mellitus, but this has rarely been borne out [22,204–211]. Similarly, the occurrence of pregnancy usually does not alter the course of acromegaly, apart from occasional occurrences of pituitary tumor enlargement during pregnancy [212,213]; it is not clear if patients with concurrent tumor production of PRL are particularly vulnerable to this complication.

In most pregnant patients with untreated acromegaly, therapy for the acromegaly can be safely deferred until after delivery. If treatment is necessary during gestation because of significant tumor enlargement or serious complications of GH excess, transsphenoidal surgery can be performed or bromocriptine may be administered safely [22,204,207,209]. To date, several acromegalic patients have received octreotide or lanreotide therapy during pregnancy, but only a few for the entire gestation; administration of these drugs has had no apparent deleterious effect on the course of the pregnancy [204,208,210,214–221]. Because of limited experience with somatostatin receptor agonists during pregnancy, it is recommended that they be discontinued once pregnancy is confirmed. Two acromegalic patients have been treated during pregnancy with the GH-receptor antagonist, pegvisomant, without apparent problems [222,223]; further experience is needed before pegvisomant can be recommended for use during gestation.

TSH-SECRETING TUMORS

To date, there have been four reports of pregnancy in patients with TSH-secreting pituitary tumors [224–227]. Two of the patients [225,226] were treated with octreotide during pregnancy without any deleterious effects. One patient had transsphenoidal surgery at 27 weeks' gestation [226]. Propylthiouracil was given to three of the patients [224,226,227] with adequate control of the hyperthyroidism in two [224,227].

POSTERIOR PITUITARY DISORDERS

DI may occur for the first time during pregnancy or the postpartum period, or may be exacerbated by pregnancy. Additionally, a unique form of transient DI may occur during pregnancy in the apparent absence of any true defect in vasopressin secretion [100,228].

Pre-existing DI

Patients with idiopathic central DI generally have normal fertility, normal pregnancies and normal deliveries [100,228]. Oxytocin secretion is usually normal [229,230]. Most women with central DI require larger doses of arginine vasopressin (AVP) to control polyuria during pregnancy, with a return to normal AVP requirements after delivery [100,228]. This increased vasopressin requirement during pregnancy is primarily due to the presence in pregnancy plasma of large amounts of vasopressinase, an enzyme which rapidly degrades vasopressin and oxytocin. Vasopressinase is a cystine aminopeptidase which is produced by the placenta and cleared by the liver; plasma levels increase throughout pregnancy, peak at term and disappear rapidly (over 2–4 weeks) following delivery. Thus, in normal third-trimester pregnant women, AVP clearance from plasma is about three times faster than in the postpartum period [100,228].

Postpartum, breast-feeding may be associated with an amelioration of central DI [100]. Since breast-feeding briskly releases oxytocin but not vasopressin [126], this suggests that high oxytocin levels may have some antidiuretic effect in these patients.

Transient DI of Pregnancy

Three forms of transient DI of pregnancy have been distinguished. A vasopressin (AVP)-responsive form probably occurs only in patients with mild or subclinical central DI; in these subjects, the normal pregnancy increase in vasopressin requirements due to placental vasopressinase cannot be met because of a limitation in AVP secretory capacity [100,228,231]. Vasopressin (AVP)-resistant forms may be due either to true renal vasopressin resistance (rare) or to abnormally high vasopressin clearance due to unusually elevated plasma vasopressinase activity [100,228,232–235]. These AVP-resistant forms can be distinguished by the presence or absence of a renal response to the vasopressin analogue desamino-D-arginine vasopressin (DDAVP). Patients with true renal resistance (nephrogenic DI) do not respond to either AVP or DDAVP; in contrast, patients with transient DI due to abnormally high vasopressinase activity do not respond to exogenous AVP, but do respond normally to DDAVP, which is resistant to degradation by vasopressinase [100,228]. Thus, DDAVP is the preparation of choice for treating either central DI or transient DI in pregnancy. True nephrogenic DI may be managed with thiazide diuretics [100,228].

Several interesting features of transient DI of pregnancy due to excess vasopressinase have been pointed out in prior reviews. Symptoms always appeared in the third trimester. Several patients have had twins or triplets. Hypertension, proteinuria, hyperuricemia and elevated liver enzymes were commonly seen. Both excessive vasopressinase production (due to large placentas, as in multiple gestations) and decreased vasopressinase clearance (probably due to liver abnormalities) may play a role in elevated plasma vasopressinase in these patients [228,235].

Postpartum DI

Central diabetes insipidus appearing in the immediate postpartum period is most likely to be due to Sheehan's syndrome [100,228]; much less commonly, DI may occur in lymphocytic hypophysitis [182–184].

References

[1] J. Erdheim, E. Stumme, Über die schwangerschaftsveranderung der hypophyse, Beitr Z Pathol Anat 46 (1909) 1–132.
[2] B.W. Scheithauer, T. Sano, K.T. Kovacs, et al., The pituitary gland in pregnancy: A clinico-pathologic and immunohistochemical study of 69 cases, Mayo Clin Proc 65 (1990) 461–474.
[3] H. Dinc, F. Esen, A. Demirci, et al., Pituitary dimensions and volume measurements in pregnancy and post partum. MR assessment, Acta Radiol 39 (1998) 64–69.
[4] Y. Miki, R. Asato, R. Okumura, et al., Anterior pituitary gland in pregnancy: Hyperintensity at MR, Radiology 187 (1993) 229–231.
[5] S.L. Asa, G. Penz, K. Kovacs, C. Ezrin, Prolactin cells in the human pituitary: A quantitative immunocytochemical analysis, Arch Pathol Lab Med 106 (1982) 360–363.
[6] L. Stefaneanu, K. Kovacs, R.V. Lloyd, et al., Pituitary lactotrophs and somatotrophs in pregnancy: A correlative in situ hybridization and immunocytochemical study, Virchows Archiv B Cell Pathol 62 (1992) 291–296.
[7] M. Visser, D.F. Swaab, Life span changes in the presence of α-melanocyte-stimulating-hormone-containing cells in the human pituitary, J Dev Physiol 1 (1979) 161–178.
[8] J.E. Tyson, P. Hwang, H. Guyda, H.G. Friesen, Studies of prolactin secretion in human pregnancy, Am J Obstet Gynecol 113 (1972) 14–20.
[9] L.A. Rigg, A. Lein, S.S.C. Yen, Pattern of increase in circulating prolactin levels during human gestation, Am J Obstet Gynecol 129 (1977) 454–456.
[10] P. Hwang, H. Guyda, H. Friesen, et al., A radioimmunoassay for human prolactin, Proc Nat Acad Sci USA 68 (1971) 1902–1906.
[11] H.M. Lloyd, J.D. Meares, J. Jacobi, Effects of oestrogen and bromocriptine on in vivo secretion and mitosis in prolactin cells, Nature 255 (1975) 497–498.
[12] H. Nogami, F. Yoshimura, A.J. Carrillo, et al., Estrogen induced prolactin mRNA accumulation in adult male rat pituitary as revealed by in situ hybridization, Endocrinol Jpn 32 (1985) 625–634.
[13] R.A. Prysor-Jones, J.J. Silverlight, S.J. Kennedy, J.S. Jenkins, Vasoactive intestinal peptide and the stimulation of lactotroph growth by oestradiol in situ, J Endocrinol 116 (1988) 259–265.
[14] K.A. Elias, R.I. Weiner, Direct arterial vascularization of estrogen-induced prolactin-secreting anterior pituitary tumors, Proc Nat Acad Sci USA 81 (1984) 4549–4553.
[15] A. Golander, T. Hurley, J. Barrett, et al., Prolactin synthesis by human-chorion decidual tissue: A possible source of amniotic fluid prolactin, Science 202 (1978) 311–313.
[16] D.H. Riddick, A.A. Luciano, W.F. Kusmik, I.A. Maslar, De novo synthesis of prolactin by human decidua, Life Sci 23 (1978) 1913–1922.
[17] V.S. Fang, M.H. Kim, Study on maternal, fetal, and amniotic human prolactin at term, J Clin Endocrinol Metab 41 (1975) 1030–1034.
[18] S.M. Rosenberg, I.A. Maslar, D.H. Riddick, Decidual production of prolactin in late gestation: Further evidence for a decidual source of amniotic fluid prolactin, Am J Obstet Gynecol 138 (1980) 681–685.
[19] D.H. Riddick, A.A. Luciano, W.F. Kusmik, I.A. Maslar, Evidence for a nonpituitary source of amniotic fluid prolactin, Fertil Steril 31 (1979) 35–39.
[20] A. Kauppila, P. Chatelain, P. Kirkinen, et al., Isolated prolactin deficiency in a woman with puerperal alactogenesis, J Endocrinol Metab 64 (1987) 309–312.
[21] D. Lee, C. Leon, B.A. Milanes, Serum prolactin during pregnancy induced by pituitary gonadotropins in a patient with post partum hypopituitarism (Sheehan's syndrome), Arch Invest Med 12 (1981) 29–41.
[22] M. Bigazzi, R. Ronga, I. Lancranjan, et al., A pregnancy in an acromegalic woman during bromocriptine treatment: Effects on growth hormone and prolactin in the maternal, fetal, and amniotic compartments, J Clin Endocrinol Metab 48 (1979) 9–12.
[23] T. Bergh, S.J. Nillius, P. Enoksson, L. Wide, Bromocriptine-induced regression of a suprasellar extending prolactinoma during pregnancy, J Endocrinol Invest 7 (1984) 133–137.
[24] A.N. Anderson, H. Pedersen, J.G. Westergaard, et al., Normal and abnormal prolactin levels during human pregnancy, Acta Obstet Gynecol Scand 63 (1984) 145–148.
[25] J.E. Tyson, H.G. Friesen, Factors influencing the secretion of human prolactin and growth hormone in menstrual and gestational women, Am J Obstet Gynecol 116 (1973) 377–387.
[26] O. Ylikorkala, S. Kivinen, M. Reinila, Serial prolactin and thyrotropin responses to thyrotropin-releasing hormone throughout normal human pregnancy, J Clin Endocrinol Metab 48 (1979) 288–292.
[27] O.A. Kletzky, R.P. Marrs, W.F. Howard, et al., Prolactin synthesis and release during pregnancy and puerperium, Am J Obstet Gynecol 136 (1980) 545–550.
[28] R.M. Boyar, J.W. Finkelstein, S. Kapen, L. Hellman, Twenty-four hour prolactin (PRL) secretory patterns during pregnancy, J Clin Endocrinol Metab 40 (1975) 1117–1120.
[29] M.E. Quigley, B. Ishizuka, J.F. Ropert, S.S.C. Yen, The food-entrained prolactin and cortisol release in late pregnancy and prolactinoma patients, J Clin Endocrinol Metab 54 (1982) 1109–1112.
[30] S. Diaz, H. Cardenas, A. Brandeis, et al., Early difference in the endocrine profile of long and short lactational amenorrhea, J Clin Endocrinol Metab 72 (1991) 196–201.
[31] A. Glasier, A.S. McNeilly, P.W. Howie, The prolactin response to suckling, Clin Endocrinol 21 (1984) 109–116.
[32] P.W. Howie, A.S. McNeilly, Effect of breast feeding patterns on human birth intervals, J Reprod Fertil 65 (1982) 545–557.
[33] V.C. Musey, D.C. Collins, P.I. Musey, et al., Long-term effect of a first pregnancy on the secretion of prolactin, N Engl J Med 316 (1987) 229–234.
[34] P.E. Garnier, M.L. Aubert, S.L. Kaplan, M.M. Grumbach, Heterogeneity of pituitary and plasma prolactin in man: Decreased affinity of "big" prolactin in a radioreceptor assay and evidence for its secretion, J Clin Endocrinol Metab 47 (1978) 1273–1281.

[35] M.D. Whitaker, G.G. Klee, P.C. Kao, et al., Demonstration of biological activity of prolactin molecular weight variants in human sera, J Clin Endocrinol Metab 58 (1984) 826–830.
[36] R.D. Jackson, J. Wortsman, W.B. Malarkey, Persistence of large molecular weight prolactin secretion during pregnancy in women with macroprolactinemia and its presence in fetal cord blood, J Clin Endocrinol Metab 68 (1989) 1046–1050.
[37] F. Pansini, C.M. Bergamini, M. Malfaccini, et al., Multiple molecular forms of prolactin during pregnancy, J Endocrinol 106 (1985) 81–85.
[38] E. Markoff, D.W. Lee, Glycosylated prolactin is a major circulating variant in human serum, J Clin Endocrinol Metab 65 (1987) 1102–1106.
[39] E. Markoff, D.W. Lee, D.R. Hollingsworth, Glycosylated and non-glycosylated prolactin in serum during pregnancy, J Clin Endocrinol Metab 67 (1988) 519–523.
[40] I.A. Hashim, R. Aston, J. Butler, et al., The proportion of glycosylated prolactin in serum is decreased in hyperprolactinemic states, J Clin Endocrinol Metab 71 (1990) 111–115.
[41] Y.N. Sinha, Structural variants of prolactin: Occurrence and physiological significance, Endocr Rev 16 (1995) 354–369.
[42] M. De la Lastra, C. Llados, Luteinizing hormone content of the pituitary gland in pregnant and non-pregnant women, J Clin Endocrinol Metab 44 (1977) 921–923.
[43] S. Jeppsson, G. Rannevik, S. Kullander, Studies on the decreased gonadotropin response after administration of LH/FSH-releasing hormone during pregnancy and the puerperum, Am J Obstet Gynecol 120 (1974) 1029–1034.
[44] J.L. Vandalem, G. Pirens, G. Hennen, U. Gaspard, Thyroliberin and gonadoliberin tests during pregnancy and the puerperium, Acta Endocrinol 86 (1977) 695–703.
[45] L.M. Rubinstein, A.F. Parlow, C. Derzko, J.M. Hershman, Pituitary gonadotropin response to LHRH in human pregnancy, Obstet Gynecol 52 (1978) 172–175.
[46] R.P. Marrs, O.A. Kletzky, D.R. Mishell Jr., A separate mechanism of gonadotropin recovery after pregnancy termination, J Clin Endocrinol Metab 52 (1981) 545–548.
[47] N. Santoro, A.L. Schneyer, J. Ibrahim, C.L. Schmidt, Gonadotropin and inhibin concentrations in early pregnancy in women with and without corpora lutea, Obstet Gynecol 79 (1992) 579–585.
[48] Y. Abe, Y. Hasegawa, K. Miyamoto, et al., High concentrations of plasma immunoreactive inhibin during normal pregnancy in women, J Clin Endocrinol Metab 71 (1990) 133–137.
[49] F. Petraglia, L. Calza, G.C. Garuti, et al., Presence and synthesis of inhibin subunits in human decidua, J Clin Endocrinol Metab 71 (1990) 487–492.
[50] A. Miyake, O. Tanizawa, T. Aono, et al., Suppression of luteinizing hormone in castrated women by the administration of human chorionic gonadotropin, J Clin Endocrinol Metab 43 (1976) 928–932.
[51] E.S. Canales, A. Zarate, J. Garrido, et al., Study on the recovery of pituitary FSH function during puerperium using synthetic LRH, J Clin Endocrinol Metab 38 (1974) 1140–1142.
[52] W.R. Keye Jr., R.B. Jaffe, Changing patterns of FSH and LH response to gonadotropin-releasing hormone in the puerperium, J Clin Endocrinol Metab 42 (1976) 1133–1138.
[53] S.L. Kaplan, M.M. Grumbach, M.L. Aubert, The ontogenesis of pituitary hormones and hypothalamic factors in the human fetus: Maturation of central nervous system regulation of anterior pituitary function, Recent Prog Horm Res 32 (1976) 161–243.
[54] J.S.D. Winter, Hypothalamic–pituitary function in the fetus and infant, Clin Endocrinol Metab 11 (1982) 41–55.
[55] J.J. Mulchahey, A.M. DiBlasio, M.C. Martin, et al., Hormone production and peptide regulation of the human fetal pituitary gland, Endocr Rev 8 (1987) 406–425.
[56] J.A. Clements, F.I. Reyes, J.S.D. Winter, C. Faiman, Studies on human sexual development. III. Fetal pituitary and serum, and amniotic fluid concentrations of LH, CG, and FSH, J Clin Endocrinol Metab 42 (1976) 9–19.
[57] D. Glinoer, The regulation of thyroid function in pregnancy: Pathways of endocrine adaptation from physiology to pathology, Endocr Rev 18 (1997) 404–433.
[58] S.O. LeBeau, S.J. Mandel, Thyroid disorders during pregnancy, Endocrinol Metab Clin N Am 35 (2006) 117–136.
[59] A. Harada, J.M. Hershman, A.W. Reed, et al., Comparison of thyroid stimulators and thyroid hormone concentrations in the sera of pregnant women, J Clin Endocrinol Metab 48 (1979) 793–797.
[60] J.E. Haddow, M.R. McClain, G. Lambert-Messerlian, et al., Variability in thyroid-stimulating hormone suppression by human chorionic gonadotropin during early pregnancy, J Clin Endocrinol Metab 93 (2008) 3341–3347.
[61] J.M. Hershman, Editorial: The role of human chorionic gonadotropin as a thyroid stimulator in normal pregnancy, J Clin Endocrinol Metab 93 (2008) 3305–3306.
[62] F. Pekonen, H. Alfthan, U.-H. Stenman, O. Ylikorkala, Human chorionic gonadotropin (hCG) and thyroid function in early human pregnancy: Circadian variation and evidence for intrinsic thyrotropic activity of hCG, J Clin Endocrinol Metab 66 (1988) 853–856.
[63] N. Yoshikawa, M. Nishikawa, M. Horimoto, et al., Thyroid-stimulating activity in sera of normal pregnant women, J Clin Endocrinol Metab 69 (1989) 891–895.
[64] J.M. Hershman, G.N. Burrow, Lack of release of human chorionic gonadotropin by thyrotropin-releasing hormone, J Clin Endocrinol Metab 42 (1976) 970–972.
[65] D.A. Fisher, A.H. Klein, Thyroid development and disorders of thyroid function in the newborn, N Engl J Med 304 (1981) 702–712.
[66] T. Vulsma, M.H. Gons, J.J.M. DeVijlder, Maternal–fetal transfer of thyroxine in congenital hypothyroidism due to a total organification defect or thyroid agenesis, N Engl J Med 321 (1989) 13–16.
[67] R.S. Goland, S. Jozak, I. Conwell, Placental corticotropin-releasing hormone and the hypercortisolism of pregnancy, Am J Obstet Gynecol 171 (1994) 1287–1291.
[68] W.E. Nolten, M.D. Lindheimer, P.A. Rueckert, et al., Diurnal patterns and regulation of cortisol secretion in pregnancy, J Clin Endocrinol Metab 51 (1980) 466–472.
[69] B.R. Carr, C.R. Parker Jr., J.D. Madden, et al., Maternal plasma adrenocorticotropin and cortisol relationships throughout human pregnancy, Am J Obstet Gynecol 139 (1981) 416–422.
[70] L. Cousins, L. Rigg, D. Hollingsworth, et al., Qualitative and quantitative assessment of the circadian rhythm of cortisol in pregnancy, Am J Obstet Gynecol 145 (1983) 411–416.
[71] A.B. Abou-samra, M. Pugeat, H. Dechaud, et al., Increased plasma concentration of N-terminal β-lipotropin and unbound cortisol during pregnancy, Clin Endocrinol 20 (1984) 221–228.
[72] W. Jeske, P. Soszynski, W. Rogozinski, et al., Plasma GHRH, CRH, ACTH, β-endorphin, human placental lactogen, GH and cortisol concentrations at the third trimester of pregnancy, Acta Endocrinol 120 (1989) 785–789.
[73] T. Suda, M. Iwashita, T. Ushiyama, et al., Responses to corticotropin-releasing hormone and its bound and free forms in pregnant and non-pregnant women, J Clin Endocrinol Metab 69 (1989) 38–42.

[74] B. Allolio, J. Hoffman, E.A. Linton, et al., Diurnal salivary cortisol pattern during pregnancy and after delivery: Relationship to plasma corticotrophin-releasing hormone, Clin Endocrinol 33 (1990) 279–289.
[75] J. Lindholm, N. Schultz-Moller, Plasma and urinary cortisol in pregnancy and during estrogen-gestagen treatment, Scand J Clin Lab Invest 31 (1973) 119–122.
[76] E. Demey-Ponsart, J.M. Foidar, J. Sulon, J.C. Sodeyez, Serum CBG, free and total cortisol and circadian patterns of adrenal function in normal pregnancy, J Steroid Biochem 16 (1982) 165–169.
[77] E.M. Scott, H.H.G. McGarrigle, G.C.L. Lachelin, The increase in plasma and saliva cortisol levels in pregnancy is not due to the increase in corticosteroid-binding globulin levels, J Clin Endocrinol Metab 71 (1990) 639–644.
[78] W.E. Rainey, K.S. Rehman, B.R. Carr, Fetal and maternal adrenals in human pregnancy, Obstet Gynecol Clin N Am 31 (2004) 817–835.
[79] J.R. Lindsay, L.K. Nieman, The hypothalamic–pituitary–adrenal axis in pregnancy: Challenges in disease detection and treatment, Endocr Rev 26 (2005) 775–799.
[80] D.E. Moore, S. Kawagoe, V. Davajan, et al., An in vivo system in man for quantitation of estrogenicity. II. Pharmacologic changes in binding capacity of serum corticosteroid-binding globulin induced by conjugated estrogens, mestranol, and ethinyl estradiol, Am J Obstet Gynecol 130 (1978) 482–486.
[81] B.R. Carr, C.R. Parker Jr., J.D. Madden, et al., Plasma levels of adrenocorticotropin and cortisol in women receiving oral contraceptive steroid treatment, J Clin Endocrinol Metab 49 (1979) 346–349.
[82] W.E. Nolten, P.A. Ruekert, Elevated free cortisol index in pregnancy: Possible regulatory mechanisms, Am J Obstet Gynecol 139 (1981) 492–498.
[83] D.L. Wilcox, J.L. Yovich, S.C. McColm, L.H. Schmitt, Changes in total and free concentrations of steroid hormones in the plasma of women throughout pregnancy: Effects of medroxyprogesterone acetate in the first trimester, J Endocrinol 107 (1985) 293–300.
[84] L.H. Rees, C.W. Burke, T. Chard, et al., Possible placental origin of ACTH in normal human pregnancy, Nature 254 (1975) 620–622.
[85] S.C. Chattoraj, A.K. Turner, J.L. Pincus, D. Charles, The significance of urinary free cortisol and progesterone in normal and anencephalic pregnancy, Am J Obstet Gynecol 124 (1976) 848–853.
[86] K. Mukherjee, G.I.M. Swyer, Plasma cortisol and adrenocorticotropic hormone in normal men and non-pregnant women, normal pregnant women and women with preeclampsia, J Obstet Gynecol Brit Commonw 79 (1972) 504–512.
[87] A. Liotta, D.T. Krieger, In vitro biosynthesis and comparative post-translational processing of immunoreactive precursor corticotropin/β-endorphin by human placental and pituitary cells, Endocrinology 106 (1980) 1504–1511.
[88] F. Petraglia, P.E. Sawchenko, J. Rivier, W. Vale, Evidence for local stimulation of ACTH secretion by corticotropin-releasing factor in human placenta, Nature 328 (1987) 717–719.
[89] D.M. Frim, R.L. Emanuel, B.G. Robinson, et al., Characterization and gestational regulation of corticotropin releasing hormone messenger RNA in human placenta, J Clin Invest 82 (1988) 287–292.
[90] S.A. Jones, A.N. Brooks, J.R.G. Challis, Steroids modulate corticotropin-releasing hormone production in human fetal membranes and placenta, J Clin Endocrinol Metab 68 (1989) 825–830.
[91] T. Usui, Y. Nakai, T. Tsukada, et al., Expression of adrenocorticotropin-releasing hormone precursor gene in placenta and other nonhypothalamic tissues, Mol Endocrinol 2 (1988) 871–875.
[92] A. Sasaki, A.S. Liotta, M.M. Luckey, et al., Immunoreactive corticotropin releasing factor is present in human maternal plasma during the third trimester of pregnancy, J Clin Endocrinol Metab 59 (1984) 812–814.
[93] R.S. Goland, S.L. Wardlaw, R.I. Stark, et al., High levels of corticotropin-releasing hormone immunoreactivity in maternal and fetal plasma during pregnancy, J Clin Endocrinol Metab 63 (1986) 1199–1203.
[94] E.A. Campbell, E.A. Linton, C.D.A. Wolfe, et al., Plasma corticotropin-releasing hormone concentrations during pregnancy and parturition, J Clin Endocrinol Metab 64 (1987) 1054–1059.
[95] T. Suda, M. Iwashita, M. Tozawa, et al., Characterization of corticotropin-releasing hormone binding protein in human plasma by chemical cross-linking and its binding during pregnancy, J Clin Endocrinol Metab 67 (1988) 1278–1283.
[96] E.A. Linton, D.P. Behan, P.W. Saphier, P.J. Lowry, Corticotropin-releasing hormone (CRH)-binding protein: Reduction in the adrenocorticotropin-releasing activity of placental but not hypothalamic CRH, J Clin Endocrinol Metab 70 (1990) 1574–1580.
[97] D. Suri, J. Moran, J.U. Hibbard, et al., Assessment of adrenal reserve in pregnancy: Defining the normal response to the adrenocorticotropin stimulation test, J Clin Endocrinol Metab 91 (2006) 3866–3872.
[98] A.B. Abou-Samra, B. Loras, M. Pugeat, et al., Demonstration of an antigluco-corticoid action of progesterone on the corticosterone inhibition of β-endorphin release by rat anterior pituitary in primary culture, Endocrinology 115 (1984) 1471–1475.
[99] U. Von Bardeleben, F. Holsboer, G.K. Stalla, O.A. Muller, Combined administration of human corticotropin-releasing factor and lysine vasopressin induces cortisol escape from dexamethasone suppression in healthy subjects, Life Sci 37 (1985) 1613–1618.
[100] J.A. Durr, Diabetes insipidus in pregnancy, Am J Kidney Dis 9 (1987) 276–283.
[101] G. Mastorakos, I. Ilias, Maternal and fetal hypothalamic–pituitary–adrenal axes during pregnancy and postpartum, Ann NY Acad Sci 997 (2003) 136–149.
[102] S.S.C. Yen, P. Vela, C.C. Tsai, Impairment of growth hormone secretion in response to hypoglycemia during early and late pregnancy, J Clin Endocrinol Metab 31 (1970) 29–32.
[103] A.C. Artenisio, A. Volpe, F. Rayonese, et al., Behavior of hPL and GH plasmatic rate in pregnant women at different times of their pregnancy during dynamic tests, Horm Metab Res 12 (1980) 205–208.
[104] F. Frankenne, J. Closset, F. Gomez, et al., The physiology of growth hormones (GHs) in pregnant women and partial characterization of the placental GH variant, J Clin Endocrinol Metab 66 (1988) 1171–1180.
[105] W.H. Daughaday, B. Trivedi, H.N. Winn, H. Yan, Hypersomatotropism in pregnant women, as measured by a human liver radioreceptor assay, J Clin Endocrinol Metab 70 (1990) 215–221.
[106] A. Caufriez, F. Frankenne, G. Hennen, G. Copinschi, Regulation of maternal IGF-I by placental GH in normal and abnormal human pregnancies, Am J Physiol 265 (1993) E572–E577.
[107] J. Fuglsang, P. Ovesen, Aspects of placental growth hormone physiology, Growth Horm IGF Res 16 (2006) 67–85.

[108] Z. Wu, M. Bidlingmaier, S. Friess, et al., A new nonisotopic, highly sensitive assay for the measurement of human placental growth hormone: Development and clinical implications, J Clin Endocrinol Metab 88 (2003) 804–811.
[109] T.J. Merimee, J. Zapf, E.R. Froesch, Insulin-like growth factor in pregnancy: Studies in a growth hormone-deficient dwarf, J Clin Endocrinol Metab 54 (1982) 1101–1103.
[110] K. Hall, G. Enberg, E. Hellem, et al., Somatomedin levels in pregnancy: Longitudinal study in healthy subjects and patients with growth hormone deficiency, J Clin Endocrinol Metab 59 (1984) 589–594.
[111] J. Verhaeghe, M. Bougoussa, E. Van Herck, et al., Placental growth hormone and IGF-I in a pregnant woman with Pit-1 deficiency, Clin Endocrinol 53 (2000) 645–647.
[112] J. Fuglsang, F. Lauszus, H. Ørskov, P. Ovesen, Placental growth hormone during pregnancy in a growth hormone deficient woman with type 1 diabetes compared to a matching diabetic control group, Growth Horm IGF Res 14 (2004) 66–70.
[113] P. Wiesli, C. Zwimpfer, J. Zapf, C. Schmid, Pregnancy-induced changes in insulin-like growth factor I (IGF-I), insulin-like growth factor binding protein 3 (IGFBP-3), and acid-labile subunit (ALS) in patients with growth hormone (GH) deficiency and excess, Acta Obstet Gynecol 85 (2006) 900–905.
[114] G. Hennen, F. Frankenne, J. Closset, et al., A human placental GH: Increasing levels during second half of pregnancy with pituitary GH suppression as revealed by monoclonal antibody radioimmunoassays, Int J Fertil 30 (1985) 27–33.
[115] F. Frankenne, F. Rentier-Delrue, M.-L. Scippo, et al., Expression of growth hormone variant gene in human placenta, J Clin Endocrinol Metab 64 (1987) 635–637.
[116] S.A. Liebhaber, M. Urbanek, J. Ray, et al., Characterization and histologic localization of human growth hormone-variant gene expression in the placenta, J Clin Invest 83 (1989) 1985–1991.
[117] F. Frankenne, M.-L. Scippo, J. Van Beeumen, et al., Identification of placental growth hormone as the growth hormone-V gene expression product, J Clin Endocrinol Metab 71 (1990) 15–18.
[118] E. Wiedemann, E. Schwartz, A.G. Frantz, Acute and chronic estrogen effects upon serum somatomedin activity, growth hormone and prolactin in man, J Clin Endocrinol Metab 42 (1976) 942–952.
[119] D.R. Clemmons, L.E. Underwood, E.C. Ridgway, et al., Estradiol treatment of acromegaly: Reduction of immunoreactive somatomedin-C and improvement of metabolic status, Am J Med 69 (1980) 571–575.
[120] S.A. Berry, C.H. Srivastava, L.R. Rubin, et al., Growth hormone-releasing hormone-like messenger ribonucleic acid and immunoreactive peptide are present in human testis and placenta, J Clin Endocrinol Metab 75 (1992) 281–284.
[121] A.L. Fowden, The insulin-like growth factors and feto-placental growth, Placenta 24 (2003) 803–812.
[122] J.J. Mulchahey, A.M. DiBlasio, M.C. Martin, et al., Hormone production and peptide regulation of the human fetal pituitary gland, Endocr Rev 8 (1987) 406–425.
[123] I.K. Ashton, J. Zapf, I. Einschenk, I.Z. Mackenzie, Insulin-like growth factors (IGF) 1 and 2 in human fetal plasma and relationship to gestational age and foetal size during mid-pregnancy, Acta Endocrinol 110 (1985) 558–563.
[124] M.D. Lindheimer, J.M. Davison, Osmoregulation, the secretion of arginine vasopressin and its metabolism during pregnancy, Eur J Endocrinol 132 (1995) 133–143.
[125] J.J. Evans, Oxytocin in the human – regulation of derivations and destinations, Eur J Endocrinol 137 (1997) 559–571.
[126] G.G. Zeeman, F.S. Khan-Dawood, M.Y. Dawood, Oxytocin and its receptor in pregnancy and parturition: Current concepts and clinical implications, Obstet Gynecol 89 (1997) 873–883.
[127] J.A. Russell, G. Leng, Sex, parturition and motherhood without oxytocin? J Endocrinol 157 (1998) 343–359.
[128] K. Kovacs, Necrosis of anterior pituitary in humans, Neuroendocrinology 4 (1969) 170–241.
[129] H.L. Sheehan, Simmonds's disease due to post-partum necrosis of the anterior pituitary, Quart J Med 8 (1939) 277–309.
[130] A.H. Zargar, B. Singh, B.A. Laway, et al., Epidemiologic aspects of postpartum pituitary hypofunction (Sheehan's syndrome), Fertil Steril 84 (2005) 523–528.
[131] G. Agostinis, Sheehan's syndrome due to very grave hemorrhagic shock caused by rupture of the splenic artery in pregnancy; pathogenesis and resuscitational therapeutic consideration, Acta Anesth (Padova) 20 (1969) 187–193.
[132] D.S. Taylor, Massive gastric hemorrhage in late pregnancy followed by hypopituitarism, J Obstet Gynecol Br Comm 79 (1972) 476–478.
[133] H.L. Sheehan, J.P. Stanfield, The pathogenesis of post-partum necrosis of the anterior lobe of the pituitary gland, Acta Endocrinol 37 (1961) 479–510.
[134] K. Kovacs, Sheehan syndrome, Lancet 361 (2003) 520–522.
[135] F. Kelestimur, Sheehan's syndrome, Pituitary 6 (2003) 181–188.
[136] M.H. Samuels, Sheehan's syndrome, Endocrinologist 14 (2004) 25–30.
[137] M.L. Collins, P. O'Brien, A. Cline, Diabetes insipidus following obstetric shock, Obstet Gynecol 53 (1979) 16S–17S.
[138] R.L. Barbieri, R.W. Randall, D.H. Saltzman, Diabetes insipidus occurring in a patient with Sheehan's syndrome during a gonadotropin-induced pregnancy, Fertil Steril 44 (1985) 529–531.
[139] G. Weston, N. Chaves, J. Bowditch, Sheehan's syndrome presenting post-partum with diabetes insipidus, Australia NZ J Obstet Gynecol 45 (2005) 249–250.
[140] F. Bakiri, M. Benmiloud, M.B. Vallotton, Arginine-vasopressin in postpartum panhypopituitarism: Urinary excretion and kidney response to osmolar load, J Clin Endocrinol Metab 58 (1984) 511–515.
[141] I. Jialal, R.K. Desai, M.C. Rajput, An assessment of posterior pituitary function in patients with Sheehan's syndrome, Clin Endocrinol 27 (1987) 91–95.
[142] Y. Iwasaki, Y. Oiso, K. Yamaguchi, et al., Neurohypophyseal function in postpartum hypopituitarism: Impaired plasma vasopressin response to osmotic stimuli, J Clin Endocrinol Metab 68 (1989) 560–565.
[143] H. Atmaca, F. Tanriverdi, C. Gokce, et al., Posterior pituitary function in Sheehan's syndrome, Eur J Endocrinol 156 (2007) 563–567.
[144] H.L. Sheehan, R. Whitehead, The neurohypophysis in post-partum hypopituitarism, J Pathol Bacteriol 85 (1963) 145–169.
[145] R. Whitehead, The hypothalamus in postpartum hypopituitarism, J Pathol Bacteriol 86 (1963) 55–67.
[146] W. Oelkers, Hyponatremia and inappropriate secretion of vasopressin (antidiuretic hormone) in patients with hypopituitarism, N Engl J Med 321 (1989) 492–496.
[147] C.R. Kleeman, J.W. Czaczkes, R. Cutler, Mechanisms of impaired water excretion in adrenal and pituitary insufficiency. IV. Antidiuretic hormone in primary and secondary adrenal insufficiency, J Clin Invest 43 (1964) 1641–1648.
[148] M. Bahemkura, P.H. Rees, Sheehan's syndrome presenting with psychosis, E Afr Med J 58 (1981) 324–329.
[149] M.J. Thomas, A.S.M. Iqbal, Sheehan's syndrome with psychosis, J Assoc Phys India 33 (1985) 175–176.

[150] S. Khanna, A. Ammini, S. Saxena, D. Mohan, Hypopituitarism presenting as delirium, Int J Psychiat Med 18 (1988) 89–92.
[151] F. Bakiri, M. Benmiloud, M.B. Vallotton, The renin–angiotensin system in panhypopituitarism: Dynamic studies and therapeutic effects in Sheehan's syndrome, J Clin Endocrinol Metab 56 (1983) 1042–1047.
[152] F. Bakiri, A.M. Riondel, M. Benmiloud, M.B. Vallotton, Aldosterone in panhypopituitarism: Dynamic studies and therapeutic effects in Sheehan's syndrome, Acta Endocrinol 112 (1986) 329–335.
[153] S. Ishibashi, T. Murase, N. Yamada, et al., Hyperlipidemia in patients with hypopituitarism, Acta Endocrinol 110 (1985) 456–460.
[154] D. Carr, H.M. Thornes, A.C. Rutter, et al., Sheehan's syndrome presenting with type III hyperlipoproteinemia, Postgrad Med J 63 (1987) 1099–1100.
[155] B.A. Laway, J.R. Bhat, S.A. Mir, et al., Sheehan's syndrome with pancytopenia – complete recovery after hormone replacement (case series with review), Ann Hematol 89 (2010) 305–308.
[156] S. Nunoda, K. Ueda, S. Kameda, H. Nakabayashi, Sheehan's syndrome with hypomagnesemia and polymorphous ventricular tachycardia, Jpn Heart J 30 (1989) 251–256.
[157] P.W. Stacpoole, T.W. Kandell, W.R. Fisher, Primary empty sella, hyperprolactinemia, and isolated ACTH deficiency after postpartum hemorrhage, Am J Med 74 (1983) 905–908.
[158] D.A. Westbrock, L.S. Srivastava, H.C. Knowles Jr., Preservation of normal menstrual cycles in a patient with Sheehan's syndrome, South Med J 76 (1983) 1065–1067.
[159] I. Jialal, C. Naidoo, R.J. Norman, et al., Pituitary function in Sheehan's syndrome, Obstet Gynecol 63 (1984) 15–19.
[160] S. Ishikawa, M. Furuse, T. Saito, et al., Empty sella in control subjects and patients with hypopituitarism, Endocrinol Jpn 35 (1988) 665–674.
[161] N. Ozbey, S. Inanc, F. Aral, et al., Clinical and laboratory evaluation of 40 patients with Sheehan's syndrome, Isr J Med Sci 30 (1994) 826–829.
[162] H.G. Grimes, M.H. Brooks, Pregnancy in Sheehan's syndrome. Report of a case and review, Obstet Gynecol Surv 35 (1980) 481–488.
[163] A.C. Moreira, L.M.Z. Maciel, M.C. Foss, et al., Gonadotropin secretory capacity in a patient with Sheehan's syndrome with successful pregnancies, Fertil Steril 42 (1984) 303–305.
[164] G. Giustina, F. Zuccato, A. Salvi, R. Candrina, Pregnancy in Sheehan's syndrome corrected by adrenal replacement therapy. Case report, Brit J Obstet Gynecol 92 (1985) 1061–1063.
[165] S. Pattanaungkul, S. Chandraprasert, Pregnancy in Sheehan's syndrome, J Med Assoc Thailand 72 (1989) 48–51.
[166] E. Algün, H. Ayakta, M. Harman, et al., Spontaneous pregnancy in a patient with Sheehan's syndrome, Eur J Obstet Gynecol 110 (2003) 242–244.
[167] C.F. Brennan, R.G.S. Malone, J.A. Weaver, Pituitary necrosis in diabetes mellitus, Lancet 2 (1956) 12–16.
[168] G. Herbai, I. Werner, Sheehan's syndrome of hypothalamic origin in a woman with juvenile diabetes mellitus, Acta Med Scand 199 (1976) 539–541.
[169] R.G. Wieland, J.M. Wieland, Isolated adrenocorticotropic hormone deficiency with antepartum pituitary infarction in a Type I diabetic, Obstet Gynecol 65 (1985) 58S–59S.
[170] M.D. Flynn, T.F. Cundy, P.J. Watkins, Antepartum pituitary necrosis in diabetes mellitus, Diab Med 5 (1988) 295–297.
[171] R. Goswami, N. Kochupillai, P.A. Crock, et al., Pituitary autoimmunity in patients with Sheehan's syndrome, J Clin Endocrinol Metab 87 (2002) 4137–4141.
[172] A. DeBellis, F. Kelestimur, A.A. Sinisi, et al., Anti-hypothalamus and anti-pituitary antibodies may contribute to perpetuate the hypopituitarism in patients with Sheehan's syndrome, Eur J Endocrinol 158 (2008) 147–152.
[173] P.A. Singer, J.H. Mestman, P.R. Manning, et al., Hypothalamic hypothyroidism secondary to Sheehan's syndrome, West J Med 120 (1974) 416–418.
[174] A.M. Fleckman, U.K. Schubart, A. Danziger, N. Fleischer, Empty sella of normal size in Sheehan's syndrome, Am J Med 75 (1983) 585–591.
[175] S. Dejager, S. Gerber, L. Foubert, G. Turpin, Sheehan's syndrome: Differential diagnosis in the acute phase, J Intern Med 244 (1998) 261–266.
[176] J. Kaplun, C. Fratila, A. Ferenczi, et al., Sequential pituitary MR imaging in Sheehan syndrome: Report of 2 cases, Am J Neuroradiol 29 (2008) 941–943.
[177] B. Knobel, S. Ben-Yosef, P. Rosman, Sheehan's syndrome and empty sella turcica, Israel J Med Sci 20 (1984) 232–235.
[178] A. Barkan, Case report: Pituitary atrophy in patients with Sheehan's syndrome, Am J Med Sci 298 (1989) 38–40.
[179] I.H. Sherif, C.M. Vanderley, S. Beshyah, S. Bosairi, Sella size and contents in Sheehan's syndrome, Clin Endocrinol 30 (1989) 613–618.
[180] H.C. Gotshalk, I.L. Tilden, Necrosis of the anterior pituitary following parturition, JAMA 114 (1940) 33–35.
[181] A. Bellastella, A. Bizzarro, C. Coronella, et al., Lymphocytic hypophysitis: A rare or underestimated disease? Eur J Endocrinol 149 (2003) 363–376.
[182] P. Caturegli, C. Newschaffer, A. Olivi, et al., Autoimmune hypophysitis, Endocr Rev 26 (2005) 599–614.
[183] J.A. Rivera, Lymphocytic hypophysitis: Disease spectrum and approach to diagnosis and therapy, Pituitary 9 (2006) 35–45.
[184] M.E. Molitch, M.P. Gillam, Lymphocytic hypophysitis, Horm Res 68 (suppl 5) (2007) 145–150.
[185] J.K. Powrie, M. Powell, A.B. Ayers, et al., Lymphocytic adenohypophysitis: Magnetic resonance imaging features of two new cases and a review of the literature, Clin Endocrinol 42 (1995) 315–322.
[186] S. Saiwai, Y. Inoue, T. Ishihara, et al., Lymphocytic adenohypophysitis: Skull radiographs and MRI, Neuroradiol 40 (1998) 114–120.
[187] P. Caturegli, I. Lupi, M. Landek-Salgado, et al., Pituitary autoimmunity: 30 years later, Autoimmunity Rev 7 (2008) 631–638.
[188] A. DeBellis, G. Ruocco, M. Battaglia, et al., Immunological and clinical aspects of lymphocytic hypophysitis, Clin Sci 114 (2008) 413–421.
[189] M.T. Selch, A.A.F. DeSalles, D.F. Kelly, et al., Stereotactic radiotherapy for the treatment of lymphocytic hypophysitis, J Neurosurg 99 (2003) 591–596.
[190] G.B. Melis, V. Mais, M. Gambacciani, et al., Dexamethasone reduces the postcastration gonadotropin rise in women, J Clin Endocrinol Metab 65 (1987) 237–241.
[191] J. Lado-Abeal, J. Rodriguez-Arnao, J.D.C. Newell-Price, et al., Menstrual abnormalities in women with Cushing's disease are correlated with hypercortisolemia rather than raised circulating androgen levels, J Clin Endocrinol Metab 83 (1998) 3083–3088.
[192] R. Pivonello, M.C. DeMartino, M. DeLeo, et al., Cushing's syndrome, Endocrinol Metab Clin N Am 37 (2008) 135–149.
[193] M. Boscaro, G. Arnaldi, Approach to the patient with possible Cushing's syndrome, J Clin Endocrinol Metab 94 (2009) 3121–3131.
[194] L.R. Sheeler, Cushing's syndrome and pregnancy, Endocrinol Metab Clin North Am 23 (1994) 619–627.

[195] J.R. Lindsay, J. Jonklaas, E.H. Oldfield, L.K. Nieman, Cushing's syndrome during pregnancy: Personal experience and review of the literature, J Clin Endocrinol Metab 90 (2005) 3077–3083.
[196] C.F. Close, M.C. Mann, J.F. Watts, K.C. Taylor, ACTH-independent Cushing's syndrome in pregnancy with spontaneous resolution after delivery: Control of the hypercortisolism with metyrapone, Clin Endocrinol 39 (1993) 375–379.
[197] C. Wallace, E.L. Toth, R.Z. Lewanczuk, K. Siminoski, Pregnancy-induced Cushing's syndrome in multiple pregnancies, J Clin Endocrinol Metab 81 (1996) 15–21.
[198] A. Lacroix, N. N'Diaye, J. Tremblay, P. Hamet, Ectopic and abnormal hormone receptors in adrenal Cushing's syndrome, Endocrine Rev 22 (2001) 75–110.
[199] L.A. Wy, H.E. Carlson, P. Kane, et al., Pregnancy-associated Cushing's syndrome secondary to a luteinizing hormone/human chorionic gonadotropin receptor-positive adrenal carcinoma, Gynecol Endocrinol 16 (2002) 413–417.
[200] K. Kreines, E. Perin, R. Salzer, Pregnancy in Cushing's syndrome, J Clin Endocrinol Metab 24 (1964) 75–79.
[201] N. Polli, F.P. Giraldi, F. Cavagnini, Cushing's disease and pregnancy, Pituitary 7 (2004) 237–241.
[202] H. Tejura, J. Weiner, O. Gibby, et al., Cushing's syndrome in pregnancy, J Obstet Gynaecol 25 (2005) 713–718.
[203] K.P. Terhune, S. Jagasia, L.S. Blevins, J.E. Phay, Diagnostic and therapeutic dilemmas of hypercortisolism during pregnancy: A case report, Am Surgeon 75 (2009) 232–234.
[204] V. Herman-Bonert, M. Seliverstov, S. Melmed, Pregnancy in acromegaly: Successful therapeutic outcome, J Clin Endocrinol Metab 83 (1998) 727–731.
[205] G.A. Kaltsas, J.J. Mukherjee, P.J. Jenkins, et al., Menstrual irregularity in women with acromegaly, J Clin Endocrinol Metab 84 (1999) 2731–2735.
[206] A. Colao, B. Merola, D. Ferone, G. Lombardi, Acromegaly, J Clin Endocrinol Metab 82 (1997) 2777–2781.
[207] M. Hisano, M. Sakata, N. Watanabe, et al., An acromegalic woman first diagnosed in pregnancy, Arch Gynecol Obstet 274 (2006) 171–173.
[208] T. Takano, J. Saito, A. Soyama, et al., Normal delivery following an uneventful pregnancy in a Japanese acromegalic patient after discontinuation of octreotide long acting release formulation at an early phase of pregnancy, Endocr J 53 (2006) 209–212.
[209] A. Atmaca, S. Dagdelen, T. Erbas, Followup of pregnancy in acromegalic women: Different presentations and outcomes, Exp Clin Endocrinol Diab 114 (2006) 135–139.
[210] R. Cozzi, R. Attanasio, M. Barausse, Pregnancy in acromegaly: A one-center experience, Eur J Endocrinol 155 (2006) 279–284.
[211] A. Beckers, A. Stevenaert, J.-M. Foidart, et al., Placental and pituitary growth hormone secretion during pregnancy in acromegalic women, J Clin Endocrinol Metab 71 (1990) 725–731.
[212] Y. Okada, I. Morimoto, K. Ejima, et al., A case of active acromegalic woman with a marked increase in serum insulin-like growth factor-1 levels after delivery, Endocr J 44 (1997) 117–120.
[213] M.J. Kupersmith, C. Rosenberg, D. Kleinberg, Visual loss in pregnant women with pituitary adenomas, Ann Intern Med 121 (1994) 473–477.
[214] E. DeMenis, D. Billeci, E. Marton, G. Gussoni, Uneventful pregnancy in an acromegalic patient treated with slow-release lanreotide: A case report, J Clin Endocrinol Metab 84 (1999) 1489.
[215] K. Takeuchi, T. Funakoshi, S. Oomori, T. Maruo, Successful pregnancy in an acromegalic woman treated with octreotide, Obstet Gynecol 93 (1999) 848.
[216] J. Mozas, E. Ocón, M. López de la Torre, et al., Successful pregnancy in a woman with acromegaly treated with somatostatin analog prior to surgical resection, Int J Gynecol Obstet 65 (1999) 71–73.
[217] T. Hierl, R. Ziegler, C. Kasperk, Pregnancy in persistent acromegaly, Clin Endocrinol 53 (2000) 262–263.
[218] M. Fassnacht, B. Capeller, W. Arlt, et al., Octreotide LAR treatment throughout pregnancy in an acromegalic woman, Clin Endocrinol 55 (2001) 411–415.
[219] O. Serri, G. Lanoie, Successful pregnancy in a woman with acromegaly treated with octreotide long-acting release, Endocrinologist 13 (2003) 17–19.
[220] P. Maffei, G. Tamagno, G.B. Nardelli, et al., Effects of octreotide exposure during pregnancy in acromegaly, Clin Endocrinol (2010) 668–677.
[221] N. Mikhail, Octreotide treatment of acromegaly during pregnancy, Mayo Clin Proc 77 (2002) 297–298.
[222] A. Qureshi, E. Kalu, G. Ramanathan, et al., IVF/ICSI in a woman with active acromegaly: Successful outcome following treatment with pegvisomant, J Assist Reprod Genet 23 (2006) 439–442.
[223] S.R. Brian, M. Bidlingmaier, M.P. Wajnrajch, et al., Treatment of acromegaly with pegvisomant during pregnancy: Maternal and fetal effects, J Clin Endocrinol Metab 92 (2007) 3374–3377.
[224] T.B. Francis, R.C. Smallridge, J. Kane, J.A. Magner, Octreotide changes serum thyrotropin (TSH) glycoisomer distribution as assessed by lectin chromatography in a TSH macroadenoma patient, J Clin Endocrinol Metab 77 (1993) 183–187.
[225] P. Caron, C. Gerbeau, L. Pradayrol, et al., Successful pregnancy in an infertile woman with a thyrotropin-secreting macroadenoma treated with somatostatin analog (octreotide), J Clin Endocrinol Metab 81 (1996) 1164–1168.
[226] G. Blackhurst, M.W. Strachan, D. Collie, et al., The treatment of a thyrotropin-secreting pituitary macroadenoma with octreotide in twin pregnancy, Clin Endocrinol 56 (2002) 401–404.
[227] S. Chaiamnuay, M. Moster, M.R. Katz, Y.N. Kim, Successful management of a pregnant woman with a TSH secreting pituitary adenoma with surgical and medical therapy, Pituitary 6 (2008) 109–113.
[228] S. Ananthakrishnan, Diabetes insipidus in pregnancy: Etiology, evaluation and management, Endocr Practice 15 (2009) 377–382.
[229] R. Rubens, M. Thiery, Diabetes insipidus and pregnancy, Eur J Obstet Gynecol Reprod Biol 26 (1987) 265–270.
[230] M.M. Shangold, R. Freeman, P. Kumaresan, et al., Plasma oxytocin concentrations in a pregnant woman with total vasopressin deficiency, Obstet Gynecol 61 (1983) 662–667.
[231] J.M. Hughes, W.M. Barron, M.L. Vance, Recurrent diabetes insipidus associated with pregnancy: Pathophysiology and therapy, Obstet Gynecol 73 (1989) 462–464.
[232] S.M. Ford, Transient vasopressin-resistant diabetes insipidus of pregnancy, Obstet Gynecol 68 (1986) 288–289.
[233] J.A. Durr, J.G. Hoggard, J.M. Hunt, R.W. Schrier, Diabetes insipidus in pregnancy associated with abnormally high circulating vasopressinase activity, N Engl J Med 361 (1987) 1070–1074.
[234] Y. Iwasaki, Y. Oiso, K. Kondo, et al., Aggravation of subclinical diabetes insipidus during pregnancy, N Engl J Med 324 (1991) 522–526.
[235] J. Krege, V.L. Katz, W.A. Bowes Jr., Transient diabetes insipidus of pregnancy, Obstet Gynecol Surv 44 (1989) 789–795.

CHAPTER

13

Drugs and Pituitary Function

Harold E. Carlson

Stony Brook University, Stony Brook, NY, USA

INTRODUCTION

Many drugs, both therapeutic and recreational, alter the function of the pituitary gland, usually as a side effect unrelated to the primary indication for which the drug was given. Tables 13.1–13.7 summarize the most important drug-related changes in pituitary hormone secretion.

ALCOHOLIC BEVERAGES

Consumption of beverages containing ethanol may alter pituitary function in several ways: (1) by direct effects on the brain or pituitary gland; (2) by altering the function of end organs (e.g., testis) and provoking feedback-mediated changes in pituitary hormone secretion; and (3) by modifying the peripheral metabolism or action of hormones with resulting effects on pituitary function.

In some studies, the acute administration of ethanol has been reported to stimulate adrenocorticotropic hormone (ACTH) and cortisol secretion [1–3]; however,

TABLE 13.1 Recreational Drugs that Alter Pituitary Function

Alcoholic beverages
Cigarettes and nicotine
Marijuana
Opiates
Cocaine
Amphetamines and methylphenidate
Caffeine
Benzodiazepines

TABLE 13.2 Drugs that Alter Prolactin Secretion

Increase	Decrease
Risperidone	
Beer	Apomorphine
Nicotine	Dopamine agonists
Opiates	
Cocaine (?)	Bromocriptine
Amphetamines (i.v.)	Cabergoline
Imipramine (±)	Aripiprazole
Desipramine (±)	
Chlorimipramine	
Amoxapine	
Monoamine oxidase inhibitors	
Antipsychotics	
Buspirone	
Metoclopramide	
Sulpiride	
Domperidone	
Physostigmine	
Reserpine (±)	
Methyldopa (±)	
Labetalol	
Verapamil (±)	
Cimetidine (i.v.)	
Ranitidine (i.v.)	
Estrogens (±)	

i.v., intravenous administration.

The Pituitary, Third Edition, DOI: 10.1016/B978-0-12-380926-1.10013-6

TABLE 13.3 Drugs that Alter Growth Hormone Secretion

Increase	Decrease
Nicotine	Atropine
Opiates	Pirenzepine
Amphetamines	Yohimbine
Methylphenidate	Phentolamine
Benzodiazepines (±)	Cimetidine (?)
Imipramine	Glucocorticoids
Desipramine	
Chlorimipramine	
Apomorphine	
Dopamine	
L-Dopa	
Bromocriptine	
Physostigmine	
Propranolol	
Clonidine	
Estrogens	
Androgens	

TABLE 13.4 Drugs that Alter Gonadotropin (Luteinizing Hormone/Follicle-Stimulating Hormone) Secretion

Increase	Decrease
Opiate antagonists	Opiates
Cocaine	Dopamine
Cancer chemotherapy	Bromocriptine
Estrogen receptor antagonists	Verapamil
Aromatase inhibitors (in men)	Estrogens
Flutamide (in men)	Androgens
Ketoconazole	Glucocorticoids
	Megestrol

these findings have not been confirmed by others [4–10]. The reasons for these discrepancies are unclear, but may in part be related to dose of ethanol [7], the presence or absence of nausea [9], the subjects' alcohol dehydrogenase genotype [8], or family history of alcoholism [2]. Chronic consumption of ethanol may lead to persistent elevation of serum cortisol [11–13], and a small number of alcoholics may develop physical stigmata of Cushing's syndrome along with nonsuppression of plasma ACTH and cortisol by dexamethasone, the so-called "alcohol-induced pseudo-Cushing's syndrome"

TABLE 13.5 Drugs that Alter Thyrotropin Secretion

Increase	Decrease
Lithium	Dopamine
Metoclopramide	L-dopa
Sulpiride	Bromocriptine
Domperidone	Verapamil
Estrogens (±)	Androgens (±)
Sunitinib	Glucocorticoids
Sorafenib	Metformin

[14,15]. The syndrome usually resolves after days to months of abstinence [11,13]. Paradoxically, the ACTH and cortisol responses to insulin-induced hypoglycemia and other stimuli are frequently blunted in alcoholics [12,14,16]. Ethanol may also stimulate the secretion of β-endorphin in some subjects [1,10].

In the absence of liver disease or malnutrition, growth hormone (GH) secretion is minimally affected by ethanol. Acute administration of alcohol produces little change in serum GH [17–19].

Daytime serum concentrations of thyrotropin (thyroid-stimulating hormone; TSH) and thyroid hormones are not altered by acute ethanol consumption [18,20], although the nocturnal TSH surge has been reported to be suppressed [19]. Chronic alcoholics may have a blunted TSH response to thyrotropin-releasing hormone (TRH), although the basal TSH level is normal [21]. Alcohol-induced liver damage can result in the "euthyroid sick" or "nonthyroidal illness" syndrome, generally with low serum triiodothyronine (T_3), elevated reverse T_3, normal or low thyroxine (T_4) and normal or slightly elevated TSH [22].

Reports concerning the effects of ethanol on gonadal function have yielded conflicting data. These inconsistencies may result from the use of different study populations, varying doses of alcohol, performing studies at different times of the day with blood sampling at varying intervals, the development of tolerance to the effects of alcohol, and the presence of variable degrees of hepatic dysfunction in chronic studies [23]. Acute ingestion of ethanol in males has been reported to increase, decrease, or have no effect on plasma testosterone and luteinizing hormone (LH) [6,18,20,23–25]. Chronic alcohol consumption, in the apparent absence of liver disease, may lower serum testosterone concentrations by inhibiting testicular synthesis and increasing hepatic metabolism of testosterone [26–28]; serum LH may rise, at least transiently, as a consequence. A later fall in LH may occur as a response to rising serum estrogen levels produced

TABLE 13.6 Drugs that Alter Adrenocorticotropin Secretion

Increase	Decrease
Nicotine	Opiates
Opiate antagonists	Glucocorticoids
Amphetamines	Megestrol
Methylphenidate	
Imipramine	
Desipramine	
Chlorimipramine	
Physostigmine	
Ketoconazole	

TABLE 13.7 Drugs that Alter Vasopressin Secretion

Increase	Decrease
Nicotine	Opiates
Lithium	Glucocorticoids

by increased hepatic aromatase activity [26–28]. Additionally, plant-derived phytoestrogens are present in alcoholic beverages and could also contribute to gonadotropin suppression [29]. Ethanol is also toxic to the seminiferous tubules, and may produce testicular atrophy and elevated serum follicle-stimulating hormone (FSH) levels [27,30].

In women, acute administration of ethanol has generally been reported to be without effect on serum LH or estradiol concentrations [31,32], although one study reported a small rise in estradiol following alcohol ingestion [33]. Chronic administration, however, has produced a variety of disturbances in the menstrual cycle [34,35]. In postmenopausal women, serum gonadotropins are altered minimally by ethanol [36].

The effects of alcohol on prolactin (PRL) are controversial. Most studies have reported no acute effect of ethanol ingestion on serum PRL concentrations [3,18–20,32,37,38]. One study reported an acute decrease in serum PRL following ethanol ingestion [31], while several studies have found a small but statistically significant dose-related rise in serum PRL following ethanol administration [1,2,4–6,39,40]. Interestingly, beer is a fairly potent stimulus to PRL secretion [38,41], an effect that appears to be independent of its ethanol content [38,42]. Serum PRL is mildly elevated in a minority of patients with alcoholic liver disease [43].

In some studies ethanol has had a transient suppressive effect on oxytocin and vasopressin secretion [3,44–46], while in others vasopressin has been unchanged or even increased [9,47,48]. Chronic alcoholics have been reported to have a decrease in the number of vasopressin-containing neurons in the supraoptic and paraventricular nucleus of the hypothalamus [49].

SMOKING

Cigarette Smoking and Nicotine

Cigarette smoking results in the acute release of several pituitary hormones, and the effects appear to be due to nicotine. Several studies have reported increases in plasma cortisol, DHEA, ACTH and β-endorphin/β-lipotropin in response to smoking one or more medium- or high-nicotine cigarettes; sham smoking or smoking low-nicotine cigarettes had no such effect [50–59]. Administration of nicotine by intravenous infusion or nasal spray also stimulates ACTH and cortisol secretion [55,60]. Chronic habitual smoking appears to result in small but significant increases in morning serum cortisol and DHEA as well as salivary cortisol over the entire day [61–63]. Similarly, a rise in serum GH following smoking has been fairly consistently observed [50,52,56,57], and several studies have reported a rise in serum PRL induced by smoking [50,52,56,64]. Although some reports [52,54] have ascribed these hormonal changes to nausea induced by rapid smoking, other studies have noted similar hormonal increments in subjects who did not experience nausea [50,51,53,57,59]. Serum IGF-1 is similar in chronic smokers and nonsmokers [65]. Studies of baseline PRL in smokers have been inconsistent. In humans, serum TSH and FSH are not acutely altered by smoking [52]. Chronic smokers and individuals exposed to second-hand smoke may have slightly lower serum levels of TSH than nonsmokers, a situation that may reflect direct or indirect nicotine effects on thyroid hormone secretion, metabolism, or action [66–68]. Serum FSH has been reported to be slightly higher in chronic smokers than in nonsmokers in some studies [69,70]. Serum LH was reported to acutely increase or decrease after smoking or nicotine administration [64,71]; no consistent changes in serum LH have been reported in chronic smokers.

Release of vasopressin and its precursor protein, neurophysin I, is stimulated by smoking or nicotine infusion [51,55,57,72,73], while oxytocin is not affected [72,73].

Marijuana

Although animal studies have shown a wide variety of effects of marijuana on hormonal systems, it has been difficult to show consistent changes in human studies, in which lower doses of marijuana or tetrahydrocannabinol are given. Additional experimental difficulties in some studies involve possible inaccuracies of reported intake, uncertainty regarding concurrent use of alcohol or other drugs, and the development of tolerance to the effects of marijuana.

In both men and women, no consistent changes have been seen in serum gonadotropins or sex steroids [74]. Serum PRL is slightly decreased or unchanged in chronic marijuana users [74,75]. Serum cortisol rose slightly after intravenous tetrahydrocannabinol or smoking marijuana [74,75]; however, this effect was blunted in chronic smokers [75]. Both growth hormone and cortisol responses to insulin-induced hypoglycemia were blunted following oral administration of tetrahydrocannabinol; however, responses were still within the normal range [76].

In a single study, serum T_4 and TSH were not altered by chronic marijuana smoking, though serum T_3 was slightly decreased [77].

OPIATES AND OPIATE ANTAGONISTS

Opiates

Acute administration of opiates (e.g., morphine, heroin, codeine, fentanyl, β-endorphin, enkephalins) has profound and generally consistent effects on human pituitary function. In males, serum LH is lowered, followed by a fall in serum testosterone [78,79]. In females, opiates suppress serum LH in premenopausal subjects, often resulting in irregular menses or amenorrhea [78]. Both morphine and an enkephalin analogue suppressed LH in postmenopausal women [80,81]. Serum FSH is also acutely decreased by opiates, but to a lesser degree [78]. Based primarily on animal studies, it appears that opiates suppress gonadotropin secretion by inhibiting GnRH release [78]; opiates do not impair the gonadotropin response to GnRH in humans [81].

PRL secretion is stimulated by all opiates, in both sexes [78,82,83]. This effect may be due to a decrease in tuberoinfundibular dopamine (DA) release [78,84].

Several human studies have reported small but significant increases in TSH in response to opiates [78]. One group has reported that TSH is decreased in chronic opium smokers [83]. Morphine and other opiates acutely stimulate GH secretion [78,85]. There is some evidence that stimulation of GH release by enkephalin analogues may involve a reduction in somatostatin secretion [86].

Opiates suppress ACTH and cortisol secretion [78]. This effect may be exerted at the pituitary level, since opiates blunt the ACTH response to lysine vasopressin and corticotropin-releasing hormone (CRH) [87,88] and since loperamide, an opiate agonist which does not cross the blood–brain barrier, suppresses cortisol secretion [89]. Alternatively, since opiates do not directly alter ACTH secretion in vitro [88], the suppressive effect of opiates may involve other suprapituitary factors.

Although conflicting data have been obtained, opiates, on balance, appear to inhibit vasopressin secretion [78]. Plasma oxytocin concentrations were decreased by opiate administration during labor, but not in late pregnancy before the onset of labor [78], and were also suppressed by opiates during breast-feeding [78].

Chronic administration of opiates, as in narcotic addiction, results in partial tolerance to their euphoric and endocrine effects. Nevertheless, chronic heroin or methadone administration may result in decreased serum LH, FSH and testosterone [78]. Thyroid function and serum TSH are normal [90], as is GH secretion [90]. Serum PRL is mildly elevated [78,83,90]. Serum cortisol is normal or slightly decreased, but may show exaggerated responses to hypoglycemia or meals [90]. Occasional cases of adrenal insufficiency have been seen in patients receiving chronic opiate therapy [91,92]. Chronic methadone maintenance has been reported to produce a mild impairment in renal concentrating ability that responds to vasopressin administration, suggesting decreased endogenous vasopressin secretion [90]. Men with chronic heroin and cocaine dependence have been reported to have mild pituitary enlargement, perhaps due to lactotroph hyperplasia [93].

Opiate Antagonists

Naloxone, naltrexone and nalmefene are opiate antagonists, nearly devoid of agonist activity, that have proved invaluable in exploring the role of endogenous opiates in human pituitary function. All three drugs cause an acute increase in serum LH in men and luteal-phase women, with little or no effect in the early follicular phase of the menstrual cycle or in postmenopausal women; smaller changes are generally seen in serum FSH [78]. Most investigators have found no effect of naloxone or nalmefene on basal serum TSH, GH and PRL [78], although one group has reported a small rise in serum PRL following naloxone administration during the luteal phase [94] and another study reported that naloxone decreased nocturnal TSH secretion [95]. Cortisol and ACTH secretion are acutely stimulated by opiate antagonists [78]. Chronic naltrexone administration, however, did not alter serum testosterone or gonadotropins [78,97], in contrast to the acute response. Taken together, these data suggest that endogenous opiates may play a significant inhibitory role in the physiologic regulation of ACTH and gonadotropin secretion.

Naloxone has little or no effect on vasopressin secretion [98], but may bring out an oxytocin response to nicotine [98] and inhibit the oxytocin response to orgasm [99]. Naloxone had no effect on plasma oxytocin concentrations in males, in females during late pregnancy or labor, or during breast-feeding [78].

COCAINE

Several studies have reported that cocaine acutely increases serum LH, FSH and cortisol, and suppresses prolactin, but does not change serum testosterone or GH [64,100–103]. Plasma oxytocin levels are suppressed in postpartum women who abuse cocaine [104]. In newly abstinent cocaine abusers, the only finding of note has been the observation that some individuals have mild or moderate hyperprolactinemia which lasts for weeks after withdrawal [105–108]. Hyperprolactinemia, if present, may result from disordered dopaminergic or opioidergic neurotransmission induced by the drug [109]. There are no data on serum thyroid hormone or TSH concentrations in cocaine abusers.

Intranasal abuse of cocaine can result in destructive lesions in the nasal septum and sinuses, often associated with antineutrophil cytoplasma antibodies; in one such case, involvement of the sella led to hypopituitarism [110].

AMPHETAMINES AND METHYLPHENIDATE

These stimulant drugs act by promoting the release and/or inhibiting the neuronal reuptake of DA, norepinephrine and, to a lesser extent, serotonin [111,112]. Acute oral administration of dextroamphetamine consistently stimulates GH and cortisol release [113,114] but has either no effect [114] or a suppressive action [115] on serum PRL. Intravenous amphetamine stimulates GH and cortisol secretion [111,116,117] but, in contrast, also appears to slightly stimulate PRL release [111,118], suggesting that high serum amphetamine concentrations achieved by bolus intravenous administration may activate additional neurotransmitter systems (e.g., serotonergic mechanisms). This interpretation is supported by the finding that a slower, prolonged intravenous infusion of amphetamine suppresses rather than stimulates serum PRL [119].

Acute oral administration of methylphenidate probably stimulates GH [113] and cortisol [120] secretion, although there is some disagreement on both of these points [113,120]. Plasma β-endorphin rose following oral methylphenidate in one study [120]. Intravenous methylphenidate raises serum GH, ACTH and cortisol [112,121,122], while serum PRL is either suppressed [112] or unchanged [121,123].

Chronic treatment of children with attention deficit disorder with stimulant drugs commonly produces slowing of linear growth [127]. The mechanism of this growth retardation is unclear, but probably relates to anorexia and decreased food intake; GH secretion, serum IGF-I and serum GH-binding protein are all normal [128,129].

CAFFEINE

Caffeine, a widely consumed stimulant, exerts its major actions through antagonism at adenosine receptors [130]; metabolites generated in vivo, such as theophylline and theobromine, may also contribute to the drug's effects [130]. Acute administration of large doses (500 mg, equivalent to five cups of coffee) to naïve normal subjects has minimal effect on pituitary function, producing only slight increases in plasma ACTH, cortisol, β-endorphin/β-lipotropin and GH; TSH and PRL are unchanged [131–135]. There are no data regarding caffeine effects on gonadotropin secretion in humans, although theophylline, a related methylxanthine, has been reported to have no effect on serum LH concentrations [136]. Theophylline has also been reported to cause the syndrome of inappropriate ADH secretion [137]. Chronic consumption of caffeine produces tolerance to most of the drug's actions, suggesting that long-term endocrine sequelae are unlikely [130,131].

BENZODIAZEPINES

Several studies have reported that acute administration of benzodiazepines (diazepam, bromazepam, metaclazepam and alprazolam) stimulates GH secretion in some normal males [138–144]. The response is seen in one-third to one-half of normal men and even less frequently in women [139,141,145]. Intravenous drug administration is generally more effective than oral dosing [141]. Serum PRL, TSH, LH and FSH are not affected [138–140,142,143,146]. Basal secretion of cortisol, β-endorphin and β-lipotropin is not altered by diazepam [145,147], but alprazolam and temazepam appear to modestly suppress serum cortisol [140,146,148]; additionally, diazepam blocks the cortisol, β-endorphin and β-lipotropin responses to hypoglycemia [147] and alprazolam blunts the ACTH and cortisol responses to social stress [149]. It is not clear whether these effects on cortisol are due to specific actions at hormone regulatory centers or reflect a more general relief of anxiety and stress by the drugs. In favor of a specific action on hormone regulation are observations that diazepam suppresses nocturnal release of cortisol and GH [150], and that alprazolam suppresses the release of ACTH and cortisol induced by naloxone or metyrapone administration [151,152].

With chronic benzodiazepine administration, basal serum GH and PRL levels are normal and the GH response to diazepam appears to be blunted [153]. Thus, signs and symptoms of GH excess do not develop in patients receiving long-term benzodiazepine therapy.

Flumazenil, a benzodiazepine receptor antagonist, had no effect on basal or naloxone-stimulated release of ACTH or cortisol, suggesting endogenous benzodiazepine-like ligands do not tonically regulate ACTH secretion [154].

ANTIDEPRESSANTS

Acute oral or intravenous administration of imipramine, desipramine and clomipramine has been reported to stimulate GH, PRL, cortisol and ACTH in normal subjects [155–158], although others have not confirmed these effects [156,159]. Many of these discrepancies appear to be due to the use of different drug doses [155,157]. Amitriptyline has little effect on any of these hormones [156,159]. A single study has reported that acute administration of chlorimipramine had no effect on serum LH and TSH concentrations [160] and oral fluvoxamine did not alter basal or stimulated secretion of LH, FSH, PRL, GH, TSH, or cortisol [161]. Oral nefazodone and intravenous citalopram have been reported to modestly stimulate PRL release [162,163].

Chronic administration of chlorimipramine modestly raised serum PRL to about twice baseline [160,164], while chronic treatment with desipramine, imipramine, nortriptyline and amitriptyline had little or no effect on serum PRL [159,160,165–168]. Chronic treatment with fluvoxamine or fluoxetine modestly raised serum prolactin in a minority of depressed patients [169,170]. There is probably little or no change in serum cortisol, TSH, or GH during chronic treatment with the tricyclic antidepressants, selective serotonin reuptake inhibitors, or monoamine oxidase inhibitors [164,167,171,172].

Amoxapine, an antidepressant structurally related to the antipsychotic agent, loxapine, has DA antagonist activity and is a modest stimulator (three to four times basal) of PRL secretion [166]. Bupropion, a nontricyclic antidepressant, has no effect on serum PRL or GH [173]. Monoamine oxidase inhibitors such as chlorgyline and pargyline also double basal PRL concentrations when given chronically [174]. Thus, with the exception of amoxapine, chlorimipramine and the monoamine oxidase inhibitors, most antidepressants have either no effect on anterior pituitary hormone secretion or minimal effects. In particular, these drugs only occasionally cause significant hyperprolactinemia (over 30 μg/L) and rarely produce galactorrhea.

Hyponatremia, apparently due to inappropriate secretion of antidiuretic hormone (ADH), has been reported with many antidepressants, including tricyclics, monoamine oxidase inhibitors and bupropion [175–177].

LITHIUM

Used primarily in the treatment of bipolar affective disorder, lithium has only two major effects on pituitary function, both indirect. Lithium acts on the thyroid gland to inhibit hormone release, resulting in activation of feedback mechanisms and increased pituitary secretion of TSH [178]. In most normal subjects, this TSH rise is minor and transient, but in susceptible individuals (often those with pre-existing thyroid damage due to autoimmune thyroiditis or radiation) frank hypothyroidism may be produced and goiter may develop [178,179]. To detect such cases of emerging hypothyroidism, serum T_4 and TSH should be monitored every 3–4 months during the first year of lithium therapy, and yearly thereafter.

Lithium also impairs the action of vasopressin on the kidney [179,180]. This mild nephrogenic diabetes insipidus results in enhanced vasopressin release with no change in the osmotic threshold for vasopressin secretion [181]. Lithium may also mildly stimulate thirst [181], an additional action that could also contribute to the polyuria and polydipsia seen in some patients receiving lithium therapy. Treatment with amiloride has been reported to improve renal concentrating ability in patients taking lithium [182].

ANTIPSYCHOTIC DRUGS

The major antipsychotic drugs (also known as neuroleptics) act as antagonists at the D-2 DA receptor; the phenothiazines, butyrophenones and thioxanthenes all share this property, which is probably the basis of their antipsychotic action [183]. Since D-2 DA receptors participate in the regulation of pituitary hormone secretion, it is not suprising that these drugs have important effects on pituitary function.

The most consistent endocrine effect of the classic neuroleptic drugs is elevation of serum PRL. This effect is due to antagonism of the PRL-inhibitory effects of endogenous DA at the pituitary lactotroph D-2 DA receptor. There is a reasonably good correlation between antipsychotic potency, D-2 DA receptor antagonism and PRL stimulation [183,184]. The major exceptions are clozapine and quetiapine, atypical neuroleptics with weak D-2 binding affinity which produce only minimal elevations in serum PRL [127,183,184] and aripiprazole, which has partial agonist activity at D-2 DA receptors [185]. Olanzapine, another atypical neuroleptic, has a higher affinity than clozapine for D_2 receptors, and has a slightly higher incidence of mild hyperprolactinemia [127,183,184]. Chronic administration of neuroleptics may result in tolerance to the PRL-elevating effects of the drugs, with some patients demonstrating normal or near-normal serum PRL concentrations after long-term therapy [186–188]. There have been reports of PRL-secreting pituitary tumors developing during chronic neuroleptic therapy [189], but these are so infrequent as to suggest that the relationship is coincidental rather than causal, particularly when viewed in the context of a high frequency of incidental pituitary tumors in the general population [190].

Hyperprolactinemia induced by neuroleptic drugs can suppress GnRH and gonadotropin secretion with consequent hypogonadism and amenorrhea [183,184], although this effect is highly variable, and many patients have normal gonadal function despite mild hyperprolactinemia [127,183,184,191].

Neuroleptics may have an inhibitory effect on GH secretion, especially that stimulated by DA agonists [192]. Clinically, there is no evidence of GH deficiency in patients receiving neuroleptics.

Neuroleptic drugs have little or no effect on ACTH and TSH secretion [193,194], although a rare side effect of neuroleptic drugs, the syndrome of inappropriate secretion of ADH (SIADH), has been reported in about a dozen patients [195].

Other DA Antagonists

Metoclopramide and domperidone are potent D-2 DA antagonists which, like the antipsychotics, stimulate PRL secretion [196,197]. Since TSH and LH, like PRL, are also under mild tonic inhibition by DA, acute administration of these drugs produces a small, transient rise in serum TSH and LH [198,199]. Chronic endocrine effects are similar to those of the antipsychotics [197,200,201]. Acutely, metoclopramide, but not sulpiride, domperidone, or haloperidol, stimulates vasopressin secretion [202].

Buspirone, an antianxiety drug, is a D-2 DA receptor antagonist as well as a serotonin receptor agonist, and acutely elevates serum PRL, cortisol and GH in man, with no effect on oxytocin or vasopressin [203–205].

DA AGONISTS

Drugs with DA agonist activity suppress PRL secretion; these include apomorphine, DA, L-dopa, L-dopa/carbidopa combinations, and the dopaminergic ergot alkaloids, bromocriptine and cabergoline [192,206–209]. Additionally, there is also an acute suppressive effect on TSH and LH, although these effects are not seen with chronic administration [207,210,211]; DA infusions, given for hypotension, may contribute to the hypothyroxinemia seen in severe systemic illness by suppressing TSH [210]. Dopaminergic drugs acutely stimulate GH secretion [192,212,213], probably by actions on the hypothalamus. Both bromocriptine and cabergoline have occasionally been associated with pituitary apoplexy in patients with pituitary tumors [214].

CHOLINERGIC AGONISTS AND ANTAGONISTS

Muscarinic blockers such as atropine and pirenzepine appear to enhance somatostatin release from the median eminence of the hypothalamus and thereby decrease GH secretion [215]. The GH response to insulin-induced hypoglycemia is relatively less affected by these drugs than other GH-provocative tests [215]. Cholinergic agonists such as physostigmine and pyridostigmine have an opposite effect, inhibiting somatostatin and stimulating GH [215]. In addition, physostigmine has been reported to stimulate PRL, ACTH, cortisol and β-endorphin, effects which were blocked by the cholinergic antagonist scopolamine [216].

ANTIHYPERTENSIVES

Reserpine, which depletes catecholamines, and methyldopa, which both depletes catecholamines and serves as a precursor for false neurotransmitters, stimulate PRL secretion modestly, although in many patients serum PRL concentrations are still within the normal range [217,218]. Methyldopa has also been reported to cause inappropriate secretion of ADH [219].

β-Adrenergic blockade with propranolol enhances the GH response to various stimuli [213,215]; selective β_1-antagonists do not share this action [220]. Most β-blockers have little or no effect on other pituitary hormones [221]. However, intravenous labetolol, a drug with both α- and β-adrenergic blocking effects as well as β-agonist actions, stimulates PRL secretion via unknown mechanisms [222].

Clonidine and related α_2-adrenergic agonists stimulate GH secretion, particularly in children, with little or no change in other anterior pituitary hormones [223,224]; clonidine is widely used as a provocative test to diagnose GH deficiency. Yohimbine, an α_2-adrenergic antagonist, and phentolamine, a nonspecific α-blocker, blunt the GH response to a variety of stimuli, but prazosin, an α_1-antagonist, does not [215,225]. Clonidine has been reported to cause SIADH [226].

Calcium channel blockers have divergent effects on pituitary hormone secretion. Diltiazem and nifedipine appear to have little or no effect, but verapamil has been reported to decrease gonadotropin and TSH secretion and enhance PRL release [227,228]. Mild hyperprolactinemia and galactorrhea have occurred in patients receiving verapamil therapy [229,230].

ANTIHISTAMINES

H_1-antihistamines

H_1 histamine receptors appear to play little role in the regulation of human pituitary function. Intravenous diphenhydramine, an H_1-antagonist, had no effect on serum GH, PRL, or TSH [231], and did not alter the TSH and PRL response to TRH or the GH response to L-dopa [232]. However, other H_1-antihistamines (meclastine and chlorpheniramine) have been reported to blunt the GH response to arginine infusion but not the response to hypoglycemia [233]. It is possible that this effect is due to the anticholinergic properties of these drugs (see above).

H_2-antihistamines

Cimetidine, the first marketed H_2-antihistamine, stimulates PRL secretion when given as an intravenous bolus that achieves high serum drug levels [231]; other pituitary hormones are not affected [231,234]. These properties are shared by another H_2-antihistamine, ranitidine [235], but not by nizatidine, which has no effect on serum PRL [236]. Animal studies suggest that the PRL-releasing effects of cimetidine and ranitidine are not mediated by H_2-histamine antagonism [237]. Acute oral dosing with cimetidine has no effect on PRL secretion [238], probably because relatively low drug concentrations are achieved in the serum.

The endocrine effects of long-term cimetidine therapy are controversial. Most investigators have found no change in serum PRL or other pituitary hormones [238,239,240].

ANTINEOPLASTIC CHEMOTHERAPY

There is little evidence that cytotoxic drugs directly alter anterior pituitary function [241]. Cancer chemotherapy commonly produces gonadal damage, with a consequent rise in serum FSH and LH due to activation of normal feedback mechanisms; a wide variety of drugs have been implicated in this regard [241–243]. Recovery may take place spontaneously years later in some male patients, while females may show progressive ovarian failure [244,245]. Similarly, the tyrosine kinase inhibitors sunitinib and sorafenib can alter thyroid function, resulting in suppressed or, more commonly, elevated serum TSH [246].

Many cancer chemotherapeutic agents have been reported to cause SIADH [241]; these include cyclophosphamide [247], melphalan [248], vincristine [249], vinblastine [250], vinorelbine [251], cisplatin [252], imatinib [253] and combination chemotherapy [254].

ESTROGENS

Estrogens have several effects on the human pituitary gland. GH secretion is potentiated, both basally and in response to a variety of provocative tests [213,255,256]. PRL secretion is also mildly to moderately increased, and is related to the dose of estrogen given [184,255–259]. There is no evidence that exogenous estrogen is involved in the genesis of pituitary prolactinomas in humans [259–262].

Gonadotropin secretion is suppressed by estrogen, especially at high doses [256,263–265]. Estrogen also exerts a positive feedback effect on gonadotropins; this is seen most vividly in the surge of LH and FSH secretion at the midpoint of the normal menstrual cycle [246]. Males may also exhibit positive feedback of estrogens on LH release [265,266].

Serum TSH may be slightly increased by exogenous estrogens [267], although some studies have failed to show this effect [210,268].

ESTROGEN RECEPTOR ANTAGONISTS AND AROMATASE INHIBITORS

Antiestrogens can have a variety of effects on pituitary hormone secretion, depending on the ambient hormonal milieu. In premenopausal women and adult men, drugs such as clomiphene, tamoxifen and raloxifene act as estrogen antagonists and block the negative feedback effects of estrogen on gonadotropin secretion, resulting in increased serum LH and FSH [269,270]. In contrast, opposite effects are seen in postmenopausal women, where the weak estrogen-agonist activity of these compounds predominates, resulting in partial suppression of gonadotropin secretion [271]. Aromatase inhibitors such as letrozole and anastrazole also increase serum gonadotropins in males [272].

ANDROGENS

Androgens suppress gonadotropin secretion through actions on both the hypothalamus and pituitary. While part of this effect may be attributable to estrogens produced by biotransformation in vivo, nonaromatizable androgens also suppress gonadotropins [273–276].

Fluoxymesterone, a nonaromatizable androgen, exerts a modest suppressive effect on TSH secretion but does not alter PRL [277]. Studies examining the effect of testosterone on these two hormones have been confounded by the concurrent increases in serum estrogens produced by aromatization in vivo.

Spontaneous GH secretion is enhanced by testosterone administration, producing a concurrent rise in serum insulin-like growth factor-I (IGF-I); the synthetic nonaromatizable androgen, oxandrolone, did not raise either mean serum GH or IGF-I in this study [278]. In other reports, however, oxandrolone was effective in enhancing the GH response to GHRH and sleep in some children [279,280], and in increasing mean 24-hour serum GH concentrations [281].

ANTIANDROGENS

Finasteride, a 5α-reductase inhibitor, has had no consistent effect on serum LH, FSH, cortisol, TSH, or T_4 in men or women [282–285]. Flutamide, an androgen receptor blocker, has been reported to increase serum LH and testosterone in men, with no change in FSH or PRL [286,287]. In postmenopausal women, LH and FSH were unchanged by flutamide while serum testosterone fell [288]. In normal and hirsute premenopausal women, no change was observed in serum LH, FSH, or testosterone [289,290].

GLUCOCORTICOIDS

In addition to the expected feedback suppression of ACTH and β-lipotropin secretion [291], glucocorticoids in large doses also exert suppressive effects on GH [292], TSH [210], gonadotropins [293,294], PRL [295] and vasopressin [296]. By suppressing TSH, lowering serum thyroxine-binding globulin and blocking extrathyroidal conversion of T_4 to T_3, large doses of glucocorticoids may contribute to the derangements of pituitary–thyroid function seen in the "euthryoid sick" or "nonthyroidal illness" syndrome [210]. In the absence of concomitant illness, the thyroid axis changes produced by glucocorticoids are modest and usually do not result in diagnostic confusion.

MISCELLANEOUS DRUGS

Anticonvulsants may influence posterior pituitary hormone secretion. Phenytoin may inhibit the secretion of ADH [297] while carbamazepine may cause SIADH [298]. Sodium valproate inhibits the vasopressin response to hypernatremia and upright posture [299] and the oxytocin response to angiotensin II [300].

Ketoconazole, an antifungal agent, interferes with the biosynthesis of testosterone and cortisol and can lead to elevations in serum gonadotropins and, less often, ACTH, by activating feedback mechanisms [301,302]. Blockade of cortisol biosynthesis by ketoconazole has been used as adjunctive therapy in the treatment of Cushing's syndrome [303].

Heparin therapy has been reported to precipitate pituitary apoplexy in one patient [304].

Bexarotene, a retinoid X-receptor agonist used in the treatment of cutaneous T-cell lymphoma, suppresses TSH secretion and has resulted in central hypothyroidism, with no effect on serum PRL or cortisol [305].

Omeprazole, a proton pump inhibitor, has been reported to cause SIADH [306].

Megestrol, a synthetic progestin, is used clinically to stimulate appetite and promote weight gain. The drug also has glucocorticoid agonist activity and has been shown to suppress serum ACTH, cortisol, LH and testosterone, and may result in adrenal insufficiency and hypogonadism [307,308]; at high doses of megestrol, Cushing's syndrome has occurred [307].

Metformin, used in the treatment of diabetes mellitus, has been reported to modestly decrease serum TSH, occasionally to subnormal levels, in diabetic patients with primary hypothyroidism, independent of thyroid hormone treatment [309,310]; no change in TSH was seen in normal subjects [310].

Interferons may have multiple effects on the pituitary. Interferon-alpha, used in the treatment of chronic viral hepatitis, has been reported to cause hypophysitis and hypopituitarism in a small number of patients [311–313]. Interferon-beta, used to treat multiple sclerosis, acutely stimulates secretion of ACTH, cortisol, PRL and GH after each injection for the first several months of therapy; the hormonal response is blunted by indomethacin and eventually partially abates with long-term therapy [314].

References

[1] J. Frias, R. Rodriguez, J.M. Torres, et al., Effects of acute alcohol intoxication on pituitary–gonadal axis hormones, pituitary–adrenal axis hormones, β-endorphin and prolactin in human adolescents of both sexes, Life Sci 67 (2000) 1081–1086.

[2] M.A. Schuckit, J.W. Tsuang, R.M. Anthenelli, Alcohol challenges in young men from alcoholic pedigrees and control families: A report from the COGA project, J Stud Alcohol 7 (1996) 368–377.

[3] J.A. Mennella, M.Y. Pepino, K.L. Teff, Acute alcohol consumption disrupts the hormonal milieu of lactating women, J Clin Endocrinol Metab 90 (2005) 1979–1985.

[4] T. Sarkala, H. Mäkisalo, T. Fukunaga, C.J.P. Eriksson, Acute effect of alcohol on estradiol, estrone, progesterone, prolactin, cortisol and luteinizing hormone in premenopausal women, Alcohol Clin Exp Res 23 (1999) 976–982.
[5] J.A. Mennella, M.Y. Pepino, Short-term effects of alcohol consumption on the hormonal milieu and mood states in nulliparous women, Alcohol 38 (2006) 29–36.
[6] Y. Ida, S. Tsujimaru, K. Nakamaura, et al., Effects of acute and repeated alcohol ingestion on hypothalamic—pituitary—gonadal and hypothalamic—pituitary—adrenal functioning in normal males, Drug Alcohol Depend 31 (1992) 57–64.
[7] C. Waltman, L.S. Blevins Jr., G. Boyd, G.S. Wand, The effects of mild ethanol intoxication on the hypothalmic—pituitary—adrenal axis in non-alcoholic men, J Clin Endocrinol Metab 77 (1993) 518–522.
[8] T.L. Wall, C.B. Nemeroff, J.C. Ritchie, C.L. Ehlers, Cortisol responses following placebo and alcohol in Asians with different ALD H2 genotypes, J Stud Alcohol 55 (1994) 207–213.
[9] W.J. Inder, R.P. Joyce, J.E. Wells, et al., The acute effects of oral ethanol on the hypothlamic—pituitary—adrenal axis in normal human subjects, Clin Endocrinol 42 (1995) 65–71.
[10] C. Gianoulakis, B. Krishnan, J. Thavondayil, Enhanced sensitivity of pituitary β-endorphin to ethanol in subjects at high risk of alcoholism, Arch Gen Psychiatry 53 (1996) 250–257.
[11] S. Kutscher, D.J. Heise, M. Banger, et al., Concomitant endocrine and immune alterations during alcohol intoxication and acute withdrawal in alcohol-dependent subjects, Neuropsychobiol 45 (2002) 144–149.
[12] G.S. Wand, A.S. Dobs, Alterations in the hypothalamic—pituitary—adrenal axis in actively drinking alcoholics, J Clin Endocrinol Metab 72 (1991) 1290–1295.
[13] B. Adinoff, K. Ruether, S. Krebaum, et al., Increased salivary cortisol concentrations during chronic alcohol intoxication in a naturalistic clinical sample of men, Alcohol Clin Exp Res 27 (2003) 1420–1427.
[14] R.G. Veldman, A.E. Meinders, On the mechanism of alcohol-induced pseudo-Cushing's syndrome, Endocr Rev 17 (1996) 262–268.
[15] V. Coiro, R. Volpi, L. Capretti, et al., Desmopressin and hexarelin tests in alcohol-induced pseudo-Cushing's syndrome, J Intern Med 247 (2000) 667–673.
[16] J.D. Berman, D.M. Cook, M. Buchman, L.D. Keith, Diminished adrenocorticotropin response to insulin-induced hypoglycemia in nondepressed, actively drinking male alcoholics, J Clin Endocrinol Metab 71 (1990) 712–717.
[17] J. Frias, J.M. Torres, R. Rodriguez, et al., Effects of acute alcohol intoxication on growth axis in human adolescents of both sexes, Life Sci 67 (2000) 2691–2697.
[18] R.H. Ylikahri, M.O. Huttunen, M. Harkonen, et al., Acute effects of alcohol on anterior pituitary secretion of the tropic hormones, J Clin Endocrinol Metab 46 (1978) 715–720.
[19] A.-C. Ekman, O. Vakkuri, M. Ekman, J. Leppaloto, et al., Ethanol decreases nocturnal plasma levels of thyrotropin and growth hormone but not those of thyroid hormones or prolactin in man, J Clin Endocrinol Metab 81 (1996) 2627–2632.
[20] M. Linnoila, R.N. Prinz, C.J. Wonsowicz, J. Leppaluoto, Effect of moderate doses of ethanol and phenobarbital on pituitary and thyroid hormones and testosterone, Br J Addict 75 (1980) 207–212.
[21] D. Hermann, A. Heinz, K. Mann, Dysregulation of the hypothalamic—pituitary—thyroid axis in alcoholism, Addiction 97 (2002) 1369–1381.
[22] S.M. Adler, L. Wartofsky, The non-thyroidal illness syndrome, Endocrinol Metab Clin N Am 36 (2007) 657–672.
[23] T.W. Boyden, R.W. Pamenter, Effects of ethanol on the male hypothalamic—pituitary—gonadal axis, Endocr Rev 4 (1983) 389–395.
[24] P. Banister, T. Handley, C. Chapman, M.S. Losowsky, LH pulsatility following acute ethanol ingestion in men, Clin Endocrinol 25 (1986) 143–150.
[25] W.R. Phipps, S.E. Lukas, J.H. Mendelson, et al., Acute ethanol administration enhances plasma testosterone levels following gonadotropin stimulation in men, Psychoneuroendocrinol 12 (1987) 459–465.
[26] G.G. Gordon, A.L. Southren, C.S. Lieber, The effect of alcoholic liver disease and alcohol ingestion on sex hormone levels, Alcohol Clin Exp Res 2 (1978) 259–263.
[27] D.H. Van Thiel, Ethanol: Its adverse effects upon the hypothalamic—pituitary—gonadal axis, J Lab Clin Med 101 (1983) 21–33.
[28] D.H. Van Thiel, J.S. Gavaler, Hypothalamic—pituitary—gonadal function in liver disease with particular attention to the endocrine effects of chronic liver disease, Prog Liv Dis 8 (1986) 273–282.
[29] J.S. Gavaler, E.R. Rosenblum, D.H. Van Thiel, et al., Biologically active phytoestrogens are present in bourbon, Alcohol Clin Exp Res 11 (1987) 399–406.
[30] J. Villalta, J.L. Ballescá, J.M. Nicolás, et al., Testicular function in asymptomatic chronic alcoholics: Relation to ethanol intake, Alcohol Clin Exp Res 21 (1997) 128–133.
[31] M. Valimaki, M. Harkonen, R. Ylikahri, Acute effects of alcohol on female sex hormones, Alcohol Clin Exp Res 7 (1983) 289–293.
[32] U. Becker, C. Gluud, P. Bennett, et al., Effect of alcohol and glucose infusion on pituitary—gonadal hormones in normal females, Drug Alcohol Depend 22 (1988) 141–149.
[33] J.H. Mendelson, S.E. Lukas, N.K. Mello, et al., Acute alcohol effects on plasma estradiol levels in women, Psychopharmacol 94 (1988) 464–467.
[34] J.H. Mendelson, N.K. Mello, Chronic alcohol effects on anterior pituitary and ovarian hormones in healthy women, J Pharmacol Exp Therap 245 (1988) 407–412.
[35] J.N. Hugues, T. Coste, G. Perret, et al., Hypothalamo—pituitary—ovarian function in thirty-one women with chronic alcoholism, Clin Endocrinol 12 (1980) 543–551.
[36] J.S. Gavaler, Effects of alcohol on endocrine function in postmenopausal women: A review, J Stud Alcohol 46 (1985) 495–516.
[37] J.A. Mennella, M.Y. Pepino, Biphasic effects of moderate drinking on prolactin during lactation, Alcohol Clin Exp Res 32 (2008) 1899–1908.
[38] G. DeRosa, S.M. Corsello, M.P. Ruffilli, et al., Prolactin secretion after beer, Lancet 2 (1981) 934.
[39] H.B. Moss, J.K. Yao, J.M. Maddock, Responses by sons of alcoholic fathers to alcoholic and placebo drinks: Perceived mood, intoxication, and plasma prolactin, Alcohol Clin Exp Res 13 (1989) 252–257.
[40] E.S. Ginsburg, B.W. Walsh, B.F. Shea, et al., Effect of acute ethanol ingestion on prolactin in menopausal women using estradiol replacement, Gynecol Obstet Invest 39 (1995) 47–49.
[41] H.E. Carlson, H.L. Wasser, R.D. Reidelberger, Beer-induced prolactin secretion: A clinical and laboratory study of the role of salsolinol, J Clin Endocrinol Metab 60 (1985) 673–677.
[42] B. Koletzko, F. Lehner, Beer and breastfeeding, Adv Exp Med Biol 478 (2000) 23–28.
[43] B. Zietz, G. Lock, B. Plach, et al., Dysfunction of the hypothalamic—pituitary—glandular axes and relation to Child-Pugh classification in male patients with alcoholic and virus-related cirrhosis, Eur J Gastroenterol Hepatol 15 (2003) 495–501.

[44] V. Coiro, A. Alboni, D. Gramellini, et al., Inhibition by ethanol of the oxytocin response to breast stimulation in normal women and the role of endogenous opioids, Acta Endocrinol 126 (1992) 213–216.

[45] U. Zimmermann, K. Spring, H.-U. Wittchen, et al., Arginine vasopressin and adrenocorticotropin secretion in response to psychosocial stress is attenuated by ethanol in sons of alcohol-dependent fathers, J Psychiat Res 38 (2004) 385–393.

[46] V. Coiro, A. Casti, E. Volta, et al., Naloxone decreases the inhibitory effect of ethanol on the release of arginine-vasopressin induced by physical exercise in man, J Neural Transm 116 (2009) 1065–1069.

[47] H. Taivainen, K. Laitinen, R. Tahtela, et al., Role of plasma vasopressin in changes of water balance accompanying acute alcohol intoxication, Alcohol Clin Exp Res 19 (1995) 759–762.

[48] M.M. Hirschl, K. Derfler, C. Bieglmayer, et al., Hormonal derangements in patients with severe alcohol intoxication, Alcohol Clin Exp Res 18 (1994) 761–766.

[49] A.J. Harding, G.M. Halliday, J.L.F. Ng, et al., Loss of vasopressin-immunoreactive neurons in alcoholics is dose-related and time-dependent, Neurosci 72 (1996) 699–708.

[50] J.N. Wilkins, H.E. Carlson, H. Van Vunakis, et al., Nicotine from cigarette smoking increases circulating levels of cortisol, growth hormone, and prolactin in male chronic smokers, Psychopharmacol 78 (1982) 305–308.

[51] O.F. Pomerleau, J.B. Fertig, L.E. Seyler, J. Jaffe, Neuroendocrine reactivity to nicotine in smokers, Psychopharmacol 81 (1983) 61–67.

[52] L.E. Seyler, O.F. Pomerleau, J.B. Fertig, et al., Pituitary hormone response to cigarette smoking, Pharmacol Biochem Behav 24 (1986) 159–162.

[53] V.V. Gossain, N.K. Sherma, L. Srivastava, et al., Hormonal effects of smoking – II. Effects on plasma cortisol, growth hormone and prolactin, Am J Med Sci 291 (1986) 325–327.

[54] D.G. Gilbert, C.J. Meliska, C.L. Williams, R.A. Jensen, Subjective correlates of cigarette-smoking-induced elevations of peripheral beta-endorphin and cortisol, Psychopharmacology 106 (1992) 275–281.

[55] J. Stalke, O. Harder, V. Bahr, et al., The role of vasopressin in the nicotine-induced stimulation of ACTH and cortisol in men, Clin Investig 70 (1992) 218–223.

[56] C. Kirschbaum, G. Scherer, C.J. Strasburger, Pituitary and adrenal hormone responses to pharmacological, physical, and psychological stimulation in habitual smokers and nonsmokers, Clin Investig 72 (1994) 804–810.

[57] P. Chiodera, R. Volpi, L. Capretti, et al., Abnormal effect of cigarette smoking on pituitary hormone secretions in insulin-dependent diabetes mellitus, Clin Endocrinol 46 (1997) 351–357.

[58] O.F. Pomerleau, Nicotine and the central nervous system: Biobehavioral effects of cigarette smoking, Am J Med 93 (suppl 1A) (1992) 2S–7S.

[59] J.H. Mendelson, M.B. Sholar, N. Goletiani, et al., Effects of low-and high-nicotine cigarette smoking on mood states and the HPA axis in men, Neuropsychopharmacol 30 (2005) 1751–1763.

[60] O.F. Pomerleau, K.A. Flessland, C.S. Pomerleau, M. Hariharan, Controlled dosing of nicotine via an intranasal nicotine aerosol delivery device (INADD), Psychopharmacol 108 (1992) 519–526.

[61] A. Steptoe, M. Ussher, Smoking, cortisol and nicotine, Int J Psychophysiol 59 (2006) 228–235.

[62] E. Badrick, C. Kirschbaum, M. Kumari, The relationship between smoking status and cortisol secretion, J Clin Endocrinol Metab 92 (2007) 819–824.

[63] A.E. Field, G.A. Colditz, W.C. Willett, et al., The relation of smoking, age, relataive weight, and dietary intake to serum adrenal steroids, sex hormones, and sex hormone-binding globulin in middle-aged men, J Clin Endocrinol Metab 79 (1994) 1310–1316.

[64] J.H. Mendelson, M.B. Sholar, N.H. Mutschler, et al., Effects of intravenous cocaine and cigarette smoking on luteinizing hormone, testosterone, and prolactin in men, J Pharmacol Exp Therap 307 (2003) 339–348.

[65] L.M. Morimoto, P.A. Newcomb, E. White, et al., Variation in plasma insulin-like growth factor-1 and insulin-like growth factor binding protein-3: Personal and lifestyle factors, Cancer Causes Control 16 (2005) 917–927.

[66] R.M. Belin, B.C. Astor, N.R. Powe, P.W. Ladenson, Smoke exposure is associated with a lower prevalence of serum thyroid autoantibodies and thyrotropin concentration elevations and a higher prevalence of mild thyrotropin concentration suppression in the third National Health and Nutrition Examination Survey (NHANES III), J Clin Endocrinol Metab 89 (2004) 6077–6086.

[67] B.O. Åsvold, T. Bjøro, T.I.L. Nilson, L.J. Vatten, Tobacco smoking and thyroid function. A population-based study, Arch Intern Med 167 (2007) 1428–1432.

[68] O.P. Soldin, B.E. Goughenour, S.Z. Gilbert, et al., Thyroid hormone levels associated with active and passive cigarette smoking, Thyroid 19 (2009) 817–823.

[69] G.C. Windham, P. Mitchell, M. Anderson, B.L. Lasley, Cigarette smoking and effects on hormone function in premenopausal women, Environ Health Perspect 113 (2005) 1285–1290.

[70] J. Richthoff, S. Elzanaty, L. Rylander, et al., Association between tobacco exposure and reproductive parameters in adolescent males, Int J Androl 31 (2007) 31–39.

[71] T. Funabashi, A. Sano, D. Mitsushima, F. Kimura, Nicotine inhibits pulsatile luteinizing hormone secretion in human males but not in human females, and tolerance to this nicotine effect is lost within one week of quitting smoking, J Clin Endocrinol Metab 90 (2005) 3908–3913.

[72] J.R. Seckl, M. Johnson, C. Shakespear, S.L. Lightman, Endogenous opioids inhibit oxytocin release during nicotine-stimulated secretion of vasopressin in man, Clin Endocrinol 28 (1988) 509–514.

[73] P. Chiodera, R. Volpi, L. Capretti, et al., Gamma-aminobutyric acid mediation of the inhibitory effect of endogenous opioids on the arginine vasopressin and oxytocin responses to nicotine from cigarette smoking, Metabolism 42 (1993) 762–765.

[74] T.T. Brown, A.S. Dobs, Endocrine effects of marijuana, J Clin Pharmacol 42 (2002) 90S–96S.

[75] M. Ranganathan, G. Braley, B. Pittman, et al., The effects of cannabinoids on serum cortisol and prolactin in humans, Psychopharmacol 203 (2009) 737–744.

[76] N.L. Benowitz, R.T. Jones, C.B. Lerner, Depression of growth hormone and cortisol response to insulin-induced hypoglycemia after prolonged oral delta-9-tetrahydrocannabinol administration in man, J Clin Endocrinol Metab 42 (1976) 938–941.

[77] O. Parshad, M. Kumar, G.N. Melville, Thyroid-gonad relationship in marijuana smokers: A field study in Jamaica, W Ind Med J 32 (1983) 101–105.

[78] C. Vuong, S.H.M. Van Uum, L.E. O'Dell, et al., The effects of opioids and opioid analogs on animal and human endocrine systems, Endocr Rev 31 (2010) 98–132.

[79] R. Hallinan, A. Byrne, K. Agho, et al., Hypogonadism in men receiving methadone and buprenorphine maintenance treatment, Int J Androl 32 (2007) 131–139.

[80] F. Petraglia, C. Porro, F. Facchinetti, et al., Opioid control of LH secretion in humans: Menstrual cycle, menopause and aging reduce effect of naloxone but not of morphine, Life Sci 38 (1986) 2103–2110.
[81] A. Grossman, P.J. Moult, R.C. Gaillard, et al., The opioid control of LH and FSH release: Effects of a met-enkephalin analogue and naloxone, Clin Endocrinol 14 (1981) 41–47.
[82] G. Bart, L. Borg, J.H. Schluger, et al., Suppressed prolactin response to dynorphin A_{1-13} in methadone-maintained versus control subjects, J Pharmacol Exp Therap 306 (2003) 581–587.
[83] G.-R. Moshtaghi-Kashanian, F. Esmaeeli, S. Dabiri, Enhanced prolactin levels in opium smokers, Addiction Biol 10 (2005) 345–349.
[84] M.J. Reymond, C. Kaur, J.C. Porter, An inhibitory role for morphine on the release of dopamine into hypophysial portal blood and on the synthesis of dopamine in tuberoinfundibular neurons, Brain Res 262 (1983) 253–258.
[85] A. Bhansali, P. Velayutham, R. Sialy, B. Sethi, Effect of opiates on growth hormone secretion in acromegaly, Horm Metab Res 37 (2005) 425–427.
[86] G. Delitala, P.A. Tomasi, M. Palermo, et al., Opioids stimulate growth hormone (GH) release in man independently of GH-releasing hormone, J Clin Endocrinol Metab 69 (1989) 356–358.
[87] E. Del Pozo, J. Martin-Perez, A. Stadelmann, et al., Inhibitory action of a metenkephalin on ACTH release in man, J Clin Invest 65 (1980) 1531–1534.
[88] R.S. Rittmaster, G.B. Cutler, D.O. Sobel, et al., Morphine inhibits the pituitary–adrenal response to ovine corticotrophin-releasing hormone in normal subjects, J Clin Endocrinol Metab 60 (1985) 891–895.
[89] F. Buzi, A. Corna, A. Pilotta, et al., Loperamide test: A simple and highly specific screening test for hypercortisolism in children and adolescents, Acta Paediatr 86 (1997) 1177–1180.
[90] M.L. Willenbring, J.E. Morley, D.D. Krahn, et al., Psychoneuroendocrine effects of methadone maintenance, Psychoneuroendocrinol 14 (1989) 371–391.
[91] C. Lee, S. Ludwig, D.R. Duerksen, Low-serum cortisol associated with opioid use: Case report and review of the literature, Endocrinologist 12 (2002) 5–8.
[92] K.E. Schimke, P. Greminger, M. Brändle, Secondary adrenal insufficiency due to opiate therapy – another differential diagnosis worth consideration, Exp Clin Endocrinol Diab 117 (2009) 649–651.
[93] S.K. Teoh, J.H. Mendelson, B.T. Woods, et al., Pituitary volume in men with concurrent heroin and cocaine dependence, J Clin Endocrinol Metab 76 (1993) 1529–1532.
[94] E.U. Snowden, F.S. Khan-Dawood, M.Y. Dawood, The effect of naloxone on endogenous opioid regulation of pituitary gonadotropins and prolactin during the menstrual cycle, J Clin Endocrinol Metab 59 (1984) 298–302.
[95] M.H. Samuels, P. Kramer, D. Wilson, G. Sexton, Effects of naloxone infusions on pulsatile thyrotropin secretion, J Clin Endocrinol Metab 78 (1994) 1249–1252.
[96] A.G. Ambrogio, F.P. Giraldi, F. Casagnini, Drugs and HPA axis, Pituitary 11 (2008) 219–229.
[97] A. Fabbri, E.A. Jannini, L. Gnessi, et al., Endorphins in male impotence: Evidence for naltrexone stimulation of erectile activity in patient therapy, Psychoneuroendocrinol 14 (1989) 103–111.
[98] J.R. Seckl, M. Johnson, C. Shakespear, S.L. Lightman, Endogenous opioids inhibit oxytocin release during nicotine-stimulated secretion of vasopressin in man, Clin Endocrinol 28 (1988) 509–514.
[99] M.R. Murphy, S.A. Checkley, J.R. Seckl, S.L. Lightman, Naloxone inhibits oxytocin release at orgasm in man, J Clin Endocrinol Metab 71 (1990) 1056–1058.
[100] C.M. Heesch, B.H. Negus, J.E. Bost, et al., Effects of cocaine on anterior pituitary and gonadal hormones, J Pharmacol Exp Therap 278 (1996) 1195–1200.
[101] M. Farré, R. De la Torre, M.L. González, et al., Cocaine and alcohol interactions in humans: Neuroendocrine effects and cocaethylene metabolism, J Pharmacol Exp Therap 283 (1997) 164–176.
[102] I. Elman, S.E. Lukas, Effects of cortisol and cocaine on plasma prolactin and growth hormone levels in cocaine-dependent volunteers, Addictive Behav 30 (2005) 859–864.
[103] N.V. Goletiani, J.H. Mendelson, M.B. Sholar, et al., Opioid and cocaine combined effect on cocaine-induced changes in HPA and HPG axes hormones in men, Pharmacol Biochem Behav 91 (2009) 526–536.
[104] K.C. Light, K.M. Grewen, J.A. Amico, et al., Deficits in plasma oxytocin responses and increased negative affect, stress, and blood pressure in mothers with cocaine exposure during pregnancy, Addictive Behav 29 (2004) 1541–1564.
[105] J.H. Mendelson, S.K. Teoh, U. Lange, et al., Anterior pituitary, adrenal and gonadal hormones during cocaine withdrawal, Am J Psychiatry 145 (1988) 1094–1098.
[106] C. Contoreggi, R.I. Herning, B. Koeppl, et al., Treatment-seeking inpatient cocaine abusers show hypothalamic dysregulation of both basal prolactin and cortisol secretion, Neuroendocrinology 78 (2003) 154–162.
[107] S.L. Walsh, W.W. Stoops, D.E. Moody, et al., Repeated dosing with oral cocaine in humans: Assessment of direct effects, withdrawal, and pharmacokinetics, Exp Clin Psychopharmacol 17 (2009) 205–216.
[108] R.D. Weiss, C. Hufford, J.H. Mendelson, Serum prolactin levels and treatment outcome in cocaine dependence, Biol Psychiatry 35 (1994) 573–574.
[109] E.M. Dax, Endocrine alterations associated with the abuse of cocaine, Trends Endocrinol Metab 1 (1989) 55–56.
[110] T.E. DeLange, S. Simsek, M.H.H. Kramer, P.W.B. Nanayakkarau, A case of cocaine-induced panhypopituitarism with human neutrophil elastase-specific anti-neutrophil cytoplasmic antibodies, Eur J Endocrinol 160 (2009) 499–502.
[111] J.I. Nurnberger, E.S. Gershon, S. Simmons, et al., Behavioral, biochemical and neuroendocrine responses to amphetamine in normal twins and "well-state" bipolar patients, Psychoneuroendocrinol 7 (1982) 163–176.
[112] P.R. Joyce, R.A. Donald, M.G. Nicholls, et al., Endocrine and behavioral responses to methylphenidate in normal subjects, Biol Psychiatry 21 (1986) 1015–1023.
[113] W.A. Brown, D.P. Corriveau, M.H. Ebert, Acute psychologic and neuroendocrine effects of dextroamphetamine and methylphenidate, Psychopharmacology 58 (1978) 189–195.
[114] T.L. White, V.K. Grover, H. DeWit, Cortisol effects of d-amphetamine relate to traits of fearlessness and aggression but not anxiety in healthy humans, Pharmacol Biochem Behav 85 (2006) 123–131.
[115] B. Wells, T. Silverstone, L. Rees, The effect of oral dextroamphetamine on prolactin secretion in man, Neuropharmacol 17 (1978) 1060–1061.
[116] L. Rees, P.W.P. Butler, C. Gosling, G.M. Besser, Adrenergic blockade and the corticosteroid and growth hormone responses to methylamphetamine, Nature 228 (1970) 565–566.
[117] U. Halbreich, G.M. Asnis, F. Halpern, et al., Diurnal growth hormone responses to dextroamphetamine in normal young men and post-menopausal women, Psychoneuroendocrinol 5 (1980) 339–344.

[118] U. Halbreich, E.J. Sachar, G.M. Asnis, et al., The prolactin response to intravenous dextroamphetamine in normal young men and postmenopausal women, Life Sci 28 (1981) 2337–2342.

[119] V. DeLeo, S.G. Cella, F. Camanni, et al., Prolactin lowering effect of amphetamine in normoprolactinemic subjects and in physiological and pathological hyperprolactinemia, Horm Metab Res 15 (1983) 439–443.

[120] R. Weizman, J. Dick, I. Gil-Ad, et al., Effects of acute and chronic methylphenidate administration on β-endorphin, growth hormone, prolactin and cortisol in children with attention deficit disorder and hyperactivity, Life Sci 40 (1987) 2247–2252.

[121] P.R. Joyce, R.A. Donald, M.G. Nicholls, Physostigmine reduces the plasma cortisol response to methylphenidate in normal subjects, J Psychiat Res 20 (1986) 151–157.

[122] D.S. Janowsky, D. Parker, P.P. Leichner, et al., Growth hormone and prolactin response to methylphenidate, Psychopharmacol Bull 12 (1976) 27–28.

[123] D.S. Janowsky, P. Leichner, D. Parker, et al., Methylphenidate and serum prolactin in man, Psychopharmacol 58 (1978) 43–47.

[124] M. Mas, M. Farré, R. De la Torre, et al., Cardiovascular and neuroendocrine effects and pharmacokinetics of 3,4-methylenedioxymethamphetamine in humans, J Pharmacol Exp Therap 290 (1999) 136–145.

[125] T. Passie, U. Hartmann, U. Schneider, et al., Ecstasy (MDMA) mimics the post-orgasmic state: Impairment of sexual drive and function during acute MDMA-effects may be due to increased prolactin secretion, Med Hypotheses 64 (2005) 899–903.

[126] K. Wolff, E.M. Tsapakis, A.R. Winstock, et al., Vasopressin and oxytocin secretion in response to the consumption of ecstasy in a clubbing population, J Psychopharmacol 20 (2006) 400–410.

[127] C.U. Correll, H.E. Carlson, Endocrine and metabolic adverse effects of psychotropic medications in children and adolescents, J Am Acad Child Adolesc Psychiatry 45 (2006) 771–791.

[128] A. Bereket, S. Turan, M.G. Karaman, et al., Height, weight, IGF-1, IGF-BP3 and thyroid functions in prepubertal children with attention deficit hyperactivity disorder: Effect of methylphenidate treatment, Horm Res 63 (2005) 159–164.

[129] P. Toren, A. Silbergeld, S. Eldar, et al., Lack of effect of methylphenidate on serum growth hormone (GH), GH-binding protein, and insulin-like growth factor I, Clin Neuropharmacol 20 (1997) 264–269.

[130] L.M. Grosso, M.B. Bracken, Caffeine metabolism, genetics and perinatal outcomes: A review of exposure assessment considerations during pregnancy, Ann Epidemiol 15 (2005) 460–466.

[131] E.R. Spindel, R.J. Wurtman, A. McCall, et al., Neuroendocrine effects of caffeine in normal subjects, Clin Pharmacol Therap 36 (1984) 402–407.

[132] D.S. Charney, G.R. Heninger, P.I. Jatlow, Increased anxiogenic effects of caffeine in panic disorders, Arch Gen Psychiatry 42 (1985) 233–243.

[133] W.R. Lovallo, M. Al'Absi, K. Blick, et al., Stress-like adrenocorticotropin responses to caffeine in young healthy men, Pharmacol Biochem Behav 55 (1996) 365–369.

[134] J.-C. Daubresse, A. Luyckx, E. Demey-Ponsart, et al., Effects of coffee and caffeine on carbohydrate metabolism, free fatty acid, insulin, growth hormone and cortisol plasma levels in man, Acta Diabet Lat 10 (1973) 1069–1084.

[135] T.W. Uhde, M.E. Tancer, D.R. Rubinow, et al., Evidence for hypothalamo-growth hormone dysfunction in panic disorder: profile of growth hormone (GH) responses to clonidine, yohimbine, caffeine, glucose, GRF and TRH in panic disorder patients versus healthy volunteers, Neuropsychopharmacol 6 (1992) 101–118.

[136] J.W. Ensinck, R.W. Stoll, C.C. Gale, et al., Effect of aminophylline on the secretion of insulin, glucagon, luteinizing hormone and growth hormone in humans, J Clin Endocrinol Metab 31 (1970) 153–161.

[137] E.N. Liberopoulos, G.H. Alexandridis, D.S. Christidis, M.S. Elisaf, SIADH and hyponatremia with theophylline, Ann Pharmacother 36 (2002) 1180–1182.

[138] K. Ajlouni, M. El-Khateeb, Effect of glucose on growth hormone, prolactin and thyroid-stimulating hormone response to diazepam in normal subjects, Horm Res 13 (1980) 160–164.

[139] M. D'Armiento, G. Bisignani, G. Reda, Effect of bromazepam on growth hormone and prolactin secretion in normal subjects, Horm Res 15 (1981) 224–227.

[140] E.D. Risby, J.K. Hsiao, R.N. Golden, W.Z. Potter, Intravenous alprazolam challenge in normal subjects. Biochemical, cardiovascular and behavioral effects, Psychopharmacol 99 (1989) 508–514.

[141] G. Laakmann, J. Treusch, M. Schmauss, et al., Comparison of growth hormone stimulation induced by desipramine, diazepam and metaclazepam in man, Psychoneuroendocrinol 7 (1982) 141–146.

[142] G. Laakmann, J. Treusch, A. Eichmer, et al., Inhibitory effect of phentolamine on diazepam-induced growth hormone secretion and lack of effect of diazepam on prolactin secretion in man, Psychoneuroendocrinol 7 (1982) 135–139.

[143] M. D'Armiento, F. Bigi, A. Pontecorvi, et al., Diazepam-stimulated GH secretion in normal subjects: Relation to oestradiol plasma levels, Horm Metab Res J Bone Joint Surg Br 16 (1984) 155.

[144] M.G. Monteiro, M.A. Schuckit, R. Hauger, et al., Growth hormone response to intravenous diazepam and placebo in 82 healthy men, Biol Psychiatry 27 (1990) 702–710.

[145] A. Breier, D.S. Charney, G.R. Heninger, Intravenous diazepam fails to change growth hormone and cortisol secretion in humans, Psychiatr Res 18 (1986) 293–299.

[146] M.D. Beary, J.H. Lacey, A.V. Bhat, The neuro-endocrine impact of 3-hydroxy-diazepam (temazepam) in women, Psychopharmacol 79 (1983) 295–297.

[147] F. Petraglia, S. Bakalakis, F. Facchinetti, et al., Effects of sodium valproate and diazepam on beta-endorphin, beta-lipotropin and cortisol secretion induced by hypoglycemic stress in humans, Neuroendocrinology 44 (1986) 320–325.

[148] D.S. Charney, A. Breier, P.I. Jatlow, G.R. Heninger, Behavioral, biochemical, and blood pressure responses to alprazolam in healthy subjects: Interactions with yohimbine, Psychopharmacol 88 (1986) 133–140.

[149] E. Fries, D.H. Hellhammer, J. Hellhammer, Attenuation of the hypothalamic–pituitary–adrenal axis responsivity to the Trier Social Stress Test by the benzodiazepine alprazolam, Psychoneuroendocrinol 31 (2006) 1278–1288.

[150] W.P. Tormey, C. Dolphin, A.S. Darragh, The effects of diazepam on sleep, and on the nocturnal release of growth hormone, prolactin, ACTH and cortisol, Br J Clin Pharmacol 8 (1979) 90–92.

[151] D.J. Torpy, J.E. Grice, G.I. Hockings, et al., Alprazolam blocks the naloxone-stimulated hypothalamo–pituitary–adrenal axis in man, J Clin Endocrinol Metab 76 (1993) 388–391.

[152] E. Arvat, B. Macagno, J. Ramunni, et al., The inhibitory effects of alprazolam, a benzodiazepine, overrides the stimulatory effect of metyrapone-induced lack of negative cortisol feedback on corticotroph secretion in humans, J Clin Endocrinol Metab 84 (1999) 2611–2615.

[153] E. Shur, H. Petursson, S. Checkley, M. Lader, Long-term benzodiazepine administration blunts growth hormone response to diazepam, Arch Gen Psychiatry 40 (1983) 1105–1108.

[154] D.J. Torpy, R.V. Jackson, J.E. Grice, et al., Effect of flumazenil on basal and naloxone-stimulated ACTH and cortisol release in humans, Clin Exp Pharmacol Physiol 21 (1994) 157–161.

[155] D. Nutt, H. Middleton, M. Franklin, The neuroendocrine effects of oral imipramine, Psychoneuroendocrinol 12 (1987) 367–375.

[156] J.N. Wilkins, J.E. Spar, H.E. Carlson, Desipramine increases circulating growth hormone in elderly depressed patients: A pilot study, Psychoneuroendocrinol 14 (1989) 195–202.

[157] G. Laakmann, H.W. Schoen, D. Blaschke, M. Wittmann, Dose-dependent growth hormone, prolactin and cortisol stimulation after i.v. administration of desipramine in human subjects, Psychoneuroendocrinol 10 (1985) 83–93.

[158] J.H. Lacey, A.H. Crisp, G.V. Groom, J. Seldrup, The impact of clomipramine and its withdrawal on some nocturnal hormonal profiles — a preliminary report, Postgrad Med J 53 (Suppl. 4) (1977) 182–189.

[159] H.Y. Meltzer, S. Piyakamala, P. Schyve, V.S. Fang, Lack of effect of tricyclic antidepressants on serum prolactin levels, Psychopharmacol 51 (1977) 185–187.

[160] A.F. Francis, R. Williams, E.N. Cole, et al., The effect of clomipramine on prolactin levels — pilot studies, Postgrad Med J 52 (Suppl 3) (1976) 87–91.

[161] O.A. Kletzky, P. St-Michel, C.A. Mashchak, B.S. Coleman, Lack of effect of fluvoxamine, a new serotonin reuptake inhibitor, on hypothalamic—pituitary function, Curr Therap Res 33 (1983) 394–400.

[162] A.E.S. Walsh, R.A. Hockney, G. Campling, P.J. Cowen, Neuroendocrine and temperature effects of nefazodone in healthy volunteers, Biol Psychiatry 33 (1993) 115–119.

[163] M.-J. Attenburrow, P.R. Mitter, R. Whale, et al., Low-dose citalopram as a 5-HT neuroendocrine probe, Psychopharmacol 155 (2001) 323–326.

[164] J. Zohar, T.R. Insel, R.C. Zohar-Kadouch, et al., Serotonergic responsivity in obsessive-compulsive disorder, Arch Gen Psychiatry 45 (1988) 167–172.

[165] J.L. Nielsen, Plasma prolactin during treatment with nortriptyline, Neuropsychobiol 6 (1980) 52–55.

[166] D.S. Cooper, A.J. Gelenberg, J.C. Wojcik, et al., The effect of amoxapine and imipramine on serum prolactin levels, Arch Intern Med 141 (1981) 1023–1025.

[167] P.J. Cowen, D.P. Geaney, M. Schacter, et al., Desipramine treatment in normal subjects, Arch Gen Psychiatry 43 (1986) 61–67.

[168] D.S. Charney, G.R. Heninger, D.E. Sternberg, Serotonin function and mechanism of action of antidepressant treatment, Arch Gen Psychiatry 41 (1984) 359–365.

[169] O. Spigset, T. Mjorndal, The effect of fluvoxamine on serum prolactin and serum sodium concentrations: Relation to platelet 5-HT_{2A} receptor status, J Clin Psychopharmacol 17 (1997) 292–297.

[170] G.I. Papakostas, K.K. Miller, T. Petersen, et al., Serum prolactin levels among outpatients with major depressive disorder during the acute phase of treatment with fluoxetine, J Clin Psychiatry 67 (2006) 952–957.

[171] S.S. Eker, C. Akkaya, A. Sarandol, et al., Effects of various antidepressants on serum thyroid hormone levels in patients with major depressive disorder, Prog in Neuro-psychopharmacol Biol Psychiatry 32 (2008) 955–961.

[172] F. Duval, M.-C. Modrani, M.-A. Crocq, et al., Effect of antidepressant medication on morning and evening thyroid function tests during a major depressive episode, Arch Gen Psychiatry 53 (1996) 833–840.

[173] P.D. Whiteman, A.W. Peck, A.S.E. Fowle, P.R. Smith, Failure of bupropion to affect prolactin or growth hormone in man, J Clin Psychiatry 44 (1983) 209–210.

[174] S.I. Slater, D.J. Shiling, S. Lipper, D.L. Murphy, Elevation of plasma prolactin by monoamine oxidase inhibitors, Lancet 2 (1977) 275–276.

[175] D. Kirby, S. Harrigan, D. Ames, Hyponatremia in elderly psychiatric patients treated with selective serotonin reuptake inhibitors and venlafaxine: A retrospective controlled study in an inpatient unit, Int J Geriatr Psychiatry 17 (2002) 231–237.

[176] S.C. Bagley, D. Yaeger, Hyponatremia associated with bupropion, a case verified by rechallenge, J Clin Psychopharmacol 25 (2005) 98–99.

[177] S. Romero, L. Pintor, M. Serra, et al., Syndrome of inappropriate secretion of antidiuretic hormone due to citalopram and venlafaxine, Gen Hosp Psychiatry 29 (2007) 81–84.

[178] J.H. Lazarus, Lithium and thyroid, Best Pract Res Clin Endocrinol Metab 23 (2009) 723–733.

[179] E.M. Grandjean, M.J. Aubry, Lithium: Updated human knowledge using an evidence-based approach. Part III: Clinical safety, CNS Drugs 23 (2009) 397–418.

[180] C. Livingstone, H. Rampes, Lithium: A review of its metabolic adverse effects, J Psychopharmacol 20 (2006) 347–355.

[181] M.D. Penney, D. Hampton, The effect of lithium therapy on arginine vasopressin secretion and thirst in man, Clin Biochem 23 (1990) 233–236.

[182] J.J. Bedford, S. Weggery, G. Ellis, et al., Lithium-induced nephrogenic diabetes insipidus: Renal effects of amiloride, Clin J Am Soc Nephrol 3 (2008) 1324–1331.

[183] P.M. Haddad, A. Wieck, Antipsychotic-induced hyperprolactinemia. Mechanisms, clinical features and management, Drugs 64 (2004) 2291–2314.

[184] M.E. Molitch, Drugs and prolactin, Pituitary 11 (2008) 209–218.

[185] B.-H. Lee, Y.-K. Kim, S.-H. Park, Using aripiprazole to resolve antipsychotic-induced symptomatic hyperprolactinemia: A pilot study, Prog Neuro-psychopharmacol Biol Psychiatry 30 (2006) 714–717.

[186] N.M. Zelaschi, G.A. Delucchi, J.L. Rodriguez, High plasma prolactin levels after long-term neuroleptic treatment, Biol Psychiatry 39 (1996) 900–901.

[187] R.L. Findling, V. Kusumakar, D. Daneman, et al., Prolactin levels during long-term risperidone treatment in children and adolescents, J Clin Psychiatry 64 (2004) 1362–1369.

[188] J. Eberhard, E. Lindström, M. Holstad, S. Levander, Prolactin level during 5 years of risperidone treatment in patients with psychotic disorders, Acta Psychiatr Scand 115 (2007) 268–276.

[189] A. Szarfman, J.M. Tonning, J.G. Levine, P.M. Doraiswamy, Atypical antipsytchotics and pituitary tumors: A pharmacovigilance study, Pharmacotherapy 26 (2006) 748–758.

[190] P. Chanson, J. Young, Pituitary incidentalomas, Endocrinologist 13 (2003) 124–135.

[191] D.L. Kleinberg, J.M. Davis, R. DeCoster, et al., Prolactin levels and adverse events in patients treated with risperidone, J Clin Psychopharmacol 19 (1999) 57–61.

[192] S. Lai, C.E. De la Vega, T.L. Sourkes, H.G. Friesen, Effect of apomorphine on growth hormone, prolactin, luteinizing hormone and follicle-stimulating hormone levels in human serum, J Clin Endocrinol Metab 37 (1973) 719–724.

[193] D. Naber, H. Steinbock, W. Greil, Effects of short- and long-term neuroleptic treatment on thyroid function, Prog Neuro-psychopharmacol 4 (1980) 199–206.

[194] J.H. Meador-Woodruff, J.F. Greden, Effects of psychotropic medications on hypothalamic—pituitary—adrenal regulation, Endocrinol Metab Clin North Am 17 (1988) 225–234.

[195] J. Ananth, K-M. Lin, SIADH: A serious side effect of psychotropic drugs, Int J Psychiatry Med 16 (1986–87) 401–407.

[196] J.S. Cunha-Filho, J.L. Gross, D. Vettori, et al., Growth hormone and prolactin secretion after metoclopramide administration

(DA2 receptor blockade) in fertile women, Horm Metab Res 33 (2001) 536–539.
[197] I. Soykan, I. Sarosiek, R.W. McCallum, The effect of chronic oral domperidone therapy on gastrointestinal symptoms, gastric emptying, and quality of life in patients with gastroparesis, Am J Gastroenterol 92 (1997) 976–980.
[198] E. Ghigo, S. Goffi, G.M. Molinatti, et al., Prolactin and TSH responses to both domperidone and TRH in normal and hyperprolactinemic women after dopamine synthesis blockade, Clin Endocrinol 23 (1985) 155–160.
[199] K. Seki, I. Nagata, Effects of a dopamine antagonist (metoclopramide) on the release of LH, FSH, TSH and PRL in normal women throughout the menstrual cycle, Acta Endocrinol 122 (1990) 211–216.
[200] P. Falaschi, G. Frajese, F. Sciarra, et al., Influence of hyperprolactinaemia due to metoclopramide on gonadal function in men, Clin Endocrinol 8 (1978) 427–433.
[201] E.I. Tamagna, W. Lane, J.M. Hershman, et al., Effect of chronic metoclopramide therapy on serum pituitary hormone concentrations, Horm Res 11 (1979) 161–169.
[202] G. Norbiato, M. Bevilacqua, E. Chebat, et al., Metoclopramide increases vasopressin secretion, J Clin Endocrinol Metab 63 (1986) 747–750.
[203] P.J. Cowen, I.M. Anderson, D.G. Grahame-Smith, Neuroendocrine effects of azapirones, J Clin Psychopharmacol 10 (3 Suppl) (1990) 21S–25S.
[204] P. Chiodera, R. Volpi, L. Capretti, et al., Different effects of the serotonergic agonists buspirone and sumatriptan on the posterior pituitary responses to hypoglycemia in humans, Neuropeptides 30 (1996) 187–192.
[205] Y.-H. Kim, J.-C. Shim, D.L. Kelly, et al., Cortisol response to buspirone in extended abstinent alcoholics, Alcohol Alcoholism 39 (2004) 287–289.
[206] M.L. Vance, W.S. Evans, M.O. Thorner, Bromocriptine. Ann Intern Med 100 (1984) 78–91.
[207] V. De Leo, F. Petraglia, M.G. Bruno, et al., Different dopaminergic control of plasma luteinizing hormone, follicle-stimulating hormone and prolactin in ovulatory and postmenopausal women: Effect of ovariectomy, Gynecol Obstet Invest 27 (1989) 94–98.
[208] P.G. Crosignani, C. Ferrari, A. Malinverni, et al., Effect of central nervous system dopaminergic activation on prolactin secretion in man: Evidence for a common central defect in hyperprolactinemic patients with and without radiological signs of pituitary tumors, J Clin Endocrinol Metab 51 (1980) 1068–1073.
[209] H.E. Carlson, Carbidopa plus L-dopa pretreatment inhibits the prolactin (PRL) response to thyrotropin-releasing hormone and thus cannot distinguish central from pituitary sites of prolactin stimulation, J Clin Endocrinol Metab 63 (1986) 249–251.
[210] J.E. Morley, Neuroendocrine control of thyrotropin secretion, Endocr Rev 2 (1981) 396–436.
[211] D.G. Johnston, R.W.G. Prescott, P. Kendall-Taylor, et al., Hyperprolactinemia. Long-term effects of bromocriptine, Am J Med 75 (1983) 868–874.
[212] M.L. Vance, D.L. Kaiser, L.A. Frohman, et al., Role of dopamine in the regulation of growth hormone secretion: Dopamine and bromocriptine augment growth hormone (GH)-releasing hormone-stimulated GH secretion in normal man, J Clin Endocrinol Metab 64 (1987) 1136–1141.
[213] C. Dieguez, M.D. Page, M.F. Scanlon, Growth hormone neuroregulation and its alterations in disease states, Clin Endocrinol 28 (1988) 109–143.
[214] G.A.B. Lima, E.D. Machado, C.M.D. Silva, et al., Pituitary apoplexy during treatment of cystic macroprolactinomas with cabergoline, Pituitary 11 (2008) 287–292.
[215] A. Giustina, J.D. Veldhuis, Pathophysiology of the neuroregulation of growth hormone secretion in experimental animals and the human, Endocr Rev 19 (1998) 717–797.
[216] S.C. Risch, D.S. Janowsky, M.A. Mott, et al., Central and peripheral cholinesterase inhibition: Effects on anterior pituitary and sympathomimetic function, Psychoneuroendocrinol 11 (1986) 221–230.
[217] R.K. Ross, A. Paganini-Hill, M.D. Krailo, et al., Effects of reserpine on prolactin levels and incidence of breast cancer in postmenopausal women, Cancer Res 44 (1984) 3106–3108.
[218] M. Baldini, U. Cornelli, M. Molinari, L. Cantalamessa, Effect of methyldopa on prolactin serum concentration, Eur J Clin Pharmacol 34 (1988) 513–515.
[219] Y. Varkel, A. Braaester, D. Nusem, T. Shkolnik, Methyldopa-induced syndrome of inappropriate antidiuretic hormone secretion and bone marrow granulomatosis, Drug Intell Clin Pharmacy 22 (1988) 700–702.
[220] U.B. Lauridsen, N.J. Christensen, J. Lyngsoe, Effects of nonselective and β_1-selective blockade on glucose metabolism and hormone responses during insulin-induced hypoglycemia in normal man, J Clin Endocrinol Metab 56 (1983) 876–882.
[221] C.A. Saxton, J.K. Faulkner, G.V. Groom, The effect on plasma prolactin, growth hormone and luteinising hormone concentrations of single oral doses of propranolol and tolamolol in normal man, Eur J Clin Pharmacol 21 (1981) 103–108.
[222] C. Barbieri, M.T. Larovere, G. Mariotti, et al., Prolactin stimulation by intravenous labetalol is mediated inside the central nervous system, Clin Endocrinol 16 (1982) 615–619.
[223] F. Galluzzi, S. Stagi, M. Parpagnoli, et al., Oral clonidine provocative test in the diagnosis of growth hormone deficiency in childhood: Should we make the timing uniform? Horm Res 66 (2006) 285–288.
[224] M.-C. Mokrani, F. Duval, T.S. Diep, et al., Multihormonal responses to clonidine in patients with affective and psychotic symptoms, Psychoneuroendocrinology 25 (2000) 741–752.
[225] P. Tatar, M. Vigas, Role of alpha-1 and alpha-2 adrenergic receptors in the growth hormone and prolactin response to insulin-induced hypoglycaemia in man, Neuroendocrinol 39 (1984) 275–280.
[226] A.W. Burrows, B. Gribbin, Clonidine-induced dilutional hyponatremia, Postgrad Med J 55 (1979) 42–44.
[227] R.E. Schoen, W.H. Frishman, H. Shamoon, Hormonal and metabolic effects of calcium channel antagonists in man, Am J Med 84 (1988) 492–504.
[228] S.R. Kelley, T.J. Kamal, M.E. Molitch, Mechanism of verapamil calcium channel blockade-induced hyperprolactinemia, Am J Physiol 270 (1996) E96–E100.
[229] E.L. Fearrington, C.H. Rand, J.D. Rose, Hyperprolactinemia—galactorrhea induced by verapamil, Am J Cardiol 51 (1983) 1466–1467.
[230] L.A. Tanner, L.A. Bosco, Gynecomastia associated with calcium channel blocker therapy, Arch Intern Med 148 (1988) 379–380.
[231] H.E. Carlson, A.F. Ippoliti, Cimetidine, an H_2-antihistamine, stimulates prolactin secretion in man, J Clin Endocrinol Metab 45 (1977) 367–370.
[232] H.E. Carlson, R.J. Chang, Studies on the role of histamine in human pituitary function, Clin Endocrinol 12 (1980) 461–466.
[233] A.E. Pontiroli, G. Viberti, A. Vicari, G. Pozza, Effect of the antihistaminic agents meclastine and dexchlorpheniramine on the response of human growth hormone to arginine infusion and insulin hypoglycemia, J Clin Endocrinol Metab 43 (1976) 582–586.
[234] H.E. Carlson, R.J. Chang, N.V. Meyer, et al., Effect of cimetidine on serum prolactin in normal women and patients with hyperprolactinemia, Clin Endocrinol 15 (1981) 491–498.

[235] G. Delitala, L. Devilla, A. Pende, A. Canessa, Effects of the H_2-receptor antagonist ranitidine on anterior pituitary hormone secretion in man, Eur J Clin Pharmacol 22 (1982) 207–211.

[236] J.T. Callaghan, R.F. Bergstrom, A. Rubin, et al., A pharmacokinetic profile of nizatidine in man, Scand J Gastroenterol 22 (Suppl 136) (1987) 9–17.

[237] U. Knigge, S. Matzen, J. Warberg, Effects of H_2-receptor antagonists on prolactin secretion: Specificity and mediation of the response, Acta Endocrinol 115 (1987) 461–468.

[238] H.E. Carlson, A.F. Ippoliti, R.S. Swerdloff, Endocrine effects of acute and chronic cimetidine administration, Dig Dis Sci 26 (1981) 428–432.

[239] T.W. Valk, B.G. England, J.C. Marshall, Effects of cimetidine on pituitary function: Alterations in hormone secretion profiles, Clin Endocrinol 15 (1981) 139–149.

[240] G.N.J. Tytgat, W. Hameeteman, C.J.J. Mulder, et al., Five-year cimetidine maintenance trial for peptic ulcer disease, Scand J Gastroenterol 25 (1990) 974–980.

[241] S.-C.J. Yeung, A.C. Chiu, R. Vassilopoulou-Sellin, R.F. Gagel, The endocrine effects of nonhormonal antineoplastic therapy, Endocr Rev 19 (1998) 144–172.

[242] M. Brydøy, S.D. Fosså, O. Dahl, T. Bjøro, Gonadal dysfunction and fertility problems in cancer survivors, Acta Oncologia 46 (2007) 480–489.

[243] C.E. Kisserud, A. Fosså, T. Bjøro, et al., Gonadal function in male patients after treatment for malignant lymphomas, with emphasis on chemotherapy, Brit J Cancer 100 (2009) 455–463.

[244] S.J. Howell, S.M. Shalet, Spermatogenesis after cancer treatment: Damage and recovery, J Natl Cancer Inst Monogr 34 (2005) 12–17.

[245] C. Sklar, Maintenance of ovarian function and risk of premature menopause related to cancer treatment, J Natl Cancer Inst Monogr 34 (2005) 25–27.

[246] F. Illouz, S. Laboureau-Soares, S. Dubois, et al., Tyrosine kinase inhibitors and modifications of thyroid function tests: A review, Eur J Endocrinol 160 (2009) 331–336.

[247] N.V. Jayachandran, P.K.S. Chandrasekhara, J. Thomas, et al., Cyclophosphamide-associated complications: We need to be aware of SIADH and central pontine myelinolysis, Rheumatology 48 (2009) 89–90.

[248] B. Greenbaum-Lefkoe, J.G. Rosenstock, J.B. Belasco, et al., Syndrome of inappropriate antidiuretic hormone secretion. A complication of high-dose intravenous melphalan, Cancer 55 (1985) 44–46.

[249] I.W. Hammond, J.A. Ferguson, K. Kwong, et al., Hyponatremia and syndrome of inappropriate anti-diuretic hormone reported with the use of vincristine®: An over-representation of Asians? Pharmacoepidemiol Drug Safety 11 (2002) 229–234.

[250] G. Fraschini, F. Recchia, F.A. Holmes, Syndrome of inappropriate antidiuretic hormone secretion associated with hepatic arterial infusion of vinblastine in three patients with breast cancer, Tumori 73 (1987) 513–516.

[251] H. Kuroda, M. Kawamura, T. Hato, et al., Syndrome of inappropriate secretion of antidiuretic hormone after chemotherapy with vinorelbine, Cancer Chemother Pharmacol 62 (2008) 331–333.

[252] K. Kagawa, K. Fujitaka, T. Isobe, et al., Syndrome of inappropriate secretion of ADH (SIADH) following cisplatin administration in a pulmonary adenocarcinoma patient with a malignant pleural effusion, Intern Med 40 (2001) 1020–1023.

[253] K. Liapis, J. Apostolidis, E. Charitaki, et al., Syndrome of inappropriate secretion of antidiuretic hormone associated with imatinib, Ann Pharmacother 42 (2008) 1882–1886.

[254] D.F. Hayes, R.M. Lechan, M.R. Posner, et al., The syndrome of inappropriate antidiuretic hormone secretion associated with induction chemotherapy for squamous cell carcinoma of the head and neck, J Surg Oncol 32 (1986) 150–152.

[255] N. Kalleinen, P. Polo-Kantola, K. Irjala, et al., 24-hour serum levels of growth hormone, prolactin and cortisol in pre- and postmenopausal women: The effect of combined estrogen and progestin treatment, J Clin Endocrinol Metab 93 (2008) 1655–1661.

[256] M. Cosma, J. Bailey, J.M. Miles, et al., Pituitary and/or peripheral estrogen-receptor α regulates follicle-stimulating hormone secretion, whereas central estrogenic pathways direct growth hormone and prolactin secretion in post-menopausal women, J Clin Endocrinol Metab 93 (2008) 951–958.

[257] P.L.H. Hwang, C.S.A. Ng, S.T. Cheong, Effect of oral contraceptives on serum prolactin: A longitudinal study in 126 normal premenopausal women, Clin Endocrinol 24 (1986) 127–133.

[258] J.B. Josimovich, M.A. Lavenhar, M.M. Devanesan, et al., Heterogeneous distribution of serum prolactin values in apparently healthy young women, and the effects of oral contraceptive medication, Fertil Steril 47 (1987) 785–791.

[259] L.J.G. Gooren, W. Harmsen-Louman, H. Van Kessel, Follow-up of prolactin levels in long-term oestrogen-treated male-to-female transsexuals with regard to prolactinoma induction, Clin Endocrinol 22 (1985) 201–207.

[260] K.K. Shy, A.M. McTiernan, J.R. Daling, N.S. Weiss, Oral contraceptive use and the occurrence of pituitary prolactinoma, JAMA 249 (1983) 2204–2207.

[261] Pituitary adenoma study group, Pituitary adenomas and oral contraceptives: A multicenter case-control study, Fertil Steril 39 (1983) 753–760.

[262] B.W. Scheithauer, K.T. Kovacs, R.V. Randall, N. Ryan, Effects of estrogen on the human pituitary: A clinicopathologic study, Mayo Clin Proc 64 (1989) 1077–1084.

[263] G. Raven, F.H. DeJong, J.-M. Kaufman, W. DeRonde, In men, peripheral estradiol levels directly reflect the action of estrogens at the hypothalamo–pituitary level to inhibit gonadotropin secretion, J Clin Endocrinol Metab 91 (2006) 3324–3328.

[264] N.D. Shaw, S.N. Histed, S.S. Srouji, et al., Estrogen negative feedback on gonadotropin secretion: Evidence for a direct pituitary effect in women, J Clin Endocrinol Metab 95 (2010) 1955–1961.

[265] S.E. Hendricks, B. Graber, J.F. Rodriguez-Sierra, Neuroendocrine responses to exogenous estrogen: No differences between heterosexual and homosexual men, Psychoneuroendocrinol 14 (1989) 177–185.

[266] L. Gooren, The neuroendocrine response of luteinizing hormone to estrogen administration in heterosexual, homosexual, and transsexual subjects, J Clin Endocrinol Metab 63 (1986) 583–588.

[267] D.D. Abech, H.B. Moratelli, S.C.B.F.S. Leite, M.C. Oliveira, Effects of estrogen replacement therapy on pituitary size, prolactin and thyroid-stimulating hormone concentrations in menopausal women, Gynecological Endocrinol 21 (2005) 223–226.

[268] P.H. Bisschop, A.W. Toorians, E. Endert, et al., The effects of sex-steroid administration on the pituitary–thyroid axis in transsexuals, Eur J Endocrinol 155 (2006) 11–16.

[269] V.L. Baker, M. Draper, S. Paul, et al., Reproductive endocrine and endometrial effects of raloxifene hydrochloride, a selective estrogen receptor modulator, in women with regular menstrual cycles, J Clin Endocrinol Metab 83 (1998) 6–13.

[270] M.W. Draper, D.E. Flowers, J.A. Neild, et al., Antiestrogenic properties of raloxifene, Pharmacology 50 (1995) 209–217.

[271] V.C. Jordan, N.F. Fritz, D.C. Torney, Endocrine effects of adjuvant chemotherapy and long-term tamoxifen administration on node-positive patients with breast cancer, Cancer Res 47 (1987) 624–630.

[272] G.G. T'Sjoen, V.A. Giagulli, H. Delva, et al., Comparative assessment in young and elderly men of the gonadotropin response to aromatase inhibition, J Clin Endocrinol Metab 90 (2005) 5717–5722.
[273] P.J. Snyder, Clinical use of androgens, Annual Rev Med 35 (1984) 207–217.
[274] C.B. Scheckter, A.M. Matsumoto, W.J. Bremner, Testosterone administration inhibits gonadotropin secretion by an effect directly on the human pituitary, J Clin Endocrinol Metab 68 (1989) 397–401.
[275] J.D. Wilson, Androgen abuse by athletes, Endocr Rev 9 (1988) 181–199.
[276] A.M. Matsumoto, Effects of chronic testosterone administration in normal men: Safety and efficacy of high dosage testosterone and parallel dose-dependent suppression of luteinizing hormone, follicle-stimulating hormone, and sperm production, J Clin Endocrinol Metab 70 (1990) 282–287.
[277] J.E. Morley, C.T. Sawin, H.E. Carlson, et al., The relationship of androgen to the thyrotropin and prolactin responses to thyrotropin-releasing hormone in hypogonadal and normal men, J Clin Endocrinol Metab 52 (1981) 173–176.
[278] K. Link, R.M. Blizzard, W.S. Evans, et al., The effect of androgens on the pulsatile release and the twenty-four-hour mean concentration of growth hormone in peripubertal males, J Clin Endocrinol Metab 62 (1986) 159–164.
[279] S. Loche, R. Corda, A. Lampis, et al., The effect of oxandrolone on the growth hormone response to growth hormone-releasing hormone in children with constitutional growth delay, Clin Endocrinol 25 (1986) 195–200.
[280] P.E. Clayton, S.M. Shalet, D.A. Price, G.M. Addison, Growth and growth hormone responses to oxandrolone in boys with constitutional delay of growth and puberty (CDGP), Clin Endocrinol 29 (1988) 123–130.
[281] A. Ulloa-Aguirre, R.M. Blizzard, E. Garcia-Rubi, et al., Testosterone and oxandrolone, a nonaromatizable androgen, specifically amplify the mass and rate of growth hormone (GH) secreted per burst without altering GH secretory burst duration or frequency or the GH half-life, J Clin Endocrinol Metab 71 (1990) 846–854.
[282] M.C. Uygur, A.I. Arik, U. Altug, D. Erol, Effects of the 5α-reductase inhibitor finasteride on serum levels of gonadal, adrenal and hypophyseal hormones and its clinical significance: A prospective clinical study, Steroids 63 (1998) 208–213.
[283] R.S. Rittmaster, A. Lemay, H. Zwicker, et al., Effect of finasteride, a 5α-reductase inhibitor, on serum gonadotropins in normal men, J Clin Endocrinol Metab 75 (1992) 484–488.
[284] F. Bayram, I.I. Müderris, M. Güven, F. Kelestimur, Comparison of high-dose finasteride (5 mg/day) versus low dose finasteride (2.5 mg/day) in the treatment of hirsutism, Eur J Endocrinol 147 (2002) 467–471.
[285] P. Moghetti, R. Castello, C.M. Magnani, et al., Clinical and hormonal effects of the 5α-reductase inhibitor finasteride in idiopathic hirsutism, J Clin Endocrinol Metab 79 (1994) 1115–1121.
[286] U.A. Knuth, R. Hano, E. Nieschlag, Effects of flutamide or cyproterone acetate on pituitary and testicular hormones in normal men, J Clin Endocrinol Metab 59 (1984) 963–969.
[287] R.J. Urban, M.R. Davis, A.D. Rogol, et al., Acute androgen receptor blockade increases luteinizing hormone secretory activity in men, J Clin Endocrinol Metab 67 (1988) 1149–1155.
[288] W.G. Rossmanith, M. Beuter, R. Benz, C. Lauritzen, How do androgens affect episodic gonadotrophin secretion in postmenopausal women? Maturitas 13 (1991) 325–335.
[289] C. Taner, M. Inal, Ö Basogul, et al., Comparison of the clinical efficacy and safety of flutamide versus flutamide plus an oral contraceptive in the treatment of hirsutism, Gynecol Obstet Invest 54 (2002) 105–108.
[290] B. Couzinet, M. Pholsena, J. Young, G. Schaison, The impact of a pure anti-androgen (flutamide) on LH, FSH, androgens and clinical status in idiopathic hirsutism, Clin Endocrinol 39 (1993) 157–162.
[291] A.B. Abou Samra, H. Dechaud, B. Estour, et al., β-lipotropin and cortisol responses to an intravenous infusion dexamethasone suppression test in Cushing's syndrome and obesity, J Clin Endocrinol Metab 61 (1985) 116–119.
[292] Z. Hochberg, Mechanisms of steroid impairment of growth, Horm Res 58 (Suppl 1) (2002) 33–38.
[293] M.R. MacAdams, R.H. White, B.E. Chipps, Reduction of serum testosterone levels during chronic glucocorticoid therapy, Ann Intern Med 104 (1986) 648–651.
[294] M. Saketos, N. Sharma, N.F. Santoro, Suppression of the hypothalamic—pituitary—ovarian axis in normal women by glucocorticoids, Biol Reprod 49 (1993) 1270–1276.
[295] A. LaMarca, M. Torricelli, G. Morgante, et al., Effects of dexamethasone and dexamethasone plus naltrexone on pituitary responses to GnRH and TRH in normal women, Horm Res 51 (1999) 85–90.
[296] W. Oelkers, Hyponatremia and inappropriate secretion of vasopressin (antidiuretic hormone) in patients with hypopituitarism, N Engl J Med 321 (1989) 492–496.
[297] A.M. Landolt, Treatment of acute post-operative inappropriate antidiuretic hormone secretion with diphenylhydantoin, Acta Endocrinol 76 (1974) 625–628.
[298] L. Appleby, Rapid development of hyponatraemia during low-dose carbamazepine therapy, J Neurol Neurosurg Psychiat 47 (1984) 1138.
[299] P. Chiodera, A. Gnudi, R. Volpi, et al., Effects of the GABAergic agent sodium valproate on the arginine vasopressin responses to hypertonic stimulation and upright posture in man, Clin Endocrinol 30 (1989) 389–395.
[300] P. Chiodera, V. Coiro, Different effects of the GABAergic agent sodium valproate on the oxytocin responses to angiotensin II and insulin-induced hypoglycemia in normal men, Horm Res 36 (1991) 27–31.
[301] A.R. Glass, Ketoconazole-induced stimulation of gonadotropin output in men: Basis for a potential test of gonadotropin reserve, J Clin Endocrinol Metab 63 (1986) 1121–1125.
[302] W.S. Tucker, B.B. Snell, D.P. Island, et al., Reversible adrenal insufficiency induced by ketoconazole, JAMA 253 (1983) 2413–2414.
[303] F.A. Shepherd, B. Hoffert, W.K. Evans, et al., Ketoconazole. Use in the treatment of ectopic adrenocorticotropic hormone production and Cushing's syndrome in small-cell lung cancer, Arch Intern Med 145 (1985) 863–864.
[304] M.M. Oo, A.Y. Krishna, G.J. Bonavita, G.W. Rutecki, Heparin therapy for myocardial infarction: An unusual trigger for pituitary apoplexy, Am J Med Sci 314 (1997) 351–353.
[305] W.M. Golden, K.B. Weber, T.L. Hernandez, et al., Single-dose rexinoid rapidly and specifically suppresses serum thyrotropin in normal subjects, J Clin Endocrinol Metab 92 (2007) 124–130.
[306] V.S. Bebarta, J.A. King, M. McDonough, Proton pump inhibitor-induced rhabdomyolysis and hyponatremic delirium, Am J Emerg Med 26 (2008) 519 e1-e2.
[307] M. Mann, E. Koller, A. Murgo, et al., Glucocorticoidlike activity of megestrol, Arch Intern Med 157 (1997) 1651–1656.
[308] D.L. Bodenner, M. Medhi, W.J. Evans, et al., Effects of megestrol acetate on pituitary function and end-organ hormone secretion: A post hoc analysis of serum samples from a 12-week study in healthy older men, Am J Geriatr Pharmacother 3 (2005) 160–167.

[309] R.A. Vigersky, A. Filmore-Nassar, A.R. Glass, Thyrotropin suppression by metformin, J Clin Endocrinol Metab 91 (2006) 225–227.
[310] C. Capelli, M. Rotondi, I. Pirola, et al., TSH-lowering effect of metformin in type 2 diabetic patients, Diab Care 32 (2009) 1589–1590.
[311] L.B. Concha, H.E. Carlson, A. Heimann, et al., Interferon-induced hypopituitarism, Am J Med 114 (2003) 161–163.
[312] W.B. Chan, C.S. Cockram, Panhypopituitarism in association with interferon-alpha treatment, Singapore Med J 45 (2004) 93–94.
[313] P.J. Tebben, J.L.D. Atkinson, B.W. Scheithauer, D. Erickson, Granulomatous adenohypophysitis after interferon and ribavirin therapy, Endocr Pract 13 (2007) 169–175.
[314] F. Then Bergh, T. Kümpfel, A. Yassouridis, et al., Acute and chronic neuroendocrine effects of interferon-β_{1a} in multiple sclerosis, Clin Endocrinol 66 (2007) 295–303.

SECTION III

PITUITARY TUMORS

CHAPTER

14

Acromegaly

Shlomo Melmed

Pituitary Center, Cedars-Sinai Medical Center, Los Angeles, USA

INTRODUCTION

Acromegaly, a spectacular clinical syndrome of disordered somatic growth and proportion, has intrigued physicians since earliest recorded history. It was, however, only in 1886 that Pierre Marie published the first clinical description of the disorder based on observing two of his patients, and his recognition of five other cases previously described by others [1]. He described the features distinguishing the disorder from myxedema and osteodystrophy and proposed the name "acromegaly." Marie did not recognize the relation of a pituitary tumor to this syndrome until 5 years later when an adenohypophyseal tumor was observed in a patient with acromegaly. In 1900, Benda recognized that pituitary adenomas in patients with acromegaly consisted mainly of adenohypophyseal eosinophilic cells, which he proposed to be hyperfunctioning [2]. Subsequent careful clinicopathologic studies by Cushing, Davidoff and Bailey were supplemented by demonstrating clinical remission of soft tissue signs of acromegaly after surgical resection of eosinophilic pituitary adenomas [3–5]. The experiments of Evans and Long demonstrating features of gigantism in rats injected with anterior pituitary extracts confirmed the association of a pituitary factor with somatic growth [6]. Establishment of the unequivocal link between hyperfunctioning adenoma and acromegaly was the earliest example of a pituitary disorder to be clinically and pathologically recognized and appropriately managed.

Incidence of Acromegaly

Acromegaly is caused by unrestrained secretion of GH and IGF-I (Figure 14.1). Several studies have undertaken a comprehensive ascertainment of acromegaly in the community. In a retrospective survey of the Newcastle region, the prevalence of acromegaly was 38 cases/million, while the annual incidence of new patients was almost 3 cases/million [7]. In Sweden, the annual incidence of new cases was reported at 3.3/million people with a prevalence of 69 cases/million people [8]. In Northern Ireland, the prevalence of acromegaly in 1984 was 63 cases/million, while the annual incidence of newly diagnosed acromegaly was 4 cases/million during the preceding 25 years [9]. More recent studies have indicated an annual incidence rate of up to 10 cases/million population, with a prevalence of more than 75 cases/million in Belgium [10] and in the United Kingdom [11]. Based upon these figures, it is apparent that ~2000 new cases of acromegaly are diagnosed annually in the USA.

Animal Models of Hypersomatotrophism

Transgenic mouse strains bearing either growth-hormone-releasing hormone (GHRH), GH, or IGF-I *trans* genes have enabled elucidation of the respective roles for these three hormones in the development of hypersomatotrophism [12–14]. Expression of a GHRH *trans* gene in mice results in increased somatic growth [14], mammosomatotroph hyperplasia [15] and GH-cell adenomas [16]. In mice bearing a *GH-trans* gene, heterologous GH mRNA is detectable from day 13 of gestation, and marked growth acceleration is evident at about 3 weeks of age [12]. All body organs, except the brain, exhibit increased growth but the liver and spleen undergo disproportionate allometric growth [12]. Therefore, although both GH and IGF-I levels are elevated in these animals, overall body growth and individual organ growth respond in different relative proportions. These observations imply that the pattern of hypersomatotrophic body and organ growth is dependent on at least two variables: external growth factors (e.g., GH

The Pituitary, Third Edition, DOI: 10.1016/B978-0-12-380926-1.10014-8

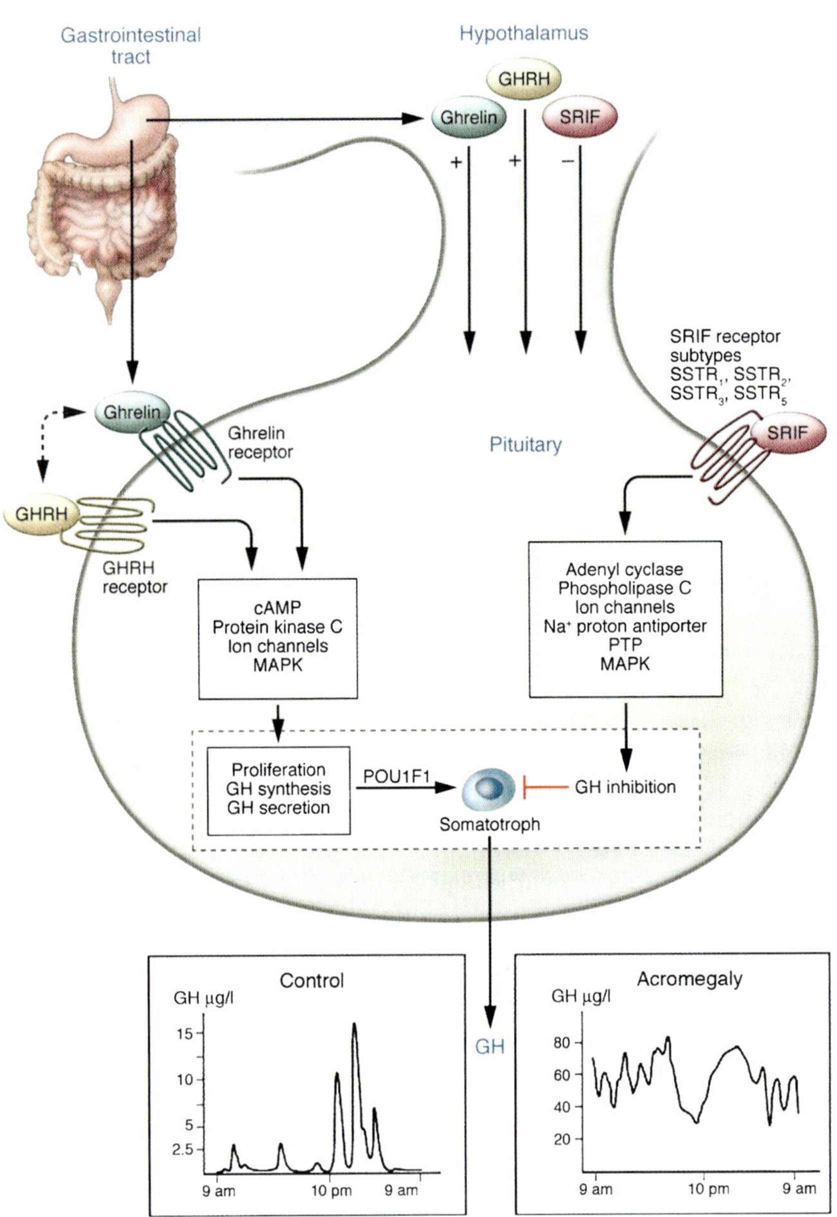

FIGURE 14.1 Normal and disrupted GHRH-GH-IGF-I axis. Pituitary somatotroph cell gene expression and GH synthesis are determined by the POU1F1 transcription factor. Net GH secretion is determined by integration of hypothalamic, nutritional, hormonal and intrapituitary signals. GH synthesis and secretion are induced by hypothalamic GHRH and gut-derived ghrelin. GHRH may also act as a coagonist for the ghrelin receptor [329]. Hypothalamic SRIF suppresses GH secretion mainly by high-affinity binding to somatotroph $SSTR_2$ and $SSTR_5$ receptor subtypes [262]. Somatostatin receptor ligands (SRLs) signal through $SSTR_2$ and $SSTR_5$ to control GH hypersecretion and shrink the tumor mass. GH secretion patterns in a normal subject and in acromegaly are depicted in the insets showing secretory bursts (mainly at night) and daytime secretion troughs. GH receptor antagonist blocks peripheral GH signaling and suppresses IGF-I generation. *Insets modified with permission from Figure 1 in [330]. Reproduced with permission from [21].*

and IGF-1) which stimulate cell division, organ and body weight, while each organ appears to possess specific intrinsic growth potentials that respond to the hormonal environment in achieving final size outcome. In contrast, transgenic mice expressing the human IGF-I gene exhibit selective organomegaly without a profound increase in longitudinal skeletal growth [13]. As these mice had suppressed endogenous GH levels, GH and IGF-I therefore appear to act both independently and synergistically in inducing clinical hypersomatotrophism. Both GH and GHRH transgenic mice also display renal glomerulosclerosis, which is not observed in animals bearing the IGF-I transgene, suggesting that GH acts directly to cause renal mesangial changes. Interestingly, IGF-1, when administered to hypophysectomized rats, does in fact mimic most of the somatic effects of GH by restoring growth [17]. These observations suggest that both GH and IGF-I may independently contribute to the pathologic findings of hypersomatotrophism [18]. Nevertheless, IGF-I is required for GH to achieve a maximally robust bone and tissue response [19].

PATHOGENESIS

Acromegaly may be caused by pituitary tumors or by extrapituitary disorders (Figures 14.1 and 14.2) [20,21].

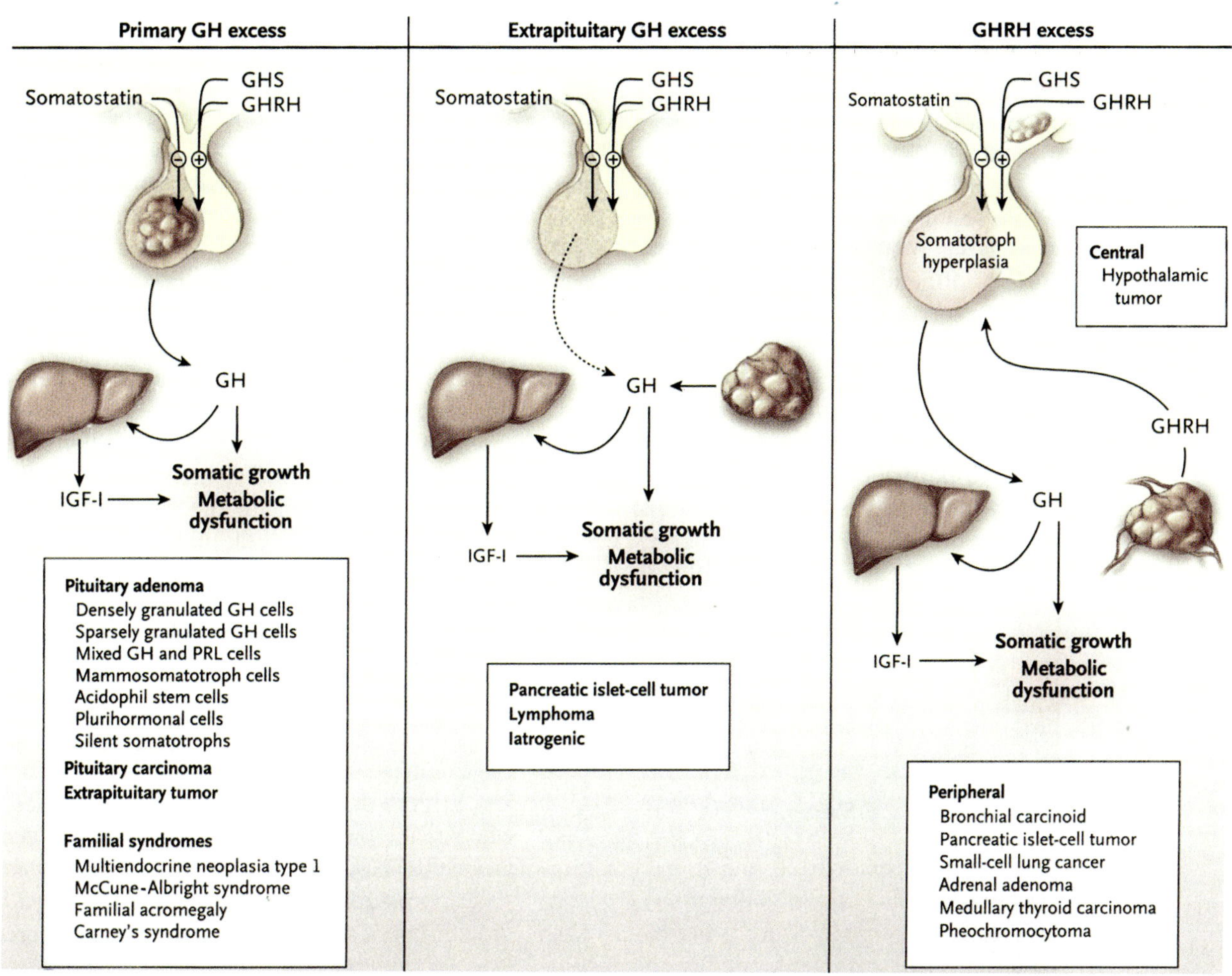

FIGURE 14.2 Causes of acromegaly. Acromegaly is caused by excessive production of growth hormone (GH) or GH-releasing hormone (GHRH). Rarely, the disease is associated with familial syndromes, including multiple endocrine neoplasisa type 1, the McCune-Albright syndrome, familial acromegaly and Carney's syndrome. GHS denotes growth hormone secretagogues and PRL prolactin. *Adapted from [20].*

Regardless of the etiology of the disorder, the disease is characterized by elevated levels of both GH and IGF-I with resultant signs and symptoms of hypersomatotrophism [22].

Pituitary Acromegaly

Over 95% of patients with acromegaly harbor a specific pituitary adenoma type responsible for unrestrained GH secretion, and these are classified according to hormone gene expression, ultrastructural features and cytogenesis [23,24]. These tumors, accounting for ~60% of GH-secreting adenomas, contain either densely or sparsely staining cytoplasmic GH granules. These variants are either slow (densely granulated) or rapidly growing (sparsely granulated) [25]. Mixed GH-cell and prolactin (PRL)-cell adenomas are composed of two distinct cell types, somatotrophs expressing GH and lactotrophs expressing PRL [26,27]. These bimorphous tumors cause acromegaly with moderately elevated serum PRL levels. Acidophil stem cell adenomas are monomorphous tumors arising from the common GH and PRL stem cell expressing both hormones [28], and often contain giant mitochondria and misplaced exocytosis of GH granules. They are often rapidly growing and invasive, and hyperprolactinemia rather than acromegaly may be the predominant presenting feature.

In contrast, monomorphous mammosomatotroph cell adenomas consist of a single mature cell expressing both GH and PRL. Serum PRL levels are usually normal or moderately elevated. Plurihormonal tumors, which are either monomorphous or plurimorphous, may express GH with any combination of PRL, thyroid-stimulating hormone (TSH), adrenocorticotrophic hormone (ACTH), or α-subunit [29,30]. Often, little correlation exists between specific hormone staining of the tumor and peripheral hormone levels. These patients may present with clinical features of acromegaly as well as the effects of the respective elevation of other pituitary trophic hormones. GH cell carcinomas with well-documented distant metastases are exceedingly rare [31]. Despite exhibiting hypercellularity, necrosis, nuclear pleomorphism and mitotic figures, they very rarely metastasize. Although locally invasive somatotropinomas are occasionally aggressive and rapidly growing, they should not be classed as malignant unless definitive proof of distant metastases is present [32].

GH cell hyperplasia is difficult to distinguish histologically from a GH cell adenoma. Hyperplasias usually consist of more than one cell type and silver staining reveals the presence of a well-preserved reticulin network without a surrounding pseudocapsule. The rigid morphologic diagnosis of GH cell hyperplasia has usually been associated with extrapituitary stimulation by GHRH from an extrapituitary tumor causing acromegaly [33].

These tumors [29], while staining positively for the presence of GH, are apparently clinically nonfunctional. Features of acromegaly are absent, although GH and/or PRL levels may in fact be elevated in some of these patients [34]. A putative peripheral GH receptor signaling defect has been postulated to explain the observed absence of hypersomatotrophic signs.

Pathogenesis of Somatotroph Cell Adenomas

Both the hypothalamus and the pituitary contribute to development of acromegaly. Disordered secretion of GHRH or SRIF, with without an intrinsic pituitary cellular defect, may result in adenoma formation [32,35].

DISORDERED GHRH SECRETION OR ACTION

GHRH induces GH gene expression and also induces somatotroph DNA synthesis, cell replication and *c-fos* expression [36]. These growth-promoting actions of GHRH are prevented by SRIF. Somatotroph GHRH action is mediated by activation of adenylate cyclase and increased cyclic adenosine monophosphate (cAMP) levels which stimulate both GH synthesis and adenoma formation. Somatotroph hyperplasia, increased GH secretion and gigantism were observed in mice expressing a pituitary-directed cholera toxin *trans* gene which induced intracellular cAMP [37]. In contrast, mice with inactivated cAMP responses developed dwarfism and low GH secretion [38].

Excess GHRH production by functional hypothalamic tumors or by abdominal or chest neuroendocrine tumors causes somatotroph hyperplasia and occasionally adenoma with resultant unrestrained GH secretion [39], implying hypothalamic hormone involvement in the pathogenesis of GH-cell adenomas and acromegaly. However, histology of most GH-cell adenoma tissue specimens does not reveal hyperplastic somatotroph tissue surrounding the adenoma [40], implying no exogenous hypothalamic overstimulation of the pituitary. GHRH production by extrapituitary tumors causing acromegaly is usually associated with somatotroph cell hyperplasia and elevated GH levels, and paradoxical responses of GH to glucose, thyrotropin-releasing hormone (TRH) and dopamine [41]. These biochemical perturbations revert to normal when the ectopic source of GHRH is removed, suggesting that exposure to high levels of GHRH alters the somatotroph response to other factors regulating GH secretion. Espression of adenoma GHRH receptors, and the failure of GH down-regulation during prolonged GHRH stimulation, also points to a possible role for GHRH in maintaining persistent GH hypersecretion. Intrapituitary and adenoma-derived GHRH correlates with tumor size and activity, implying a paracrine role for GHRH in mediating adenoma pathogenesis [42]. GHRH also modestly stimulates PRL secretion in most acromegaly patients [41]. These observations, coupled with the fact that up to 40% of these patients also have hyperprolactinemia, imply a role for GHRH in the pathogenesis of the disorder. Although SRIF secretion may theoretically be attenuated, thus giving rise to unrestrained GH secretion, TSH responses to TRH in acromegaly are either normal or in fact blunted, suggesting intact SRIF activity. Alternatively, high GH levels in these patients may abnormally autoregulate the somatotroph.

SURGICAL RESPONSES

Postoperative GH testing often remains disordered after initial pituitary tumor resection, suggesting that the hypothalamus is primarily responsible for altered GH secretion and tumor development. However, surgical resection of well-defined GH-secreting tumors (<5 mm) results in a definitive cure of excess hormone secretion in most patients [43,44]. Low postoperative tumor recurrence rates in these patients, together with restoration of most dynamic GH responses after surgery, however, is strongly suggestive of intact hypothalamic function in these patients.

GH SECRETORY PATTERNS

Although basal GH levels are usually high in acromegaly, episodic pulsatile patterns of GH release are apparent, and the nocturnal GH surge is usually preserved [45]. Patients receiving long-acting somatostatin analogues also retain GH pulsatility, suggesting persistent GHRH secretion [46]. Paradoxical GH responses to glucose, dopamine and TRH, and loss of pituitary desensitization to hypothalamic GHRH, however, point to an intrinsic somatotroph abnormality.

DISORDERED SOMATOTROPH CELL FUNCTION

In vitro responses of somatotroph tumor cell cultures exposed to physiologic levels of GHRH, SRIF and IGF-1, are similar to those observed in the limited number of similar studies in normal cultured human pituitary tissue [47]. GH gene expression is stimulated in vitro by GHRH and inhibited by IGF-1, as evidenced by changes in adenoma cells' GH mRNA content [48]. Adenoma tissue also expresses receptors for GHRH, Ghrelin [49] and SRIF [50], but activating mutations of either the GHRH or SRIF receptor have not been reported. Ghrelin also induces proliferation of rat somatotroph tumor cells [51]. These apparently physiologic responses imply intact control of GH gene expression in tumor cells and favor disordered hypothalamic etiology for clinically abnormal GH hypersecretion.

A pre-existing somatotroph cell mutation may be a prerequisite for the abnormal growth response to disordered GHRH secretion or action (Table 14.1). The monoclonal origin of somatotroph adenomas, as determined by X chromosome inactivation analysis of somatotroph tumor DNA [52], suggests that a somatic somatotroph mutation leads to clonal expansion and tumor formation. Autonomous GH secretion by the transformed somatotroph likely ensues as a result of several pathogenetic mechanisms including intrinsic cell cycle dysfunction, altered hormonal and paracrine factors regulating both GH gene expression and secretion, and somatotroph cell growth [21]. An altered Gs (α) protein identified in a subset of GH-secreting pituitary adenomas is characterized by high levels of intracellular cAMP and GH hypersecretion [53]. Point mutations in two critical sites, Arg_{201}, the site for ADP-ribosylation, and Gly_{227}, the GTP-binding domain of Gs (α) proteins, prevent GTPase activity and result in constitutive adenylyl cyclase activation. The tumor contains a dominant mutant Gs (α), termed *gsp*, which recapitulates the effects of GHRH and results in elevated cAMP levels [53]. These activating gsp mutations are present in about 30% of GH-secreting tumors with enhanced tumor adenylyl cyclase activity and lower GH levels than nonmutant-bearing tumors.

Dysregulated pituitary signaling of numerous neurotransmitters and growth factors, including FGF, dopamine, estrogen, FGF and NGF have been identified in pituitary adenomas, but have not uniformly been observed in acromegaly [54]. Overexpressed oncogenes, inactivated tumor suppressor genes, or epigenetic changes associated with GH-secreting adenomas are shown in Table 14.1. Pituitary tumor-transforming gene (PTTG) [55,56] is over-expressed in GH-secreting and other functional pituitary tumors, and its abundance correlates with tumor size and invasiveness [55]. PTTG is the index securin protein, regulating sister

TABLE 14.1 Genes that Contribute to the Molecular Pathogenesis of GH-Secreting Adenomas

Gene	Function	Mode of Activation/ Inactivation	Clinical Context	Specificity for GH-Secreting Pituitary Adenoma
GNAS	Oncogene	Activating, imprinting	Nonfamilial, syndromic or sporadic	Relatively specific
CREB	Transcription factor	Constitutive phosphorylation	Sporadic	Relatively specific
AIP	Tumor suppressor	Inactivating	Familial, syndromic	Relatively specific
MEN1	Tumor suppressor	Inactivating	Familal, syndromic	Not specific
PRKAR1A	Tumor suppressor	Inactivating	Familial, syndromic	Not specific
H-RAS (Harvey rat sarcoma virus oncogene)	Oncogene	Activating	Invasive or malignant	Not specific
CCNB2	Cyclin	Induced by HMGA	Sporadic	Not specific
CCND1 (cyclin D1)	Oncogene	Over-expression	Sporadic	Not specific
HMGA2	Oncogene	Over-expression	Sporadic	Not specific
FGFR4 (FGF receptor 4)	Oncogene	Alternative transcription	Sporadic	Not specific
PTTG	Securin	Over-expression	Sporadic	Not specific
Rb	Tumor suppressor	Epigenetic silencing	Sporadic	Not specific
CDKN1B	CDK inhibitor	Nonsense mutation	Sporadic	Not specific
GADD45γ	Proliferation inhibitor	Epigenetic silencing	Sporadic	Not specific
MEG3	Proliferation inhibitor	Epigenetic silencing	Sporadic	Not specific

Adapted from [21].

chromatid separation during the cell cycle [56], and its over-expression leads to aneuploidy. In contrast, expression of a proapoptotic and growth arrest factor, GADD45γ, is lost in GH-secreting adenomas [57]. Thus, a spectrum of genetic events appears to culminate in somatotroph transformation and adenoma pathogenesis.

Although the somatotroph is clearly transformed, the sequence of events leading to clonal expansion is multifactorial. An activated oncogene(s) may be required for initiating tumorigenesis, while promotion of tumor growth may require permissive GHRH and other growth factor (e.g., bFGF) stimulation. Nevertheless, GH-secreting tumors rarely transform to true malignancy, and their growth restraint is likely reflective of lineage-specific pituitary cell growth arrest and senescence mediated by p21, a CDK inhibitor [58].

EXTRAPITUITARY ACROMEGALY

The source of excessive GH secretion in acromegaly may not necessarily be pituitary in origin [21]. Patients with extrapituitary acromegaly include those with excess ectopic GHRH or GH secretion, and very rarely a putative growth factor disorder termed acromegaloidism (Figure 14.2).

Criteria for Diagnosis of Ectopic Acromegaly

Because ectopic acromegaly requires a different management approach than that recommended for classic pituitary GH hypersecretion, stringent clinical and biochemical criteria should be fulfilled to confirm this diagnosis [59]. These include the demonstration of elevated circulating GHRH or GH levels in the absence of a primary lesion of the pituitary gland, as well as a significant arteriovenous hormone gradient across the ectopic tumor source (Figure 14.3). Excision or functional ablation of the ectopic hormone-producing tumor source should ideally result in biochemical and clinical cure of acromegaly. Tumor tissue should also be shown to express the GHRH or GH gene product by demonstrating specific mRNA expression, hormone biosynthesis and polypeptide immunoreactivity. Patients with nonconventional biochemical, imaging, or clinical features of pituitary acromegaly may inadvertently be diagnosed as harboring a nonpituitary source of excess GHRH or GH secretion, and be inappropriately treated. A definitive diagnosis of the etiology of

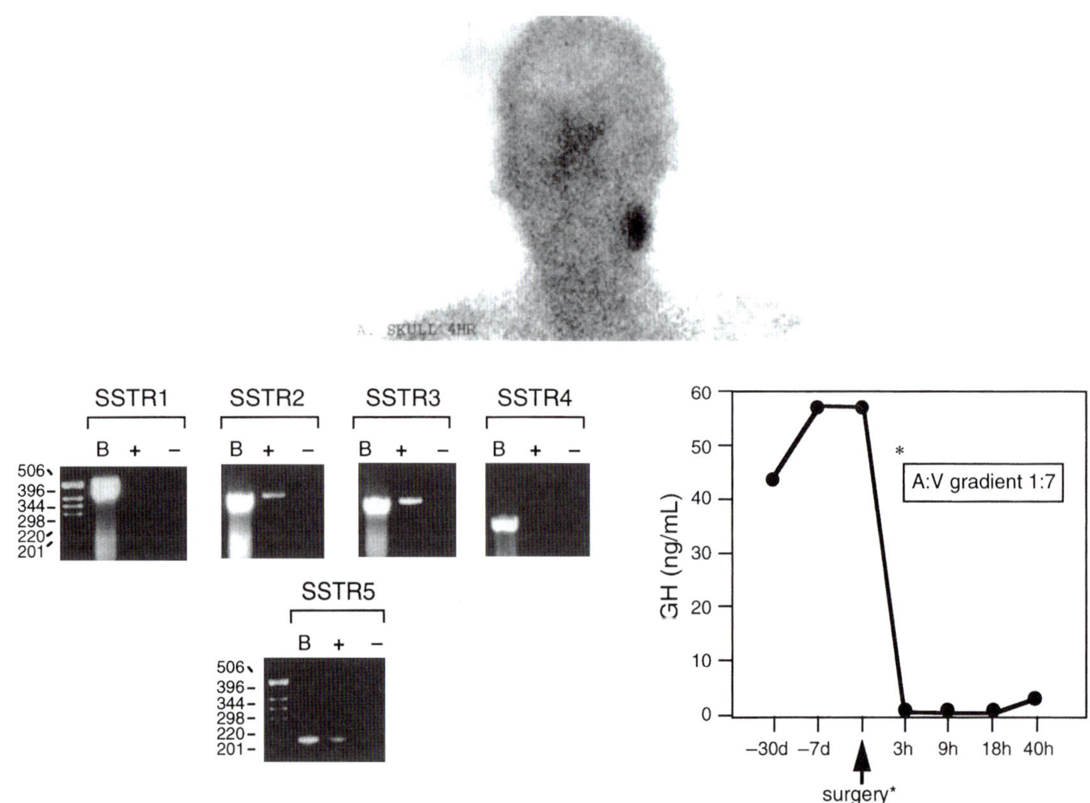

FIGURE 14.3 SSTR receptor scan for diagnosis of ectopic acromegaly. Radiolabeled octreoscan reveals metastatic neck GH-secreting carcinoma which expresses SSTR2, SSTR3 and SSTR5 receptors. Mass resection normalizes GH levels within 3 hours. *From [89].*

hypersomatotrophism should therefore be made prior to instituting acromegaly therapy.

GHRH Hypersecretion

HYPOTHALAMIC

Hypothalamic GHRH is secreted into the portal system, impinges upon the somatotroph cells, binds to specific surface receptors, and elicits intracellular signals that modulate pituitary GH synthesis and/or secretion [60]. Hypothalamic tumors, including hamartomas, choristomas, gliomas and gangliocytomas may produce excessive GHRH with subsequent GH hypersecretion and resultant acromegaly [40]. These patients may have somatotroph hyperplasia, or very rarely a pituitary GH-cell adenoma, supporting the notion that excess hypothalamic GHRH leads to pituitary hyperplasia and subsequent adenoma formation. As patients reported with hypothalamic acromegaly have all usually undergone resection of the adenomatous or hyperplastic pituitary, definitive proof of a primary hypothalamic tumor causing acromegaly may be elusive. Pituitary mammosomatotroph hyperplasia with no evidence for pituitary adenoma or an extrapituitary tumor source of GHRH has been described in a young child with gigantism [61].

PERIPHERAL

GHRH is synthesized and expressed in multiple extrapituitary tissues [62–64]. Excessive peripheral production of GHRH by a tumor source would therefore be expected to cause somatotroph cell hyperstimulation and increased GH secretion. The structure of hypothalamic GHRH was in fact elucidated from material extracted from pancreatic GHRH-secreting tumors in two patients with acromegaly [33,65]. Immunoreactive GHRH is present in several tumors, including carcinoid tumors, pancreatic cell tumors, small-cell lung cancers, adrenal adenomas and pheochromocytomas which have been reported to secrete GHRH. Acromegaly in these patients, however, is uncommon. In a retrospective survey of 177 patients with acromegaly only a single patient was identified with elevated plasma GHRH levels [66]. The association of acromegaly with carcinoid tumors had been recognized prior to the characterization of hypothalamic GHRH [67–69]. Carcinoid tumors comprise most of the tumors associated with ectopic GHRH secretion, the majority bronchial in origin [70–77]. Pancreatic cell tumors, small-cell lung cancers, adrenal adenoma, pheochromocytoma, medullary thyroid, endometrial and breast cancer have also rarely been described to express GHRH and cause acromegaly [33,74–80]. Although most patients with carcinoid tumors do not exhibit clinical features of acromegaly, many of these tumors do in fact express immunoreactive GHRH and manifest abnormal GH-secretory dynamics [78]. The observed high incidence of GHRH expression and low incidence of acromegaly in these patients may be due to disordered GHRH tissue processing, or to impaired GHRH bioactivity.

Most carcinoid tumors are slow-growing, with insidious development of acromegaly. These patients present with features of classical acromegaly, accompanied by elevated circulating GH and IGF-I levels. Patients also often experience systemic effects, obvious metastatic disease, or other humoral effects of the carcinoid syndrome [76]. Following surgical removal, GH levels fall and soft tissue signs of acromegaly regress. The pituitary often shows evidence of somatotroph hyperplasia with preserved reticulin network. A true GH-cell adenoma with distorted reticulin network may also occassionally be present.

TREATMENT

Surgical resection of the tumor secreting ectopic GHRH should reverse GH hypersecretion, and pituitary surgery should not be required in these patients. Nonresectable, disseminated, or recurrent carcinoid syndrome with ectopic GHRH secretion can also be managed medically with long-acting somatostatin analogues [81]. Administration of the analogue lowers circulating GH and IGF-I levels, and also suppresses ectopic tumor elaboration of GHRH [74–76,82–85]. The drug suppresses both pituitary GH as well as the peripheral tumor source of GHRH, thus attenuating the deleterious effects of chronic hypersomatotrophism [86].

GH Hypersecretion

ECTOPIC PITUITARY ADENOMAS

Embryonal pituitary development involves dorsal migration of fetal adenohypophyseal cells. Functional pituitary adenomas secreting GH may arise from ectopic pituitary remnants in the sphenoid sinus and wing, petrous temporal bone and the nasopharyngeal cavity [87,88]. Residual tumor cells may also be dislodged after neurosurgical resection of invasive pituitary adenomas and give rise to subsequent recurrent ectopic adenomas. Very rarely, pituitary carcinoma may spread to the meninges, cerebrospinal fluid, or cervical lymph nodes, resulting in functional GH-secreting metastases which may also be diagnosed by radiolabeled octreotide imaging (octreoscan) (Figure 14.3) [89].

PERIPHERAL GH-SECRETING TUMORS

Immunoreactive GH has been identified in normal human tissues, including liver, kidney, lung, colon, stomach and brain [90]. Extracts of lung adenocarcinoma, breast cancer and ovarian tissues also contain immunoreactive GH without clinical evidence of acromegaly [91]. A GH-secreting intramesenteric pancreatic islet cell tumor was associated with acromegaly [59], as was a non-Hodgkins lymphoma [92]. Ectopic GH secretion by the pancreatic tumor was unambiguously confirmed by high arteriovenous tumor gradient of GH, normalization of GH and IGF-I after tumor resection, positive GH immunoperoxidase staining, demonstration of in vitro GH synthesis and release, and expression of GH mRNA. Postoperative GH suppression after glucose and stimulation by GHRH were intact. Based on the features of this unique case, the very rare patients with ectopic GH secretion would be expected to exhibit a normal-sized or small pituitary gland and normal GHRH levels.

Acromegaloidism

Patients who manifest clinical features of acromegaly but do not harbor a demonstrable pituitary or extrapituitary tumor have been termed "acromegaloid." An exhaustive evaluation for acromegaly should be undertaken prior to patients being diagnosed as acromegaloid. These patients exhibit soft tissue and skin changes usually associated with acromegaly and some may even have bony features of the disorder, and occasionally hyperglycemia. GH and IGF-I levels are apparently normal and respond appropriately to dynamic pituitary testing. Pachydermoperiostosis should be considered in the differential diagnosis. Unique growth factor activity, partially characterized by bioassay, was described in the sera of these patients [93], and insulin resistance and defective IGF-I binding were demonstrated in cells derived from two patients with acromegaloidism and acanthosis nigricans [94].

Genetic Syndromes

Several genetic syndromes associated with acromegaly or gigantism have been described (Table 14.2).

McCune-Albright Syndrome

Polyostotic fibrous dysplasia, cutaneous cafe-au-lait pigmentation, sexual precocity, hyperthyroidism, hypercortisolism, hyperprolactinemia and acromegaly comprise a rare hypersecretory endocrinopathy [95], McCune-Albright syndrome (OMIM 1748000). Postzygotic *GNAS* mutations lead to a mosaic tissue-specificity which results in GH, and rarely TSH, hypersecretion. Few of these patients exhibit definitive evidence for a pituitary adenoma, although most dynamic GH responses are indistinguishable from patients harboring GH-secreting somatotroph adenomas. In four of eight patients, Gα mutations were detected in both endocrine and nonendocrine organs [96]. Management of GH

TABLE 14.2 Familial Pituitary Tumor Syndromes

Syndrome	Gene (locus)	Most Frequent Mutation(s)	Pituitary Features	Other Key Features
MEN1	MEN1 (11q13)	c.249-252delGTCT, an exon 2 predicted frameshift, in 4.5%	Pituitary adenoma in 30–40% (PRL 60%, NFA 15% GH, 10%, ACTH 5%, TSH rare)	Primary hyperparathyroidism, pancreatic tumors, foregut carcinoid tumors, adrenocrotical tumors (usually nonfunctional), rarely pheochromocytomas, skin lesions (facial angiomas, collagenomas and lipomas)
MEN1-like (MEN4)	CDKN1B (12p13)	Only two reported cases	Pituitary adenoma	Primary hyperparathyroidism and single cases reported of renal angiomyolipoma, neuroendocrine cervical carcinoma
Carney complex	PRKAR1A (17q23-24)	c.491-492delTG in exon 5	Pituitary hyperplasia in most patients, adenoma in ~10% (GH and PRL)	Atrial myxomas, lentigines, Schwann-cell tumors, adrenal hyperplasia
Familial, isolated pituitary adenomas	AIP[c] (11q13.3)	Gln14X nonsense mutation[e]	Pituitary adenoma (majority GH, PRL or mixed GH and PRL)	NR

Only two reported cases to date: one GH-secreting and on ACTH-secreting adenoma.
[c]AIP mutations reported in 15% of individuals with familial isolated pituitary adenoma and 50% of those with isolated familial somatotrophinomas. [e]This is the most commonly identified mutation, but is likely to be over-represented secondary to a Finnish founder effect.
Adapted from [322].

hypersecretion in these patients includes medical treatment with somatostatin analogues, or pituitary irradiation.

MULTIPLE ENDOCRINE NEOPLASIA

GH-cell pituitary adenoma causing acromegaly is a well-documented component of the autosomal dominant multiple endocrine neoplasia I (MEN I) syndrome which also includes parathyroid and pancreatic tumors (OMIM131100). The disorder is associated with germ cell inactivation of the MENIN tumor suppressor gene which maps to chromosome 11q13 [97,98], leading to development of endocrine tumors. About 40% of these patients harbor pituitary tumors including prolactinomas or GH-secreting adenomas, and rarely ACTH- or TSH-secreting adenomas [99]. Rarely, functional pancreatic tumors in MENI also express excess circulating GHRH [100]. A germline mutation in the *CDK 1B* inhibitor has also been described in a family with features of a recessive MEN-1-like phenotype [101], which includes acromegaly and parathyroid adenomas.

Carney Complex

This syndrome, which comprises spotty skin pigmentation, mucosal and cardiac myxomas, and acromegaly (OMIM160908), is associated with elevated somatotroph protein kinase A levels. These patients usually harbor an inactivating *PRKARIA* mutation on chromosome 2p16 [102].

Familial Acromegaly

In rarely encountered families with familial isolated pituitary adenomas, gigantism or acromegaly may affect young patients with mostly macroadenomas (Table 14.5) [103–105]. These families, which predispose to isolated cases of acromegaly and/or gigantism, harbor a mutation in chromosome 11q13, which has been mapped to the aryl hydrocarbon receptor-interacting protein (AIP) gene in ~15% of such patients [106–108].

Gigantism

The diagnosis of pituitary gigantism should be considered in children who are >3 standard deviations (SD) above normal mean height for age, or >2 SDs over their adjusted mean parental height. The biochemical diagnosis is similar to that for acromegaly, i.e., GH levels are in excess of 1 μg/L after a glucose load and serum IGF-I concentrations are elevated. Gigantism may be caused by a variety of conditons (Table 14.3) [109]. Familial tall stature, redundancy of Y chromosomes, Marfan's syndrome and homocystinuria should be excluded prior to considering the endocrine causes of tall stature. About 20% of patients with gigantism are associated with the McCune-Albright syndrome, with somatotroph hyperplasia or true pituitary adenomas. Somatotroph hyperplasia and acidophilic stem cell adenomas have been reported in cases of gigantism beginning in infancy or early childhood, suggesting early hypersecretion of GHRH or disordered pituicyte cell differentiation accounts for the hypersomatotrophism [61,109]. In children undergoing pubertal growth spurts, however, GH response to glucose may be paradoxical and serum IGF-I concentrations are often physiologically elevated. If pituitary imaging reveals the presence of an adenoma, it should be resected surgically. Somatostatin analogues with or without dopamine agonists and pegvisomant have successfully been employed in treating these children [110–113]. Radiation therapy should be considered for failed responses to surgery and medical treatment.

CLINICAL FEATURES OF ACROMEGALY

Acromegaly manifestations may be due to either central pressure effects of the pituitary mass or peripheral actions of excess GH and IGF-1 (Table 14.4). Central features of the expanding pituitary mass are common to all pituitary masses. They include headache, visual dysfunction due to chiasmal compression, and rarely hypothalamic and frontal lobe dysfunction. The headache is often severe and sometimes debilitating. Lateral extension may impinge upon cranial nerves III, IV and VI with diplopia, or nerve V leading to facial pain; temporal lobe invasion may also occur. Inferior extension of the mass may cause cerebrospinal fluid rhinorrhea and nasopharyngeal sinus invasion [114]. These local signs are especially important in acromegaly, as

TABLE 14.3 Causes of Tall Stature

Genetic
Familial
Sex chromosome redundancy
Marfan's syndrome
Homocystinuria
Neurofibromatosis
Endocrine – metabolic
Growth hormone-secreting pituitary adenomas or hyperplasia
Hyperinsulinism
Lipoatrophic diabetes
Hyperthyroidism
Prepubertal sex steroid excess
Unclassified – cerebral gigantism

Adapted from [109].

TABLE 14.4 Clinical Features of Acromegaly

Local tumor effects	Visceromegaly
Pituitary enlargement	Tongue
Visual-field defects	Thyroid gland
Cranial-nerve palsy	Salivary glands
Headache	Liver
Somatic systems	Spleen
Acral enlargement, including thickness of	Kidney
soft tissue of hands and feet	Prostate
Musculoskeletal system	Endocrine-metabolic
Gigantism	Reproduction
Prognathism	Menstrual abnormalities
Jaw malocclusion	Galactorrhea
Arthralgias and arthritis	Decreased libido, impotence, low sex-hormone-binding globulin
Carpal tunnel syndrome	Multiple endocrine neoplasia type 1
Acroparesthesia	Hyperparathyroidism
Proximal myopathy	Pancreatic islet cell tumors
Hypertrophy of frontal bones	Carbohydrate
Skin and gastrointestinal system	Impaired glucose tolerance
Hyperhidrosis	Insulin resistance and hyperinsulinemia
Oily texture	Diabetes mellitus
Skin tags	Lipid
Colon polyps	Hypertriglyceridemia
Cardiovascular system	Minerals
Left ventricular hypertrophy	Hypercalciuria, increased levels of 25-hydroxyvitamin D_3
Asymmetric septal hypertrophy	Urinary hydroxyproline
Cardiomyopathy	Electrolyte
Hypertension	Low renin levels
Congestive heart failure	Increased aldosterone
Pulmonary system	Thyroid
Sleep disturbances	Low thyroxine binding-globulin levels
Sleep apnea (central and obstructive)	Goiter
Narcolepsy	

Adapted from [20].

most series report a relatively higher preponderance of macroadenomas (>65%) in acromegaly [115].

GH Action in Acromegaly

Although several intracellular mechanisms act to attenuate GH receptor signaling [116,117], high GH levels observed in acromegaly overwhelm these intracellular buffers and lead to complex gene expression patterns controlling cell proliferation, glucose metabolism and growth factor functions.

An inframe deletion of exon 3 in the GH receptor (d3-GHR) appears to enable increased intracellular signaling and accelerated growth ensuing from enhanced GH responsiveness [118]. Acromegaly patients harboring this polymorphism exhibit a more florid clinical phenotype with increased prevalence of osteoarthritis, dolichocolon and polyps [119]. The polymorphism also correlates with discordant GH/IGF-I treatment responses [120] and persistent biochemical resistance to pituitary-directed treatment [121]. Conversely, responsiveness to the GH receptor antagonist appears to be enhanced by the presence of the deletion [122].

Effects of Excessive GH Secretion

The protean clinical manifestations of hypersomatotrophism are caused by elevated GH and/or IGF-I levels (Table 14.4). Effects of hypersomatotrophism on acral and soft tissue growth, as well as metabolic function, may occur insidiously over several years (Table 14.5) (Figures 14.4–14.6) [123,124]. The elusiveness of the symptomatology often results in the disease being diagnosed only when patients seek care for dental, orthopedic, or rheumatologic disorders. Only 13% of 256 acromegalic patients diagnosed during a 20-year period presented with primary symptoms of altered facial appearance or enlargement of extremities [125]. In a review of several hundred patients worldwide, 98% were reported with acral enlargement, while hyperhidrosis was prominent in 70% [123]. Morever, the time between onset of symptoms and diagnosis of acromegaly ranges from 6.6–10.2 years, with a mean delay of almost 9 years [7]. The latency period to time of diagnosis appears to have shortened, likely reflective of enhanced physician awareness, availability of more sensitive diagnostic tools, and increased use of MRI which unmasks incidentally discovered pituitary adenomas [124].

TABLE 14.5 Presentation of Acromegaly

Presenting Chief Complaint	Frequency (%)
Menstrual disturbance	13
Change in appearance/acral growth	11
Headaches	8
Paresthesias/carpal tunnel syndrome	6
Diabetes mellitus/impaired glucose tolerance	5
Heart disease	3
Visual impairment	3
Decreased libido/impotence	3
Arthropathy	3
Thyroid disorder	2
Hypertension	1
Gigantism	1
Fatigue	0.3
Hyperhidrosis	0.3
Somnolence	0.3
Other	5
Chance (detected by unrelated physical or dental examination or X-ray)	40
Total	100

From [123] based on 310 patients.

Generalized visceromegaly occurs with enlargement of the tongue, bones, salivary glands, thyroid, heart, liver and spleen. Clinically apparent hepatosplenomegaly, however, is rare. Patients have characteristic facial features, large fleshy nose, spade-like hands and frontal bossing. Some patients, if presenting early, may have subtle facial and peripheral features. Serial review of old photographs often accentuates the progress of these subtle physical changes [126]. Increase in shoe, ring, or hat size is commonly reported. Although skeletal muscle mass is largely unchanged in acromegaly, the nonsmooth-muscle lean compartment is increased [127]. Mechanisms underlying metabolic adaptation to maintaining steady state protein mass include enhanced protein breakdown synthesis rates, with intact protein oxidation [128].

Skeletal Changes

Progressive acral changes, if untreated, lead to severe facial and skeletal disfigurement especially if the excess GH secretion begins prior to closure of the epiphyses [129–131] (Figure 14.6).

Periosteal new bone formation in response to IGF-I [132] results in skeletal overgrowth leading to mandibular overgrowth with prognathism, maxillary widening, teeth separation, frontal bossing, jaw malocclusion and overbite, and nasal bone hypertrophy. Characteristic voice deepening with a sonorous resonance occurs because of laryngeal hypertrophy and enlarged paranasal sinuses.

Arthropathy occurs in about 70% of patients, most of whom exhibit objective signs of joint swelling, hypermobility and cartilaginous thickening [133,134]. Up to half of patients experience joint symptoms severe enough to limit or impair daily activities [135,136]. Severe joint pain unusually signifies irreversible joint degeneration. Knees, hips, shoulders, lumbosacral joints, elbows and ankles are affected in decreasing order of frequency. Joint involvement may be mono- or polyarticular and although crepitus, stiffness, tenderness and hypermobility are common, joint effusions are rarely encountered [137].

Local periarticular fibrous tissue thickening may cause subsequent joint stiffening, deformities and nerve entrapment. Neural enlargement, local fluid retention and swelling of wrist soft tissues may lead to carpal tunnel syndrome, a painful edematous entrapment median neuropathy, which occurs in up to half of all patients. This condition generally resolves early after treatment [138]. In patients with uncontrolled GH and

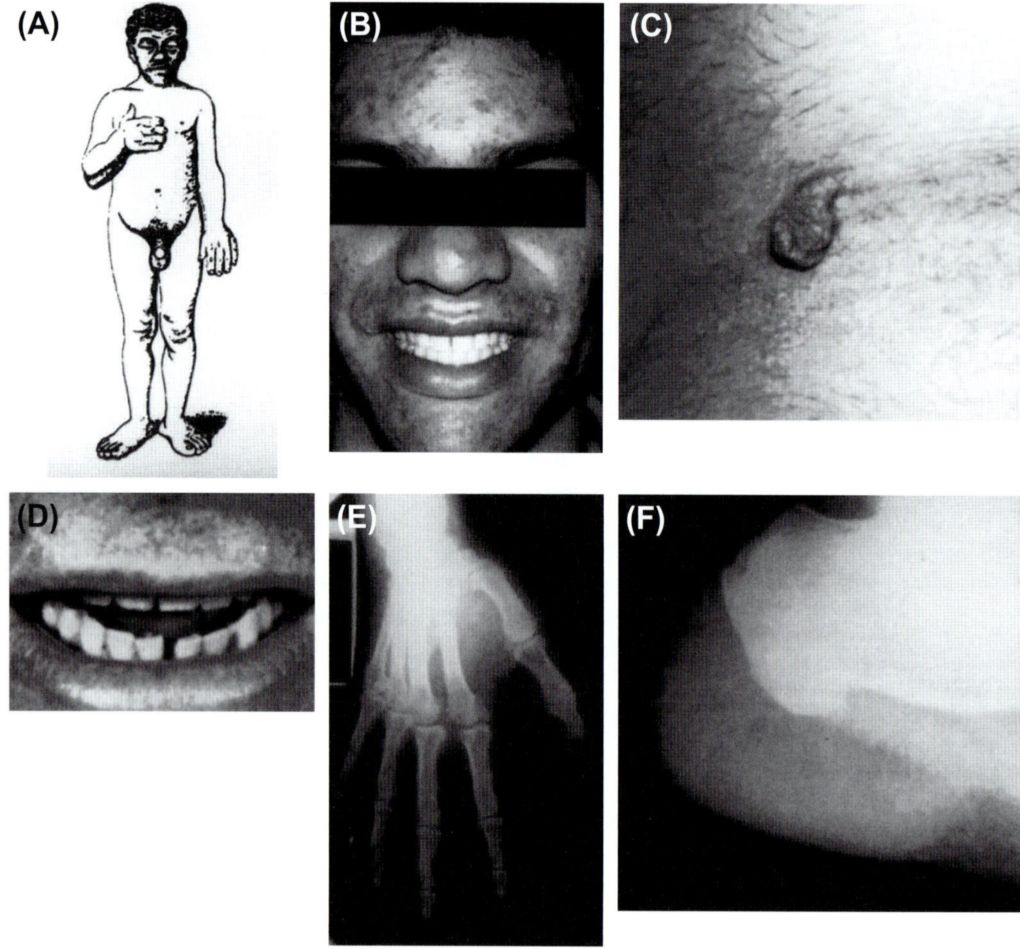

FIGURE 14.4 Clinical signs of acromegaly. (A) Original figure depicting earliest illustration of clinical features of acromegaly by Minkowski in 1887. Note acromegalic facies, fleshy fingers and toes, and frontal bossing. (B) Acromegaly in a young male with active perspiration, oily skin, acne and widened tooth gap. (C) Prominent skin tags may be associated with the presence of colon polyps. (D) Jaw overbite and widening of spaces between incisors due to mandibular growth in acromegaly. (E) X-ray image of bony "tufting" seen at ends of terminal phalanges indicates bony overgrowth. (F) Increased heel pad thickness. *(D) and (F) from [331].*

IGF-I levels, spinal involvement including osteophytosis, disc space widening and increased anteroposterior vertebral length may lead to dorsal kyphosis scoliosis, and vertebral fractures [139]. About 70% of patients exhibit large-joint and axial arthropathy, including synovitis and periarticular calcifications [134,140,141]. Vertebral fractures in men appear to ensue on a background of prolonged osteoporosis [142].

PATHOLOGY OF ARTHROPATHY

Uneven chondrocyte proliferation with subsequent increased joint space occurs early in response to increased GH and IGF-I levels. Ulcerations and fissures on the weight-bearing areas of new cartilage are often accompanied by new bone formation. This process eventually results in debilitating osteoarthritis associated with bone remodeling, osteophyte formation, subchondral cysts, narrowed joint spaces and lax periarticular ligaments. Osteophytes are seen at the tufts of the phalanges and over the anterior aspects of spinal vertebrae. Ossification of ligaments and periarticular calcium pyrophosphate deposition are also found [134]. The duration of hypersomatotrophism appears to directly correlate with the severity of the joint changes [143], and responses to therapy (see below) will usually depend upon the degree of irreversible cartilage degeneration already in place.

Skin Changes

Hyperhidrosis and oily skin with an unpleasant odor are common early signs, occurring in up to 70% of patients. Patients often relate the need to increase their use of deodorant or cosmetic powders. Facial wrinkles, nasolabial folds and heel pads are increased in thickness, and body hair may become coarsened [144,145]. These effects may correlate with IGF-1 levels and improve after treatment. Thickening of the skin has been attributed to glycosaminoglycan deposition [146], while connective

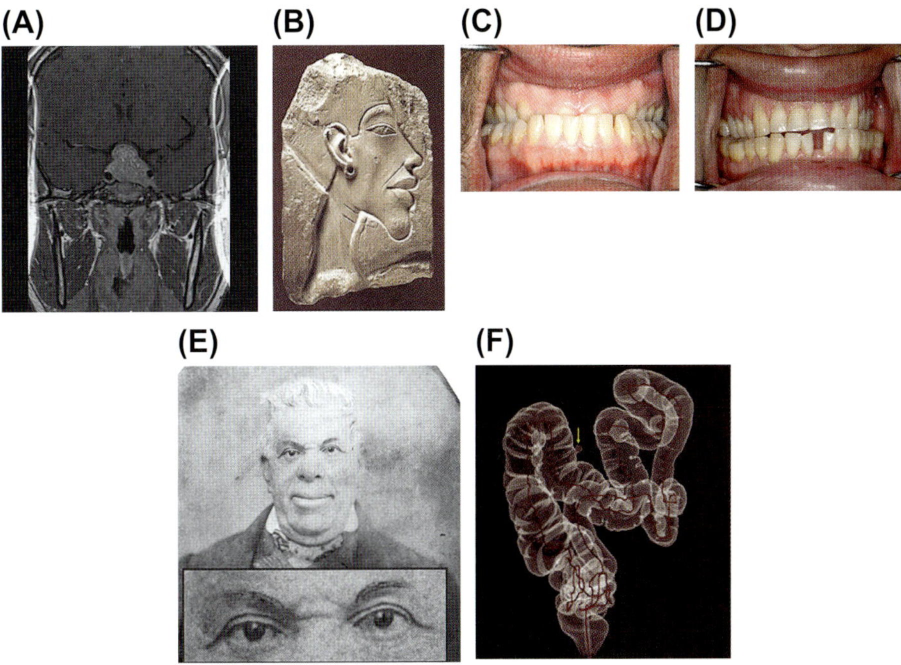

FIGURE 14.5 Clinical signs of acromegaly. (A) MRI of GH-secreting pituitary macroadenoma depicting lateral tumor extension into cavernous sinus, and dorsal elevation of optic chiasm (coronal image). (B) Limestone portrait of Egyptian Akhenaten ca. 1365 BC showing jaw prognathism and thickened lips. *Reproduced with permission from http://commons.wikimedia.org/wiki/file:reliefportraitofakhenaten01.png and source: Staatliche Museen Zu Berlin-Preufsicher Kulturbesitz, Agyptisches Museum.* (C) Jaw prognathism and mandibular overbite and (D) widened incisor tooth gap in two acromegaly patients. (E) Governor Pio Pico of California in 1858. Note acromegaly facial features and mild left proptosis consistent with cavernous sinus tumor invasion [332]. (F) Dolicomegacolon in acromegaly as visualized by CT colonography. Colonic centerline is red, and yellow arrow indicates a diverticulum of the transverse colon. *Reproduced with permission [191], and from Melmed [21].*

tissue collagen production is also increased [147,148]. Skin tags are common and these may be important markers for the concomitant presence of adenomatous colonic polyps [149]. Raynaud's phenomenon may also be present in up to one-third of patients.

Cardiovascular Complications

Cardiovascular disease is a major cause of morbidity and mortality [147,150–152] with symptomatic cardiac disease present in up to 60% of patients. Arrhythmias, hypertension, valvular disease, and sodium and fluid

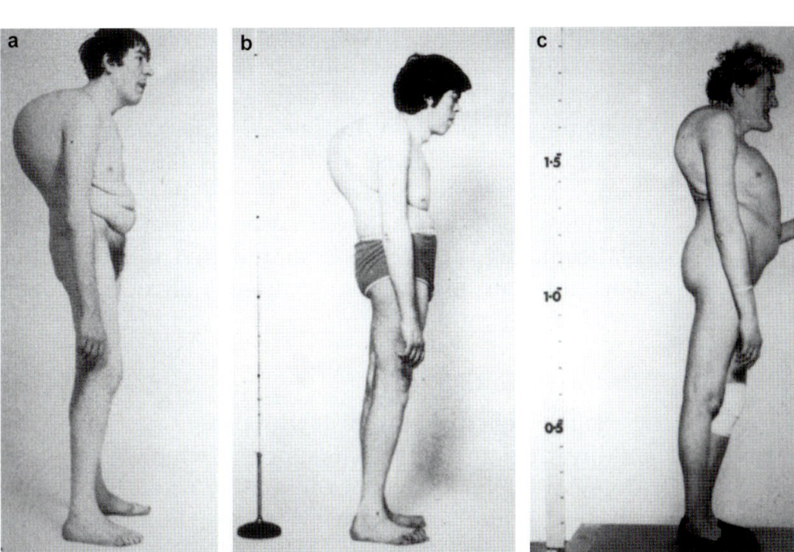

FIGURE 14.6 Severe skeletal disfigurement in three patients with growth hormone-secreting pituitary tumors. *From [129].*

retention leading to expanded extracellular fluid volume, are common manifestations. Overall, the constellation of glucose intolerance, hypertension, arrhythmias and diastolic overload may lead to intractable heart failure, especially if rigorous biochemical acromegaly control is not achieved [21]. About half of all patients are at "intermediate-to-high" risk for coronary atherosclerosis [153]. Nevertheless, in a 5-year prospective report of 52 patients, calcium scores and results of myocardial SPECT perfusion indicated no major coronary arterial changes from expected controls. Furthermore, acute ischemic events were not observed in this cohort [154].

About half of patients with active acromegaly have hypertension, and 50% of these have evidence of left ventricular dysfunction [155]. Interestingly, left ventricular hypertrophy is also reported in 20% of young normotensive patients, and in up to 90% of those with longstanding disease. Increased postexercise ventricular ejection fraction is observed in ~70% of patients [151,156]. Assymmetric septal hypertrophy is common and concentric myocardial hypertrophy develops, with associated diastolic heart failure if GH levels are not controlled [157]. Subclinical left ventricular diastolic dysfunction is consistent with unique pathologic findings including myocardial hypertrophy, interstitial fibrosis and lymphocytic myocardial infiltrates. Electrocardiograms are abnormal in about 50% of patients, with S-T segment, T-wave abnormalities, conduction defects and arrhythmias accounting for most changes. Hypertension has been ascribed to plasma volume expansion and increased cardiac output [158], and GH also exerts direct antinatriuretic effects. GH acts to induce transepithelial sodium transport at the aldosterone-sensitive distal nephron, and induces transcription of the cortical collecting duct epithelial sodium channel α-subunit [159]. Although heart failure is usually reversible with SRIF analogue treatment, aortic and mitral valve regurgitation and hypertension usually persist despite biochemical disease control [160].

Cardiovascular disease is the most important cause of mortality in acromegaly, accounting for ~60% of deaths [150]. The presence of cardiovascular disease at the time of diagnosis is associated with high mortality rates, and effective control of GH and IGF-I levels improves cardiac function [156].

Respiratory Complications

Prognathism, thick lips, macroglossia and hypertrophied nasal structures may result in significant airway obstruction [161,162]. Additional clinical features of acromegaly contribute to impaired upper respiratory function. Irregular hypertrophy of laryngeal mucosa and cartilage may lead to unilateral or bilateral vocal cord fixation or laryngeal stenosis with accompanying voice changes [161]. Tracheal calcification and cricoarytenoid joint arthropathy may also be present. These obstructive features may necessitate tracheostomy either to maintain adequate baseline airway function, or especially at the time of surgical anesthesia. Difficulty in tracheal intubation is often encountered in patients undergoing anesthesia. Central respiratory center depression as well as upper airway obstruction may contribute to the development of paroxysmal daytime sleep (narcolepsy), sleep apnea and habitual excessive snoring. Obstructive sleep apnea, characterized by excessive daytime sleepiness with at least five nocturnal episodes of obstructive apnea per hour has been documented in >50% of patients [163–165]. These patients may also have a ventilation–perfusion defect with hypoxemia. The sleep apnea of acromegaly may be due to either obstruction of the respiratory tract, or may be central in origin [166]. Interestingly, the central form of sleep apnea is associated with higher GH and IGF-I levels, possibly reflecting a loss of central somatostatin tone accounting for the disorder [163,167].

Neuromuscular Changes

Peripheral acroparesthesias occur in almost half of all patients. Synovial edema and hyperplastic wrist ligaments and tendons contribute to painful median nerve compression with resultant carpal tunnel syndrome [168]. A true symmetrical peripheral neuropathy occurs, and this rare mixed motor and sensory impairment should be distinguished from diabetic neuropathy which may occur secondarily to acromegaly. The pathologic features of median neuropathy have been ascribed to increased edema, rather than extrinsic compression [138]. About half of all patients develop proximal myopathy which may be accompanied by myalgias and cramps and nonspecific electromyogram (EMG) myopathic changes. Histologic examination reveals hypertrophy and necrosis of skeletal muscle fiber in patients with proximal muscle weakness and elevated creatine phosphokinase (CPK) levels [169]. Although bony overgrowth of frontal bones may mask eye changes, true exophthalmos may be present. Open angle glaucoma may also result from impaired aqueous filtration through hypertrophied tissue surrounding the canal of Schlemm.

Psychologic Changes

Self-esteem may diminish with progressive facial and bodily disfigurement. It is unclear whether reported depression, mood swings and apathy result from these physical effects or whether they are intrinsic central effects of high GH levels. There is no clear evidence for an increased incidence of psychologic disorders in acromegaly [170,171].

ACROMEGALY AND DEVELOPMENT OF NEOPLASMS

Several benign and malignant tumors have been reported in association with acromegaly and retrospective studies have indicated a three-fold increased risk for gastrointestinal malignancies [172,173]. Nevertheless, a compelling cause–effect relationship of acromegaly with cancer has not been established [174–188]. Although coexistence of acromegaly and meningioma has been reported, meningiomas are known to develop at sites of previous head trauma, inflammation, or irradiation [189]. No association has been reported between acromegaly and other intracranial neoplasms.

Reports of a high prevalence of colonic polyps in acromegaly may reflect increased physician awareness in screening for these tumors, as well as the use of diagnostic colonoscopy. Prospectively, ~45% of patients with acromegaly harbor colonic polyps, but a controlled study in 161 patients revealed no increased polyp incidence in acromegaly [187]. Acrochordons (skin tags) have been noted in most patients found to harbor colonic lesions [149,175]. However, serum levels of GH or IGF-I and the presence of colonic polyps do not correlate [175]. Hypertrophic mucosal folds, colonic hypertrophy, dolichocolon and slow colonic transit times are commonly encountered, and intestinal bacterial overgrowth has been attributed to autonomic dysfunction [190]. Colonoscopy is warranted in these patients once every 3–5 years after diagnosis, depending on the presence of other risk factors. Timely diagnosis and resection of premalignant polyps is therefore prudent for improved morbidity in this relatively high-risk group of patients. On repeat colonoscopy, colon polyp prevalence correlated with IGF-I levels [188]. Computed tomography has also been advocated in light of the technical challenges posed by colonoscopy in acromegaly [191].

Thus, the body of evidence suggests that mortality from colon cancer is largely related to GH levels, rather than the observed enhanced incidence of the disease in acromegaly (Tables 14.6 and 14.7). In a large survey of 1362 patients in the UK, cancer incidence was in fact lower than expected, and the observed enhanced colon cancer mortality in acromegaly correlated with GH levels [192]. As patients with acromegaly are living longer due to improved biochemical control, it is apparent that long-term prospective controlled studies are required to resolve this question, as the incidence of malignancy increases with aging.

TABLE 14.6 Predictors of Mortality

Predictors of Mortality
Growth hormone level >2.5 μg/L
Elevated insulin-like growth factor 1 level
Hypertension
Age
Time of delay from diagnosis
Male gender
Prior pituitary radiotherapy
ACTH-dependent adrenal insufficiency
Treatment with hydrocortisone >25 mg per day

Adapted from [262].

TABLE 14.7

Acromegaly and cancer incidence: Multicenter analysis

			Person-years	Cancers		
A.		n	at risk	Observed	O/E	p
	Females	95	1351	8	1.33	ns
	Males	128	1630	5	1.30	ns
	Total	223	2981	13	1.3	
B.		4822	21740	178	0.76–3.4	na

A. Multicenter analysis of cancer incidence in patients with acromegaly ranging in age from 1–79 years. *Adapted from [185].*
B. Analysis of nine retrospective published reports (1956–1998) of cancer incidence in patients with acromegaly. *Included are data from [7,8,125,173,185,201,323,324].* O/E, Observed/expected ratio.

Endocrine Complications

Elevated serum PRL levels, with or without galactorrhea, occur in about one-third of patients, some of whom present with PRL levels >100 μg/L [115,193]. Several mechanisms may underlie hyperprolactinemia in acromegaly. Functional pituitary stalk compression by an adenoma may prevent hypothalamic dopamine from impinging upon pituitary lactotrophs, resulting in release from tonic hypothalamic inhibition [193]. GH-secreting adenoma types may also concomitantly secrete PRL, including mixed GH-cell and PRL-cell plurihormonal adenomas, monomorphous mammosomatotroph adenomas, and acidophilic stem cell adenomas [29]. In patients with galactorrhea and normal PRL levels, elevated GH concentrations may crossreact and behave as an agonist for PRL-binding sites in the breast. Hypopituitarism, which develops as a result of the tumor mass compressing surrounding normal pituitary tissue, leads to amenorrhea or impotence [115,194], while up to 20% of patients may also have secondary thyroid or adrenal failure. Gonadal function is also an important determinant of bone density in these patients.

Carbohydrate intolerance is caused by direct anti-insulin effects of GH, and patients may develop insulin-requiring diabetes mellitus or microalbuminuria [195]. Carbohydrate intolerance and insulin requirements improve remarkably after lowering of GH by surgery or somatostatin analogue therapy. Hypertriglyceridemia (type IV), hypercalciuria and hypercalcemia are commonly found [196]. Pituitary hypersecretion of associated hormones by mixed somatotroph tumors commonly results in hyperprolactinemia, and rarely in Cushing's disease (ACTH hypersecretion) or hyperthyroidism (TSH hypersecretion). IGF-I is a determinant of thyroid cell growth [197] leading to diffuse or nodular toxic or nontoxic goiter, or Graves' disease [198].

Associated manifestations of MEN I may be present in affected individuals. These include hypercalcemia with hyperparathyroidism or pancreatic tumors. Benign prostatic hypertrophy has been documented with no apparent increase in prostate cancer rates [199].

Morbidity and Mortality

Increased acromegaly mortality (~ three-fold), is mostly attributed to cardiovascular, cerebrovascular and respiratory abnormalities [200] has been reported [7,8,147,150, 192,201–205]. In a retrospective study reported in 1966, 50% of patients were reported who succumbed before the age of 50, with cardiovascular disease being the most common cause of death (Table 14.8). In 194 patients with acromegaly, a reduced life expectancy was found, with cardiovascular disorders accounting for 24% of deaths followed by respiratory (18%) and cerebrovascular disease (14%). Diabetes mellitus, found in 20% of patients, was associated with 2.5 times the predicted risk of death, while hypertension had been present in 45% of patients with acromegaly [7,8,150]. Significant independent determinants of mortality include serum GH levels >2.5 μg/L, elevated age-matched serum IGF-1 levels, and the presence of pre-existing heart disease [206]. As achieving optimal biochemical control may be challenging, rigorous diagnosis and treatment of comorbidities that contribute to mortality is important. Hypertension and diabetes mellitus are amenable to early interventions, which have likely contributed to the observed trend of reduction in mortality rates more recently reported [207]. Other variables which increase mortality include hypertension, age at diagnosis, time delay for diagnosis, male gender, previous pituitary irradiation and the presence of pituitary failure, especially ACTH insufficiency. In the West Midlands Acromegaly database, mortality rates were increased in 226 men and 275 women with acromegaly over a 14-year median follow-up period (SMR 1.7, 95% CI 1.4–2.0, $p < 0.001$) as compared with the general population [208]. Mortality rates were also higher in patients who had received radiotherapy (SMR 2.1, 95% CI 1.7–2.6, $p = 0.006$). While cardiovascular and cerebrosvascular diseases contributed to overall increased mortality, cerebrovascular disease was the major cause of death in patients who had undergone radiotherapy (Table 14.8). In another study, 211 acromegaly patients receiving

TABLE 14.8 Studies Assessing the Role of Pituitary Radiotherapy in Mortality in Patients with Acromegaly

First Author, Year	No. of Patients	RR	SMR	RR	Comments
Biermasz, 2004	164	57 CRt	NA	1.73 (0.77–3.86); age and sex adjusted, 1.169 (0.52–2.65)	Cause of death not known
Holdaway, 2004	208	143 CRT, 35 Yttrium	NA	NA	No increase in stroke mortality
Ayuk, 2004	419	211 CRT	DXT group, 1.58 (1.22–2.04); $p = 0.005$	1.67 (1.1–2.56); $p = 0.02$	Cerebrovascular SMR = 4.42
Kauppinen-Makelin, 2005	334	116 CRT	DXT group, 1.69 (1.05–2.58); non-DXT, 0.94 (0.62–1.37); $p < 0.001$	2.27 ($p = 0/08$)	6/8 stroke deaths
Mestron, 2005	1219	504 CRT, 27 stereotactic radiotherapy, 9 radiosurgery	HR 2.29 (1.03–5.08)	NA	Cerebrovascular mortality data NA
Sherlock, 2009	501	220 CRT, 17 Yttrium/ radiosurgery	2.1 vs. 1.4 for non-DXT ($p = 0.006$)	1.8 ($p = 0.008$)	Cerebrovascular SMR 4.1

RR,risk ratio; SMR, standardized mortality rate; HR, hazard ratio; CRT, conventional radiotherapy.
Adapted from [325].

TABLE 14.9

Post-treatment GH Levels and Mortality in Acromegaly

Mortality	Post-treatment GH (ng/mL) <2.5 n=541	2.5–9.9 n=493	>10 n=207	p
Overall	1.10 (0.89–1.15)	1.41 (1.16–1.69)	*2.12* (1.70–2.62)	<0.0001
Cancer-related	0.96 (0.63–1.41)	0.81 (0.50–1.24)	*1.81* (1.13–2.74)	<0.05

Post-treatment GH levels correlate with mortality in acromegaly. Standardized mortality ratios are depicted for overall mortality and for cancer-related mortality.
Adapted from Orme et al J Clin Endocrinol Metab 1998 [192].

pituitary-directed radiotherapy were shown to exhibit high mortality rates (SMR 1.58, 95% CI 1.22–204, p = 0.005), predominately as a result of cerebrovascular disease (SMR 4.42, 95% CI 2.71–7.22, p = 0.005) [209]. Both ACTH deficiency and use of high doses of hydrocortisone replacement (>25 mg per day) increased mortality relative risk, mostly attributed to increased cardiovascular disease [208]. Thus, multiple factors independently increasing mortality rates (Table 14.6) should be considered at diagnosis and follow-up of a patient with acromegaly. Early diagnosis of comorbidities, tight biochemical control of growth hormone and IGF-I levels, normalization of blood pressure, early detection and treatment of adrenal insufficiency with doses of hydrocortisone <25 mg per day should contribute to reduced mortality rates. Cerebrovascular and cardiovascular disorders and diabetes mellitus should be addressed early and aggressively.

Control of GH levels to <2.5 μg/L after surgery or medical treatments appears to generally reverse adverse mortality rates [202,203] and it is apparent that tight biochemical control of acromegaly significantly reduces both morbidity and mortality (Table 14.9).

DIAGNOSIS

The biochemical diagnosis of acromegaly requires demonstration of central autonomous GH hypersecretion, as well as elevated IGF-I levels reflecting systemic peripheral exposure to tonically elevated GH levels [210]. Basal a.m. and random GH levels are elevated in acromegaly [211–213]. Because of the episodic nature of GH secretion, however, serum concentrations may normally fluctuate from "undetectable" up to 30 μg/L [214]. When GH is sampled every 5 minutes, GH levels are undetectable in about half of samples collected over 24 hours [213,215]. In acromegaly, however, samples collected over 24 hours contain detectable levels of GH (>2 μg/L) [171,201], while mean 24-h integrated GH levels <2.5 μg/L usually exclude the diagnosis of acromegaly [216].

Although episodic basal GH secretion patterns are sustained in acromegaly, normal diurnal variation is absent with a loss of sleep-related rise in GH [217]. These patients exhibit a higher episodic GH pulse frequency which often persists after surgical adenoma resection. In acromegaly, serum GH levels invariably do not suppress to <1 μg/L within 1–2 hours of an oral glucose (75 g) load; glucose may actually stimulate GH secretion in about 10% of patients [197]. Thus, biochemical exclusion of acromegaly requires a random GH <0.4 μg/L or a GH nadir during OGTT of <1 μg/L, both of with measured normal IGF-I levels (Table 14.10) [217–219].

Using ultrasensitive GH assays, nadir GH levels <0.3 μg/L after a glucose load accurately distinguish patients with active acromegaly from those controlled, or those without disease [220,221]. With these highly sensitive assays, random GH levels in patients with acromegaly may be <1.0 μg/L, and even as low as 0.37 μg/L when IGF-I levels are still elevated postoperatively (Figure 14.7) [222]. Serum IGF-I levels are invariably high in acromegaly [223] and are reflective of a biomarker for integrated GH secretion. Age-matched IGF-I elevations may persist for several months postoperatively when GH levels are apparently controlled [224]. As pregnancy and late puberty are associated with elevated IGF-I levels, a high IGF-I value is highly specific for acromegaly in the nonpregnant adult and correlates with clinical indices of disease activity (Figures 14.8 and 14.9) [223]. IGFBP-3 levels are usually elevated, but provide little added diagnostic value [225,226].

In summary, the challenges of accurate biochemical diagnosis include the pulsatile pattern of GH secretion, sleep-related GH elevations, age, BMI and nutritional-related changes in GH levels. Patients with malnutrition, liver disease, renal failure, or uncontrolled diabetes may all fail to suppress GH after a glucose load. GH and IGF-I measurements are also beset by poor reproducibility and standardization (Table 14.11) [227–229]. These challenges were exemplified in a study which reported that nadir GH levels after OGTT varied widely by ~50%, and in 30% of subjects the diagnosis of acromegaly was inconsistently validated [230].

TABLE 14.10 Diagnosis of Acromegaly

Random GH >0.4 μg/L and elevated age-matched IGF-I levels
OR
GH nadir during OGTT >1 μg/L

From [197].

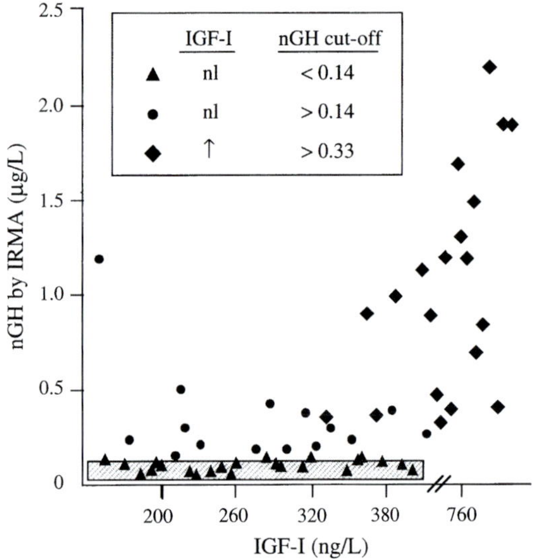

FIGURE 14.7 Ultrasensitive GH immunoradiometric assay distinguishes acromegaly status in postoperative patients. *Adapted from [222].*

TABLE 14.11 Factors Resulting in Discordant Circulating IGF-I and GH Values

Unreliable or imprecise definition of "normal" GH values
Delayed normalization of IGF-I levels following therapeutic intervention
GH secretory pattern that more effectively stimulates IGF-I production
Persistently elevated and erratic GH pulse frequency following treatment
Contribution of local IGF-I production to circulating IGF-I levels
Variable sensitivity and reproducibility of assays employed

Adapted from [224].

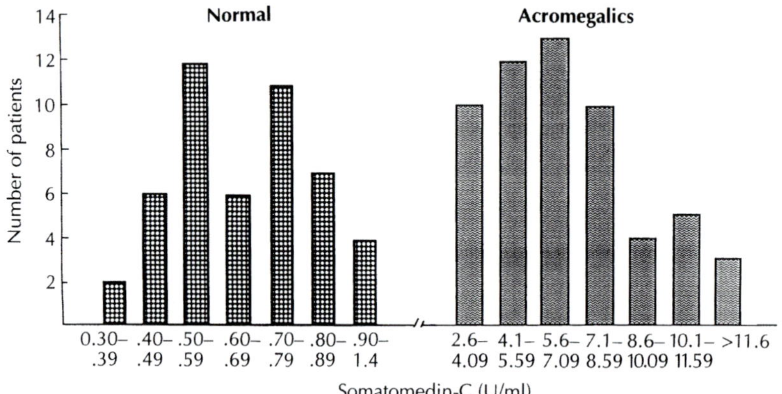

FIGURE 14.8 Circulating insulin-like growth factor-I levels in acromegaly. *From [202].*

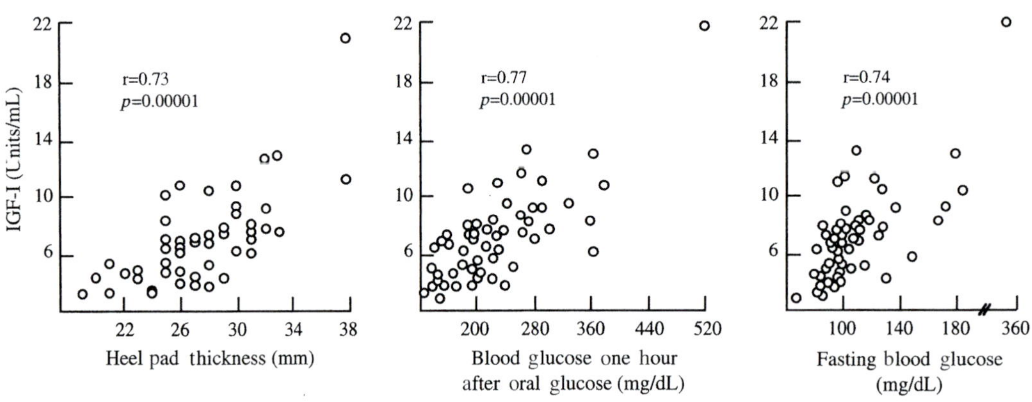

FIGURE 14.9 IGF-I levels correlate with indices of clinical activity in acromegaly. *Adapted from [223].*

Once the biochemical diagnosis of autonomous GH hypersecretion has been established, a pituitary MRI with administration of contrast material should be performed.

Differential Diagnosis of Acromegaly

The approach to diagnosis of the various forms of acromegaly [22] is outlined in Figure 14.10. Over 95% of patients harbor a GH-secreting pituitary adenoma [22]. The very rare diagnosis of extrapituitary acromegaly should only be considered in a small number of patients, but is important in planning effective management. Regardless of the cause, GH and IGF-I levels are invariably elevated and GH levels fail to suppress (<1 μg/L) after an oral glucose load in all forms of acromegaly [231]. Patients with clinical features of acromegaly, normal GH and IGF-I levels and no evidence for extrapituitary tumor likely represent "burned out" acromegaly associated with an infarcted pituitary adenoma, often with resultant empty sella. Discordant circulating IGF-I and GH levels may be encountered (Table 14.12), and these may reflect poor assay precision, or persistently elevated bioactive GH levels despite apparent appropriate glucose suppression [218]. Dynamic pituitary tests are not helpful in distinguishing GH-secreting pituitary tumors from extrapituitary tumors [232]. However, measuring GHRH plasma

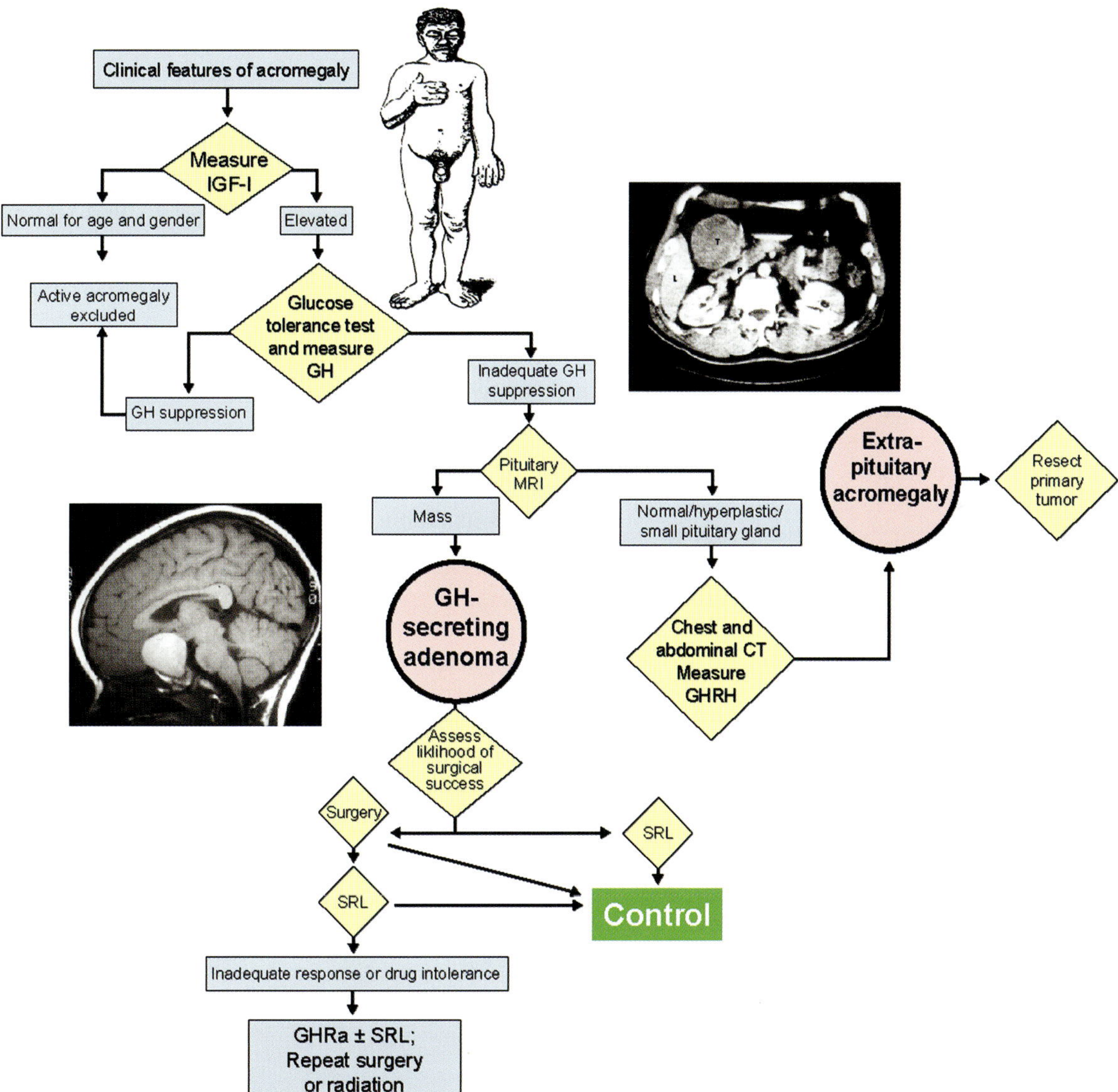

FIGURE 14.10 Diagnosis and treatment of acromegaly. The oral glucose-tolerance test is performed with 75 g of glucose and growth hormone (GH) measured over a period of 2 hours. Disease control implies a nadir level of less than 1 ug of GH per liter after the glucose-tolerance test and an age-adjusted normal IGF-I level. IGF-I, insulin-like growth factor I; MRI, magnetic resonance imaging; CT, computed tomography; SRL, somatostatin receptor ligand; GHRa, GH receptor antagonist; SRL, SRIF receptor ligand. *Modified from [20].*

TABLE 14.12 Effective Management of Growth Hormone-secreting Adenomas

Suppress autonomous GH secretion to <1 ng/ml after a glucose load
Normalize IGF-I levels to age- and gender-matched controls
Remove or reduce pituitary tumor mass
Correct visual and neurologic defects
Preserve pituitary trophic hormone function
Treat acral, cardiovascular, pulmonary and metabolic complications
Prevent systemic sequelae of long-term hypersomatotrophism
Prevent biochemical or local recurrence
Restore mortality rates to expected age-matched controls

is precise and cost-effective for the diagnosis of ectopic acromegaly.

Unique and unexpected clinical features in acromegaly, including respiratory wheezing or dyspnea, facial flushing, peptic ulcers, or renal stones will sometimes be helpful in alerting the physician to diagnosing associated nonpituitary endocrine tumors. Specific biochemical markers of an underlying ectopic tumor (including hypoglycemia, hyperinsulinemia, hypergastrinemia and rarely hypercortisolism) are not usually encountered in pituitary acromegaly, and their presence should alert the physician to search for an extrapituitary source of GH excess.

Anatomical localization of the pituitary or extrapituitary tumor is achieved using imaging techniques, including magnetic resonance imaging (MRI) and computed tomography (CT) scanning. As routine abdominal or chest imaging will yield a very low incidence of true positive cases of ectopic tumor, such screening of these patients is not recommended as being cost-effective. Elevated circulating GHRH levels, a normal- or small-sized pituitary gland, or clinical and biochemical features of other tumors known to be associated with extrapituitary acromegaly are indications for extrapituitary imaging. An enlarged pituitary is, however, often found on the MRI of patients with peripheral GHRH-secreting tumors, and the radiological diagnosis of a pituitary adenoma may be difficult to exclude.

Exceedingly rare miscellaneous conditions associated with acromegaly, including acromegaloidism and McCune-Albright syndrome should be considered only after definitive exclusion of pituitary and extrapituitary tumors.

TREATMENT OF ACROMEGALY

Aims

A strategy for managing patients with acromegaly should aim to comprehensively manage the pituitary mass, suppress hypersecretion of GH and IGF-I, and prevent long-term sequelae of hypersomatotrophism (Table 14.12) [231]. The mortality associated with untreated or partially treated acromegaly is about double the expected mortality rate of age-matched healthy subjects, and it is therefore important to achieve optimally effective GH control. Elevated GH levels per se are associated with increased morbidity and account for the single most important determinant of mortality (Figures 14.11–14.13) [150,192,202,203].

Goals of Therapy

An effective management strategy for patients with acromegaly should address the comprehensive goals of eliminating morbidity and reducing mortality rates to those expected for age- and sex-adjusted control populations (Table 14.12).

1. Selective resection or shrinkage of the pituitary tumor should be accompanied by correction of associated parasellar local pressure effects, and growth recurrence of the pituitary mass should ideally be prevented.
2. Anatomic or functional ablation of the disordered pituitary mass should not compromise residual

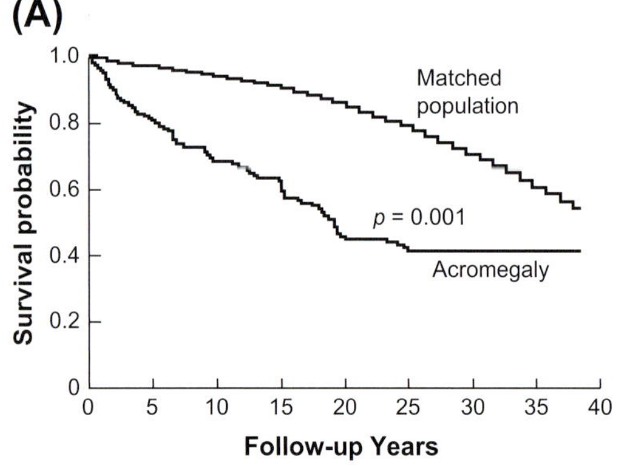

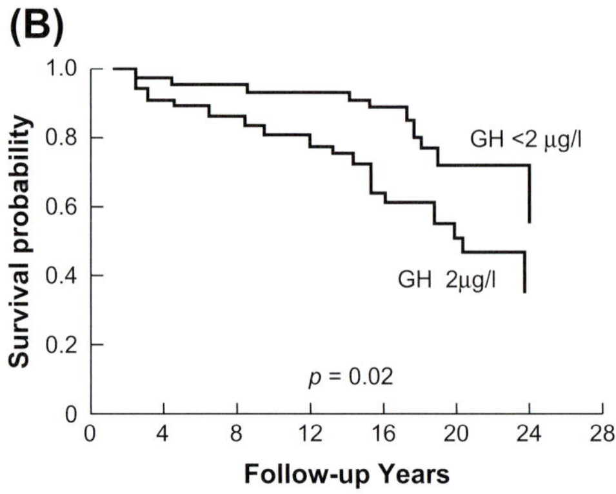

FIGURE 14.11 Survival of patients with acromegaly is diminished (A), and is largely determined by GH levels (B). *Adapted from [333].*

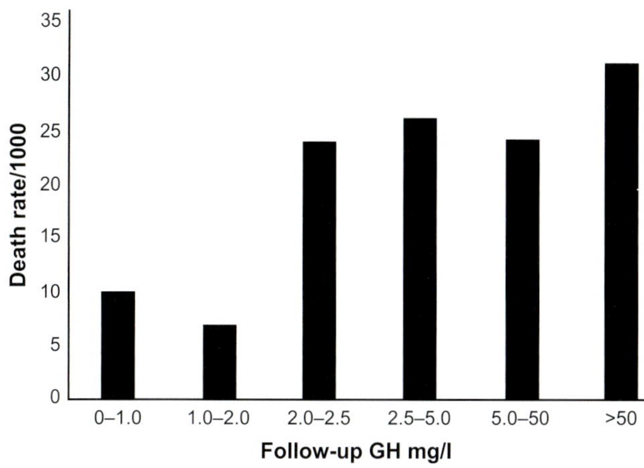

FIGURE 14.12 Death rates per 1000 in patients with acromegaly related to post-treatment GH levels. *Adapted from [209].*

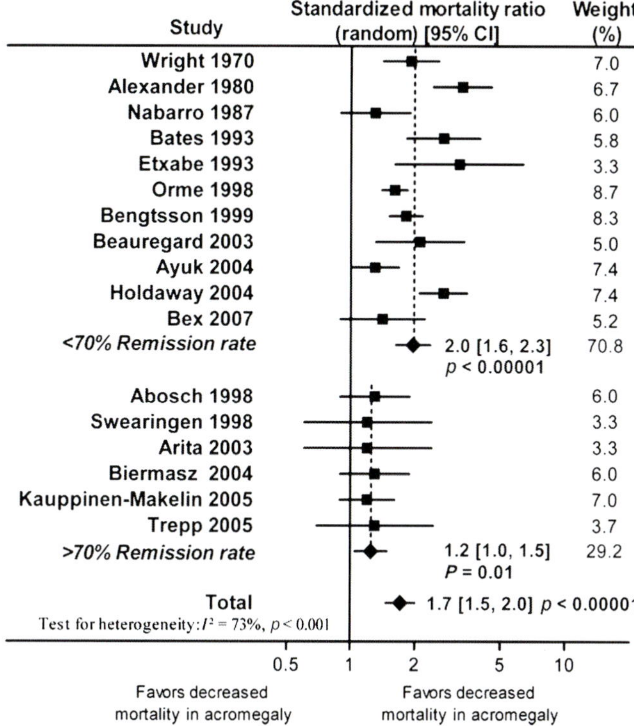

FIGURE 14.13 Pooled standardized mortality ratios (SMRs) in studies of acromegaly. Data are SMR (95% confidence interval). *Reproduced from [200].*

anterior pituitary trophic function, especially the adrenal, thyroid and gonadal axes.

3. The morbid effects of hypersomatotrophism, including glucose intolerance, hypertension, soft tissue swellings, nerve entrapments and arthritis should be ameliorated or reversed. These disorders are often neglected in the context of specialized neurosurgical or endocrine management, which tends to rely on objective radioimaging or hormone assay criteria. As patients with acromegaly are living longer, their metabolic, acral and soft tissue manifestations require rigorous diagnosis and management, if they cannot in fact be prevented.
4. Integrated 24-hour GH secretion and IGF-I levels should be normalized, and postoperatively, serum GH levels should be suppressed to <1 ng/ml after an oral glucose load. Ideally, a "cured" patient should have "normal" 24-hour integrated GH secretion of GH, restored circadian rhythm and exhibit appropriate responses of GH to provocative stimuli. Long-term adverse implications of mildly elevated (1–2.5 μg/L) integrated GH levels are presently unclear.
5. Long-term follow-up should ideally be aimed at preventing both biochemical and anatomical recurrences. Early detection of undesirable late sequelae of hypersomatotrophism is essential to prevent irreversible systemic changes including cardiovascular disorders, debilitating arthritis and diabetes mellitus.

The three therapeutic modes currently available for management of acromegaly, including surgery, irradiation and medical treatment, in and of themselves do not comprehensively fulfill these goals. Their respective side effects and complications also require careful consideration when choosing an appropriate therapeutic strategy (Table 14.13).

Surgical Management

Selective transsphenoidal surgical resection often with minimally invasive endoscopic techniques, is the indicated treatment for well-circumscribed somatotroph cell adenomas (Figure 14.14) [1]. The uses of the operative microscope, microinstrumentation, sophisticated head immobilization techniques and accurate MRI localization have all combined to achieve a high level of expert success with this procedure [233]. Residual pituitary function is usually intact after resection of well-encapsulated tumors that are totally confined within the pituitary fossa. These resections are technically challenging, compounded by microscopic lesions situated in anatomically inaccessible confined sellar spaces, the proximity of vital vascular and brain structures, and the location of dural tumor microfoci, which persistently hypersecrete GH. Safe surgical access may also be impeded by internal carotid artery tortuosity or microaneurysms. Surgery reverses the signs of preoperative compression and the compromised trophic hormone secretion is often restored. The success of surgery is largely dependent upon the expertise and experience of the neurosurgeon. The skilled surgeon will balance the extent of maximal tumor tissue removal with the need to preserve anterior pituitary function, especially when resecting large invasive tumors. Metabolic

TABLE 14.13 Acromegaly Management. The Goals of Acromegaly Management Include: (1) The Control of GH and IGF1 Secretion and Tumor Growth; (2) Relief of Compressive Effects on Central Nervous System and Vascular Structures, if Present; (3) Preserve or Restore Pituitary Hormone Reserve Function; and (4) Treat Comorbidities and Normalize Mortality Rates

	Surgery	Radiotherapy	SRL	GHR Antagonist
Mode	Transsphenoidal resection	Non-invasive	Monthly injection	Daily injection
Biochemical control – GH<2.5 μg/L	Macroadenomas <50% Microadenomas >80%	~50% in 10 years	~65%	0
– IGF1 normalized	Macroadenomas <50%	<30%	~65%	90%
Onset	Microadenomas >80%	Slow (yrs)	Rapid	Rapid
Tumor mass	Rapid Debulked or resected	Ablated	Growth constrained or tumor shrinks ~50%	Unknown
Disadvantages:				
Hypopituitarism	~10%	>50%	None	Low IGF1
Other	Tumor persistence or recurrence, diabetes insipidus, local complications	Local nerve damage, 2nd brain tumor, visual and CNS disorders, cerebrovascular risk	Gallstones, nausea, diarrhea	Elevated liver enzymes

Adapted with permission from [20,21].

dysfunction and soft tissue swelling start improving almost immediately, as GH levels return to normal levels within hours of successful tumor resection. Surgical outcome can usually be correlated with the size of the adenoma and preoperative serum GH level. In patients with tumors less than 5 mm in diameter and totally confined to the sella, and in whom preoperative serum GH levels are <40 ng/ml, a favorable surgical response is portended. Overall, long-term biochemical control is achieved in ~70% of patients undergoing surgical resection of well-circumscribed microadenomas <10 mm in diameter [43]. In constrast, <50% of all-sized macroadenomas had postoperative GH levels <2 ng/ml after glucose (Table 14.14) [44,234]. Unique surgical problems encountered in acromegaly include difficulties in endotracheal intubation due to macroglossia and/or kyphosis [235]. Rarely, tracheostomy may be required for anesthesia.

Side Effects of Surgery

New hypopituitarism develops in up to ~30% of patients undergoing transsphenoidal surgery, reflecting operative damage to the surrounding normal pituitary tissue [236]. Although often transient, these complications may require lifelong pituitary hormone replacement. Permanent diabetes insipidus, cerebrospinal fluid leaks, hemorrhage and meningitis occur in up to 10% of patients. Secondary empty sella may also develop postoperatively. The incidence of local complications depends upon the size of the tumor and the extent of local invasiveness. Experienced pituitary surgeons report significantly lower postoperative complication rates [236]. Recurrence (~7% over 10 years) or persistence of acromegaly after surgery usually indicates incomplete surgical removal of adenomatous tissue, inaccessible cavernous sinus tissue, or nesting of functional tumor tissue within the dural sellar lining which is difficult to visualize and resect. Rarely, surgical "failures" may require reoperation.

Radiation Treatment

Conventional external deep X-ray therapy as well as heavy-particle (proton-beam) irradiation is employed as primary or adjuvant therapies for acromegaly [237]. High-energy ionizing radiation can be delivered to the pituitary tumor by megavoltage radiation sources [238–243]. Factors important in balancing maximal tumor radiation with minimal soft tissue damage include precise MR image localization, effective simulation and isocentral rotational techniques, and high-voltage (6–15 MeV) delivery. Indications for use of radiation as primary therapy is a highly individualized choice, depending upon the expertise and experience of the treating radiotherapist, as well as the willingness of the patient to choose the benefits of the therapy vs. its potential risks. Patients undergoing conventional radiation therapy are administered up to 5000 rads in split doses of 180 rad fractions divided over 6 weeks. Tumor growth is invariably arrested and most pituitary adenomas shrink [243]. GH levels begin falling gradually during the first year after treatment. After 10 years, ~50% of patients having undergone radiation achieve GH levels <2 μg/L and normalized IGF-I levels [237].

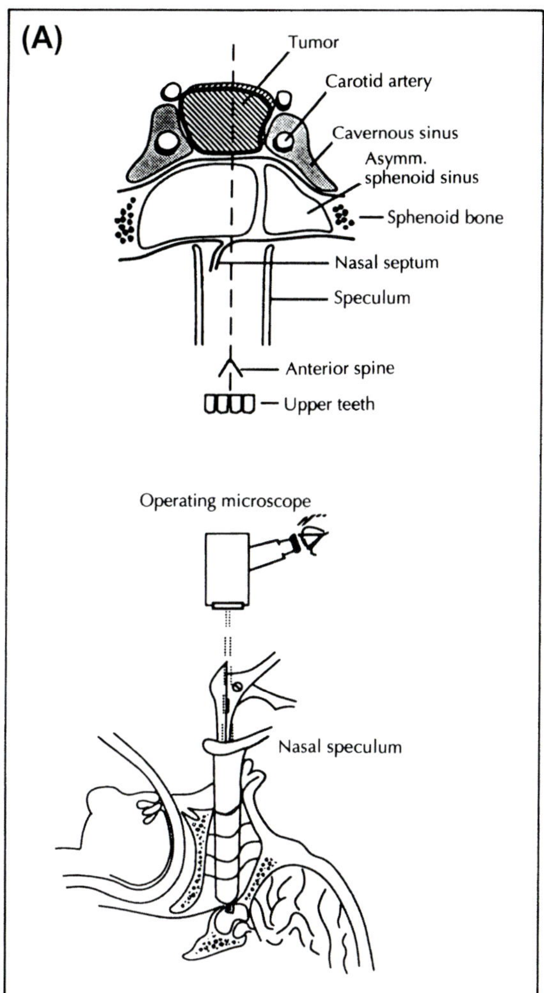

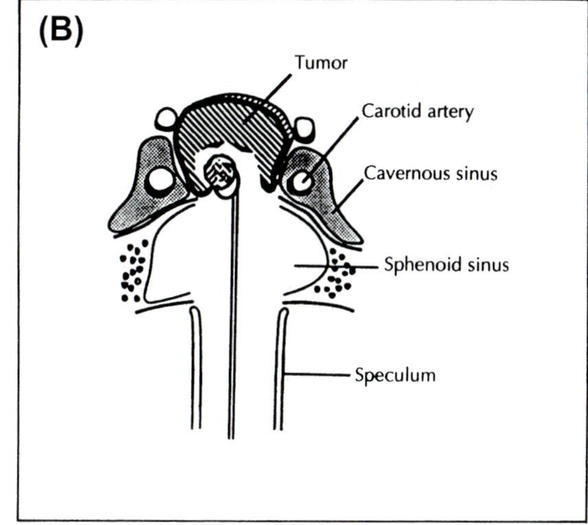

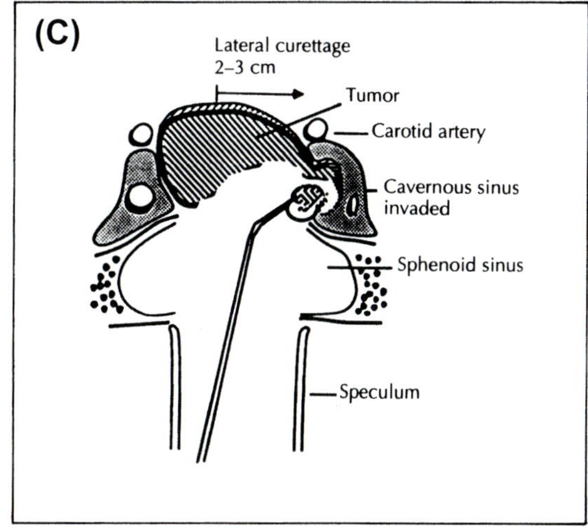

FIGURE 14.14 Transsphenoidal surgery in acromegaly. (A) Depiction of standard transsphenoidal midline approach to secreting pituitary tumors; (B) schematic depiction of midline tumor curettage; (C) schematic depiction of lateral parasellar curettage. *From [234].*

Biochemical response to radiation correlates with pretreatment GH levels. When these were >100 ng/ml, only 60% of patients had GH <5 ng/ml after 18 years. This slow rate of biochemical response is the major disadvantage of this form of treatment. During the initial years after irradiation, over half of all patients may continue to be exposed to unacceptably high levels of circulating GH and IGF-1. During the first 7 years after irradiation, <5% of patients normalize IGF-I levels [240], while ~70% of patients exhibit normal IGF-I levels when tested after longer follow-up (Figure 14.15) [241].

TABLE 14.14 Surgical Remission Rates

	% Cured Micros/Macros	Criteria
Swearingen (N=149)	91/48	NL IGF-I and/or GH <2.5 OGTT
Fred (N=99)	88/53	NL IGF-I and/or GH <2.0 OGTT
Beauregard (N=103)	82/47	NL IGF-I and GH <1.0 OGTT
Shimon (N=98)	84/64	NL IGF-I and GH <2.0 OGTT
Krieger (N=181)	80/31	Random GH <2.0

Swearingen B, et al J Clin Endocrinol Metab 1998 83:3419-3426 [202], Freda PU et al J Neurosurg 1998, 89:353-358 [204]; Beauregard C, et al Clin Endocrinol 2003; 58:86-91 [326]; Shimon I et al Neurosurgery 2001 48:1239-1243 [44]; Krieger MD et al J Neurosurg 2003 98:719-724 [327].

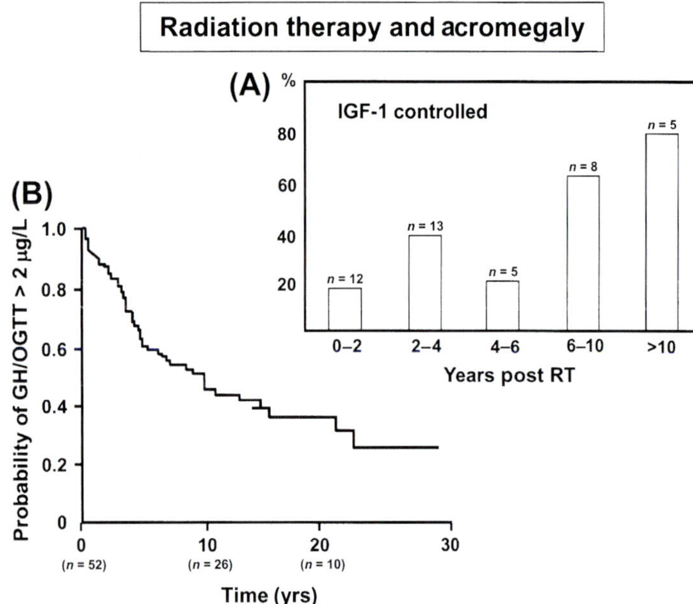

FIGURE 14.15 (A) Long-term effect of radiation therapy on GH secretion using a GH nadir after oral glucose load below 2 μg/L as the cure criterion and the probability of not being cured with time after radiotherapy. The numbers of patients not cured at 5, 10 and 20 years after pituitary irradiation are indicated in parentheses. Each step represents one cure; each cross (+) denotes a patient not cured at the latest follow-up. *From Barrande [242].* (B) Percentage of patients who were not receiving medical therapy with a normal IGF-I level according to years after RT. N, The total number of patients who had IGF-I measured in that time interval after RT. *From [241].*

Stereotactic Radiosurgery

Focused γ radiation derived from a ^{60}Cobalt source can be delivered with stereotactic precision and is especially useful for microadenomas <3 cm in diameter and distant from the optic tracts. Five years after gamma knife irradiation, about half of 82 acromegaly patients exhibited post-OGTT GH levels <1 μg/L, while pituitary failure developed in about a quarter of all patients (Figure 14.16) [244].

Side Effects of Radiotherapy

About 50% of all patients receiving radiotherapy develop pituitary trophic hormone disruption within the first 10 years of the treatment (Figure 14.15) [238], and this incidence increases annually thereafter [245]. Replacement of gonadal steroids, thyroid hormone, and/or cortisone are necessary in these patients. Side effects of conventional radiation include hair loss, cranial nerve palsies, tumor necrosis with hemorrhage, and rarely loss of vision due to optic nerve damage or pituitary apoplexy. These effects have been documented in 1–2% of patients [245–249]. Lethargy, impaired memory and personality changes may also occur [250]. The incidence of local complications have been markedly diminished by use of highly reproducible simulators, precise rotational isocentric arc capability and doses of <5000 rad [251]. Proton-beam therapy [252] is performed in a limited number of specialized centers and is contraindicated in patients with suprasellar extension of their tumors due to exposure of the optic tracts to the radiation field. After stereotactic ablation of pituitary tumors by the gamma knife in 1567 patients, 13 developed cerebral radionecrosis [253]. Secondary brain neoplasms occurring following conventional radiation are very rare [254,255] and arise within the radiation field region at a cumulative risk frequency of 1.9% over 20 years.

In summary, radiation therapy is highly effective in shrinking most GH-cell adenomas and in effectively lowering GH levels over 20 years in ~90% of patients. Overall, determinants of radiation-induced hypopituitarism include prior surgery, the precision of stereotactic tumor focus, and pituitary stalk exposure to the radiation field [21]. Because of the relatively commonly observed side effects, radiation should be indicated as adjuvant therapy for patients who are not clinically and biochemically controlled by surgical or medical management, or for those who refuse surgery or medical therapy.

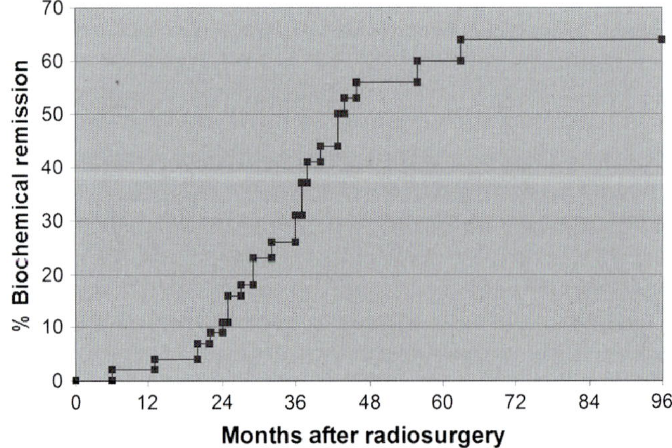

FIGURE 14.16 Acromegaly response to radiosurgery. Biochemical remission rate after radiosurgery for 46 patients with GH-producing pituitary adenomas. *Adapted from [334].*

Medical Treatment

Several medications are available to treat acromegaly (Table 14.15). These molecules are largely developed based on understanding receptor signaling and their respective dysfunctions in the disorder (Figure 14.17).

Dopamine Agonists

Dopamine inhibits GH secretion in about one-third of patients with acromegaly. Bromocriptine, a dopamine agonist, or cabergoline (a longer-acting analogue) have been used as either a primary or adjuvant therapy for acromegaly [256]. Usually, up to 20 mg/day bromocriptine is required to suppress GH in these patients, a dose higher than required to suppress PRL in patients harboring prolactinomas [257]. Side effects of bromocriptine especially with the high doses required, include gastrointestinal upset, transient nausea and vomiting, headache, transient postural hypotension with dizziness, nasal stuffiness and, rarely, cold-induced peripheral vasospasm. Cabergoline, a long-acting dopamine agonist, has been reported to suppress GH to <2 ng/ml, and normalize IGF-I in up to a third of patients with acromegaly [258]. In 198 acromegaly patients receiving dopamine agonists, GH and IGF levels were reduced by ~30%, and this effect appeared to correlate with prior radiotherapy, but not with pretreatment prolactin levels [256]. Side effects of cabergoline include gastrointestinal symptoms, dizziness, headache and mood disorders [259]. High doses of cabergoline used in patients with Parkinson's disease have been associated with cardiac valvular dysfunctions [260].

SRIF Receptor Ligands

Endogenous SRIF inhibits pituitary GH secretion, attenuates insulin secretion, and regulates multiple gastrointestinal secretions and functions [126]. SRIF action is mediated by five receptor subtypes expressed in a cell- and tissue-specific pattern which confers both functional and therapeutic ligand specificity [261,262]. The SSTR2 and SSTR5 subtypes are preferentially expressed on somatotroph and thyrotroph cell surfaces and mediate GH, TSH and ACTH secretion by suppressing intracellular cAMP levels [263–266]. As most GH-secreting adenomas abundantly express SSTR2 and SSTR5, SRIF receptor ligands (SRLs) have been successfully employed for treating acromegaly.

Both octreotide and lanreotide preparations exhibit selective affinity for SSTR2 and SSTR5 and have proven safe and effective for long-term acromegaly treatment. Octreotide, an octapeptide SRIF analogue [267,268], inhibits GH secretion with a potency 45 times greater than native SRIF, while its potency for inhibiting insulin release is only 1.3-fold that of SRIF. Because of its relative resistance to enzymatic degradation, the in vivo half life of the analogue is prolonged (up to 2 hours) after subcutaneous injection [269]. Lantreotide is an 8-amino acid cyclic peptide [270], and drug responsiveness correlates with GH-secreting adenoma SST2 expression [271,272]. Rebound GH hypersecretion seen following SRIF infusion does not occur after octreotide or lanreotide administration. These pharmacologic differences provide unique advantages for using the analogues in long-term acromegaly therapy [273,274].

TABLE 14.15 Acromegaly Medical Treatments

Drug	Dose
SRL	
Octreotide	50–400 μg sc every 8 h
Somatuline	60–120 mg deep sc every 4 wks
Octreotide LAR	10–40 mg im every 4 wks
GH antagonist	
Pegvisomant	10–40 mg sc daily
Dopamine agonist	
Cabergoline	1–4 mg orally weekly

Effects of SRLs on Biochemical Control

A single subcutaneous administration of 50 or 100 μg subcutaneous octreotide suppresses both basal and stimulated GH secretion for up to 5 hours [268]. In a double-blind, placebo-controlled trial, subcutaneous octreotide administered as 8-hourly injections significantly attenuated GH and IGF-I levels in over 90% of patients (Figure 14.18) [275] and the medication normalizes IGF-I levels in about 70% of patients. In patients with GH-secreting microadenomas, integrated GH and pooled IGF-I levels are almost invariably normalized [275], while the response in larger tumors is less pronounced. Tumors derived from patients not responding to SRLs do not express SSTR2 [276,277] and this effect is also evident in vivo (Figure 14.19). Insufficient adenoma SRIF-binding sites, or possibly a postreceptor defect, may be present in the minority (~5%) of patients not responding to SRIF analogues. Some patients appear to benefit from combined treatment with both SRIF analogues and dopamine agonists [278]. Combination therapy induces additive GH and IGF-I suppression compared with separate administration of similar doses of either drug [256,258].

Long-acting somatostatin analogue formulations provide a safe therapy that faciliates patient acceptance, enhances compliance and enables maximal biochemical control of the disorder. Sandostatin LAR is a sustained-release intramuscular depot preparation of octreotide microspheres [279,280]. Injection of 20–30 mg results

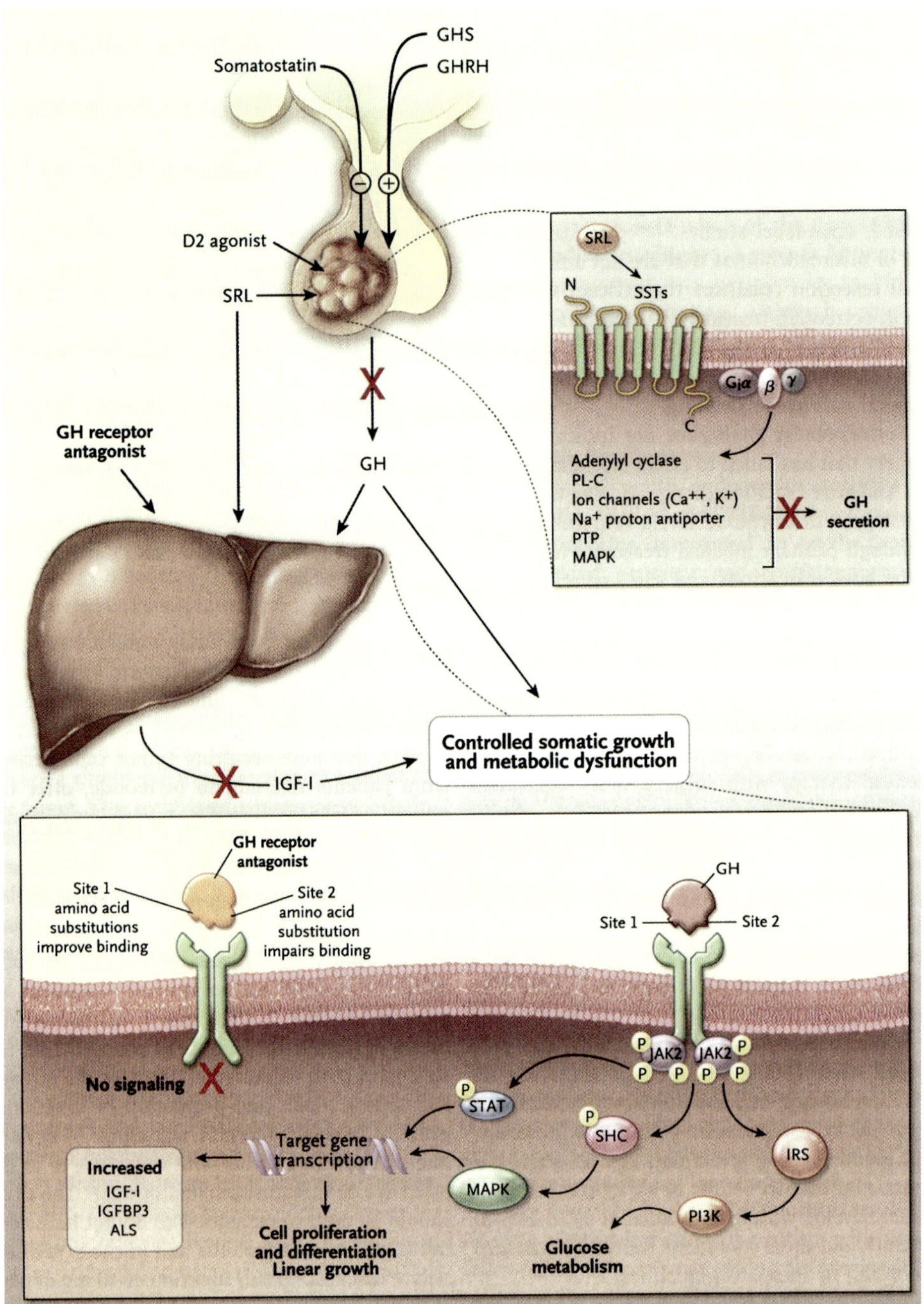

FIGURE 14.17 Receptor targets for treatment of acromegaly. Pituitary somatostatin receptor subtypes and D2 receptors and peripheral growth hormone (GH) receptors are targets for therapeutic ligands. Clinically approved and investigational drugs with ligand affinities for human somatostatin receptors are dually selective (cotreotide and lanreotide), panselective, monoselective, or chimeric (for the D2 dopamine receptors). A somatostatin receptor ligand (SRL) suppresses levels of both GH and IGF-I, constrains tumor growth, and inhibits hepatic GH-receptor binding and action. GH-receptor antagonists prevent GH receptor signaling, which attenuates peripheral IGF-I levels. SST, somatostatin receptor subtype; G, α, β and γ, G protein alpha, beta and gamma subunits; PL-C, phospholipase C; PTP, protein tyrosine phosphatase; MAPK, mitogen-activated protein kinase; IGFBP3, insulin-like growth factor-binding protein 3; ALS, acid-labile subunit; STAT, signal transducers and activators of transcription; JAK2, Janus kinase 2; P13K, phosphoinositide 3 kinase; IRS, insulin receptor substrate. *Reproduced with permission from [20].*

in peak drug level at 28 days, with integrated GH levels effectively suppressed for up to 49 days (Figure 14.20). In an open-label study of 151 patients responsive to octreotide, the drug suppressed serum GH levels to <2.5 ng/ml in ~70% of all patients [280]. GH levels were suppressed to <2.5 μg/L and IGF-I levels normalized in ~80% of patients followed for up to 9 years treatment with SRIF analogues [281,282]. In another study, GH <2 μg/L and normal IGF-I levels were achieved in 70% of 36 patients followed for 3–18 years [283].

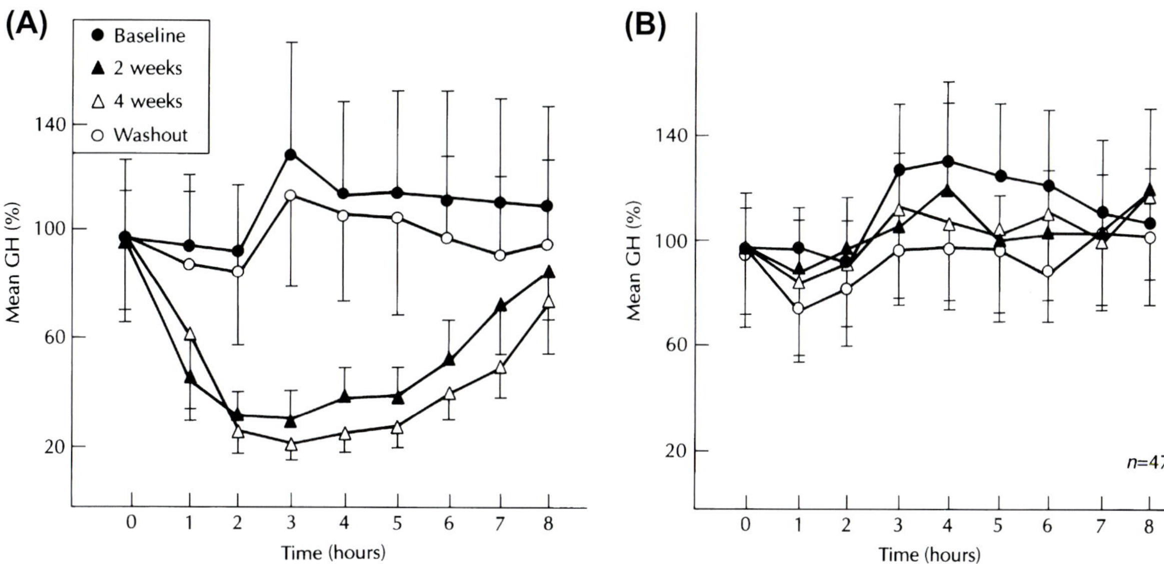

FIGURE 14.18 Effect of octreotide on hourly growth hormone levels in acromegaly. Mean percentage changes (± SE of basal values) of serum growth hormone (GH) concentrations in patients with acromegaly treated with 100 μg octreotide subcutaneously every 8 hours ($n = 52$). Blood was sampled before an injection and every hour for 8 subsequent hours before treatment ("baseline"), at the end of weeks 2 and 4 of treatment, and 4 weeks after discontinuation of treatment ("washout"). Octreotide was administered just after the 0-hour sampling. *From [275].*

Lanreotide autogel is a water-soluble gel (Somatuline in the USA) administered by deep subcutaneous injection every 28 days. Sixty-eight percent of 130 patients receiving 60, 90, or 120 mg somatuline for 1 year suppressed GH levels to <2.5 μg/L (Figure 14.21) [284].

Effects of SRLs on Pituitary Adenoma Size

About 50% of all patients receiving SRIF analogues experience a reduction of pituitary adenoma size (Figure 14.22) [285–287]. The magnitude of this shrinkage ranges from 20–80% and at least in some studies appears dose-related. If shrinkage occurs, it is evident relatively rapidly, and if the mass is not visibly smaller on MRI within 16 weeks of initiating therapy, further treatment will likely not impact adenoma size. Tumor shrinkage caused by SRLs is also associated with restoration of eugonadism in over half of patients with acromegaly and hypogonadism [281,282], likely due to relief of pituitary compression. In a randomized prospective controlled study, patients received preoperative SRIF analogues for 3–6 months and demonstrated improved postoperative biochemical control for those with macroadenomas [288]. Preoperative SRIF analogue therapy may also facilitate safer anesthesia by reducing tracheal soft tissue swelling and macroglossia [289], and by improving incipient cardiac failure.

Effects of Octreotide on Clinical Features of Acromegaly

Attenuated GH and IGF-I levels observed during chronic SRL administration are accompanied by marked improvements in many signs and symptoms

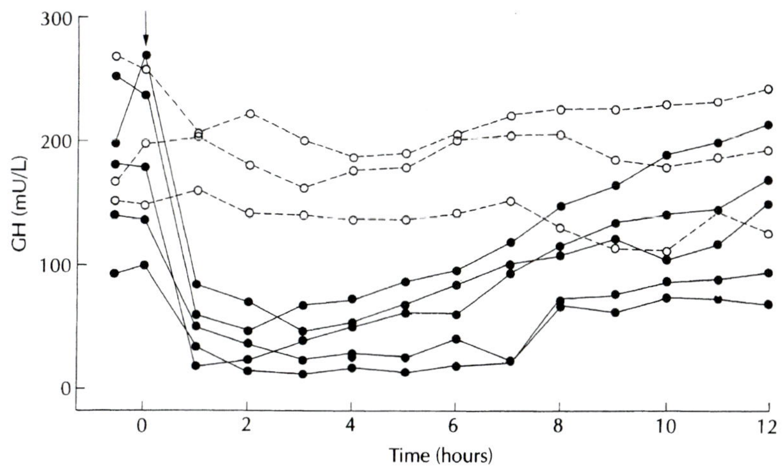

FIGURE 14.19 Pituitary tumor SSTR expression determines therapeutic responsiveness. Growth hormone (GH) responses to a single 100 μg subcutaneous dose of octreotide in eight acromegalic patients. All patients were imaged with in vivo radiolabeled octreotide. -o = scan negative; -● = scan positive. *From [335].*

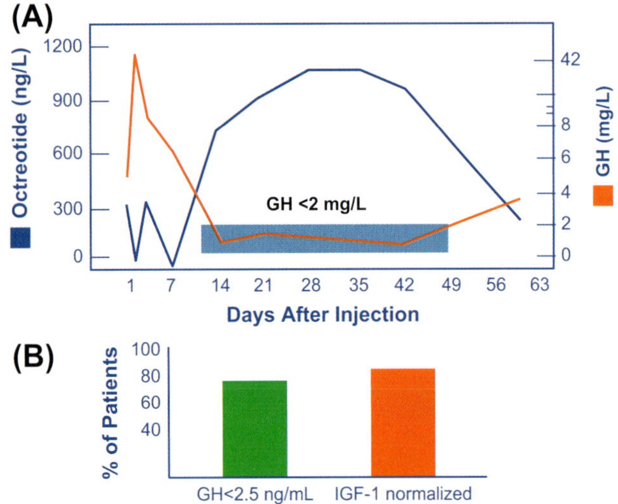

FIGURE 14.20 (A) Pharmacodynamics of octreotide LAR injection in acromegaly. *From [336].* (B) Long-term GH responses to monthly LAR injections in 12 patients. *From [337].*

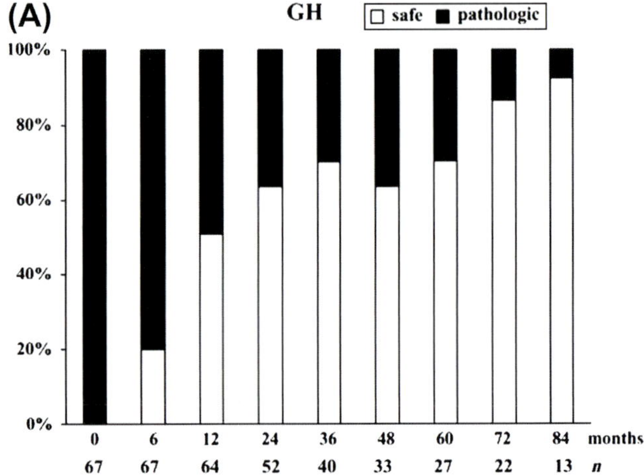

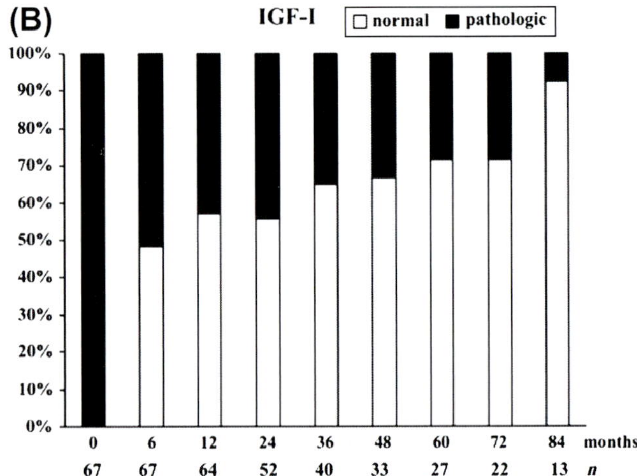

FIGURE 14.21 Percentage of patients achieving GH <2.5 μg/L and normal IGF-I. Percentage of patients achieving or not achieving (white and black bars, respectively) safe GH (top) and normal age-matched IGF-I (bottom) levels during treatment. Shown on the horizontal axis (for both panels) are months (upper line) elapsed after treatment start and number of patients (lower line) evaluated at each period. *Adapted from [282].*

of acromegaly [290]. Patients experience a general feeling of well-being and features associated with soft tissue swelling resolve within several days of initiating treatment in over 70% of patients (Figure 14.23). Paresthesias, numbness and tenderness due to nerve entrapments disappear, swollen facial features improve, and swelling of feet and hands resolves. Increased oily perspiration at rest also diminishes. Headache, a common symptom in acromegaly, usually resolves rapidly [291,292] often within minutes of injection. Asymptomatic patients experienced decrease heart rate and left ventricular wall thickness [156]. SRIF analogues reduce systemic arterial resistance, oxygen consumption and fluid volume, and restore functional activity. Importantly, persistently elevated GH levels after a year of SRL treatment were associated with increased systolic blood pressure [156]. After 1 year of treatment with SRIF analogues, left ventricular mass index, mitral flow velocity, diastolic blood pressure, heart rate and left ventricular ejection fraction improved significantly in 56 patients [293]. Joint function and crepitus improve during therapy [135], and ultrasound evidence of bone or cartilage repair has been demonstrated [294]. Sleep apnea improves after sustained treatment with octreotide.

Factors that determine SRIF analogue efficacy include tumor SSTR2 expression, frequency of drug administration, total dose, the size of the tumor and pretreatment GH levels. Smaller tumors secreting less GH may in fact express higher numbers of SRIF receptors which enable enhanced drug action. Surgical debulking of large adenomas also leads to enhanced postoperative drug effectiveness [295,296]. In the long term, patients are not desensitized to SRIF analogues and GH suppression is effectively maintained [282].

Side Effects

Although SRIF analogues are costly, they are generally safe and well-tolerated [273]. SRIF suppresses pancreatic secretions, gastrointestinal motility and splanchnic blood flow, leading to predominantly gastrointestinal side effects (Table 14.13). These include transient loose stools, nausea, mild malabsorption and flatulence in about one-third of all patients. Hypoglycemia or hyperglycemia are not commonly encountered [297] and insulin requirements in diabetic patients with acromegaly are dramatically reduced within hours of receiving SRIF analogues. SRIF analogues attenuate gallbladder contractility and delay emptying, leading to

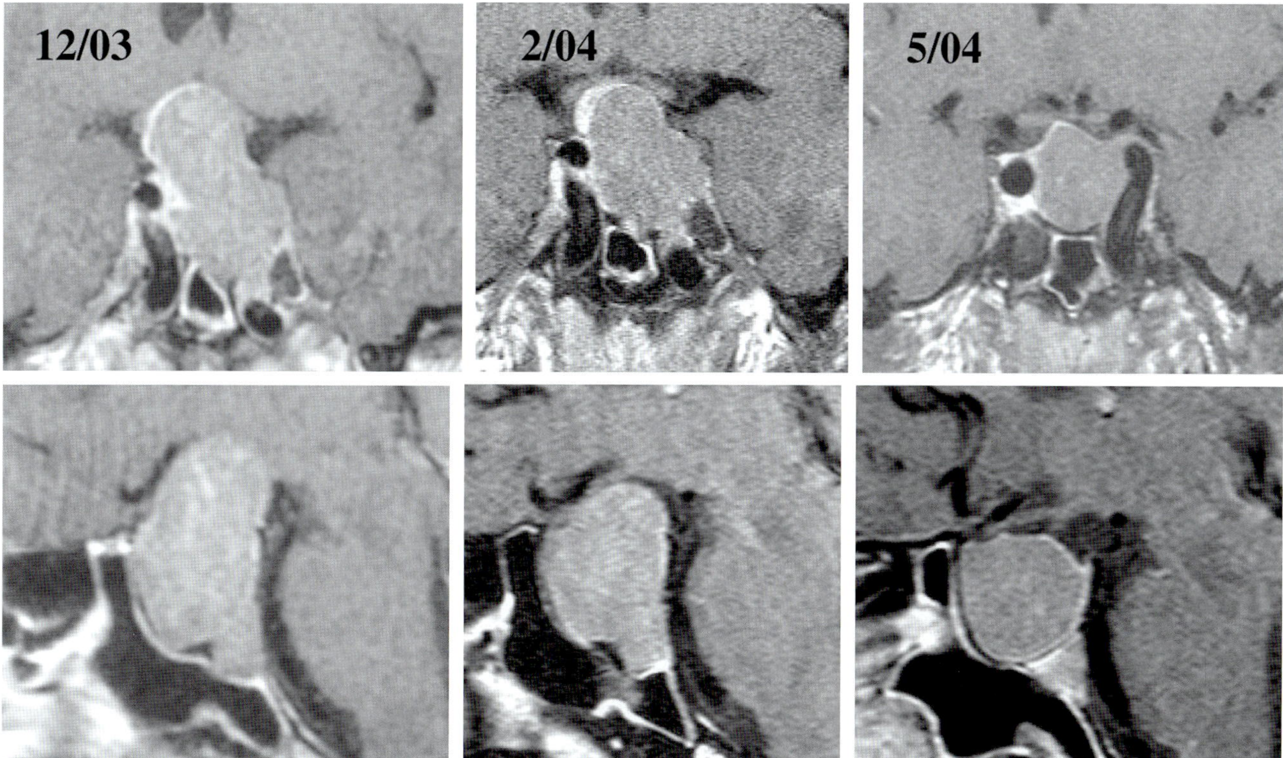

FIGURE 14.22 Example of pituitary tumor shrinkage due to primary medical therapy as evidenced by serial MRI. Acromegaly patient aged 27 years received octreotide LAR 20 mg im every 4 weeks, and MRI performed at the indicated dates.

sludge formation, as evidenced by ultrasonography in up to 25% of patients [298,299]. These are usually cholesterol deposits and disappear within 30 days of stopping the medication. Frank cholecystitis is not commonly encountered. The incidence of gallbladder sludge or stones appears to be geographically variable, with higher rates reported in China [299], Australia [274] and the UK [300]. In the USA, up to 30% of patients will likely exhibit ultrasonographic evidence of echogenic gallbladder deposits within the first 18 months of treatment. Thereafter, further episodes of sludge formation are not usually encountered [301].

GH Receptor Antagonist

Abrogation of GH receptor signaling leads to inactivation of postreceptor GH signal transduction, a pegvisomant, PEGylated mutant GH molecule, blocks functional receptor signaling and subsequent IGF-I generation [302,303]. The drug thus effectively blocks peripheral GH action. Daily injections of pegvisomant (20 mg) normalize IGF-I levels in over 90% of patients, and result in dose-dependent decreased soft tissue swelling, as assessed by ring size and improved perspiration [304].

Pegvisomant treatment resulted in IGF-I normalization in 95% of 57 patients followed for up to 91 months [305]. The drug is particularly useful in patients resistant to, or intolerant of, SRL therapy, as it effectively normalizes IGF-I levels in these patients [306]. Pegvisomant is also particularly useful in patients with associated resistant diabetes [307]. In patients resistant to SRIF analogues, pegvisomant may be used in combination management. Addition of weekly pegvisomant injections to maximal monthly SRL doses normalized IGF-I levels in 95% of such patients (Figure 14.24) [308]. As GH levels remain elevated, patients receiving pegvisomant should be monitored by measuring IGF-I levels.

Side Effects

As a precaution, an MRI should be performed every 6 months to exclude possible continued pituitary tumor growth, especially for macroadenomas during the first year of treatment [309]. Increased liver transaminase levels were noted in ~5% of patients [310], and the incidence of reversible liver enzyme alterations may be higher in patients receiving long-term combined therapy with SRLs [311]. Injection site reactions, lipohypertrophy, or lipoatrophy have also been reported. Intuitively, lowering of IGF-I to below normal levels by excessive pegvisomant dosing may lead to features of adult GH deficiency.

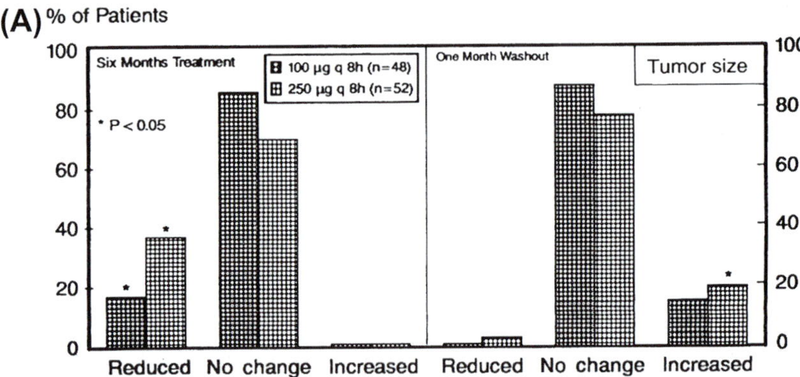

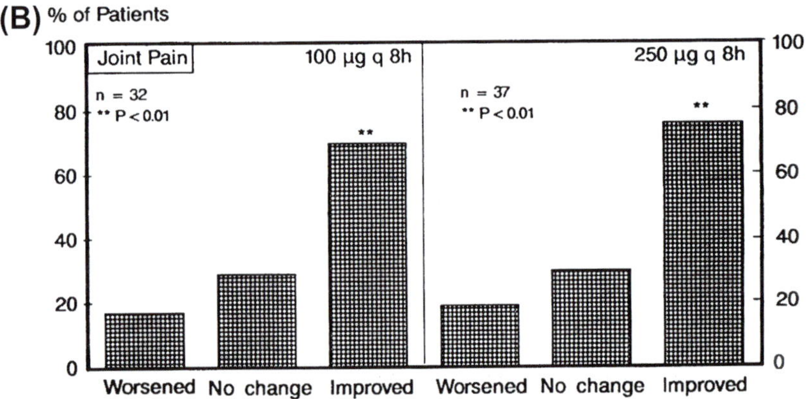

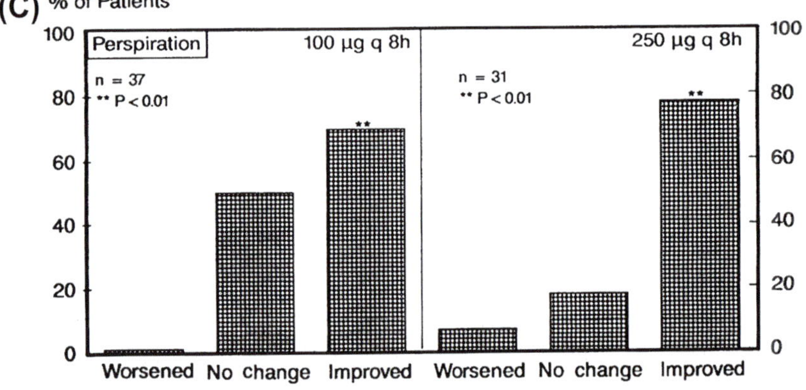

FIGURE 14.23 Clinical effects of octreotide on (A) tumor size; (B) joint pain; (C) perspiration; in acromegalic patients after 6 months' treatment with octreotide (100 or 250 µg 8-hourly). *From [275].*

Choice of Therapy

The goal of therapy is tight control of GH secretion as adverse mortality rates correlate strongly with GH levels. A suggested approach to decision-making for therapy of the patient with acromegaly is shown in Figure 14.25. Each treatment modality has its respective advantages and disadvantages (Table 14.14) and these should be weighed carefully to individualize patient care. Selective surgical excision of a well-defined pituitary microadenoma is the primary treatment of choice for most patients. Because of the invariably favorable biochemical response of small GH-secreting adenomas to octreotide, this option, with its potential side effects described, should be offered to patients. Macroadenomas and locally invasive tumors present a difficult surgical challenge, as remission rates in these patients are unacceptably low. Successful medical debulking of the sellar or parasellar mass prior to surgery would therefore be highly desirable [312]. Preoperative SRIF analogue treatment for up to 16 weeks to shrink the pituitary adenoma appears to be warranted in these patients, up to 50% of patients exhibit some degree of tumor shrinkage, thus potentially improving surgical morbidity and possibly enhancing subsequent postoperative results. This is especially important for those patients with relatively inaccessible tumor tissue and cavernous sinus invasion. These patients will invariably

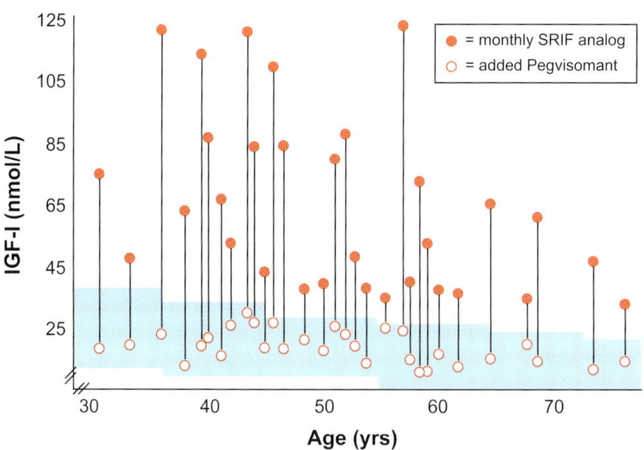

FIGURE 14.24 IGF-I concentration in serum of 31 patients with acromegaly before (filled circles) and after (open circles) 138 [35–149] weeks of combined therapy. Shaded area indicates age-dependent normal range for IGF-I. *Adapted from [338].*

require postoperative medical treatment, and octreotide and lanreotide preparations exhibit similar efficacy and safety results [313].

Primary therapy with SRIF receptor ligands may be offered to those patients who refuse surgery or who find the risks of surgery or anesthesia unacceptable. Patients with invasive macroadenomas will invariably have persistently elevated postoperative GH levels and will require postoperative somatostatin analogue treatment. Biochemical control achieved by primary SRL therapy is no different from that achieved by surgery alone [314]. Five years of primary SRIF analogue therapy in 45 patients resulted in GH control to <2.5 μg/L in 100%, and IGF-I normalization in 98%, of responsive patients [315]. Therefore, in patients whose pituitary lesion does not impinge on vital structures, primary medical management may be an informed therapeutic option (Figure 14.26) [282,316,317].

Radiation therapy should be administered to patients who fail to respond to medical therapy, who cannot tolerate the medication, or who prefer not to receive long-term injections. After external irradiation, patients require medication for several years until GH levels are effectively lowered. GH-secreting pituitary tumors that recur despite medical therapy or irradiation may rarely require reoperation.

Treatment of acromegaly should be focused on the myriad of patient concerns outlined in Table 14.16. Importantly, patients require careful counseling for anxiety and interpretation of laboratory test results. Although tight GH control is critical, these additional clinical issues must also be addressed. The criteria for effective control of hypersomatotrophism include a suppressed GH of less than 1 ng/ml after oral glucose for postoperative patients, and normalized IGF-I levels for those receiving SRLs [318]. There appears to be a strong correlation between fasting basal GH levels suppressed to <2.5 μg/L, and nadir GH levels of <2.5 μg/L after OGTT during follow-up. Radiation therapy and SRL

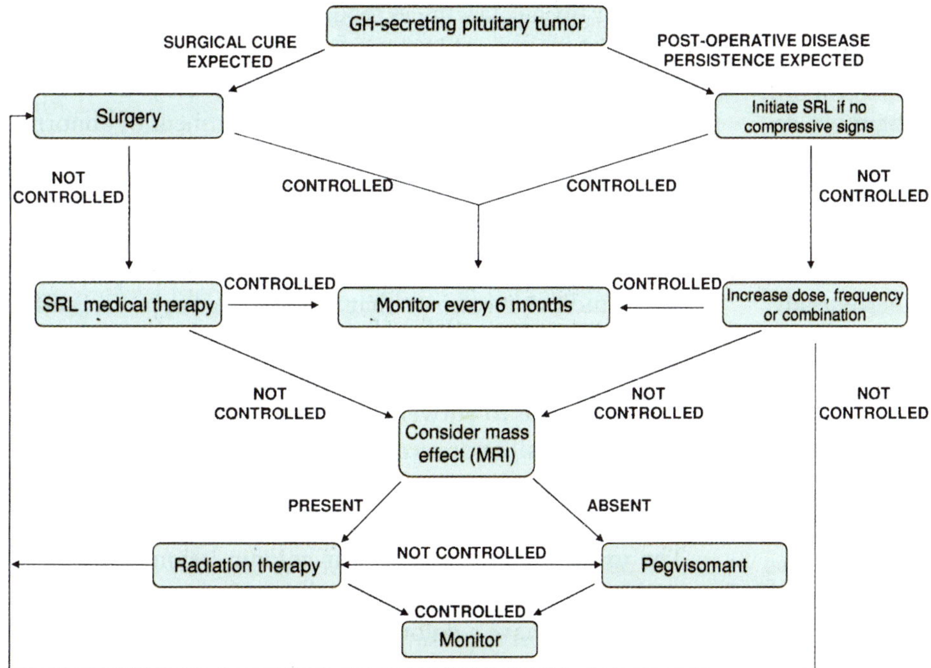

FIGURE 14.25 Flowchart for decision-making in the treatment of acromegaly. Summary of management strategy for patients with acromegaly. First level, surgery SR; SRL DR. Second level, SRL SR; monitor SR; increase dose DR. Third level, MRI DR. Fourth level, Radiation DR; Pegvisomant DR. Fifth level, Monitor SR; back to surgery SR. Control is defined by GH and IGF-I measurements as outlined in the text. *Adapted from [231].*

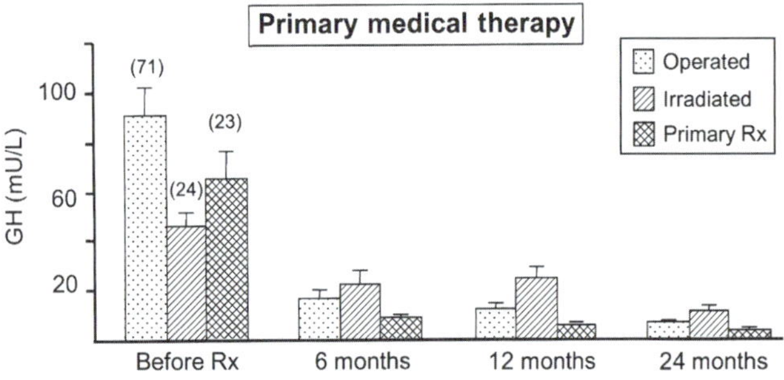

FIGURE 14.26 Primary medical therapy. GH and IGF-I levels before and during lanreotide therapy (mean + SEM) in separately groups of operated, irradiated, and de novo patients. *From [339].*

treatments both exacerbate the discordance of GH and IGF-I responses [318,319]. Patients should be followed quarterly until biochemical control is achieved. Thereafter, hormone evaluation should be performed semiannually, while in those patients who are biochemically in remission and in whom no residual tumor tissue is present, MRI should be repeated every 1–2 years [320]. Comprehensive physical examination should include evaluations of new skin tag and lipoma growth, as well as nerve entrapments and jaw overbites. Rheumatologic, dental and cardiac evaluations will usually be required in addition to the metabolic follow-up. In patients with evidence of residual tumor, or in those requiring hormone replacement or medical treatment, visual field perimetry and reserve testing of the adrenal, gonadal and thyroid axes should be repeated semiannually and pituitary MRI annually. Mammography and colonoscopy should be performed annually in patients over the age of 50, especially in those harboring skin tags.

An integrated approach to therapy and biochemical and clinical control takes advantage of the benefits of available therapeutic options, while balancing potential side effects of the treatments (Table 14.17). Maximal and sustained long-term control of GH and IGF-I should ameliorate the deleterious clinical effects of these hormones. This control can be achieved by judicious use of the treatment modalities described. Novel peptide delivery systems [321] and new stereotactic neurosurgical techniques will provide improved therapeutic choices offering optimal long-term biochemical and clinical cure.

TABLE 14.16 Patient-focused Treatment Targets for Acromegaly

Arthralgias and headache
Cardiac failure and hypertension
Diabetes
Sleep apnea
Endocrine replacement
Side effects of therapy
Patient self-image
Maxillofacial surgery
Anxiety
Fertility
Interpret laboratory testing

Adapted from [328].

TABLE 14.17 Treatment Outcomes. Each Patient Requires a Distinct Individualized Treatment Plan. Measurement of Basal GH, GH after OGTT, and IGF1 Levels will Determine the Degree of Biochemical Control. Clinical Comorbidities Require Rigorous Proactive Evaluation and Management to Achieve Optimal Mortality Outcomes.

	Management
Biochemical and clinical control: Nadir GH <1 μg/L post OGTT Age-matched normal IGF1 level Tumor stable No comorbidities	None, or no change in current treatment Evaluate pituitary axes Annual MRI
Biochemical abnormality: Basal GH >0.4 μg/L Nadir GH >1 μg/L post OGTT Elevated IGF1 level Tumor stable No comorbidities	Weigh treatment benefit vs. risks Consider new treatment if being treated Evaluate pituitary axes MRI as indicated
Biochemically and clinically active: Basal GH >0.4 μg/L Nadir GH >1 μg/L Elevated IGF1 level Tumor growing Active comorbidities	Actively treat or change treatment Evaluate pituitary function Assess cardiovascular, metabolic and tumoral comorbidity MRI as indicated

Based on Recommendations Published in [231]

References

[1] P. Marie, On two cases of acromegaly: Marked hypertrophy of the upper and lower limbs and the head, Rev Med 6 (1886) 297–333.

[2] C. Benda, Beitrage zur normalen und pathologischen histologic der menschhchen hypophysis cerebri, Klin Wochenschr 36 (1900) 1205.

[3] L.M. Davidoff, Studies in acromegaly. II Historical note, Endocrinology 10 (1926) 453.

[4] H. Cushing, Partial hypophysectomy for acromegaly: With remarks on the function of the hypophysis, Ann Surg 50 (1909) 1002–1017.

[5] P. Bailey, L.M. Davidoff, Concerning the microscopic structure of the hypophysis cerebri in acromegaly: (based on a study of tissues removed at operation from 35 patients), Am J Pathol 1 (2) (1925) 185–208.

[6] H.M. Evans, J.A. Long, The effect of the anterior lobe of the pituitary administered intra-peritoneally upon growth, maturity and oestrus cycle of the rat, Anat Rev 21 (1921) 62.

[7] L. Alexander, D. Appleton, R. Hall, W.M. Ross, R. Wilkinson, Epidemiology of acromegaly in the Newcastle region, Clin Endocrinol (Oxf) 12 (1) (1980) 71–79.

[8] B.A. Bengtsson, S. Eden, I. Ernest, A. Oden, B. Sjogren, Epidemiology and long-term survival in acromegaly. A study of 166 cases diagnosed between 1955 and 1984, Acta Med Scand 223 (4) (1988) 327–335.

[9] C.M. Ritchie, A.B. Atkinson, A.L. Kennedy, A.R. Lyons, D.S. Gordon, T. Fannin, et al., Ascertainment and natural history of treated acromegaly in Northern Ireland, Ulster Med J 59 (1) (1990) 55–62.

[10] A.F. Daly, M. Rixhon, C. Adam, A. Dempegioti, M.A. Tichomirowa, A. Beckers, High prevalence of pituitary adenomas: A cross-sectional study in the province of Liege, Belgium. J Clin Endocrinol Metab 91 (12) (2006) 4769–4775.

[11] A. Fernandez, N. Karavitaki, J.A. Wass, Prevalence of pituitary adenomas: A community-based, cross-sectional study in Banbury (Oxfordshire, UK), Clin Endocrinol (Oxf) 72 (2009) 377–382.

[12] B.T. Shea, R.E. Hammer, R.L. Brinster, Growth allometry of the organs in giant transgenic mice, Endocrinology 121 (6) (1987) 1924–1930.

[13] L.S. Mathews, R.E. Hammer, R.R. Behringer, A.J. D'Ercole, G.I. Bell, R.L. Brinster, et al., Growth enhancement of transgenic mice expressing human insulin-like growth factor I, Endocrinology 123 (6) (1988) 2827–2833.

[14] K.E. Mayo, R.E. Hammer, L.W. Swanson, R.L. Brinster, M.G. Rosenfeld, R.M. Evans, Dramatic pituitary hyperplasia in transgenic mice expressing a human growth hormone-releasing factor gene, Mol Endocrinol 2 (7) (1988) 606–612.

[15] L. Stefaneanu, K. Kovacs, E. Horvath, S.L. Asa, N.E. Losinski, N. Billestrup, et al., Adenohypophysial changes in mice transgenic for human growth hormone-releasing factor: A histological, immunocytochemical, and electron microscopic investigation, Endocrinology 125 (5) (1989) 2710–2718.

[16] S.L. Asa, K. Kovacs, L. Stefaneanu, E. Horvath, N. Billestrup, C. Gonzalez-Manchon, et al., Pituitary adenomas in mice transgenic for growth hormone-releasing hormone, Endocrinology 131 (5) (1992) 2083–2089.

[17] H.P. Guler, J. Zapf, E. Scheiwiller, E.R. Froesch, Recombinant human insulin-like growth factor I stimulates growth and has distinct effects on organ size in hypophysectomized rats, Proc Nat Acad Sci USA 85 (13) (1988) 4889–4893.

[18] A.A. Butler, D. Le Roith, Control of growth by the somatropic axis: Growth hormone and the insulin-like growth factors have related and independent roles, Annu Rev Physiol 63 (2001) 141–164.

[19] H. Kim, E. Barton, N. Muja, S. Yakar, P. Pennisi, D. Leroith, Intact insulin and insulin-like growth factor-I receptor signaling is required for growth hormone effects on skeletal muscle growth and function in vivo, Endocrinology 146 (4) (2005) 1772–1779.

[20] S. Melmed, Medical progress: Acromegaly, N Engl J Med 355 (24) (2006) 2558–2573.

[21] S. Melmed, Acromegaly pathogenesis and treatment, J Clin Invest 119 (11) (2009) 3189–3202.

[22] S. Melmed, Acromegaly [see comments], N Engl J Med 322 (14) (1990) 966–977.

[23] S. Melmed, G.D. Braunstein, E. Horvath, C. Ezrin, K. Kovacs, Pathophysiology of acromegaly, Endocr Rev 4 (3) (1983) 271–290.

[24] M. Al-Shraim, S.L. Asa, The 2004 World Health Organization classification of pituitary tumors: What is new? Acta Neuropathol 111 (1) (2006) 1–7.

[25] S.L. Asa, K. Kovacs, Pituitary pathology in acromegaly, Endocrinol Metab Clin North Am 21 (3) (1992) 553–574.

[26] R.V. Lloyd, M. Cano, W.F. Chandler, A.L. Barkan, E. Horvath, K. Kovacs, Human growth hormone and prolactin secreting pituitary adenomas analyzed by in situ hybridization, Am J Pathol 134 (3) (1989) 605–613.

[27] N.S. Halmi, Occurrence of both growth hormone- and prolactin-immunoreactive material in the cells of human somatotropic pituitary adenomas containing mammotropic elements, Virchows Arch A Pathol Anat Histopathol 398 (1) (1982) 19–31.

[28] E. Horvath, K. Kovacs, W. Singer, C. Ezrin, N.A. Kerenyi, Acidophil stem cell adenoma of the human pituitary, Arch Pathol Lab Med 101 (11) (1977) 594–599.

[29] K. Kovacs, E. Horvath, S.L. Asa, et al., Pituitary cells producing more than one hormone, Trends Endocrinol Metab 1 (1989) 104–108.

[30] R.Y. Osamura, K. Watanabe, Immunohistochemical colocalization of growth hormone (GH) and alpha subunit in human GH secreting pituitary adenomas, Virchows Arch A Pathol Anat Histopathol 411 (4) (1987) 323–330.

[31] P.M. Stewart, M.P. Carey, C.T. Graham, A.D. Wright, D.R. London, Growth hormone secreting pituitary carcinoma: A case report and literature review, Clin Endocrinol (Oxf) 37 (2) (1992) 189–194.

[32] B.W. Scheithauer, T.A. Gaffey, R.V. Lloyd, T.J. Sebo, K.T. Kovacs, E. Horvath, et al., Pathobiology of pituitary adenomas and carcinomas, Neurosurgery 59 (2) (2006) 341–353. discussion 353.

[33] M.O. Thorner, R.L. Perryman, M.J. Cronin, A.D. Rogol, M. Draznin, A. Johanson, et al., Somatotroph hyperplasia. Successful treatment of acromegaly by removal of a pancreatic islet tumor secreting a growth hormone-releasing factor, J Clin Invest 70 (5) (1982) 965–977.

[34] A.A. Sakharova, E.V. Dimaraki, W.F. Chandler, A.L. Barkan, Clinically silent somatotropinomas may be biochemically active, J Clin Endocrinol Metab 90 (4) (2005) 2117–2121.

[35] S. Melmed, Mechanisms for pituitary tumorigenesis: The plastic pituitary, J Clin Invest 112 (11) (2003) 1603–1618.

[36] N. Billestrup, L.W. Swanson, W. Vale, Growth hormone-releasing factor stimulates proliferation of somatotrophs in vitro, Proc Nat Acad Sci USA 83 (18) (1986) 6854–6857.

[37] F.H. Burton, K.W. Hasel, F.E. Bloom, J.G. Sutcliffe, Pituitary hyperplasia and gigantism in mice caused by a cholera toxin transgene, Nature 350 (6313) (1991) 74–77.

[38] R.S. Struthers, W.W. Vale, C. Arias, P.E. Sawchenko, M.R. Montminy, Somatotroph hypoplasia and dwarfism in transgenic mice expressing a non-phosphorylatable CREB mutant, Nature 350 (6319) (1991) 622–624.

[39] S.L. Asa, J.M. Bilbao, K. Kovacs, J.A. Linfoot, Hypothalamic neuronal hamartoma associated with pituitary growth hormone cell adenoma and acromegaly, Acta Neuropathol 52 (3) (1980) 231–234.

[40] S.L. Asa, B.W. Scheithauer, J.M. Bilbao, E. Horvath, N. Ryan, K. Kovacs, et al., A case for hypothalamic acromegaly: A clinicopathological study of six patients with hypothalamic gangliocytomas producing growth hormone-releasing factor, J Clin Endocrinol Metab 58 (5) (1984) 796–803.

[41] T. Sano, S.L. Asa, K. Kovacs, Growth hormone-releasing hormone-producing tumors: Clinical, biochemical, and morphological manifestations, Endocr Rev 9 (3) (1988) 357–373.

[42] K. Thapar, K. Kovacs, L. Stefaneanu, B. Scheithauer, D.W. Killinger, R.V. Lloyd, et al., Overexpression of the growth-hormone-releasing hormone gene in acromegaly-associated pituitary tumors. An event associated with neoplastic progression and aggressive behavior, Am J Pathol 151 (3) (1997) 769–784.

[43] J. Kreutzer, M.L. Vance, M.B. Lopes, E.R. Laws Jr., Surgical management of GH-secreting pituitary adenomas: An outcome study using modern remission criteria, J Clin Endocrinol Metab 86 (9) (2001) 4072–4077.
[44] I. Shimon, Z.R. Cohen, Z. Ram, M. Hadani, Transsphenoidal surgery for acromegaly: Endocrinological follow-up of 98 patients, Neurosurgery 48 (6) (2001) 1239–1243, discussion 44–5.
[45] K. Bajuk Studen, A. Barkan, Assessment of the magnitude of growth hormone hypersecretion in active acromegaly: Reliability of different sampling models, J Clin Endocrinol Metab 93 (2) (2008) 491–496.
[46] S.W. Lamberts, J.C. Reubi, E.P. Krenning, Somatostatin analogs in the treatment of acromegaly, Endocrinol Metab Clin North Am 21 (3) (1992) 737–752.
[47] M. Ishibashi, T. Yamaji, Direct effects of catecholamines, thyrotropin-releasing hormone, and somatostatin on growth hormone and prolactin secretion from adenomatous and non-adenomatous human pituitary cells in culture, J Clin Invest 73 (1) (1984) 66–78.
[48] S. Yamashita, M. Weiss, S. Melmed, Insulin-like growth factor I regulates growth hormone secretion and messenger ribonucleic acid levels in human pituitary tumor cells, J Clin Endocrinol Metab 63 (3) (1986) 730–735.
[49] A.D. Howard, S.D. Feighner, D.F. Cully, J.P. Arena, P.A. Liberator, C.I. Rosenblum, et al., A receptor in pituitary and hypothalamus that functions in growth hormone release, Science 273 (5277) (1996) 974–977.
[50] I. Shimon, S. Melmed, Genetic basis of endocrine disease: Pituitary tumor pathogenesis, J Clin Endocrinol Metab 82 (6) (1997) 1675–1681.
[51] A.M. Nanzer, S. Khalaf, A.M. Mozid, R.C. Fowkes, M.V. Patel, J.M. Burrin, et al., Ghrelin exerts a proliferative effect on a rat pituitary somatotroph cell line via the mitogen-activated protein kinase pathway, Eur J Endocrinol 151 (2) (2004) 233–240.
[52] V. Herman, J. Fagin, R. Gonsky, K. Kovacs, S. Melmed, Clonal origin of pituitary adenomas, J Clin Endocrinol Metab 71 (1990) 1427–1433.
[53] L. Vallar, A. Spada, G. Giannattasio, Altered Gs and adenylate cyclase activity in human GH-secreting pituitary adenomas, Nature 330 (6148) (1987) 566–568.
[54] S.L. Asa, S. Ezzat, The pathogenesis of pituitary tumors, Annu Rev Pathol 4 (2009) 97–126.
[55] A.P. Heaney, G.A. Horwitz, Z. Wang, R. Singson, S. Melmed, Early involvement of estrogen-induced pituitary tumor transforming gene and fibroblast growth factor expression in prolactinoma pathogenesis, Nat Med 5 (11) (1999) 1317–1321.
[56] H. Zou, T.J. McGarry, T. Bernal, M.W. Kirschner, Identification of a vertebrate sister-chromatid separation inhibitor involved in transformation and tumorigenesis, Science 285 (5426) (1999) 418–422.
[57] X. Zhang, H. Sun, D.C. Danila, S.R. Johnson, Y. Zhou, B. Swearingen, et al., Loss of expression of GADD45 gamma, a growth inhibitory gene, in human pituitary adenomas: Implications for tumorigenesis, J Clin Endocrinol Metab 87 (3) (2002) 1262–1267.
[58] V. Chesnokova, S. Zonis, K. Kovacs, A. Ben-Shlomo, K. Wawrowsky, S. Bannykh, et al., p21(Cip1) restrains pituitary tumor growth, Proc Nat Acad Sci USA 105 (45) (2008) 17498–17503.
[59] S. Melmed, C. Ezrin, K. Kovacs, R.S. Goodman, L.A. Frohman, Acromegaly due to secretion of growth hormone by an ectopic pancreatic islet-cell tumor, N Engl J Med 312 (1) (1985) 9–17.
[60] L.A. Frohman, J.O. Jansson, Growth hormone-releasing hormone, Endocr Rev 7 (3) (1986) 223–253.
[61] A. Moran, S.L. Asa, K. Kovacs, E. Horvath, W. Singer, U. Sagman, et al., Gigantism due to pituitary mammosomatotroph hyperplasia, N Engl J Med 323 (5) (1990) 322–327.
[62] N.D. Christofides, A. Stephanou, H. Suzuki, Y. Yiangou, S.R. Bloom, Distribution of immunoreactive growth hormone-releasing hormone in the human brain and intestine and its production by tumors, J Clin Endocrinol Metab 59 (4) (1984) 747–751.
[63] S.L. Asa, K. Kovacs, M.O. Thorner, D.A. Leong, J. Rivier, W. Vale, Immunohistological localization of growth hormone-releasing hormone in human tumors, J Clin Endocrinol Metab 60 (3) (1985) 423–427.
[64] A. Sasaki, S. Sato, S. Yumita, K. Hanew, Y. Miura, K. Yoshinaga, Multiple forms of immunoreactive growth hormone-releasing hormone in human plasma, hypothalamus, and tumor tissues, J Clin Endocrinol Metab 68 (1) (1989) 180–185.
[65] R. Guillemin, P. Brazeau, P. Bohlen, F. Esch, N. Ling, W.B. Wehrenberg, Growth hormone-releasing factor from a human pancreatic tumor that caused acromegaly, Science 218 (4572) (1982) 585–587.
[66] M.O. Thorner, L.A. Frohman, D.A. Leong, J. Thominet, T. Downs, P. Hellmann, et al., Extrahypothalamic growth-hormone-releasing factor (GRF) secretion is a rare cause of acromegaly: Plasma GRF levels in 177 acromegalic patients, J Clin Endocrinol Metab 59 (5) (1984) 846–849.
[67] P.H. Sonksen, A.B. Ayres, M. Braimbridge, B. Corrin, D.R. Davies, G.M. Jeremiah, et al., Acromegaly caused by pulmonary carcinoid tumours, Clin Endocrinol (Oxf) 5 (5) (1976) 503–513.
[68] F.T. Dabek, Bronchial carcinoid tumour with acromegaly in two patients, J Clin Endocrinol Metab 38 (2) (1974) 329–333.
[69] L.A. Frohman, M. Szabo, M. Berelowitz, M.E. Stachura, Partial purification and characterization of a peptide with growth hormone-releasing activity from extrapituitary tumors in patients with acromegaly, J Clin Invest 65 (1) (1980) 43–54.
[70] P.P. Garcia-Luna, A. Leal-Cerro, C. Montero, B.W. Scheithauer, A. Campanario, C. Dieguez, et al., A rare cause of acromegaly: Ectopic production of growth hormone-releasing factor by a bronchial carcinoid tumor, Surg Neurol 27 (6) (1987) 563–568.
[71] D.M. Wilson, G.P. Ceda, D.G. Bostwick, R.J. Webber, J.R. Minkoff, A. Pont, et al., Acromegaly and Zollinger-Ellison syndrome secondary to an islet cell tumor: Characterization and quantification of plasma and tumor human growth hormone-releasing factor, J Clin Endocrinol Metab 59 (5) (1984) 1002–1005.
[72] R. Boizel, S. Halimi, F. Labat, R. Cohen, I. Bachelot, Acromegaly due to a growth hormone-releasing hormone-secreting bronchial carcinoid tumor: Further information on the abnormal responsiveness of the somatotroph cells and their recovery after successful treatment, J Clin Endocrinol Metab 64 (2) (1987) 304–308.
[73] G. Sassolas, J.A. Chayvialle, C. Partensky, G. Berger, J. Trouillas, F. Berger, et al., [Acromegaly, clinical expression of the production of growth hormone releasing factor in pancreatic tumors], Ann Endocrinol (Paris) 44 (6) (1983) 347–354.
[74] A.L. Barkan, Y. Shenker, R.J. Grekin, W.W. Vale, Acromegaly from ectopic growth hormone-releasing hormone secretion by a malignant carcinoid tumor. Successful treatment with long-acting somatostatin analogue SMS 201-995, Cancer 61 (2) (1988) 221–226.
[75] S. Melmed, F.H. Ziel, G.D. Braunstein, T. Downs, L.A. Frohman, Medical management of acromegaly due to ectopic production of growth hormone-releasing hormone by a carcinoid tumor, J Clin Endocrinol Metab 67 (2) (1988) 395–399.

[76] M.R. Drange, S. Melmed, Long-acting lanreotide induces clinical and biochemical remission of acromegaly caused by disseminated growth hormone-releasing hormone-secreting carcinoid [see comments], J Clin Endocrinol Metab 83 (9) (1998) 3104–3109.

[77] J. Rivier, J. Spiess, M. Thorner, W. Vale, Characterization of a growth hormone-releasing factor from a human pancreatic islet tumour, Nature 300 (5889) (1982) 276–278.

[78] K. Oberg, I. Norheim, L. Wide, Serum growth hormone in patients with carcinoid tumours; basal levels and response to glucose and thyrotrophin releasing hormone, Acta Endocrinol (Copenh) 109 (1) (1985) 13–18.

[79] C. Nasr, A. Mason, M. Mayberg, S.M. Staugaitis, S.L. Asa, Acromegaly and somatotroph hyperplasia with adenomatous transformation due to pituitary metastasis of a growth hormone-releasing hormone-secreting pulmonary endocrine carcinoma, J Clin Endocrinol Metab 91 (12) (2006) 4776–4780.

[80] Y. Dayal, H.D. Lin, K. Tallberg, S. Reichlin, R.A. DeLellis, H.J. Wolfe, Immunocytochemical demonstration of growth hormone-releasing factor in gastrointestinal and pancreatic endocrine tumors, Am J Clin Pathol 85 (1) (1986) 13–20.

[81] N.R. Biermasz, J.W. Smit, A.M. Pereira, M. Frolich, J.A. Romijn, F. Roelfsema, Acromegaly caused by growth hormone-releasing hormone-producing tumors: Long-term observational studies in three patients, Pituitary 10 (3) (2007) 237–249.

[82] J.A. Ramsay, K. Kovacs, S.L. Asa, M.J. Pike, M.O. Thorner, Reversible sellar enlargement due to growth hormone-releasing hormone production by pancreatic endocrine tumors in an acromegalic patient with multiple endocrine neoplasia type I syndrome, Cancer 62 (2) (1988) 445–450.

[83] D.M. Wilson, A.R. Hoffman, Reduction of pituitary size by the somatostatin analogue SMS 201-995 in a patient with an islet cell tumour secreting growth hormone releasing factor, Acta Endocrinol (Copenh) 113 (1) (1986) 23–28.

[84] K. von Werder, M. Losa, O.A. Muller, L. Schweiberer, R. Fahlbusch, E. Del Pozo, Treatment of metastasising GRF-producing tumour with a long-acting somatostatin analogue, Lancet 2 (8397) (1984) 282–283.

[85] D.E. Moller, A.C. Moses, K. Jones, M.O. Thorner, M.L. Vance, Octreotide suppresses both growth hormone (GH) and GH-releasing hormone (GHRH) in acromegaly due to ectopic GHRH secretion, J Clin Endocrinol Metab 68 (2) (1989) 499–504.

[86] M.C. Zatelli, P. Maffei, D. Piccin, C. Martini, F. Rea, D. Rubello, et al., Somatostatin analogs in vitro effects in a growth hormone-releasing hormone-secreting bronchial carcinoid, J Clin Endocrinol Metab 90 (4) (2005) 2104–2109.

[87] R.V. Lloyd, W.F. Chandler, K. Kovacs, et al., Ectopic pituitary adenomas with normal anterior pituitary glands, Am J Surg Pathol 10 (1986) 546–552.

[88] B. Corenblum, F.E. LeBlanc, M. Watanabe, Acromegaly with an adenomatous pharyngeal pituitary, JAMA 243 (14) (1980) 1456–1457.

[89] Y. Greenman, P. Woolf, J. Coniglio, R. O'Mara, L. Pei, J.W. Said, et al., Remission of acromegaly caused by pituitary carcinoma after surgical excision of growth hormone-secreting metastasis detected by 111-indium pentetreotide scan, J Clin Endocrinol Metab 81 (4) (1996) 1628–1633.

[90] C.V. Kyle, M.C. Evans, W.D. Odell, Growth hormone-like material in normal human tissues, J Clin Endocrinol Metab 53 (6) (1981) 1138–1144.

[91] A. Kaganowicz, N.H. Farkouh, A.G. Frantz, A.U. Blaustein, Ectopic human growth hormone in ovaries and breast cancer, J Clin Endocrinol Metab 48 (1) (1979) 5–8.

[92] F. Beuschlein, C.J. Strasburger, V. Siegerstetter, D. Moradpour, P. Lichter, M. Bidlingmaier, et al., Acromegaly caused by secretion of growth hormone by a non-Hodgkin's lymphoma, N Engl J Med 342 (25) (2000) 1871–1876.

[93] M.W. Ashcraft, P.I. Hartzband, A.J. Van Herle, N. Bersch, D.W. Golde, A unique growth factor in patients with acromegaloidism, J Clin Endocrinol Metab 57 (2) (1983) 272–276.

[94] L. Low, S.D. Chernausek, M.A. Sperling, Acromegaloid patients with type A insulin resistance: Parallel defects in insulin and insulin-like growth factor-I receptors and biological responses in cultured fibroblasts, J Clin Endocrinol Metab 69 (2) (1989) 329–337.

[95] L. Cuttler, J.A. Jackson, M. Saeed uz-Zafar, L.L. Levitsky, R.C. Mellinger, L.A. Frohman, Hypersecretion of growth hormone and prolactin in McCune-Albright syndrome, J Clin Endocrinol Metab 68 (6) (1989) 1148–1154.

[96] L.S. Weinstein, A. Shenker, P.V. Gejman, M.J. Merino, E. Friedman, A.M. Spiegel, Activating mutations of the stimulatory G protein in the McCune-Albright syndrome, N Engl J Med 325 (24) (1991) 1688–1695.

[97] S.C. Chandrasekharappa, S.C. Guru, P. Manickam, S.E. Olufemi, F.S. Collins, M.R. Emmert-Buck, et al., Positional cloning of the gene for multiple endocrine neoplasia-type 1, Science 276 (5311) (1997) 404–407.

[98] B.T. Teh, S. Kytola, F. Farnebo, L. Bergman, F.K. Wong, G. Weber, et al., Mutation analysis of the MEN1 gene in multiple endocrine neoplasia type 1, familial acromegaly and familial isolated hyperparathyroidism, J Clin Endocrinol Metab 83 (8) (1998) 2621–2626.

[99] S.J. Marx, S.K. Agarwal, M.B. Kester, C. Heppner, Y.S. Kim, M.C. Skarulis, et al., Multiple endocrine neoplasia type 1: Clinical and genetic features of the hereditary endocrine neoplasias, Recent Prog Horm Res 54 (1999) 397–438, discussion 439.

[100] T. Sano, R. Yamasaki, H. Saito, T. Hirose, E. Kudo, K. Kameyama, et al., Growth hormone-releasing hormone (GHRH)-secreting pancreatic tumor in a patient with multiple endocrine neoplasia type I, Am J Surg Pathol 11 (10) (1987) 810–819.

[101] N.S. Pellegata, L. Quintanilla-Martinez, H. Siggelkow, E. Samson, K. Bink, H. Hofler, et al., Germ-line mutations in p27Kip1 cause a multiple endocrine neoplasia syndrome in rats and humans, Proc Nat Acad Sci USA 103 (42) (2006) 15558–15563.

[102] S.A. Boikos, C.A. Stratakis, Carney complex: The first 20 years, Curr Opin Oncol 19 (1) (2007) 24–29.

[103] M.R. Gadelha, T.R. Prezant, K.N. Une, R.P. Glick, S.F. Moskal, M. Vaisman, et al., Loss of heterozygosity on chromosome 11q13 in two families with acromegaly/gigantism is independent of mutations of the multiple endocrine neoplasia type I gene, J Clin Endocrinol Metab 84 (1) (1999) 249–256.

[104] S. Yamada, K. Yoshimoto, T. Sano, K. Takada, M. Itakura, M. Usui, et al., Inactivation of the tumor suppressor gene on 11q13 in brothers with familial acrogigantism without multiple endocrine neoplasia type 1, J Clin Endocrinol Metab 82 (1) (1997) 239–242.

[105] M.R. Gadelha, K.N. Une, K. Rohde, M. Vaisman, R.D. Kineman, L.A. Frohman, Isolated familial somatotropinomas: Establishment of linkage to chromosome 11q13.1-11q13.3 and evidence for a potential second locus at chromosome 2p16-12, J Clin Endocrinol Metab 85 (2) (2000) 707–714.

[106] M. Georgitsi, A. Raitila, A. Karhu, K. Tuppurainen, M.J. Makinen, O. Vierimaa, et al., Molecular diagnosis of pituitary adenoma predisposition caused by aryl hydrocarbon receptor-interacting protein gene mutations, Proc Nat Acad Sci USA 104 (10) (2007) 4101–4105.

[107] C.A. Leontiou, M. Gueorguiev, J. van der Spuy, R. Quinton, F. Lolli, S. Hassan, et al., The role of the aryl hydrocarbon receptor-interacting protein gene in familial and sporadic pituitary adenomas, J Clin Endocrinol Metab 93 (6) (2008) 2390–2401.

[108] M.L. Jaffrain-Rea, M. Angelini, D. Gargano, M.A. Tichomirowa, A.F. Daly, J.F. Vanbellinghen, et al., Expression of aryl hydrocarbon receptor (AHR) and AHR-interacting protein in pituitary adenomas: Pathological and clinical implications, Endocr Relat Cancer 16 (3) (2009) 1029–1043.

[109] W.H. Daughaday, Pituitary gigantism, Endocrinol Metab Clin North Am 21 (3) (1992) 633–647.

[110] D. Zimmerman, W.F. Young Jr., M.J. Ebersold, B.W. Scheithauer, K. Kovacs, E. Horvath, et al., Congenital gigantism due to growth hormone-releasing hormone excess and pituitary hyperplasia with adenomatous transformation, J Clin Endocrinol Metab 76 (1) (1993) 216–222.

[111] S.J. Gelber, D.S. Heffez, P.A. Donohoue, Pituitary gigantism caused by growth hormone excess from infancy, J Pediatr 120 (6) (1992) 931–934.

[112] H.G. Maheshwari, T.R. Prezant, V. Herman-Bonert, H. Shahinian, K. Kovacs, S. Melmed, Long-acting peptidomimergic control of gigantism caused by pituitary acidophilic stem cell adenoma, J Clin Endocrinol Metab 85 (9) (2000) 3409–3416.

[113] N. Goldenberg, M.S. Racine, P. Thomas, B. Degnan, W. Chandler, A. Barkan, Treatment of pituitary gigantism with the growth hormone receptor antagonist pegvisomant, J Clin Endocrinol Metab 93 (8) (2008) 2953–2956.

[114] S. Melmed, G.D. Braunstein, R.J. Chang, D.P. Becker, Pituitary tumors secreting growth hormone and prolactin [clinical conference], Ann Intern Med 105 (2) (1986) 238–253.

[115] M.R. Drange, N.R. Fram, V. Herman-Bonert, S. Melmed, Pituitary tumor registry: A novel clinical resource, J Clin Endocrinol Metab 85 (1) (2000) 168–174.

[116] N.J. Lanning, C. Carter-Su, Recent advances in growth hormone signaling, Rev Endocr Metab Disord 7 (4) (2006) 225–235.

[117] A.J. Brooks, J.W. Wooh, K.A. Tunny, M.J. Waters, Growth hormone receptor; mechanism of action, Int J Biochem Cell Biol 40 (10) (2008) 1984–1989.

[118] C. Dos Santos, L. Essioux, C. Teinturier, M. Tauber, V. Goffin, P. Bougneres, A common polymorphism of the growth hormone receptor is associated with increased responsiveness to growth hormone, Nat Genet 36 (7) (2004) 720–724.

[119] M.J. Wassenaar, N.R. Biermasz, A.M. Pereira, A.A. van der Klaauw, J.W. Smit, F. Roelfsema, et al., The exon-3 deleted growth hormone receptor polymorphism predisposes to long-term complications of acromegaly, J Clin Endocrinol Metab 94 (12) (2009) 4671–4678.

[120] A. Bianchi, A. Giustina, V. Cimino, R. Pola, F. Angelini, A. Pontecorvi, et al., Influence of growth hormone receptor d3 and full-length isoforms on biochemical treatment outcomes in acromegaly, J Clin Endocrinol Metab 94 (6) (2009) 2015–2022.

[121] M. Mercado, B. Gonzalez, C. Sandoval, Y. Esquenazi, F. Mier, G. Vargas, et al., Clinical and biochemical impact of the d3 growth hormone receptor genotype in acromegaly, J Clin Endocrinol Metab 93 (9) (2008) 3411–3415.

[122] I. Bernabeu, C. Alvarez-Escola, C. Quinteiro, T. Lucas, M. Puig-Domingo, M. Luque-Ramirez, et al., The exon 3-deleted growth hormone receptor is associated with better response to pegvisomant therapy in acromegaly, J Clin Endocrinol Metab 95 (1) (2010) 222–229.

[123] M.E. Molitch, Clinical manifestations of acromegaly, Endocrinol Metab Clin North Am 21 (3) (1992) 597–614.

[124] L. Nachtigall, A. Delgado, B. Swearingen, H. Lee, R. Zerikly, A. Klibanski, Changing patterns in diagnosis and therapy of acromegaly over two decades, J Clin Endocrinol Metab 93 (6) (2008) 2035–2041.

[125] J.D. Nabarro, Acromegaly, Clin Endocrinol (Oxf) 26 (4) (1987) 481–512.

[126] S. Reichlin, Somatostatin, N Engl J Med 309 (24) (1983) 1495–1501.

[127] P.U. Freda, W. Shen, C.M. Reyes-Vidal, E.B. Geer, F. Arias-Mendoza, D. Gallagher, et al., Skeletal muscle mass in acromegaly assessed by magnetic resonance imaging and dual-photon x-ray absorptiometry, J Clin Endocrinol Metab 94 (8) (2009) 2880–2886.

[128] J. Gibney, T. Wolthers, M.G. Burt, K.C. Leung, A.M. Umpleby, K.K. Ho, Protein metabolism in acromegaly: Differential effects of short- and long-term treatment, J Clin Endocrinol Metab 92 (4) (2007) 1479–1484.

[129] E.M. Whitehead, S.M. Shalet, D. Davies, B.A. Enoch, D.A. Price, C.G. Beardwell, Pituitary gigantism: A disabling condition, Clin Endocrinol (Oxf) 17 (3) (1982) 271–277.

[130] S.A. Lieberman, A.R. Hoffman, Sequelae to acromegaly: Reversibility with treatment of the primary disease, Horm Metab Res 22 (6) (1990) 313–318.

[131] A. Colao, P. Marzullo, G. Vallone, V. Marino, M. Annecchino, D. Ferone, et al., Reversibility of joint thickening in acromegalic patients: An ultrasonography study, J Clin Endocrinol Metab 83 (6) (1998) 2121–2125.

[132] T.L. McCarthy, M. Centrella, E. Canalis, Regulatory effects of insulin-like growth factors I and II on bone collagen synthesis in rat calvarial cultures, Endocrinology 124 (1) (1989) 301–309.

[133] L.M. Davidoff, Studies in acromegaly. III. The anamnesis and symptomatology in one hundred cases, Endocrinology 10 (1926) 461–476.

[134] S.A. Lieberman, A.G. Bjorkengren, A.R. Hoffman, Rheumatologic and skeletal changes in acromegaly, Endocrinol Metab Clin North Am 21 (3) (1992) 615–631.

[135] M.W. Layton, E.J. Fudman, A. Barkan, E.M. Braunstein, I.H. Fox, Acromegalic arthropathy. Characteristics and response to therapy, Arthritis Rheum 31 (8) (1988) 1022–1027.

[136] H.K. Ibbertson, P.J. Manning, I.M. Holdaway, G. Gamble, B.J. Synek, The acromegalic rosary, Lancet 337 (8734) (1991) 154–156.

[137] A. Colao, P. Marzullo, D. Ferone, S. Spiezia, G. Cerbone, V. Marino, et al., Prostatic hyperplasia: An unknown feature of acromegaly, J Clin Endocrinol Metab 83 (3) (1998) 775–779.

[138] P.J. Jenkins, S.A. Sohaib, S. Akker, R.R. Phillips, K. Spillane, J.A. Wass, et al., The pathology of median neuropathy in acromegaly, Ann Intern Med 133 (3) (2000) 197–201.

[139] M.J. Wassenaar, N.R. Biermasz, N. van Duinen, A.A. van der Klaauw, A.M. Pereira, F. Roelfsema, et al., High prevalence of arthropathy, according to the definitions of radiological and clinical osteoarthritis, in patients with long-term cure of acromegaly: A case-control study, Eur J Endocrinol 160 (3) (2009) 357–365.

[140] A. Colao, S. Cannavo, P. Marzullo, R. Pivonello, S. Squadrito, G. Vallone, et al., Twelve months of treatment with octreotide-LAR reduces joint thickness in acromegaly, Eur J Endocrinol 148 (1) (2003) 31–38.

[141] S. Bonadonna, G. Mazziotti, M. Nuzzo, A. Bianchi, A. Fusco, L. De Marinis, et al., Increased prevalence of radiological spinal deformities in active acromegaly: A cross-sectional study in postmenopausal women, J Bone Miner Res 20 (10) (2005) 1837–1844.

[142] G. Mazziotti, A. Bianchi, S. Bonadonna, V. Cimino, I. Patelli, A. Fusco, et al., Prevalence of vertebral fractures in men with acromegaly, J Clin Endocrinol Metab 93 (12) (2008) 4649–4655.
[143] R.F. Dons, P. Rosselet, B. Pastakia, J. Doppman, P. Gorden, Arthropathy in acromegalic patients before and after treatment: A long-term follow-up study, Clin Endocrinol (Oxf) 28 (5) (1988) 515–524.
[144] K.M. Kho, A.D. Wright, F.H. Doyle, Heel pad thickness in acromegaly, Br J Radiol 43 (506) (1970) 119–125.
[145] J.E. MacSweeney, M.A. Baxter, G.F. Joplin, Heel pad thickness is an insensitive index of biochemical remission in acromegaly, Clin Radiol 42 (5) (1990) 348–350.
[146] L.Y. Matsuoka, J. Wortsman, C.E. Kupchella, A. Eng, J.E. Dietrich, Histochemical characterization of the cutaneous involvement of acromegaly, Arch Intern Med 142 (10) (1982) 1820–1823.
[147] A.S. Bates, W. Van't Hoff, J.M. Jones, R.N. Clayton, An audit of outcome of treatment in acromegaly, Q J Med 86 (5) (1993) 293–299.
[148] A. Ben-Shlomo, S. Melmed, Skin manifestations in acromegaly, Clin Dermatol 24 (4) (2006) 256–259.
[149] J. Leavitt, I. Klein, F. Kendricks, J. Gavaler, D.H. VanThiel, Skin tags: A cutaneous marker for colonic polyps, Ann Intern Med 98 (6) (1983) 928–930.
[150] C. Rajasoorya, I.M. Holdaway, P. Wrightson, D.J. Scott, H.K. Ibbertson, Determinants of clinical outcome and survival in acromegaly, Clin Endocrinol (Oxf) 41 (1) (1994) 95–102.
[151] A. Colao, A. Cuocolo, P. Marzullo, E. Nicolai, D. Ferone, A.M. Della Morte, et al., Impact of patient's age and disease duration on cardiac performance in acromegaly: A radionuclide angiography study, J Clin Endocrinol Metab 84 (5) (1999) 1518–1523.
[152] R. Lopez-Velasco, H.F. Escobar-Morreale, B. Vega, E. Villa, J.M. Sancho, J.L. Moya-Mur, et al., Cardiac involvement in acromegaly: Specific myocardiopathy or consequence of systemic hypertension? J Clin Endocrinol Metab 82 (4) (1997) 1047–1053.
[153] S. Cannavo, B. Almoto, G. Cavalli, S. Squadrito, G. Romanello, M.T. Vigo, et al., Acromegaly and coronary disease: An integrated evaluation of conventional coronary risk factors and coronary calcifications detected by computed tomography, J Clin Endocrinol Metab 91 (10) (2006) 3766–3772.
[154] F. Bogazzi, L. Battolla, C. Spinelli, G. Rossi, S. Gavioli, V. Di Bello, et al., Risk factors for development of coronary heart disease in patients with acromegaly: A five-year prospective study, J Clin Endocrinol Metab 92 (11) (2007) 4271–4277.
[155] R. Luboshitzki, H. Hammerman, D. Barzilai, W. Markiewicz, The heart in acromegaly: Correlation of echocardiographic and clinical findings, Isr J Med Sci 16 (5) (1980) 378–383.
[156] A. Colao, A. Cuocolo, P. Marzullo, E. Nicolai, D. Ferone, L. Florimonte, et al., Effects of 1-year treatment with octreotide on cardiac performance in patients with acromegaly, J Clin Endocrinol Metab 84 (1) (1999) 17–23.
[157] A. Giustina, E. Boni, G. Romanelli, V. Grassi, G. Giustina, Cardiopulmonary performance during exercise in acromegaly, and the effects of acute suppression of growth hormone hypersecretion with octreotide, Am J Cardiol 75 (15) (1995) 1042–1047.
[158] P. Chanson, J. Timsit, C. Masquet, A. Warnet, P.J. Guillausseau, P. Birman, et al., Cardiovascular effects of the somatostatin analog octreotide in acromegaly, Ann Intern Med 113 (12) (1990) 921–925.
[159] P. Kamenicky, S. Viengchareun, A. Blanchard, G. Meduri, P. Zizzari, M. Imbert-Teboul, et al., Epithelial sodium channel is a key mediator of growth hormone-induced sodium retention in acromegaly, Endocrinology 149 (7) (2008) 3294–3305.
[160] A.M. Pereira, S.W. van Thiel, J.R. Lindner, F. Roelfsema, E.E. van der Wall, H. Morreau, et al., Increased prevalence of regurgitant valvular heart disease in acromegaly, J Clin Endocrinol Metab 89 (1) (2004) 71–75.
[161] B. Trotman-Dickenson, A.P. Weetman, J.M. Hughes, Upper airflow obstruction and pulmonary function in acromegaly: Relationship to disease activity, Q J Med 79 (290) (1991) 527–538.
[162] T. Pekkarinen, M. Partinen, R. Pelkonen, M. Iivanainen, Sleep apnoea and daytime sleepiness in acromegaly: Relationship to endocrinological factors, Clin Endocrinol (Oxf) 27 (6) (1987) 649–654.
[163] F. Rosenow, S. Reuter, U. Deuss, B. Szelies, R.D. Hilgers, W. Winkelmann, et al., Sleep apnoea in treated acromegaly: Relative frequency and predisposing factors, Clin Endocrinol (Oxf) 45 (5) (1996) 563–569.
[164] M.V. Davi, L. Dalle Carbonare, A. Giustina, M. Ferrari, A. Frigo, V. Lo Cascio, et al., Sleep apnoea syndrome is highly prevalent in acromegaly and only partially reversible after biochemical control of the disease, Eur J Endocrinol 159 (5) (2008) 533–540.
[165] F.R. van Haute, G.F. Taboada, L.L. Correa, G.A. Lima, R. Fontes, A.P. Riello, et al., Prevalence of sleep apnea and metabolic abnormalities in patients with acromegaly and analysis of cephalometric parameters by magnetic resonance imaging, Eur J Endocrinol 158 (4) (2008) 459–465.
[166] P. Attal, P. Chanson, Endocrine aspects of obstructive sleep apnea, J Clin Endocrinol Metab 95 (2) (2010) 483–495.
[167] R.R. Grunstein, K.Y. Ho, M. Berthon-Jones, D. Stewart, C.E. Sullivan, Central sleep apnea is associated with increased ventilatory response to carbon dioxide and hypersecretion of growth hormone in patients with acromegaly, Am J Respir Crit Care Med 150 (2) (1994) 496–502.
[168] J.D. O'Duffy, R.V. Randall, C.S. MacCarty, Median neuropathy (carpal-tunnel syndrome) in acromegaly. A sign of endocrine overactivity, Ann Intern Med 78 (3) (1973) 379–383.
[169] M. Nagulesparen, R. Trickey, M.J. Davies, J.S. Jenkins, Muscle changes in acromegaly, Br Med J 2 (6041) (1976) 914–915.
[170] R.T. Abed, J. Clark, M.H. Elbadawy, M.J. Cliffe, Psychiatric morbidity in acromegaly, Acta Psychiatr Scand 75 (6) (1987) 635–639.
[171] K. Furman, S. Ezzat, Psychological features of acromegaly, Psychother Psychosom 67 (3) (1998) 147–153.
[172] E. Ron, G. Gridley, Z. Hrubec, W. Page, S. Arora, J.F. Fraumeni, Acromegaly and gastrointestinal cancer, Cancer 68 (8) (1991) 1673–1677.
[173] N.W. Cheung, S.C. Boyages, Increased incidence of neoplasia in females with acromegaly, Clin Endocrinol (Oxf) 47 (3) (1997) 323–327.
[174] J.E. Brunner, C.C. Johnson, S. Zafar, E.L. Peterson, J.F. Brunner, R.C. Mellinger, Colon cancer and polyps in acromegaly: Increased risk associated with family history of colon cancer, Clin Endocrinol (Oxf) 32 (1) (1990) 65–71.
[175] S. Ezzat, C. Strom, S. Melmed, Colon polyps in acromegaly, Ann Intern Med 114 (9) (1991) 754–755.
[176] E.A. Ituarte, J. Petrini, J.M. Hershman, Acromegaly and colon cancer, Ann Intern Med 101 (5) (1984) 627–628.
[177] A. Pines, P. Rozen, E. Ron, T. Gilat, Gastrointestinal tumors in acromegalic patients, Am J Gastroenterol 80 (4) (1985) 266–269.
[178] S. Ezzat, S. Melmed, Clinical review 18: Are patients with acromegaly at increased risk for neoplasia? J Clin Endocrinol Metab 72 (2) (1991) 245–249.
[179] B. Delhougne, C. Deneux, R. Abs, P. Chanson, H. Fierens, P. Laurent-Puig, et al., The prevalence of colonic polyps in acromegaly: A colonoscopic and pathological study in 103 patients, J Clin Endocrinol Metab 80 (11) (1995) 3223–3226.

[180] S.D. Ladas, N.C. Thalassinos, G. Ioannides, S.A. Raptis, Does acromegaly really predispose to an increased prevalence of gastrointestinal tumours? Clin Endocrinol (Oxf) 41 (5) (1994) 597–601.
[181] M. Terzolo, G. Tappero, G. Borretta, G. Asnaghi, A. Pia, G. Reimondo, et al., High prevalence of colonic polyps in patients with acromegaly. Influence of sex and age, Arch Intern Med 154 (11) (1994) 1272–1276.
[182] H.F. Vasen, K.J. van Erpecum, F. Roelfsema, F. Raue, H. Koppeschaar, G. Griffioen, et al., Increased prevalence of colonic adenomas in patients with acromegaly, Eur J Endocrinol 131 (3) (1994) 235–237.
[183] A. Colao, A. Balzano, D. Ferone, N. Panza, G. Grande, P. Marzullo, et al., Increased prevalence of colonic polyps and altered lymphocyte subset pattern in the colonic lamina propria in acromegaly, Clin Endocrinol (Oxf) 47 (1) (1997) 23–28.
[184] P.J. Jenkins, P.D. Fairclough, T. Richards, D.G. Lowe, J. Monson, A. Grossman, et al., Acromegaly, colonic polyps and carcinoma, Clin Endocrinol (Oxf) 47 (1) (1997) 17–22.
[185] P. Mustacchi, M.B. Shimkin, Occurrence of cancer in acromegaly and in hypopituitarism, Cancer 10 (1) (1957) 100–104.
[186] P.J. Jenkins, Acromegaly and colon cancer, Growth Horm IGF Res 10 (Suppl A) (2000) S35–S36.
[187] A.G. Renehan, P. Bhaskar, J.E. Painter, S.T. O'Dwyer, N. Haboubi, J. Varma, et al., The prevalence and characteristics of colorectal neoplasia in acromegaly, J Clin Endocrinol Metab 85 (9) (2000) 3417–3424.
[188] P.J. Jenkins, V. Frajese, A.M. Jones, C. Camacho-Hubner, D.G. Lowe, P.D. Fairclough, et al., Insulin-like growth factor I and the development of colorectal neoplasia in acromegaly, J Clin Endocrinol Metab 85 (9) (2000) 3218–3221.
[189] E.M. Bunick, L.C. Mills, L.I. Rose, Association of acromegaly and meningiomas, JAMA 240 (12) (1978) 1267–1268.
[190] E. Resmini, A. Parodi, V. Savarino, A. Greco, A. Rebora, F. Minuto, et al., Evidence of prolonged orocecal transit time and small intestinal bacterial overgrowth in acromegalic patients, J Clin Endocrinol Metab 92 (6) (2007) 2119–2124.
[191] E. Resmini, A. Tagliafico, L. Bacigalupo, G. Giordano, E. Melani, A. Rebora, et al., Computed tomography colonography in acromegaly, J Clin Endocrinol Metab 94 (1) (2009) 218–222.
[192] S. Orme, R.J.Q. McNally, R.A. Cartwright, P.E. Belchetz, Mortality and cancer incidence in acromegaly: A retrospective cohort study, J Clin Endo Metab 83 (1998) 2730–2734.
[193] A.L. Barkan, Acromegaly. Diagnosis and therapy, Endocrinol Metab Clin North Am 18 (2) (1989) 277–310.
[194] G.A. Kaltsas, J.J. Mukherjee, P.J. Jenkins, M.A. Satta, N. Islam, J.P. Monson, et al., Menstrual irregularity in women with acromegaly, J Clin Endocrinol Metab 84 (8) (1999) 2731–2735.
[195] R. Baldelli, L. De Marinis, A. Bianchi, R. Pivonello, V. Gasco, R. Auriemma, et al., Microalbuminuria in insulin sensitivity in patients with growth hormone-secreting pituitary tumor, J Clin Endocrinol Metab 93 (3) (2008) 710–714.
[196] R.A. James, N. Moller, S. Chatterjee, M. White, P. Kendall-Taylor, Carbohydrate tolerance and serum lipids in acromegaly before and during treatment with high dose octreotide, Diabet Med 8 (6) (1991) 517–523.
[197] A. Giustina, A. Barkan, F.F. Casanueva, F. Cavagnini, L. Frohman, K. Ho, et al., Criteria for cure of acromegaly: A consensus statement, J Clin Endocrinol Metab 85 (2) (2000) 526–529.
[198] R.J. Robbins, S. Melmed (Eds.), Acromegaly: A century of scientific progress, Plenum Press, New York, 1987.
[199] A. Colao, P. Marzullo, S. Spiezia, D. Ferone, A. Giaccio, G. Cerbone, et al., Effect of growth hormone (GH) and insulin-like growth factor I on prostate diseases: An ultrasonographic and endocrine study in acromegaly, GH deficiency, and healthy subjects, J Clin Endocrinol Metab 84 (6) (1999) 1986–1991.
[200] I.M. Holdaway, M.J. Bolland, G.D. Gamble, A meta-analysis of the effect of lowering serum levels of GH and IGF-I on mortality in acromegaly, Eur J Endocrinol 159 (2) (2008) 89–95.
[201] A.D. Wright, D.M. Hill, C. Lowy, T.R. Fraser, Mortality in acromegaly, Q J Med 39 (153) (1970) 1–16.
[202] B. Swearingen, F.G. Barker, L. Katznelson, B.M. Biller, S. Grinspoon, A. Klibanski, et al., Long-term mortality after transsphenoidal surgery and adjunctive therapy for acromegaly, J Clin Endocrinol Metab 83 (10) (1998) 3419–3426.
[203] A. Abosch, J.B. Tyrrell, K.R. Lamborn, L.T. Hannegan, C.B. Applebury, C.B. Wilson, Transsphenoidal microsurgery for growth hormone-secreting pituitary adenomas: Initial outcome and long-term results, J Clin Endocrinol Metab 83 (10) (1998) 3411–3418.
[204] P.U. Freda, S.L. Wardlaw, K.D. Post, Long-term endocrinological follow-up evaluation in 115 patients who underwent transsphenoidal surgery for acromegaly, J Neurosurg 89 (3) (1998) 353–358.
[205] D. Jenkins, I. O'Brien, A. Johnson, R. Shakespear, M.C. Sheppard, P.M. Stewart, The Birmingham pituitary database: Auditing the outcome of the treatment of acromegaly, Clin Endocrinol (Oxf) 43 (5) (1995) 517–522.
[206] A. Ben-Shlomo, Pituitary gland: Predictors of acromegaly-associated mortality, Nat Rev Endocrinol 6 (2) (2010) 67–69.
[207] O.M. Dekkers, N.R. Biermasz, A.M. Pereira, J.A. Romijn, J.P. Vandenbroucke, Mortality in acromegaly: A metaanalysis, J Clin Endocrinol Metab 93 (1) (2008) 61–67.
[208] M. Sherlock, R.C. Reulen, A.A. Alonso, J. Ayuk, R.N. Clayton, M.C. Sheppard, et al., ACTH deficiency, higher doses of hydrocortisone replacement, and radiotherapy are independent predictors of mortality in patients with acromegaly, J Clin Endocrinol Metab 94 (11) (2009) 4216–4223.
[209] J. Ayuk, R.N. Clayton, G. Holder, M.C. Sheppard, P.M. Stewart, A.S. Bates, Growth hormone and pituitary radiotherapy, but not serum insulin-like growth factor-I concentrations, predict excess mortality in patients with acromegaly, J Clin Endocrinol Metab 89 (4) (2004) 1613–1617.
[210] A. Sata, K.K. Ho, Growth hormone measurements in the diagnosis and monitoring of acromegaly, Pituitary 10 (2) (2007) 165–172.
[211] A.L. Barkan, I.Z. Beitins, R.P. Kelch, Plasma insulin-like growth factor-I/somatomedin-C in acromegaly: Correlation with the degree of growth hormone hypersecretion, J Clin Endocrinol Metab 67 (1) (1988) 69–73.
[212] B.M. Chang-DeMoranville, I.M. Jackson, Diagnosis and endocrine testing in acromegaly, Endocrinol Metab Clin North Am 21 (3) (1992) 649–668.
[213] K.Y. Ho, J.D. Veldhuis, M.L. Johnson, R. Furlanetto, W.S. Evans, K.G. Alberti, et al., Fasting enhances growth hormone secretion and amplifies the complex rhythms of growth hormone secretion in man, J Clin Invest 81 (4) (1988) 968–975.
[214] M.L. Hartman, J.D. Veldhuis, M.L. Vance, A.C. Faria, R.W. Furlanetto, M.O. Thorner, Somatotropin pulse frequency and basal concentrations are increased in acromegaly and are reduced by successful therapy, J Clin Endocrinol Metab 70 (5) (1990) 1375–1384.

[215] K.Y. Ho, W.S. Evans, R.M. Blizzard, J.D. Veldhuis, G.R. Merriam, E. Samojlik, et al., Effects of sex and age on the 24-hour profile of growth hormone secretion in man: Importance of endogenous estradiol concentrations, Journal of Clinical Endocrinology and Metabolism 64 (1987) 51–58.
[216] E. Duncan, J.A. Wass, Investigation protocol: Acromegaly and its investigation, Clin Endocrinol (Oxf) 50 (3) (1999) 285–293.
[217] A.L. Barkan, S.E. Stred, K. Reno, M. Markovs, N.J. Hopwood, R.P. Kelch, et al., Increased growth hormone pulse frequency in acromegaly, J Clin Endocrinol Metab 69 (6) (1989) 1225–1233.
[218] E.V. Dimaraki, C.A. Jaffe, R. DeMott-Friberg, W.F. Chandler, A.L. Barkan, Acromegaly with apparently normal GH secretion: Implications for diagnosis and follow-up, J Clin Endocrinol Metab 87 (8) (2002) 3537–3542.
[219] P.U. Freda, C.M. Reyes, A.T. Nuruzzaman, R.E. Sundeen, J.N. Bruce, Basal and glucose-suppressed GH levels less than 1 microg/L in newly diagnosed acromegaly, Pituitary 6 (4) (2003) 175–180.
[220] P.U. Freda, A.T. Nuruzzaman, C.M. Reyes, R.E. Sundeen, K.D. Post, Significance of "abnormal" nadir growth hormone levels after oral glucose in postoperative patients with acromegaly in remission with normal insulin-like growth factor-I levels, J Clin Endocrinol Metab 89 (2) (2004) 495–500.
[221] A.C. Costa, A. Rossi, C.E. Martinelli Jr., H.R. Machado, A.C. Moreira, Assessment of disease activity in treated acromegalic patients using a sensitive GH assay: Should we achieve strict normal GH levels for a biochemical cure? J Clin Endocrinol Metab 87 (7) (2002) 3142–3147.
[222] P.U. Freda, K.D. Post, J.S. Powell, S.L. Wardlaw, Evaluation of disease status with sensitive measures of growth hormone secretion in 60 postoperative patients with acromegaly, J Clin Endocrinol Metab 83 (11) (1998) 3808–3816.
[223] D.R. Clemmons, J.J. Van Wyk, E.C. Ridgway, B. Kliman, R.N. Kjellberg, L.E. Underwood, Evaluation of acromegaly by radioimmunoassay of somatomedin-C, N Eng J Med 301 (1979) 1138–1142.
[224] M.R. Drange, IGFs in the evaluation of acromegaly, in: R.G. Rosenfeld, C.T. Roberts (Eds.), Contemporary Endocrinology The IGF System: Molecular Biology, Physiology, and Clinical Applications, Humana Press, 1999, pp. 699–720.
[225] D.R. Clemmons, Clinical utility of measurements of insulin-like growth factor 1, Nat Clin Pract Endocrinol Metab 2 (8) (2006) 436–446.
[226] D. Le Roith, The insulin-like growth factor system, Exp Diab Res 4 (4) (2003) 205–212.
[227] C.J. Strasburger, M. Bidlingmaier, How robust are laboratory measures of growth hormone status? Horm Res 64 (Suppl 2) (2005) 1–5.
[228] M. Bidlingmaier, Problems with GH assays and strategies toward standardization, Eur J Endocrinol 159 (Suppl 1) (2008) S41–S44.
[229] T.V. Nguyen, A.E. Nelson, C.J. Howe, M.J. Seibel, R.C. Baxter, D.J. Handelsman, et al., Within-subject variability and analytic imprecision of insulin-like growth factor axis and collagen markers: Implications for clinical diagnosis and doping tests, Clin Chem 54 (8) (2008) 1268–1276.
[230] A. Pokrajac, G. Wark, A.R. Ellis, J. Wear, G.E. Wieringa, P.J. Trainer, Variation in GH and IGF-I assays limits the applicability of international consensus criteria to local practice, Clin Endocrinol (Oxf) 67 (1) (2007) 65–70.
[231] S. Melmed, A. Colao, A. Barkan, M. Molitch, A.B. Grossman, D. Kleinberg, et al., Guidelines for acromegaly management: An update, J Clin Endocrinol Metab 94 (5) (2009) 1509–1517.
[232] S. Melmed, Extrapituitary acromegaly, Endocrinol Metab Clin North Am 20 (1991) 1–9.
[233] E.R. Laws, Surgery for acromegaly: Evolution of the techniques and outcomes, Rev Endocr Metab Disord 9 (1) (2008) 67–70.
[234] R. Fahlbusch, J. Honegger, M. Buchfelder, Surgical management of acromegaly, Endocrinol Metab Clin North Am 21 (3) (1992) 669–692.
[235] J.D. Law-Koune, N. Liu, B. Szekely, M. Fischler, Using the intubating laryngeal mask airway for ventilation and endotracheal intubation in anesthetized and unparalyzed acromegalic patients, J Neurosurg Anesthesiol 16 (1) (2004) 11–13.
[236] I. Ciric, A. Ragin, C. Baumgartner, D. Pierce, Complications of transsphenoidal surgery: Results of a national survey, review of the literature, and personal experience, Neurosurgery 40 (2) (1997) 225–236, discussion 36–7.
[237] P.J. Jenkins, P. Bates, M.N. Carson, P.M. Stewart, J.A. Wass, Conventional pituitary irradiation is effective in lowering serum growth hormone and insulin-like growth factor-I in patients with acromegaly, J Clin Endocrinol Metab 91 (4) (2006) 1239–1245.
[238] R.C. Eastman, P. Gorden, E. Glatstein, J. Roth, Radiation therapy of acromegaly, Endocrinol Metab Clin North Am 21 (3) (1992) 693–712.
[239] C.M. Feek, J. McLelland, J. Seth, A.D. Toft, W.J. Irvine, P.L. Padfield, et al., How effective is external pituitary irradiation for growth hormone-secreting pituitary tumors? Clin Endocrinol (Oxf) 20 (4) (1984) 401–408.
[240] A.L. Barkan, I. Halasz, K.J. Dornfeld, C.A. Jaffe, R.D. Friberg, W.F. Chandler, et al., Pituitary irradiation is ineffective in normalizing plasma insulin-like growth factor I in patients with acromegaly, J Clin Endocrinol Metab 82 (10) (1997) 3187–3191.
[241] J.S. Powell, S.L. Wardlaw, K.D. Post, P.U. Freda, Outcome of radiotherapy for acromegaly using normalization of insulin-like growth factor I to define cure, J Clin Endocrinol Metab 85 (5) (2000) 2068–2071.
[242] G. Barrande, M. Pittino-Lungo, J. Coste, D. Ponvert, X. Bertagna, J.P. Luton, et al., Hormonal and metabolic effects of radiotherapy in acromegaly: Long-term results in 128 patients followed in a single center, J Clin Endocrinol Metab 85 (10) (2000) 3779–3785.
[243] N.R. Biermasz, H. van Dulken, F. Roelfsema, Long-term follow-up results of postoperative radiotherapy in 36 patients with acromegaly, J Clin Endocrinol Metab 85 (7) (2000) 2476–2482.
[244] F. Castinetti, D. Taieb, J.M. Kuhn, P. Chanson, M. Tamura, P. Jaquet, et al., Outcome of gamma knife radiosurgery in 82 patients with acromegaly: Correlation with initial hypersecretion, J Clin Endocrinol Metab 90 (8) (2005) 4483–4488.
[245] A.J. van der Lely, W.W. de Herder, J.A. Janssen, S.W. Lamberts, Acromegaly: The significance of serum total and free IGF-I and IGF-binding protein-3 in diagnosis, J Endocrinol 155 (Suppl 1) (1997) S9–13, discussion S5–6.
[246] J.L. Millar, N.A. Spry, D.S. Lamb, J. Delahunt, Blindness in patients after external beam irradiation for pituitary adenomas: Two cases occurring after small daily fractional doses, Clin Oncol (R Coll Radiol) 3 (5) (1991) 291–294.
[247] M.J. Alexander, A.A. DeSalles, U. Tomiyasu, Multiple radiation-induced intracranial lesions after treatment for pituitary adenoma. Case report, J Neurosurg 88 (1) (1998) 111–115.
[248] M. Ahmed, I. Kanaan, A. Rifai, A. Tulbah, N. Ghannam, An unusual treatment-related complication in a patient with growth hormone-secreting pituitary tumor, J Clin Endocrinol Metab 82 (9) (1997) 2816–2820.

[249] O. al-Mefty, J.E. Kersh, A. Routh, R.R. Smith, The long-term side effects of radiation therapy for benign brain tumors in adults, J Neurosurg 73 (4) (1990) 502–512.
[250] J.R. Crossen, D. Garwood, E. Glatstein, E.A. Neuwelt, Neurobehavioral sequelae of cranial irradiation in adults: A review of radiation-induced encephalopathy, J Clin Oncol 12 (3) (1994) 627–642.
[251] A.J. van der Lely, W.W. de Herder, S.W. Lamberts, The role of radiotherapy in acromegaly, J Clin Endocrinol Metab 82 (10) (1997) 3185–3186.
[252] R.N. Kjellberg, B. Kliman, B.J. Swisher, Radiosurgery for pituitary adenoma with bragg peak proton beam, Asclepios Publishing, Paris, 1980.
[253] M. Brada, T.V. Ajithkumar, G. Minniti, Radiosurgery for pituitary adenomas, Clin Endocrinol (Oxf) 61 (5) (2004) 531–543.
[254] M. Brada, D. Ford, S. Ashley, J.M. Bliss, S. Crowley, M. Mason, et al., Risk of second brain tumour after conservative surgery and radiotherapy for pituitary adenoma, B Med J 304 (6838) (1992) 1343–1346.
[255] R.W. Tsang, N.J. Laperriere, W.J. Simpson, J. Brierley, T. Panzarella, H.S. Smyth, Glioma arising after radiation therapy for pituitary adenoma. A report of four patients and estimation of risk, Cancer 72 (7) (1993) 2227–2233.
[256] M. Sherlock, E. Fernandez-Rodriguez, A.A. Alonso, R.C. Reulen, J. Ayuk, R.N. Clayton, et al., Medical therapy in patients with acromegaly: Predictors of response and comparison of efficacy of dopamine agonists and somatostatin analogues, J Clin Endocrinol Metab 94 (4) (2009) 1255–1263.
[257] C.A. Jaffe, A.L. Barkan, Treatment of acromegaly with dopamine agonists, Endocrinol Metab Clin North Am 21 (3) (1992) 713–735.
[258] V.J. Moyes, K.A. Metcalfe, W.M. Drake, Clinical use of cabergoline as primary and adjunctive treatment for acromegaly, Eur J Endocrinol 159 (5) (2008) 541–545.
[259] R. Abs, J. Verhelst, D. Maiter, K. Van Acker, F. Nobels, J.L. Coolens, et al., Cabergoline in the treatment of acromegaly: A study in 64 patients, J Clin Endocrinol Metab 83 (2) (1998) 374–378.
[260] R. Schade, F. Andersohn, S. Suissa, W. Haverkamp, E. Garbe, Dopamine agonists and the risk of cardiac-valve regurgitation, N Engl J Med 356 (1) (2007) 29–38.
[261] G. Weckbecker, I. Lewis, R. Albert, H.A. Schmid, D. Hoyer, C. Bruns, Opportunities in somatostatin research: Biological, chemical and therapeutic aspects, Nat Rev Drug Discov 2 (12) (2003) 999–1017.
[262] A. Ben-Shlomo, S. Melmed, Pituitary somatostatin receptor signaling, Trends Endocrinol Metab 21 (2010) 123–133.
[263] Y. Greenman, S. Melmed, Heterogeneous expression of two somatostatin receptor subtypes in pituitary tumors, J Clin Endocrinol Metab 78 (2) (1994) 398–403.
[264] Y. Greenman, S. Melmed, Expression of three somatostatin receptor subtypes in pituitary adenomas: Evidence for preferential SSTR5 expression in the mammosomatotroph lineage, J Clin Endocrinol Metab 79 (3) (1994) 724–729.
[265] I. Shimon, X. Yan, J.E. Taylor, M.H. Weiss, M.D. Culler, S. Melmed, Somatostatin receptor (SSTR) subtype-selective analogues differentially suppress in vitro growth hormone and prolactin in human pituitary adenomas. Novel potential therapy for functional pituitary tumors, J Clin Invest 100 (9) (1997) 2386–2392.
[266] A. Ben-Shlomo, K.A. Wawrowsky, I. Proekt, N.M. Wolkenfeld, S.G. Ren, J. Taylor, et al., Somatostatin receptor type 5 modulates somatostatin receptor type 2 regulation of adrenocorticotropin secretion, J Biol Chem 280 (25) (2005) 24011–24021.
[267] G. Plewe, J. Beyer, U. Krause, M. Neufeld, E. del Pozo, Long-acting and selective suppression of growth hormone secretion by somatostatin analogue SMS 201-995 in acromegaly, Lancet 2 (8406) (1984) 782–784.
[268] S.W. Lamberts, The role of somatostatin in the regulation of anterior pituitary hormone secretion and the use of its analogs in the treatment of human pituitary tumors, Endocr Rev 9 (4) (1988) 417–436.
[269] J.A. Wass, M.O. Thorner, D.V. Morris, L.H. Rees, A.S. Mason, A.E. Jones, et al., Long-term treatment of acromegaly with bromocriptine, Br Med J 1 (6065) (1977) 875–878.
[270] F. Castinetti, A. Saveanu, I. Morange, T. Brue, Lanreotide for the treatment of acromegaly, Adv Ther 26 (6) (2009) 600–612.
[271] A.P. Casarini, R.S. Jallad, E.M. Pinto, I.C. Soares, S. Nonogaki, D. Giannella-Neto, et al., Acromegaly: Correlation between expression of somatostatin receptor subtypes and response to octreotide-lar treatment, Pituitary 12 (4) (2009) 297–303.
[272] A. Saveanu, P. Jaquet, T. Brue, A. Barlier, Relevance of coexpression of somatostatin and dopamine D2 receptors in pituitary adenomas, Mol Cell Endocrinol 286 (1–2) (2008) 206–213.
[273] S.W. Lamberts, A.J. van der Lely, W.W. de Herder, L.J. Hofland, Octreotide. N Engl J Med 334 (4) (1996) 246–254.
[274] K.Y. Ho, A.J. Weissberger, P. Marbach, L. Lazarus, Therapeutic efficacy of the somatostatin analog SMS 201-995 (octreotide) in acromegaly. Effects of dose and frequency and long-term safety, Ann Intern Med 112 (3) (1990) 173–181.
[275] S. Ezzat, P.J. Snyder, W.F. Young, L.D. Boyajy, C. Newman, A. Klibanski, et al., Octreotide treatment of acromegaly. A randomized, multicenter study, Ann Intern Med 117 (9) (1992) 711–718.
[276] S.L. Fougner, O.C. Borota, J.P. Berg, J.K. Hald, J. Ramm-Pettersen, J. Bollerslev, The clinical response to somatostatin analogues in acromegaly correlates to the somatostatin receptor subtype 2a protein expression of the adenoma, Clin Endocrinol (Oxf) 68 (3) (2008) 458–465.
[277] D. Ferone, W.W. de Herder, R. Pivonello, J.M. Kros, P.M. van Koetsveld, T. de Jong, et al., Correlation of in vitro and in vivo somatotropic adenoma responsiveness to somatostatin analogs and dopamine agonists with immunohistochemical evaluation of somatostatin and dopamine receptors and electron microscopy, J Clin Endocrinol Metab 93 (4) (2008) 1412–1417.
[278] S.W. Lamberts, M. Zweens, L. Verschoor, E. del Pozo, A comparison among the growth hormone-lowering effects in acromegaly of the somatostatin analog SMS 201-995, bromocriptine, and the combination of both drugs, J Clin Endocrinol Metab 63 (1) (1986) 16–19.
[279] A.K. Flogstad, J. Halse, S. Bakke, I. Lancranjan, P. Marbach, C. Bruns, et al., Sandostatin LAR in acromegalic patients: Long-term treatment, J Clin Endocrinol Metab 82 (1) (1997) 23–28.
[280] I. Lancranjan, A.B. Atkinson, Results of a European multicentre study with Sandostatin LAR in acromegalic patients. Sandostatin LAR Group, Pituitary 1 (2) (1999) 105–114.
[281] C.L. Ronchi, V. Varca, P. Beck Peccoz, E. Orsi, F. Donadio, A. Baccarelli, et al., Comparison between six-year therapy with long-acting somatostatin analogs and successful surgery in acromegaly: Effects on cardiovascular risk factors, J Clin Endocrinol Metab 91 (1) (2006) 121–128.
[282] R. Cozzi, M. Montini, R. Attanasio, M. Albizzi, G. Lasio, S. Lodrini, et al., Primary treatment of acromegaly with octreotide LAR: A long-term (up to nine years) prospective study of its efficacy in the control of disease activity and tumor shrinkage, J Clin Endocrinol Metab 91 (4) (2006) 1397–1403.

[283] J.C. Maiza, D. Vezzosi, M. Matta, F. Donadille, F. Loubes-Lacroix, M. Cournot, et al., Long-term (up to 18 years) effects on GH/IGF-1 hypersecretion and tumour size of primary somatostatin analogue (SSTa) therapy in patients with GH-secreting pituitary adenoma responsive to SSTa, Clin Endocrinol (Oxf) 67 (2) (2007) 282–289.

[284] P. Caron, M. Bex, D.R. Cullen, U. Feldt-Rasmussen, A.M. Pico Alfonso, S. Pynka, et al., One-year follow-up of patients with acromegaly treated with fixed or titrated doses of lanreotide autogel, Clin Endocrinol (Oxf) 60 (6) (2004) 734–740.

[285] J.S. Bevan, Clinical review: The antitumoral effects of somatostatin analog therapy in acromegaly, J Clin Endocrinol Metab 90 (3) (2005) 1856–1863.

[286] S. Melmed, R. Sternberg, D. Cook, A. Klibanski, P. Chanson, V. Bonert, et al., A critical analysis of pituitary tumor shrinkage during primary medical therapy in acromegaly, J Clin Endocrinol Metab 90 (7) (2005) 4405–4410.

[287] P.U. Freda, L. Katznelson, A.J. van der Lely, C.M. Reyes, S. Zhao, D. Rabinowitz, Long-acting somatostatin analog therapy of acromegaly: A meta-analysis, J Clin Endocrinol Metab 90 (8) (2005) 4465–4473.

[288] S.M. Carlsen, M. Lund-Johansen, T. Schreiner, S. Aanderud, O. Johannesen, J. Svartberg, et al., Preoperative octreotide treatment in newly diagnosed acromegalic patients with macroadenomas increases cure short-term postoperative rates: A prospective, randomized trial, J Clin Endocrinol Metab 93 (8) (2008) 2984–2990.

[289] E.C. Nemergut, A.S. Dumont, U.T. Barry, E.R. Laws, Perioperative management of patients undergoing transsphenoidal pituitary surgery, Anesth Analg 101 (4) (2005) 1170–1181.

[290] A. Colao, P. Marzullo, D. Ferone, L. Spinelli, A. Cuocolo, D. Bonaduce, et al., Cardiovascular effects of depot long-acting somatostatin analog Sandostatin LAR in acromegaly, J Clin Endocrinol Metab 85 (9) (2000) 3132–3140.

[291] J. Pascual, J. Freijanes, J. Berciano, C. Pesquera, Analgesic effect of octreotide in headache associated with acromegaly is not mediated by opioid mechanisms. Case report, Pain 47 (3) (1991) 341–344.

[292] M. Fleseriu, C. Yedinak, C. Campbell, J.B. Delashaw, Significant headache improvement after transsphenoidal surgery in patients with small sellar lesions, J Neurosurg 110 (2) (2009) 354–358.

[293] A. Colao, R. Pivonello, M. Galderisi, P. Cappabianca, R.S. Auriemma, M. Galdiero, et al., Impact of treating acromegaly first with surgery or somatostatin analogs on cardiomyopathy, J Clin Endocrinol Metab 93 (7) (2008) 2639–2646.

[294] A. Scillitani, I. Chiodini, V. Carnevale, G.M. Giannatempo, V. Frusciante, M. Villella, et al., Skeletal involvement in female acromegalic subjects: The effects of growth hormone excess in amenorrheal and menstruating patients, J Bone Miner Res 12 (10) (1997) 1729–1736.

[295] A. Colao, R. Attanasio, R. Pivonello, P. Cappabianca, L.M. Cavallo, G. Lasio, et al., Partial surgical removal of growth hormone-secreting pituitary tumors enhances the response to somatostatin analogs in acromegaly, J Clin Endocrinol Metab 91 (1) (2006) 85–92.

[296] N. Karavitaki, H.E. Turner, C.B. Adams, S. Cudlip, J.V. Byrne, V. Fazal-Sanderson, et al., Surgical debulking of pituitary macroadenomas causing acromegaly improves control by lanreotide, Clin Endocrinol (Oxf) 68 (6) (2008) 970–975.

[297] G. Mazziotti, I. Floriani, S. Bonadonna, V. Torri, P. Chanson, A. Giustina, Effects of somatostatin analogs on glucose homeostasis: A metaanalysis of acromegaly studies, J Clin Endocrinol Metab 94 (5) (2009) 1500–1508.

[298] S. Melmed, R.H. Dowling, L. Frohman, et al., Consensus statement: Benefits vs. risks of medical therapy for acromegaly, Am J Med 97 (1994) 468.

[299] Y.F. Shi, X.F. Zhu, A.G. Harris, J.X. Zhang, Q. Dai, Prospective study of the long-term effects of somatostatin analog (octreotide) on gallbladder function and gallstone formation in Chinese acromegalic patients, J Clin Endocrinol Metab 76 (1) (1993) 32–37.

[300] M.D. Page, M.E. Millward, A. Taylor, M. Preece, M. Hourihan, R. Hall, et al., Long-term treatment of acromegaly with a long-acting analogue of somatostatin, octreotide, Q J Med 74 (274) (1990) 189–201.

[301] C.B. Newman, S. Melmed, P.J. Snyder, W.F. Young, L.D. Boyajy, R. Levy, et al., Safety and efficacy of long-term octreotide therapy of acromegaly: Results of a multicenter trial in 103 patients – a clinical research center study, J Clin Endocrinol Metab 80 (9) (1995) 2768–2775.

[302] W.Y. Chen, D.C. Wight, T.E. Wagner, J.J. Kopchick, Expression of a mutated bovine growth hormone gene suppresses growth of transgenic mice, Proc Nat Acad Sci USA 87 (13) (1990) 5061–5065.

[303] P.J. Trainer, W.M. Drake, L. Katznelson, P.U. Freda, V. Herman-Bonert, A.J. van der Lely, et al., Treatment of acromegaly with the growth hormone-receptor antagonist pegvisomant, N Engl J Med 342 (16) (2000) 1171–1177.

[304] A.J. van der Lely, R.K. Hutson, P.J. Trainer, G.M. Besser, A.L. Barkan, L. Katznelson, et al., Long-term treatment of acromegaly with pegvisomant, a growth hormone receptor antagonist, Lancet 358 (9295) (2001) 1754–1759.

[305] C.E. Higham, T.T. Chung, J. Lawrance, W.M. Drake, P.J. Trainer, Long-term experience of pegvisomant therapy as a treatment for acromegaly, Clin Endocrinol (Oxf) 71 (1) (2009) 86–91.

[306] V.S. Herman-Bonert, K. Zib, J.A. Scarlett, S. Melmed, Growth hormone receptor antagonist therapy in acromegalic patients resistant to somatostatin analogs, J Clin Endocrinol Metab 85 (8) (2000) 2958–2961.

[307] A.L. Barkan, P. Burman, D.R. Clemmons, W.M. Drake, R.F. Gagel, P.E. Harris, et al., Glucose homeostasis and safety in patients with acromegaly converted from long-acting octreotide to pegvisomant, J Clin Endocrinol Metab 90 (10) (2005) 5684–5691.

[308] J.O. Jorgensen, U. Feldt-Rasmussen, J. Frystyk, J.W. Chen, L.O. Kristensen, C. Hagen, et al., Cotreatment of acromegaly with a somatostatin analog and a growth hormone receptor antagonist, J Clin Endocrinol Metab 90 (10) (2005) 5627–5631.

[309] J.H. Buhk, S. Jung, M.N. Psychogios, S. Goricke, S. Hartz, S. Schulz-Heise, et al., Tumor volume of growth hormone-secreting pituitary adenomas during treatment with pegvisomant: A prospective multicenter study, J Clin Endocrinol Metab 95 (2) (2010) 552–558.

[310] I. Schreiber, M. Buchfelder, M. Droste, K. Forssmann, K. Mann, B. Saller, et al., Treatment of acromegaly with the GH receptor antagonist pegvisomant in clinical practice: Safety and efficacy evaluation from the German Pegvisomant Observational Study, Eur J Endocrinol 156 (1) (2007) 75–82.

[311] S.J. Neggers, W.W. de Herder, J.A. Janssen, R.A. Feelders, A.J. van der Lely, Combined treatment for acromegaly with long-acting somatostatin analogs and pegvisomant: Long-term safety for up to 4.5 years (median 2.2 years) of follow-up in 86 patients, Eur J Endocrinol 160 (4) (2009) 529–533.

[312] R.S. Jallad, N.R. Musolino, S. Kodaira, V.A. Cescato, M.D. Bronstein, Does partial surgical tumour removal influence the response to octreotide-LAR in acromegalic patients previously resistant to the somatostatin analogue? Clin Endocrinol (Oxf) 67 (2) (2007) 310–315.

[313] R.D. Murray, S. Melmed, A critical analysis of clinically available somatostatin analog formulations for therapy of acromegaly, J Clin Endocrinol Metab 93 (8) (2008) 2957–2968.
[314] A. Colao, P. Cappabianca, P. Caron, E. De Menis, A.J. Farrall, M.R. Gadelha, et al., Octreotide LAR vs. surgery in newly diagnosed patients with acromegaly: A randomized, open-label, multicentre study, Clin Endocrinol (Oxf) 70 (5) (2009) 757–768.
[315] A. Colao, R.S. Auriemma, M. Galdiero, G. Lombardi, R. Pivonello, Effects of initial therapy for five years with somatostatin analogs for acromegaly on growth hormone and insulin-like growth factor-I levels, tumor shrinkage, and cardiovascular disease: A prospective study, J Clin Endocrinol Metab 94 (10) (2009) 3746–3756.
[316] M.C. Sheppard, Primary medical therapy for acromegaly, Clin Endocrinol (Oxf) 58 (4) (2003) 387–399.
[317] A. Colao, R.S. Auriemma, A. Rebora, M. Galdiero, E. Resmini, F. Minuto, et al., Significant tumour shrinkage after 12 months of lanreotide Autogel-120 mg treatment given first-line in acromegaly, Clin Endocrinol (Oxf) 71 (2) (2009) 237–245.
[318] J.D. Carmichael, V. Bonert, J.M. Mirocha, S. Melmed, The utility of oral glucose tolerance testing for diagnosis and assessment of treatment outcomes in 166 patients with acromegaly, J Clin Endo Metab 94 (2) (2009) 523–527.
[319] M. Sherlock, A. Aragon Alonso, R.C. Reulen, J. Ayuk, R.N. Clayton, G. Holder, et al., Monitoring disease activity using GH and IGF-I in the follow-up of 501 patients with acromegaly, Clin Endocrinol (Oxf) 71 (1) (2009) 74–81.
[320] I. Shimon, S. Melmed, Management of pituitary tumors, Ann of Intern Med 129 (6) (1998) 472–483.
[321] J. Weeke, S.E. Christensen, H. Orskov, A. Kaal, M.M. Pedersen, P. Illum, et al., A randomized comparison of intranasal and injectable octreotide administration in patients with acromegaly, J Clin Endocrinol Metab 75 (1) (1992) 163–169.
[322] M.S. Elston, K.L. McDonald, R.J. Clifton-Bligh, B.G. Robinson, Familial pituitary tumor syndromes, Nat Rev Endocrinol 5 (8) (2009) 453–461.
[323] V. Popovic, S. Damjanovic, D. Micic, M. Nesovic, M. Djurovic, M. Petakov, et al., Increased incidence of neoplasia in patients with pituitary adenomas. The Pituitary Study Group, Clin Endocrinol (Oxf) 49 (4) (1998) 441–445.
[324] J. Barzilay, G.J. Heatley, G.W. Cushing, Benign and malignant tumors in patients with acromegaly, Arch Intern Med 151 (8) (1991) 1629–1632.
[325] M. Sherlock, J. Ayuk, J.W. Tomlinson, A.A. Toogood, A. Aragon-Alonso, M.C. Sheppard, et al., Mortality in patients with pituitary disease, Endocr Rev 31 (2010) 301–342.
[326] C. Beauregard, U. Truong, J. Hardy, O. Serri, Long-term outcome and mortality after transsphenoidal adenomectomy for acromegaly, Clin Endocrinol (Oxf) 58 (1) (2003) 86–91.
[327] M.D. Krieger, W.T. Couldwell, M.H. Weiss, Assessment of long-term remission of acromegaly following surgery, J Neurosurg 98 (4) (2003) 719–724.
[328] S. Melmed, Acromegaly, second ed., Blackwell Science Publishing, Massachusetts, USA, 2002.
[329] F.F. Casanueva, J.P. Camina, M.C. Carreira, Y. Pazos, J.L. Varga, A.V. Schally, Growth hormone-releasing hormone as an agonist of the ghrelin receptor GHS-R1a, Proc Nat Acad Sci USA 105 (51) (2008) 20452–20457.
[330] F. Roelfsema, N.R. Biermasz, A.M. Pereira, J.A. Romijn, The role of pegvisomant in the treatment of acromegaly, Expert Opin Biol Ther 8 (5) (2008) 691–704.
[331] S.B. Melmed, Disorders of the Hypothalamus and Anterior Pituitary, fifth ed. Mosby Publishing, St. Louis, 1998.
[332] I.S. Login, J. Login, Governor Pio Pico, the monster of California … no more: Lessons in neuroendocrinology, Pituitary 13 (1) (2010) 80–86.
[333] I.M. Holdaway, R.C. Rajasoorya, G.D. Gamble, Factors influencing mortality in acromegaly, J Clin Endocrinol Metab 89 (2) (2004) 667–674.
[334] B.E. Pollock, J.T. Jacob, P.D. Brown, T.B. Nippoldt, Radiosurgery of growth hormone-producing pituitary adenomas: Factors associated with biochemical remission, J Neurosurg 106 (5) (2007) 833–838.
[335] E. Ur, S.J. Mather, J. Bomanji, D. Ellison, K.E. Britton, A.B. Grossman, et al., Pituitary imaging using a labelled somatostatin analogue in acromegaly, Clin Endocrinol (Oxf) 36 (2) (1992) 147–150.
[336] I. Lancranjan, C. Bruns, P. Grass, P. Jaquet, J. Jervell, P. Kendall-Taylor, et al., Sandostatin LAR: A promising therapeutic tool in the management of acromegalic patients, Metabolism 45 (8 Suppl 1) (1996) 67–71.
[337] P.M. Stewart, K.F. Kane, S.E. Stewart, I. Lancranjan, M.C. Sheppard, Depot long-acting somatostatin analog (Sandostatin-LAR) is an effective treatment for acromegaly, J Clin Endocrinol Metab 80 (11) (1995) 3267–3272.
[338] S.J. Neggers, M.O. van Aken, J.A. Janssen, R.A. Feelders, W.W. de Herder, A.J. van der Lely, Long-term efficacy and safety of combined treatment of somatostatin analogs and pegvisomant in acromegaly, J Clin Endocrinol Metab 92 (12) (2007) 4598–4601.
[339] R. Baldelli, A. Colao, P. Razzore, M.L. Jaffrain-Rea, P. Marzullo, E. Ciccarelli, et al., Two-year follow-up of acromegalic patients treated with slow release lanreotide (30 mg), J Clin Endocrinol Metab 85 (11) (2000) 4099–4103.

CHAPTER

15

Prolactinoma

Mary P. Gillam [1], Mark E. Molitch [2]

[1] Endocrinologist, Chicago, IL, USA,

[2] Northwestern University Feinberg School of Medicine, Chicago, IL, USA

INTRODUCTION

Coincident with the initial characterization of prolactin (PRL) in the early 1930s by Riddle and his colleagues (see Chapter 5) were the first clinical reports of a syndrome of amenorrhea coupled with galactorrhea [1]. However, it was not until 1972 that Friesen et al. first demonstrated elevated PRL levels in the serum of a patient with a prolactinoma, the decline in such levels with partial adenomectomy, and the production of PRL by the tumor in vitro [2]. Over the ensuing years, improvements in diagnostic radiologic procedures, advances in surgical techniques and the development of dopamine agonists as medical therapy have resulted in highly successful rates of treatment for the majority of prolactinomas. Prolactinomas are the most common subtype of the hormone-secreting pituitary tumors according to autopsy, epidemiological and surgical series [3,4].

Classification

Prolactinomas are classified on a clinical basis by size: microadenomas are defined as less than 10 mm in diameter; macroadenomas are greater than 10 mm in diameter. Giant prolactinomas are defined as greater than 4 cm in diameter and/or those with more than 2 cm of suprasellar extension. Supra-, infra- and parasellar extension occurs when adenomas grow beyond the immediate sellar region. Invasion can be detected grossly, radiologically, or microscopically. The direction and degree of extrasellar extension and invasion are of obvious clinical importance. The larger the tumor and the more invasive it is, the less likely it is that surgery or medical therapy will provide a complete cure [5–7]. The importance of radiologic demonstration of invasion is unclear, as a large proportion of macro- and microadenomas show evidence of dural invasion when examined histologically [8,9].

In general, serum PRL levels parallel the size of the tumors. However, when two-site immnunoradiometric assays (IRMA) or chemiluminometric (ICMA) assays are used, patients with very high PRL levels may appear to have PRL levels that are normal or only moderately elevated, i.e., in the order of 30–200 μg/L, due to the "hook effect" [10]. Under these circumstances, a prolactinoma may be misclassified as a clinically nonfunctioning macroadenoma, which may cause a similar moderate PRL elevation due to interference with dopamine transport to normal lactotrophs [11–13]. This confusion can be avoided by remeasuring the PRL in such patients at 1:100 dilution (see Chapter 5).

Pathologically, lactotroph adenomas are subclassified into sparsely granulated variants, densely granulated variants and acidophil stem cell adenomas [14]. Sparsely granulated prolactinomas are the most common subtype. Untreated sparsely granulated adenomas exhibit chromophobic morphology and globular juxtanuclear/golgi PRL immunoreactivity [15]. Densely granulated lactotroph adenomas, which are less common, exhibit acidophilic morphology and diffuse cytoplasmic PRL immunoreactivity [15]. Acidophil stem cell adenomas are rare, aggressive lactotroph tumors composed of oncocytic cells with large cytoplasmic vacuoles corresponding to giant mitochondria. They are marked by nuclear Pit-1 staining, diffuse PRL and scant growth hormone (GH) reactivity, and occasional fibrous bodies [15]. Other bihormonal adenomas that secrete both PRL and GH are derived from mixed GH/PRL cell adenomas or mammosomatotroph adenomas [14]. Prolactinomas that have been treated with bromocriptine exhibit fibrous changes, and may

The Pituitary, Third Edition, DOI: 10.1016/B978-0-12-380926-1.10015-X lose their characteristic histologic appearance. Usually, these lactotroph tumors will demonstrate some focal PRL reactivity and nuclear positivity for Pit-1 [15]. The new entity of "atypical adenoma" designated by the World Health Organization (WHO) is defined as an invasive tumor with elevated mitotic index, Ki67 labeling index >3% and extensive nuclear immunostaining for p53 protein [14]. Malignant prolactinomas are currently defined by the presence of distant cerebrospinal and/or systemic metastases.

Epidemiology and Natural History of Prolactinomas

Pituitary adenomas are found at autopsy in 1.5–31% of subjects not suspected of having pituitary disease while alive [4]. The average frequency of finding an adenoma for these studies, which examined a total of 18,902 pituitaries, is 10.7%. In the studies in which PRL immunohistochemistry was performed, 22–66% of such adenomas stained positively for PRL [4].

In these postmortem studies, all but seven of the tumors (99.97%) were less than 10 mm in diameter, and these seven were <15 mm in diameter. Thus, microprolactinomas are present in about 5% of the adult population. The infrequent finding of macroadenomas among these studies suggests that growth from micro- to macroadenomas is uncommon, and/or that virtually all macroadenomas come to clinical attention during life, and therefore are not included in autopsy findings.

Epidemiologic studies have found a ten-fold difference in the prevalence of pituitary tumors, ranging from 8.2–94 per 100,000. The most recent population studies report higher figures reflecting, in part, the improved diagnostic biochemical and radiologic techniques that have developed over the 30 years spanning these studies [16–19]. The highest figure of ~1:1000 may be an underestimate, as it is only about 1% of the actual frequency of tumors determined from the autopsy studies. As in the autopsy series, the most common tumors were prolactinomas, comprising 57–66% of cases in the United Kingdom [19] and Belgian series [3].

Studies examining the natural history of untreated microprolactinomas have shown that significant growth of these tumors is uncommon. Six series of patients with microadenomas who were found to have CT or tomographic evidence of prolactinomas were observed without treatment for a period of up to 8 years [20–25] (Table 15.1). Of 139 tumors followed, only 9 (7%) microprolactinomas had evidence of growth using these methods of imaging. In a similar 2–6 year follow-up of 140 patients with hyperprolactinemia and no radiologic evidence of tumor (idiopathic hyperprolactinemia), only 22 (15.7%) developed evidence of microadenomas [22,23,26–28]. It should be noted that both of these figures represent very general estimates of the likelihood of tumor growth or emergence, since the imaging methods used to detect and/or measure adenoma size changed over the surveillance period for most of these series, from one with low sensitivity and specificity (tomography) to one with better sensitivity and specificity (CT). Thus, the true rates of progression from normal sellas or those with minimal abnormalities to documentation of the presence of a tumor have not been determined accurately and it is likely that the numbers given above are overestimates rather than underestimates. Studies examining the risk of progression from normal sella to microprolactinoma, or from micro- to macroprolactinoma in untreated individuals using modern imaging techniques with greater sensitivity and specificity (i.e., pituitary-dedicated, gadolinium enhanced MRI) have not been published. Nonetheless, based upon the available data, it appears that the vast majority of microprolactinomas stay small. Hyperprolactinemia may spontaneously resolve in some untreated patients, particularly those who are eumenorrheic or postmenopausal [22,29,30].

TABLE 15.1 Studies Examining the Natural History of Prolactinomas

Study	Reference	Patients (n)	Evidence of Tumor Growth	Length of Follow-up (years)
von Werder et al.	[24]	10	1	4
March et al.	[21]	43	2	4
Weiss et al.	[25]	27	3	6
Koppleman et al.	[20]	8	1	2.5–7.5
Sisam et al.	[23]	38	0	4
Schlechte et al.	[22]	13	2	5.3
Total		**139**	**9 (6.5%)**	**2.5–8.0**

Several efforts have been made to identify prognostic markers of aggressive behavior or pituitary tumor progression [31,32], but prognostication continues to remain a major challenge for clinicians and pituitary pathologists. A number of potential markers have been analyzed, including morphologic features, dural invasion, cytogenetics, proliferative markers, p53 immunostaining and gene expression profiling. Unfortunately, none of these methods has proven to consistently correlate with invasiveness, growth, or recurrence [8,33–37]. Although a single retrospective study reported a set of genes that were differentially expressed among surgically resected stable versus clinically progressive prolactinomas, these data have not been independently replicated, nor has this gene set shown an advantage in terms of its prognostic utility over more easily assessed variables, such as radiologic invasiveness [38]. Whether the WHO-defined entity of "atypical adenoma" will predict clinical behavior is not known at this time, and future prospective studies shall determine whether this pathological classification scheme provides meaningful prognostic clinical information.

PATHOGENESIS

Scientific investigation over the last decade has produced substantial advances in delineating the etiology of prolactinomas and pituitary tumors in general. Nonetheless, the molecular mechanisms underlying most cases of prolactinomas have not been fully defined. Some of the alterations and pathophysiologic mechanisms that have been reported are observed in several or all of the pituitary lineages, while other pathways restraining pituitary tumor growth and progression are lineage-specific. While many of the described molecular defects were identified originally in human pituitary adenomas, others have been identified by their incidental discovery in transgenic or knockout mouse models, in which case the corresponding molecular changes may or may not have been verified in human samples.

Although highly differentiated, pituitary lactotrophs are capable of responding to various stimuli and reentering the cell cycle, thus permitting reversible and adaptive changes in cell growth. A prominent example of this behavior is the expansion of the lactotroph population that occurs during pregnancy, through cellular proliferation, transdifferentiation from other adenohypophyseal cell types, or possibly through stem cell replenishment [39–41]. Observation of this biological plasticity fueled early theories of pituitary tumorigenesis, which proposed that hormonal or growth factor stimulation serves as a primary etiologic factor in neoplastic transformation. However, modern techniques of molecular biology using the principle of X chromosome inactivation later proved that pituitary adenomas are monoclonal neoplasms [42,43]. As such, the initial step in pituitary tumor development involves the acquisition of a typically somatic genetic event, which subsequently confers its derivatives with a selective growth advantage. It is nonetheless likely, however, that the local hormonal milieu plays an important role in promoting the neoplastic process by enhancing the proliferative potential of tumorous tissue through permissive effects on cellular growth.

Following the scientific determination of the monoclonal nature of these tumors, an intense investigation commenced to identify those fundamental cell-autonomous events necessary and/or sufficient to transform pituitary cells. It has since been appreciated that the acquisition of several somatic genetic changes is usually required for neoplastic transformation in humans [44]. Furthermore, it has become apparent that no single factor completely underlies all pituitary oncogenesis, and the components involved and sequence of events in the tumorigenic cascade are highly variable and heterogeneous. In some tumors, gene amplifications or mutations are the primary events; in others, altered function of microRNAs or epigenetic changes may stimulate the process. Typically, initial pathogenetic events involve loss-of-function of tumor suppressors or gain-of-function of oncogenes, favoring a selection process through which additional defects may accumulate. In some cases, this may lead to more aggressive behavior marked by unrestrained proliferation, insensitivity to inhibitory signals and evasion of apoptosis [44].

Prolactinomas, like pituitary tumors in general, exhibit growth attributes that differentiate them from other types of human malignancies. For example, the vast majority of prolactinomas are pathologically benign and stable. While locally invasive growth is frequent, malignant behavior and metastatic spread are rare. This intrinsic resistance to malignant transformation has been attributed to the process of oncogene-induced cell senescence, but a heightened sensitivity of adenohypophyseal tissue specifically for this process is a biological phenomenon that remains incompletely understood on a molecular level [45,46]. As a second example, most lactotroph tumors retain some degree of sensitivity to inhibitory growth signals, as demonstrated by their frequent responsiveness to dopamine agonist medical therapy. In keeping with these unique characteristics, the scientific evidence gathered thus far has shown that the molecular defects that are routinely found in nonendocrine carcinomas have not been consistently identified in pituitary adenomas, suggesting that pituitary cells are governed by distinct mechanisms of cell cycle control.

In the present era, the search for candidate pituitary lactotroph oncogenes or tumor suppressors has largely utilized two strategies. The first involves a candidate gene approach, in which a search for causal factors is explored among components known to be important for pituitary development or homeostasis. The second employs a reverse genetics approach, using unbiased techniques such as differential display. Over the last several years, a plethora of studies have reported overexpressed putative oncogenes, or underrepresented alleged tumor suppressors in human pituitary tumor tissue. Deciphering out those findings which represent true pathophysiologic events that initiate the tumorigenic cascade versus phenomena that accompany or cooperate with the transformation process are important areas of uncertainty that require further investigation.

The pathogenetic defects associated with human prolactinomas include a diverse set of alterations encompassing one or more of the following general mechanisms: disrupted chromatin remodeling, dysregulated cell cycle control, altered hormone or growth factor signaling, aberrant expression of pituitary development factors. The specific genetic defects associated with familial prolactinomas may be unique, although the cellular signaling pathways downstream of the initial predisposing genetic defect are likely to represent mechanisms that are shared by sporadic processes of tumorigenesis.

Familial Prolactinomas

A minority of prolactinomas occur as part of an inherited predisposition syndrome. Though uncommon, single gene disorders that predispose to pituitary neoplasia afford a unique window of insight into the mechanisms that drive carcinogenesis. Prolactinomas are the most common subtype of pituitary adenoma reported in multiple endocrine neoplasia type 1 (MEN1), a disorder that behaves as an autosomal dominant trait with reduced penetrance of tumors in the anterior pituitary, parathyroids and pancreatic islets. MEN1 syndrome is caused by germline inactivating mutations in the *MEN1* gene, which encodes the tumor suppressor menin. Additional somatic loss of heterozygosity at the *MEN1* locus (11q13) inactivates the normal allele. Since LOH at 11q13 is observed in 20–30% of sporadic lactotroph tumors [47,48], a role for menin in sporadic tumorigenesis has been suggested. Mutational analysis of the coding region of the *MEN1* gene has found mutations in <2% of sporadic tumors, and levels of the mRNA transcript are not reduced [49–52]. However, a significant reduction in menin protein expression is observed in ~50% of sporadic pituitary adenomas [53], and it therefore remains possible that defects in post-translational processing of menin or alterations in the effectors of menin action could play a role in the tumorigenic process in sporadic tumors.

Validation of the tumor suppressor role of menin was achieved with the generation and phenotypic analysis of *Men1* knockout mice, as mice heterozygous for *Men1* disruption develop tumors in neuroendocrine organs (predominantly lactotroph adenomas in the pituitary) following somatic loss of the wild-type allele, around 9 months of age [54,55]. Thus, tumorigenesis in *Men1* knockout mice closely recapitulates the process that occurs in humans. The molecular mechanism(s) by which menin serves in a tumor suppressor function continue to remain enigmatic, however. Mounting evidence suggests that menin regulates gene expression at an epigenetic level by altering chromatin modifications [56,57]. For example, menin has been shown to promote histone methylation and positively regulate the expression of several cell cycle proteins, including the cyclin-dependent kinase inhibitors p18 and p27 [58,59], data which are relevant given that *Cdkn2c*$^{-/-}$;*Cdkn1b*$^{-/-}$ mice develop pituitary and pancreatic islet tumors [60,61]. These findings are consistent with a model in which menin promotes histone methylation at the promoters of p18 and p27 to up-regulate their expression. This consequently maintains an inhibitory effect on the G_1 cyclin-dependent kinases and prevents Rb phosphorylation, thereby halting cell cycle progression. Confirmation of these putative epigenetic targets of menin, and verification that alterations in them have a direct effect on the tumorigenic process in tumors of lactotrophs and/or other pituitary cell types, is awaited.

Germline mutations in the *AIP* gene were identified in a Finnish population of patients with familial isolated pituitary adenoma (FIPA) associated with somatotropinomas and prolactinomas [62]. In the initial report, 8 of 54 patients from several families with a predisposition to prolactinomas and somatotropinomas harbored one of three different *AIP* germline mutations [62]. The specificity of this finding was noted by the absence of mutations in nonaffected individuals. LOH at the *AIP* locus was found in the tumors examined, suggesting that loss of the wild-type allele led to tumor development. Moreover, of the 35 different mutations described to date, approximately 60% are nonsense or frameshifts, predicting truncation or absence of the resulting protein [63]. Hence, *AIP* appears to be a classic tumor suppressor gene with tumors in affected patients showing somatic loss of the wild-type allele. Germline *AIP* mutations have been detected in a small proportion (15%) of other FIPA kindreds [64–66], but they are rarely identified in individuals with sporadic prolactinomas [67,68] or somatotropinomas [63,64,67–70]. Similarly, somatic mutations of the *AIP* gene have thus far not been reported in tumorous adenohypophyseal tissue [71].

The *AIP* gene encodes a 630-amino acid cochaperone protein called the aryl hydrocarbon receptor interacting protein (AIP). Early nondefinitive studies employing over-expression constructs in GH3 and nonpituitary cell lines suggest that AIP might suppress cell proliferation through interactions with phosphodiesterase PDE4A5 [65]. Like menin, AIP is widely expressed, leaving unexplained the basis for the predilection to pituitary neoplasia in its functional absence. The report of an *AIP* knockout mouse model indicates that nullizygosity at the *AIP* locus leads to embryonic lethality [72]. Long-term studies evaluating the tumor potential of heterozygous or pituitary-specific *AIP* knockout mice have not been reported.

Altered Chromatin Remodeling

Recent studies have proven a causal role for the *HMGA2* gene in the process leading to the generation of human pituitary prolactinomas. The high-mobility group A (HMGA) proteins are nonhistone nuclear proteins known as architectural transcription factors that bind to the minor groove of AT-rich enhancers or promoters, and they introduce structural alterations in chromatin through complex networks of protein–DNA and protein–protein interactions [73]. These epigenetic regulators influence a diverse spectrum of biological processes, ranging from embryonic development, cell differentiation, cell cycle progression, apoptosis, senescence, to DNA repair [74]. A role for HMGA2 in pituitary oncogenesis was initially suspected based upon the observation that the majority (85% of females, 40% of males) of transgenic mice ubiquitously over-expressing a CMV-driven *HMGA2* gene (*HMGA2*^{tg}) develop aggressive lactotroph and somatotroph pituitary adenomas by 12 (female) to 18 (male) months of age [75]. This in vivo demonstration of tumorigenesis confirmed conclusions drawn from earlier in vitro experiments that revealed oncogenic properties for HMGA proteins, such as their ability to transform fibroblasts and promote anchorage-independent cell growth [76]. The *HMGA2* gene is located on chromosome 12, and polysomy and structural rearrangements of chromosome 12 are frequent cytogenetic alterations in human prolactinomas [77,78]. Cytogenetic fluorescent in situ hybridization (FISH) analysis of human prolactinoma specimens revealed an increased dosage (trisomy or tetrasomy) of chromosome 12, and an amplification of the *HMGA2* locus, which correlated with over-expression of the *HMGA2* gene (Figure 15.1) [79]. Of note, transgenic mice over-expressing the *HMGA1* gene (*HMGA1*^{tg}) also exhibit a high incidence of mammosomatotroph adenomas, but neither rearrangement nor amplification of the *HMGA1* gene has been found in human pituitary adenomas.

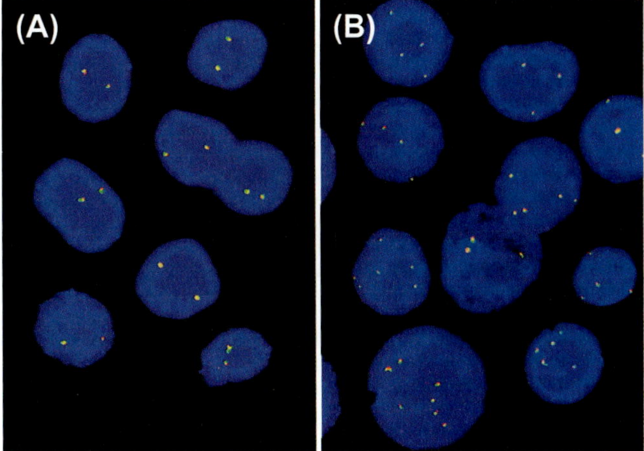

FIGURE 15.1 *HMGA2* amplification in human prolactinomas. Interphase FISH analysis of *HMGA2* dosage in human pituitary adenomas using dual-color probes (red and green), which recognize the 5′ and the 3′ regions of the gene. The nonfunctioning adenoma in panel A shows two fluorescent signals on the disomic sample, whereas the prolactinoma in panel B shows three or more signals, thus indicating overrepresentation of the *HMGA2* region. *Adapted from figure 1 from [75], with permission.*

In addition to gene amplification, there are data suggesting that alterations in post-transcriptional regulation of HMGA2 protein production by microRNAs (miRNAs) could contribute to its overexpression in some cases. The 3′ untranslated region (UTR) of the HMGA2 mRNA contains target sequences for several different miRNAs, including seven target sites for let-7 miRNA binding (Figure 15.2) [80]. Expression of HMGA2 is suppressed by let-7 in vitro [80,81] and disrupting the let-7 regulation of HMGA2 augments oncogenic transformation [81]. In fact, the separation of the regulatory 3′-UTR region from the intact *HMGA2* coding sequence has been demonstrated to have neoplastic effects in a variety of human tumors and a transgenic mouse model, suggesting that negative regulation of HMGA2 expression via the 3′-UTR is an important control mechanism [80,82]. In one pathological study of human pituitary adenomas, reduced expression of the let-7 miRNA was observed in 6 of 9 (68%) prolactinomas and this down-regulation inversely correlated with HMGA2 immunoreactivity and tumor invasion, implying that loss of let-7 expression might contribute to the aggressive phenotype of these cancers via re-expression of HMGA2 [83]. Thus, alterations in let-7 or other miRNAs targeting HMGA2 could represent an additional mechanism for HMGA2 over-expression in sporadic prolactinomas.

A series of experiments subsequently demonstrated a molecular mechanism involving disruption of signaling and cell cycle pathways known to be relevant for pituitary homeostasis to explain the process by which over-expression of HMGA2 induces the

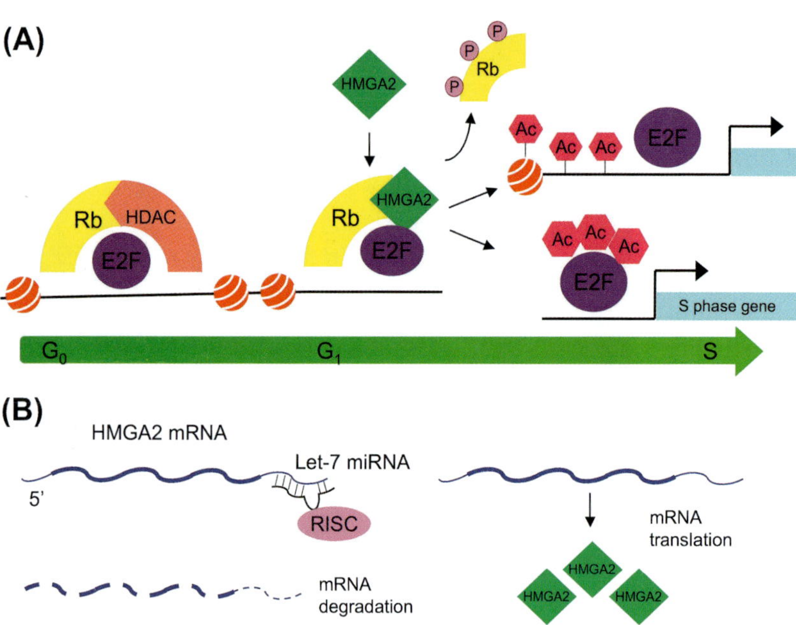

FIGURE 15.2 (A) Schematic model illustrating a molecular mechanism by which over-expression of HMGA2 protein promotes cell cycle progression through the G_1–S transition. The HMGA2 proteins displace histone deacetylase 1 (HDAC1) from the pRb/E2F1 complex. *From [84]*. This leads to both histone acetylation (upper diagonal arrow) and E2F-1 acetylation (lower diagonal arrow), and subsequent enhanced E2F1 transcriptional activity. *From [84]*. (B) Schematic diagram illustrating microRNA regulation of HMGA2 levels. On the left, the let-7 microRNA binds to the 3′ untranslated region of the *HMGA2* gene and thus down-regulates HMGA2 expression by causing the degradation of the mRNA and/or by inhibiting translation (latter not shown). *From [80,83]*. On the right, loss of let-7 miRNA results in increased HMGA2 mRNA levels.

development of mammosomatotroph adenomas (Figure 15.2). Rb is a key regulator of the G_1–S transition of the cell cycle via two processes: (1) by binding and inhibiting the activity of the E2F class of transcription factors; and (2) by recruiting histone deacetylases (HDACs) to E2F-responsive promoters. Histone acetyl transferases and HDACs acetylate and deacetylate, respectively, core histone tails that protrude from the nucleosome. Histone acetylation weakens the interaction between histone N-terminal tails and DNA, thus opening up chromatin and increasing accessibility for activating transcription factors. Immunoprecipitation studies using cell lysates from pituitary tissue of HMGA2 transgenic mice (*HMGA2^{tg}*) demonstrate that HMGA2 proteins interfere with the recruitment of HDAC1 to the Rb/E2F1 complex, resulting in greater acetylation of both E2F1 and DNA-associated histones [84]. This displacement of HDAC enhances E2F1 activity and assists in driving cells into S phase (Figure 15.2). The dependency of HMGA2 tumorigenesis on E2F1 activation was confirmed genetically by demonstrating that HMGA2 transgenic mice bred on an *E2f1*-deficient background (*HMGA^{tg};E2f1$^{-/-}$*) suppresses the development of lactotroph and somatotroph tumors by 75% [84].

An additional mechanism that could contribute to HMGA2-mediated pituitary transformation involves its role in stem cell biology. Emerging experimental data support the existence of a stem cell population in the adult adenohypophysis, a niche that could represent a potential source of transforming pituitary cells [39,40,85]. Given prior evidence that HMGA2 participates in the maintenance of the stem cell self-renewal capacity in neural stem cells [86], it is possible that dysregulation of HMGA2 could also influence the expansion of pituitary cancer stem cells.

Cell Cycle Dysregulation

Deregulation of the cell cycle represents a fundamental mechanism upon which many aspects of pituitary oncogenesis ultimately converge. A comprehensive discussion of these processes is beyond the scope of this chapter, and the reader is referred to recent reviews (reviewed in [87]). An abbreviated overview is presented here to facilitate reader understanding (Figure 15.3). The G_1 phase of the cell cycle is dominated by a complex set of interacting proteins that regulate exit from quiescence and progression into S phase. These proteins include cyclin-dependent kinases (CDKs), their regulatory cyclin subunits and CDK inhibitors. CDK4 and CDK6 activity requires D-type cyclins, the synthesis of which is regulated by mitogenic signaling pathways. In quiescent cells, hypophosphorylated forms of Rb participate in transcriptional repressor complexes with the E2F class of transcription factors, and recruit histone deacetylases and chromatin-remodeling factors to E2F-responsive promoters [88]. In early G_1 in response to mitogenic signals, CDK4/6–cyclin D complexes phosphorylate retinoblastoma protein (Rb), resulting in its partial inactivation, thereby activating the E2F/DP transcription factors that modulate the expression of genes required for cell cycle progression [89,90]. In late G_1 cyclin E pairs with CDK2 to complete phosphorylation of Rb, which further contributes to G_1 exit and S phase initiation. Two families of CDK inhibitor (CKI) proteins

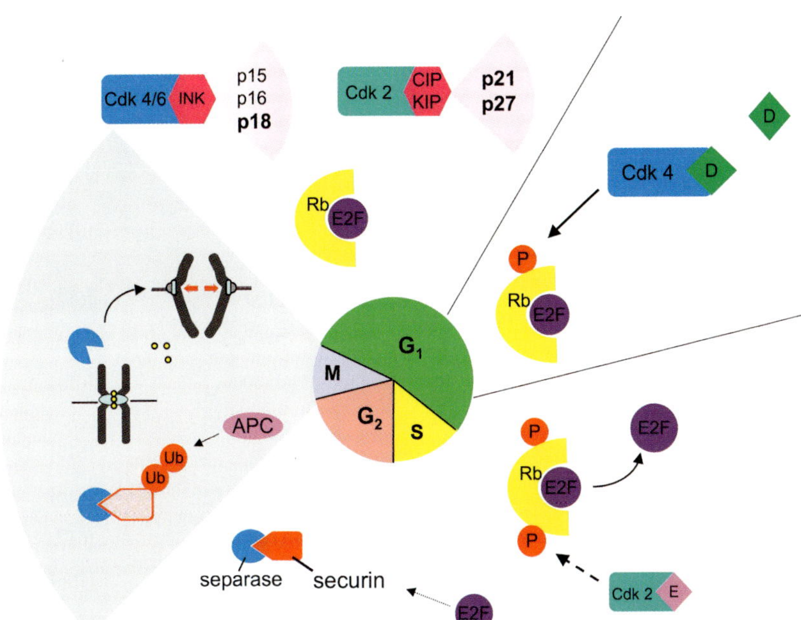

FIGURE 15.3 Schematic illustration of the major cell cycle regulators involved in lactotroph proliferation. During G_0, cyclin-dependent kinase inhibitors of the INK4 family inhibit cyclin-dependent kinase 4 or 6, while those of the Cip/Kip family inhibit CDK2. Rb remains in an un- or hypophosphorylated state. In early G_1, mitogenic signaling prompts cyclin D association with CDK4 to phosphorylate and thereby inactivate Rb. Further Rb phosphorylation by cyclin E/CDK2 complexes releases E2Fs and histone deacetylases (HDACs) (not pictured) from Rb restraint, permitting entry into S phase. Securin binds to and inhibits separase, which, when released following securin ubiquitylation and degradation, cleaves proteins that hold sister chromatids together, thereby initiating anaphase. Those cell cycle regulators that are specifically relevant to pituitary tumorigenesis include p18, p21, p27, CDK4, Rb, E2F and securin. D, cyclin D; E, cyclin E; CDK4, cyclin-dependent kinase 4; CDK2, cyclin-dependent kinase 2; APC, anaphase promoting complex; P, phosphorylation; Ub, ubiquitylation. *From [87].*

negatively regulate G_1 CDK activity [91]. Proteins of the INK4 family (p16^{INK4a}, p15^{INK4b}, p18^{INK4c} and p19^{INK4d}) negatively regulate the activities of CDK4 and CDK6, whereas the Kip/Cip family of inhibitors, which includes p27^{Kip1}, p21^{Cip1} and p57^{Kip2}, inhibits late G_1 activity of cyclin E/CDK2 complexes.

A series of studies reporting the phenotypes of mice with targeted disruption of G_1 cell cycle regulators collectively support the premise that the pathway controlling the G_1/S checkpoint in the cell cycle is central to the control of proliferation in the anterior pituitary [87]. The first of these identified was Rb itself. Mice heterozygous for Rb develop aggressive pituitary tumors by 12 months of age [92]. Although initially discovered in the intermediate lobe in the 129SV strain, anterior lobe tumors have subsequently been demonstrated in other (C57BL/6) strains [93]. Mice deficient for *Cdkn1b* (encoding p27^{kip1}) or *Cdkn2c* (encoding p18^{INK4c}) also exhibit spontaneous pituitary adenomas by 10 months [94–96]. On the other hand, *Cdk4*$^{-/-}$ mice develop postnatal pituitary lactotroph and somatotroph hypoplasia [97]. Numerous subsequent reports of mice with combined knockout of two or more cell cycle regulators have begun to define genetic pathways that are critical for mediating oncogenic processes in the pituitary. For instance, Rb$^{+/-}$ pituitary tumorigenesis is partially averted by deletion of the Rb effectors E2F1 or E2F3, indicating that deregulation of E2F and the resulting proliferation are important processes in pituitary tumorigenesis [98,99]. As another example, double deficiency of p27 and Cdk2 suppresses intermediate lobe pituitary tumors, but unexpectedly promotes the appearance of anterior lobe tumors, indicating that Cdk2 is dispensable for the inhibitory actions of p27 in the anterior pituitary [100]. These types of mouse genetic studies, which provide the most rigorous scientific evidence, demonstrate the complexity of the networks involved in the process of tumorigenesis, and will continue to be important for unraveling the fundamental molecular pathways that are essential towards this end.

Studies analyzing the expression of cell cycle proteins in human prolactinomas have shown that intragenic mutations are exceedingly rare. Instead, loss of gene expression due to epigenetic silencing appears to represent a more common mechanism of deregulation [101]. Those alterations that have been identified in human prolactinomas, and that have been validated with a corresponding assessment of protein levels, are summarized in Table 15.2. These alterations most frequently arise as a result of hypermethlyation of CpG islands in the promoter regions of CKIs, leading to reduced expression of the protein product. The causative versus permissive role of these types of epigenetic modifications in pituitary transformation has not been fully ascertained, so it remains possible that the changes in CpG island methylation status that have been identified are simply reinforcing already established gene silencing events.

Pttg (encoding the protein product securin) was initially identified by mRNA differential display from the GH4 somatolactotroph tumor cell line [102] and was subsequently found to be over-expressed in a wide variety of endocrine and nonendocrine tumors,

TABLE 15.2 Altered Cell Cycle Regulator Expression in Human Prolactinomas

Gene	Protein	Molecular or Genetic Alteration	Frequency of Finding	Reference
RB1	retinoblastoma	LOH, in highly invasive or malignant tumors	4/4, 100%	[609]
		Promoter methylation	7/9, 78%	[610]
CDKN2A	p16	CpG island methylation, correlating with reduced protein expression	8/9, 89%	[611]
		Protein expression lost	3/3, 100%	[612]
CDKN2C	p18	Reduced protein and mRNA levels	60, 70%	[613]
		LOH, promoter methylation, correlating with reduced protein expression	25%*, 100%	[614]
CDKN1A	p21	Over-expression by IHC	81%	[615]
CDKN1B	p27	Absent nuclear expression by IHC	5/9, 56%	[616]
		Germline inactivating mutation	case reports	[617,618]
PTTG1	securin	Over-expressed by IHC	12/14, 86%	[106]
		>50% increase in mRNA expression	9/10, 90%	[105]
CCND1	cyclin D1	Allelic imbalance (gene amplification)	15/60*, 25%	[619]
CCND3	cyclin D3	Over-expression by IHC	68%	[620]

LOH, loss of heterozygosity; IHC, immunchists chemistry.
* *Represent collections of all pituitary subtypes.*

including all subtypes of pituitary adenomas [103–105] and prolactinomas [106,107]. Securin is a multifunctional protein with diverse functions, including roles in mitotic regulation, DNA damage, apoptosis and angiogenesis [108]. The most widely studied function of securin concerns that of its role in the spindle assembly checkpoint. As a mitotic regulator, securin exhibits a tightly regulated, cell cycle-dependent expression pattern [109] which is modulated by cyclin B-CDK1 mediated phosphorylation, serving to stabilize securin, and Cdc14 dephosphorylation, which primes it for ubiquitin-mediated proteasomal degradation by the anaphase-promoting complex at the end of metaphase [110–113]. Although securin can act as a cochaperone for nuclear import of separase, during most of the cell cycle securin prevents separase from cleaving cohesin subunits which normally hold sister chromatids together (Figure 15.3). Following the ubiquitylation and rapid destruction of securin, separase becomes activated and cleaves the Scc1 subunit of cohesin, triggering the onset of anaphase [108].

Although the molecular mechanism to account for its over-expression in tumors remains elusive [114], a substantial body of experimental data has been generated supporting the role of *PTTG1* as a pituitary oncogene. For example, securin exhibits transforming properties in vitro and is tumorigenic in vivo [102]. In vitro, over-expression of securin induces a partial G_2/M arrest, and results in aberrant chromatid separation and aneuploidy [102,115–117]. Likewise, in vivo deletion of *pttg1* in mouse embryonic fibroblasts and pituitary tissue promotes aneuploidy, indicating the requirement for strict regulation of the levels of this protein to maintain genomic stability [118,119]. The induction of aneuploidy and chromosomal instability may subserve a potential transforming mechanism of securin over-expression in both pituitary and nonpituitary tumors [120]. Other cellular roles of securin that are consistent with participation in tumorigenesis include: (1) activation of basic fibroblast growth factor (bFGF), c-myc, and cyclin D3, with the latter function possibly indicating effects on the G_1/S checkpoint transition; (2) regulation of DNA damage/repair processes; and (3) interaction with p53, and modulation of p53-dependent or -independent apoptotic signaling pathways [116,121–123].

Phenotypic analyses of the over-expression and deletion of *PTTG1* in mice have augmented knowledge of the function of securin. Although not targeted to pituitary lactotrophs, these in vivo models have been instrumental in validating securin as a permissive pituitary oncogene, and have proven to be insightful for establishing the genetic relationships between it and other cell cycle regulators. Transgenic over-expression of human *PTTG1* driven by the alpha glycoprotein subunit (αGSU) promoter in mice (*αGSU-PTTG1*^{tg}) causes focal plurihormonal pituitary hyperplasia [124], while aged *αGSU-PTTG1*^{tg} mice develop hormone-secreting microadenomas. When bred on an Rb heterozygous background, pituitary glands of *αGSU-PTTG1*^{tg}; *Rb*$^{+/-}$ mice exhibit marked hyperplasia and a 3.5-fold higher prevalence of tumors arising from αGSU-expressing cells, compared with single *αGSU-PTTG1*^{tg} or *Rb*$^{+/-}$ mice [125]. Altogether, these findings demonstrate that over-expression of securin promotes pituitary cell proliferation, is permissive for tumorigenesis and cooperates with other oncogenic stimuli to promote adenoma formation. Correspondingly, deleting *pttg1* from Rb heterozygous mice (*Rb*$^{+/-}$; *pttg1*$^{-/-}$) delays the onset and reduces the penetrance of anterior pituitary tumors from 86% to 30% [118]. This latter finding, together with evidence that securin mRNA and protein levels are upregulated in pretumorous Rb$^{+/-}$ pituitary tissue [118], and data demonstrating securin as an E2F target [126], places securin downstream of Rb genetically. *Pttg1* deficiency is associated with a strong induction of the cyclin-dependent kinase inhibitor p21, which probably occurs in response to mitotic defects and subsequent activation of a p53 checkpoint [127]. Indeed, the protection from *Rb* tumorigenesis afforded by pttg1 deficiency is dependent upon intact p21 function, as demonstrated by the finding that the additional deletion of p21 on the compound Rb/securin deficient background (*Rb*$^{+/-}$; *pttg1*$^{-/-}$;*Cdkn1c*$^{-/-}$) restores tumor potential to these mice [128]. While a series of experiments demonstrate that securin deficiency and the induction of p21 engages a senescent, tumor-restraining response, the interpretation of these results is complicated by the fact that the relationships among securin, p21, p53 and Rb are complex and have nonlinear components outside the G_1–S transition [129]. Thus, some uncertainty remains regarding the precise point within the cell cycle that misregulated securin promotes oncogenic effects. Nonetheless, these studies collectively establish that an exquisitely tuned regulation of securin levels is important for ensuring pituitary homeostasis, and future challenges are anticipated to determine how this protein or its molecular pathways can or should be therapeutically targeted.

Growth Factor and Hormone Signaling

Pituitary lactotrophs are targets for several local growth factors and systemic hormones that influence their proliferative status. The over-expression of these mitogens or, more commonly, the constitutive activation or altered structure of their receptors may result in unscheduled proliferation and ultimately, transformation. Among the classical growth factors and hormones, abundant evidence implicates alterations in the receptors for fibroblast growth factor (FGF), estradiol (E2) and epidermal growth factor (EGF) as having pathobiological roles in prolactinomas.

A variant of the fibroblast growth factor receptor 4 (FGFR4) appears to play a causal role in the pathogenesis of a variety of pituitary adenoma subtypes including a small proportion of sporadic prolactinomas. The FGF family consists of 23 ligands which signal through transmembrane receptor tyrosine kinase receptors. These FGF receptors (FGFRs) comprise four receptor tyrosine kinases designated FGF1R–4R. Several of the FGFs and their receptors are abundantly expressed in the anterior pituitary and play key roles in adenohypophyseal development and hormone synthesis. For example, basic FGF (or FGF2) regulates the synthesis of multiple pituitary hormones [130] and is differentially expressed by pituitary tumor cells [131]. In addition, FGF 19, which selectively binds to FGFR4, potently induces PRL gene expression [132]. A comparative screen of normal and adenomatous human pituitaries to examine possible differences in FGFR expression identified an N-terminally truncated variant of FGFR4 in adenomatous pituitaries [133]. This isoform, which lacks the signal peptide and the first and second immunoglobulin-like extracellular domains, is generated by an alternative transcription initiation site that utilizes a cryptic promoter [134,135]. Unlike the normal membrane-anchored FGFR4, the pituitary-tumor-derived FGFR4 (ptd-FGFR4) is mislocalized with an expression pattern restricted to the cytoplasm. Analyses of FGFR4 expression in normal and sporadic adenomatous human pituitary specimens by immunohistochemistry indicate that cytoplasmic FGFR4 is expressed in approximately 50% of pituitary adenomas overall but it is absent from the normal pituitary, where only the secretable FGFR4 and other transmembrane FGFRs (#1–3) are found [133,136,137].

In support of an oncogenic role for the variant FGFR4, ptd-FGFR4 exhibits transforming properties in soft agar and is tumorigenic when transplanted into immunodeficient mice. The direct role of ptd-FGFR4 in pituitary lactotroph tumorigenesis was cemented by the demonstration that lactotroph-specific driven over-expression of ptd-FGFR4 (rPRLp-*ptd-FGFR4*$^{+g}$), but not the wild-type FGFR4 (rPRLp-*FGFR4*$^{+g}$), in mice leads to the development of tumors with morphologic features mimicking human prolactinomas, indicating that this oncoprotein can recapitulate the disease in an animal model [134]. The phenotype is highly penetrant such that 90% of male and female *ptd-FGFR4*$^{rPRLp\text{-}tg}$ mice develop lactotroph micro- and macroadenomas secreting PRL by 11 months of age [134]. As observed in many murine models of pituitary tumorigenesis, females display significantly larger tumors, some of which are invasive, whereas male animals develop multifocal microadenomas. All of the tumors exhibit disruption of the normal acinar structure and prominent vascularity, suggesting the possibility that FGFR4 normally plays a role in maintaining tissue architecture and/or vascularization [134].

Further investigation into the mechanism by which the variant ptd-FGFR4 promotes this invasive growth behavior led to the identification of specific alterations in the cellular localization of two cell adhesion molecules (CAMs) that are associated with the aberrant expression of ptd-FGFR4 (Figure 15.4). Typically, changes in the expression or function of CAMs can be correlated with alterations in the adhesive status of tumor cells, which allow them to acquire a more invasive phenotype [138]. The abnormal expression of ptd-FGFR4 disrupts a multiprotein complex of CAMs involving FGFR4, N-cadherin and neural cell adhesion molecule 1 (NCAM-1) [136,139]. Whereas the full-length, wild-type FGFR4 physically associates with NCAM-1 to facilitate maintenance of N-cadherin expression at the cell membrane, ptd-FGFR4 shows minimal interaction with NCAM-1, leading to the ectopic displacement of N-cadherin to the cytoplasm [139]. These changes manifest in reduced stromal adhesiveness by cells in vitro and invasive growth in vivo [139]. Such findings are consistent with other lines of evidence that show CAM interactions with FGFRs can promote the development or progression of some epithelial neoplasias [140,141]. Furthermore, the cytoplasmic sequestration of N-cadherin induced by ptd-FGFR4 destabilizes the interaction between N-cadherin and one of its downstream targets, β-catenin, resulting in diminished β-catenin expression [139]. Apart from its participation in the cadherin complex, β-catenin is a pivotal member of the canonical Wnt signaling pathway, where it modulates the transcriptional activity of lymphoid enhancer factor (Lef-1)/T cell factor proteins [142]. The precise further consequences and specific relevance of β-catenin down-regulation for the tumorigenic process in this specific setting are not known. Nonetheless, it appears that the membranous expression of a full-length FGFR4 is necessary to orchestrate signaling events that are important for normal cell adhesiveness, and the transforming properties of the variant ptd-FGFR4 may be partially attributable to disruption of this proadhesive membrane complex [136]. Inhibition of the kinase activity of ptd-FGFR4 in xenografted mice restores membranous N-cadherin expression in tumor cells [136]. Studies investigating the effects of kinase inhibitors on tumor growth have not been documented, and are necessary to determine the therapeutical potential of these agents to treat human tumors.

Several lines of evidence support the trophic role of the gonadal steroid estrogen in the proliferation of normal and transformed lactotrophs. In vitro, E2 stimulates PRL secretion, and in vivo, E2 administration induces lactotroph tumors in humans and in rodents [143–145]. Several cases of lactotroph adenoma development have been reported in male–female transsexuals given very high doses of unopposed estrogen [146–149]. Disruption of estrogen action experimentally in rodent tumor models (i.e., dominant-negative

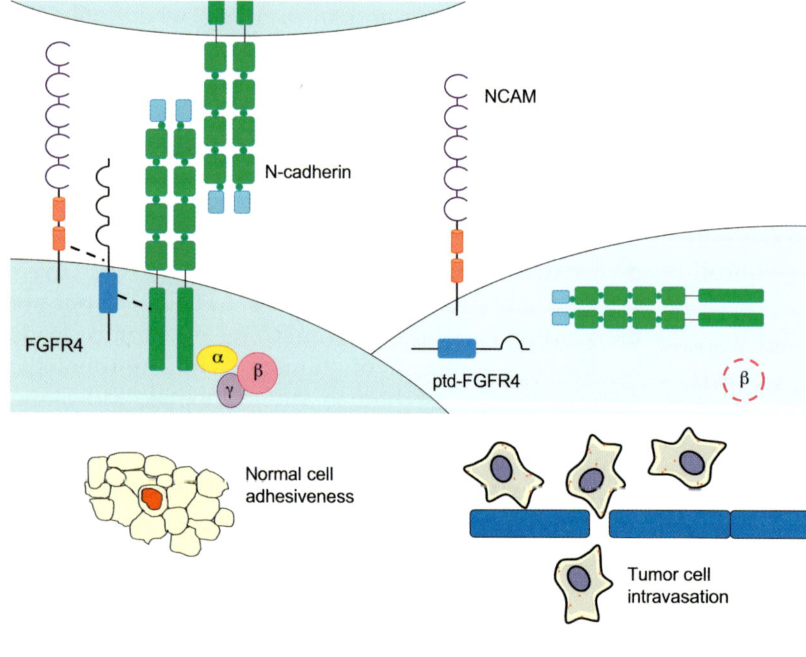

FIGURE 15.4 Schematic illustration of a proposed model for the mechanism by which alterations in fibroblast growth factor receptor 4 (FGFR4) disrupt cell–cell and cell–matrix adhesion forces in pituitary adenomas. The membrane locations of neural cell adhesion molecule 1 (NCAM-1), FGFR4 and N-cadherin are critical for the formation of a proadhesive multiprotein complex. As shown on the left, wild-type FGFR4, residing on the cell membrane, physically interacts with neural cell adhesion molecule 1 (NCAM-1) to stabilize the membranous location of N-cadherin. *From [139].* As illustrated by the dotted line, the exact nature of the interactions between FGFR4 and NCAM-1, and between FGFR4 and N-cadherin, has not been determined. The NCAM-1–FGFR4–N-cadherin complex also serves to maintain the association between N-cadherin and beta-catenin, which preserves the actin cytoskeletal structure. By contrast, as shown on the right, the pituitary-tumor-derived fibroblast growth factor receptor 4 (ptd-FGFR4) isoform is restricted to the cytoplasm, causing disassociation of FGFR4 from NCAM-1. *From [139].* The resulting disruption of the NCAM-1–FGFR4–N-cadherin complex could alter the normal cell–cell and cell–matrix adhesive properties. Potentially, this may lead to tumor cell intravasation. FGFR-4, fibroblast growth factor receptor 4; NCAM-1; neural cell adhesion molecule 1; ptd-FGFR-4, pituitary-tumor-derived fibroblast growth factor receptor 4.

estrogen receptor (ER) adenoviral transduction) suppresses tumor formation [150], whereas transgenic over-expression of the ER coactivator SRC-3 leads to the development of lactotroph adenomas in nearly half of all mice [151]. The treatment of humans with prolactinomas with selective estrogen receptor modulators or aromatase inhibitors reduces PRL levels and induces tumor regression in some cases [152,153].

In the pituitary, the mitogenic and regulatory effects of E2 are mediated, at least in part, through its two nuclear receptors, estrogen receptor-α (ER-α) and estrogen receptor-β (ER-β), which are ligand-activated transcription factors that are members of the steroid receptor superfamily. Normal human lactotrophs and lactotroph adenomas express both ER-α and ER-β isoforms, with the ER-α isoform being dominant for the action of growth [154].

Analyses of ER isoform expression in human pituitary tumors show that multiple forms of alternatively spliced ER mRNA transcripts are co-expressed with wild-type ER mRNA in a tumor phenotype-specific manner [155,156]. Prolactinomas display a diverse array of variant ER mRNAs that delete a single exon, including Δ2ER, Δ3ER, Δ4ER, Δ5ER and Δ7ER, of which only Δ4ER and Δ7ER are uniformly expressed in the normal pituitary at levels comparable to those in the tumors. In particular, Δ2ER and Δ5ER are abundantly expressed in lactotroph tumors, but are nearly undetectable in normal tissues. Δ5ER mRNA is translated inframe into a truncated protein that binds DNA but lacks the ligand binding and AF-2 domains, and it modulates the activity of wild-type ER in certain settings. The Δ5ER splice variant exhibits dominant-negative, dominant-positive, or ER-independent activity and differential effects on cellular proliferation, depending upon the cellular and promoter context [157–160]. For example, human breast or osteosarcoma cell lines that stably over-express the Δ5ER isoform exhibit E2-independent effects on ERE-regulated gene transcription and increases in cellular growth rates, suggesting that this isoform could be a target for growth factor kinase-signaling pathways that influence its interactions with other coregulatory proteins [159,161]. This may result in enhanced cellular growth in the absence of stimulation of ERE-dependent gene activation, and an E2-independent growth phenotype.

Although it may be liberal to extrapolate data from transfected cell lines to pituitary tissue, it is possible that specific ER variants could modulate E2 sensitivity in normal or adenomatous cells, or could be involved in promoting aberrant cell growth and abnormal PRL synthesis in tumors. Which ER-responsive genes are differentially activated or repressed by the isoforms in pituitary tissue, how the variants might promote neoplastic transformation or progression in lactotrophs, or whether they have tumorigenic capability in vivo has not been determined.

Other growth factor families such as the EGF family may play an important role in prolactinoma tumorigenesis. The EGF-EGFR (or ERRB) signaling network is highly complex due to a multiplicity of ligands [13] that feed into several combinations of ERBB homo- or heterodimers, which engage in lateral and cross-talk signaling cascades [162]. The EGFR (ERBB1) serves as the common receptor for EGF and TGF-alpha, and is one of four highly homologous tyrosine kinase receptors in the ERBB family that also includes ERBB2 (HER2/neu), ERBB3 and ERBB4 [162]. ERBB2 cannot bind to growth factor ligands, but functions as an amplifier and is the preferred heterodimeric partner of the other three ERBB receptors [162]. ERBB3 possesses defective kinase activity, but can be activated by neuregulins and other ERBB receptors or non-ERBB receptors, leading to downstream activation of the PI3K/AKT pathway, among others [162]. Both ERBB2 and ERBB3 up-regulation have been described in various human cancers.

EGF is expressed in normal pituitary lactotrophs, where it potently stimulates PRL gene transcription [163]. ERBB 1 and 2 have been shown to be expressed in the normal anterior pituitary and in all pituitary adenoma subtypes at variable levels [164–167]. ERBB3 expression has been documented in a subset of tumorous lactotrophs, but its precise expression level in normal lactotrophs is not known [168]. Increased expression of various ERBB family members has been reported in some histologic studies in clinically aggressively-behaving adenomas, primarily of somatotroph origin, suggesting the possibility that they play a functional role in tumor growth [166,169]. Support for a pivotal role for EGFR signaling in prolactinoma progression is demonstrated by the observation that lactotroph-targeted TGFα over-expression in transgenic mice leads to selective lactotroph hyperplasia and the development of adenomas [170]. Evidence implicating other ERBB receptor activity as permissive for lactotroph tumor progression is emerging. For example, activation of the ERBB2/ERBB3 heterodimer, which mediates heregulin-induced PRL synthesis in transformed lactotrophs, is associated with sustenance of mitogenic (ERK) and survival (AKT) pathways in human prolactinomas [168]. Moreover, treatment of GH4 cells with tyrosine kinase inhibitors that target these ERBBs can attenuate PRL secretion, though effects on proliferation have not yet been shown [168]. Further detailed studies of ERBB expression, regulation and function in normal and tumorous lactotrophs, corroborated by in vivo validation, are required to precisely clarify what role the ERRB network has, if any, in prolactinoma development or progression. At the moment, these studies provide preliminary proof of concept evidence that therapeutic targeting of ERBB2/3 may control hyperprolactinemia in tumors resistant to standard therapies.

Disruption of inhibitory and/or negative feedback signaling to pituitary lactotrophs may be involved in the promotion of lactotroph neoplasia in some circumstances. Locally, hypothalamic dopamine, acting through the D_2 receptor (D_2R), inhibits lactotroph proliferation and PRL gene expression. Thus, impaired dopamine inhibition or functional inactivation of the D_2R could theoretically contribute to the formation of prolactinomas. The indispensable role of the D_2R in restraining lactotroph growth was confirmed by findings in D_2R knockout mice. Young (<12 months) female *Drd2*$^{-/-}$ mice develop lactotroph hyperplasia and aged (>17 months) females develop massive invasive prolactinomas [171,172]. Thus, chronic loss of neurohormonal dopamine inhibition promotes a transition from hyperplasia to neoplasia in lactotrophs, possibly in part by increasing the frequency with which tumor-initiating events can occur. On the other hand, aged male *Drd2*$^{-/-}$ mice develop multifocal microadenomas without preceding hyperplasia, indicating that prolonged loss of dopamine inhibition can also promote microadenoma formation independently of hyperplastic stimulation [171,172]. Mutations of the coding sequence of the *DRD2* gene have not been reported in prolactinomas [173]. However, D_2R protein expression is reduced [174] or lost [175] in some prolactinomas that are resistant to dopamine agonist therapy (see Dopamine agonist resistance section).

PRL autoregulation has been observed in mice, and the consequences of disrupted PRL feedback on pituitary lactotrophs have been demonstrated in *Prl* and *Prlr* knockout mice. Targeted disruption of the *Prl* gene in mice causes PRL deficiency, leads to the development of lactotroph hyperplasia by 6 weeks of age and lactotroph adenomas by 8 months of age [176]. This timeframe is analogous to that which occurs in *Drd2*$^{-/-}$ mice, and is likewise accelerated in females. *Prlr* knockout mice exhibit even earlier lactotroph hyperplasia and develop larger and more invasive adenomas than those observed in the *Drd2*$^{-/-}$ mice, providing further support for the importance of this short autoregulatory loop [177]. At present, however, direct demonstration for impaired PRL feedback in human prolactinomas is lacking, as there are no reports of inactivating mutations in the *PRLR* gene in humans, or reports of prolactinomas in humans with long-standing hypoprolactinemia.

Aberrant Expression of Developmental Factors

A small but increasing body of evidence links transcription factors or signaling events that are involved in early adenohypophyseal development or lineage determination with the progression of pituitary neoplasia. Two examples of this phenomenon include the aberrant postnatal expression of bone morphogenetic protein 4 (BMP4) and p8, both of which were identified from global gene expression profiling of lactotroph adenomas derived from genetically modified mice.

BMP4 is a member of the TGF-β superfamily and exerts an important autocrine/paracrine effect in adenohypophyseal development and patterning of the pituitary, from the initial induction of Rathke's pouch to cell specification in the anterior lobe and differentiation of the lactotroph lineage [178,179]. BMP4 is expressed in adult somatotrophs and corticotrophs, but not in lactotrophs, indicating a possible role for this cytokine in maintaining pituitary lineage specification [180]. mRNA differential display identified the BMP inhibitor noggin as down-regulated and BMP4 as up-regulated in prolactinomas from *Drd2*$^{-/-}$ mice [181]. Subsequently, BMP4 was found to be over-expressed in several models of prolactinomas, including estradiol-induced rat prolactinomas and human prolactinomas, but not in normal lactotroph tissue or human pituitary adenomas of other subtypes.

Further experiments designed to interrogate the role of BMP-4 in lactotroph tumorigenesis showed that in vivo, BMP-4 stimulates GH3 cell proliferation and promotes the expression of c-myc in human prolactinomas [181]. These effects are specific to tumorous lactotrophs, as they are not observed in other subtypes of human adenohypophyseal tumors [181]. Moreover, inhibiting the action of BMP-4 in GH3 cells by stable expression of a dominant-negative SMAD4 (similar to mothers against decapentaplegic) construct inhibits the growth of tumors when injected into immunodeficient mice, indicating that the TGF-β/SMAD signaling pathway is likely to be important for tumor growth in this model [181]. Bolstering this premise is the finding that tumor growth resumes and c-myc becomes re-expressed upon loss of the stable integration of the dominant-negative SMAD4 construct from GH3 cells [181]. Mechanistically, the proliferative effects of BMP-4 appear to be mediated through overlapping intracellular signaling pathways involving ERα and SMAD4, as BMP-4 induction of cell proliferation is inhibited by reciprocal antagonists of either pathway [181]. A synergistic BMP-4 and E2 cross-talk also plays a role in regulating PRL transcription and secretion [182].

In a similar strategy, microarray studies were used to compare expression profiles from pituitary tumors in glycoprotein hormone alpha (CGA) promoter-driven transgenic mice over-expressing leutinizing hormone beta (LHβ) to wild-type pituitaries. These mice exhibit chronically elevated LH levels, leading to hyperplasia of the Pit-1 lineages at 5 months, and ultimately, ovary-dependent lactotroph adenomas in older females [183]. One of many genes shown to have altered expression levels by differential display was an HMGA-related nuclear protein called p8. Normally, p8 is transiently expressed in the developing pituitary gland, but is quiescent in the adult [184]. A 12-fold induction of the p8 gene was identified in tumorous lactotroph tissue, though an increase in its expression was not observed in the pretumorous hyperplastic gland. When clonal GH3 cell lines with reduced expression of p8 are injected into immunodeficient mice, tumor development is attenuated or abolished, as compared to tumors derived from wild-type GH3 cells, indicating that p8 is required to maintain the tumorigenic capacity of GH3 cells.

Taken together, there is insufficient evidence to validate a direct role of BMP4 or p8 in the initial stages of pituitary lactotroph transformation. However, their misexpression in postnatal neoplastic pituitaries, which is associated with enhanced proliferation, may represent examples of a common mechanism whereby the re-emergence of developmental factors plays permissive roles in sustaining the transformed status of these cells.

CLINICAL MANIFESTATIONS

Local Mass Effects

As mentioned previously, about 95% of prolactinomas are microadenomas, having a tumor diameter less than 10 mm. There may be local or even diffuse invasion of the dura and bone of the sella turcica but this does not usually give rise to clinically apparent symptoms. Local mass effects may well cause symptoms in patients with macroadenomas, depending upon the size and extent of extrasellar extension. The frequency of such symptoms is much lower than in patients with nonsecreting tumors because prolactinoma patients usually present with symptoms of reproductive/sexual dysfunction (see below). Visual field defects due to chiasmal compression depend upon the amount of suprasellar extension. In one series of macroadenoma patients of all types reported, the average amount of suprasellar extension of patients with visual disturbances was 18.5 mm, whereas the average amount of such extension without visual disturbances was 9.5 mm [185]. It should be remembered that generally there is about 10 mm between the top of the normal pituitary and the chiasm [186]. Because of the great variation in how these tumors grow superiorly with respect to the location of the chiasm, visual field defects can range from the classical complete bi-temporal hemianopsia to small, partial quadrantic defects to scotomas [186]. There are no specific types of visual field defects peculiar to prolactinomas compared to other types of tumors.

Approximately 10% of prolactinomas invade the cavernous sinus [187]. Ophthalmoplegias are relatively uncommon, being due to entrapment of cranial nerves III, IV and VI. The first and second division of the trigeminal nerve (V_1 and V_2) and the carotid artery are other major structures in the cavernous sinus that can be involved. In some patients a cavernous sinus syndrome may develop, consisting of ophthalmoplegia and pain or hyperesthesia in the distribution of V_1 [188]. The carotid artery may be encased within the tumor. Pituitary tumors are an uncommon cause of cavernous sinus syndrome, being the etiology in only six of 102 patients with this syndrome reported from the Mayo Clinic [189]. Shrinkage of these tumors with dopamine agonists can be quite dramatic [188], and surgery is rarely curative and is potentially fraught with complications [190].

Extensive invasion of the floor of the skull with massive destruction of bone occasionally occurs and may cause problems by entrapping cranial nerves and compressing vital brain structures [191,192]. Extrasellar extension in other directions may cause temporal lobe epilepsy and hydrocephalus [193]. These large, invasive tumors are uncommon but not rare (see Giant prolactinomas). Local mass effects may cause hypopituitarism because of direct pituitary compression or hypothalamic/stalk dysfunction. The larger the tumor, the more likely there is to be one or more hormonal deficits [192,194–196]. All patients with macroadenomas should be evaluated for possible deficits in pituitary function.

Symptoms

The clinical manifestations due to hyperprolactinemia and their pathophysiology are discussed extensively in Chapter 5. The frequencies with which various clinical manifestations occur in patients with prolactinomas varies depending upon referral patterns. In some centers, many patients with microadenomas are managed by gynecologists and general internists, and the endocrinologist only sees patients unresponsive to dopamine agonists or those with very large macroadenomas.

Women

The classic presentation of prolactinomas in premenopausal women includes symptoms of galactorrhea, amenorrhea and/or infertility. In older series of women with prolactinomas undergoing transsphenoidal surgery, the frequency of oligoamenorrhea is ~90% and galactorrhea is ~85%. Although the usual situation is that of secondary amenorrhea, primary amenorrhea may also occur. Presentation because of severe headaches or visual field disturbance due to large tumors is uncommon in women, who usually initially seek medical attention because of menstrual dysfunction or galactorrhea, which generally occur even with minimal PRL elevations and long before the tumors have grown large [197]. Postmenopausal women with prolactinomas usually present with mass effects from large tumors, although some are discovered simply because of a history of "premature" menopause [198].

Men

A greater proportion of males with prolactinomas that come to clinical attention have macroprolactinomas, compared to women. In most radiologic series, a macroadenoma is discovered in 80–90% of male cases [199–207]. Although symptoms of hypogonadism are still most prevalent, symptoms due to mass effects commonly serve as those that prompt medical attention. Overall, about one-third of men will typically have symptoms due to tumor size. Although the larger tumor size in men may be due to diagnostic delay, this explanation is inconsistent with the known infrequency with which small untreated tumors grow over time. Retrospective analyses report higher indices of proliferating cells by Ki67 immunoreactivity in surgically resected macroadenomas from males compared to similar tumors from females [33,204]. Thus, it remains possible that there are fundamental sex-specific biological differences in tumors found in men versus women, but these changes have not been identified on a molecular level.

The well-documented high efficacy of dopamine agonist therapy for the treatment of hyperprolactinemia and tumor shrinkage applies to prolactinomas in both female and male patients [208,209]. Furthermore, for most male patients, dopamine agonist therapy will normalize PRL levels, regardless of tumor size [210]. In one prospective study of males with prolactinomas who were treated for 24 months with cabergoline, PRL levels normalized in 76% of patients with macroadenomas and in 80% of those with microprolactinomas at mean doses of 1.5 and 1.0 mg/week, respectively [211]. These treatment outcomes are in line with results of other series of similar duration reporting the efficacy of cabergoline [209,212]. Normalization of testosterone levels in males with successful treatment of hyperprolactinemia ranges from 50–60% [210,211]. When normal testosterone levels are achieved, the sperm volume and count are also likely to normalize, albeit after a prolonged (~2 years) duration [211]. The majority of males who achieve normal PRL levels will show improvement in semen quality and sexual potency [213]. Improvement in testosterone levels is often delayed for several months following normalization of PRL levels, but testosterone replacement should be considered for males who remain hypogonadal.

Children and Adolescents

Children and adolescents with prolactinomas may present with growth arrest, pubertal delay, or primary amenorrhea, in addition to the more standard presentations of galactorrhea, oligo/amenorrhea and mass effects such as headaches or visual disturbances [214–216]. In contrast to the distribution of adult patients, there is a disproportionately larger number of pediatric patients who have macroadenomas (62%), even allowing for possible selection bias because of reporting from neurosurgical units [214,217–226]. Overall, the proportion of boys who present with macroadenomas at diagnosis is slightly greater than girls (81.3% vs. 58.8%). The reasons for the higher percentage of macroadenomas and the relative resistance to dopamine agonists among children and adolescents are not known.

Medical therapy is effective in normalizing prolactin levels and reducing tumor mass in children or adolescents with prolactinomas. However, the percentage of pediatric patients resistant to dopamine agonists may be higher than that observed in adults. Colao et al. [215] reported that PRL levels were normalized in ten of 26 (38%) children and adolescents taking bromocriptine, five of 15 (33%) taking quinagolide and 15 of 21 (71%) taking cabergoline. Poor compliance and drug intolerance very likely contributed to the lower than typical efficacies reported in this study. Children with microprolactinomas are unlikely to exhibit other anterior pituitary deficiencies, but hypopituitarism is common among children who have macroprolactinomas with or without extrasellar extension (33.3% and 77.8%, respectively). Reduction of tumor size by dopamine agonists or surgery will usually restore pituitary function [227,228]. Long-term follow-up of children and adolescents who are diagnosed and treated for prolactinomas has not found this to be associated with major adverse health consequences, aside from those specific to radiotherapy in those rare children treated with this modality [215–217]. Normal, uncomplicated pregnancies have been documented in a large number of these patients during or following treatment [215,217]. Osteopenia has been observed in young hyperprolactinemic patients. In one study, 22 patients who were diagnosed with prolactinomas before the age of 18 years had a bone mineral density at the lumbar spine that was significantly lower than in age-matched controls (0.78 ± 0.06 vs. 0.96 ± 0.02 g/cm^2) [229]. Treatment with a dopamine agonist improved, but did not normalize, bone mineral density values [229]. Whether the reduced bone mass associated with hyperprolactinemia translates into an increased risk for future osteoporotic fractures is not known.

DIAGNOSIS

Hormone Levels

The differential diagnosis of hyperprolactinemia is broad and is covered in Chapter 5, with diagnostic testing. Through a careful history and physical examination, as well as routine blood chemistry and thyroid function testing, most of these disorders can be excluded, with the exception of those related to hypothalamic–pituitary disease. Experience shows that abnormal PRL responses in a variety of stimulation and suppression tests are nonspecific and at present, dynamic testing of PRL secretion is not recommended in the differential diagnosis of hyperprolactinemia [230].

As mentioned in Chapter 5, a critical distinction to be made is between PRL-secreting macroadenomas and "nonsecreting" macroadenomas that cause a PRL elevation because of hypothalamic/stalk dysfunction. Generally, large PRL-secreting macroadenomas will have PRL levels above 250 ng/ml and virtually all micro- and macroprolactinomas will have levels above 100 ng/ml. Nonsecreting macroadenomas commonly cause PRL elevations in the 25–100 ng/ml levels [12]. Those with PRL levels between 100 and 250 ng/ml may prove troublesome in this differential diagnosis [11,13,231].

Imaging

All patients with hyperprolactinemia in whom non-hypothalamic–pituitary disorders have been excluded should be imaged with pituitary-dedicated magnetic resonance imaging (MRI) with gadolinium when available. Computed tomography (CT) with direct coronal scans provides less information about surrounding vasculature, the optic chiasm and invasion of the cavernous sinus (see Chapter 20). One potential problem in investigating patients with mild hyperprolactinemia is the finding of a false-positive CT or MRI scan. Because these techniques are now able to detect incidental nonsecreting tumors, cysts, infarcts, etc. [4], the finding of a "microprolactinoma" on a scan in a patient with elevated PRL levels may not always be a true-positive finding. Thus a patient with idiopathic hyperprolactinemia may have a "tumor" found on scan that, when removed, still leaves the patient hyperprolactinemic. For most patients with microadenomas, surgery will not be performed in any case and such lesions can then be followed with serial imaging, if necessary. In most cases, PRL levels alone can simply be followed in patients with microadenomas and imaging repeated only if PRL levels rise.

Current policy has been to perform formal visual field testing in patients whose tumors are adjacent to or pressing on the optic chiasm, as visualized on an MRI scan. If a clear distance of >2 mm is seen, then such testing is unnecessary.

TREATMENT

Observation

Asymptomatic patients with prolactinomas do not have an absolute requirement for treatment of their prolactinomas. Indications for therapy in patients with prolactinomas may be divided into two categories: (1) effects of tumor size; and (2) effects of hyperprolactinemia (Table 15.3). As noted above, studies examining the natural history of untreated microprolactinomas have shown that significant growth of these tumors is uncommon. Therefore, asymptomatic eugonadal women with microprolactinomas can go untreated as long as they are monitored closely to ensure stable tumor size. It is very unlikely for a prolactinoma to grow significantly without an increase in serum prolactin levels, although this phenomenon has been reported [232]. Therefore, most patients with microadenomas verified by imaging may be monitored with serial prolactin levels. If prolactin levels rise or symptoms of mass effects develop, then MRI is indicated to assess for possible tumor growth. Significant increases in prolactin levels usually, though not always [233], reflect tumor growth. A microadenoma with documented evidence of growth demands therapy for the size change alone, as it may be one of the 7% that will grow to be a macroadenoma.

TABLE 15.3 Indications for Therapy

MASS EFFECTS
Hypopituitarism
Visual field defects due to pressure on the optic chiasm
Cranial nerve deficits
Headaches
EFFECTS OF HYPERPROLACTINEMIA
Hypogonadism
Amenorrhea or oligoamenorrhea
Infertility
Impotence
Osteoporosis or osteopenia
Relative indications:
Bothersome hirsuitism
Bothersome galactorrhea

The presence of a macroadenoma raises the probability for the tumor in question to have biological characteristics that confer a propensity to grow. Moreover, most macroprolactinomas are associated with prolactin elevations significant enough to elicit symptoms that would warrant treatment. Therefore, therapy is usually advisable for these tumors. Local or diffuse invasion or compression of adjacent structures, such as the stalk or optic chiasm, are additional indications for therapy. Other indications for therapy are relative, being due to the hyperprolactinemia itself. These include: decreased libido, menstrual dysfunction, galactorrhea, infertility, hirsutism, impotence and premature osteoporosis. Eugonadal women with nonbothersome galactorrhea do not have specific reasons for therapy.

Hypogondal women with microprolactinomas may be treated with oral contraceptives, provided that their prolactin levels do not increase substantially and there is no evidence of tumor enlargement [234]. Series of patients with prolactinomas who are treated with oral contraceptives for hypogonadism have not shown substantial risk for tumor enlargement [235,236]. Nevertheless, individual case reports of tumor enlargement during estrogen therapy have been documented, so patients who use oral contraceptives should be followed carefully with periodic monitoring of prolactin levels [237,238].

Surgery

Surgical Indications and Approaches

Historically, surgical resection of prolactinomas was the preferred mode of therapy for prolactinomas until the 1980s, when the effectiveness of bromocriptine was demonstrated for the hormonal and growth control of these tumors. Most authorities advocate surgical treatment of prolactinomas for selected circumstances, including: (1) unstable neurological dysfunction associated with pituitary apoplexy; (2) failure of medical therapy to adequately reduce PRL levels to alleviate hypogonadism; (3) failure of medical therapy to control tumor growth (i.e., tumor enlargement); (4) tumor expansion accompanied by neuroopthalmologic deficits during pregnancy that is refractory to reinstitution of dopamine agonist therapy; (5) in preparation for planned pregnancy following a previous pregnancy complicated by worrisome tumor enlargement.

Pituitary apoplexy is a potentially life-threatening clinical syndrome caused by infarction or hemorrhage into an existing pituitary tumor [239]. Under such circumstances, patients may develop visual disturbance, associated with severe headache, altered consciousness and vascular collapse. In the setting of progressive neurological symptoms, i.e., severe and worsening visual loss, it represents the most urgent indication for surgical intervention [240]. However, when apoplexy is mild and visual field deficits are stable, this condition may be managed medically with careful monitoring by visual field assessments and serial MRI, as complete resolution of neuroophthalmologic signs and visual deficits may occur [241–243]. Efforts to medically manage patients with pituitary apoplexy are particularly advisable for prolactinomas, as surgical intervention and decompression do not ensure long-term cure of these tumors.

When surgery is undertaken, the transsphenoidal approach represents the standard of care for both microprolactinomas and the overwhelming majority of macroprolactinomas [244]. Craniotomy is reserved for tumors that are inaccessible via the transsphenoidal route. Such cases might include patients with large tumors with parasellar or unusual intracranial extensions, such as those extending towards the frontal or temporal lobes [245]. Giant and invasive prolactinomas cannot be cured by surgery, regardless of the surgical technique employed or experience of the neurosurgeon; therefore the goal of surgery under these circumstances is to debulk with the aim of alleviating symptoms related to mass effects [246] (see Special situations: giant prolactinomas).

Several recent technological advances have become available to pituitary surgeons, including endonasal endoscopy, intraoperative MRI and neuronavigation [247]. Studies performed thus far suggest that initial surgical remission rates of the endonasal endoscopic approach are comparable to those obtained using the traditional operating microscope but complication rates are slightly lower overall, and the operative duration and hospitalization lengths may be reduced [247–257]. In a single exception, one retrospective series found a higher rate of postoperative CSF leaks with the endoscopic approach [258]. Regardless of the innovative operative techniques and imaging modalities employed, the specific surgical treatment plan of a patient with a prolactinoma ultimately depends upon the availability, familiarity and expertise of these instruments for the neurosurgical center and neurosurgeon to which one refers their patients. Definitive data on the impact of these technological advances on surgical outcomes are not yet available.

Surgical Success Rates

Surgical outcomes are highly dependent upon the expertise and experience of the neurosurgeon, as well as the size of the tumor. Surgical results from 50 published series have been summarized in a recent comprehensive review, and the results of an additional three since published are herein [256,259–261]. Only results from the latest series from a given neurosurgical/endocrine team are included, omitting data from earlier studies. Criteria for inclusion in this analysis consist of the following: (1) cure or remission rates are reported with respect to size of the tumor (microadenoma vs. macroadenoma); (2) normalization of prolactin levels define surgical remission; and (3) surgical cure rates are reported on the basis of the number of patients with documented follow-up. Combining data from all 53 series, 1680/2236 (75.1%) microadenomas and 797/2318 (34.4%) macroadenomas are classified as achieving initial surgical remission, i.e., having PRL levels normalized within 1–12 weeks following surgery. Within these series the surgical success rates were highly variable. For series with at least ten patients, the surgical remission rate varies from 38% to 100% for microadenomas and from 6.7% to 80% for macroadenomas. Similar data were procured from a mail survey of 80 neurosurgeons, which found surgical cure rates of 74% of 1518 PRL-secreting "microadenomas" and 30% of 1022 PRL-secreting "macroadenomas" [262]. In this latter report, criteria for the assignment of patients to micro- or macroadenoma status was made on the basis of imaging and/or prolactin levels (< or >200 ng/ml, respectively). Clearly, for the macroadenomas the success rate in large part was dependent on the size of tumors chosen for surgery. In many series, the objective was, appropriately, debulking of a very large tumor rather than cure and in other series very large tumors were not operated upon.

Gonadal function improves in both sexes upon achievement of normoprolactinemia following successful surgical resection [196,263–265]. In young women, normal LH pulsatility is restored as early as the eighth postoperative day [265,266]. Normal reproductive function can be achieved when PRL levels are reduced to levels slightly above normal, but since such patients appear to have a much greater chance of recurrence of more significant hyperprolactinemia (see below), they cannot be regarded as definitively cured. Patients with macroadenomas of all types may be hypopituitary before surgery and, depending upon the extent of resection, may have significant changes in pituitary function postoperatively. In an analysis of 84 patients with pituitary macroadenomas (36 were prolactinomas) who underwent surgery, only 78% of those with normal preoperative pituitary function retained normal function postoperatively [267]. One-third of those with some pituitary deficits prior to surgery improved and one-third with deficits had worsened pituitary function after surgery. None of the panhypopituitary patients improved following surgery [267].

Recurrence and Long-term Cure

An area of controversy regarding the surgical efficacy of prolactinomas pertains to the likelihood of recurrence of hyperprolactinemia in patients who have undergone an initial remission. Rates of recurrence, as observed with rates of surgical remissions, are highly divergent among neurosurgical centers, ranging from 0 [268] to 50% [269]. In part, this variability reflects differences in the level of neurosurgical expertise, but it also occurs as a consequence of interstudy differences in postsurgical surveillance duration, attrition rates and the definitions of cure/recurrence employed. It is likely that surgical series with relatively short follow-up times will underestimate the true recurrence rate because the time to recurrence of hyperprolactinemia in some tumors may be lengthy [270]. As is the case for surgical cure, recurrence is most frequently defined as the discovery of an elevated prolactin level at any point in the postoperative surveillance period following an initial surgical remission. Some authors use less stringent criteria for cure, regarding patients with mild asymptomatic hyperprolactinemia as in remission [271]. Given all of these factors, a precise assessment of recurrence rates is difficult to establish.

Recurrence rates have been reported in 29 microprolactinoma series and 19 macroprolactinoma series. Using data abstracted from these studies, the recurrence rates for microadenomas (150/855 = 17.5%) and macroadenomas (105/466 = 23.5%) are roughly similar. Recurrence is most often detected biochemically (hyperprolactinemia), not necessarily with radiographic documentation of tumor regrowth. Recurrence of the hyperprolactinemia is usually accompanied by sexual or reproductive dysfunction.

Overall long-term surgical cure rates may be calculated based upon data from the surgical series that report both initial remission rates and recurrence rates, understanding that these numbers reflect a reporting bias, as they are derived from neurosurgeons who are willing to publish their data. Based on an initial remission rate of 79.2% and the recurrence rate of 17.5%, an overall long-term surgical cure rate for microadenomas among this subset of series using a normal PRL level as the criterion is 61.7%. For patients with macroadenomas, with an initial remission rate of 39.4% and a recurrence rate of 23.5%, the long-term cure rate is 15.9%. These general numbers may be given to patients when counseling them with respect to choices of therapy. Neurosurgeons who compile their own data on surgical cures and remission may provide patients with individualized estimates for remission or cure. For patients with giant prolactinomas and those with considerable cavernous sinus invasion, the chance for surgical cure is essentially zero [272–274].

Predictors of Remission and Cure

A number of studies have analyzed clinical, radiological and biochemical factors that might predict initial surgical remission and likelihood for long-term cure.

Several studies identify an inverse relationship between preoperative prolactin levels and the likelihood of initial surgical remission [6,261,271,273,275–281]. In some cases, preoperative PRL levels have been shown to be more predictive of surgical success than the actual size of the tumor. Patients with serum PRL levels >200 ng/ml were found to have a lesser chance for surgical cure even when stratified within micro- and macroadenoma groups [275,277,278,280,282,283]. Thus, PRL levels >200 ng/ml appear to be a risk factor for poor surgical outcome independent of tumor size.

Initial surgical success is also correlated with adenoma stage and the degree of tumor invasion [6,38,261,271,282]. A low immediate postoperative prolactin level has been shown to be an excellent predictor of long-term surgical cure [284,285]. For example, one large analysis of surgical outcomes of 339 surgically resected prolactinomas showed that when a postoperative PRL level of <5 ng/ml was achieved, 80.5% of the cohort remained in remission over a mean follow-up of 9.2 years [285]. In this series, the immediate postoperative PRL level was a better predictor of long-term surgical cure than the preoperative PRL level. A separate 5-year follow-up study found that a postoperative PRL <10 ng/ml predicted biochemical cure with 100% accuracy for both micro- and macroadenomas; cure was unlikely to be obtained in patients with postoperative PRL levels between 10 and 20 ng/ml [284]. Repeat transsphenoidal surgery for persistent tumor after failed surgery or radiotherapy is curative in less than 50% of the cases [285].

The impact of pretreatment with dopamine agonist therapy used preoperatively on surgical outcomes for prolactinomas is not definitive, owing to disparate results and to the lack of prospective randomized assessments. In the past, some neurosurgeons reported that prolactinomas that had been exposed to bromocriptine treatment seem to have a more fibrotic consistency that renders complete resection difficult. In two retrospective analyses, preoperative use of bromocriptine was associated with poorer surgical cure rates, as compared to rates of surgical cure in the absence of initial medical therapy [286,287]. However, the majority of other series investigating this issue have not corroborated these results [288–292], and two groups have reported better tumoral control when patients were pretreated with bromocriptine prior to surgical intervention [293,294]. Data regarding fibrosis and surgical results related to preoperative use of cabergoline are lacking. Since surgery for prolactinomas typically follows a trial, and often, subsequent failure of dopamine agonist therapy, selection biases could hamper the proper interpretation of these data. Therefore, long-term follow-up data from prospective surgical series in which patients are randomly assigned to preoperative medical therapy or placebo would be necessary to make definitive conclusions on its effects on surgical control or cure.

Complications

Complications from transsphenoidal surgery for microadenomas are infrequent. The mortality rate for transsphenoidal surgery for all types of secreting and nonsecreting macroadenomas is 0.9%, and the major morbidity rate is 6.5% (visual loss 1.5%, stroke/vascular injury 0.6%, meningitis/abscess 0.5%, oculomotor palsy 0.6%, CSF rhinorrhea 3.3% [245,262,295,296]. Transient diabetes insipidus (DI) is quite common with transsphenoidal surgery for both micro- and macroadenomas and permanent DI occurs in about 1% of surgeries on macroadenomas [262,296]. Hypopituitarism is common in patients with macroadenomas prior to surgery as a result of mass effects, occurring in more than 50% of patients. With surgery, either further worsening or improvement may occur [267]. Pituitary surgery involving craniotomy is much more hazardous. Although visual field defects and visual acuity can be improved in 74% of patients whose macroadenomas abut the optic chiasm [297], a small number of patients with normal visual fields may have visual defects after surgery due to herniation of the chiasm into an empty sella, direct injury or devascularization of the optic apparatus, fracture of the orbit, postoperative hematoma, or cerebral vasospasm [298].

Radiotherapy

Radiotherapy (RT) plays an adjunctive role in the management of prolactinomas, and is primarily used after failed transsphenoidal surgery and medical therapy for recurrent or residual disease. Rarely, it is administered postoperatively as a prophylactic measure to prevent growth of a remnant tumor. Several methodologies for the delivery of RT are available. Conventional fractionated external beam RT is delivered in doses of 200 cGy 4–5 days per week over a period of 6 weeks up to a total dose of 45–50 Gy [299]. Stereotactic radiotherapy is usually delivered as a single fraction using a multiheaded cobalt unit. This type of RT, often referred to as "gamma knife," is the most commonly used technique in the present era. Its hallmark is the sharp dose gradient of radiation at the treatment field edges, which reduces the dose of radiation to the surrounding normal brain tissue.

The two general therapeutic goals for performing RT in prolactinomas include: (1) arrest of tumor growth and prevention of adverse sequelae due to mass effects; and (2) normalization of hyperprolactinemia. On a practical level, improvement without normalization of PRL levels may be an acceptable goal for prolactinomas, since eugonadism can sometimes be restored in the setting of mild hyperprolactinemia. However, for the purpose of determining effectiveness, imprecise definitions of "mildly elevated prolactin levels" and "improvement" preclude accurate assessments of RT efficacy, and therefore most analyses of RT utilize the more stringent outcome of normoprolactinemia.

Analysis of Radiotherapy Studies

Several important caveats require consideration when interpreting data from clinical studies reporting the antitumoral efficacy of RT for the treatment of prolactinomas. The first relates to the definitions of tumor control endpoints. Tumor control may be defined with either endocrinologic (normalization of prolactin levels) or volumetric (long-term radiographic assessment of tumor size) endpoints. In some series, "tumor control" refers to stable prolactin levels or the absence of radiographic progression. The second important observation is that the majority of the studies are retrospective, single-arm analyses. Finally, and most importantly, is the reported or nonreported inclusion or exclusion of individuals who receive concomitant medical therapy. In some studies, patients who are designated as "cured" or "in remission" continue to receive dopamine agonist therapy throughout the follow-up period. Under these circumstances, it is impossible to separate out any prolactin-lowering effects of RT from the effects of dopamine agonists.

Efficacy: Conventional

Today, conventional RT is used in the management of aggressive prolactinomas that are not candidates for single-dose stereotactic radiotherapy (SDSR) (see Selecting the mode of RT, below). Prior to the availability of SDSR, conventional RT was used in patients primarily after failure of medical and/or surgical therapy and very infrequently as primary therapy [200,300–311]. In whatever clinical setting it was used, however, normalization of hyperprolactinemia was infrequent.

The use of conventional RT as primary therapy for prolactinomas has only been reported in a minority of cases. Three series report results of a total of 24 individuals treated in such a manner with follow-up ranging from 1 to 14 years [300,301,303–305,311]. Combining the outcome data from these patients, the rate of normalization of hyperprolactinemia following primary conventional RT employing no other associated therapy is 37.5% (9/24). Similarly, conventional RT following noncurative surgery rarely normalizes prolactin levels. Among three series of patients who received conventional RT for prolactinomas following incomplete surgical resection, 0 [200], 9 [304] and 23% [306] of patients achieved normal prolactin levels after mean follow up of 4, 5.8 and 3 years, respectively. Two series of patients who received LINAC-based fractionated RT after unsuccessful transsphenoidal surgery achieved modestly higher overall PRL normalization rates of 36.3% and 25% [312,313]. When normal prolactin levels were achieved it was, for the majority of cases, only with an extended latency usually beyond 10 years.

As emphasized above, the majority of series reporting RT outcomes in patients with prolactinomas include patients treated with multimodal therapy (surgery, dopamine agonists and RT). Clearly, it is not possible to dissect out what specific effect RT has in lowering prolactin levels and controlling tumor growth in these patients. Since these prolactinomas represent the most therapy-resistant tumors, normalization of hyperprolactinemia may have been infeasible, and under these circumstances, RT may have been employed primarily to attenuate further growth or to relieve mass effects on cranial nerves.

Efficacy: Single-dose Stereotactic

Almost 400 patients with prolactinomas have been reported who have undergone treatment with SDSR alone, or after failure of medical and/or surgical therapy [314–316]. Remission rates, which are variably or ill defined, among these series ranges from 0 to 83%. The study methods and outcome criteria are heterogeneous, with variables including lengths of follow-up, definitions for remission, prior or concurrent therapy, tumor volumes or degree of invasion and prescription doses. Most of these studies assess efficacy at relatively short durations following SDSR, which may underestimate the complete response rates and the incidence of RT-induced hypopituitarism. Three retrospective studies have reported outcome data with post-SDSR surveillance intervals approaching or exceeding 5 years (Table 15.4) [314,315,317]. In all three of these studies, the remission criterion for hormonal activity is defined as normalization of prolactin levels in the absence of dopamine agonist therapy [314,315,317]. In two of these studies, the effect of SDSR on the change in adenoma size was assessed by determining the number of prolactinomas that show a 20% reduction in volume after RT [315,317]. Biochemical remission was observed in 20–37% of these patients after a median follow-up of 5–8 years. Tumor volume reduction (20%) was less consistent, ranging from 46–71%. The median time to PRL normalization was 2 years in two of these studies, but a lengthy 8 years for the third study, despite its use of a higher mean marginal dose. Recurrence of hyperprolactinemia following apparent remission is not reported in these studies, but has been documented following the use of SDSR for the management of other types of functioning pituitary tumors [318].

There are limited data assessing the efficacy of SDSR as primary therapy for prolactinomas, due to the preference for dopamine agonists as first-line therapy. A single

TABLE 15.4 Long-term Outcome Data for Prolactinomas Treated with Gamma Knife Radiotherapy

Study	Margin Dose (Gy)	Number of Patients	Biochemical Remission (%)	20% Tumor Size Reduction (%)	Median Follow-up (mos)	Median Latency to Biochemical Remission (mos)	Remission Predictors
Pourtian et al. [317]	18.6	23 biochemical 28 volume	26	46	58	24.5	Tumor volume, off dopamine agonist at time of RT
Jezkova et al. [315]	34	35	37	71	75	96	None identified
Castinetti et al. [314]	26	15	20	ND	96	24	Tumor volume, initial PRL level

study reports specific data for 77 patients who did not receive pre- or post-SDSR medical therapy [319]. Normalization of prolactin in the absence of concomitant medical therapy was achieved in 16 (20.8%) of these patients at a follow-up duration of 2 years. The data obtained from this center would indicate that SDSR is not a highly effective mode of primary therapy if the goal of RT is normalization of hyperprolactinemia.

Information about pregnancy after SDSR for prolactinomas is scarce. Pan et al. report that nine infertile women became pregnant 2–13 months after SDSR and all gave birth to normal children [319]. Jezkova et al. report that six infertile women in their center who previously failed dopamine agonist therapy became pregnant after normalization of PRL levels following successful SDSR [315].

Clinical factors predictive of remission following RT vary among all the studies reported, but include volume of tissue to treat [314,317], dose of radiation [319–322] and initial prolactin level [314]. Whether discontinuation of dopamine agonist therapy should precede SDSR to improve response rates is controversial. Three retrospective studies have documented a deleterious effect of dopamine agonist therapy on the rate of PRL normalization when it is administered concomitantly with SDSR [317,321,323]. The biological mechanism underlying this attenuating effect may be related to the influence of dopamine agonists on cell cycle progression, rendering treated tumorous lactotrophs less sensitive to radiation-induced DNA damage [324]. It is possible, however, that studies which showed an association between the cessation of dopamine agonist therapy and greater SDSR efficacy were biased by the inclusion of patients with more aggressive disease who remained on drug therapy. Moreover, the ideal duration to withhold medical therapy prior to SDSR, if there is one, is not known.

Selecting the Mode of Radiotherapy

Under most circumstances, SDSR is the preferred mode of RT due to its ability to deliver a highly focused dose to the tumor in a single session, while sparing surrounding tissue from harmful effects of radiation [324]. In the early days of SDSR, high doses for large pituitary adenomas near the optic apparatus resulted in a high incidence of optic neuropathy [325]. The risk of optic nerve damage is dose-dependent, with a 78% risk of optic neuropathy in patients receiving >15 Gy, and 27% risk for those receiving 10–15 Gy to the optic apparatus [326,327]. In order to achieve an acceptable fall-off gradient with single-session therapy, current practice aims to limit irradiation of the optic apparatus to single doses less than 8 Gy [299,322,328–330]. Therefore, prolactinomas with significant suprasellar extension, or those with less than 5 mm clearance between the tumor margin and the optic apparatus are poor candidates for SDSR [322,328,329]. Although it has been reported that the cranial nerves in the cavernous sinus are relatively resistant to radiation effects, incidences of cranial neuropathy, especially after repeat SDSR, have been documented [331]. Prospective evaluations directly comparing the rates of prolactin normalization using conventional versus SDSR for the treatment of prolactinomas have not been published.

In addition to patient convenience, one of the proposed advantages of SDSR is its shorter latency to hormonal and tumor size responses. It appears likely that SDSR lowers prolactin levels more rapidly than conventional external beam RT, although this claim is not substantiated by any prospective comparative study. With the exception of one outlier study [315], most of the series that have documented mean/median latencies to biochemical remission for prolactinomas report responses that range from 2–3 years [314,317,321,329, 332–334]. The latency to normalization of hyperprolactinemia for conventional external beam RT is in the order of several years.

Complications of Conventional Radiotherapy

The most frequent long-term morbidity of conventional RT is radiation-induced hypopituitarism, with a cumulative actuarial risk of approximately 50% at 10–20 years [335–337]. Hypopituitarism is likely secondary to hypothalamic and pituitary damage, although the former is considered of primary importance [338]. The consequences of hypopituitarism may be more significant than issues related to just hormone replacement dosing and monitoring. A large prospective study from the UK showed that the standardized mortality rate was higher in patients with hypopituitarism that had been treated with RT compared with those who had not received RT [339]. A large proportion of this excess was due to a significant increase in cerebrovascular-disease-associated deaths in the RT group.

Additional complications that occur months to years after RT of pituitary adenomas include cerebrovascular accidents, optic nerve damage, neurologic dysfunction and soft tissue reactions [337,340–342]. Conventional RT is associated with an increased risk of secondary radiation-induced intracranial malignancies, with a cumulative risk of 2.0% at 10 years and 2.4% risk at 20 years [343–345].

Complications of Single-dose Stereotactic Radiotherapy

The most common complication of SDSR is hypopituitarism, which increases in incidence with longer follow-up. The reported rates of hypopituitarism range from 0–72% following SDSR [320,321,346–350]. These analyses are confounded by factors such as previous pituitary surgery in some individuals. A long-term follow-up study with a mean follow-up of 17 years determined a relatively high cumulative incidence of hypopituitarism at 72% [351]. Cranial neuropathies are uncommon, but have been reported following SDSR. The severity of these cases ranges from non-specific visual loss to blindness [321,330,352]. The risk of damage to the optic apparatus is approximately 1%. Cranial neuropathies involving nerves that traverse the cavernous sinus (III, IV, V, VI) are less common but still occur [330,331,352,353]. Radiation necrosis of surrounding brain tissue occurs in approximately 0.2–0.8% of cases [330,340]. The risk of secondary intracranial malignancies in individuals who have undergone SDSR is unknown.

Medical Therapy

Medical therapy in the form of dopamine agonists represents the primary therapy for almost all prolactinomas, including microadenomas that require treatment, macroprolactinomas and giant prolactinomas. These agents are highly effective in achieving the treatment goals outlined above with the most favorable benefit/risk profile.

Dopamine agonists inhibit prolactin synthesis and secretion by binding to and activating dopamine D_2 receptors (D_2R) on pituitary lactotrophs [354]. The D_2R belong to the 7-transmembrane domain class of G-protein-coupled receptors and exist in two molecularly distinct long and short forms that arise from alternative splicing from the same gene [354]. The long form has an additional 29-amino acids in the third intracellular loop, a region involved in the coupling to the G-proteins [354]. Activation of the D_2R results in the inhibition of prolactin synthesis and secretion through pathways mediated by several G-proteins. Gαi2 mediates D_2R -induced adenyl cyclase inhibition and a subsequent reduction in intracellular cAMP, probably the major pathway involved in the inhibition of prolactin gene transcription [355,356]. Gαo couples the D_2R to Ca^{2+} channels; dopamine agonist-mediated inhibition of inward Ca^{2+} flux also serves to inhibit phospholipase C and the phosphoinositide pathway [357]. Furthermore, Gαo also couples the D_2R to constitutive and hormone-stimulated levels of mitogen-activated protein kinase (MAPK) and extracellular signal-regulated kinases (ERK1 and ERK2) [358–361], thereby inhibiting cell proliferation. On a cellular level, dopamine agonist treatment causes an involution of the endoplasmic reticulum and Golgi apparati leading to reduction in the size of individual lactotrophs [362]. The issue as to whether dopamine agonists induce apoptosis in lactotrophs is controversial [358,363–368]

Cabergoline: Efficacy

Cabergoline (1-ethyl-3,3-[3′-dimethylamino-propyl] 3-[6′allylergoline-8β-carbonyl]urea diphosphate) is a D_2R-selective agonist with a long duration of action which permits once- or twice-weekly administration. The long duration of action stems from its slow elimination from pituitary tissue, its high affinity binding to pituitary dopamine receptors and extensive enterohepatic recycling [369]. After oral administration, PRL-lowering effects are detectable at 3 hours and gradually increase so that the prolactin-lowering effect plateaus between 48 and 120 hours [369–371]. Therapeutic doses range from 0.5 to 2.0 mg/week, although most patients are successfully treated with weekly doses less than 1.5 mg.

Cabergoline is highly effective in normalizing serum PRL levels, reducing tumor mass and restoring gonadal function. In a multicenter, prospective randomized comparative trial conducted in 459 hyperprolactinemic women (279 microadenomas, three macroadenomas, 167 idiopathic hyperprolactinemia, ten other), of those women treated with cabergoline, 83% achieved normoprolactinemia, 72% resumed ovulatory cycles and 3% discontinued the medication because of adverse effects, while of women treated with bromocriptine, 59%

achieved normoprolactinemia, 52% resumed ovulatory cycles and 12% stopped the drug because of adverse effects [372]. A large comparative retrospective study of 455 patients confirmed the high efficacy of cabergoline [209]. In the 425 patients for whom follow-up data were available, cabergoline treatment normalized PRL levels in 92% of patients with idiopathic hyperprolactinemia or microprolactinomas, 77% of patients with macroprolactinomas and 86% of the overall study population [209]. Side effects were observed in 13%, but only caused discontinuation of the drug in 4%.

About 80–90% of patients who respond to dopamine agonists will do so rapidly (within 3 months), at low doses (less than 2.0 mg/week), with good tolerability [373,374]. However, some patients who do not respond to typical doses of cabergoline will respond at higher doses, and about 10–15% of patients respond with a step-wise reduction in PRL levels with each increase in dose (see Dopamine agonist resistance section) [152,375]. A single-arm prospective study of 150 patients (93 microadenomas, 57 macroadenomas) consisting of untreated patients, patients who experienced previous dopamine agonist intolerance, and patients with previously determined dopamine agonist resistance found that PRL levels could be normalized in 99.3% of patients within 1 year using an individualized treatment protocol employing higher doses of cabergoline, when necessary, with no dropouts [374]. In this study, the achievement of normoprolactinemia led to reversal of hypogonadism in all cases. The mean weekly dose of cabergoline used to normalize hyperprolactinemia was 2.0 ± 0.3 mg in untreated patients, 0.9 mg ± 0.1 mg in bromocriptine-intolerant patients and 5.2 mg ± 0.6 mg in resistant patients. Thus, with dose escalations, cabergoline will normalize prolactin levels in the majority of prolactinomas patients (see Dopamine agonist resistance section). As long as adverse effects from higher doses do not develop, dose escalations are reasonable, with the expectation that future attempts to minimize the dose are made, and patients are notified of the association of cardiac valvular fibrosis that has been reported in patients taking large doses of cabergoline (see below).

Studies examining the effect of cabergoline on macroadenoma size have shown a high response rate, with tumor shrinkage responses of at least 25% documented in the majority of patients [209,211,212,373,376–384]. Two studies reported a semiquantitative assessment of changes in tumor size in patients with macroadenomas who were treated with cabergoline for at least 12 months [373,382]. Combining the data from these two studies which included 127 patients in total, 86 (67.7%) experienced a greater than 50% tumor size reduction, 28 (22.0%) showed a 25–50% reduction and 13 (10.2%) showed a less than 25% reduction in tumor size [373,382]. In 30 of 127 macroadenomas (23.6%), the tumors completely disappeared on MR imaging. One study compared the extent of tumor size reduction among 26 patients who were drug-naïve, 19 intolerant of other dopamine agonists, 47 resistant to other dopamine agonists, or 28 who were responsive to other dopamine agonists, but no longer using them due to poor compliance or drug unavailability [382]. The prevalence of macroprolactinoma shrinkage was greatest among drug-naïve subjects (92.3%); however, significant tumor shrinkage (>50%) still occurred in a substantial proportion of patients who had previous exposure to other dopamine agonists (38.4%) or who had experienced drug intolerance (42.1%). The group of individuals whose tumors previously displayed resistance to other dopamine agonists had the lowest prevalence of significant tumor shrinkage in response to cabergoline (30.3%) [382]. Nonetheless, cabergoline is still the dopamine agonist that has shown the greatest efficacy in the setting of dopamine agonist resistance (see Dopamine agonist resistance section).

Cabergoline: Side Effects

Adverse effects associated with the use of cabergoline are similar to those reported for the other dopamine agonists, but are generally less frequent, less severe, and of shorter duration [234]. Discontinuation of cabergoline treatment due to side effects is reported in less than 3–4% of patients [209,385,386]. Most side effects subside with dose reduction or abate with continued use [386]. The most common adverse events are nausea or vomiting, followed by headache and dizziness [385,386]. Hypotension has been reported in a few women, but is largely asymptomatic [372]. Pleuropulmonary inflammatory-fibrotic syndrome has been described in a few patients [387–389]. Constrictive pericarditis was diagnosed in one patient with Parkinson's disease receiving cabergoline therapy at a dose of 10 mg daily [390].

Cabergoline: Possible Association with Cardiac Valve Disease

The large experience with high doses of dopamine agonists in Parkinson's disease has also drawn attention to another new and potentially more serious issue, that of cardiac valvular abnormalities. This phenomenon was first reported in 2002 for pergolide [391] and in 2004 for cabergoline [392]. Subsequent reports showed a 3–6-fold increased risk of valvular abnormalities in Parkinson's disease patients treated with high doses (3–6 mg/day) of pergolide and cabergoline, and a meta-analysis demonstrated that 34% of patients treated with cabergoline had moderate to severe valvular abnormalities, 22% of those treated with pergolide had such lesions, while only 4% of patients treated with other nonergot dopaminergic agents and 5% of controls had such lesions [393]. Importantly, of the 477 patients treated with cabergoline and pergolide, only three (0.6%) were found to have severe valvulopathy [393]. In some, but not all of these studies, the cumulative dose appeared to be important as well. Because of these findings, pergolide was withdrawn from the market in the US and some other countries. Although a few cases of valvular disease have been reported with very high doses of bromocriptine in Parkinson's patients [394,395], this appears to occur much less often as compared to pergolide and cabergoline [396,397].

The findings on echocardiography consist of leaflet and chordae thickening and stiffening, with incomplete valvular closing and regurgitation [398]. Histologically, there is evidence of fibroblast proliferation with deposition of a plaque-like process on the valve leaflet surfaces that may also encase the chordae tendinae [396,398]. The abnormalities are similar to those seen in patients with carcinoid syndrome and those treated with methysergide and dexfenfluramine [396,398]. What these drugs appear to have in common is the ability to stimulate serotonin 2B receptors, which are present in heart valves and are essential for normal cardiac development [396]. Stimulation of the serotonin 2B receptor results in activation of several mitogenic pathways, ultimately causing this overgrowth valve disorder [396]. Both cabergoline and pergolide are potent serotonin 2B receptor agonists, whereas bromocriptine is only a partial agonist [396].

Echocardiographic studies of patients with hyperprolactinemia treated with cabergoline have been reported. However, one problem in evaluating such patients is the high rate of valvular abnormalities as detected by echocardiography in "normal" individuals. For example, in the Framingham Heart Study of 1696 men and 1893 women aged 54 ± 10 years, mitral regurgitation (MR) and tricuspid regurgitation (TR) of more than or equal to mild severity was seen in 19% and 17%, respectively, and aortic regurgitation (AR) of more than or equal to trace severity was seen in 11% [399]. When limited to moderate severity, the frequencies of TR and AR were about 0.8% and 0.5%, respectively. In the more recent CARDIA study of 4352 men and women aged 21–35 years, MR was found in 10.5% and AR in 0.8% [400].

Most studies that have systematically assessed cardiac valve function in patients treated with relatively low doses of dopamine agonists have not observed significant differences in the incidence of valvular heart disease. At the time of the writing of this chapter, echocardiographic data are already available on a fair number of patients treated with cabergoline along with matched controls. Lancellotti et al. found moderate MR and PR in three of 102 patients taking cabergoline and none in 51 age- and sex-matched controls [401]. Clinically relevant valvular disease was found in 8/47 (17%) patients treated with cabergoline and 13/78 (17%) controls in a study reported by Kars et al. [402]. In a study by Vallette et al. moderate valvular regurgitation was found in 4/70 (5.7%) patients treated with cabergoline and in 5/70 (7.1%) control subjects [403]. Similarly, Bogazzi et al. found that 7/100 (7%) patients treated with cabergoline and 6/100 (6%) controls had moderate regurgitation in any valve [404]. Only one of 100 cabergoline-treated patients and none of 100 matched controls had significant valvular disease in a study by Nachtigall et al. [405]; however, none of the 50 cabergoline-treated patients or the 50 controls had moderate valvular disease in a study by Herring et al. [406]. In contrast, Colao et al. found moderate TR in an astounding 27/50 (54%) of cabergoline-treated patients and 9/50 (18%) controls [407]. There are three other reports without controls of prolactinoma patients treated with cabergoline who underwent echocardiography. Collectively, these reported no clinically significant valvulopathy in the 106 patients of Ono et al. [374], none among the 44 patients in the study by Wakil et al. [408] and mild MR in 1/45 patients in the study by Devin et al. [409]. It should also be mentioned that increases in other minor abnormalities of valve thickening or calcification without significant regurgitation in cabergoline patients were seen in some studies [401,402] but not in others [403,406,407].

Therefore, of the seven studies [401–407] which included age- and sex-matched controls, only one [407] showed a significantly increased risk of clinically significant valve disease in prolactinoma patients treated with cabergoline. This study [407] also found rates in their control group of moderate TR that was more than six-fold greater than that seen in any of the other studies or in large population-based studies [399,400]. Thus, it would appear that the echocardiographers in this study [407] were perhaps using criteria for valvular abnormalities quite different from the other studies. It should further be mentioned that the prevalence of trivial or mild valvular regurgitation was high and similar in both patients and controls in these studies.

Thus, it appears that patients taking conventional doses (≤2 mg/wk) of cabergoline are not at an increased risk of valvular disease. In our practice, patients taking such conventional doses are informed of the potential risk with much larger than usual doses, are reassured, and only undergo echocardiography if they have an audible heart murmur, if they are concerned, or if there are any other cardiac symptoms or signs that are concerning. In patients taking higher than conventional doses of cabergoline, they again are reassured but echocardiography is also performed to be prudent. If valve abnormalities are then found, alternatives include: (1) continue cabergoline with annual echocardiographic monitoring to detect possible worsening; (2) switch to bromocriptine, which appears to have much lower risk of valve disease; (3) transsphenoidal surgery in those patients in whom a surgical approach has a reasonable likelihood of cure. Surgery in patients who do not respond to or are intolerant of dopamine agonists shows that 12/45 (27%) of those with macroadenomas and 10/16 (62%) with microadenomas can obtain normal PRL levels without medication [260]. However, surgery in resistant macroadenoma patients appears to have a relatively high complication rate [260]. Patients not desiring fertility could also be treated with estrogen/testosterone replacement or even bone antiresorptive agents (see above) but these will have no effect on tumor size. Thus, the patient with a prolactinoma and valvular disease represents a therapeutic challenge, but one that can be overcome. It is important not to alarm patients unduly about the very remote possibility of a potentially adverse effect of cabergoline on cardiac valvular function, but it may be prudent to evaluate and monitor patients taking larger than standard doses by echocardiography. Although some centers now perform echocardiography routinely prior to starting long-term cabergoline therapy [410], we have adopted a selective approach to echocardiographic screening at therapy initiation, and employ this testing after discussion of the risks and options with patients.

Bromocriptine: Efficacy

Bromocriptine (2-brono-α-ergocryptine mesylate) is an ergot derivative that has D_2R agonist and D_1R antagonist properties. It was the first dopamine agonist introduced into clinical practice, and is the most extensively studied. Although its use has largely been supplanted by cabergoline, some patients may use this drug in specific situations (e.g., patients with cardiac valve insufficiency). In contrast to cabergoline, bromocriptine has a relatively short elimination half life, so it is usually taken 2 or 3 times daily. After a single oral dose of 2.5 mg, serum levels peak after 3 hours and nadir at 7 hours. There is a very high first-pass effect, with 94% of a dose being metabolized and only 6% of an absorbed dose reaching the systemic circulation unchanged [411]. Only the native compound is bioactive and metabolites are inactive. Therapeutic doses range from 2.5 to 15 mg/day and most patients are successfully treated with daily doses of 7.5 mg or less.

Several series of patients have reported the efficacy of bromocriptine in lowering PRL levels for the treatment of tumoral or idiopathic hyperprolactinemia. Among ten studies that include a total of 471 microprolactinomas, bromocriptine normalized serum PRL in 365 (77.8%) [310,372,375,412–418]. Among nine studies that include a total of 225 macroprolactinomas, bromocriptine normalized serum PRL levels in 163 (72.5%) [194,210,375,419–424]. In several large, early studies, totaling more than 400 hyperprolactinemic patients treated with bromocriptine, normoprolactinemia or return of ovulatory menses occurred in 80–90% of patients. When both PRL levels and return of menses are studied in the same patients, it has been shown that reductions in PRL to levels slightly above the normal range are often sufficient to restore ovulation and menses.

Studies examining the effect of bromocriptine on macroadenoma size have shown that the majority of tumors will show some degree of reduction in size as assessed by CT scan imaging [425]. Of 21 different series examining tumor shrinkage among patients with macroadenomas totaling 302 individuals, 76.8% of tumors decreased in size in response to bromocriptine with periods of observation ranging from 6 weeks to over 10 years [194,288,292,310,421,424,426–440]. Ten studies including a total of 112 patients report a semiquantitative assessment of changes in tumor size in patients with macroadenomas who were treated with bromocriptine for 3–24 months. Among the 112 patients, 45 (40.2%) demonstrated >50% reduction in tumor size, 32 (28.6%) had 25–50% reduction in tumor size, 14 (12.5%) had <25% reduction and 21 (18.7%) had no evidence of change in tumor size [194,288,292,310,426,429,430,435,436,440]. Overall, these tumor shrinkage rates are lower than those observed in macroprolactinoma patients treated with cabergoline, although technically, the studies are not directly comparable as a result of differences in treatment duration and the imaging techniques employed. As with cabergoline, a significant proportion of microprolactinomas treated with bromocriptine will disappear completely [427].

Detailed analyses regarding the time course of tumor size reduction have been most extensively reported in macroprolactinomas treated with bromocriptine. In general, tumor shrinkage occurs at variable intervals, but importantly, some patients experience extremely rapid decreases in tumor size with significant improvement in visual fields noted within 24–72 hours, and changes apparent on imaging within 2 weeks [441]. In the prospective multicenter US trial, most patients experienced reduction in tumor size by 6 weeks but in several others, improvement was not demonstrated until the scans scheduled at the 6-month time point. A progressive decrease in tumor size was often noted between 6 months and 1 year, and in some cases, further reduction in tumor size continued for several years thereafter.

Visual field improvement generally parallels and often precedes the changes seen on pituitary imaging [194,436]. Reduction in PRL levels almost always precedes any detectable change in tumor size, and PRL nonresponders are also tumor size nonresponders. In some patients, normalization of PRL levels is accompanied by only modest changes in tumor size. Once maximum size reduction is achieved, the dose of bromocriptine can often be substantially, albeit gradually, reduced.

Bromocriptine: Side Effects

The most common and limiting side effects of bromocriptine are gastrointestinal in nature, and include nausea and vomiting [442]. Symptoms tend to occur after the initial dose and with dosage increases, but can be minimized by introducing the drug at a low dosage at bedtime, taking it with food, and by very gradual dose escalation. Most often, tolerance develops to these effects, but occasionally, therapy withdrawal or dose reduction followed by a more gradual reintroduction is required. Postural hypotension occurs in a small percentage of patients when initiating therapy [386]. Patients receiving high doses of bromocriptine (30–75 mg/day) may experience a syndrome of painless digital vasospasm in response to cold [443,444].

The most common neurological adverse effects include headache and drowsiness. Symptoms of psychosis, or exacerbation of pre-existing psychosis, have been associated with the use of bromocriptine [445–447]. Turner et al. [447] noted psychotic reactions in eight of 600 patients receiving either bromocriptine or lisuride from hyperprolactinemia or acromegaly. Rare reports of exacerbation of pre-existing schizophrenia also exist, therefore, the drug should be given cautiously to such patients. Psychotic reactions usually resolve within 72 hours of drug discontinuation.

Reversible pleuropulmonary changes consisting of pleural effusions, pleural thickening and parenchymal lung changes have been reported in patients treated with high doses of bromocriptine for Parkinson's disease [448]. These findings have not been reported with doses of bromocriptine used for the treatment of hyperprolactinemia.

Nonsurgical cerebrospinal fluid rhinorrhea has been reported during treatment of adults with macroprolactinomas using either cabergoline or bromocriptine due to tumor shrinkage, when the adenoma previously served as a "cork" for the tumor-induced defect in the skull base [449–456]. A retrospective study assessing the frequency of this complication among 114 individuals with macroprolactinomas found an overall incidence of 8.7%, with 2.6% of cases being spontaneous and 6.1% associated with dopamine agonist use [455]. Neurosurgical correction of the CSF leak may be necessary in some individuals, but spontaneous resolution has also been described [457,458]. Discontinuation of dopamine agonist therapy in patients who develop CSF rhinorrhea is not necessary.

Pergolide

Another dopamine agonist that went through early trials demonstrating efficacy in the treatment of prolactinomas is pergolide. Hyperprolactinemia can be controlled with single daily doses of 50–150 μg [459]. Several studies have shown comparability to bromocriptine with respect to tolerance and efficacy, including tumor size reduction [460–464]. Experience has shown that some patients who do not respond to bromocriptine do so to pergolide and vice versa [465]. Only 39 patients from these series [463,464,466,467] had sufficient data to quantitate tumor size reduction. Of these, 29 (75%) had a greater than 50% reduction, four (10%) had 25–50% reduction, two (5%) had less than 25% reduction and four (10%) had no change in tumor size. Because of concern regarding valvular abnormalities in patients with Parkinson's disease taking high doses of pergolide, this drug has been removed from the market in the US and some other countries [468].

Quinagolide

Quinagolide (CV 205-502) is a nonergot dopamine agonist with specific D_2R activity. Therapeutic doses range from 0.03 to 0.6 mg/day. Approximately 50% of patients who are resistant to bromocriptine respond to quinagolide. Its efficacy in reducing tumor size and normalizing PRL levels is similar to that of bromocriptine and pergolide [259].

Di Sarno et al. compared the outcome of quinagolide and cabergoline in a sequential treatment administered to 39 patients [469]. Treatment with quinagolide for 12 months was followed by a 12 months wash-out period and then cabergoline treatment was given for a further 12-month period. After treatment with quinagolide for the first 12 months, prolactin levels normalized in 100% of patients with microprolactinomas and in 88% of patients with macroprolactinomas. Following the wash-out period, cabergoline was given to the same patients. After 12 months of cabergoline treatment, prolactin levels normalized in 96% and 88% of patients with micro- and macroprolactinomas, respectively. Thus, in this particular study, both quinagolide and cabergoline treatments induced the normalization of serum PRL levels in the great majority of patients with micro- and macroprolactinomas. In a randomized, crossover study of 20 patients with hyperprolactinemia receiving once-daily quinagolide or twice-weekly cabergoline for 12 weeks, a higher percentage of patients achieved normal PRL levels with cabergoline compared with quinagolide but clinical endpoints, such as amenorrhea, oligomenorrhea, galactorrhea and impotence, were similar, as were the frequency of side effects [470]. A total of 105 patients using quinagolide have been assessed for tumor size reduction in a semiquantitative way in studies ranging from 2 to 36 months in duration [471–479]. Of these 105, 50 (48.1%) experienced a greater than 50% tumor size reduction, 21 (20.2%) experienced a 25–50% size reduction, 18 (17.3%)

experienced a less than 25% reduction and 15 (14.4%) had no change in tumor size. Adverse effects are consistent with those reported for other dopamine agonists, although they occur less frequently than with bromocriptine [259]. This drug is unavailable in the US at the present time, but is approved for use in Europe.

Discontinuation of Medical Therapy

Dopamine agonist therapy may not be a life long requirement to maintain normoprolactinemia for a subset of patients with prolactinomas. The appropriate duration of therapy, however, has not been defined. Studies dating back to the early 1980s have documented maintenance of normal prolactin levels after discontinuation of bromocriptine in a small percentage of dopamine-agonist-treated patients. The mechanism underlying sustained remission may be related to tumor necrosis and to the fibrotic changes that can occur in response to long-term dopamine agonist therapy [367,480]. The critical data needed to consider drug discontinuation include: (1) the likelihood of maintaining normoprolactinemia following withdrawal of a particular dopamine agonist; (2) the duration normoprolactinemia is sustained; (3) the risk for tumor enlargement.

After withdrawal of bromocriptine (Table 15.5) remission rates have been reported ranging from 0 to 44% [310,415,433,481–487]. In the only study restricted to patients with macroprolactinomas, van't Verlaat et al. [488] reported a remission rate in 8% of 12 patients after 12 months. Importantly, an increase in tumor volume with clear-cut re-expansion has been found in only a minority of cases [489–491] (<10%) after bromocriptine discontinuation and tumor regrowth seems to depend on

TABLE 15.5 Rates of PRL Normalization Following Dopamine Agonist Withdrawal

Author	Reference	Drug	No. Subjects				Treatment Duration (Months)	Normal PRL (%)	Follow-up Duration (Months)
			Total	Micro	Macro	NTH			
Johnston et al.	[433]	BRC	37			19	12–72	5.4	0.5
Zarate et al.	[486]	BRC	16			0	Mean 24	37.5	24
Moriondo et al.	[415]	BRC	36	36	0	0	Mean 12	22	Up to 30
Johnston et al.	[482]	BRC	13	5	6	2	Mean 44	7.7	1–12.5
Maxson et al.	[483]	BRC	7	7	0	0	>12	0	2
Wang et al.	[310]	BRC	24	15	4	5	Mean 24	21	12–48
Winkelmann et al.	[485]	BRC	40					18.4	5–25
Rasmussen et al.	[621]	BRC	75				Mean 24	44	>6
Van't Verlaat et al.	[488]	BRC	12	0	12	0	Median 60	8.3	12
Passos et al.	[484]	BRC	131				Mean 47	20.6	Mean 44
Biswas et al.	[487]	BRC	22	22	0	0	Median 36	50	>12
Ferrari et al.	[380]	CAB	65	42	7	15	Median 14	31.3 (year 1) 66.7 (year 2)	3–24
Muratori et al.	[494]	CAB	26	26	0	0	12	19	38–60
Cannavò et al.	[381]	CAB	37	26	11	0	24	13.5	12
Di Sarno et al.	[469]	CAB	39	23	16	0	12	10.2	12
Biswas et al.	[487]	CAB	67	67	0	0	Median 36	31.3	>12
Colao et al.	[622]	CAB	231	115	79	27	43 (micro) 42 (macro) 39 (NTH)	61 (micro) 47 (macro) 42 (NTH)	47 (micro) 44 (macro) 39 (NTH)
Kharlip et al.	[495]	CAB	46	31	11	4	Median 51.6	46	median 15
Johnston et al.	[482]	PER	2	1	1	0	24	0	2
Di Sarno et al.	[469]	CV	39	23	16	0	12	0	0.5–2

BRC, bromocriptine; CAB, cabergoline; PER, pegolide; CV, quinagolide; NTH, non-tumoral hyperprolactinemia.

the duration of previous treatment, although the data to this point are very sparse [310,415,433,481–488,492]. In their metaanalysis, Dekkers et al. found the average remission rate from bromocriptine to be 20% using either a fixed- or random-effects model [493].

As noted above, cabergoline has a substantially greater success rate in shrinking macroadenomas. Following withdrawal from cabergoline treatment, persistent normoprolactinemia was found by Ferrari et al. [380] in 31.2% of 32 patients; by Muratori et al. [494] in 24% of 25 patients; by Cannavò et al. [381] in one macro- (11%) and four microprolactinomas (22%) and by Biswas et al. [487] in 31.3% of 67 patients with microadenomas (Table 15.5). In a sequential study aiming at comparing the efficacy of a 12-month course of treatment with quinagolide and cabergoline in 39 patients (23 with microprolactinoma and 16 with macroprolactinoma), Di Sarno et al. [469] also found persistent normoprolactinemia in none of the patients during the treatment with quinagolide and in 10.2% (17.4% of 23 microprolactinomas) treated with cabergoline (Table 15.5). Colao et al. [492] reported a Kaplan-Meier estimate of recurrence rate of hyperprolactinemia after 5 years of cabergoline withdrawal of only 24% in patients with nontumoral hyperprolactinemia, 32.6% in patients with micro- and 43.3% in those with macroprolactinomas. MRI evidence of tumor regrowth was not found in any patient; only ten women (22.2%) and seven men (38.9%) with recurrent hyperprolactinemia redeveloped gonadal dysfunction. The patients showing small remnant tumors on MRI at treatment withdrawal, either with macro- or microprolactinomas at their diagnosis, had a higher estimated recurrence rate after 5 years than those without evident tumor (macroprolactinomas 77.5 vs. 32.6%, $p = 0.001$; microprolactinomas 41.5 vs. 26.2%, $p = 0.02$). Age, basal prolactin levels, nadir prolactin levels, percent prolactin suppression, nadir tumor diameter after cabergoline, treatment duration, and cabergoline dose were all higher before treatment withdrawal in patients developing a recurrence of hyperprolactinemia as compared to those achieving persistent control [492]. More recently, Kharlip et al. found rates of recurrence of 52% in 31 patients with microadenomas and 55% in 11 patients with macroadenomas [495]. They also noted that the larger the size of the tumor remnant at the time of withdrawal, the greater the chance of recurrence [495].

Based on the data reported from these studies, it appears that clinicians should only attempt dopamine agonist withdrawal when its success is probable. Factors favoring success include: (1) use of cabergoline vs. bromocriptine; (2) normalization of PRL for at least 2 years; (3) maintenance of normoprolactinemia for at least 1 year after tapering to a dose of 0.5 mg cabergoline per week; and (4) tumor no longer visible on MRI. When these criteria are met, 48–76% of patients with microadenomas and 42–75% of patients with macroadenomas can end treatment with cabergoline successfully. If, however, a substantial tumor remnant is still visible on MRI, then these success rates decrease to 48–60% for patients with microadenomas and 42% for those with macroadenomas. Nevertheless, if the tumor is still visible, the more pronounced the reduction in tumor size with treatment, the greater the chance of success with treatment after cabergoline withdrawal. Although studies on bromocriptine have not been analyzed in the same fashion, the same predictive factors potentially hold true, albeit the overall success rates will most probably be considerably lower [496].

Dopamine Agonist Resistance

Dopamine agonists are highly effective in normalizing prolactin levels, alleviating symptoms of hyperprolactinemia and reducing tumor size. Nonetheless, a small subset of individuals with prolactinomas does not respond satisfactorily to these agents [497]. Prolactinomas exhibit varying degrees of responsiveness to the class of dopamine agonists, ranging from complete response at one end of the spectrum to total resistance at the other. In addition, individual prolactinomas may respond poorly or incompletely to one dopamine agonist, but well to another. Patients who initially respond to a dopamine agonist and later become secondarily resistant are rare; reasons for this acquired nonresponsiveness include noncompliance, institution of gonadal steroid replacement, and rarely, transformation to carcinoma [498–503]. Under most circumstances, the normalization of prolactin levels achieved with a dopamine agonist is accompanied by substantial tumor size reduction. However, unusual cases of "selective" dopamine agonist resistance have been reported in a few patients exhibiting discordant responses to prolactin-lowering and tumor size-reducing effects [497,504]. Finally, the concept of dopamine agonist resistance must be distinguished from that of dopamine agonist intolerance, in which adverse effects of the medication prevent the achievement of an effective response.

DEFINITION OF DOPAMINE AGONIST RESISTANCE

Three caveats should be recognized when analyzing data regarding the prevalence of dopamine agonist resistance and the effectiveness of the individual dopamine agonist agents in this specific situation. First, varying definitions of dopamine agonist responsiveness and resistance are used throughout the literature, including failure to normalize prolactin levels, failure to reduce prolactin levels sufficiently to achieve ovulation, or failure to enable a 50% reduction of hyperprolactinemia [375,378,505,506]. Second, the absence of standardized dose limits to which a dopamine agonist should be escalated to classify a tumor as having resistance confounds the literature. Recent publications have attempted to address the continuous nature of pharmacologic resistance by classifying patients categorically according to their sensitivity to cabergoline [373]. Finally, the intensity of the effort to increase the dose may play a determining role in achieving a complete response. Therefore, the percentage of patients deemed responsive or resistant to a particular dopamine agonist will depend upon both the aggressiveness and dose threshold set by the practitioner.

The desired biological response in the treatment of hyperprolactinemia in women is the achievement of ovulation. A reduction of hyperprolactinemia, rather than complete normalization, may be sufficient to achieve this goal. Using this threshold is impractical for study purposes, however, as it represents a level that varies on an individual basis and is frequently not specified in the medical literature. Therefore, the authors prefer to define dopamine agonist resistance with respect to hormone levels as the failure to achieve normoprolactinemia.

Dopamine agonist resistance also occurs in cases where drug therapy has little or no impact on tumor size reduction. The frequency of this outcome is also dependent upon the threshold set as "significant" tumor size reduction. Throughout the literature, tumor size reduction is generally reported in terms of various percentages, ranging from 80%, 75%, 50%, 25%, 10% and no change. Although seemingly arbitrary, it is the authors' practice to define dopamine agonist resistance with respect to tumor size as the failure to achieve tumor size reduction of 50%.

MECHANISMS OF DOPAMINE AGONIST RESISTANCE

Dopamine agonists inhibit prolactin synthesis and secretion by binding to and activating dopamine D2 receptors (D_2R) on pituitary lactotrophs [507]. The D_2R exists as two isoforms, referred to as the long and short isoforms [354,508,509]. The long form has an additional 29-amino acids in the third intracellular loop, which is a region involved in the coupling to the G-proteins [510,511]. The existence of these two variants may have implications for the mechanisms of dopamine agonist resistance (see below).

Molecular mechanisms implicated in dopamine agonist resistance in human prolactinomas are incompletely understood. These mechanisms are likely to encompass a complex, diverse set of alterations, and the substantial genetic heterogeneity among the paucity of available surgical specimens complicates the assessment of individual factors that are responsible for aggressive behavior and drug resistance (Figure 15.5) [512]. The obvious candidate for a molecular alteration leading to dopamine agonist resistance is the lactotroph D_2R itself. As previously discussed, disruption of the *Drd2* gene in mice leads to the delayed development of lactotroph adenomas. However, somatic mutations in the coding sequence of the *DRD2* gene do not appear to account for the development of human prolactinomas

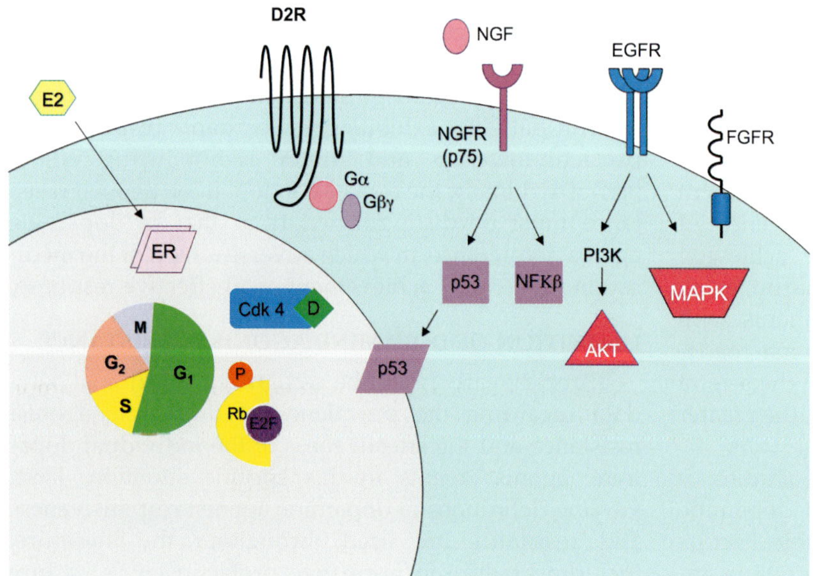

FIGURE 15.5 Schematic illustration of the alterations implicated in dopamine agonist resistance or progression in prolactinomas. The expression of the dopamine receptor 2 (D_2R) is reduced in some resistant prolactinomas, and may be lost in processes leading to malignant transformation. A reduced proportion of short to long D_2R isoforms may also contribute to reduced dopamine agonist responsiveness. Alterations in nerve growth factor (NGF) signaling and an autocrine loop which maintains D_2R expression have been identified in human prolactinoma specimens. NGF appears to regulate D_2R expression by inducing $p75^{NGFR}$ receptor-mediated nuclear translocation of p53 and activation of NF-κB. Alterations in EGFR signaling may be permissive for lactotroph tumor progression, possibly through sustenance of mitogenic (MAPK) and survival (AKT) pathways. Estradiol promotes the proliferation of both benign and adenomatous lactotrophs. (*See text for references.*) D_2R, dopamine 2 receptor; NGF, nerve growth factor; NGFR, nerve growth factor receptor; E2, estradiol; ER, estrogen receptor; MAPK, mitogen-activated protein kinase; PI3K, phosphatidylinositol-3 kinase; AKT, protein kinase B; EGFR, epidermal growth factor receptor; FGFR4, fibroblast growth factor receptor; Cdk4, cyclin-dependent kinase 4; Rb, retinoblastoma protein.

[173]. Studies that have examined pathogenetic mechanisms of drug-resistant, aggressive prolactinoma behavior focus on the three areas of investigation: (1) studies of D_2R expression/affinity; (2) studies of D_2R isoforms and their relationship to G-protein activation; and (3) studies involving regulation of D_2R expression.

There is experimental evidence that some dopamine-agonist-resistant prolactinomas have a reduced density of D_2Rs [175,506,513,514]. A comparison of D_2R density and affinity in primary cell cultures of prolactinomas derived from bromocriptine-sensitive ($n = 10$) and -resistant ($n = 8$) patients [506] found that the density of dopaminergic binding sites, as assessed by [^{3}H]-spiroperidol (a selective D_2R antagonist), was reduced by 50% in the group of resistant prolactinomas overall as compared to the group of bromocriptine-sensitive adenomas. The binding affinity, nonetheless, was similar. Perhaps more significantly, five of the resistant prolactinomas that grew during therapy showed a dramatic reduction in D_2R sites, exhibiting only 10% of dopaminergic binding sites found in normally responsive tumors. In the majority of tumors, adenyl cyclase activity within the cells paralleled the changes in D_2R number proportionately, demonstrating that the D_2Rs from the resistant prolactinomas couple normally to adenyl cyclase, despite the overall reduction in D_2R number. However, for the tumors that grew during therapy, dopamine paradoxically stimulated adenyl cyclase activity. For this subset of resistant tumors, the possibility of abnormal coupling of the D_2R to second messengers (Gαi2 proteins), in addition to an overall reduction in D_2R expression, remains a possibility.

Since this initial report, additional studies examining D_2R expression in dopamine-agonist-resistant prolactinomas have yielded conflicting results. [174,175,515, 516]. The variable findings are probably related to tumor heterogeneity, as well as to the specific methods and sensitivities of techniques employed (i.e., assessment of mRNA vs. protein expression). In contrast to the results reported above, Kovacs et al. demonstrated preservation of both D_2R mRNA and protein expression in their group of prolactinomas resistant to dopamine agonist therapy [515]. Progressive reduction or loss of D_2R expression may, however, be associated with tumor evolution to a more dedifferentiated state. For example, Winkelmann et al. reported a clinical case with molecular analysis of D_2R expression in a malignant prolactinoma that was initially responsive to bromocriptine, but gradually became resistant to dopamine agonist therapy and eventually developed intra- and extracranial metastases [501]. Intact D_2R mRNA transcripts were found in the original tumor and metastatic tissues, whereas D_2R protein was expressed only in the initial neurosurgical specimens and lost in the metastases obtained post-mortem. The loss of D_2R protein expression despite the retention of the transcript suggests that alterations in post-transcriptional processing of the D_2R may contribute to the development of dopamine resistance and aggressive behavior in some prolactinomas.

A second area of investigation into the mechanism of dopamine agonist resistance has focused on differences in the proportion of short (D_2S) and long (D_2L) dopamine receptor variants, and correlating this with the degree of dopamine agonist responsiveness. The two molecular isoforms of the D_2R display comparable binding characteristics, but they are regulated differently [513,517] and they may exhibit differential coupling to selective G-proteins [356,510]. The D_2S receptor appears to be more efficient than the D_2L at coupling to adenyl cyclase [518,519]. Using quantitative RT-PCR, both the short and long isoforms were found in sensitive prolactinomas, in equivalent proportions to that reported for normal pituitary lactotrophs [174]. By contrast, the proportion of mRNA corresponding to the D_2S was lower in resistance compared to responsive prolactinomas (D_2S/D_2L ratio $= 0.74$ and 1.00, respectively). The significance of this altered ratio is uncertain, however, since the magnitude of the decrease in D_2S receptor expression is modest. Consequently, alterations in the ratio of the receptor variants may contribute to, but are unlikely to solely determine, the spectrum of dopamine agonist responsiveness observed among prolactinomas [520].

The third major area of investigation has focused on the role of autocrine pathways of inhibitory growth signaling in the development of dopamine agonist resistance in human prolactinomas. A nerve growth factor (NGF)-mediated autocrine loop has been identified in pituitary lactotrophs that influences cell proliferation and differentiation [521]. This autocrine loop has been shown to be present in a human cell line derived from a dopaminergic-sensitive prolactinoma, but lost in a second cell line derived from a dopaminergic-resistant tumor [175]. The cell line generated from the "sensitive" tumor maintains D_2R expression, is more differentiated and is nontumorigenic. The other "resistant" cell line, obtained from a human prolactinoma refractory to dopaminergic therapy, lacks D_2R expression, has transforming capability and is tumorigenic in vivo. An analysis of the NGF system in each of these two tumor cell lines has revealed that the dopamine-agonist-sensitive cell line secretes high levels of NGF and expresses both the $p75^{NGFR}$ and trkA receptors for NGF [522]. In contrast, the resistant cell line does not produce NGF, and expresses only the trkA, but not the $p75^{NGFR}$, receptor [522]. Exposure of the resistant cells to exogenous NGF induces expression and secretion of biologically active NGF and the expression of $p75^{NGFR}$ receptors, thus restoring the autocrine loop. Furthermore, NGF treatment of the resistant cells results in decreased proliferation in vitro, reduced capacity to form colonies in soft agar and loss of tumorigenic activity in nude mice [175,523]. Consistent with these effects, the ablation of NGF production in the responsive cells leads to transformation and loss of D_2R expression [522]. The exact mechanism by which NGF regulates D_2R expression has not been conclusively identified, but initial studies suggest that it may involve activation of NF-κB signaling pathways and/or p53-dependent induction of p21. For example, in one study, exposure of NGF to a dopamine-agonist-resistant prolactinoma cell line promoted D_2R expression by inducing $p75^{NGFR}$-receptor-mediated nuclear translocation and activation of NF-κB complexes, which subsequently increased the transcriptional activity of a D_2R promoter-driven reporter gene [524]. In a second study, the disruption of NGF-mediated autocrine signaling loop in resistant cells was shown to result in nuclear exclusion of the p53 tumor suppressor, while treatment with exogenous NGF promoted a conformational change in p53 that permitted its nuclear translocation and reconstituted its DNA-binding activity [525].

In summary, there is a line of evidence demonstrating that a subset of dopamine-agonist-resistant prolactinomas are associated with a reduction in D_2R expression, but not an alteration in binding affinity. In some cases of dopamine agonist resistance, disruptions in the autocrine growth factor signaling pathway mediated by NGF may accompany or lead to D_2R down-regulation. Whether D_2R receptor isoform ratios are altered, are related to differences in G-protein specificity, or have a major impact on promoting dopamine agonist resistance is unresolved. It should be emphasized that additional undiscovered molecular alterations further downstream of the D_2R may contribute to their insensitivity to inhibitory dopaminergic influence. Finally, as yet unidentified alterations altogether unrelated to D_2R signaling (i.e., ERBB up-regulation) are likely to influence dopamine agonist sensitivity [168], and these may play a role in the aggressive behavior of more dedifferentiated tumors.

RESISTANCE TO PROLACTIN-LOWERING EFFECTS OF DOPAMINE AGONISTS

On the basis of the efficacy data compiled in published analyses, it is possible to estimate the prevalence of resistance to the specific dopamine agonists, with respect to the normalization of prolactin. Overall, approximately 24%, 13% and 11% of patients demonstrate resistance to bromocriptine, pergolide and cabergoline, respectively [259]. Resistance to quinagolide is difficult to ascertain, since there are no large published series in which quinagolide was given to totally drug-naïve patients, which would allow determination of the percentage of patients responding with a normalization of prolactin levels in the absence of any prior drug therapy. Virtually all of the studies testing the efficacy of quinagolide were conducted in patients who had previously been treated with bromocriptine.

Most of the clinical data regarding dopamine agonist resistance involve studies investigating whether another dopamine agonist may be effective in patients previously treated with and found to be resistant to bromocriptine. Of all the dopamine agonists, cabergoline has been shown to be most effective in normalizing prolactin levels in patients who demonstrate resistance to bromocriptine. Approximately 80% of bromocriptine-resistant patients will achieve a normal prolactin level using cabergoline [209,526]. Colao et al. showed that 85% of 20 patients resistant to both bromocriptine and quinagolide responded to cabergoline with a normalization of PRL levels, and 70% responded with some change in tumor size [526]. In close agreement with these results, a subgroup analysis from a large study of patients treated with cabergoline found that 70% of 58 patients in whom bromocriptine failed to normalize PRL were controlled with cabergoline [209]. Of note, these patients did require higher doses of cabergoline (1.5 mg/week) compared to the overall cohort (0.5 mg/week). Only seven (12%) of the patients previously found to be resistant to bromocriptine were completely resistant to cabergoline (<50% decrease in prolactin levels). Two large, prospective randomized studies directly compared bromocriptine to cabergoline with respect to drug efficacy, thus allowing a comparison of the prevalence of resistance to each drug within the same study. In the European Cabergoline Collaborative Study, prolactin was normalized in 48 of 74 (65%) women taking bromocriptine and in 66 of 72 (92%) women taking cabergoline [372]. In a multicenter study conducted in France, 27 of 58 (48%) women taking bromocriptine and 56 of 60 (93%) women taking cabergoline normalized their prolactin levels [527].

Complete resistance to cabergoline is extraordinarily uncommon, and most "partial" resistance can often be overcome by increasing the dose. Ono et al. found that 11/60 (18.3%) previously untreated patients required a greater than usual dose, i.e., greater than 2 mg/week, of cabergoline to normalize PRL levels [374]. Of these, four required 3 mg/week, two required 6 mg/week, four required 9 mg per week and one required 11 mg/week to normalize PRL levels. Of their total 150 patients, normalization of PRL could eventually be achieved in all but one, but doses had to be raised to higher than standard levels in ~15% [374]. In another study, DiSarno et al. found that ten of 56 (17.9%) patients with macroadenomas and six of 60 (10%) patients with microadenomas required larger than usual doses of cabergoline, but they only increased the dosages to a maximum of 7 mg/week and did not achieve PRL normalization in any of these resistant patients [375]. We have also encountered a number of resistant patients and reported one who had small, continued, stepwise reductions in PRL as we gradually increased his dose of cabergoline to 3 mg per day [152]. Thus, true nonresponsiveness to cabergoline is very rare, less than 1% in the authors' experience.

Quinagolide (CV 205-502) has been shown to be effective in improving hyperprolactinemia in some patients resistant to bromocriptine, but this effect is highly variable among the available studies [528–533]. This drug is not available in the US. Sporadic reports of the use of pergolide in bromocriptine-resistant patients have demonstrated only modest efficacy [534,535].

RESISTANCE TO MASS-REDUCING EFFECTS OF DOPAMINE AGONISTS

There are no prospective, randomized series that have compared one dopamine agonist to another with respect to their abilities to decrease tumor size. An analysis of three comparable series of patients treated with bromocriptine, pergolide and cabergoline in separate studies shows that prolactin levels could be lowered to normal in 66%, 68% and 100%, and tumor size decreased by at least 50% in 64%, 86% and 96% of patients receiving bromocriptine [194], pergolide [466] and cabergoline [382], respectively. The final time points for the assessment of the efficacy of these drugs were different; the effects of pergolide and cabergoline were assessed at 24–27 months, whereas the effects of bromocriptine were assessed at 12 months. Since the process of tumor mass reduction will continue after 1 year in some cases, it is possible that the efficacy of bromocriptine in reducing tumor size is underestimated by these data.

On the basis of the studies cited above for prolactin level reduction and tumor size reduction it is possible to make a rough, overall comparison of the three evaluable dopamine agonists. With respect to lack of normalization of prolactin levels, resistance can be expected in 25–50% of patients taking bromocriptine, 10–30% taking pergolide and 5–18% taking cabergoline. With respect to failure to achieve at least a 50% decrease in tumor size, resistance can be expected in about one-third of those taking bromocriptine, about 15% of those taking pergolide and 5–10% of those taking cabergoline.

TREATMENT APPROACHES FOR DOPAMINE-AGONIST-RESISTANT PROLACTINOMAS

The possible treatment approaches for patients with prolactinomas that demonstrate dopamine agonist resistance include: (1) trial of an alternative dopamine agonist; (2) escalation of the dopamine agonist beyond conventional doses; (3) surgical adenomectomy; (4) radiotherapy; and (5) experimental therapy. As noted above, some patients who do not respond to one dopamine agonist will respond to another, and vice versa. For the patient resistant to cabergoline, the most common approach is simply to continue to increase the dose of cabergoline, as long as a reduction in PRL levels can be demonstrated with each stepwise increase. Most patients tolerate such dose increases quite well, although echocardiographic monitoring may be prudent.

Transsphenoidal surgery remains an option if the tumor is potentially resectable and an experienced neurosurgeon is available. Radiotherapy may be effective in controlling tumor growth, although its efficacy in restoring PRL levels to normal is limited. If fertility is a major concern, induction of ovulation is possible in hyperprolactinemic patients even without lowering prolactin levels, using clomiphene citrate, gonadotropins and pulsatile GnRH [536–538]. Of the experimental therapies, an ongoing phase II clinical trial assessing the effectiveness of temozolomide (Temodar®) is active. A number of potential molecular targets have been identified and shown variable effectiveness in vitro or in isolated case reports, but these alternative methods are in preclinical stages and should be reserved for situations in which all other standard therapies have failed [152].

Medical Therapy: Conclusions

By far, the greatest experience in treating patients with prolactinomas has been with bromocriptine and cabergoline. In head-to-head randomized, prospective comparison studies [539], retrospective analyses [375] and general clinical experience, cabergoline has been shown to be substantially more effective in normalizing PRL levels and more successful in reducing tumor size, while maintaining a more favorable side effect profile. Patients are less likely to be resistant to the therapeutic effects of cabergoline; furthermore, most patients found to be resistant to bromocriptine subsequently respond to cabergoline. Finally, treatment with cabergoline affords a greater chance of obtaining permanent remission and successful withdrawal of medication, compared to treatment with bromocriptine. Thus, in general, cabergoline is preferable to bromocriptine as an initial therapeutic agent.

There is much less experience with pergolide and quinagolide in the primary treatment of patients with prolactinomas. However, these drugs appear to have similar efficacy and adverse event profiles compared to bromocriptine. Use of very high doses of pergolide has been associated with organ fibrosis, including cardiac valve fibrosis. Therefore, pergolide should be avoided if high doses are needed. Depending upon pricing in some countries, pergolide may be less expensive than other dopamine agonists and this may factor into its use. Pergolide is not available in the US. Quinagolide is currently available in several European countries and in Canada but is not available in the US. In patients who do not achieve acceptable biochemical or tumor size changes in response to dopamine agonists, transsphenoidal surgery remains an option if the tumor is potentially resectable and an experienced neurosurgeon is available. Radiotherapy may be effective in controlling tumor growth, although its efficacy in restoring PRL levels to normal is limited. If fertility is a major concern, induction of ovulation is possible in hyperprolactinemic patients even without lowering PRL levels, using clomiphene citrate, gonadotropins and pulsatile GnRH [540].

Conclusions Regarding Treatment

MICROADENOMAS

Treatment of patients with microprolactinomas is not mandatory for those who are asymptomatic, eugonadal and do not desire fertility. The risk of progression of microadenoma to macroadenoma is probably under 5%; therefore, these patients can be followed carefully with pituitary MRI and observed as long as there is no evidence of tumor enlargement. Women and men who are hypogonadal should be treated, however, since long-term hypogonadism due to hyperprolactinemia is associated with premature osteoporosis in both sexes. Women who are eugonadal and continue to have ovulatory menses do not have an elevated risk of osteoporosis. For women, if fertility is not a concern, then the options are to use either estrogen replacement therapy (oral contraceptive) or a dopamine agonist. If the main concern is osteoporosis, an antiresorptive agent may be sufficient. Because of its efficacy in reducing PRL levels, favorable adverse effect profile and convenient dosing, cabergoline appears to be the initial drug of choice for most patients with prolactinomas. If fertility is the primary reason to restore ovulation, then some consider bromocriptine to be preferable because of its more established safety profile (see below). For some individuals, the cost of treatment and requirement of having to take a medication for many years make them prefer to undergo transsphenoidal surgery as their primary option. This may also be the primary treatment option for the ~10% of patients who either just cannot tolerate or do not respond to dopamine agonists. Most studies have not corroborated very early reports of reduced surgical success rates associated with prior bromocriptine-induced tumor fibrosis, so this argument should not preclude an indecisive patient from undergoing a trial of dopamine agonist therapy. Based on a comprehensive analysis of surgical outcome data, the initial surgical cure rates for microadenomas appear to be in the 65–85% range, with a later recurrence for hyperprolactinemia of about 20%. Thus the ultimate surgical cure rate for microadenomas is in the 60% range. Radiation therapy has an extremely limited role in patients with microadenomas, and is only advised for those who do not respond to dopamine agonists and who are not cured by surgery.

MACROADENOMAS

Dopamine agonists are universally recommended as the initial therapy for patients with PRL-secreting macroadenomas because of their high efficacy and the poor results of surgery in most patients. Surgery can be performed later in patients whose tumor responses to such medications are not optimal. Even if this subsequent surgery is necessary for tumor debulking, it is rarely curative and a dopamine agonist is usually necessary postoperatively for treatment of the hyperprolactinemia. Cabergoline is the dopamine agonist of choice for macroprolactinomas due to its better tolerability and greater efficacy. For the small proportion of patients whose tumors are relatively resistant and require larger than standard doses of cabergoline to normalize prolactin levels and/or control tumor mass, echocardiographic monitoring may be prudent. Radiation therapy has a very limited role and is only recommended for those who have no response to dopamine agonists or whose tumor exhibits documented growth while taking a dopamine agonist after incomplete adenomectomy. Stereotactic radiotherapy appears to be the ideal form of radiotherapy at this point, although long-term complications remain to be assessed fully.

Whether surgery should be considered for removal of a shrunken tumor during dopamine agonist treatment is controversial. However, as complete surgical removal is rarely achieved and dopamine agonists will continue to be necessary to control the hyperprolactinemia, there seems to be little rationale for surgical intervention if the tumor mass is adequately reduced. In fact, a study comparing the outcomes of patients treated with bromocriptine alone versus surgery plus bromocriptine found that there were no differences between the groups with respect to final PRL levels and tumor size, but the surgical intervention group had the additional adverse effects of surgery now imposed [232].

When dopamine agonist therapy is stopped, the prolactinoma may expand to its original size, often within days to weeks. However, several series have now shown that dopamine agonists may be successfully tapered and discontinued in a subset of patients, in particular those patients with prolactinomas who have received at least 2 years of treatment, whose PRL has remained normal with tapering and whose tumors are no longer visible on MRI. Recurrence of hyperprolactinemia following dopamine agonist withdrawal can occur even in patients who meet these narrow criteria, so patients whose therapy has been tapered or withdrawn must be monitored closely for symptoms, PRL levels and serial MRI scans.

The anatomic response of tumors to dopamine agonist treatment should be monitored carefully by MRI and visual field examinations to detect tumors that do not respond or enlarge, as they may represent a rare case of pituitary carcinoma.

PREGNANCY IN WOMEN WITH PROLACTINOMAS

As discussed in Chapter 5, hyperprolactinemia is usually associated with anovulation and infertility, and correction of the hyperprolactinemia with dopamine agonists restores ovulation in about 90% of cases. When a woman harbors a prolactinoma as the cause of the hyperprolactinemia, two major issues arise when ovulation and fertility are restored: (1) the effects of the dopamine agonist on early fetal development occurring before a pregnancy is diagnosed; and (2) the effect of the pregnancy itself on the prolactinoma.

Effects of Bromocriptine on the Developing Fetus

As a general principle, it is advised that fetal exposure to dopamine agonists be limited to as short a period as possible. Most advise that mechanical contraception be used until the first two to three cycles have occurred, so that an intermenstrual interval can be established. In this way, a woman will know when she has missed a menstrual period, a pregnancy test can be performed quickly, and the dopamine agonist stopped. Thus, the dopamine agonist will have been given for only about 3–4 weeks of the gestation. When used in this fashion, bromocriptine has not been found to cause any increase in spontaneous abortions, ectopic pregnancies, trophoblastic disease, multiple pregnancies, or congenital malformations (Table 15.6) [541,542]. Long-term follow-up studies of 64 children between the ages of 6 months and 9 years whose mothers took bromocriptine in this fashion have shown no ill effects [543]. Experience is limited to only just over 100 women, however, with the use of bromocriptine throughout the gestation, but no abnormalities were noted in the infants except one with an undescended testicle and one with a talipes deformity [542,544–546].

Experience with the use of cabergoline in pregnancy is accumulating. Data on exposure of the fetus or embryo during the first several weeks of pregnancy have been reported in over 700 cases and such use has not shown an increased percentage of spontaneous abortion, premature delivery, or multiple births (Table 15.6) [547–557]. Outcome data with respect to malformations are available for 628 pregnancies [547–557]. Major

TABLE 15.6 Effect of Bromocriptine and Cabergoline on Pregnancies*

	Bromocriptine (N)	Bromocriptine (%)	Cabergoline (N)	Cabergoline (%)	Normal (%)
Pregnancies	6.239	100	760	100	100
– Spontaneous abortions	620	9.9	59	7.8	10–15
– Terminations	75	1.2	60[†]	9.0	20
– Ectopic	31	0.5	2	0.3	1.0–1.5
– Hydatidiform moles	11	0.2	1	0.2	0.1–0.15%
Deliveries (known duration)	4139	100	547	100	100
– At term (>37 weeks)	3620	87.5	480[††]	87.1	87.3
– Preterm (<37 weeks)	519	12.5	67	12.9	12.7
Deliveries (known outcome)	5120	100	428	100	100
– Single births	5031	98.3	416	97.2	96.8
– Multiple births	89	1.7	12	2.8	3.2
Babies (known details)	5213	100	628	100	100
– Normal	5030	98.2	615	97.9	97
– With malformations	93	1.8	13	2.1	3.0

** Data for bromocriptine from references [541,542]; data for cabergoline from references [372,380,381,549,554,557,558,561,623–625]. Data for normals from references [626,627].*
[†]11 of these terminations were for malformations.
[††]5 of these births were stillbirths.

malformations were found in only two of these series. The total frequency of malformations in pregnancies that went to term was 2.2% (13/628). However, in addition there were six pregnancy terminations because of malformations in the series of Colao et al. [558]. There was also one termination for a fetal malformation in the series of 23 pregnancies reported by Webster et al. [372]. In the series of 91 pregnancies in 80 women treated with cabergoline reported by Ono et al., there was one stillbirth, one spontaneous abortion and one elective termination for an unspecified reason [554]. In the series of 100 pregnancies reported by Lebbe et al., there were three terminations for fetal malformations (one case of trisomy 21, one case of rhomencephalo-synapsis and one severe hydrocephaly with extended spina bifida) [549]. If the 11 elective terminations for malformations are added to the above numbers for pregnancy outcomes, then there were 24 malformations out of 639 pregnancies, or 3.8%. Short-term follow-up studies of 177 infants born to mothers who used cabergoline during pregnancy indicate normal neonatal physical and mental development [549,559].

Quinagolide does not appear to be safe during pregnancy. A review of 176 pregnancies, in which quinagolide was maintained for a median duration of 37 days, reported 24 spontaneous abortions, one ectopic pregnancy and one stillbirth at 31 weeks of gestation [386]. Furthermore, nine fetal malformations were reported in this group, including spina bifida, trisomy 13, Down syndrome, talipes, cleft lip, arrhinencephaly and Zellweger syndrome [386].

Thus, bromocriptine has the largest safety database and has a proven safety record for pregnancy. The database for the use of cabergoline in pregnancy is much smaller, but there is no evidence at present indicating that it exerts deleterious effects on the developing fetus. The incidence of malformation in the offspring of women treated with either drug is not greater than that found in the general population. The numbers of abortions and malformations associated with the use of quinagolide during pregnancy raise serious concern. Therefore, quinagolide should not be used when fertility is desired. If reinstitution of a dopamine agonist is needed later in gestation to control tumor growth, either drug could be used.

Effect of Pregnancy on Prolactinoma Size

Estrogens have a marked stimulatory effect on PRL synthesis and secretion and the high estrogen levels of pregnancy can stimulate lactotroph cell hyperplasia (see Chapter 5). Those autopsy studies showing lactotroph cell hyperplasia during pregnancy have now been corroborated in vivo, MRI scans showing a gradual increase in pituitary volume over the course of gestation, beginning by the second month and peaking the first week postpartum with a final height reaching to almost 12 mm in some cases [560]. As noted above, a dopamine agonist used to facilitate ovulation and control tumor size is generally stopped when pregnancy is diagnosed. Prolactinoma enlargement during pregnancy (Figure 15.6) therefore results from both the stimulatory effect of these high estrogen levels and the discontinuation of the dopamine agonist that had been responsible for tumor shrinkage.

Data analyzing the risk of symptomatic tumor enlargement in pregnant women with prolactinomas, divided according to their status as micro- or macroprolactinomas, have been analyzed (Table 15.7) [259,540,554,561]. The risk of symptomatic tumor enlargement for microadenomas is only 2.2% (13/584 pregnancies). Surgical intervention was not required in any and therapy with bromocriptine in six individuals was followed by the resolution of their symptoms. Fifty-six of 201 pregnancies (27.9%) in patients with macroadenomas were complicated by symptomatic tumor enlargement; surgical intervention was carried out in 12 of these cases and bromocriptine therapy in 17, leading to resolution of their symptoms. No ill effects of these interventions on the infant were observed in these cases. A total of 161 women with macroadenomas had undergone surgery or radiation prior to pregnancy; for these, the risk for tumor enlargement was only 4.3% [259,540]. Lebbe et al. also reported information on MRI scans done routinely between 24 and 32 weeks of

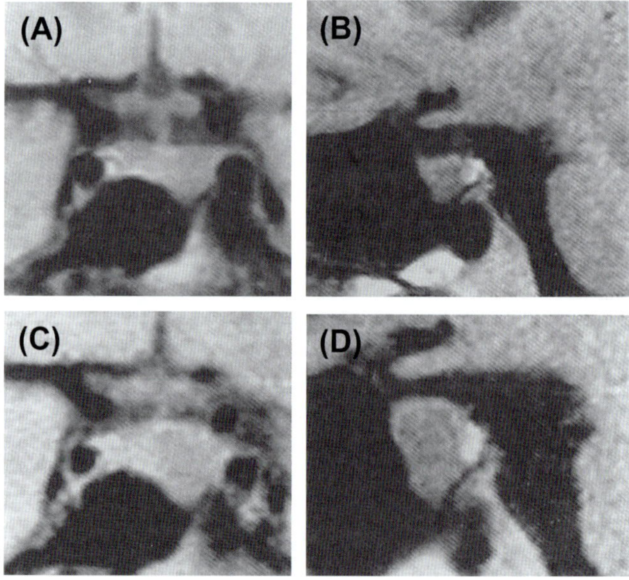

FIGURE 15.6 Coronal (left) and sagittal (right) MRI scans of an intrasellar prolactin-secreting macroadenoma in a woman prior to conception (above) and at 7 months of gestation (below). Note the marked tumor enlargement at the latter point, at which time the patient was complaining of headaches.

TABLE 15.7 Effect of Pregnancy on Prolactinomas

	Total no. Patients	Symptomatic Enlargement	% Symptomatic Enlargement
Microadenomas	528	13	2.5
Macroadenomas	172	56	32.6
Macroadenomas – prior surgery or radiation	161	7	4.3

Data from references [540,554,561].

gestation in 34 women in whom the cabergoline had been stopped shortly after the pregnancy was diagnosed [549]. Compared to prepregnancy scans, of the 12 with macroadenomas, five had no change in tumor size, none had a decrease in tumor size, three had an increase of <5 mm and four had an increase of >5 mm in size; of the 22 with microadenomas, nine had no change in tumor size, three had a decrease in tumor size, eight had an increase of <5 mm in size and two had an increase of >5 mm in size [549]. Cabergoline was restarted in five of the patients because the adenomas reached the chiasm with reduction in tumor size in each case but because cabergoline was not restarted because of symptomatic regrowth, they are not included in the summary of all cases discussed above and given in Table 15.7.

As stated above, no teratogenic or other untoward effects of bromocriptine cabergoline on pregnancy have been noted when bromocriptine was stopped within a few weeks of conception. Experience is limited, however, with the use of bromocriptine or cabergoline given throughout the gestation (see above) [259,562]. In two studies in which bromocriptine was given before elective therapeutic abortions at 6–9 weeks [563] or 20 weeks [564] of gestation, there were no effects on estradiol, estriol, progesterone, testosterone, dehydroepiandrosterone, dehydroepiandrosterone sulfate, androstenedione, cortisol, or human placental lactogen. In all studies maternal and fetal PRL levels were suppressed but in the three cases in which amniotic fluid PRL was measured, it was suppressed in two [564] and normal in the third [565]. Thus, these few studies of bromocriptine treatment late in gestation suggest that such use is probably safe, but there have been no large-scale or long-term studies. Laloi-Michelin et al. reported on two patients with macroadenomas treated throughout gestation with cabergoline and two additional macroadenoma patients treated with cabergoline only for tumor growth near term, finding successful reduction of the enlarged tumor in these two cases and no adverse effects of cabergoline on fetal outcomes in any [562]. Liu and Tyrrell [566] also found no problems with the late reintroduction of cabergoline for tumor growth and Banerjee et al. [567] reported no problems in a woman treated with cabergoline throughout three pregnancies. The use of prophylactic bromocriptine or cabergoline throughout the pregnancy likely prevents tumor regrowth during the pregnancy in most cases, but such use must be balanced against the potential risks of continuing the medication.

In some patients, postpartum PRL levels and tumor sizes are actually reduced as compared with values before pregnancy [568], but this has not been observed in all series [569]. Ikegami et al. [570] found that patients previously treated by transsphenoidal surgery had lower postpartum PRL levels than patients not cured by surgery and subsequently treated with bromocriptine, and also those just treated with bromocriptine. These lower levels of PRL then contributed to decreased milk production and poorer breast-feeding. In their study no nursing patient showed a sharp increase in PRL levels or complained of symptoms suggestive of tumor enlargement, such as headaches or visual disturbances.

Recommendations for Management of Pregnancy

For the hyperprolactinemic woman with a microadenoma there are three possible choices to restore fertility: dopamine agonist alone, transsphenoidal selective adenomectomy, or dopamine agonist after surgery. Although bromocriptine had been preferred as the primary treatment for such patients because of its efficacy in restoring ovulation and very low (1–2%) risk of clinically serious tumor enlargement, accumulating data for cabergoline suggests that its safety record is equal to that of bromocriptine and generally it is better tolerated and more efficacious. Transsphenoidal surgery causes a permanent reduction in PRL levels in only 60% of cases and entails morbidity and mortality, albeit at the low rates discussed above. Pregnancy can generally be achieved in over 85% of patients with dopamine agonists or surgery [554,569,571,572]. Rare patients who do not respond to either modality may need additional hormonal maneuvers to facilitate ovulation, such as clomiphene citrate plus human chorionic gonadotropin [538,573] or in vitro fertilization (IVF). Although radiotherapy has been advocated by some for patients with microadenomas before bromocriptine-induced pregnancy, it does not appear to be warranted, as the risk of tumor enlargement without radiotherapy is much lower than the risk of known, long-term sequelae of pituitary radiotherapy – viz. hypopituitarism (see above).

A patient with a microadenoma treated only with a dopamine agonist should be carefully followed throughout gestation. PRL levels do not always rise during pregnancy in women with prolactinomas, as they do in normal women. Usually PRL levels rise over the first 6–10 weeks after stopping the drug and then do not increase further [574]. PRL levels may also not rise with tumor enlargement [575]. Therefore, periodic checking of PRL levels is of no benefit. Because of the low incidence of tumor enlargement, routine, periodic visual field testing is not cost-effective. Visual field testing and MRI scanning (without contrast) are performed only in patients who become symptomatic. In the patient with tumor enlargement who does not respond to reinstitution of a dopamine agonist, surgery or early delivery may be required. For the patient with a small intrasellar or inferiorly extending macroadenoma, dopamine agonists are also favored as the primary therapy. The likelihood that such a tumor will enlarge sufficiently to cause clinically serious complications is probably only marginally higher than the likelihood in patients with microadenomas.

In a woman with a larger macroadenoma that may have suprasellar extension, there is a 28% risk of clinically serious tumor enlargement during pregnancy when only dopamine agonists are used. There is no clear-cut answer as to the best therapeutic approach and this has to be a highly individualized decision that the patient has to make after a clear, documented discussion of the various therapeutic alternatives. One approach is to perform a prepregnancy transsphenoidal surgical debulking of the tumor. This should greatly reduce the risk of serious tumor enlargement, but cases with massive tumor expansion during pregnancy after such surgery have been reported [576]. After surgical debulking, a dopamine agonist is required to restore normal PRL levels and allow ovulation. Although radiotherapy before pregnancy, followed by bromocriptine, also reduces the risk of tumor enlargement, it is rarely curative (see above). Radiotherapy may also result in long-term hypopituitarism (see above), so that this approach seems less acceptable than transsphenoidal surgery plus bromocriptine. A third approach, that of giving bromocriptine continuously throughout gestation, has been advocated [546]. At this point, however, data regarding the effects of continuous bromocriptine therapy on the developing fetus are still quite meager, and such therapy cannot be recommended without reservation. Data regarding the effects of continuous cabergoline therapy on the developing fetus are even fewer [562,567] and such treatment also cannot be recommended without reservation. Should pregnancy at an advanced stage be discovered in a woman taking bromocriptine or cabergoline, however, the data that exist are reassuring and would not justify therapeutic abortion. A fourth approach, and the one most commonly employed, is to stop the dopamine agonist after pregnancy is diagnosed.

For patients with macroadenomas treated with a dopamine agonist alone or after surgery or irradiation, careful follow-up with 1–3-monthly formal visual field testing is warranted. Repeat MRI scanning, done without contrast, is reserved for patients with symptoms of tumor enlargement and/or evidence of a developing visual field defect or both. Repeat scanning after delivery to detect asymptomatic tumor enlargement may be useful as well.

Should symptomatic tumor enlargement occur with any of these approaches, reinstitution of the dopamine agonist is probably less harmful to the mother and child than surgery. There have been a number of cases reported where such reinstitution of the dopamine agonist has worked quite satisfactorily, causing rapid tumor size reduction with no adverse effects on the infant (see above). Any type of surgery during pregnancy results in a 1.5-fold increase in fetal loss in the first trimester and a five-fold increase in fetal loss in the second trimester, although there is no risk of congenital malformations from such surgery [577,578]. Thus, dopamine agonist reinstitution would appear to be preferable to surgical decompression. However, such medical therapy must be very closely monitored, and transsphenoidal surgery or delivery (if the pregnancy is far enough advanced) should be performed if there is no response to the dopamine agonist and vision is progressively worsening.

OTHER SPECIAL SITUATIONS

Giant Prolactinomas

Giant prolactinomas are traditionally defined as prolactin-secreting adenomas greater than 4 cm in diameter and/or those with more than 2 cm of suprasellar extension [191,273,579–581]. They are usually associated with very high serum PRL concentrations, in the range of 20,000–100,000 ng/ml when measured with two-site monoclonal immunoradiometric or chemiluminometric assays. The exact prevalence of giant prolactinomas is not known for certain, but two retrospective analyses of prolactinomas at single institutions indicate that they are uncommon, reporting prevalences of 0.5% and 4.4% among all pituitary tumors [274,582].

Giant prolactinomas represent a special management situation for two reasons. First, the therapeutic goals for these tumors often differ from those established for more common macroprolactinomas. Second, specific complications may arise during the treatment of giant prolactinomas which may alter initial therapeutic plans, requiring alternative or additional modes of therapy. Whereas the therapeutic goals for most micro- and macroprolactinomas include normalization of hyperprolactinemia, restoration of eugonadism and reduction in tumor size, these goals may not be realistic for some giant prolactinomas. Since prolactin levels must be reduced to near normal levels to restore normal reproductive function, a reduction of 50% or even 90% (though substantial) may not be great enough to restore sexual and reproductive function in severe hyperprolactinemia. Rather, neurological effects, such as encroachment upon or invasion into critical neural structures, take priority. Furthermore, in some situations, particularly in long-standing tumors, reduction of tumor size may not reverse visual field defects or hypopituitarism, and a more feasible goal may be prevention of further growth. The benefits of any form of treatment designed to achieve these goals must be balanced against risks associated with the specific therapy [583].

Patients with giant prolactinomas are at risk for pituitary apoplexy, intratumoral hematoma and nonsurgical CSF rhinorrhea [274,449,452–454,582]. Any of these complications may require timely surgical intervention and correction, though this does not obviate the need for further medical and/or radiotherapy postoperatively. The absolute indications for surgical intervention in patients with giant prolactinomas are the same for all prolactinomas, and include continued tumor growth on medical therapy, acute neurologic defects that do not respond rapidly to medical therapy and unstable pituitary apoplexy. Surgical cure is not a realistic attainable goal for giant prolactinomas, but tumor debulking may be necessary in the aforementioned specific situations.

Surgical response rates have been reported in a limited number of patients with giant pituitary tumors operated via the transsphenoidal, craniotomy and combined transsphenoidal–craniotomy routes. Improvement, rather than normalization of prolactin, usually defines a response in these circumstances. Mohr et al. reported that six of 14 patients with giant prolactinomas who underwent transsphenoidal surgery required bromocriptine for persistent hyperprolactinemia postoperatively [579]. Whether the eight remaining patients in this series achieved remission or cure cannot be ascertained from their data [579]. There have been no other series restricted to patients with giant prolactinomas treated with surgery alone that has reported hormonal cure or complete resection of tumor mass in a single patient [190,191,273].

The morbidity and mortality rates associated with surgical intervention are considerably higher for giant pituitary adenomas than for smaller, noninvasive adenomas, especially those that require transfrontal approaches. Complication rates specific to surgery for giant prolactinomas are not available, but may be estimated on the basis of complication rates found after surgical resection of giant pituitary adenomas in general. Of 16 cases of giant pituitary adenoma operated via craniotomy by Symon et al., three died in the immediate postoperative period and two others died within 6 months of surgery [581]. In a series of 77 patients operated upon by Pia et al., there were eight operative deaths and considerable morbidity, including increased visual loss in four, oculomotor disturbances in eight, diabetes insipidus in 15, mental deterioration in 14 and CSF fistulas in five [580]. Even the most recent surgical series still report significant complication rates. In a series of 92 giant pituitary tumors operated on via the transsphenoidal or combined transsphenoidal/transfrontal routes, surgical morbidity was 3.3%, CSF leak was 5.4% and worsening vision on follow-up was 7.6% [584]. Another recent surgical series of 43 giant pituitary adenomas reported by Garibi et al. found a mortality of 4.7%, with permanent diabetes insipidus in 9.3% and meningitis with CSF fistula formation in 14.0% [585]. Thus, surgery for giant prolactinomas can be successful in debulking tumors but actual cure is uncommon, and complication rates are high, with mortality rates ranging from 3.3% [584] to 31.2% [581] and the major morbidity rates ranging from 10% [579] to 62% [581].

Radiotherapy has been utilized as adjunctive therapy in patients with giant prolactinomas; however, the effects of radiotherapy alone are difficult to discern from the effects of either prior surgery or concomitant medical therapy. One study of four giant prolactinomas that were treated initially with conventional radiotherapy (41.4–50 Gy) prior to medical therapy reported that no patient had been endocrinologically or radiologically cured with radiotherapy after an interval varying between 1 month and 7 years [586]. Nevertheless, radiotherapy may be indicated for those demonstrating absolutely no response to dopamine agonists or whose tumor was documented to actually grow on dopamine agonists or after incomplete surgical removal [587].

Normalization of prolactin and even radiologic disappearance of tumor is possible in some giant prolactinomas. Data on the efficacy of medical therapy for giant prolactinomas have been reported in 11 series that reported results of at least two patients (Table 15.8). Some of these patients underwent prior surgery

TABLE 15.8 Medical Therapy for Giant Prolactinomas

Series	Reference	Drug	Number of Patients	Previous Surgery	Mean DA Dose	Normal Prolactin	50% Tumor Reduction
Murphy et al.	[273]	BRC	2	2	NR	1	2
Davis et al.	[191]	BRC	9	NR	NR	4	7
Grebe et al.	[586]	BRC	4	0*	NR	3	NR
Saeki et al.	[588]	BRC	10	4	NR	7	NR
Minniti et al.	[628]	CAB	4	1	1.6 mg/wk	3	1
Shrivastava et al.	[274]	BRC	10	1	NR	9	10
Corsello et al.	[582]	CAB	10	4	3.3 mg/wk	5	7
Wu ZB et al.	[629]	BRC	20	6	NR	8	11
Mascarell S et al.	[630]	BRC, CAB	3	1, 1	40 mg/d BRC, CAB 2.5 mg/wk	0	1 (BRC) 1 (CAB)
Shimon I et al.	[631]	CAB	12	2	4.3 mg/wk	10	6
Cho et al.	[632]	CAB	10	0	< 3 mg/wk	5	10
Total			**94**			**55 (59%)**	**56 (80%)**

BRC, bromocriptine; CAB, cabergoline; NR, not reported.
** All four underwent prior RT.*

or radiotherapy, which in most cases was associated with little change in prolactin levels or tumor mass. Of 94 patients reported in these series who were treated with either bromocriptine or cabergoline, 55 (59%) achieved a normal prolactin level and 56 of 80 (70%) experienced at least a 50% reduction in tumor size. In the 41% of patients who did not normalize prolactin levels with medical therapy, partial responses (prolactin reductions ~95%) were possible in many cases. Thus, medical therapy should always be attempted first line in these patients.

Because of the excellent potential results with dopamine agonists and poor results of surgery in most patients, the authors recommend dopamine agonists as initial therapy for patients with giant prolactinomas, and reserve surgery for those patients who demonstrate inadequate responses to medical therapy. Even if subsequent surgery is necessary for tumor debulking, it rarely is curative and a dopamine agonist is usually necessary for treatment of the hyperprolactinemia. In some extreme cases, complete tumor removal may not be achievable by any means and control of further tumor growth may be acceptable. Given the relatively high complication rates associated with surgery in these patients, it is important to balance the benefits of therapy with potential complications. A reduction in dopamine agonist doses may be possible in patients taking large doses of dopamine agonists after normoprolactinemia has been achieved and sustained for a duration sufficient enough to ascertain a reasonable chance for success. Successful dopamine agonist withdrawal has been reported in a few patients [588]. However, when therapy is discontinued, the prolactinoma may return to its original size, often within days to weeks [489]. This potential return to pretherapy size dictates extreme caution when withdrawing dopamine agonists in giant prolactinomas, as rapid tumor expansion may produce more severe clinical symptoms than slow tumor enlargement.

Malignant Prolactinomas

Malignant prolactinomas are rare tumors. Their exact incidence is not known for certain, but overall pituitary carcinomas represent less than 0.2% of symptomatic pituitary tumors, and prolactinomas comprise approximately one-third of these [589]. Approximately 53 cases of malignant prolactinoma have been published in the English literature [590–595]. Most commonly, malignant prolactinomas are indistinguishable from invasive macroadenomas at presentation [589]. The diagnosis of pituitary carcinoma can only be made upon demonstration of metastastic spread; reliable distinction between carcinoma and adenoma cannot be made on the basis of standard histologic or molecular criteria [589]. Although gene expression profiling of prolactinomas has identified a subset genes that are up-regulated at the mRNA level in highly invasive tumors [38], at this time, there are no reliable methods to accurately identify those invasive pituitary tumors most likely to metastasize, thus permitting early aggressive treatment before progression to pituitary carcinomas [589,594,596].

Typically, the primary tumor is treated with medical, surgical and/or radiotherapy, followed by a long latency (years) before recurrence or progression of residual tumor occurs and metastases become apparent [589,594]. Less commonly, a malignant prolactinoma will exhibit early aggressive behavior with multiple recurrences and early development of metastases [589,594]. For malignant prolactinomas the latent period between initial diagnosis and detection of metastases is reported to range from 2 to 228 months [597]. Once metastases are diagnosed, survival is usually very short with a mean survival time of approximately 10 months [589,594]. The vast majority (80%) die within 18 months [597]. However, prolonged, asymptomatic survival has been reported in a few patients [594]. Where possible, dopamine agonists should be employed, as they can sometimes be effective in reducing the mass of tumor [594]. Unfortunately, once craniospinal or systemic metastases become obvious, therapeutic options are limited in efficacy, and treatment is mainly palliative [589,594]. Surgery may be useful in debulking the lesion and relieving local compressive effects [589,594]. Chemotherapy with somatostatin infusion, procarbazine, vincristine, cisplatine, lomustine, carboplatin and etoposide has been attempted but as yet has not been demonstrated to be effective [589,594]. With the exception of a single case [598], there is no evidence that either radiotherapy or chemotherapy prolongs survival to any major extent [589].

Recently the alkylating agent, temozolomide, has been found to be effective in four cases of patients with malignant prolactinomas [590–592,595]. In each case primary tumor volume, size of metastases and prolactin levels were significantly reduced [590–592, 595]. On the other hand, we have treated one case of malignant prolactinoma for whom temozolomide was ineffective. Three additional cases with giant prolactinomas that were progressing in size and refractory to dopamine agonists, surgery and irradiation have also responded to temozolomide [515,592,599]. Follow-up for these cases is limited to only a few years, so that at this point it is uncertain the extent to which this agent can potentially prolong life. Temozolomide is actively being studied in a US multicenter phase II clinical trial in functioning and nonsecreting invasive pituitary adenomas to assess its effect on tumor growth, response and duration of response (NIH clinical trial #NCT0060128).

Prolactinomas in Multiple Endocrine Neoplasia

Prolactinomas occur in about 20% of patients with multiple endocrine neoplasia type 1 (MEN-1), and represent the most frequent type of pituitary adenoma observed in this syndrome [600–602]. Genotype–phenotype correlations have not been identified for most mutations of the *MEN-1* gene. However, one nonsense mutation, R460X, has been identified in four kindreds from the Burin peninsula of Newfoundland which is associated with a very high incidence of prolactinomas and hyperparathyroidism (90% each) [603–605].

Prolactinomas arising in patients with MEN-1 are larger and behave more aggressively than those that develop sporadically [600,602,606]. In the France–Belgium multicenter study of 136 individuals with MEN-1-harboring pituitary adenomas [602], macroprolactinomas were found much more frequently in MEN-1 patients than in non-MEN-1 subjects (84% vs. 24%), and a high proportion of the MEN-1 prolactinomas were classified as invasive (24%). Over a median of 11.4 years of follow-up, the response to treatment was less efficacious in the MEN-1 adenomas, with prolactin level normalization achieved in 44% of MEN-1 cases as compared to 90% in sporadic cases. These and other data suggest that prolactinomas in MEN-1 may be relatively resistant to treatment [602,607,608]. The general treatment strategy for prolactinomas in patients with MEN-1 does not differ from that for sporadic prolactinomas, but more intensive pharmacologic therapy or the use of multiple therapeutic modalities may be required to achieve satisfactory outcomes.

References

[1] O. Riddle, W.R. Bates, W.S. Dykshorn, A new hormone of the anterior pituitary, Proc Soc Exptl Biol Med 29 (1932) 1211–1212.

[2] H. Friesen, B.R. Webster, P. Hwang, H. Guyda, R.E. Munro, L. Read, Prolactin synthesis and secretion in a patient with the Forbes-Albright syndrome, J Clin Endocrinol Metab 34 (1) (1972) 192–199.

[3] A.F. Daly, M.A. Tichomirowa, A. Beckers, The epidemiology and genetics of pituitary adenomas, Best Pract Res Clin Endocrinol Metab 23 (5) (2009) 543–554.

[4] M.E. Molitch, Pituitary tumours: Pituitary incidentalomas, Best Pract Res Clin Endocrinol Metab 23 (5) (2009) 667–675.

[5] E. Delgrange, T. Duprez, D. Maiter, Influence of parasellar extension of macroprolactinomas defined by magnetic resonance imaging on their responsiveness to dopamine agonist therapy, Clin Endocrinol (Oxf) 64 (4) (2006) 456–462.

[6] M. Losa, P. Mortini, R. Barzaghi, L. Gioia, M. Giovanelli, Surgical treatment of prolactin-secreting pituitary adenomas: Early results and long-term outcome, J Clin Endocrinol Metab 87 (7) (2002) 3180–3186.

[7] Z.B. Wu, Z.P. Su, J.S. Wu, W.M. Zheng, Q.C. Zhuge, M. Zhong, Five years follow-up of invasive prolactinomas with special reference to the control of cavernous sinus invasion, Pituitary 11 (1) (2008) 63–70.

[8] B.P. Meij, M.B. Lopes, D.B. Ellegala, T.D. Alden, E.R. Laws Jr., The long-term significance of microscopic dural invasion in 354 patients with pituitary adenomas treated with transsphenoidal surgery, J Neurosurg 96 (2) (2002) 195–208.

[9] W.R. Selman, E.R. Laws Jr., B.W. Scheithauer, S.M. Carpenter, The occurrence of dural invasion in pituitary adenomas, J Neurosurg 64 (3) (1986) 402–407.

[10] E. St-Jean, F. Blain, R. Comtois, High prolactin levels may be missed by immunoradiometric assay in patients with macroprolactinomas, Clin Endocrinol (Oxf) 44 (3) (1996) 305–309.

[11] J.S. Bevan, C.W. Burke, M.M. Esiri, C.B. Adams, Misinterpretation of prolactin levels leading to management errors in patients with sellar enlargement, Am J Med 82 (1) (1987) 29–32.

[12] N. Karavitaki, G. Thanabalasingham, H.C. Shore, R. Trifanescu, O. Ansorge, N. Meston, et al., Do the limits of serum prolactin in disconnection hyperprolactinaemia need re-definition? A study of 226 patients with histologically verified non-functioning pituitary macroadenoma, Clin Endocrinol (Oxf) 65 (4) (2006) 524–529.

[13] M.E. Molitch, S. Reichlin, Hypothalamic hyperprolactinemia: Neuroendocrine regulation of prolactin secretion in patients with lesions of the hypothalamus and pituitary stalk, in: R.M. MacLeod, M.O. Thorner, U. Scapagnini (Eds.), Prolactin Basic and Clinical Correlates, Liviana Press, Padova, 1985, pp. 709–719.

[14] R.J. Lloyd, K. Kovacs, W.F. Young, W.E. Farrell, S.L. Asa, J. Trouillas, et al., Tumours of the pituitary gland, in: R.A. DeLellis, R.V. Lloyd, P.U. Heitz (Eds.), WHO classification of tumours: Pathology and genetics of tumours of endocrine organs, IARC Press, Lyon, 2004, pp. 9–48.

[15] N.Y. Al-Brahim, S.L. Asa, My approach to pathology of the pituitary gland, J Clin Pathol 59 (12) (2006) 1245–1253.

[16] J.F. Annegers, C.B. Coulam, C.F. Abboud, E.R. Laws Jr., L.T. Kurland, Pituitary adenoma in Olmsted County, Minnesota, 1935–1977. A report of an increasing incidence of diagnosis in women of childbearing age, Mayo Clin Proc 53 (10) (1978) 641–643.

[17] R.N. Clayton, Sporadic pituitary tumours: From epidemiology to use of databases, Baillieres Best Pract Res Clin Endocrinol Metab 13 (3) (1999) 451–460.

[18] A.F. Daly, M. Rixhon, C. Adam, A. Dempegioti, M.A. Tichomirowa, A. Beckers, High prevalence of pituitary adenomas: A cross-sectional study in the province of Liege, Belgium J Clin Endocrinol Metab 91 (12) (2006) 4769–4775.

[19] A. Fernandez, N. Karavitaki, J.A. Wass, Prevalence of pituitary adenomas: A community-based, cross-sectional study in Banbury (Oxfordshire, UK), Clin Endocrinol (Oxf) 72 (3) (2010) 377–382.

[20] M.C. Koppelman, M.J. Jaffe, K.G. Rieth, R.C. Caruso, D.L. Loriaux, Hyperprolactinemia, amenorrhea, and galactorrhea. A retrospective assessment of twenty-five cases, Ann Intern Med 100 (1) (1984) 115–121.

[21] C.M. March, O.A. Kletzky, V. Davajan, J. Teal, M. Weiss, M.L. Apuzzo, et al., Longitudinal evaluation of patients with untreated prolactin-secreting pituitary adenomas, Am J Obstet Gynecol 139 (7) (1981) 835–844.

[22] J. Schlechte, K. Dolan, B. Sherman, F. Chapler, A. Luciano, The natural history of untreated hyperprolactinemia: A prospective analysis, J Clin Endocrinol Metab 68 (2) (1989) 412–418.

[23] D.A. Sisam, J.P. Sheehan, L.R. Sheeler, The natural history of untreated microprolactinomas, Fertil Steril 48 (1) (1987) 67–71.

[24] K. Von Werder, T. Eversmann, R. Fahlbusch, H-K. Rjosk, Development of hyperprolactinemia in patients with adenomas with and without prior operative treatment, Excerpta Med Int Congr Ser 584 (1982) 175–188.

[25] M.H. Weiss, J. Teal, P. Gott, R. Wycoff, R. Yadley, M.L. Apuzzo, et al., Natural history of microprolactinomas: Six-year follow-up, Neurosurgery 12 (2) (1983) 180–183.

[26] T.L. Martin, M. Kim, W.B. Malarkey, The natural history of idiopathic hyperprolactinemia, J Clin Endocrinol Metab 60 (5) (1985) 855–858.

[27] A.E. Pontiroli, L. Falsetti, Development of pituitary adenoma in women with hyperprolactinaemia: Clinical, endocrine, and radiological characteristics, Br Med J (Clin Res Ed) 288 (6416) (1984) 515–518.

[28] H.K. Rjosk, R. Fahlbusch, K. von Werder, Spontaneous development of hyperprolactinaemia, Acta Endocrinol (Copenh) 100 (3) (1982) 333–336.

[29] W.J. Jeffcoate, N. Pound, N.D. Sturrock, J. Lambourne, Long-term follow-up of patients with hyperprolactinaemia, Clin Endocrinol (Oxf) 45 (3) (1996) 299–303.

[30] S. Karunakaran, R.C. Page, J.A. Wass, The effect of the menopause on prolactin levels in patients with hyperprolactinaemia, Clin Endocrinol (Oxf) 54 (3) (2001) 295–300.

[31] A. Gurlek, N. Karavitaki, O. Ansorge, J.A. Wass, What are the markers of aggressiveness in prolactinomas? Changes in cell biology, extracellular matrix components, angiogenesis and genetics, Eur J Endocrinol 156 (2) (2007) 143–153.

[32] G. Kontogeorgos, Predictive markers of pituitary adenoma behavior, Neuroendocrinology 83 (3-4) (2006) 179–188.

[33] E. Delgrange, J. Trouillas, D. Maiter, J. Donckier, J. Tourniaire, Sex-related difference in the growth of prolactinomas: A clinical and proliferation marker study, J Clin Endocrinol Metab 82 (7) (1997) 2102–2107.

[34] W. Ma, H. Ikeda, T. Yoshimoto, Clinicopathologic study of 123 cases of prolactin-secreting pituitary adenomas with special reference to multihormone production and clonality of the adenomas, Cancer 95 (2) (2002) 258–266.

[35] W. Saeger, D.K. Ludecke, M. Buchfelder, R. Fahlbusch, H.J. Quabbe, S. Petersenn, Pathohistological classification of pituitary tumors: 10 years of experience with the German Pituitary Tumor Registry, Eur J Endocrinol 156 (2) (2007) 203–216.

[36] B.W. Scheithauer, T.A. Gaffey, R.V. Lloyd, T.J. Sebo, K.T. Kovacs, E. Horvath, et al., Pathobiology of pituitary adenomas and carcinomas, Neurosurgery 59 (2) (2006) 341–353, discussion 53.

[37] K. Thapar, B.W. Scheithauer, K. Kovacs, P.J. Pernicone, E.R. Laws Jr., p53 expression in pituitary adenomas and carcinomas: Correlation with invasiveness and tumor growth fractions, Neurosurgery 38 (4) (1996) 765–770, discussion 70–71.

[38] G. Raverot, A. Wierinckx, E. Dantony, C. Auger, G. Chapas, L. Villeneuve, et al., Prognostic factors in prolactin pituitary tumors: Clinical, histological, and molecular data from a series of 94 patients with a long postoperative follow-up, J Clin Endocrinol Metab 95 (4) (2010) 1708–1716.

[39] T. Fauquier, K. Rizzoti, M. Dattani, R. Lovell-Badge, I.C. Robinson, SOX2-expressing progenitor cells generate all of the major cell types in the adult mouse pituitary gland, Proc Nat Acad Sci USA 105 (8) (2008) 2907–2912.

[40] A.S. Gleiberman, T. Michurina, J.M. Encinas, J.L. Roig, P. Krasnov, F. Balordi, et al., Genetic approaches identify adult pituitary stem cells, Proc Nat Acad Sci USA 105 (17) (2008) 6332–6337.

[41] B.W. Scheithauer, T. Sano, K.T. Kovacs, W.F. Young Jr., N. Ryan, R.V. Randall, The pituitary gland in pregnancy: A clinicopathologic and immunohistochemical study of 69 cases, Mayo Clin Proc 65 (4) (1990) 461–474.

[42] J.M. Alexander, B.M. Biller, H. Bikkal, N.T. Zervas, A. Arnold, A. Klibanski, Clinically nonfunctioning pituitary tumors are monoclonal in origin, J Clin Invest 86 (1) (1990) 336–340.

[43] V. Herman, J. Fagin, R. Gonsky, K. Kovacs, S. Melmed, Clonal origin of pituitary adenomas, J Clin Endocrinol Metab 71 (6) (1990) 1427–1433.

[44] D. Hanahan, R.A. Weinberg, The hallmarks of cancer, Cell 100 (1) (2000) 57–70.
[45] W.J. Mooi, D.S. Peeper, Oncogene-induced cell senescence – halting on the road to cancer, N Engl J Med 355 (10) (2006) 1037–1046.
[46] N.E. Sharpless, R.A. DePinho, Cancer: Crime and punishment, Nature 436 (7051) (2005) 636–637.
[47] M.D. Boggild, S. Jenkinson, M. Pistorello, M. Boscaro, M. Scanarini, P. McTernan, et al., Molecular genetic studies of sporadic pituitary tumors, J Clin Endocrinol Metab 78 (2) (1994) 387–392.
[48] Q. Dong, L.V. Debelenko, S.C. Chandrasekharappa, M.R. Emmert-Buck, Z. Zhuang, S.C. Guru, et al., Loss of heterozygosity at 11q13: Analysis of pituitary tumors, lung carcinoids, lipomas, and other uncommon tumors in subjects with familial multiple endocrine neoplasia type 1, J Clin Endocrinol Metab 82 (5) (1997) 1416–1420.
[49] S.L. Asa, K. Somers, S. Ezzat, The MEN-1 gene is rarely down-regulated in pituitary adenomas, J Clin Endocrinol Metab 83 (9) (1998) 3210–3212.
[50] T.R. Prezant, J. Levine, S. Melmed, Molecular characterization of the Men1 tumor suppressor gene in sporadic pituitary tumors, J Clin Endocrinol Metab 83 (4) (1998) 1388–1391.
[51] C. Wenbin, A. Asai, A. Teramoto, N. Sanno, T. Kirino, Mutations of the MEN1 tumor suppressor gene in sporadic pituitary tumors, Cancer Lett 142 (1) (1999) 43–47.
[52] Z. Zhuang, S.Z. Ezzat, A.O. Vortmeyer, R. Weil, E.H. Oldfield, W.S. Park, et al., Mutations of the MEN1 tumor suppressor gene in pituitary tumors, Cancer Res 57 (24) (1997) 5446–5451.
[53] M. Theodoropoulou, I. Cavallari, L. Barzon, D.M. D'Agostino, T. Ferro, T. Arzberger, et al., Differential expression of menin in sporadic pituitary adenomas, Endocr Relat Cancer 11 (2) (2004) 333–344.
[54] P. Bertolino, W.M. Tong, D. Galendo, Z.Q. Wang, C.X. Zhang, Heterozygous Men1 mutant mice develop a range of endocrine tumors mimicking multiple endocrine neoplasia type 1, Mol Endocrinol 17 (9) (2003) 1880–1892.
[55] J.S. Crabtree, P.C. Scacheri, J.M. Ward, L. Garrett-Beal, M.R. Emmert-Buck, K.A. Edgemon, et al., A mouse model of multiple endocrine neoplasia, type 1, develops multiple endocrine tumors, Proc Nat Acad Sci USA 98 (3) (2001) 1118–1123.
[56] C.M. Hughes, O. Rozenblatt-Rosen, T.A. Milne, T.D. Copeland, S.S. Levine, J.C. Lee, et al., Menin associates with a trithorax family histone methyltransferase complex and with the hoxc8 locus, Mol Cell 13 (4) (2004) 587–597.
[57] A. Yokoyama, T.C. Somervaille, K.S. Smith, O. Rozenblatt-Rosen, M. Meyerson, M.L. Cleary, The menin tumor suppressor protein is an essential oncogenic cofactor for MLL-associated leukemogenesis, Cell 123 (2) (2005) 207–218.
[58] S.K. Karnik, C.M. Hughes, X. Gu, O. Rozenblatt-Rosen, G.W. McLean, Y. Xiong, et al., Menin regulates pancreatic islet growth by promoting histone methylation and expression of genes encoding p27Kip1 and p18INK4c, Proc Nat Acad Sci USA 102 (41) (2005) 14659–14664.
[59] T.A. Milne, C.M. Hughes, R. Lloyd, Z. Yang, O. Rozenblatt-Rosen, Y. Dou, et al., Menin and MLL cooperatively regulate expression of cyclin-dependent kinase inhibitors, Proc Nat Acad Sci USA 102 (3) (2005) 749–754.
[60] D.S. Franklin, V.L. Godfrey, H. Lee, G.I. Kovalev, R. Schoonhoven, S. Chen-Kiang, et al., CDK inhibitors p18(INK4c) and p27(Kip1) mediate two separate pathways to collaboratively suppress pituitary tumorigenesis, Genes Dev 12 (18) (1998) 2899–2911.
[61] D.S. Franklin, V.L. Godfrey, D.A. O'Brien, C. Deng, Y. Xiong, Functional collaboration between different cyclin-dependent kinase inhibitors suppresses tumor growth with distinct tissue specificity, Mol Cell Biol 20 (16) (2000) 6147–6158.
[62] O. Vierimaa, M. Georgitsi, R. Lehtonen, P. Vahteristo, A. Kokko, A. Raitila, et al., Pituitary adenoma predisposition caused by germline mutations in the AIP gene, Science 312 (5777) (2006) 1228–1230.
[63] M.S. Elston, K.L. McDonald, R.J. Clifton-Bligh, B.G. Robinson, Familial pituitary tumor syndromes, Nat Rev Endocrinol 5 (8) (2009) 453–461.
[64] T. Iwata, S. Yamada, N. Mizusawa, H.M. Golam, T. Sano, K. Yoshimoto, The aryl hydrocarbon receptor-interacting protein gene is rarely mutated in sporadic GH-secreting adenomas, Clin Endocrinol (Oxf) 66 (4) (2007) 499–502.
[65] C.A. Leontiou, M. Gueorguiev, J. van der Spuy, R. Quinton, F. Lolli, S. Hassan, et al., The role of the aryl hydrocarbon receptor-interacting protein gene in familial and sporadic pituitary adenomas, J Clin Endocrinol Metab 93 (6) (2008) 2390–2401.
[66] R.A. Toledo, D.M. Lourenco Jr., B. Liberman, M.B. Cunha-Neto, M.G. Cavalcanti, C.B. Moyses, et al., Germline mutation in the aryl hydrocarbon receptor interacting protein gene in familial somatotropinoma, J Clin Endocrinol Metab 92 (5) (2007) 1934–1937.
[67] M. Georgitsi, A. Raitila, A. Karhu, K. Tuppurainen, M.J. Makinen, O. Vierimaa, et al., Molecular diagnosis of pituitary adenoma predisposition caused by aryl hydrocarbon receptor-interacting protein gene mutations, Proc Nat Acad Sci USA 104 (10) (2007) 4101–4105.
[68] A. Raitila, M. Georgitsi, A. Karhu, K. Tuppurainen, M.J. Makinen, K. Birkenkamp-Demtroder, et al., No evidence of somatic aryl hydrocarbon receptor interacting protein mutations in sporadic endocrine neoplasia, Endocr Relat Cancer 14 (3) (2007) 901–906.
[69] L.A. Aaltonen, Aryl hydrocarbon receptor-interacting protein and acromegaly, Horm Res 68 (Suppl 5) (2007) 127–131.
[70] L. Cazabat, R. Libe, K. Perlemoine, F. Rene-Corail, N. Burnichon, A.P. Gimenez-Roqueplo, et al., Germline inactivating mutations of the aryl hydrocarbon receptor-interacting protein gene in a large cohort of sporadic acromegaly: Mutations are found in a subset of young patients with macroadenomas, Eur J Endocrinol 157 (1) (2007) 1–8.
[71] A. Barlier, J.F. Vanbellinghen, A.F. Daly, M. Silvy, M.L. Jaffrain-Rea, J. Trouillas, et al., Mutations in the aryl hydrocarbon receptor interacting protein gene are not highly prevalent among subjects with sporadic pituitary adenomas, J Clin Endocrinol Metab 92 (5) (2007) 1952–1955.
[72] B.C. Lin, R. Sullivan, Y. Lee, S. Moran, E. Glover, C.A. Bradfield, Deletion of the aryl hydrocarbon receptor-associated protein 9 leads to cardiac malformation and embryonic lethality, J Biol Chem 282 (49) (2007) 35924–35932.
[73] A. Fusco, M. Fedele, Roles of HMGA proteins in cancer, Nat Rev Cancer 7 (12) (2007) 899–910.
[74] R. Sgarra, S. Zammitti, A. Lo Sardo, E. Maurizio, L. Arnoldo, S. Pegoraro, et al., HMGA molecular network: From transcriptional regulation to chromatin remodeling, Biochim Biophys Acta 1799 (1–2) (2010) 37–47.
[75] M. Fedele, S. Battista, L. Kenyon, G. Baldassarre, V. Fidanza, A.J. Klein-Szanto, et al., Overexpression of the HMGA2 gene in transgenic mice leads to the onset of pituitary adenomas, Oncogene 21 (20) (2002) 3190–3198.
[76] L.J. Wood, J.F. Maher, T.E. Bunton, L.M. Resar, The oncogenic properties of the HMG-I gene family, Cancer Res 60 (15) (2000) 4256–4261.
[77] D. Bettio, N. Rizzi, D. Giardino, L. Persani, F. Pecori-Giraldi, M. Losa, et al., Cytogenetic study of pituitary adenomas, Cancer Genet Cytogenet 98 (2) (1997) 131–136.

[78] P. Finelli, D. Giardino, N. Rizzi, S. Buiatiotis, T. Virduci, A. Franzin, et al., Non-random trisomies of chromosomes 5, 8 and 12 in the prolactinoma sub-type of pituitary adenomas: Conventional cytogenetics and interphase FISH study, Int J Cancer 86 (3) (2000) 344–350.

[79] P. Finelli, G.M. Pierantoni, D. Giardino, M. Losa, O. Rodeschini, M. Fedele, et al., The high mobility group A2 gene is amplified and overexpressed in human prolactinomas, Cancer Res 62 (8) (2002) 2398–2405.

[80] Y.S. Lee, A. Dutta, The tumor suppressor microRNA let-7 represses the HMGA2 oncogene, Genes Dev 21 (9) (2007) 1025–1030.

[81] C. Mayr, M.T. Hemann, D.P. Bartel, Disrupting the pairing between let-7 and Hmga2 enhances oncogenic transformation, Science 315 (5818) (2007) 1576–1579.

[82] S. Battista, V. Fidanza, M. Fedele, A.J. Klein-Szanto, E. Outwater, H. Brunner, et al., The expression of a truncated HMGI-C gene induces gigantism associated with lipomatosis, Cancer Res 59 (19) (1999) 4793–4797.

[83] Z.R. Qian, S.L. Asa, H. Siomi, M.C. Siomi, K. Yoshimoto, S. Yamada, et al., Overexpression of HMGA2 relates to reduction of the let-7 and its relationship to clinicopathological features in pituitary adenomas, Mod Pathol 22 (3) (2009) 431–441.

[84] M. Fedele, R. Visone, I. De Martino, G. Troncone, D. Palmieri, S. Battista, et al., HMGA2 induces pituitary tumorigenesis by enhancing E2F1 activity, Cancer Cell 9 (6) (2006) 459–471.

[85] J. Chen, N. Hersmus, V. Van Duppen, P. Caesens, C. Denef, H. Vankelecom, The adult pituitary contains a cell population displaying stem/progenitor cell and early embryonic characteristics, Endocrinology 146 (9) (2005) 3985–3998.

[86] J. Nishino, I. Kim, K. Chada, S.J. Morrison, HMGA2 promotes neural stem cell self-renewal in young but not old mice by reducing p16Ink4a and p19Arf expression, Cell 135 (2) (2008) 227–239.

[87] V. Quereda, M. Malumbres, Cell cycle control of pituitary development and disease, J Mol Endocrinol 42 (2) (2009) 75–86.

[88] O. Stevaux, N.J. Dyson, A revised picture of the E2F transcriptional network and RB function, Curr Opin Cell Biol 14 (6) (2002) 684–691.

[89] A. Blais, B.D. Dynlacht, E2F-associated chromatin modifiers and cell cycle control, Curr Opin Cell Biol 19 (6) (2007) 658–662.

[90] A. Sun, L. Bagella, S. Tutton, G. Romano, A. Giordano, From G_0 to S phase: A view of the roles played by the retinoblastoma (Rb) family members in the Rb-E2F pathway, J Cell Biochem 102 (6) (2007) 1400–1404.

[91] C.J. Sherr, J.M. Roberts, CDK inhibitors: Positive and negative regulators of G_1-phase progression, Genes Dev 13 (12) (1999) 1501–1512.

[92] T. Jacks, A. Fazeli, E.M. Schmitt, R.T. Bronson, M.A. Goodell, R.A. Weinberg, Effects of an Rb mutation in the mouse, Nature 359 (6393) (1992) 295–300.

[93] S.W. Leung, E.H. Wloga, A.F. Castro, T. Nguyen, R.T. Bronson, L. Yamasaki, A dynamic switch in $Rb^{+/-}$ mediated neuroendocrine tumorigenesis, Oncogene 23 (19) (2004) 3296–3307.

[94] M.L. Fero, M. Rivkin, M. Tasch, P. Porter, C.E. Carow, E. Firpo, et al., A syndrome of multiorgan hyperplasia with features of gigantism, tumorigenesis, and female sterility in p27(Kip1)-deficient mice, Cell 85 (5) (1996) 733–744.

[95] H. Kiyokawa, R.D. Kineman, K.O. Manova-Todorova, V.C. Soares, E.S. Hoffman, M. Ono, et al., Enhanced growth of mice lacking the cyclin-dependent kinase inhibitor function of p27(Kip1), Cell 85 (5) (1996) 721–732.

[96] K. Nakayama, N. Ishida, M. Shirane, A. Inomata, T. Inoue, N. Shishido, et al., Mice lacking p27(Kip1) display increased body size, multiple organ hyperplasia, retinal dysplasia, and pituitary tumors, Cell 85 (5) (1996) 707–720.

[97] S. Jirawatnotai, A. Aziyu, E.C. Osmundson, D.S. Moons, X. Zou, R.D. Kineman, et al., Cdk4 is indispensable for postnatal proliferation of the anterior pituitary, J Biol Chem 279 (49) (2004) 51100–51106.

[98] E.Y. Lee, H. Cam, U. Ziebold, J.B. Rayman, J.A. Lees, B.D. Dynlacht, E2F4 loss suppresses tumorigenesis in Rb mutant mice, Cancer Cell 2 (6) (2002) 463–472.

[99] L. Yamasaki, R. Bronson, B.O. Williams, N.J. Dyson, E. Harlow, T. Jacks, Loss of E2F-1 reduces tumorigenesis and extends the lifespan of $Rb1(^{+/-})$mice, Nat Genet 18 (4) (1998) 360–364.

[100] E. Aleem, H. Kiyokawa, P. Kaldis, Cdc2-cyclin E complexes regulate the G_1/S phase transition, Nat Cell Biol 7 (8) (2005) 831–836.

[101] T. Tateno, X. Zhu, S.L. Asa, S. Ezzat, Chromatin remodeling and histone modifications in pituitary tumors, Mol Cell Endocrinol 326 (2010) 1–21.

[102] L. Pei, S. Melmed, Isolation and characterization of a pituitary tumor-transforming gene (PTTG), Mol Endocrinol 11 (4) (1997) 433–441.

[103] A.P. Heaney, R. Singson, C.J. McCabe, V. Nelson, M. Nakashima, S. Melmed, Expression of pituitary-tumour transforming gene in colorectal tumours, Lancet 355 (9205) (2000) 716–719.

[104] C. Saez, M.A. Japon, F. Ramos-Morales, F. Romero, D.I. Segura, M. Tortolero, et al., hpttg is over-expressed in pituitary adenomas and other primary epithelial neoplasias, Oncogene 18 (39) (1999) 5473–5476.

[105] X. Zhang, G.A. Horwitz, A.P. Heaney, M. Nakashima, T.R. Prezant, M.D. Bronstein, et al., Pituitary tumor transforming gene (PTTG) expression in pituitary adenomas, J Clin Endocrinol Metab 84 (2) (1999) 761–767.

[106] M. Filippella, F. Galland, M. Kujas, J. Young, A. Faggiano, G. Lombardi, et al., Pituitary tumour transforming gene (PTTG) expression correlates with the proliferative activity and recurrence status of pituitary adenomas: A clinical and immunohistochemical study, Clin Endocrinol (Oxf) 65 (4) (2006) 536–543.

[107] C.J. McCabe, J.S. Khaira, K. Boelaert, A.P. Heaney, L.A. Tannahill, S. Hussain, et al., Expression of pituitary tumour transforming gene (PTTG) and fibroblast growth factor-2 (FGF-2) in human pituitary adenomas: Relationships to clinical tumour behaviour, Clin Endocrinol (Oxf) 58 (2) (2003) 141–150.

[108] G. Vlotides, T. Eigler, S. Melmed, Pituitary tumor-transforming gene: Physiology and implications for tumorigenesis, Endocr Rev 28 (2) (2007) 165–186.

[109] F. Ramos-Morales, A. Dominguez, F. Romero, R. Luna, M.C. Multon, J.A. Pintor-Toro, et al., Cell cycle regulated expression and phosphorylation of hpttg proto-oncogene product, Oncogene 19 (3) (2000) 403–409.

[110] L.J. Holt, A.N. Krutchinsky, D.O. Morgan, Positive feedback sharpens the anaphase switch, Nature 454 (7202) (2008) 353–357.

[111] O. Stemmann, H. Zou, S.A. Gerber, S.P. Gygi, M.W. Kirschner, Dual inhibition of sister chromatid separation at metaphase, Cell 107 (6) (2001) 715–726.

[112] H. Zou, T.J. McGarry, T. Bernal, M.W. Kirschner, Identification of a vertebrate sister-chromatid separation inhibitor involved in transformation and tumorigenesis, Science 285 (5426) (1999) 418–422.

[113] A. Zur, M. Brandeis, Securin degradation is mediated by fzy and fzr, and is required for complete chromatid separation but not for cytokinesis, EMBO J 20 (4) (2001) 792–801.

[114] S. Melmed, Acromegaly pathogenesis and treatment, J Clin Invest 119 (11) (2009) 3189–3202.

[115] P.V. Jallepalli, I.C. Waizenegger, F. Bunz, S. Langer, M.R. Speicher, J.M. Peters, et al., Securin is required for chromosomal stability in human cells, Cell 105 (4) (2001) 445–457.

[116] D.S. Kim, J.A. Franklyn, V.E. Smith, A.L. Stratford, H.N. Pemberton, A. Warfield, et al., Securin induces genetic instability in colorectal cancer by inhibiting double-stranded DNA repair activity, Carcinogenesis 28 (3) (2007) 749–759.

[117] R. Yu, W. Lu, J. Chen, C.J. McCabe, S. Melmed, Overexpressed pituitary tumor-transforming gene causes aneuploidy in live human cells, Endocrinology 144 (11) (2003) 4991–4998.

[118] V. Chesnokova, K. Kovacs, A.V. Castro, S. Zonis, S. Melmed, Pituitary hypoplasia in $Pttg^{-/-}$ mice is protective for $Rb^{+/-}$ pituitary tumorigenesis, Mol Endocrinol 19 (9) (2005) 2371–2379.

[119] Z. Wang, R. Yu, S. Melmed, Mice lacking pituitary tumor transforming gene show testicular and splenic hypoplasia, thymic hyperplasia, thrombocytopenia, aberrant cell cycle progression, and premature centromere division, Mol Endocrinol 15 (11) (2001) 1870–1879.

[120] J.M. Schvartzman, R. Sotillo, R. Benezra, Mitotic chromosomal instability and cancer: Mouse modelling of the human disease, Nat Rev Cancer 10 (2) (2010) 102–115.

[121] J.A. Bernal, R. Luna, A. Espina, I. Lazaro, F. Ramos-Morales, F. Romero, et al., Human securin interacts with p53 and modulates p53-mediated transcriptional activity and apoptosis, Nat Genet 32 (2) (2002) 306–311.

[122] J.A. Bernal, M. Roche, C. Mendez-Vidal, A. Espina, M. Tortolero, J.A. Pintor-Toro, Proliferative potential after DNA damage and non-homologous end joining are affected by loss of securin, Cell Death Differ 15 (1) (2008) 202–212.

[123] F. Romero, A.M. Gil-Bernabe, C. Saez, M.A. Japon, J.A. Pintor-Toro, M. Tortolero, Securin is a target of the UV response pathway in mammalian cells, Mol Cell Biol 24 (7) (2004) 2720–2733.

[124] R.A. Abbud, I. Takumi, E.M. Barker, S.G. Ren, D.Y. Chen, K. Wawrowsky, et al., Early multipotential pituitary focal hyperplasia in the alpha-subunit of glycoprotein hormone-driven pituitary tumor-transforming gene transgenic mice, Mol Endocrinol 19 (5) (2005) 1383–1391.

[125] I. Donangelo, S. Gutman, E. Horvath, K. Kovacs, K. Wawrowsky, M. Mount, et al., Pituitary tumor transforming gene overexpression facilitates pituitary tumor development, Endocrinology 147 (10) (2006) 4781–4791.

[126] C. Zhou, K. Wawrowsky, S. Bannykh, S. Gutman, S. Melmed, E2F1 induces pituitary tumor transforming gene (PTTG1) expression in human pituitary tumors, Mol Endocrinol 23 (12) (2009) 2000–2012.

[127] V. Chesnokova, S. Zonis, T. Rubinek, R. Yu, A. Ben-Shlomo, K. Kovacs, et al., Senescence mediates pituitary hypoplasia and restrains pituitary tumor growth, Cancer Res 67 (21) (2007) 10564–10572.

[128] V. Chesnokova, S. Zonis, K. Kovacs, A. Ben-Shlomo, K. Wawrowsky, S. Bannykh, et al., p21(Cip1) restrains pituitary tumor growth, Proc Nat Acad Sci USA 105 (45) (2008) 17498–17503.

[129] D.L. Burkhart, J. Sage, Cellular mechanisms of tumour suppression by the retinoblastoma gene, Nat Rev Cancer 8 (9) (2008) 671–682.

[130] D. Gospodarowicz, J.A. Abraham, J. Schilling, Isolation and characterization of a vascular endothelial cell mitogen produced by pituitary-derived folliculo stellate cells, Proc Nat Acad Sci USA 86 (19) (1989) 7311–7315.

[131] S. Ezzat, H.S. Smyth, L. Ramyar, S.L. Asa, Heterogenous in vivo and in vitro expression of basic fibroblast growth factor by human pituitary adenomas, J Clin Endocrinol Metab 80 (3) (1995) 878–884.

[132] S. Yu, L. Zheng, S.L. Asa, S. Ezzat, Fibroblast growth factor receptor 4 (FGFR4) mediates signaling to the prolactin but not the FGFR4 promoter, Am J Physiol Endocrinol Metab 283 (3) (2002) E490–E495.

[133] S.A. Abbass, S.L. Asa, S. Ezzat, Altered expression of fibroblast growth factor receptors in human pituitary adenomas, J Clin Endocrinol Metab 82 (4) (1997) 1160–1166.

[134] S. Ezzat, L. Zheng, X.F. Zhu, G.E. Wu, S.L. Asa, Targeted expression of a human pituitary tumor-derived isoform of FGF receptor-4 recapitulates pituitary tumorigenesis, J Clin Invest 109 (1) (2002) 69–78.

[135] S. Yu, S.L. Asa, R.J. Weigel, S. Ezzat, Pituitary tumor AP-2alpha recognizes a cryptic promoter in intron 4 of fibroblast growth factor receptor 4, J Biol Chem 278 (22) (2003) 19597–19602.

[136] S. Ezzat, L. Zheng, D. Winer, S.L. Asa, Targeting N-cadherin through fibroblast growth factor receptor-4: Distinct pathogenetic and therapeutic implications, Mol Endocrinol 20 (11) (2006) 2965–2975.

[137] Z.R. Qian, T. Sano, S.L. Asa, S. Yamada, H. Horiguchi, T. Tashiro, et al., Cytoplasmic expression of fibroblast growth factor receptor-4 in human pituitary adenomas: Relation to tumor type, size, proliferation, and invasiveness, J Clin Endocrinol Metab 89 (4) (2004) 1904–1911.

[138] U. Cavallaro, G. Christofori, Multitasking in tumor progression: Signaling functions of cell adhesion molecules, Ann NY Acad Sci 1014 (2004) 58–66.

[139] S. Ezzat, L. Zheng, S.L. Asa, Pituitary tumor-derived fibroblast growth factor receptor 4 isoform disrupts neural cell-adhesion molecule/N-cadherin signaling to diminish cell adhesiveness: A mechanism underlying pituitary neoplasia, Mol Endocrinol 18 (10) (2004) 2543–2552.

[140] U. Cavallaro, J. Niedermeyer, M. Fuxa, G. Christofori, N-CAM modulates tumour-cell adhesion to matrix by inducing FGF-receptor signalling, Nat Cell Biol 3 (7) (2001) 650–657.

[141] K. Suyama, I. Shapiro, M. Guttman, R.B. Hazan, A signaling pathway leading to metastasis is controlled by N-cadherin and the FGF receptor, Cancer Cell 2 (4) (2002) 301–314.

[142] H. Clevers, Wnt/beta-catenin signaling in development and disease, Cell 127 (3) (2006) 469–480.

[143] J. Gorski, D. Wendell, D. Gregg, T.Y. Chun, Estrogens and the genetic control of tumor growth, Prog Clin Biol Res 396 (1997) 233–243.

[144] S.W. Lamberts, T. Verleun, L. Hofland, R. Oosterom, Differences in the interaction between dopamine and estradiol on prolactin release by cultured normal and tumorous human pituitary cells, J Clin Endocrinol Metab 63 (6) (1986) 1342–1347.

[145] M.E. Lieberman, R.A. Maurer, J. Gorski, Estrogen control of prolactin synthesis in vitro, Proc Nat Acad Sci USA 75 (12) (1978) 5946–5949.

[146] K. Garcia-Malpartida, A. Martin-Gorgojo, M. Rocha, M. Gomez-Balaguer, A. Hernandez-Mijares, Prolactinoma induced by estrogen and cyproterone acetate in a male-to-female transsexual, Fertil Steril 94 (3) (2010) 1097.

[147] L.J. Gooren, J. Assies, H. Asscheman, R. de Slegte, H. van Kessel, Estrogen-induced prolactinoma in a man, J Clin Endocrinol Metab 66 (2) (1988) 444–446.

[148] K. Kovacs, L. Stefaneanu, S. Ezzat, H.S. Smyth, Prolactin-producing pituitary adenoma in a male-to-female transsexual patient with protracted estrogen administration. A morphologic study, Arch Pathol Lab Med 118 (5) (1994) 562–565.

[149] O. Serri, D. Noiseux, F. Robert, J. Hardy, Lactotroph hyperplasia in an estrogen treated male-to-female transsexual patient, J Clin Endocrinol Metab 81 (9) (1996) 3177–3179.
[150] E.J. Lee, W.R. Duan, M. Jakacka, B.D. Gehm, J.L. Jameson, Dominant negative ER induces apoptosis in GH(4) pituitary lactotrope cells and inhibits tumor growth in nude mice, Endocrinology 142 (9) (2001) 3756–3763.
[151] M.I. Torres-Arzayus, J. Font de Mora, J. Yuan, F. Vazquez, R. Bronson, M. Rue, et al., High tumor incidence and activation of the PI3K/AKT pathway in transgenic mice define AIB1 as an oncogene, Cancer Cell 6 (3) (2004) 263–274.
[152] M.P. Gillam, S. Middler, D.J. Freed, M.E. Molitch, The novel use of very high doses of cabergoline and a combination of testosterone and an aromatase inhibitor in the treatment of a giant prolactinoma, J Clin Endocrinol Metab 87 (10) (2002) 4447–4451.
[153] S.W. Lamberts, T. Verleun, R. Oosterom, Effect of tamoxifen administration on prolactin release by invasive prolactin-secreting pituitary adenomas, Neuroendocrinology 34 (5) (1982) 339–342.
[154] K.E. Friend, Y.K. Chiou, M.B. Lopes, E.R. Laws Jr., K.M. Hughes, M.A. Shupnik, Estrogen receptor expression in human pituitary: Correlation with immunohistochemistry in normal tissue, and immunohistochemistry and morphology in macroadenomas, J Clin Endocrinol Metab 78 (6) (1994) 1497–1504.
[155] S.S. Chaidarun, A. Klibanski, J.M. Alexander, Tumor-specific expression of alternatively spliced estrogen receptor messenger ribonucleic acid variants in human pituitary adenomas, J Clin Endocrinol Metab 82 (4) (1997) 1058–1065.
[156] M.A. Shupnik, L.K. Pitt, A.Y. Soh, A. Anderson, M.B. Lopes, E.R. Laws Jr., Selective expression of estrogen receptor alpha and beta isoforms in human pituitary tumors, J Clin Endocrinol Metab 83 (11) (1998) 3965–3972.
[157] A. Bollig, R.J. Miksicek, An estrogen receptor-alpha splicing variant mediates both positive and negative effects on gene transcription, Mol Endocrinol 14 (5) (2000) 634–649.
[158] W. Bryant, A.E. Snowhite, L.W. Rice, M.A. Shupnik, The estrogen receptor (ER)alpha variant Delta5 exhibits dominant positive activity on ER-regulated promoters in endometrial carcinoma cells, Endocrinology 146 (2) (2005) 751–759.
[159] S.S. Chaidarun, B. Swearingen, J.M. Alexander, Differential expression of estrogen receptor-beta (ER beta) in human pituitary tumors: Functional interactions with ER alpha and a tumor-specific splice variant, J Clin Endocrinol Metab 83 (9) (1998) 3308–3315.
[160] H. Ohlsson, A.E. Lykkesfeldt, M.W. Madsen, P. Briand, The estrogen receptor variant lacking exon 5 has dominant negative activity in the human breast epithelial cell line HMT-3522S1, Cancer Res 58 (19) (1998) 4264–4268.
[161] S.A. Fuqua, D.M. Wolf, Molecular aspects of estrogen receptor variants in breast cancer, Breast Cancer Res Treat 35 (3) (1995) 233–241.
[162] A. Citri, Y. Yarden, EGF-ERBB signalling: Towards the systems level, Nat Rev Mol Cell Biol 7 (7) (2006) 505–516.
[163] G.H. Murdoch, E. Potter, A.K. Nicolaisen, R.M. Evans, M.G. Rosenfeld, Epidermal growth factor rapidly stimulates prolactin gene transcription, Nature 300 (5888) (1982) 192–194.
[164] S.S. Chaidarun, M.C. Eggo, M.C. Sheppard, P.M. Stewart, Expression of epidermal growth factor (EGF), its receptor, and related oncoprotein (erbB-2) in human pituitary tumors and response to EGF in vitro, Endocrinology 135 (5) (1994) 2012–2021.
[165] S. Ezzat, L. Zheng, H.S. Smyth, S.L. Asa, The c-erbB-2/neu proto-oncogene in human pituitary tumours, Clin Endocrinol (Oxf) 46 (5) (1997) 599–606.
[166] V.K. LeRiche, S.L. Asa, S. Ezzat, Epidermal growth factor and its receptor (EGF-R) in human pituitary adenomas: EGF-R correlates with tumor aggressiveness, J Clin Endocrinol Metab 81 (2) (1996) 656–662.
[167] O. Onguru, B.W. Scheithauer, K. Kovacs, S. Vidal, L. Jin, S. Zhang, et al., Analysis of epidermal growth factor receptor and activated epidermal growth factor receptor expression in pituitary adenomas and carcinomas, Mod Pathol 17 (7) (2004) 772–780.
[168] G. Vlotides, O. Cooper, Y.H. Chen, S.G. Ren, Y. Greenman, S. Melmed, Heregulin regulates prolactinoma gene expression, Cancer Res 69 (10) (2009) 4209–4216.
[169] M.L. Jaffrain-Rea, E. Petrangeli, C. Lubrano, G. Minniti, D. Di Stefano, F. Sciarra, et al., Epidermal growth factor binding sites in human pituitary macroadenomas, J Endocrinol 158 (3) (1998) 425–433.
[170] J. McAndrew, A.J. Paterson, S.L. Asa, K.J. McCarthy, J.E. Kudlow, Targeting of transforming growth factor-alpha expression to pituitary lactotrophs in transgenic mice results in selective lactotroph proliferation and adenomas, Endocrinology 136 (10) (1995) 4479–4488.
[171] S.L. Asa, M.A. Kelly, D.K. Grandy, M.J. Low, Pituitary lactotroph adenomas develop after prolonged lactotroph hyperplasia in dopamine D_2 receptor-deficient mice, Endocrinology 140 (11) (1999) 5348–5355.
[172] M.A. Kelly, M. Rubinstein, S.L. Asa, G. Zhang, C. Saez, J.R. Bunzow, et al., Pituitary lactotroph hyperplasia and chronic hyperprolactinemia in dopamine D_2 receptor-deficient mice, Neuron 19 (1) (1997) 103–113.
[173] E. Friedman, E.F. Adams, A. Hoog, P.V. Gejman, E. Carson, C. Larsson, et al., Normal structural dopamine type 2 receptor gene in prolactin-secreting and other pituitary tumors, J Clin Endocrinol Metab 78 (3) (1994) 568–574.
[174] L. Caccavelli, F. Feron, I. Morange, E. Rouer, R. Benarous, D. Dewailly, et al., Decreased expression of the two D_2 dopamine receptor isoforms in bromocriptine-resistant prolactinomas, Neuroendocrinology 60 (3) (1994) 314–322.
[175] C. Missale, F. Boroni, M. Losa, M. Giovanelli, A. Zanellato, R. Dal Toso, et al., Nerve growth factor suppresses the transforming phenotype of human prolactinomas, Proc Nat Acad Sci USA 90 (17) (1993) 7961–7965.
[176] M.E. Cruz-Soto, M.D. Scheiber, K.A. Gregerson, G.P. Boivin, N.D. Horseman, Pituitary tumorigenesis in prolactin gene-disrupted mice, Endocrinology 143 (11) (2002) 4429–4436.
[177] K.G. Schuff, S.T. Hentges, M.A. Kelly, N. Binart, P.A. Kelly, P.M. Iuvone, et al., Lack of prolactin receptor signaling in mice results in lactotroph proliferation and prolactinomas by dopamine-dependent and -independent mechanisms, J Clin Invest 110 (7) (2002) 973–981.
[178] S.W. Davis, S.A. Camper, Noggin regulates Bmp4 activity during pituitary induction, Dev Biol 305 (1) (2007) 145–160.
[179] K.M. Scully, M.G. Rosenfeld, Pituitary development: Regulatory codes in mammalian organogenesis, Science 295 (5563) (2002) 2231–2235.
[180] D. Giacomini, M. Paez-Pereda, M. Theodoropoulou, M. Labeur, D. Refojo, J. Gerez, et al., Bone morphogenetic protein-4 inhibits corticotroph tumor cells: Involvement in the retinoic acid inhibitory action, Endocrinology 147 (1) (2006) 247–256.
[181] M. Paez-Pereda, D. Giacomini, D. Refojo, A.C. Nagashima, U. Hopfner, Y. Grubler, et al., Involvement of bone morphogenetic protein 4 (BMP-4) in pituitary prolactinoma pathogenesis through a Smad/estrogen receptor crosstalk, Proc Nat Acad Sci USA 100 (3) (2003) 1034–1039.

[182] D. Giacomini, M. Paez-Pereda, J. Stalla, G.K. Stalla, E. Arzt, Molecular interaction of BMP-4, TGF-beta, and estrogens in lactotrophs: Impact on the PRL promoter, Mol Endocrinol 23 (7) (2009) 1102–1114.

[183] H.P. Mohammad, R.A. Abbud, A.F. Parlow, J.S. Lewin, J.H. Nilson, Targeted overexpression of luteinizing hormone causes ovary-dependent functional adenomas restricted to cells of the Pit-1 lineage, Endocrinology 144 (10) (2003) 4626–4636.

[184] C.C. Quirk, D.D. Seachrist, J.H. Nilson, Embryonic expression of the luteinizing hormone beta gene appears to be coupled to the transient appearance of p8, a high mobility group-related transcription factor, J Biol Chem 278 (3) (2003) 1680–1685.

[185] I. Ciric, M. Mikhael, T. Stafford, L. Lawson, R. Garces, Transsphenoidal microsurgery of pituitary macroadenomas with long-term follow-up results, J Neurosurg 59 (3) (1983) 395–401.

[186] O. Melen, Neuro-ophthalmologic features of pituitary tumors, Endocrinol Metab Clin North Am 16 (3) (1987) 585–608.

[187] J.P. Cottier, C. Destrieux, L. Brunereau, P. Bertrand, L. Moreau, M. Jan, et al., Cavernous sinus invasion by pituitary adenoma: MR imaging, Radiology 215 (2) (2000) 463–469.

[188] L.W. King, M.E. Molitch, J.W. Gittinger Jr., S.M. Wolpert, J. Stern, Cavernous sinus syndrome due to prolactinoma: Resolution with bromocriptine, Surg Neurol 19 (3) (1983) 280–284.

[189] J.E. Thomas, R.E. Yoss, The parasellar syndrome: Problems in determining etiology, Mayo Clin Proc 45 (9) (1970) 617–623.

[190] B. Guidetti, B. Fraioli, G.P. Cantore, Results of surgical management of 319 pituitary adenomas, Acta Neurochir (Wien) 85 (3-4) (1987) 117–124.

[191] J.R. Davis, M.C. Sheppard, D.A. Heath, Giant invasive prolactinoma: A case report and review of nine further cases, Q J Med 74 (275) (1990) 227–238.

[192] P.O. Lundberg, B. Drettner, A. Hemmingsson, B. Stenkvist, L. Wide, The invasive pituitary adenoma. A prolactin-producing tumor, Arch Neurol 34 (12) (1977) 742–749.

[193] O.M. Zikel, J.L. Atkinson, D.L. Hurley, Prolactinoma manifesting with symptomatic hydrocephalus, Mayo Clin Proc 74 (5) (1999) 475–477.

[194] M.E. Molitch, R.L. Elton, R.E. Blackwell, B. Caldwell, R.J. Chang, R. Jaffe, et al., Bromocriptine as primary therapy for prolactin-secreting macroadenomas: Results of a prospective multicenter study, J Clin Endocrinol Metab 60 (4) (1985) 698–705.

[195] P.B. Nelson, M. Goodman, J.C. Maroon, A.J. Martinez, J. Moossy, A.G. Robinson, Factors in predicting outcome from operation in patients with prolactin-secreting pituitary adenomas, Neurosurgery 13 (6) (1983) 634–641.

[196] K.D. Post, B.J. Biller, L.S. Adelman, M.E. Molitch, S.M. Wolpert, S. Reichlin, Selective transsphenoidal adenomectomy in women with galactorrhea-amenorrhea, JAMA 242 (2) (1979) 158–162.

[197] S. Franks, J.D. Nabarro, Prevalence and presentation of hyperprolactinaemia in patients with "functionless" pituitary tumours, Lancet 1 (8015) (1977) 778–780.

[198] Y. Maor, M. Berezin, Hyperprolactinemia in postmenopausal women, Fertil Steril 67 (4) (1997) 693–696.

[199] M. Berezin, I. Shimon, M. Hadani, Prolactinoma in 53 men: Clinical characteristics and modes of treatment (male prolactinoma), J Endocrinol Invest 18 (6) (1995) 436–441.

[200] J.N. Carter, J.E. Tyson, G. Tolis, S. Van Vliet, C. Faiman, H.G. Friesen, Prolactin-screening tumors and hypogonadism in 22 men, N Engl J Med 299 (16) (1978) 847–852.

[201] R.H. Goodman, M.E. Molitch, K.D. Post, I.M.D. Jackson, Prolactin secreting tumors in the male, in: K.D. Post, I.M.D. Jackson, S. Reichlin (Eds.), The Pituitary Adenoma., Plenum Press, New York, 1980, pp. 91–108.

[202] F. Grisoli, F. Vincentelli, P. Jaquet, M. Guibout, J. Hassoun, P. Farnarier, Prolactin secreting adenoma in 22 men, Surg Neurol 13 (4) (1980) 241–247.

[203] A.L. Hulting, C. Muhr, P.O. Lundberg, S. Werner, Prolactinomas in men: Clinical characteristics and the effect of bromocriptine treatment, Acta Med Scand 217 (1) (1985) 101–109.

[204] H. Nishioka, J. Haraoka, K. Akada, Growth potential of prolactinomas in men: Is it really different from women? Surg Neurol 59 (5) (2003) 386–390, discussion 390–391.

[205] Y. Ramot, M.J. Rapoport, P. Hagag, A.J. Wysenbeek, A study of the clinical differences between women and men with hyperprolactinemia, Gynecol Endocrinol 10 (6) (1996) 397–400.

[206] R.F. Spark, C.A. Wills, G. O'Reilly, B.J. Ransil, R. Bergland, Hyperprolactinaemia in males with and without pituitary macroadenomas, Lancet 2 (8290) (1982) 129–132.

[207] J.P. Walsh, P.T. Pullan, Hyperprolactinaemia in males: A heterogeneous disorder, Aust NZ J Med 27 (4) (1997) 385–390.

[208] A. Colao, A.D. Sarno, P. Cappabianca, F. Briganti, R. Pivonello, C.D. Somma, et al., Gender differences in the prevalence, clinical features and response to cabergoline in hyperprolactinemia, Eur J Endocrinol 148 (3) (2003) 325–331.

[209] J. Verhelst, R. Abs, D. Maiter, A. van den Bruel, M. Vandeweghe, B. Velkeniers, et al., Cabergoline in the treatment of hyperprolactinemia: A study in 455 patients, J Clin Endocrinol Metab 84 (7) (1999) 2518–2522.

[210] J.J. Pinzone, L. Katznelson, D.C. Danila, D.K. Pauler, C.S. Miller, A. Klibanski, Primary medical therapy of micro- and macroprolactinomas in men, J Clin Endocrinol Metab 85 (9) (2000) 3053–3057.

[211] A. Colao, G. Vitale, P. Cappabianca, F. Briganti, A. Ciccarelli, M. De Rosa, et al., Outcome of cabergoline treatment in men with prolactinoma: Effects of a 24-month treatment on prolactin levels, tumor mass, recovery of pituitary function, and semen analysis, J Clin Endocrinol Metab 89 (4) (2004) 1704–1711.

[212] B.M. Biller, M.E. Molitch, M.L. Vance, K.B. Cannistraro, K.R. Davis, J.A. Simons, et al., Treatment of prolactin-secreting macroadenomas with the once-weekly dopamine agonist cabergoline, J Clin Endocrinol Metab 81 (6) (1996) 2338–2343.

[213] M. De Rosa, S. Zarrilli, G. Vitale, C. Di Somma, F. Orio, L. Tauchmanova, et al., Six months of treatment with cabergoline restores sexual potency in hyperprolactinemic males: An open longitudinal study monitoring nocturnal penile tumescence, J Clin Endocrinol Metab 89 (2) (2004) 621–625.

[214] S. Cannavo, M. Venturino, L. Curto, E. De Menis, C. D'Arrigo, P. Tita, et al., Clinical presentation and outcome of pituitary adenomas in teenagers, Clin Endocrinol (Oxf) 58 (4) (2003) 519–527.

[215] A. Colao, S. Loche, M. Cappa, A. Di Sarno, M.L. Landi, F. Sarnacchiaro, et al., Prolactinomas in children and adolescents. Clinical presentation and long-term follow-up, J Clin Endocrinol Metab 83 (8) (1998) 2777–2780.

[216] L.H. Duntas, Prolactinomas in children and adolescents – consequences in adult life, J Pediatr Endocrinol Metab 14 (Suppl 5) (2001) 1227–1232, discussion 1261–1262.

[217] S.V. Acharya, R.A. Gopal, T.R. Bandgar, S.R. Joshi, P.S. Menon, N.S. Shah, Clinical profile and long term follow up of children and adolescents with prolactinomas, Pituitary 12 (3) (2009) 186–189.

[218] R. Artese, D.H. D'Osvaldo, I. Molocznik, H. Benencia, J. Oviedo, J.A. Burdman, et al., Pituitary tumors in adolescent patients, Neurol Res 20 (5) (1998) 415–417.

[219] E.H. Dyer, T. Civit, A. Visot, O. Delalande, P. Derome, Transsphenoidal surgery for pituitary adenomas in children, Neurosurgery 34 (2) (1994) 207–212, discussion 212.

[220] H.L. Fideleff, H.R. Boquete, A. Sequera, M. Suarez, P. Sobrado, A. Giaccio, Peripubertal prolactinomas: Clinical presentation and long-term outcome with different therapeutic approaches, J Pediatr Endocrinol Metab 13 (3) (2000) 261−267.
[221] B. Fraioli, L. Ferrante, P. Celli, Pituitary adenomas with onset during puberty. Features and treatment, J Neurosurg 59 (4) (1983) 590−595.
[222] S.F. Haddad, J.C. VanGilder, A.H. Menezes, Pediatric pituitary tumors, Neurosurgery 29 (4) (1991) 509−514.
[223] T.A. Howlett, J.A. Wass, A. Grossman, P.N. Plowman, M. Charlesworth, R. Touzel, et al., Prolactinomas presenting as primary amenorrhoea and delayed or arrested puberty: Response to medical therapy, Clin Endocrinol (Oxf) 30 (2) (1989) 131−140.
[224] G. Maira, C. Anile, Pituitary adenomas in childhood and adolescence, Can J Neurol Sci 17 (1) (1990) 83−87.
[225] T. Mindermann, C.B. Wilson, Pediatric pituitary adenomas, Neurosurgery 36 (2) (1995) 259−268, discussion 269.
[226] M.D. Partington, D.H. Davis, E.R. Laws Jr., B.W. Scheithauer, Pituitary adenomas in childhood and adolescence. Results of transsphenoidal surgery, J Neurosurg 80 (2) (1994) 209−216.
[227] A. Colao, Pituitary tumors in childhood, Endotextorg (2004). Available from, www.endotext.org.
[228] L.D. George, N. Nicolau, M.F. Scanlon, J.S. Davies, Recovery of growth hormone secretion following cabergoline treatment of macroprolactinomas, Clin Endocrinol (Oxf) 53 (5) (2000) 595−599.
[229] A. Colao, C. Di Somma, S. Loche, A. Di Sarno, M. Klain, R. Pivonello, et al., Prolactinomas in adolescents: Persistent bone loss after 2 years of prolactin normalization, Clin Endocrinol (Oxf) 52 (3) (2000) 319−327.
[230] F.F. Casanueva, M.E. Molitch, J.A. Schlechte, R. Abs, V. Bonert, M.D. Bronstein, et al., Guidelines of the Pituitary Society for the diagnosis and management of prolactinomas, Clinical Endocrinol (2006) 65.
[231] A. Kruse, J. Astrup, C. Gyldensted, G.E. Cold, Hyperprolactinaemia in patients with pituitary adenomas. The pituitary stalk compression syndrome, Br J Neurosurg 9 (4) (1995) 453−457.
[232] G. Hofle, R. Gasser, I. Mohsenipour, G. Finkenstedt, Surgery combined with dopamine agonists versus dopamine agonists alone in long-term treatment of macroprolactinoma: A retrospective study, Exp Clin Endocrinol Diabetes 106 (3) (1998) 211−216.
[233] D.A. Sisam, J.P. Sheehan, O.P. Schumacher, Lack of demonstrable tumor growth in progressive hyperprolactinemia, Am J Med 80 (2) (1986) 279−280.
[234] M.E. Molitch, Medical treatment of prolactinomas, Endocrinol Metab Clin North Am 28 (1) (1999) 143−169.
[235] B. Corenblum, L. Donovan, The safety of physiological estrogen plus progestin replacement therapy with oral contraceptive therapy in women with pathological hyperprolactinemia, Fertil Steril 59 (3) (1993) 671−673.
[236] S.L. Tan, H.S. Jacobs, Rapid regression through bromocriptine therapy of a suprasellar extending prolactinoma during pregnancy, Int J Gynaecol Obstet 24 (3) (1986) 209−215.
[237] U.M. Fahy, P.A. Foster, H.W. Torode, M. Hartog, M.G. Hull, The effect of combined estrogen/progestogen treatment in women with hyperprolactinemic amenorrhea, Gynecol Endocrinol 6 (3) (1992) 183−188.
[238] M.M. Garcia, L.P. Kapcala, Growth of a microprolactinoma to a macroprolactinoma during estrogen therapy, J Endocrinol Invest 18 (6) (1995) 450−455.
[239] H.S. Randeva, J. Schoebel, J. Byrne, M. Esiri, C.B. Adams, J.A. Wass, Classical pituitary apoplexy: Clinical features, management and outcome, Clin Endocrinol (Oxf) 51 (2) (1999) 181−188.
[240] E.R. Laws, Pituitary tumor apoplexy: A review, J Intensive Care Med 23 (2) (2008) 146−147.
[241] L. Sibal, S.G. Ball, V. Connolly, R.A. James, P. Kane, W.F. Kelly, et al., Pituitary apoplexy: A review of clinical presentation, management and outcome in 45 cases, Pituitary 7 (2004) 157−163.
[242] P. Maccagnan, C.L. Macedo, M.J. Kayath, R.G. Nogueira, J. Abucham, Conservative management of pituitary apoplexy: A prospective study, J Clin Endocrinol Metab 80 (7) (1995) 2190−2197.
[243] S.T. Onesti, T. Wisniewski, K.D. Post, Clinical versus subclinical pituitary apoplexy: Presentation, surgical management, and outcome in 21 patients, Neurosurgery 26 (6) (1990) 980−986.
[244] J.A. Jane, Surgical techniques in transsphenoidal surgery: What is the standard of care in pituitary adenoma surgery? Curr Opin Endocrinol Diabetes 14 (2004) 264−270.
[245] E.R. Laws Jr., K. Thapar, Pituitary surgery, Endocrinol Metab Clin North Am 28 (1) (1999) 119−131.
[246] M. Jan, H. Dufour, T. Brue, P. Jaquet, Prolactinoma surgery, Ann Endocrinol (Paris) 68 (2−3) (2007) 118−119.
[247] M. Buchfelder, S. Schlaffer, Surgical treatment of pituitary tumours, Best Pract Res Clin Endocrinol Metab 23 (5) (2009) 677−692.
[248] P. Cappabianca, L.M. Cavallo, A. Colao, E. de Divitiis, Surgical complications associated with the endoscopic endonasal transsphenoidal approach for pituitary adenomas, J Neurosurg 97 (2) (2002) 293−298.
[249] M.T. Sheehan, J.L. Atkinson, J.L. Kasperbauer, B.J. Erickson, T.B. Nippoldt, Preliminary comparison of the endoscopic transnasal vs the sublabial transseptal approach for clinically nonfunctioning pituitary macroadenomas, Mayo Clin Proc 74 (7) (1999) 661−670.
[250] D.R. White, R.E. Sonnenburg, M.G. Ewend, B.A. Senior, Safety of minimally invasive pituitary surgery (MIPS) compared with a traditional approach, Laryngoscope 114 (11) (2004) 1945−1948.
[251] A. Kuroki, T. Kayama, Endoscopic approach to the pituitary lesions: Contemporary method and review of the literature, Biomed Pharmacother 56 (Suppl 1) (2002) 158s−164s.
[252] G. Zada, D.F. Kelly, P. Cohan, C. Wang, R. Swerdloff, Endonasal transsphenoidal approach for pituitary adenomas and other sellar lesions: An assessment of efficacy, safety, and patient impressions, J Neurosurg 98 (2) (2003) 350−358.
[253] D.Y. Cho, W.R. Liau, Comparison of endonasal endoscopic surgery and sublabial microsurgery for prolactinomas, Surg Neurol 58 (6) (2002) 371−375, discussion 375−376.
[254] T. Kawamata, H. Iseki, R. Ishizaki, T. Hori, Minimally invasive endoscope-assisted endonasal trans-sphenoidal microsurgery for pituitary tumors: Experience with 215 cases comparing with sublabial trans-sphenoidal approach, Neurol Res 24 (3) (2002) 259−265.
[255] H.D. Jho, Endoscopic pituitary surgery, Pituitary 2 (2) (1999) 139−154.
[256] G. Frank, E. Pasquini, G. Farneti, D. Mazzatenta, V. Sciarretta, V. Grasso, et al., The endoscopic versus the traditional approach in pituitary surgery, Neuroendocrinology 83 (3−4) (2006) 240−248.
[257] A.K. Jain, A.K. Gupta, A. Pathak, A. Bhansali, J.R. Bapuraj, Excision of pituitary adenomas: Randomized comparison of surgical modalities, Br J Neurosurg 21 (4) (2007) 328−331.
[258] J. D'Haens, K. Van Rompaey, T. Stadnik, P. Haentjens, K. Poppe, B. Velkeniers, Fully endoscopic transsphenoidal surgery for functioning pituitary adenomas: A retrospective comparison with traditional transsphenoidal microsurgery in the same institution, Surg Neurol 72 (4) (2009) 336−340.

[259] M.P. Gillam, M.E. Molitch, G. Lombardi, A. Colao, Advances in the treatment of prolactinomas, Endocr Rev 27 (2006) 485–534.
[260] D.K. Hamilton, M.L. Vance, P.T. Boulos, E.R. Laws, Surgical outcomes in hyporesponsive prolactinomas: Analysis of patients with resistance or intolerance to dopamine agonists, Pituitary 8 (1) (2005) 53–60.
[261] J. Kreutzer, R. Buslei, H. Wallaschofski, B. Hofmann, C. Nimsky, R. Fahlbusch, et al., Operative treatment of prolactinomas: Indications and results in a current consecutive series of 212 patients, Eur J Endocrinol 158 (1) (2008) 11–18.
[262] N.T. Zervas, Surgical results for pituitary adenomas: Results of an international survey, in: P.M. Black, N.T. Zervas, E.C. Ridgway, J.B. Martin (Eds.), Secretory tumors of the pituitary gland., Raven Press, New York, 1984, pp. 377–385.
[263] B.M. Arafah, A. Manni, J.S. Brodkey, B. Kaufman, M. Velasco, O.H. Pearson, Cure of hypogonadism after removal of prolactin-secreting adenomas in men, J Clin Endocrinol Metab 52 (1) (1981) 91–94.
[264] F.T. Murray, D.F. Cameron, C. Ketchum, Return of gonadal function in men with prolactin-secreting pituitary tumors, J Clin Endocrinol Metab 59 (1) (1984) 79–85.
[265] A. Stevenaert, A. Beckers, J.L. Vandalem, G. Hennen, Early normalization of luteinizing hormone pulsatility after successful transsphenoidal surgery in women with microprolactinomas, J Clin Endocrinol Metab 62 (5) (1986) 1044–1047.
[266] K. Koizumi, T. Aono, K. Koike, K. Kurachi, Restoration of LH pulsatility in patients with prolactinomas after trans-sphenoidal surgery, Acta Endocrinol (Copenh) 107 (4) (1984) 433–438.
[267] A.T. Nelson Jr., H.S. Tucker Jr., D.P. Becker, Residual anterior pituitary function following transsphenoidal resection of pituitary macroadenomas, J Neurosurg 61 (3) (1984) 577–580.
[268] M.F. Scanlon, J.R. Peters, J.P. Thomas, S.H. Richards, W.H. Morton, S. Howell, et al., Management of selected patients with hyperprolactinaemia by partial hypophysectomy, Br Med J (Clin Res Ed) 291 (6508) (1985) 1547–1550.
[269] O. Serri, E. Rasio, H. Beauregard, J. Hardy, M. Somma, Recurrence of hyperprolactinemia after selective transsphenoidal adenomectomy in women with prolactinoma, N Engl J Med 309 (5) (1983) 280–283.
[270] E. Ciccarelli, E. Ghigo, C. Miola, G. Gandini, E.E. Muller, F. Camanni, Long-term follow-up of "cured" prolactinoma patients after successful adenomectomy, Clin Endocrinol (Oxf) 32 (5) (1990) 583–592.
[271] J.B. Tyrrell, K.R. Lamborn, L.T. Hannegan, C.B. Applebury, C.B. Wilson, Transsphenoidal microsurgical therapy of prolactinomas: Initial outcomes and long-term results, Neurosurgery 44 (2) (1999) 254–261, discussion 61–63.
[272] H.Z. Gokalp, H. Deda, A. Attar, H.C. Ugur, E. Arasil, N. Egemen, The neurosurgical management of prolactinomas, J Neurosurg Sci 44 (3) (2000) 128–132.
[273] F.Y. Murphy, D.L. Vesely, R.M. Jordan, S. Flanigan, P.O. Kohler, Giant invasive prolactinomas, Am J Med 83 (5) (1987) 995–1002.
[274] R.K. Shrivastava, M.S. Arginteanu, W.A. King, K.D. Post, Giant prolactinomas: Clinical management and long-term follow up, J Neurosurg 97 (2) (2002) 299–306.
[275] G. Charpentier, T. de Plunkett, P. Jedynak, F. Peillon, P. Le Gentil, J. Racadot, et al., Surgical treatment of prolactinomas. Short- and long-term results, prognostic factors, Horm Res 22 (3) (1985) 222–227.
[276] R.A. Kristof, J. Schramm, L. Redel, G. Neuloh, M. Wichers, D. Klingmuller, Endocrinological outcome following first time transsphenoidal surgery for GH-, ACTH-, and PRL-secreting pituitary adenomas, Acta Neurochir (Wien) 144 (6) (2002) 555–561, discussion 561.
[277] R.V. Randall, E.R. Laws Jr., C.F. Abboud, M.J. Ebersold, P.C. Kao, B.W. Scheithauer, Transsphenoidal microsurgical treatment of prolactin-producing pituitary adenomas. Results in 100 patients, Mayo Clin Proc 58 (2) (1983) 108–121.
[278] S.E. Rawe, H.O. Williamson, J.H. Levine, S.A. Phansey, D. Hungerford, W.Y. Adkins, Prolactinomas: Surgical therapy, indications and results, Surg Neurol 14 (3) (1980) 161–167.
[279] J. Webster, M.D. Page, J.S. Bevan, S.H. Richards, A.G. Douglas-Jones, M.F. Scanlon, Low recurrence rate after partial hypophysectomy for prolactinoma: The predictive value of dynamic prolactin function tests, Clin Endocrinol (Oxf) 36 (1) (1992) 35–44.
[280] R.H. Wiebe, R.S. Kramer, C.B. Hammond, Surgical treatment of prolactin-secreting microadenomas, Am J Obstet Gynecol 134 (1) (1979) 49–55.
[281] S. Wolfsberger, T. Czech, H. Vierhapper, R. Benavente, E. Knosp, Microprolactinomas in males treated by transsphenoidal surgery, Acta Neurochir (Wien) 145 (11) (2003) 935–940, discussion 940–941.
[282] R. Fahlbusch, M. Buchfelder, Present status of neurosurgery in the treatment of prolactinomas, Neurosurg Rev 8 (3–4) (1985) 195–205.
[283] A.M. Landolt, Surgical treatment of pituitary prolactinomas: Postoperative prolactin and fertility in seventy patients, Fertil Steril 35 (6) (1981) 620–625.
[284] A.P. Amar, W.T. Couldwell, J.C. Chen, M.H. Weiss, Predictive value of serum prolactin levels measured immediately after transsphenoidal surgery, J Neurosurg 97 (2) (2002) 307–314.
[285] S.L. Feigenbaum, D.E. Downey, C.B. Wilson, R.B. Jaffe, Transsphenoidal pituitary resection for preoperative diagnosis of prolactin-secreting pituitary adenoma in women: Long term follow-up, J Clin Endocrinol Metab 81 (5) (1996) 1711–1719.
[286] A.M. Landolt, P.J. Keller, E.R. Froesch, J. Mueller, Bromocriptine: Does it jeopardise the result of later surgery for prolactinomas? Lancet 2 (8299) (1982) 657–658.
[287] S.G. Soule, J. Farhi, G.S. Conway, H.S. Jacobs, M. Powell, The outcome of hypophysectomy for prolactinomas in the era of dopamine agonist therapy, Clin Endocrinol (Oxf) 44 (6) (1996) 711–716.
[288] J.S. Bevan, C.B. Adams, C.W. Burke, K.E. Morton, A.J. Molyneux, R.A. Moore, et al., Factors in the outcome of transsphenoidal surgery for prolactinoma and non-functioning pituitary tumour, including pre-operative bromocriptine therapy, Clin Endocrinol (Oxf) 26 (5) (1987) 541–556.
[289] G. Faglia, P. Moriondo, P. Travaglini, M.A. Giovanelli, Influence of previous bromocriptine therapy on surgery for microprolactinoma, Lancet 1 (8316) (1983) 133–134.
[290] R. Fahlbusch, M. Buchfelder, H.K. Rjosk, K. von Werder, Influence of preoperative bromocriptine therapy on success of surgery for microprolactinoma, Lancet 2 (8401) (1984) 520.
[291] M. Giovanelli, M. Losa, P. Mortini, S. Acerno, E. Giugni, Surgical results in microadenomas, Acta Neurochir Suppl 65 (1996) 11–12.
[292] M.H. Weiss, R.R. Wycoff, R. Yadley, P. Gott, S. Feldon, Bromocriptine treatment of prolactin-secreting tumors: Surgical implications, Neurosurgery 12 (6) (1983) 640–642.
[293] M.E. Sughrue, E.F. Chang, J.B. Tyrell, S. Kunwar, C.B. Wilson, L.S. Blevins Jr., Pre-operative dopamine agonist therapy improves post-operative tumor control following prolactinoma resection, Pituitary 12 (3) (2009) 158–164.
[294] J.A. Thomson, D.L. Davies, E.H. McLaren, G.M. Teasdale, Ten year follow up of microprolactinoma treated by transsphenoidal surgery, Br Med J 309 (6966) (1994) 1409–1410.

[295] F.G. Barker 2nd, A. Klibanski, B. Swearingen, Transsphenoidal surgery for pituitary tumors in the United States, 1996–2000: Mortality, morbidity, and the effects of hospital and surgeon volume, J Clin Endocrinol Metab 88 (10) (2003) 4709–4719.
[296] N. Sudhakar, A. Ray, J.A. Vafidis, Complications after transsphenoidal surgery: Our experience and a review of the literature, Br J Neurosurg 18 (5) (2004) 507–512.
[297] A.R. Cohen, P.R. Cooper, M.J. Kupersmith, E.S. Flamm, J. Ransohoff, Visual recovery after transsphenoidal removal of pituitary adenomas, Neurosurgery 17 (3) (1985) 446–452.
[298] D.L. Barrow, G.T. Tindall, Loss of vision after transsphenoidal surgery, Neurosurgery 27 (1) (1990) 60–68.
[299] F. Castinetti, J. Regis, H. Dufour, T. Brue, Role of stereotactic radiosurgery in the management of pituitary adenomas, Nat Rev Endocrinol 6 (4) (2010) 214–223.
[300] J.L. Antunes, E.M. Housepian, A.G. Frantz, Prolactin-secreting pituitary tumors, Ann Neurol 2 (1977) 148–153.
[301] F. Gomez, F.I. Reyes, C. Faiman, Nonpuerperal galactorrhea and hyperprolactinemia. Clinical findings, endocrine features and therapeutic responses in 56 cases, Am J Med 62 (5) (1977) 648–660.
[302] A. Grossman, B.L. Cohen, M. Charlesworth, P.N. Plowman, L.H. Rees, J.A. Wass, et al., Treatment of prolactinomas with megavoltage radiotherapy, Br Med J (Clin Res Ed) 288 (6424) (1984) 1105–1109.
[303] D.G. Johnston, K. Hall, P. Kendall-Taylor, W.M. Ross, A.L. Crombie, D.B. Cook, et al., The long-term effects of megavoltage radiotherapy as sole or combined therapy for large prolactinomas: Studies with high definition computerized tomography, Clin Endocrinol (Oxf) 24 (6) (1986) 675–685.
[304] D.L. Kleinberg, G.L. Noel, A.G. Frantz, Galactorrhea: A study of 235 cases, including 48 with pituitary tumors, N Engl J Med 296 (11) (1977) 589–600.
[305] A.E. Mehta, F.I. Reyes, C. Faiman, Primary radiotherapy of prolactinomas. Eight- to 15-year follow-up, Am J Med 83 (1) (1987) 49–58.
[306] G.E. Sheline, A. Grossman, A.E. Jones, G.M. Besser, Radiation therapy for prolactinomas, in: P.M. Black, N.T. Zervas, E.C. Ridgway, J.B. Martin (Eds.), Secretory tumors of the pituitary gland., Raven Press, New York, 1984.
[307] S. Tsagarakis, A. Grossman, P.N. Plowman, A.E. Jones, R. Touzel, L.H. Rees, et al., Megavoltage pituitary irradiation in the management of prolactinomas: Long-term follow-up, Clin Endocrinol (Oxf) 34 (5) (1991) 399–406.
[308] R.W. Tsang, J.D. Brierley, T. Panzarella, M.K. Gospodarowicz, S.B. Sutcliffe, W.J. Simpson, Role of radiation therapy in clinical hormonally-active pituitary adenomas, Radiother Oncol 41 (1) (1996) 45–53.
[309] E.A. Wallace, I.M. Holdaway, Treatment of macroprolactinomas at Auckland Hospital 1975–91, NZ Med J 108 (994) (1995) 50–52.
[310] C. Wang, K.S. Lam, J.T. Ma, T. Chan, M.Y. Liu, R.T. Yeung, Long-term treatment of hyperprolactinaemia with bromocriptine: Effect of drug withdrawal, Clin Endocrinol (Oxf) 27 (3) (1987) 363–371.
[311] D. Zierhut, M. Flentje, J. Adolph, J. Erdmann, F. Raue, M. Wannenmacher, External radiotherapy of pituitary adenomas, Int J Radiat Oncol Biol Phys 33 (2) (1995) 307–314.
[312] M. Mitsumori, D.C. Shrieve, E. Alexander 3rd, U.B. Kaiser, G.E. Richardson, P.M. Black, et al., Initial clinical results of LINAC-based stereotactic radiosurgery and stereotactic radiotherapy for pituitary adenomas, Int J Radiat Oncol Biol Phys 42 (3) (1998) 573–580.
[313] P. Colin, N. Jovenin, B. Delemer, J. Caron, H. Grulet, A.C. Hecart, et al., Treatment of pituitary adenomas by fractionated stereotactic radiotherapy: A prospective study of 110 patients, Int J Radiat Oncol Biol Phys 62 (2) (2005) 333–341.
[314] F. Castinetti, M. Nagai, I. Morange, H. Dufour, P. Caron, P. Chanson, et al., Long-term results of stereotactic radiosurgery in secretory pituitary adenomas, J Clin Endocrinol Metab 94 (9) (2009) 3400–3407.
[315] J. Jezkova, V. Hana, M. Krsek, V. Weiss, V. Vladyka, R. Liscak, et al., Use of the Leksell gamma knife in the treatment of prolactinoma patients, Clin Endocrinol (Oxf) 70 (5) (2009) 732–741.
[316] M.N. Pamir, T. Kilic, M. Belirgen, U. Abacioglu, N. Karabekiroglu, Pituitary adenomas treated with gamma knife radiosurgery: Volumetric analysis of 100 cases with minimum 3 year follow-up, Neurosurgery 61 (2) (2007) 270–280, discussion 280.
[317] N. Pouratian, J. Sheehan, J. Jagannathan, E.R. Laws Jr., L. Steiner, M.L. Vance, Gamma knife radiosurgery for medically and surgically refractory prolactinomas, Neurosurgery 59 (2) (2006) 255–266, discussion 266.
[318] F. Castinetti, M. Martinie, I. Morange, H. Dufour, N. Sturm, J.G. Passagia, et al., A combined dexamethasone desmopressin test as an early marker of postsurgical recurrence in Cushing's disease, J Clin Endocrinol Metab 94 (6) (2009) 1897–1903.
[319] L. Pan, N. Zhang, E.M. Wang, B.J. Wang, J.Z. Dai, P.W. Cai, Gamma knife radiosurgery as a primary treatment for prolactinomas, J Neurosurg 93 (Suppl 3) (2000) 10–13.
[320] S.H. Kim, R. Huh, J.W. Chang, Y.G. Park, S.S. Chung, Gamma knife radiosurgery for functioning pituitary adenomas, Stereotact Funct Neurosurg 72 (Suppl 1) (1999) 101–110.
[321] B.E. Pollock, T.B. Nippoldt, S.L. Stafford, R.L. Foote, C.F. Abboud, Results of stereotactic radiosurgery in patients with hormone-producing pituitary adenomas: Factors associated with endocrine normalization, J Neurosurg 97 (3) (2002) 525–530.
[322] M. Thoren, C. Hoybye, E. Grenback, M. Degerblad, T. Rahn, A.L. Hulting, The role of gamma knife radiosurgery in the management of pituitary adenomas, J Neurooncol 54 (2) (2001) 197–203.
[323] A.M. Landolt, N. Lomax, Gamma knife radiosurgery for prolactinomas, J Neurosurg 93 (Suppl 3) (2000) 14–18.
[324] J. Jagannathan, C.P. Yen, N. Pouratian, E.R. Laws, J.P. Sheehan, Stereotactic radiosurgery for pituitary adenomas: A comprehensive review of indications, techniques and long-term results using the gamma knife, J Neurooncol 92 (3) (2009) 345–356.
[325] F.P. Rocher, I. Sentenac, C. Berger, I. Marquis, P. Romestaing, J.P. Gerard, Stereotactic radiosurgery: The Lyon experience, Acta Neurochir Suppl 63 (1995) 109–114.
[326] K.A. Leber, J. Bergloff, G. Pendl, Dose-response tolerance of the visual pathways and cranial nerves of the cavernous sinus to stereotactic radiosurgery, J Neurosurg 88 (1) (1998) 43–50.
[327] R.B. Tishler, J.S. Loeffler, L.D. Lunsford, C. Duma, E. Alexander 3rd, H.M. Kooy, et al., Tolerance of cranial nerves of the cavernous sinus to radiosurgery, Int J Radiat Oncol Biol Phys 27 (2) (1993) 215–221.
[328] M. Brada, T.V. Ajithkumar, G. Minniti, Radiosurgery for pituitary adenomas, Clin Endocrinol (Oxf) 61 (5) (2004) 531–543.
[329] E.R. Laws Jr., M.L. Vance, Radiosurgery for pituitary tumors and craniopharyngiomas, Neurosurg Clin N Am. 10 (2) (1999) 327–336.
[330] T.C. Witt, Stereotactic radiosurgery for pituitary tumors, Neurosurg Focus 14 (5) (2003) e10.
[331] J. Jagannathan, J.P. Sheehan, N. Pouratian, E.R. Laws, L. Steiner, M.L. Vance, Gamma knife surgery for Cushing's disease, J Neurosurg 106 (6) (2007) 980–987.

[332] J.Y. Choi, J.H. Chang, J.W. Chang, Y. Ha, Y.G. Park, S.S. Chung, Radiological and hormonal responses of functioning pituitary adenomas after gamma knife radiosurgery, Yonsei Med J 44 (4) (2003) 602–607.

[333] Z. Petrovich, C. Yu, S.L. Giannotta, C.S. Zee, M.L. Apuzzo, Gamma knife radiosurgery for pituitary adenoma: Early results, Neurosurgery 53 (1) (2003) 51–59, discussion 59–61.

[334] S.C. Yoon, T.S. Suh, H.S. Jang, S.M. Chung, Y.S. Kim, M.R. Ryu, et al., Clinical results of 24 pituitary macroadenomas with linac-based stereotactic radiosurgery, Int J Radiat Oncol Biol Phys 41 (4) (1998) 849–853.

[335] M.D. Littley, S.M. Shalet, C.G. Beardwell, E.L. Robinson, M.L. Sutton, Radiation-induced hypopituitarism is dose-dependent, Clin Endocrinol (Oxf) 31 (3) (1989) 363–373.

[336] P.J. Snyder, B.F. Fowble, N.J. Schatz, P.J. Savino, T.A. Gennarelli, Hypopituitarism following radiation therapy of pituitary adenomas, Am J Med 81 (3) (1986) 457–462.

[337] R.W. Tsang, J.D. Brierley, T. Panzarella, M.K. Gospodarowicz, S.B. Sutcliffe, W.J. Simpson, Radiation therapy for pituitary adenoma: Treatment outcome and prognostic factors, Int J Radiat Oncol Biol Phys 30 (3) (1994) 557–565.

[338] N.A. Samaan, M.M. Bakdash, J.B. Caderao, A. Cangir, R.H. Jesse Jr., A.J. Ballantyne, Hypopituitarism after external irradiation. Evidence for both hypothalamic and pituitary origin, Ann Intern Med 83 (6) (1975) 771–777.

[339] J.W. Tomlinson, N. Holden, R.K. Hills, K. Wheatley, R.N. Clayton, A.S. Bates, et al., Association between premature mortality and hypopituitarism. West Midlands Prospective Hypopituitary Study Group, Lancet 357 (9254) (2001) 425–431.

[340] G. Becker, M. Kocher, R.D. Kortmann, F. Paulsen, B. Jeremic, R.P. Muller, et al., Radiation therapy in the multimodal treatment approach of pituitary adenoma, Strahlenther Onkol 178 (4) (2002) 173–186.

[341] M. Brada, L. Burchell, S. Ashley, D. Traish, The incidence of cerebrovascular accidents in patients with pituitary adenoma, Int J Radiat Oncol Biol Phys 45 (3) (1999) 693–698.

[342] S.C. Rush, M.J. Kupersmith, I. Lerch, P. Cooper, J. Ransohoff, J. Newall, Neuro-ophthalmological assessment of vision before and after radiation therapy alone for pituitary macroadenomas, J Neurosurg 72 (4) (1990) 594–599.

[343] E.M. Erfurth, B. Bulow, Z. Mikoczy, G. Svahn-Tapper, L. Hagmar, Is there an increase in second brain tumours after surgery and irradiation for a pituitary tumour? Clin Endocrinol (Oxf) 55 (5) (2001) 613–616.

[344] G. Minniti, D. Traish, S. Ashley, A. Gonsalves, M. Brada, Risk of second brain tumor after conservative surgery and radiotherapy for pituitary adenoma: Update after an additional 10 years, J Clin Endocrinol Metab 90 (2) (2005) 800–804.

[345] R.W. Tsang, N.J. Laperriere, W.J. Simpson, J. Brierley, T. Panzarella, H.S. Smyth, Glioma arising after radiation therapy for pituitary adenoma. A report of four patients and estimation of risk, Cancer 72 (7) (1993) 2227–2233.

[346] M. Hayashi, M. Izawa, H. Hiyama, S. Nakamura, S. Atsuchi, H. Sato, et al., Gamma knife radiosurgery for pituitary adenomas, Stereotact Funct Neurosurg 72 (Suppl 1) (1999) 111–118.

[347] M. Izawa, M. Hayashi, K. Nakaya, H. Satoh, T. Ochiai, T. Hori, et al., Gamma knife radiosurgery for pituitary adenomas, J Neurosurg 93 (Suppl 3) (2000) 19–22.

[348] Y.L. Lim, W. Leem, T.S. Kim, B.A. Rhee, G.K. Kim, Four years' experiences in the treatment of pituitary adenomas with gamma knife radiosurgery, Stereotact Funct Neurosurg 70 (Suppl 1) (1998) 95–109.

[349] R. Martinez, G. Bravo, J. Burzaco, G. Rey, Pituitary tumors and gamma knife surgery. Clinical experience with more than two years of follow-up, Stereotact Funct Neurosurg 70 (Suppl 1) (1998) 110–118.

[350] M. Mokry, S. Ramschak-Schwarzer, J. Simbrunner, J.C. Ganz, G. Pendl, A six year experience with the postoperative radiosurgical management of pituitary adenomas, Stereotact Funct Neurosurg 72 (Suppl 1) (1999) 88–100.

[351] C. Hoybye, E. Grenback, T. Rahn, M. Degerblad, M. Thoren, A.L. Hulting, Adrenocorticotropic hormone-producing pituitary tumors: 12- to 22-year follow-up after treatment with stereotactic radiosurgery, Neurosurgery 49 (2) (2001) 284–291, discussion 291–292.

[352] J.P. Sheehan, A. Niranjan, J.M. Sheehan, J.A. Jane Jr., E.R. Laws, D. Kondziolka, et al., Stereotactic radiosurgery for pituitary adenomas: An intermediate review of its safety, efficacy, and role in the neurosurgical treatment armamentarium, J Neurosurg 102 (4) (2005) 678–691.

[353] J.C. Chen, S.L. Giannotta, C. Yu, Z. Petrovich, M.L. Levy, M.L. Apuzzo, Radiosurgical management of benign cavernous sinus tumors: Dose profiles and acute complications, Neurosurgery 48 (5) (2001) 1022–1030, discussion 1030–1032.

[354] F.J. Monsma Jr., L.D. McVittie, C.R. Gerfen, L.C. Mahan, D.R. Sibley, Multiple D_2 dopamine receptors produced by alternative RNA splicing, Nature 342 (6252) (1989) 926–929.

[355] P. De Camilli, D. Macconi, A. Spada, Dopamine inhibits adenylate cyclase in human prolactin-secreting pituitary adenomas, Nature 278 (5701) (1979) 252–254.

[356] S.E. Senogles, The D_2 dopamine receptor isoforms signal through distinct Gi alpha proteins to inhibit adenylyl cyclase. A study with site-directed mutant Gi alpha proteins, J Biol Chem 269 (37) (1994) 23120–23127.

[357] L. Vallar, L.M. Vicentini, J. Meldolesi, Inhibition of inositol phosphate production is a late, Ca^{2+}-dependent effect of D_2 dopaminergic receptor activation in rat lactotroph cells, J Biol Chem 263 (21) (1988) 10127–10134.

[358] J.J. An, S.R. Cho, D.W. Jeong, K.W. Park, Y.S. Ahn, J.H. Baik, Anti-proliferative effects and cell death mediated by two isoforms of dopamine D_2 receptors in pituitary tumor cells, Mol Cell Endocrinol 206 (1–2) (2003) 49–62.

[359] B. Banihashemi, P.R. Albert, Dopamine-D_2S receptor inhibition of calcium influx, adenylyl cyclase, and mitogen-activated protein kinase in pituitary cells: Distinct G-alpha and G-betagamma requirements, Mol Endocrinol 16 (10) (2002) 2393–2404.

[360] C. Iaccarino, T.A. Samad, C. Mathis, H. Kercret, R. Picetti, E. Borrelli, Control of lactotrop proliferation by dopamine: Essential role of signaling through D_2 receptors and ERKs, Proc Nat Acad Sci USA 99 (22) (2002) 14530–14535.

[361] J.C. Liu, R.E. Baker, C. Sun, V.C. Sundmark, H.P. Elsholtz, Activation of Go-coupled dopamine D_2 receptors inhibits ERK1/ERK2 in pituitary cells. A key step in the transcriptional suppression of the prolactin gene, J Biol Chem 277 (39) (2002) 35819–35825.

[362] G.T. Tindall, K. Kovacs, E. Horvath, M.O. Thorner, Human prolactin-producing adenomas and bromocriptine: A histological, immunocytochemical, ultrastructural, and morphometric study, J Clin Endocrinol Metab 55 (6) (1982) 1178–1183.

[363] M.P. Aoki, A. Aoki, C.A. Maldonado, Sexual dimorphism of apoptosis in lactotrophs induced by bromocryptine, Histochem Cell Biol 116 (3) (2001) 215–222.

[364] A. Gruszka, J. Kunert-Radek, M. Pawlikowski, The effect of octreotide and bromocriptine on expression of a pro-apoptotic Bax protein in rat prolactinoma, Folia Histochem Cytobiol 42 (1) (2004) 35–39.

[365] A. Jaubert, F. Ichas, L. Bresson-Bepoldin, Signaling pathway involved in the pro-apoptotic effect of dopamine in the GH3 pituitary cell line, Neuroendocrinology 83 (2) (2006) 77–88.
[366] H. Kanasaki, K. Fukunaga, K. Takahashi, K. Miyazaki, E. Miyamoto, Involvement of p38 mitogen-activated protein kinase activation in bromocriptine-induced apoptosis in rat pituitary GH3 cells, Biol Reprod 62 (6) (2000) 1486–1494.
[367] L. Stefaneanu, K. Kovacs, B.W. Scheithauer, G. Kontogeorgos, D.L. Riehle, T.J. Sebo, et al., Effect of dopamine agonists on lactotroph adenomas of the human pituitary, Endocr Pathol 11 (4) (2000) 341–352.
[368] R. Wasko, M. Wolun-Cholewa, P. Bolko, M. Kotwicka, Effect of bromocriptine on cell apoptosis and proliferation in GH3 cell culture, Neuro Endocrinol Lett 25 (3) (2004) 223–228.
[369] A.C. Andreotti, E. Pianezzola, S. Persiani, M.A. Pacciarini, M. Strolin Benedetti, A.E. Pontiroli, Pharmacokinetics, pharmacodynamics, and tolerability of cabergoline, a prolactin-lowering drug, after administration of increasing oral doses (0.5, 1.0, and 1.5 milligrams) in healthy male volunteers, J Clin Endocrinol Metab 80 (3) (1995) 841–845.
[370] C. Ferrari, C. Barbieri, R. Caldara, M. Mucci, F. Codecasa, A. Paracchi, et al., Long-lasting prolactin-lowering effect of cabergoline, a new dopamine agonist, in hyperprolactinemic patients, J Clin Endocrinol Metab 63 (4) (1986) 941–945.
[371] G.B. Melis, M. Gambacciani, A.M. Paoletti, F. Beneventi, V. Mais, P. Baroldi, et al., Dose-related prolactin inhibitory effect of the new long-acting dopamine receptor agonist cabergoline in normal cycling, puerperal, and hyperprolactinemic women, J Clin Endocrinol Metab 65 (3) (1987) 541–545.
[372] J. Webster, G. Piscitelli, A. Polli, C.I. Ferrari, I. Ismail, M.F. Scanlon, A comparison of cabergoline and bromocriptine in the treatment of hyperprolactinemic amenorrhea. Cabergoline Comparative Study Group, N Engl J Med 331 (14) (1994) 904–909.
[373] E. Delgrange, T. Daems, J. Verhelst, R. Abs, D. Maiter, Characterization of resistance to the prolactin-lowering effects of cabergoline in macroprolactinomas: A study in 122 patients, Eur J Endocrinol 160 (5) (2009) 747–752.
[374] M. Ono, N. Miki, T. Kawamata, R. Makino, K. Amano, T. Seki, et al., Prospective study of high-dose cabergoline treatment of prolactinomas in 150 patients, J Clin Endocrinol Metab 93 (12) (2008) 4721–4727.
[375] A. Di Sarno, M.L. Landi, P. Cappabianca, F. Di Salle, F.W. Rossi, R. Pivonello, et al., Resistance to cabergoline as compared with bromocriptine in hyperprolactinemia: Prevalence, clinical definition, and therapeutic strategy, J Clin Endocrinol Metab 86 (11) (2001) 5256–5261.
[376] E. Ciccarelli, M. Giusti, C. Miola, F. Potenzoni, D. Sghedoni, F. Camanni, et al., Effectiveness and tolerability of long term treatment with cabergoline, a new long-lasting ergoline derivative, in hyperprolactinemic patients, J Clin Endocrinol Metab 69 (4) (1989) 725–728.
[377] A. Colao, A. Di Sarno, M.L. Landi, S. Cirillo, F. Sarnacchiaro, G. Facciolli, et al., Long-term and low-dose treatment with cabergoline induces macroprolactinoma shrinkage, J Clin Endocrinol Metab 82 (11) (1997) 3574–3579.
[378] E. Delgrange, D. Maiter, J. Donckier, Effects of the dopamine agonist cabergoline in patients with prolactinoma intolerant or resistant to bromocriptine, Eur J Endocrinol 134 (4) (1996) 454–456.
[379] C. Ferrari, A. Mattei, G.B. Melis, A. Paracchi, M. Muratori, G. Faglia, et al., Cabergoline: Long-acting oral treatment of hyperprolactinemic disorders, J Clin Endocrinol Metab 68 (6) (1989) 1201–1206.
[380] C. Ferrari, A. Paracchi, A.M. Mattei, S. de Vincentiis, A. D'Alberton, P. Crosignani, Cabergoline in the long-term therapy of hyperprolactinemic disorders, Acta Endocrinol (Copenh) 126 (6) (1992) 489–494.
[381] S. Cannavo, L. Curto, S. Squadrito, B. Almoto, A. Vieni, F. Trimarchi, Cabergoline: A first-choice treatment in patients with previously untreated prolactin-secreting pituitary adenoma, J Endocrinol Invest 22 (5) (1999) 354–359.
[382] A. Colao, A. Di Sarno, M.L. Landi, F. Scavuzzo, P. Cappabianca, R. Pivonello, et al., Macroprolactinoma shrinkage during cabergoline treatment is greater in naive patients than in patients pretreated with other dopamine agonists: A prospective study in 110 patients, J Clin Endocrinol Metab 85 (6) (2000) 2247–2252.
[383] C.I. Ferrari, R. Abs, J.S. Bevan, G. Brabant, E. Ciccarelli, T. Motta, et al., Treatment of macroprolactinoma with cabergoline: A study of 85 patients, Clin Endocrinol (Oxf) 46 (4) (1997) 409–413.
[384] N. Pontikides, G.E. Krassas, E. Nikopoulou, T. Kaltsas, Cabergoline as a first-line treatment in newly diagnosed macroprolactinomas, Pituitary 2 (4) (2000) 277–281.
[385] C.P. Rains, H.M. Bryson, A. Fitton, Cabergoline, A review of its pharmacological properties and therapeutic potential in the treatment of hyperprolactinaemia and inhibition of lactation, Drugs 49 (2) (1995) 255–279.
[386] J. Webster, A comparative review of the tolerability profiles of dopamine agonists in the treatment of hyperprolactinaemia and inhibition of lactation, Drug Saf 14 (4) (1996) 228–238.
[387] M.H. Bhatt, S.P. Keenan, J.A. Fleetham, D.B. Calne, Pleuropulmonary disease associated with dopamine agonist therapy, Ann Neurol 30 (4) (1991) 613–616.
[388] E. Frans, R. Dom, M. Demedts, Pleuropulmonary changes during treatment of Parkinson's disease with a long-acting ergot derivative, cabergoline, Eur Respir J 5 (2) (1992) 263–265.
[389] S.H. Guptha, A.D. Promnitz, Pleural effusion and thickening due to cabergoline use in a patient with Parkinson's disease, Eur J Intern Med 16 (2) (2005) 129–131.
[390] L.H. Ling, J.E. Ahlskog, T.M. Munger, A.H. Limper, J.K. Oh, Constrictive pericarditis and pleuropulmonary disease linked to ergot dopamine agonist therapy (cabergoline) for Parkinson's disease, Mayo Clin Proc 74 (4) (1999) 371–375.
[391] A.M. Pritchett, J.F. Morrison, W.D. Edwards, H.V. Schaff, H.M. Connolly, R.E. Espinosa, Valvular heart disease in patients taking pergolide, Mayo Clin Proc 77 (12) (2002) 1280–1286.
[392] J. Horvath, R.D. Fross, G. Kleiner-Fisman, R. Lerch, H. Stalder, S. Liaudat, et al., Severe multivalvular heart disease: A new complication of the ergot derivative dopamine agonists, Mov Disord 19 (6) (2004) 656–662.
[393] G. Simonis, J.T. Fuhrmann, R.H. Strasser, Meta-analysis of heart valve abnormalities in Parkinson's disease patients treated with dopamine agonists, Mov Disord 22 (13) (2007) 1936–1942.
[394] J. Serratrice, P. Disdier, G. Habib, F. Viallet, P.J. Weiller, Fibrotic valvular heart disease subsequent to bromocriptine treatment, Cardiol Rev 10 (6) (2002) 334–336.
[395] K. Yamashiro, M. Komine-Kobayashi, T. Hatano, T. Urabe, H. Mochizuki, N. Hattori, et al., The frequency of cardiac valvular regurgitation in Parkinson's disease, Mov Disord 23 (7) (2008) 935–941.
[396] B.L. Roth, Drugs and valvular heart disease, N Engl J Med 356 (1) (2007) 6–9.
[397] R. Schade, F. Andersohn, S. Suissa, W. Haverkamp, E. Garbe, Dopamine agonists and the risk of cardiac-valve regurgitation, N Engl J Med 356 (1) (2007) 29–38.

[398] A. Antonini, W. Poewe, Fibrotic heart-valve reactions to dopamine-agonist treatment in Parkinson's disease, Lancet Neurol 6 (9) (2007) 826–829.
[399] J.P. Singh, J.C. Evans, D. Levy, M.G. Larson, L.A. Freed, D.L. Fuller, et al., Prevalence and clinical determinants of mitral, tricuspid, and aortic regurgitation (the Framingham Heart Study), Am J Cardiol 83 (6) (1999) 897–902.
[400] C.L. Reid, H. Anton-Culver, C. Yunis, J.M. Gardin, Prevalence and clinical correlates of isolated mitral, isolated aortic regurgitation, and both in adults aged 21 to 35 years (from the CARDIA study), Am J Cardiol 99 (6) (2007) 830–834.
[401] P. Lancellotti, E. Livadariu, M. Markov, A.F. Daly, M.C. Burlacu, D. Betea, et al., Cabergoline and the risk of valvular lesions in endocrine disease, Eur J Endocrinol 159 (1) (2008) 1–5.
[402] M. Kars, V. Delgado, E.R. Holman, R.A. Feelders, J.W. Smit, J.A. Romijn, et al., Aortic valve calcification and mild tricuspid regurgitation but no clinical heart disease after 8 years of dopamine agonist therapy for prolactinoma, J Clin Endocrinol Metab 93 (9) (2008) 3348–3356.
[403] S. Vallette, K. Serri, J. Rivera, P. Santagata, S. Delorme, N. Garfield, et al., Long-term cabergoline therapy is not associated with valvular heart disease in patients with prolactinomas, Pituitary 12 (3) (2009) 153–157.
[404] F. Bogazzi, S. Buralli, L. Manetti, V. Raffaelli, T. Cigni, M. Lombardi, et al., Treatment with low doses of cabergoline is not associated with increased prevalence of cardiac valve regurgitation in patients with hyperprolactinaemia, Int J Clin Pract 62 (12) (2008) 1864–1869.
[405] L.B. Nachtigall, E. Valassi, J. Lo, D. McCarty, J. Passeri, B.M. Biller, et al., Gender effects on cardiac valvular function in hyperprolactinaemic patients receiving cabergoline: A retrospective study, Clin Endocrinol (Oxf) 72 (1) (2010) 53–58.
[406] N. Herring, C. Szmigielski, H. Becher, N. Karavitaki, J.A. Wass, Valvular heart disease and the use of cabergoline for the treatment of prolactinoma, Clin Endocrinol (Oxf) 70 (1) (2009) 104–108.
[407] A. Colao, M. Galderisi, A. Di Sarno, M. Pardo, M. Gaccione, M. D'Andrea, et al., Increased prevalence of tricuspid regurgitation in patients with prolactinomas chronically treated with cabergoline, J Clin Endocrinol Metab 93 (10) (2008) 3777–3784.
[408] A. Wakil, A.S. Rigby, A.L. Clark, A. Kallvikbacka-Bennett, S.L. Atkin, Low dose cabergoline for hyperprolactinaemia is not associated with clinically significant valvular heart disease, Eur J Endocrinol 159 (4) (2008) R11–R14.
[409] J.K. Devin, V.T. Lakhani, B.F. Byrd 3rd, L.S. Blevins Jr., Prevalence of valvular heart disease in a cohort of patients taking cabergoline for management of hyperprolactinemia, Endocr Pract 14 (6) (2008) 672–677.
[410] E. Valassi, A. Klibanski, B.M. Biller, Clinical review: Potential cardiac valve effects of dopamine agonists in hyperprolactinemia, J Clin Endocrinol Metab 95 (3) (2010) 1025–1033.
[411] H.F. Schran, S.I. Bhuta, H.J. Schwarz, M.O. Thorner, The pharmacokinetics of bromocriptine in man, Adv Biochem Psychopharmacol 23 (1980) 125–139.
[412] A.R. Badano, H.R. Miechi, A. Mirkin, O.A. Arcangeli, N.J. Aparicio, A. Rodriguez, et al., Bromocriptine in the treatment of hyperprolactinemic amenorrhea, Fertil Steril 31 (2) (1979) 124–129.
[413] T. Bergh, S.J. Nillius, L. Wide, Bromocriptine treatment of 42 hyperprolactinaemic women with secondary amenorrhoea, Acta Endocrinol (Copenh) 88 (3) (1978) 435–451.
[414] P.G. Crosignani, C. Ferrari, A. Liuzzi, R. Benco, A. Mattei, P. Rampini, et al., Treatment of hyperprolactinemic states with different drugs: A study with bromocriptine, metergoline, and lisuride, Fertil Steril 37 (1) (1982) 61–67.
[415] P. Moriondo, P. Travaglini, M. Nissim, A. Conti, G. Faglia, Bromocriptine treatment of microprolactinomas: Evidence of stable prolactin decrease after drug withdrawal, J Clin Endocrinol Metab 60 (4) (1985) 764–772.
[416] M. Moro, C. Maraschini, P. Toja, A. Masala, S. Alagna, P.P. Rovasio, et al., Comparison between a slow-release oral preparation of bromocriptine and regular bromocriptine in patients with hyperprolactinemia: A double blind, double dummy study, Horm Res 35 (3-4) (1991) 137–141.
[417] T. Sabuncu, E. Arikan, E. Tasan, H. Hatemi, Comparison of the effects of cabergoline and bromocriptine on prolactin levels in hyperprolactinemic patients, Intern Med 40 (9) (2001) 857–861.
[418] M.O. Thorner, H.F. Schran, W.S. Evans, A.D. Rogol, J.L. Morris, R.M. MacLeod, A broad spectrum of prolactin suppression by bromocriptine in hyperprolactinemic women: A study of serum prolactin and bromocriptine levels after acute and chronic administration of bromocriptine, J Clin Endocrinol Metab 50 (6) (1980) 1026–1033.
[419] P.G. Crosignani, A.M. Mattei, V. Severini, V. Cavioni, P. Maggioni, G. Testa, Long-term effects of time, medical treatment and pregnancy in 176 hyperprolactinemic women, Eur J Obstet Gynecol Reprod Biol 44 (3) (1992) 175–180.
[420] O. Essais, R. Bouguerra, J. Hamzaoui, Z. Marrakchi, S. Hadjri, S. Chamakhi, et al., Efficacy and safety of bromocriptine in the treatment of macroprolactinomas, Ann Endocrinol (Paris) 63 (6 Pt 1) (2002) 524–531.
[421] A. Liuzzi, D. Dallabonzana, G. Oppizzi, G.G. Verde, R. Cozzi, P. Chiodini, et al., Low doses of dopamine agonists in the long-term treatment of macroprolactinomas, N Engl J Med 313 (11) (1985) 656–659.
[422] J.O. Sieck, N.L. Niles, J.R. Jinkins, O. Al-Mefty, S. el-Akkad, N. Woodhouse, Extrasellar prolactinomas: Successful management of 24 patients using bromocriptine, Horm Res 23 (3) (1986) 167–176.
[423] J.W. van't Verlaat, I. Lancranjan, M.J. Hendriks, R.J. Croughs, Primary treatment of macroprolactinomas with Parlodel LAR, Acta Endocrinol (Copenh) 119 (1) (1988) 51–55.
[424] J.A. Wass, J. Williams, M. Charlesworth, D.P. Kingsley, A.M. Halliday, I. Doniach, et al., Bromocriptine in management of large pituitary tumours, Br Med J (Clin Res Ed) 284 (6333) (1982) 1908–1911.
[425] J.S. Bevan, J. Webster, C.W. Burke, M.F. Scanlon, Dopamine agonists and pituitary tumor shrinkage, Endocr Rev 13 (2) (1992) 220–240.
[426] D.L. Barrow, G.T. Tindall, K. Kovacs, M.O. Thorner, E. Horvath, J.C. Hoffman Jr., Clinical and pathological effects of bromocriptine on prolactin-secreting and other pituitary tumors, J Neurosurg 60 (1) (1984) 1–7.
[427] J.F. Bonneville, D. Poulignot, F. Cattin, M. Couturier, E. Mollet, J.L. Dietemann, Computed tomographic demonstration of the effects of bromocriptine on pituitary microadenoma size, Radiology 143 (2) (1982) 451–455.
[428] B. Corenblum, P.J. Taylor, Long-term follow-up of hyperprolactinemic women treated with bromocriptine, Fertil Steril 40 (5) (1983) 596–599.
[429] R. Demura, O. Kubo, H. Demura, K. Shizume, K. Kitamura, Changes in computed tomographic findings in microprolactinomas before and after bromocriptine, Acta Endocrinol (Copenh) 110 (3) (1985) 308–312.
[430] R. Fahlbusch, M. Buchfelder, U. Schrell, Short-term preoperative treatment of macroprolactinomas by dopamine agonists, J Neurosurg 67 (6) (1987) 807–815.

[431] R.W. Gasser, E. Mueller-Holzner, F. Skrabal, G. Finkenstedt, U. Mayr, M. Tabarelli, et al., Macroprolactinomas and functionless pituitary tumours. Immunostaining and effect of dopamine agonist therapy, Acta Endocrinol (Copenh) 116 (2) (1987) 253–259.

[432] B.L. Horowitz, D.J. Hamilton, C.J. Sommers, R.N. Bryan, A.E. Boyd 3rd, Effect of bromocriptine and pergolide on pituitary tumor size and serum prolactin, Am J Neuroradiol 4 (3) (1983) 415–417.

[433] D.G. Johnston, R.W. Prescott, P. Kendall-Taylor, K. Hall, A.L. Crombie, R. Hall, et al., Hyperprolactinemia. Long-term effects of bromocriptine, Am J Med 75 (5) (1983) 868–874.

[434] A.M. McGregor, M.F. Scanlon, R. Hall, K. Hall, Effects of bromocriptine on pituitary tumour size, Br Med J 2 (6192) (1979) 700–703.

[435] M. Nissim, B. Ambrosi, V. Bernasconi, G. Giannattasio, M.A. Giovanelli, M. Bassetti, et al., Bromocriptine treatment of macroprolactinomas: Studies on the time course of tumor shrinkage and morphology, J Endocrinol Invest 5 (6) (1982) 409–415.

[436] P.T. Pullan, W.M. Carroll, T.M. Chakera, M.S. Khangure, R.J. Vaughan, Management of extra-sellar pituitary tumours with bromocriptine: Comparison of prolactin secreting and non-functioning tumours using half-field visual evoked potentials and computerised tomography, Aust NZ J Med 15 (2) (1985) 203–208.

[437] L.G. Sobrinho, M.C. Nunes, C. Calhaz-Jorge, J.C. Mauricio, M.A. Santos, Effect of treatment with bromocriptine on the size and activity of prolactin producing pituitary tumours, Acta Endocrinol (Copenh) 96 (1) (1981) 24–29.

[438] R.F. Spark, R. Baker, D.C. Bienfang, R. Bergland, Bromocriptine reduces pituitary tumor size and hypersection. Requiem for pituitary surgery? JAMA 247 (3) (1982) 311–316.

[439] A. Warfield, D.M. Finkel, N.J. Schatz, P.J. Savino, P.J. Snyder, Bromocriptine treatment of prolactin-secreting pituitary adenomas may restore pituitary function, Ann Intern Med 101 (6) (1984) 783–785.

[440] F. Wollesen, T. Andersen, A. Karle, Size reduction of extrasellar pituitary tumors during bromocriptine treatment, Ann Intern Med 96 (3) (1982) 281–286.

[441] M.O. Thorner, W.H. Martin, A.D. Rogol, J.L. Morris, R.L. Perryman, B.P. Conway, et al., Rapid regression of pituitary prolactinomas during bromocriptine treatment, J Clin Endocrinol Metab 51 (3) (1980) 438–445.

[442] D.G. Kissner, J.C. Jarrett, Side effects of bromocriptine, N Engl J Med 302 (13) (1980) 749–750.

[443] W. Dutz, Drugs stimulion dopamine receptors, in: M.N.G. Dukes (Ed.), Meylers side effects of drugs, an encyclopedia of adverse reactions and interactions, (twelfth ed.), Elsevier, Amsterdam, 1992, pp. 317–318.

[444] J.A. Wass, M.O. Thorner, G.M. Besser, Letter: Digital vasospasm with bromocriptine, Lancet 1 (7969) (1976) 1135.

[445] C.M. Le Feuvre, A.J. Isaacs, O.S. Frank, Bromocriptine-induced psychosis in acromegaly, Br Med J (Clin Res Ed) 285 (6351) (1982) 1315.

[446] K.C. Pearson, Mental disorders from low-dose bromocriptine, N Engl J Med 305 (3) (1981) 173.

[447] T.H. Turner, J.C. Cookson, J.A. Wass, P.L. Drury, P.A. Price, G.M. Besser, Psychotic reactions during treatment of pituitary tumours with dopamine agonists, Br Med J (Clin Res Ed) 289 (6452) (1984) 1101–1103.

[448] N.G. McElvaney, P.G. Wilcox, A. Churg, J.A. Fleetham, Pleuropulmonary disease during bromocriptine treatment of Parkinson's disease, Arch Intern Med 148 (10) (1988) 2231–2236.

[449] F. Afshar, A. Thomas, Bromocriptine-induced cerebrospinal fluid rhinorrhea, Surg Neurol 18 (1) (1982) 61–63.

[450] S.L. Aronoff, W.H. Daughaday, E.R. Laws Jr., Bromocriptine treatment of prolactinomas, N Engl J Med 300 (24) (1979) 1391.

[451] D.S. Baskin, C.B. Wilson, CSF rhinorrhea after bromocriptine for prolactinoma, N Engl J Med 306 (3) (1982) 178.

[452] J.G. Kok, A.K. Bartelink, B.P. Schulte, A. Smals, G. Pieters, E. Meyer, et al., Cerebrospinal fluid rhinorrhea during treatment with bromocriptine for prolactinoma, Neurology 35 (8) (1985) 1193–1195.

[453] A.M. Landolt, Cerebrospinal fluid rhinorrhea: A complication of therapy for invasive prolactinomas, Neurosurgery 11 (3) (1982) 395–401.

[454] K.S. Leong, P.M. Foy, A.C. Swift, S.L. Atkin, D.R. Hadden, I.A. MacFarlane, CSF rhinorrhoea following treatment with dopamine agonists for massive invasive prolactinomas, Clin Endocrinol (Oxf) 52 (1) (2000) 43–49.

[455] S.G. Suliman, A. Gurlek, J.V. Byrne, N. Sullivan, G. Thanabalasingham, S. Cudlip, et al., Nonsurgical cerebrospinal fluid rhinorrhea in invasive macroprolactinoma: Incidence, radiological, and clinicopathological features, J Clin Endocrinol Metab 92 (10) (2007) 3829–3835.

[456] P. Cappabianca, S. Lodrini, G. Felisati, C. Peca, R. Cozzi, A. Di Sarno, et al., Cabergoline-induced CSF rhinorrhea in patients with macroprolactinoma. Report of three cases, J Endocrinol Invest 24 (3) (2001) 183–187.

[457] O. Barlas, C. Bayindir, K. Hepgul, M. Can, T. Kiris, E. Sencer, et al., Bromocriptine-induced cerebrospinal fluid fistula in patients with macroprolactinomas: Report of three cases and a review of the literature, Surg Neurol 41 (6) (1994) 486–489.

[458] R.T. Netea-Maier, E.J. van Lindert, H. Timmers, E.L. Schakenraad, J.A. Grotenhuis, A.R. Hermus, Cerebrospinal fluid leakage as a complication of treatment with cabergoline for macroprolactinomas, J Endocrinol Invest 29 (11) (2006) 1001–1005.

[459] L. Lemberger, R. Crabtree, J.T. Callaghan, Pergolide, a potent long-acting dopamine-receptor agonist, Clin Pharmacol Ther 27 (5) (1980) 642–651.

[460] R.E. Blackwell, E.L. Bradley Jr., L.B. Kline, E.R. Duvall, J.J. Vitek, G.W. DeVane, et al., Comparison of dopamine agonists in the treatment of hyperprolactinemic syndromes: A multicenter study, Fertil Steril 39 (6) (1983) 744–748.

[461] S. Franks, P.M. Horrocks, S.S. Lynch, W.R. Butt, D.R. London, Treatment of hyperprolactinaemia with pergolide mesylate: Acute effects and preliminary evaluation of long-term treatment, Lancet 2 (8248) (1981) 659–661.

[462] A. Grossman, P.M. Bouloux, R. Loneragan, L.H. Rees, J.A. Wass, G.M. Besser, Comparison of the clinical activity of mesulergine and pergolide in the treatment of hyperprolactinaemia, Clin Endocrinol (Oxf) 22 (5) (1985) 611–616.

[463] P. Kendall-Taylor, K. Hall, D.G. Johnston, R.W. Prescott, Reduction in size of prolactin-secreting tumours in men treated with pergolide, Br Med J (Clin Res Ed) 285 (6340) (1982) 465–467.

[464] D.L. Kleinberg, A.E. Boyd 3rd, S. Wardlaw, A.G. Frantz, A. George, N. Bryan, et al., Pergolide for the treatment of pituitary tumors secreting prolactin or growth hormone, N Engl J Med 309 (12) (1983) 704–709.

[465] O.A. Kletzky, R. Borenstein, G.N. Mileikowsky, Pergolide and bromocriptine for the treatment of patients with hyperprolactinemia, Am J Obstet Gynecol 154 (2) (1986) 431–435.

[466] P.U. Freda, C.I. Andreadis, A.G. Khandji, M. Khoury, J.N. Bruce, T.P. Jacobs, et al., Long-term treatment of prolactin-secreting macroadenomas with pergolide, J Clin Endocrinol Metab 85 (1) (2000) 8–13.

[467] S.W. Lamberts, R.F. Quik, A comparison of the efficacy and safety of pergolide and bromocriptine in the treatment of hyperprolactinemia, J Clin Endocrinol Metab 72 (3) (1991) 635–641.

[468] M.E. Molitch, The cabergoline-resistant prolactinoma patient: New challenges, J Clin Endocrinol Metab 93 (12) (2008) 4643–4645.

[469] A. Di Sarno, M.L. Landi, P. Marzullo, C. Di Somma, R. Pivonello, G. Cerbone, et al., The effect of quinagolide and cabergoline, two selective dopamine receptor type 2 agonists, in the treatment of prolactinomas, Clin Endocrinol (Oxf) 53 (1) (2000) 53–60.

[470] D.A. De Luis, A. Becerra, M. Lahera, J.I. Botella, V.C. Valero, A randomized cross-over study comparing cabergoline and quinagolide in the treatment of hyperprolactinemic patients, J Endocrinol Invest 23 (7) (2000) 428–434.

[471] B. Crottaz, A. Uske, M.J. Reymond, F. Rey, R.A. Siegel, J. Brownell, et al., CV 205-502 treatment of macroprolactinomas, J Endocrinol Invest 14 (9) (1991) 757–762.

[472] Y. Khalfallah, B. Claustrat, M. Grochowicki, F. Flocard, S. Horlait, P. Serusclat, et al., Effects of a new prolactin inhibitor, CV 205-502, in the treatment of human macroprolactinomas, J Clin Endocrinol Metab 71 (2) (1990) 354–359.

[473] A. Kvistborg, J. Halse, S. Bakke, T. Bjoro, E. Hansen, O. Djoseland, et al., Long-term treatment of macroprolactinomas with CV 205-502, Acta Endocrinol (Copenh) 128 (4) (1993) 301–307.

[474] O. Serri, H. Beauregard, J. Lesage, L. Pedneault, R. Comtois, N. Jilwan, et al., Long term treatment with CV 205-502 in patients with prolactin-secreting pituitary macroadenomas, J Clin Endocrinol Metab 71 (3) (1990) 682–687.

[475] T. Svoboda, A. Luger, E. Knosp, G. Geyer, [Treatment of prolactinoma with a new dopamine agonist], Dtsch Med Wochenschr 116 (33) (1991) 1224–1227.

[476] A.J. van der Lely, J. Brownell, S.W. Lamberts, The efficacy and tolerability of CV 205-502 (a nonergot dopaminergic drug) in macroprolactinoma patients and in prolactinoma patients intolerant to bromocriptine, J Clin Endocrinol Metab 72 (5) (1991) 1136–1141.

[477] J.W. van't Verlaat, R.J. Croughs, J. Brownell, Treatment of macroprolactinomas with a new non-ergot, long-acting dopaminergic drug, CV 205-502, Clin Endocrinol (Oxf) 33 (5) (1990) 619–624.

[478] M.L. Vance, J.R. Cragun, C. Reimnitz, R.J. Chang, E. Rashef, R.E. Blackwell, et al., CV 205-502 treatment of hyperprolactinemia, J Clin Endocrinol Metab 68 (2) (1989) 336–339.

[479] P.S. Barnett, E. Palazidou, J.P. Miell, P.B. Coskeran, J. Butler, J.M. Dawson, et al., Endocrine function, psychiatric and clinical consequences in patients with macroprolactinomas after long-term treatment with the new non-ergot dopamine agonist CV205-502, Q J Med 81 (295) (1991) 891–906.

[480] M.M. Esiri, J.S. Bevan, C.W. Burke, C.B. Adams, Effect of bromocriptine treatment on the fibrous tissue content of prolactin-secreting and nonfunctioning macroadenomas of the pituitary gland, J Clin Endocrinol Metab 63 (2) (1986) 383–388.

[481] T. Bergh, S.J. Nillius, L. Wide, Menstrual function and serum prolactin levels after long-term bromocriptine treatment of hyperprolactinaemic amenorrhoea, Clin Endocrinol (Oxf) 16 (6) (1982) 587–593.

[482] D.G. Johnston, K. Hall, P. Kendall-Taylor, D. Patrick, M. Watson, D.B. Cook, Effect of dopamine agonist withdrawal after long-term therapy in prolactinomas. Studies with high-definition computerised tomography, Lancet 2 (8396) (1984) 187–192.

[483] W.S. Maxson, M. Dudzinski, S.H. Handwerger, C.B. Hammond, Hyperprolactinemic response after bromocriptine withdrawal in women with prolactin-secreting pituitary tumors, Fertil Steril 41 (2) (1984) 218–223.

[484] V.Q. Passos, J.J. Souza, N.R. Musolino, M.D. Bronstein, Long-term follow-up of prolactinomas: Normoprolactinemia after bromocriptine withdrawal, J Clin Endocrinol Metab 87 (8) (2002) 3578–3582.

[485] W. Winkelmann, B. Allolio, U. Deuss, D. Heesen, D. Kaulen, Persisting normoprolactinemia after withdrawal of bromocriptine long-term therapy in patients with prolactinomas, in: R.M. MacLeod, M.O. Thorner, U. Scapagnini (Eds.), Basic and Clinical Correlates, Liviana Press, Padova, 1985, pp. 817–822.

[486] A. Zarate, E.S. Canales, C. Cano, C.J. Pilonieta, Follow-up of patients with prolactinomas after discontinuation of long-term therapy with bromocriptine, Acta Endocrinol (Copenh) 104 (2) (1983) 139–142.

[487] M. Biswas, J. Smith, D. Jadon, P. McEwan, D.A. Rees, L.M. Evans, et al., Long-term remission following withdrawal of dopamine agonist therapy in subjects with microprolactinomas, Clin Endocrinol (Oxf) 63 (1) (2005) 26–31.

[488] J.W. van't Verlaat, R.J. Croughs, Withdrawal of bromocriptine after long-term therapy for macroprolactinomas; effect on plasma prolactin and tumour size, Clin Endocrinol (Oxf) 34 (3) (1991) 175–178.

[489] J.J. Orrego, W.F. Chandler, A.L. Barkan, Rapid re-expansion of a macroprolactinoma after early discontinuation of bromocriptine, Pituitary 3 (3) (2000) 189–192.

[490] M.O. Thorner, R.L. Perryman, A.D. Rogol, B.P. Conway, R.M. Macleod, I.S. Login, et al., Rapid changes of prolactinoma volume after withdrawal and reinstitution of bromocriptine, J Clin Endocrinol Metab 53 (3) (1981) 480–483.

[491] M.L. Vance, W.S. Evans, M.O. Thorner, Drugs five years later: Bromocriptine. Ann Intern Med 100 (1) (1984) 78–91.

[492] A. Colao, A. Di Sarno, P. Cappabianca, C. Di Somma, R. Pivonello, G. Lombardi, Withdrawal of long-term cabergoline therapy for tumoral and nontumoral hyperprolactinemia, N Engl J Med 349 (21) (2003) 2023–2033.

[493] O.M. Dekkers, J. Lagro, P. Burman, J.O. Jorgensen, J.A. Romijn, A.M. Pereira, Recurrence of hyperprolactinemia after withdrawal of dopamine agonists: Systematic review and meta-analysis, J Clin Endocrinol Metab 95 (1) (2010) 43–51.

[494] M. Muratori, M. Arosio, G. Gambino, C. Romano, O. Biella, G. Faglia, Use of cabergoline in the long-term treatment of hyperprolactinemic and acromegalic patients, J Endocrinol Invest 20 (9) (1997) 537–546.

[495] J. Kharlip, R. Salvatori, G. Yenokyan, G.S. Wand, Recurrence of hyperprolactinemia after withdrawal of long-term cabergoline therapy, J Clin Endocrinol Metab 94 (7) (2009) 2428–2436.

[496] M.E. Molitch, Pituitary gland: Can prolactinomas be cured medically? Nat Rev Endocrinol 6 (4) (2010) 186–188.

[497] M.E. Molitch, Dopamine resistance of prolactinomas, Pituitary 6 (1) (2003) 19–27.

[498] S.J. Hurel, P.E. Harris, A.M. McNicol, S. Foster, W.F. Kelly, P.H. Baylis, Metastatic prolactinoma: Effect of octreotide, cabergoline, carboplatin and etoposide; immunocytochemical analysis of proto-oncogene expression, J Clin Endocrinol Metab 82 (9) (1997) 2962–2965.

[499] D. Dallabonzana, B. Spelta, G. Oppizzi, C. Tonon, G. Luccarelli, P.G. Chiodini, et al., Reenlargement of macroprolactinomas during bromocriptine treatment: Report of two cases, J Endocrinol Invest 6 (1) (1983) 47–50.

[500] H.D. Breidahl, D.J. Topliss, J.W. Pike, Failure of bromocriptine to maintain reduction in size of a macroprolactinoma, Br Med J (Clin Res Ed) 287 (6390) (1983) 451–452.

[501] J. Winkelmann, U. Pagotto, M. Theodoropoulou, K. Tatsch, W. Saeger, A. Muller, et al., Retention of dopamine 2 receptor mRNA and absence of the protein in craniospinal and extracranial metastasis of a malignant prolactinoma: A case report, Eur J Endocrinol 146 (1) (2002) 81–88.

[502] E. Delgrange, J. Crabbe, J. Donckier, Late development of resistance to bromocriptine in a patient with macroprolactinoma, Horm Res 49 (5) (1998) 250–253.

[503] M.S. Mallea-Gil, C. Cristina, M.I. Perez-Millan, A.M. Villafane, C. Ballarino, G. Stalldecker, et al., Invasive giant prolactinoma with loss of therapeutic response to cabergoline: Expression of angiogenic markers, Endocr Pathol 20 (1) (2009) 35–40.

[504] S. Cannavo, L. Bartolone, A. Blandino, S. Spinella, S. Galatioto, F. Trimarchi, Shrinkage of a PRL-secreting pituitary macroadenoma resistant to cabergoline, J Endocrinol Invest 22 (4) (1999) 306–309.

[505] T. Brue, I. Pellegrini, A. Priou, I. Morange, P. Jaquet, Prolactinomas and resistance to dopamine agonists, Horm Res 38 (1-2) (1992) 84–89.

[506] I. Pellegrini, R. Rasolonjanahary, G. Gunz, P. Bertrand, S. Delivet, C.P. Jedynak, et al., Resistance to bromocriptine in prolactinomas, J Clin Endocrinol Metab 69 (3) (1989) 500–509.

[507] A. Mansour, J.H. Meador-Woodruff, J.R. Bunzow, O. Civelli, H. Akil, S.J. Watson, Localization of dopamine D2 receptor mRNA and D1 and D2 receptor binding in the rat brain and pituitary: An in situ hybridization-receptor autoradiographic analysis, J Neurosci 10 (8) (1990) 2587–2600.

[508] R. Dal Toso, B. Sommer, M. Ewert, A. Herb, D.B. Pritchett, A. Bach, et al., The dopamine D2 receptor: Two molecular forms generated by alternative splicing, Embo J 8 (13) (1989) 4025–4034.

[509] B. Giros, P. Sokoloff, M.P. Martres, J.F. Riou, L.J. Emorine, J.C. Schwartz, Alternative splicing directs the expression of two D2 dopamine receptor isoforms, Nature 342 (6252) (1989) 923–926.

[510] S.E. Senogles, T.L. Heimert, E.R. Odife, M.W. Quasney, A region of the third intracellular loop of the short form of the D2 dopamine receptor dictates Gi coupling specificity, J Biol Chem 279 (3) (2004) 1601–1606.

[511] J. Guiramand, J.P. Montmayeur, J. Ceraline, M. Bhatia, E. Borrelli, Alternative splicing of the dopamine D2 receptor directs specificity of coupling to G-proteins, J Biol Chem 270 (13) (1995) 7354–7358.

[512] S. Melmed, Mechanisms for pituitary tumorigenesis: The plastic pituitary, J Clin Invest 112 (11) (2003) 1603–1618.

[513] L.A. Kukstas, C. Domec, L. Bascles, J. Bonnet, D. Verrier, J.M. Israel, et al., Different expression of the two dopaminergic D2 receptors, D2415 and D2444, in two types of lactotroph each characterised by their response to dopamine, and modification of expression by sex steroids, Endocrinology 129 (2) (1991) 1101–1103.

[514] V.Q. Passos, M.A. Fortes, D. Giannella-Neto, M.D. Bronstein, Genes differentially expressed in prolactinomas responsive and resistant to dopamine agonists, Neuroendocrinology 89 (2) (2009) 163–170.

[515] K. Kovacs, L. Stefaneanu, E. Horvath, M. Buchfelder, R. Fahlbusch, W. Becker, Prolactin-producing pituitary tumor: Resistance to dopamine agonist therapy. Case report, J Neurosurg 82 (5) (1995) 886–890.

[516] P. Petrossians, W. de Herder, D. Kwekkeboom, G. Lamberigts, A. Stevenaert, A. Beckers, Malignant prolactinoma discovered by D2 receptor imaging, J Clin Endocrinol Metab 85 (1) (2000) 398–401.

[517] D. Guivarc'h, J.D. Vincent, P. Vernier, Alternative splicing of the D2 dopamine receptor messenger ribonucleic acid is modulated by activated sex steroid receptors in the MMQ prolactin cell line, Endocrinology 139 (10) (1998) 4213–4221.

[518] G. Hayes, T.J. Biden, L.A. Selbie, J. Shine, Structural subtypes of the dopamine D2 receptor are functionally distinct: Expression of the cloned D2A and D2B subtypes in a heterologous cell line, Mol Endocrinol 6 (6) (1992) 920–926.

[519] J.P. Montmayeur, J. Guiramand, E. Borrelli, Preferential coupling between dopamine D2 receptors and G-proteins, Mol Endocrinol 7 (2) (1993) 161–170.

[520] A. Barlier, I. Pellegrini-Bouiller, L. Caccavelli, G. Gunz, I. Morange-Ramos, P. Jaquet, et al., Abnormal transduction mechanisms in pituitary adenomas, Horm Res 47 (4–6) (1997) 227–234.

[521] C. Missale, P. Spano, Nerve growth factor in pituitary development and pituitary tumors, Front Neuroendocrinol 19 (2) (1998) 128–150.

[522] C. Missale, M. Losa, S. Sigala, A. Balsari, M. Giovanelli, P.F. Spano, Nerve growth factor controls proliferation and progression of human prolactinoma cell lines through an autocrine mechanism, Mol Endocrinol 10 (3) (1996) 272–285.

[523] C. Missale, F. Boroni, M. Frassine, A. Caruso, P. Spano, Nerve growth factor promotes the differentiation of pituitary mammotroph cells in vitro, Endocrinology 136 (3) (1995) 1205–1213.

[524] C. Fiorentini, N. Guerra, M. Facchetti, A. Finardi, L. Tiberio, L. Schiaffonati, et al., Nerve growth factor regulates dopamine D(2) receptor expression in prolactinoma cell lines via p75 (NGFR)-mediated activation of nuclear factor-kappaB, Mol Endocrinol 16 (2) (2002) 353–366.

[525] M. Facchetti, D. Uberti, M. Memo, C. Missale, Nerve growth factor restores p53 function in pituitary tumor cell lines via trkA-mediated activation of phosphatidylinositol 3-kinase, Mol Endocrinol 18 (1) (2004) 162–172.

[526] A. Colao, A. Di Sarno, F. Sarnacchiaro, D. Ferone, G. Di Renzo, B. Merola, et al., Prolactinomas resistant to standard dopamine agonists respond to chronic cabergoline treatment, J Clin Endocrinol Metab 82 (3) (1997) 876–883.

[527] V. Pascal-Vigneron, G. Weryha, M. Bosc, J. Leclere, [Hyperprolactinemic amenorrhea: Treatment with cabergoline versus bromocriptine. Results of a national multicenter randomized double-blind study], Presse Med 24 (16) (1995) 753–757.

[528] T. Brue, I. Pellegrini, G. Gunz, I. Morange, D. Dewailly, J. Brownell, et al., Effects of the dopamine agonist CV 205-502 in human prolactinomas resistant to bromocriptine, J Clin Endocrinol Metab 74 (3) (1992) 577–584.

[529] L. Duranteau, P. Chanson, A. Lavoinne, S. Horlait, J. Lubetzki, J.M. Kuhn, Effect of the new dopaminergic agonist CV 205-502 on plasma prolactin levels and tumour size in bromocriptine-resistant prolactinomas, Clin Endocrinol (Oxf) 34 (1) (1991) 25–29.

[530] B. Merola, F. Sarnacchiaro, A. Colao, C. Di Somma, A. Di Sarno, D. Ferone, et al., Positive response to compound CV 205-502 in hyperprolactinemic patients resistant to or intolerant of bromocriptine, Gynecol Endocrinol 8 (3) (1994) 175–181.

[531] R. Razzaq, D.J. O'Halloran, C.G. Beardwell, S.M. Shalet, The effects of CV205-502 in patients with hyperprolactinaemia intolerant and/or resistant to bromocriptine, Horm Res 39 (5–6) (1993) 218–222.

[532] V. Rohmer, E. Freneau, I. Morange, C. Simonetta, Efficacy of quinagolide in resistance to dopamine agonists: Results of a multicenter study. Club de l'Hypophyse, Ann Endocrinol (Paris) 61 (5) (2000) 411–417.

[533] Z. Shoham, R. Homburg, H.S. Jacobs, CV 205-502—effectiveness, tolerability, and safety over 24-month study, Fertil Steril 55 (3) (1991) 501—506.
[534] S.R. Ahmed, S.M. Shalet, Discordant responses of prolactinoma to two different dopamine agonists, Clin Endocrinol (Oxf) 24 (4) (1986) 421—426.
[535] M. Berezin, D. Avidan, E. Baron, Long-term pergolide treatment of hyperprolactinemic patients previously unsuccessfully treated with dopaminergic drugs, Isr J Med Sci 27 (7) (1991) 375—379.
[536] P.G. Crosignani, C. Ferrari, C. Scarduelli, M.C. Picciotti, R. Caldara, A. Malinverni, Spontaneous and induced pregnancies in hyperprolactinemic women, Obstet Gynecol 58 (6) (1981) 708—713.
[537] G. Leyendecker, T. Struve, E.J. Plotz, Induction of ovulation with chronic intermittent (pulsatile) administration of LH-RH in women with hypothalamic and hyperprolactinemic amenorrhea, Arch Gynecol 229 (3) (1980) 177—190.
[538] E. Radwanska, H.H. McGarrigle, V. Little, D. Lawrence, S. Sarris, G.I. Swyer, Induction of ovulation in women with hyperprolactinemic amenorrhea using clomiphene and human chorionic gonadotropin of bromocriptine, Fertil Steril 32 (2) (1979) 187—192.
[539] J. Webster, G. Piscitelli, A. Polli, A. D'Alberton, L. Falsetti, C. Ferrari, et al., The efficacy and tolerability of long-term cabergoline therapy in hyperprolactinaemic disorders: An open, uncontrolled, multicentre study. European Multicentre Cabergoline Study Group, Clin Endocrinol (Oxf) 39 (3) (1993) 323—329.
[540] M.E. Molitch, Pituitary disorders during pregnancy, Endocrinol Metab Clin North Am 35 (1) (2006) 99—116.
[541] P. Krupp, C. Monka, Bromocriptine in pregnancy: Safety aspects, Klin Wochenschr 65 (17) (1987) 823—827.
[542] P. Krupp, C. Monka, K. Richter, The safety aspects of infertility treatments. Second World Congress of Gynecology and Obstetrics; 1988; Rio de Janeiro, Brazil 1988 p. 9.
[543] J.P. Raymond, E. Goldstein, P. Konopka, M.F. Leleu, R.E. Merceron, Y. Loria, Follow-up of children born of bromocriptine-treated mothers, Horm Res 22 (3) (1985) 239—246.
[544] E.S. Canales, I.C. Garcia, J.E. Ruiz, A. Zarate, Bromocriptine as prophylactic therapy in prolactinoma during pregnancy, Fertil Steril 36 (4) (1981) 524—526.
[545] P. Konopka, J.P. Raymond, R.E. Merceron, J. Seneze, Continuous administration of bromocriptine in the prevention of neurological complications in pregnant women with prolactinomas, Am J Obstet Gynecol 146 (8) (1983) 935—938.
[546] V. Ruiz-Velasco, G. Tolis, Pregnancy in hyperprolactinemic women, Fertil Steril 41 (6) (1984) 793—805.
[547] S. Abu-Fadil, G. DeVane, T.M. Siler, S.S. Yen, Effects of oral contraceptive steroids on pituitary prolactin secretion, Contraception 13 (1) (1976) 79—85.
[548] E.B. Gold, Epidemiology of pituitary adenomas, Epidemiol Rev 3 (1981) 163—183.
[549] M. Lebbe, C. Hubinont, P. Bernard, D. Maiter, Outcome of 100 pregnancies initiated under treatment with cabergoline in hyperprolactinaemic women, Clin Endocrinol (Oxf) 73 (2) (2010) 147—148.
[550] R. Maheux, M. Jenicek, R. Cleroux, H. Beauregard, X. De Muylder, N.M. Gratton, et al., Oral contraceptives and prolactinomas: A case-control study, Am J Obstet Gynecol 143 (2) (1982) 134—138.
[551] F. Marin, K.T. Kovacs, B.W. Scheithauer, W.F. Young Jr., The pituitary gland in patients with breast carcinoma: A histologic and immunocytochemical study of 125 cases, Mayo Clin Proc. 67 (10) (1992) 949—956.
[552] M.E. Molitch, Clinical features and epidemiology of prolactinomas in women, in: J.M. Olefsky, R.J. Robbins (Eds.), Prolactinomas: Practical diagnosis and management, Churchill Livingstone, New York, 1986, pp. 67—95.
[553] M.E. Molitch, S. Reichlin, The amenorrhea, galactorrhea and hyperprolactinemia syndromes, in: G. Stollerman (Ed.), Advances in internal medicine, Year Book Medical Publishers, Chicago, 1980, pp. 37—65.
[554] M. Ono, N. Miki, K. Amano, T. Kawamata, T. Seki, R. Makino, et al., Individualized high-dose cabergoline therapy for hyperprolactinemic infertility in women with micro- and macroprolactinomas, J Clin Endocrinol Metab 95 (6) (2010) 2672—2679.
[555] B.M. Sherman, C.E. Harris, J. Schlechte, T.M. Duello, N.S. Halmi, J. VanGilder, et al., Pathogenesis of prolactin-secreting pituitary adenomas, Lancet 2 (8098) (1978) 1019—1021.
[556] L. Teperman, W. Futterweit, R. Zappulla, L.I. Malis, Oral contraceptive history as a risk indicator in patients with pituitary tumors with hyperprolactinemia: A case comparison study of twenty patients, Neurosurgery 7 (6) (1980) 571—573.
[557] G. Stalldecker, M.S.M. Gil, M.A. Guitelman, A. Alfieri, M.C. Ballarino, L. Boero, et al., Effects of cabergoline on pregnancy and embryo-fetal development: Retrospective study on 103 pregnancies and a review of the literature, Pituitary (2010). in press.
[558] A. Colao, R. Abs, D.G. Barcena, P. Chanson, W. Paulus, D.L. Kleinberg, Pregnancy outcomes following cabergoline treatment: Extended results from a 12-year observational study, Clin Endocrinol (Oxf) 68 (1) (2008) 66—71.
[559] E. Robert, L. Musatti, G. Piscitelli, C.I. Ferrari, Pregnancy outcome after treatment with the ergot derivative, cabergoline, Reprod Toxicol 10 (4) (1996) 333—337.
[560] H. Dinc, F. Esen, A. Demirci, A. Sari, H. Resit Gumele, Pituitary dimensions and volume measurements in pregnancy and post partum. MR assessment, Acta Radiol 39 (1) (1998) 64—69.
[561] M.D. Bronstein, Prolactinomas and pregnancy, Pituitary 8 (1) (2005) 31—38.
[562] M. Laloi-Michelin, N. Ciraru-Vigneron, T. Meas, Cabergoline treatment of pregnant women with macroprolactinomas, Int J Gynaecol Obstet 99 (1) (2007) 61—62.
[563] O. Ylikorkala, S. Kivinen, L. Ronnberg, Bromocriptine treatment during early human pregnancy: Effect on the levels of prolactin, sex steroids and placental lactogen, Acta Endocrinol (Copenh) 95 (3) (1980) 412—415.
[564] W.D. Lehmann, K. Musch, A.S. Wolf, Influence of bromocriptine on plasma levels of prolactin and steroid hormones in the 20th week of pregnancy, J Endocrinol Invest 2 (3) (1979) 251—255.
[565] T. Espersen, J. Ditzel, Pregnancy and delivery under bromocriptine therapy, Lancet 2 (8045) (1977) 985—986.
[566] C. Liu, J.B. Tyrrell, Successful treatment of a large macroprolactinoma with cabergoline during pregnancy, Pituitary 4 (3) (2001) 179—185.
[567] A. Banerjee, K. Wynne, T. Tan, E.C. Hatfield, N.M. Martin, C. Williamson, et al., High dose cabergoline therapy for a resistant macroprolactinoma during pregnancy, Clin Endocrinol (Oxf) 70 (5) (2009) 812—813.
[568] P.G. Crosignani, A.M. Mattei, C. Scarduelli, V. Cavioni, P. Boracchi, Is pregnancy the best treatment for hyperprolactinaemia? Hum Reprod 4 (8) (1989) 910—912.
[569] N.A. Samaan, P.N. Schultz, T.A. Leavens, M.E. Leavens, Y.Y. Lee, Pregnancy after treatment in patients with prolactinoma: Operation versus bromocriptine, Am J Obstet Gynecol 155 (6) (1986) 1300—1305.

[570] H. Ikegami, T. Aono, K. Koizumi, K. Koike, H. Fukui, O. Tanizawa, Relationship between the methods of treatment for prolactinomas and the puerperal lactation, Fertil Steril 47 (5) (1987) 867–869.
[571] E.R. Laws Jr., N.C. Fode, R.V. Randall, C.F. Abboud, C.B. Coulam, Pregnancy following transsphenoidal resection of prolactin-secreting pituitary tumors, J Neurosurg 58 (5) (1983) 685–688.
[572] M.E. Molitch, Pregnancy and the hyperprolactinemic woman, N Engl J Med 312 (21) (1985) 1364–1370.
[573] H.H. McGarrigle, S. Sarris, V. Little, D. Lawrence, E. Radwanska, G.I. Swyer, Induction of ovulation with clomiphene and human chorionic gonadotrophin in women with hyperprolactinaemic amenorrhoea, Br J Obstet Gynaecol 85 (9) (1978) 692–697.
[574] O. Narita, T. Kimura, N. Suganuma, M. Osawa, S. Mizutani, T. Masahashi, et al., Relationship between maternal prolactin levels during pregnancy and lactation in women with pituitary adenoma, Nippon Sanka Fujinka Gakkai Zasshi 37 (5) (1985) 758–762.
[575] W.A. Divers Jr., S.S. Yen, Prolactin-producing microadenomas in pregnancy, Obstet Gynecol 62 (4) (1983) 425–429.
[576] P.E. Belchetz, A. Carty, L.G. Clearkin, J.C. Davis, R.V. Jeffreys, P.G. Rae, Failure of prophylactic surgery to avert massive pituitary expansion in pregnancy, Clin Endocrinol (Oxf) 25 (3) (1986) 325–330.
[577] J.B. Brodsky, E.N. Cohen, B.W. Brown Jr., M.L. Wu, C. Whitcher, Surgery during pregnancy and fetal outcome, Am J Obstet Gynecol 138 (8) (1980) 1165–1167.
[578] R. Cohen-Kerem, C. Railton, D. Oren, M. Lishner, G. Koren, Pregnancy outcome following non-obstetric surgical intervention, Am J Surg 190 (3) (2005) 467–473.
[579] G. Mohr, J. Hardy, R. Comtois, H. Beauregard, Surgical management of giant pituitary adenomas, Can J Neurol Sci 17 (1) (1990) 62–66.
[580] H.W. Pia, E. Grote, G. Hildebrandt, Giant pituitary adenomas, Neurosurg Rev 8 (3–4) (1985) 207–220.
[581] L. Symon, J. Jakubowski, B. Kendall, Surgical treatment of giant pituitary adenomas, J Neurol Neurosurg Psychiatry 42 (11) (1979) 973–982.
[582] S.M. Corsello, G. Ubertini, M. Altomare, R.M. Lovicu, M.G. Migneco, C.A. Rota, et al., Giant prolactinomas in men: Efficacy of cabergoline treatment, Clin Endocrinol (Oxf) 58 (5) (2003) 662–670.
[583] M.E. Molitch, Medical treatment of giant prolactinomas, in: O. Al-Mefty, T. Origitano, H.L. Harkey (Eds.), Controversies in neurosurgery, Thieme Medical Publishers, New York, 1996, pp. 2–10.
[584] A. Goel, T. Nadkarni, D. Muzumdar, K. Desai, U. Phalke, P. Sharma, Giant pituitary tumors: A study based on surgical treatment of 118 cases, Surg Neurol 61 (5) (2004) 436–445, discussion 445–446.
[585] J. Garibi, I. Pomposo, G. Villar, S. Gaztambide, Giant pituitary adenomas: Clinical characteristics and surgical results, Br J Neurosurg 16 (2) (2002) 133–139.
[586] S.K. Grebe, J.W. Delahunt, C.M. Feek, Treatment of extensively invasive (giant) prolactinomas with bromocriptine, NZ Med J 105 (931) (1992) 129–131.
[587] M.Y. Yang, C.C. Shen, W.L. Ho, Treatments of multi-invasive giant prolactinoma, J Clin Neurosci 11 (1) (2004) 70–75.
[588] N. Saeki, M. Nakamura, K. Sunami, A. Yamaura, Surgical indication after bromocriptine therapy on giant prolactinomas: Effects and limitations of the medical treatment, Endocr J 45 (4) (1998) 529–537.
[589] G.A. Kaltsas, P. Nomikos, G. Kontogeorgos, M. Buchfelder, A.B. Grossman, Clinical review: Diagnosis and management of pituitary carcinomas, J Clin Endocrinol Metab 90 (5) (2005) 3089–3099.
[590] S. Byrne, C. Karapetis, N. Vrodos, A novel use of temozolomide in a patient with malignant prolactinoma, J Clin Neurosci 16 (12) (2009) 1694–1696.
[591] C.E. Fadul, A.L. Kominsky, L.P. Meyer, L.S. Kingman, W.B. Kinlaw, C.H. Rhodes, et al., Long-term response of pituitary carcinoma to temozolomide. Report of two cases, J Neurosurg 105 (4) (2006) 621–626.
[592] C. Hagen, H.D. Schroeder, S. Hansen, M. Andersen, Temozolomide treatment of a pituitary carcinoma and two pituitary macroadenomas resistant to conventional therapy, Eur J Endocrinol 161 (4) (2009) 631–637.
[593] A.P. Huang, S.H. Yang, C.C. Yang, M.F. Kuo, M.Z. Wu, Y.K. Tu, Malignant prolactinoma with craniospinal metastasis in a 12-year-old boy, J Neurooncol 90 (1) (2008) 41–46.
[594] M. Kars, F. Roelfsema, J.A. Romijn, A.M. Pereira, Malignant prolactinoma: Case report and review of the literature, Eur J Endocrinol 155 (4) (2006) 523–534.
[595] S. Lim, H. Shahinian, M.M. Maya, W. Yong, A.P. Heaney, Temozolomide: A novel treatment for pituitary carcinoma, Lancet Oncol 7 (6) (2006) 518–520.
[596] S.L. Asa, Practical pituitary pathology: What does the pathologist need to know? Arch Pathol Lab Med 132 (8) (2008) 1231–1240.
[597] P.J. Pernicone, B.W. Scheithauer, T.J. Sebo, K.T. Kovacs, E. Horvath, W.F. Young Jr., et al., Pituitary carcinoma: A clinicopathologic study of 15 cases, Cancer 79 (4) (1997) 804–812.
[598] A. Popadic, A. Witzmann, M. Buchfelder, H. Eiter, P. Komminoth, Malignant prolactinoma: Case report and review of the literature, Surg Neurol 51 (1) (1999) 47–54, discussion -55.
[599] L.M. Neff, M. Weil, A. Cole, T.R. Hedges, W. Shucart, D. Lawrence, et al., Temozolomide in the treatment of an invasive prolactinoma resistant to dopamine agonists, Pituitary 10 (1) (2007) 81–86.
[600] J.R. Burgess, J.J. Shepherd, V. Parameswaran, L. Hoffman, T.M. Greenaway, Spectrum of pituitary disease in multiple endocrine neoplasia type 1 (MEN 1): Clinical, biochemical, and radiological features of pituitary disease in a large MEN 1 kindred, J Clin Endocrinol Metab 81 (7) (1996) 2642–2646.
[601] T. O'Brien, D.S. O'Riordan, H. Gharib, B.W. Scheithauer, M.J. Ebersold, J.A. van Heerden, Results of treatment of pituitary disease in multiple endocrine neoplasia, type I, Neurosurgery 39 (2) (1996) 273–278, discussion 278–279.
[602] B. Verges, F. Boureille, P. Goudet, A. Murat, A. Beckers, G. Sassolas, et al., Pituitary disease in MEN type 1 (MEN1): Data from the France–Belgium MEN1 multicenter study, J Clin Endocrinol Metab 87 (2) (2002) 457–465.
[603] W. Hao, M.C. Skarulis, W.F. Simonds, L.S. Weinstein, S.K. Agarwal, C. Mateo, et al., Multiple endocrine neoplasia type 1 variant with frequent prolactinoma and rare gastrinoma, J Clin Endocrinol Metab 89 (8) (2004) 3776–3784.
[604] S.E. Olufemi, J.S. Green, P. Manickam, S.C. Guru, S.K. Agarwal, M.B. Kester, et al., Common ancestral mutation in the MEN1 gene is likely responsible for the prolactinoma variant of MEN1 (MEN1Burin) in four kindreds from Newfoundland, Hum Mutat 11 (4) (1998) 264–269.
[605] E.M. Petty, J.S. Green, S.J. Marx, R.T. Taggart, N. Farid, A.E. Bale, Mapping the gene for hereditary hyperparathyroidism and prolactinoma (MEN1Burin) to chromosome 11q: Evidence for a founder effect in patients from Newfoundland, Am J Hum Genet 54 (6) (1994) 1060–1066.

[606] J. Trouillas, F. Labat-Moleur, N. Sturm, M. Kujas, M.F. Heymann, D. Figarella-Branger, et al., Pituitary tumors and hyperplasia in multiple endocrine neoplasia type 1 syndrome (MEN1): A case-control study in a series of 77 patients versus 2509 non-MEN1 patients, Am J Surg Pathol 32 (4) (2008) 534–543.

[607] A. Beckers, D. Betea, H.V. Socin, A. Stevenaert, The treatment of sporadic versus MEN1-related pituitary adenomas, J Intern Med 253 (6) (2003) 599–605.

[608] S. Corbetta, A. Pizzocaro, M. Peracchi, P. Beck-Peccoz, G. Faglia, A. Spada, Multiple endocrine neoplasia type 1 in patients with recognized pituitary tumours of different types, Clin Endocrinol (Oxf) 47 (5) (1997) 507–512.

[609] L. Pei, S. Melmed, B. Scheithauer, K. Kovacs, W.F. Benedict, D. Prager, Frequent loss of heterozygosity at the retinoblastoma susceptibility gene (RB) locus in aggressive pituitary tumors: Evidence for a chromosome 13 tumor suppressor gene other than RB, Cancer Res 55 (8) (1995) 1613–1616.

[610] A. Ogino, A. Yoshino, Y. Katayama, T. Watanabe, T. Ota, C. Komine, et al., The p15(INK4b)/p16(INK4a)/RB1 pathway is frequently deregulated in human pituitary adenomas, J Neuropathol Exp Neurol 64 (5) (2005) 398–403.

[611] N. Seemann, D. Kuhn, C. Wrocklage, K. Keyvani, W. Hackl, M. Buchfelder, et al., CDKN2A/p16 inactivation is related to pituitary adenoma type and size, J Pathol 193 (4) (2001) 491–497.

[612] M. Woloschak, A. Yu, J. Xiao, K.D. Post, Frequent loss of the P16INK4a gene product in human pituitary tumors, Cancer Res 56 (11) (1996) 2493–2496.

[613] M.G. Hossain, T. Iwata, N. Mizusawa, Z.R. Qian, S.W. Shima, T. Okutsu, et al., Expression of p18(INK4C) is down-regulated in human pituitary adenomas, Endocr Pathol 20 (2) (2009) 114–121.

[614] M. Kirsch, M. Morz, T. Pinzer, H.K. Schackert, G. Schackert, Frequent loss of the CDKN2C (p18INK4c) gene product in pituitary adenomas, Genes Chromosomes Cancer 48 (2) (2009) 143–154.

[615] A.G. Neto, I.E. McCutcheon, R. Vang, M.L. Spencer, W. Zhang, G.N. Fuller, Elevated expression of p21 (WAF1/Cip1) in hormonally active pituitary adenomas, Ann Diagn Pathol 9 (1) (2005) 6–10.

[616] C.M. Bamberger, M. Fehn, A.M. Bamberger, D.K. Ludecke, F.U. Beil, W. Saeger, et al., Reduced expression levels of the cell-cycle inhibitor p27Kip1 in human pituitary adenomas, Eur J Endocrinol 140 (3) (1999) 250–255.

[617] M. Georgitsi, A. Raitila, A. Karhu, R.B. van der Luijt, C.M. Aalfs, T. Sane, et al., Germline CDKN1B/p27Kip1 mutation in multiple endocrine neoplasia, J Clin Endocrinol Metab 92 (8) (2007) 3321–3325.

[618] N.S. Pellegata, L. Quintanilla-Martinez, H. Siggelkow, E. Samson, K. Bink, H. Hofler, et al., Germ-line mutations in p27Kip1 cause a multiple endocrine neoplasia syndrome in rats and humans, Proc Nat Acad Sci USA 103 (42) (2006) 15558–15563.

[619] N.A. Hibberts, D.J. Simpson, J.E. Bicknell, J.C. Broome, P.R. Hoban, R.N. Clayton, et al., Analysis of cyclin D1 (CCND1) allelic imbalance and overexpression in sporadic human pituitary tumors, Clin Cancer Res 5 (8) (1999) 2133–2139.

[620] W. Saeger, S. Schreiber, D.K. Ludecke, Cyclins D1 and D3 and topoisomerase II alpha in inactive pituitary adenomas, Endocr Pathol 12 (1) (2001) 39–47.

[621] C. Rasmussen, J. Brownell, T. Bergh, Clinical response and prolactin concentration in hyperprolactinemic women during and after treatment for 24 months with the new dopamine agonist, CV 205-502, Acta Endocrinol (Copenh) 125 (2) (1991) 170–176.

[622] A. Colao, A. Di Sarno, E. Guerra, R. Pivonello, P. Cappabianca, F. Caranci, et al., Predictors of remission of hyperprolactinaemia after long-term withdrawal of cabergoline therapy, Clin Endocrinol (Oxf) 67 (3) (2007) 426–433.

[623] E. Ciccarelli, S. Grottoli, P. Razzore, D. Gaia, A. Bertagna, S. Cirillo, et al., Long-term treatment with cabergoline, a new long-lasting ergoline derivate, in idiopathic or tumorous hyperprolactinaemia and outcome of drug-induced pregnancy, J Endocrinol Invest 20 (9) (1997) 547–551.

[624] E. Ricci, F. Parazzini, T. Motta, C.I. Ferrari, A. Colao, A. Clavenna, et al., Pregnancy outcome after cabergoline treatment in early weeks of gestation, Reprod Toxicol 16 (6) (2002) 791–793.

[625] J.A. Verhelst, Toward the establishment of a clinical prediction rule for response of prolactinomas to cabergoline, J Clin Endocrinol Metab 84 (12) (1999) 4747.

[626] M.A. Canfield, M.A. Honein, N. Yuskiv, J. Xing, C.T. Mai, J.S. Collins, et al., National estimates and race/ethnic-specific variation of selected birth defects in the United States, 1999–2001, Birth Defects Res A Clin Mol Teratol 76 (11) (2006) 747–756.

[627] J.A. Martin, H.C. Kung, T.J. Mathews, D.L. Hoyert, D.M. Strobino, B. Guyer, et al., Annual summary of vital statistics 2006, Pediatrics 121 (4) (2008) 788–801.

[628] G. Minniti, M.L. Jaffrain-Rea, A. Santoro, V. Esposito, L. Ferrante, R. Delfini, et al., Giant prolactinomas presenting as skull base tumors, Surg Neurol 57 (2) (2002) 99–103, discussion 104.

[629] Z.B. Wu, C.J. Yu, Z.P. Su, Q.C. Zhuge, J.S. Wu, W.M. Zheng, Bromocriptine treatment of invasive giant prolactinomas involving the cavernous sinus: Results of a long-term follow up, J Neurosurg 104 (1) (2006) 54–61.

[630] S. Mascarell, D.H. Sarne, Clinical presentation and response to therapy in patients with massive prolactin hypersecretion, Pituitary 10 (1) (2007) 95–101.

[631] I. Shimon, C. Benbassat, M. Hadani, Effectiveness of long-term cabergoline treatment for giant prolactinoma: Study of 12 men, Eur J Endocrinol 156 (2) (2007) 225–231.

[632] E.H. Cho, S.A. Lee, J.Y. Chung, E.H. Koh, Y.H. Cho, J.H. Kim, et al., Efficacy and safety of cabergoline as first line treatment for invasive giant prolactinoma, J Korean Med Sci 24 (5) (2009) 874–878.

CHAPTER

16

Cushing's disease

Xavier Bertagna [1,2], *Laurence Guignat* [1], *Marie-Charles Raux-Demay* [3], *Brigitte Guilhaume* [1], *François Girard* [3]

[1] Service des Maladies Endocriniennes et Métaboliques, Centre de Référence des Maladies Rares de la Surrénale, hôpital Cochin, Paris, France [2] Département Endocrinologie-Diabète, INSERM U-1016, Institut Cochin, Faculté de Médecine Paris Descartes, Université Paris 5, Paris, France, [3] Explorations Fonctionelles Endocriniennes, hôpital Trousseau, Paris, France.

PATHOPHYSIOLOGY

Cushing's syndrome refers to the manifestations of chronic glucocorticoid excess and may result from various causes (Table 16.1). In Cushing's disease pituitary adrenocorticotropic hormone (ACTH) oversecretion induces bilateral adrenocortical hyperplasia and excess production of cortisol, adrenal androgens and 11-deoxycorticosterone, which together provoke the clinical and biologic features of the disease.

EPIDEMIOLOGY

Cushing's disease is the most frequent cause of spontaneous Cushing's syndrome in adults. In most series its prevalence is approximately 70% with a definite female preponderance, the female/male ratio ranging between 3:1 and 10:1 [1–4]. In our series of 809 adult patients with spontaneous Cushing's syndromes, Cushing's disease accounts for 68% of the cases, and the female/male ratio is 2.8 (Table 16.2). Distribution of the age at diagnosis shows a peak in adult females in the 25–45-year range (Figure 16.1).

In children, the causes of Cushing's syndrome have a different distribution. Primary adrenocortical tumors are more frequent and Cushing's disease accounts for about 50% of the cases. Children with this condition are usually older than 9 with an equal sex ratio [5–9]. Cushing's disease accounts for 50% of Cushing's syndrome and is almost always caused by a pituitary microadenoma. The commonest age of presentation of pediatric Cushing's disease is during adolescence, and there is a strong predominance of males in prepubertal patients. Ectopic ACTH syndrome is extremely rare, occurring much less frequently than in adults. Unilateral adrenal tumors are an important cause of pediatric Cushing's syndrome (about 40%) and are almost always adrenal carcinoma in children, with rarely a pure hypercortisolism, but usually associated virilization. Primary bilateral adrenocortical hyperplasia is a rare but important cause of pediatric Cushing's syndrome, usually associated with the Carney complex, and typically occurs in adolescence or early adulthood. A total of 398 cases of pediatric Cushing's syndrome are reported in the literature, with 182 Cushing's disease, 11 ectopic ACTH syndrome, 164 adrenocortical tumors, 16 McCune Albright syndrome and 11 primary bilateral adrenocortical hyperplasia. The peak incidence was 14.1 years in Cushing's disease, 10.1 years in ectopic ACTH syndrome, 4.5 years in adrenocortical tumors, 1.2 in McCune-Albright syndrome and 13 in primary bilateral adrenocortical hyperplasia [8].

Cushing's disease is rare; its true incidence, which varies with age and sex, is difficult to evaluate. Incidence data are available on pituitary [10,11] and adrenocortical [12,13] tumors. The prevalence of corticotroph tumors in the former [14] and that of Cushing's syndrome in the latter [15–17] provide an indirect means whereby the incidence of Cushing's disease may be roughly estimated to be in the range of 1–10 new cases per million per year. European population-based studies reported an incidence of newly diagnosed Cushing's disease of 0.7 to 2.4 cases per 1 million inhabitants per year [18,19]. In Vizcaya (Spain), the prevalence of known cases of Cushing's disease at the end of 1992 was

The Pituitary, Third Edition, DOI: 10.1016/B978-0-12-380926-1.10016-1

TABLE 16.1 Causes of Cushing's Syndrome

SPONTANEOUS
ACTH-dependent
Pituitary ACTH oversecretion
Cushing's disease
Primary corticotroph
Anterior pituitary adenoma
Anterior pituitary mixed adenoma
Anterior pituitary cancer
Ectopic corticotroph adenoma
Multiple endocrine neoplasia type 1
Intermediate lobe pituitary adenoma?
Primary hypothalamic dysfunction
CRH-producing tumor
Hypothalamic CRH-producing tumor
Ectopic CRH-producing tumor
Nonpituitary ACTH oversection
Ectopic ACTH syndrome
Endocrine tumors
Mononuclear cells
Cortisol hyperreactive syndrome?
ACTH-independent (Adrenal Cushing's Syndrome)
Unilateral adrenocortical tumors
Adrenocortical adenoma
Adrenocortical carcinoma
Bilateral adrenocortical disorders
Primary pigmented nodular adrenal disease
ACTH-independent macronodular adrenal hyperplasia (AI-MAH)
Gonadal tumors
IATROGENIC
Exogenous Glucocorticoids
Exogenous Cortrosyn

CRH, corticotropin-releasing hormone.

39.1 per million inhabitants [18]. According to the Nationwide Inpatient Sample database, the largest all-payer inpatient care database in the US which contains data from approximately 8 million discharges annually from 1004 hospitals located in 37 states, there were an estimated 3525 cases of transsphenoidal resection of Cushing's disease between 1993 and 2002 [20].

Recent data suggest that Cushing's syndrome is more common than had previously been thought. In addition to the classical overt Cushing's syndrome, mild forms of Cushing's syndrome (named subclinical Cushing's syndrome or occult Cushing's syndrome) have been identified in patients with type 2 diabetes [21–24], hypertension [25], osteoporosis [26], and subjects with an adrenal incidentaloma. The reported prevalence of Cushing's syndrome is between 2% and 9.4 % in overweight type 2 diabetic patients and reaches 10.8% in patients with T-scores of 2.5 or less and vertebral fractures, although a final diagnosis could not to be confirmed in all patients. For instance, definitive mild Cushing's syndrome was identified in four patients (2%) among 200 overweight, type-2 diabetic patients with poor metabolic control (HbA1C > 8%), with three Cushing's disease and one surgically proven adrenal adenoma. Definitive diagnosis remains to be established in seven additional patients (3.5%) [21].

TABLE 16.2 Etiology of 809 Spontaneous Cushing's Syndromes in Adults

	Number of Patients (%)	Female/Male Ratio
Cushing's disease	550 (68)	2.8
Primary adrenocortical tumor	199 (25)	4.2
Benign adrenocortical adenoma	111 (14)	0.5
Adrenocortical carcinoma	88 (11)	3.6
Ectopic ACTH syndrome	58 (7)	1.4
Primary adrenocortical nodular dysplasia	2 (0.2)	–

CHRONIC ACTH AND PROOPIOMELANOCORTIN (POMC) PEPTIDE OVERSECRETION BY THE PITUITARY

Normal Synthesis and Secretion of ACTH

Mechanisms of ACTH Biosynthesis

The mechanisms of ACTH biosynthesis have been fully elucidated in the last 30 years; a high-molecular-weight ACTH-precursor molecule was identified and characterized in the ACTH-producing AtT-20/D16-v mouse tumor cell line [27]. Recombinant DNA methods unravelled the primary structure of this precursor [28] – called POMC – in many species including humans [29–31]. This is fully described in Chapter 2.

The overall mechanism of POMC gene expression in man is shown schematically in Figure 16.2; a single POMC gene per haploid genome is present on the distal region (2p23–25) of the short arm of chromosome 2 [32,33]; it consists of three exons, the coding regions

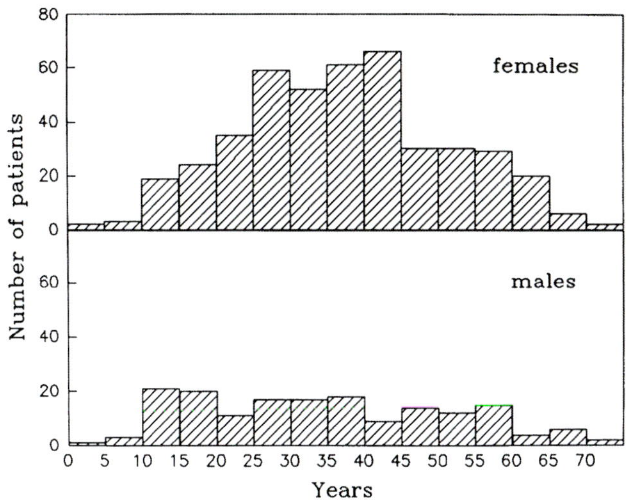

FIGURE 16.1 Patient age at the time of diagnosis of Cushing's disease.

(in black) being present only on exons 2 and 3. After the splicing of the primary transcript a mature messenger RNA (mRNA) of 1072 nucleotides (nt) is generated and a poly (A)+ tail of about 200 nt is added. A pre-POMC molecule is first translated starting with a 26-amino acid signal peptide necessary for the translocation of the nascent protein through the membrane of the rough endoplasmic reticulum. Within the Golgi apparatus and the secretory granule the POMC molecule undergoes a series of proteolytic cleavages and chemical transformations which together result in the maturation or processing of the precursor [34]: proteolysis occurs at pairs of basic amino acids. Among the nine potential cleavage sites of the human POMC only four are utilized in the anterior pituitary, generating the N-terminal fragment [35,36], the joining peptide [37–39], ACTH [40–42], β-lipotropin (β-LPH), and a small amount of γ-LPH and β-endorphin (β-end) [42,43]. Other chemical transformations include glycosylation of the N-terminal fragment [44], C-terminal amidation of the joining peptide [38,39,45,46], and partial phosphorylation of ACTH on Ser_{31} [47,48]. An alternate mode of nonprimate POMC processing takes place in the intermediate lobe of the pituitary, releasing smaller peptides such as β-melanocyte-stimulating hormone (β-MSH), corticotrophin-like intermediate lobe peptide (CLIP) and α-MSH [49,50]. It does not normally occur in the human pituitary where the intermediate lobe is only fully present in the fetus [51].

POMC gene expression also occurs in many normal nonpituitary tissues [52,53]; it does so at a very low level and predominantly through an alternate mode of gene transcription [54–56], generating negligible amounts of POMC peptide [57–59]. It is assumed that the highly predominant, if not the sole, source of circulating

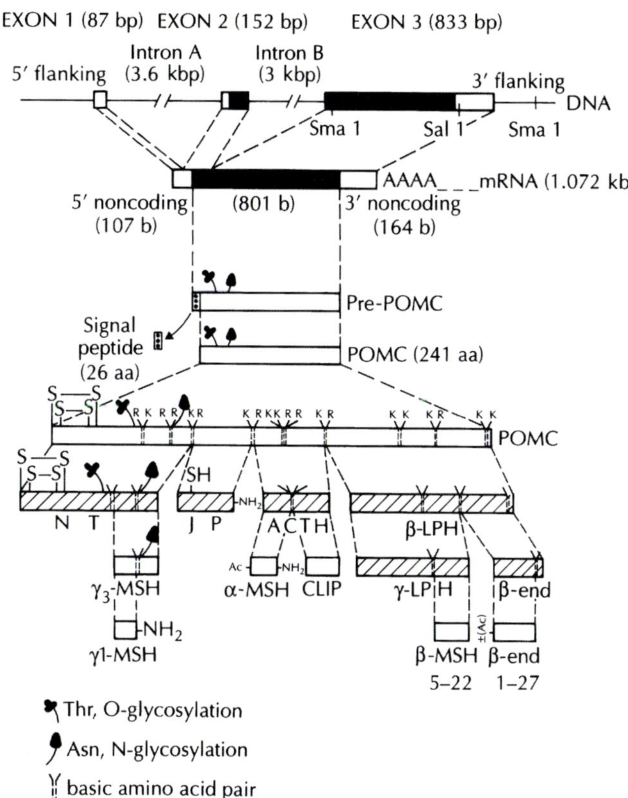

FIGURE 16.2 Schematic view of human proopiomelanocortin (POMC) gene expression. Black bars denote the protein-coding regions of the DNA and messenger RNA (mRNA). Hatched bars denote the peptide fragments found in the human anterior pituitary.

ACTH and POMC peptides in humans, under normal circumstances, is the anterior pituitary corticotroph cell.

The coordinate proteolysis of POMC and the equimolar secretion of the various POMC peptides has two implications: any of the non-ACTH POMC peptides can be assayed in blood as an alternate marker of the overall pituitary corticotroph activity; a specific pattern of POMC peptides is associated with the pituitary corticotroph, and any qualitative abnormality suggests a pathologic nonpituitary source [60–62]. Yet, in highly aggressive, poorly differentiated pituitary corticotroph adenomas, decreased expression of convertases indicates that intact POMC may be secreted; these adenomas are therefore often "silent" [61,63].

Regulation of ACTH Secretion

The normal circadian rhythm of plasma cortisol is directly driven by pituitary corticotroph activity [64–66]. Its pattern is derived from variations in the number and amplitude of episodic ACTH bursts [67,68]. Pituitary corticotroph activity increases in the second half of the night, around 2–4 a.m., peaks on waking and gradually falls during the morning [69]. Various physical and psychologic stresses can interrupt this normal rhythm, at any time, with an acute rise in

ACTH. Both the normal circadian rhythm and the stress-induced changes are central nervous system (CNS) mediated under the primary – although not exclusive – control of hypothalamic corticotropin-releasing hormone (CRH) [70].

CRH [71] acts directly on the corticotroph cell through specific receptors that activate the adenylyl cyclase and increase intracellular cyclic adenosine monophosphate (cAMP) formation [72,73]. Arginine vasopressin (AVP), through its own specific V_1 type receptors, also acts on the corticotroph cell to activate phospholipase C, leading to increased phosphoinositide turnover, Ca^{2+} release and protein kinase C activation [74]. The action of AVP potentiates that of CRH [75] by further increasing cAMP formation [76–78]; cross-talk between the two transducing systems provides the synergistic action that promotes the maximal ACTH response by increasing both POMC gene transcription and secretory granule exocytosis [79–81]. This phenomenon, thoroughly studied in vitro on animal models, is also observed in humans; the simultaneous administration of CRH and AVP (or its analogue lysine vasopressin, LVP) induces a maximal ACTH rise, higher than that obtained by either secretagogue alone or their sum [82–84]. The specific AVP receptor of the corticotroph cell was recently cloned; this V3 (or V1b) receptor is closely analogous to the V1a receptor [85,86]. Interestingly, the AVP analogue, DDAVP or desmopressin, also has definite affinity for the V3 receptor, explaining that it is a powerful stimulator of ACTH secretion in a vast majority (ca. 85%) of patients with Cushing's disease [87].

Glucocorticoids exert a negative feedback on pituitary ACTH [88]. In patients with primary adrenal deficiency, basal and stimulated ACTH are increased. On the other hand, excess glucocorticoid administration or secretion by a primary adrenocortical tumor inhibits basal and stimulated ACTH. Prolonged glucocorticoid suppression of the hypothalamic–corticotroph axis characteristically induces long-lasting unresponsiveness, which may extend for months or years after the source of excess glucocorticoid has been withdrawn. Glucocorticoids inhibit hypothalamic CRH production [89] and also act directly at the corticotroph cell, as demonstrated in various animal models. They inhibit basal and stimulated ACTH release [90,91], as well as POMC gene transcription in a dose-dependent manner [92]. Interestingly this inhibition is not complete and a small proportion of POMC transcription is not suppressed, even by very high amounts of glucocorticoids [80,93].

A proposed neuro–immuno–endocrine loop is emerging which suggests that corticotroph function not only acts on immunocompetent cells – through cortisol production – but is itself the target of various immunomodulators [94]. Data obtained in the rat show that interleukin-1 and -6 both exert a stimulatory action on ACTH release at the hypothalamic and pituitary levels [95–97]. It is suggested that they participate in the physiologic ACTH rise in acute infectious stress, as they experimentally mediate that which occurs after bacterial lipopolysaccharide injections. Both cytokines are normally present in the rat anterior pituitary, apparently in a subpopulation of thyroid-stimulating hormone (TSH) cells and in folliculostellate cells for interleukin-1 and interleukin-6, respectively, thus raising the possibility that they act as local paracrine factors [98,99]. The role of the gp130-related cytokines, particularly LIF (leukemia inhibitory factor), has been convincingly established in the regulation of POMC expression and corticotroph cell development [100]. Further studies are obviously needed to establish the exact significance of these data, the effects of other regulatory peptides found in the pituitary [101] and their possible implication on the physiology and pathophysiology of ACTH release in humans [102,103].

Similarly PPAR gamma [104] and retinoic acid [105] play a role in POMC gene regulation, at least in animal models.

Oversecretion of ACTH in Cushing's Disease

Cushing's Hypothesis

The proposition that the pituitary was responsible for the clinical features of Cushing's disease was convincingly expressed for the first time in Harvey Cushing's classic monograph of 1932; the basophil adenomas of the pituitary body and their clinical manifestations (pituitary basophilism) [106]. Cushing was recognizing that...

> ... striking clinical effects might be produced by minute, symptomatically predictable (pituitary) adenomas. So it is the degree of secretory activity of an adenoma which may be out of all proportion to its dimension, that evokes the recognizable symptom-complex in all hypersecretory states...

he was still wondering however:

> ... if the polyglandular features of the disorder are partly due, as premised, to a secondary hyperplasia of adrenal cortex ...

Much uncertainty remained at that time on the fine pathophysiologic mechanism of this disorder, yet the crucial clinical and pathologic observations had been made and the pertinent questions had been asked. Today it is recognized that chronic oversecretion of cortisol, androgens and 11-deoxycorticosterone by hyperplastic adrenocortical glands is directly responsible for the clinical features of Cushing's disease, a phenomenon which is primarily driven by pituitary ACTH oversecretion.

Demonstrating ACTH Oversecretion

When plasma ACTH became measurable by bioassay [107] it was found to be normal or slightly elevated in patients with Cushing's disease [108–110]. ACTH radioimmunoassay [64] came as an illuminating tool for the fine exploration of these patients.

A majority of patients with Cushing's disease have normal plasma ACTH values in the morning, although as a group their mean ACTH value is significantly higher than that of normal subjects [109,111–113]. However, even a normal ACTH value is inappropriately high or not normally restrained in view of the hypercortisolic state; repeated ACTH measurements over 24 hours show that patients with Cushing's disease have high evening values with a lack of the normal circadian rhythm [65,66,114]. Continuous sampling with a persistaltic pump has not been performed to study 24-hour integrated plasma ACTH, as has been done for cortisol [115,116]. The fragility of the molecule in blood probably precluded this approach, which might be performed by measuring other, more stable, POMC peptides such as β- and γ-LPHs [117].

ACTH Secretion is Dysregulated, not Autonomous

Besides being increased, corticotroph activity has acquired altered regulatory mechanisms that are the hallmark of Cushing's disease. Plasma ACTH – and cortisol – classically have lost their normal circadian periodicity; yet episodic fluctuations occur and in some cases a significant circadian variation may still be present (Figure 16.3) [66,118–120]. They are unresponsive to stress [121,122]; they have become partially resistant to the suppressive action of glucocorticoids [123]; they are – inappropriately – sensitive to the stimulatory action of CRH and/or AVP in spite of the hypercortisolic state [111,124,125].

These observations are of utmost importance. Not only do they provide the basis for pathophysiologic understanding of ACTH oversecretion, but they also support the rationale of the diagnostic procedures [126].

The Source and Mechanism of ACTH Oversecretion in Cushing's Disease

The Classic Anterior Pituitary Corticotroph Adenoma

That Cushing's disease is a primary pituitary disorder caused by a corticotroph adenoma is based on the frequency with which such adenomas are found at surgery and the histologic, biochemical and clinical evidences for a suppressed hypothalamic CRH.

PREVALENCE

Since the late 1970s many groups have reported the high frequency of pituitary microadenomas found at surgery in patients who were systematically subjected to sellar exploration by the transsphenoidal route, whether or not a pituitary tumor had been suspected by prior X-ray, computed tomography (CT) scanning, or, more recently, magnetic resonance imaging (MRI). As a rule such tumors are found in more than 80% of the cases [127–135]. Although small, and "silent," corticotroph tumors are sometimes found at autopsy of nonCushing's patients, the prevalence of such adenomas is definitively higher in patients with Cushing's disease [136].

HISTOLOGY

The basophilic adenomas of Cushing's disease have variable sizes; a large majority of them are microadenomas arbitrarily defined as being less than 10 mm with a mean of approximately 5 mm (Figure 16.4) [14,130,137]. Most are localized to a primary right- or

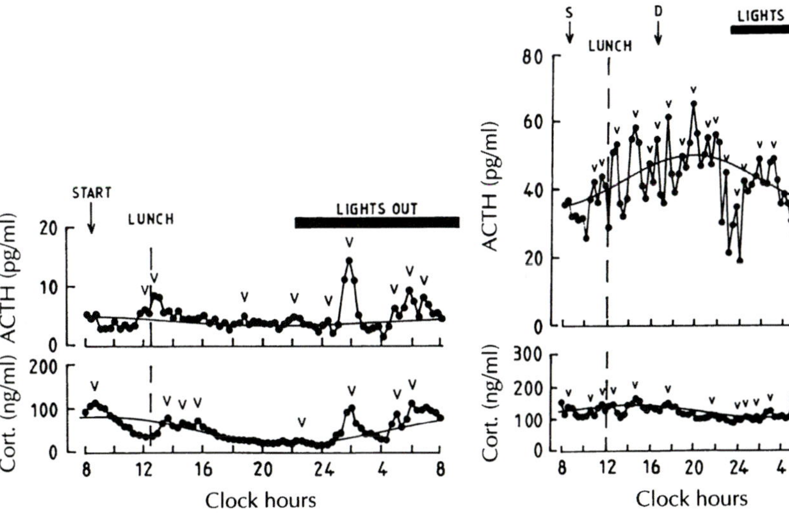

FIGURE 16.3 Twenty-four-hour profile of cortisol (Cort.) and adrenocorticotrophic hormone (ACTH) in a normal woman (left panel) and a woman with Cushing's disease (right panel). *From Liu et al. (54).*

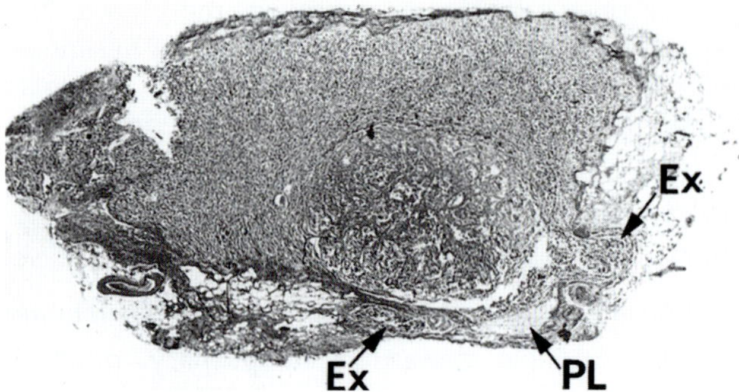

FIGURE 16.4 Pituitary gland from a necropsy in a patient with Cushing's disease (horizontal section x 10). A prominent microadenoma is located within the anterior lobe, in the vicinity of the posterior lobe (only a small portion of which is recognizable on this section: PL). Two invasive extensions (Ex) of the tumor are progressing within the neighboring tissues of the sella turcica. *Courtesy of L. Olivier.*

left-sided position within the gland, but a significant proportion (ca. 15%) are situated centrally [130]. Some are found outside the pituitary fossa and develop from the uppermost part of the pituitary gland (pars tuberalis), above the diaphragma, out of reach of the neurosurgeon via the transsphenoidal route, and several cases of Cushing's disease have been reported with an ectopic corticotroph adenoma [138–140] in the mucosa of the sphenoidal sinus [141], and even in an ovarian teratoma [142].

The classic basophilic adenoma is not encapsulated and is composed of compact cords of more or less homogeneous cells. The granule content is responsible for its basophilic and PAS-staining properties; the latter is now explained since non-ACTH POMC peptides (the N-terminal fragment) are glycosylated [44]. Electron microscopy shows secretory granules which are highly variable in size (from 100 to 700 nm) and in amount (Figure 16.5) [143]. Occasionally the paucity of the granule content explains why some adenomas appear chromophobe at the light microscope. Within the same tumor a variable pattern of granule load and size may be observed. In some adenomas [144] tumor cells show characteristic features of Crooke's cell [145], as depicted in the normal corticotroph of patients treated with corticosteroids: a ring-shaped homogeneous dense hyaline area constitutes an amorphous zone that repels the granules to the margin of the cell and close to the nucleus; ultrastructural studies show that it is made of filaments [146].

Immunocytochemistry has recently provided the ultimate means to recognize corticotroph cells by specific immunodetection of their content [143,148]. For a given antibody the signal is generally correlated to the cell granule load (Figure 16.6A, B). The sensitivity of the method sometimes allows the detection of an immune signal in what appeared to be a chromophobe adenoma [143]. Many adenomas will, unsurprisingly, react with different antisera directed against different POMC fragments, though some will respond only to a given antiserum. Although this type of observation may point to some peculiar mode of POMC processing in a particular tumor which would not generate a generally accessible epitope to the antibody, as has been described for example in endorphin adenomas [148], it should be kept in mind that different antisera may show variable sensitivities. More recently the specific recognizition of POMC RNA by in situ hybridization has been achieved in human corticotroph adenomas (Figure 16.6C).

The periadenomatous tissue shows a variable density of corticotroph cells, with frequent and typical Crooke's cells [146]. The coexistence of corticotroph hyperplasia and adenoma has been reported [149–152].

SUPPRESSED HYPOTHALAMIC CRH

A crucial clue to the pathophysiologic mechanism of ACTH oversecretion in Cushing's disease is that pituitary corticotroph adenomas are associated with a series of histologic, biochemical and clinical arguments that hypothalamic CRH is chronically suppressed: (1) histologically, examination of the periadenomatous tissue does not show – in the vast majority of the cases –

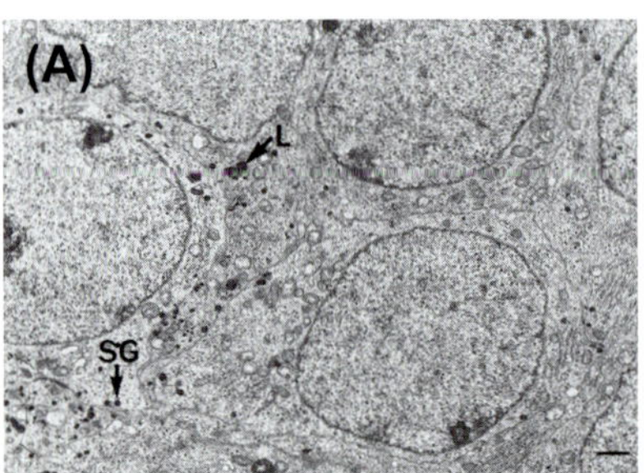

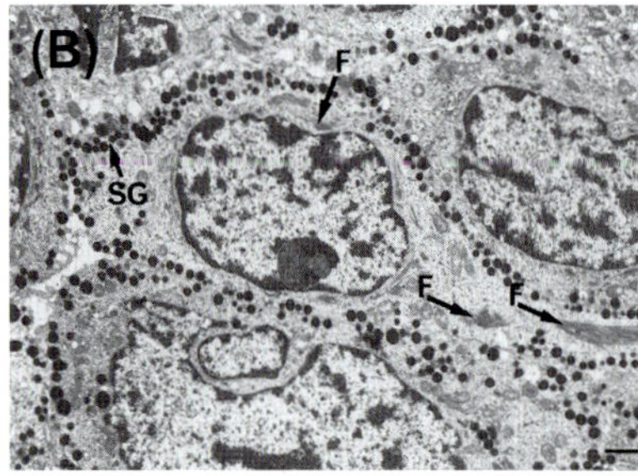

FIGURE 16.5 Ultrastructural study of two surgically removed microadenomas, exhibiting completely different cytological features (same magnification, bars = 1 μm). (A) This tumor is homogeneously constituted of poorly granulated cells (SG, secretory granules; L, lysosomal formations) with a large clear nucleus and a narrow ring of cytoplasm. (B) On the contrary, the second tumor is composed of granulated cells. The secretory granules (SG) vary in size, and are generally distributed along the plasma membrane. The tumor cells harbor a dense nucleus with a prominent nucleolus, and more or less developed bundles of filaments (F). *Courtesy of E. Vila-Porcile.*

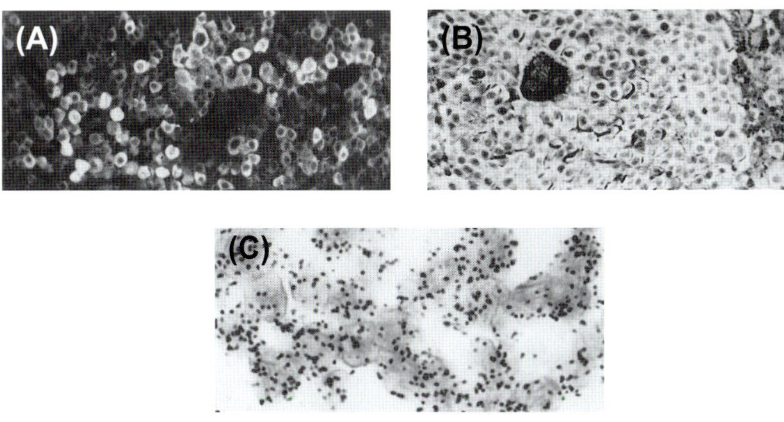

FIGURE 16.6 Cytologic study of surgically removed corticotroph microadenomas. (A) Immunofluorescence with an anti-$ACTH_{25-39}$ antibody; in this tumor, immunoreactive cells are scattered among unlabeled cells. Immunoreaction varies from cell to cell, and only concerns the cytoplasm, the nuclei thus appearing as dark dots (x350). (B) Immunofluorescence with an anti-β-endorphin antibody; in this second tumor, all the cells are heavily immunoreactive, and are densely clustered around a capillary (large dark area). The bright immunofluorescent labeling is homogeneous and is restricted to the cytoplasm (x350). *Courtesy of L. Olivier.* (C) In situ hybridization of human corticotroph tumor cells with a ^{32}P-labeled proopiomelanocortin (POMC) DNA probe. Diffuse hybridization signal indicated by the black silver grains localize high concentrations of POMC mRNA in the tumor cells. *Courtesy of P. L. Texier.*

specific evidence of corticotroph cell hyperplasia [153–155]; (2) biochemically, measurement of POMC peptides by various radioimmunoassays (RIAs) reveals low concentrations in periadenomatous tissue in comparison with the adenoma and also with normal human pituitaries [156,157]; and (3) clinically, suppressed hypothalamic CRH is supported by the lack of response to stress (insulin-induced hypoglycemia) in Cushing's disease in contrast to other situations of ACTH hypersecretion which are thought to be CRH-dependent (e.g., depression) [121,122]. It is supported also by clinical evaluation after selective pituitary surgery in case of both success and failure. In the former case, successful removal of the adenoma results in a state of selective pituitary corticotroph deficiency that spontaneously resumes its activity over months or years; all parameters of normality will be restored including perfect conservation of circadian rhythm [129,158–163]. Even the cases of failure are interesting; in such patients it was found that 24-hour urinary cortisol excretion and plasma ACTH were unchanged from preoperative values despite removal of a significant, generally half, portion of the anterior pituitary. This was taken as an indication that an adenoma was present but missed since, if the disease were due to diffuse corticotroph hyperplasia, it would be expected that partial hypophysectomy would have induced at least a partial decrease in ACTH and cortisol production [129].

POMC Gene Expression is Qualitatively Unaltered

Numerous studies performed in vitro show that in the vast majority of corticotroph adenomas the products of POMC gene transcription and of POMC processing are identical with those in the normal human anterior pituitary.

The gene transcription shows no gross abnormality and the POMC transcripts in pituitary tumors are similar to those in the normal pituitary [60,164–166]; a 1200-nt POMC mRNA is the highly predominant, if not sole, transcript (Figure 16.7). A small percentage (<5%) of transcripts result from an alternate mode of RNA splicing adding 30 nt at the 5′ end of the second exon. It has no implication on the open reading frame, which is not modified. Fewer than 1% of transcripts result from the use of an upstream promoter at −369 nt [167].

The N-terminal fragment [168], the joining peptide [38], authentic ACTH1–39 [40,41,61,62], β-LPH and variable amounts of γ-LPH and β-endorphin [62,169, 170] are the normal end-products of POMC processing

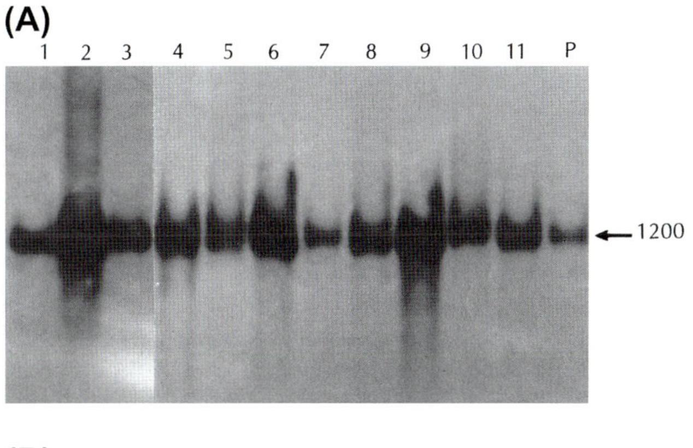

FIGURE 16.7 Northern blot analysis of RNAs from human pituitary corticotroph adenomas. (A) Lanes 1–11, 1 μg total RNA from pituitary tumors; lane P, 2 μg total RNA from a normal human pituitary. (B) In black, the pHOX3 probe used for hybridization corresponding to most of the coding region of exon 3.

found both in tumor extracts and in culture media. A somewhat higher proportion of β-endorphin over β-LPH – and γ-LPH over β-LPH – has been reported [60,158], yet the recruitment of proteolytic sites that are not normally activated in the normal pituitary is not observed and peptides like CLIP and α-MSH are neither produced nor released. This general finding supports the use of highly specific immunoradiometric assays (IRMAs) for plasma ACTH detection as a valid and significant means to evaluate patients with Cushing's disease [171]. In rare instances qualitative alterations of POMC gene expression have been described, in silent corticotroph adenomas and in pituitary cancers [172–174]; as already mentioned, poorly differentiated corticotroph adenomas may preferentially secrete intact POMC [63].

Thus, tumor POMC peptides, including ACTH, usually show no peculiar or unexpected molecular forms, in contrast with what is often found when POMC expression occurs in a nonpituitary tumor (Figure 16.8). Any of them can be used alternatively for clinical investigation, all their plasma values being highly correlated [175].

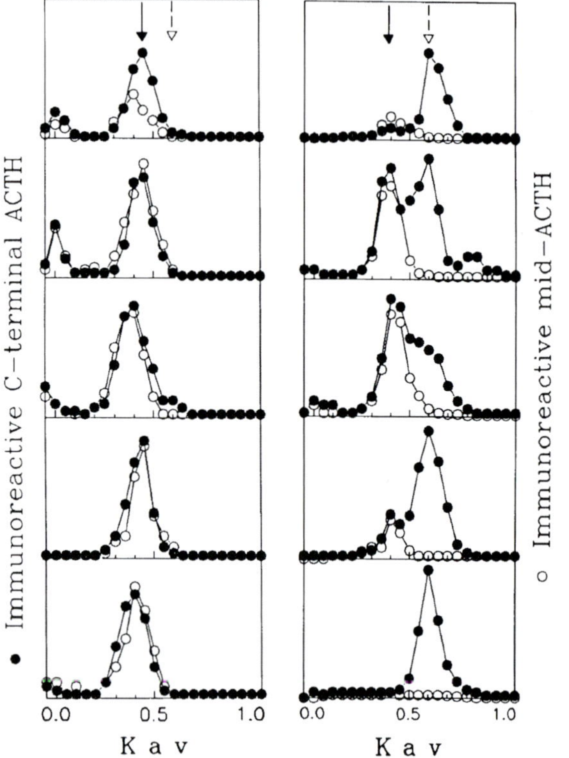

FIGURE 16.8 Immunodetection of adrenocorticotropic hormone (ACTH)-like peptides after Sephadex G-50 gel exclusion chromatography of tissue extracts. Left panel: only $ACTH_{1-39}$ is detected (↓) in one normal pituitary and four corticotroph adenomas. Right panel: variable amounts of corticotrophin-like intermediate lobe peptides (CLIP) (¦) are present in five nonpituitary tumors responsible for the ectopic ACTH syndrome.

POMC Gene Expression is not Normally Restrained

THE DETERMINANTS OF ACTH OVERSECRETION

In a system normally regulated by a negative feedback loop, two determinants which are not exclusive of each other may theoretically provoke and maintain unrestrained hormone production: (1) the set-point defect at the cell level; and (2) the tumoral mass at the tissue level. These pathophysiologic mechanisms have been thoroughly studied in vivo and in vitro in various models such as primary hyperparathyroidism where the two determinants cooperate [176]. In the case of human corticotroph tumors, in vitro studies offer obvious difficulties: the latter tumors are much rarer, and direct comparison between the tumoral and the normal corticotroph cell is seldom achieved, yet a number of experimental and human studies provide insight for a pathophysiologic explanation of the phenomenon.

The Set-point Defect or Partial Resistance to Glucocorticoid

The hallmark of ACTH oversecretion in Cushing's disease is its partial resistance to the normal suppressive effect of glucocorticoids [123,177]. The dose–response curve between administered dexamethasone and plasma ACTH or endogenous cortisol production is shifted to the right (Figure 16.9). Because ACTH secretion by the pituitary tumor is not normally restrained, ACTH is overproduced, with subsequent chronic hypercortisolism. Since peripheral tissues have retained their normal sensitivity to the action of cortisol [178,179] they appropriately develop the features of Cushing's disease.

In vitro studies have confirmed that pituitary corticotroph adenomas are not autonomous and have indeed retained some sensitivity to the suppressive effect of glucocorticoids which invariably decrease basal and/or stimulated ACTH release [180–186]. A direct comparison between the responses of normal and tumoral cells in vitro is lacking most of the time. A single study measured the effects of two doses of dexamethasone (1 and 10 μg/dl) on both ACTH release and POMC mRNA content in cultured cells obtained either from corticotroph adenomas or from their (presumably normal) periadenomatous tissues. Whereas dexamethasone efficiently reduced both parameters in the periadenomatous cells, its suppressive effect was reduced in the tumoral cells [164].

Schematically, normal secretion of ACTH results from a fine equilibrium within the corticotroph cell between two opposite regulators with stimulatory (cAMP and protein kinase C pathways driven by CRH and AVP) and inhibitory (glucocorticoid pathway) actions. A subtle imbalance between the two regulators should lead to ACTH dysregulation and, in the case

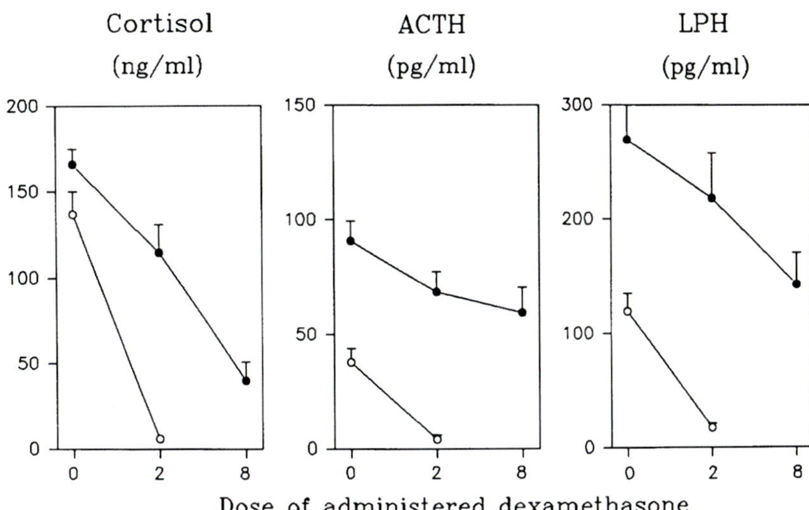

FIGURE 16.9 Variations (mean ± SEM) of plasma cortisol, adrenocortcotropic hormone (ACTH) and lipotropin (LPH) in response to increasing daily doses of dexamethasone administered for 2 days in 15 normal subjects (○) and in 16 patients with Cushing's disease (•).

overproduction, to an apparent state of resistance to glucocorticoids. Thus variable, and probably numerous, mechanisms may provoke a set-point defect. Other pathways may also play a role [100,104,105].

A gross abnormality in the nature of the glucocorticoid receptor in the tumoral corticotroph cell has not yet been demonstrated [187], although loss of heterozygozity at the glucocorticoid receptor gene locus may be frequent [188]. The recent elucidation of a molecular alteration responsible for the syndrome of general resistance to glucocorticoids [189] may pinpoint more precise targets for future studies on the DNA and/or mRNA coding for the human glucocorticoid receptor in the tumor. Alternatively, the functional activity of a structurally normal glucocorticoid receptor may be reduced by a variety of intracellular defects. Among many other causes, it is decreased in experimental animal models where v-mos and Ha-ras oncoproteins are overexpressed [190,191]; recent data have elucidated a general mechanism whereby the activated glucocorticoid receptor and the products of the protooncogenes c-*fos* and c-*jun* inhibit each other's action at the gene level [192,193].

A set-point defect might also be caused by the exaggerated activation of cAMP and/or protein kinase C pathways. In vitro studies on rat anterior pituitary cells show that whenever one of these two pathways is stimulated, ACTH suppression by glucocorticoids is diminished [80,90,194]. Increased cAMP formation in AtT-20 cells directly blunts the suppressive effect of glucocorticoids on POMC synthesis through the inhibition of glucocorticoid receptor binding to DNA [195]. A subset of human growth hormone (GH)-producing pituitary tumors is associated with increased production of cAMP [196]; it has been shown to result from the intrinsic activation of their G-protein by a single base mutation which suppresses the GTPase activity of the α-subunit [197]. This precise type of acquired generic alteration has so far not been found in corticotroph tumors [198]. Similarly, although a number of endocrine tumors occur in the Carney complex, including pituitary GH adenomas, no patient with Cushing's disease has ever been described; in that situation, increased activity of the cAMP pathway is induced by mutations of PRKAR1A, the regulatory subunit of PKA. This may be another indication that, in contrast with other types of pituitary adenomas, the cAMP pathway does not actually play a pathogenetic role in the origin of pituitary corticotroph adenomas [199]. An alternate hypothesis, already suggested for other types of endocrine tumors, is that the tumoral cell acquires an abnormal sensitivity to non-CRH hypothalamic neurohormones [136]. In vivo studies have claimed that various hypothalamic factors like thyrotropin-releasing hormone (TRH) and luteinizing hormone (LH)-releasing hormone (LHRH) would increase ACTH release in occasional patients [200–202]. The significance of these results suffers from the inescapable drawback of uncontrolled trials. Very few studies reported the data in vivo and in vitro in the same patient. Few cases, however, have been described which still make it possible that some rare tumor has acquired this unexpected sensitivity [182,203,204]. More and more growth factors also seem to play a role in an autocrine or paracrine fashion within the pituitary [101]; their involvement in the pathogenesis of tumor formation is not yet established.

Recent studies of growth factors, or using the transcriptome approach might hopefully shed some light on the still elusive pathophysiology of these tumors [205,206].

In the context of familial pituitary adenoma syndrome, corticotroph adenomas can be observed in some patients with MEN1 or mutated AIP (see below). These syndromes point to different, specific cell signaling pathways.

THE TUMOR MASS

At the tissue level, the mass of the tumor is another determinant of the final level of ACTH oversecretion. In vitro studies on rat anterior pituitary cells show that increasing glucocorticoids cannot totally suppress the rate of POMC gene transcription [80,93]. Although these studies should not be simply transposed to a pathologic human condition, it should not be totally ruled out that some inescapable POMC gene expression contributes to the unrestrained ACTH secretion, especially when the tumor mass becomes important.

Both clinical and experimental observations show that situations where maximal ACTH secretion is chronically solicited induce an increase in corticotroph cell mass. Rare cases of poorly controlled Addisonian patients have apparently developed pituitary enlargement [207–210]. A large increase in corticotroph cell area is observed in the anterior pituitary of adrenalectomized rats [211,212]. It is possible that glucocorticoids exert a direct inhibitory action on the growth of corticotroph cells [213], their deprivation being a direct stimulus for growth. It is thought, however, that corticotroph cell growth is driven by the action of CRH. Indeed the growth-promoting effect of various hypothalamic neurohormones is well documented, like that of GHRH on GH cells for example, which may proceed through the activation of cellular oncogenes [214]. Long-term administration of CRH in experimental animals also leads to corticotroph cell hyperplasia [215,216] and hypertrophy [211].

To explain the growth of a pituitary corticotroph adenoma on these grounds would imply two necessary conditions: (1) that the adenoma be sensitive to the action of CRH and (2) that CRH be present, as least at some time of the development of the adenoma. Pituitary corticotroph adenomas remain sensitive to the stimulatory actions of CRH [124,125,217,218] and AVP [110,219] in vivo. These actions are used as investigational tools to target the pituitary origin of ACTH oversecretion. In vitro studies have largely confirmed that the tumoral cells are the direct target of these secretagogues [180–184,220]. A synergistic effect of AVP has also been observed [183]. Quantitatively the responses of the tumor cells have rarely been compared to that of normal human corticotroph cells. A single study reported that nine of 16 such tumors had identical sensitivity to CRH as the paired nonadenomatous tissue, and seven had a lower sensitivity [182]. In addition to its action on adenylyl cyclase, CRH has been shown to modulate action potential firing and to increase intracellular calcium on cultured cells obtained from human corticotroph adenomas [221,222].

It may seem paradoxical to invoke a role for CRH in the growth of a corticotroph adenoma when much evidence suggests that it is suppressed in Cushing's disease. This contradiction is only apparent. It is conceivable that, although it is not originally responsible, CRH contributes, at least at the beginning of the disease, to the progression of a pituitary tumor resulting from a clonal event primarily responsible for a set-point defect with secondary tumor growth (Figure 16.10).

DOES A PITUITARY CLONAL EVENT LEAD TO BOTH A SET-POINT DEFECT AND TUMOR GROWTH?

The clonal origin of various human endocrine tumors has been recognized, based on the study of genetic markers borne by the X chromosome in female heterozygous patients. Recent techniques using DNA probes directed at various genetic markers (hypoxanthine phosphoribosyl transferase and/or phosphoglycerate kinase) studied the X-inactivation pattern in peripheral and tumoral tissues through the combined DNA digestion

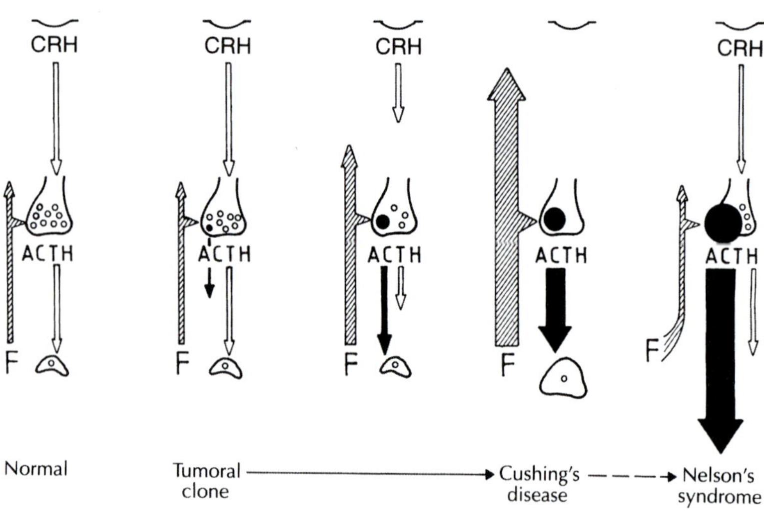

FIGURE 16.10 Pathogenesis of Cushing's disease. Schematic view of a tentative pituitary hypothesis. ACTH, adrenocorticotropic hormone; CRH, corticotropin-releasing hormone; F, cortisol.

with a methylation-specific enzyme and the restriction enzyme giving rise to a restriction fragment length polymorphism. They have shown the monoclonal nature of all nonfunctioning pituitary tumors [223,224]. Recent studies performed on functioning tumors [225] showed a monoclonal pattern in three of three GH-secreting adenomas, four of four PRL-secreting adenomas, and three of four corticotroph adenomas; the fourth corticotroph adenoma was substantially contaminated by interspersed normal adenohypophyseal tissue that may have induced an apparent polyclonal pattern. More recent studies using another anonymous marker of the X chromosome, the M27β probe, have confirmed these results in pituitary corticotroph adenomas [226–228].

Whatever its mechanism, the occurrence of a state of partial resistance to glucocorticoids in a clone of pituitary corticotroph cells could theoretically have the following consequences (Figure 16.10).

1. At the beginning the small tumoral clone would secrete only a minor amount of ACTH with no subsequent increase in cortisol. Persistent CRH action on "cortisol-deprived" clonal cells would constitute an ideal stimulatory condition for their further growth. Thus the adenoma would develop and tumoral ACTH would progressively override nontumoral ACTH with subsequent increased cortisol production and ultimate extinction of hypothalamic CRH.
2. The full-blown expression of Cushing's disease would be attained. This scheme could be extended to the situation where bilateral total adrenalectomy would constitute a further stimulus for tumor progression by restoring normal cortisol (exogenously administered) and eventually CRH.
3. Two conditions that would concur again to stimulate the growth of the tumor, possibly leading to Nelson's syndrome. The set-point defect and the tumor growth potential would be linked. This scheme explains how CRH could have a transient role in the progression of the adenoma. It shows how at some time a pituitary might contain both an adenoma and still normal corticotroph cells, as has been occasionally seen on histologic examination [149–152].

Variants of the Anterior Pituitary Corticotroph Adenoma

PITUITARY CARCINOMAS

Although corticotroph adenomas often show invasive features and sometimes a high mitotic index, the existence of primary pituitary carcinomas is still a subject of debate. The presence of extraneural metastases is required for this diagnosis. Several such patients have been reported [229–232], including cases where immunocytochemistry of distant metastases (liver, bone) proved the presence of POMC peptides [232]. This situation is more frequently, but not exclusively, associated with Nelson's syndrome, occurs equally in males and females, and the mean age is relatively low. Caution should be exerted to eliminate the possibility that an occult nonpituitary tumor secreting ACTH has metastasized to different sites, including the pituitary. Because the growth aggressiveness of the pituitary tumor may be the ultimate prognostic factor [233], methods to predict it via the mitotic index, nuclear aneuploidy, or other means would certainly be helpful.

MIXED ADENOMAS

Concurrent secretion of another pituitary hormone by corticotroph adenomas, although rare, has been reported. It is seldom of clinical significance and most often a chance discovery through global immunocytochemical testing of the surgically removed tissue. Prolactin (PRL) [234], TSH, LH and α-subunits have been found to coexist in an occasional corticotroph adenoma [235].

Curiously, cholecystokinin (CCK) [236], neuromedin U [237], and more recently galanin [238], have been found to be specifically present in corticotroph adenomas as well as in normal human corticotrophs. The significance of this colocalization is unknown. Not unexpectedly other proteins which are ubiquitous biochemical markers of neurosecretory granules such as chromogranin A [239], secretogranin I and II, and 7B2 are present in all pituitary tumors, including corticotroph adenomas [240,241]. Whether they exert any peripheral, autocrine, or paracrine function also needs to be demonstrated. Some of them, like chromogranin A and secretogranin I, have numerous potential proteolytic sites that may be natural substrates for maturation enzymes. In several systems [242,243] including AtT-20 cells [244] a maturation product of chromogranin A, pancreastatin [242], exerts an inhibitory effect on the resident hormone release and may be part of an ultrashort autocrine negative feedback.

Other peptides such as parathyroid hormone (PTH)-related protein [245] and bombesin [246] have been occasionally found associated with pituitary corticotroph adenomas. Again the significance of these associations is not known. Because bombesin has been attributed to a growth effect it may be of pathophysiologic relevance.

SILENT CORTICOTROPH ADENOMAS

The development of immunhistochemistry revealed that some pituitary tumors unexpectedly contained immunoreactive ACTH, although the patients had no clinical or biologic evidence of hypercortisolism [247–250]; hence the name "silent" corticotroph adenomas. Most often these tumors present as macroadenomas, revealed clinically because of their space-occupying effect. Thorough studies through electron microscopy have separated various subtypes; some are morphologically indistinguishable from the classical basophilic adenoma, others show subtle differences in granule size and loss of some type of microfilaments. In some tumors immunoreactive ACTH cells are rare and associated with other cell populations containing GH, PRL, LH, FSH and TSH [251].

No abnormality has been observed that would alter the quality of the POMC message [166]. The most likely explanation for the clinical silence relies on two molecular bases: the low levels of POMC mRNA on the one hand and the occasional alteration in POMC processing on the other [63,172,173]. However, some tumors show no evidence of any such abnormality. It is then speculated that an intrinsic traffic or export defect is responsible, as suggested by reports of increased lysosomal activity [248].

These tumors emphasize the notion that the growth and secretory activities of a corticotroph tumor need not be concordant. They raise the possibility that growth-promoting factors are operating which are not linked to POMC over-expression. Different types of mutations of Gαs have already been described in a subset of GH-secreting pituitary adenomas [197]. Thus it is likely that variability in the genetic causes of pituitary corticotroph adenomas will be the rule, with a range of consequences. At one end of the spectrum, a given mutation may essentially alter the sensitivity to glucocorticoid; at the other end another mutation may alter mainly the growth regulation leading to a silent corticotroph tumor.

It should be kept in mind that the clinical silence of these tumors should only be asserted after a well-designed hormonal investigation. The secondary occurrence of florid Cushing's disease has indeed been reported in patients who have harbored such tumors for many years [252–254].

Familial Pituitary Adenomas and Cushing's Disease

The multiple endocrine neoplasia type I (MEN I) is a familial disease transmitted as an autosomal dominant trait which combines the occurrence of tumoral lesions in the parathyroid, the pancreas and the pituitary, although all endocrine tissues may not be simultaneously involved [255]. Pituitary lesions have been reported to occur in 15–50% of the cases with a high predominance of PRL and GH hypersecretory syndromes and nonfunctional tumors [256,257]. In a recent study of 16 patients with Zollinger-Ellison syndrome and MEN I, three (19%) were found to have Cushing's disease with biologic and imaging evidence of a pituitary origin [258]. In the three cases the hypercortisolism was mild and might have escaped diagnosis had it not been systematically looked for. This is a unique situation where familial cases of Cushing's disease have recently been reported [259]. Cushing's disease of MEN I must be distinguished from Cushing's syndrome, which often occurs in the sporadic form of Zollinger-Ellison syndrome where an ectopic ACTH syndrome originates from the pancreatic tumoral lesion. The interesting feature of MEN I is the insight on tumor formation that has recently emerged. The pancreatic lesions are also characterized by islet-cell hyperplasia but with concomitant multifocal clonal tumors. Tumor transformation in the pancreas was associated with the deletion of specific DNA regions on chromosome 11, pointing to a possible new antioncogene responsible for endocrine tumor formation induced by the loss of its two alleles [260]. This specific gene alteration, also found in occasional sporadic pituitary tumors, was absent in four examined corticotroph adenomas [261].

The gene coding for aryl hydrocarbon-receptor interacting protein (AIP) was recently found to be involved in familial pituitary adenomas, predominantly GH-secreting [262]; yet, a minor subset of corticotroph adenomas may occur in mutated patients [263,264].

Interestingly, and as already mentioned, no Cushing's disease has been reported in patients with Carney complex [199], or in patients with CDKN1B mutations [264].

Intermediate Lobe Pituitary Adenoma

Besides the classic anterior pituitary corticotroph cells, a second type of POMC-producing cells form clusters of α-MSH immunoreactive cells arranged in follicles in the colloid cyst region in the human gland. They are thought to be the remnants of the fetal intermediary lobe and may generate the cellular cords that penetrate the pituitary posterior lobe [265]. The diversity of POMC-producing cells in the normal human pituitary logically suggested that each of them could give rise to a different subtype of pituitary adenoma with specific localization and secretory pattern, both in terms of POMC peptide molecular forms and dynamic regulation.

Supporting the hypothesis that some human corticotroph adenomas arise from remnants of the pars intermedia are two animal models of Cushing's disease: the dog and the horse both develop the disease spontaneously in association with tumors of the pars intermedia (in at least 30% of the dogs and in all cases of the horses) [136,266,267]. These tumors logically process POMC into essentially intermediate-like peptides; although ACTH is only a minor product, its plasma concentrations reach abnormal levels because of the high biosynthetic activity and the mass of the tumor. The tumoral secretion is unresponsive to the classical regulators of anterior pituitary corticotroph-like dexamethasone, CRH and vasopressin. As expected, dopaminergic agonists are effective therapeutic agents [268,269].

Evidence for an identical subtype of intermediate-like pituitary adenoma in man has been advanced in a single study [270]. Based on histologic data showing the close association of argyrophil fibers with nests of tumoral cells, and the hormonal work-up showing responses more like those expected of an intermediate lobe tumor, it was suggested that these tumors arose from intermediate lobe remnants, were more often associated with hyperplastic lesions, were less amenable to surgical cure, and were driven by a general hypothalamic defect with decreased dopamine turnover. Investigation of a specific POMC peptide pattern was not performed, and others could not confirm these data [271,272].

Dopaminergic agents have long been claimed to be effective in an occasional patient [203,273], although controlled studies had rather shown that this condition was rare [274,275] and these patients did not necessarily harbor an intermediate lobe pituitary adenoma [276]. Yet more recent studies have added new insight on the presence of dopamine receptors in corticotroph adenomas, using direct assessment by in situ hybridization, quantitative evaluation of mRNA, and direct immunohistochemistry; functional D2 receptors are indeed present in a majority of corticotroph adenomas [277].

Hypothalamus-dependent Cushing's Disease

Although it is becoming increasingly clear that a vast majority of the patients with Cushing's disease harbor a corticotroph adenoma in their pituitary there are still some cases – including patients from Cushing's monograph of 1932 [106] – where pituitary lesions were apparently absent. Therefore two questions remain to be solved: (1) is there a subset of patients with Cushing's disease where pituitary ACTH oversecretion is caused by a primary hypothalamic dysfunction creating simple diffuse corticotroph hyperplasia? and (2) in the vast majority of patients who harbor a pituitary corticotroph adenoma, does the lesion result from prior hyperplasia caused by a primary hypothalamic dysfunction?

IS THERE A SUBSET OF PATIENTS WITH CUSHING'S DISEASE DUE TO PRIMARY HYPOTHALAMIC DYSFUNCTION?

Abnormalities in the quantitative and qualitative aspects of various CNS and anterior pituitary functions have been interpreted as evidence for a primary (and general?) hypothalamic dysfunction that would include CRH overproduction with subsequent ACTH oversecretion. Classically cited are the loss of normal ACTH circadian rhythm, the decreased suppressive effect of glucocorticoids, altered secretory patterns of GH, TSH, PRL and gonadotropins, and modified sleep electroencephalography (EEG) patterns [2,136,278]. A detailed statistical analysis (performed retrospectively on already published studies) showed that the distribution of parameters of plasma cortisol fluctuations was compatible with the existence of two populations of patients with Cushing's disease. It was hypothesized that highly fluctuating cortisol concentrations were of hypothalamic origin, low fluctuations of primary pituitary origin [279]. Also in favor of a primary hypothalamic disorder was the apparent, and sometimes persistent, cure of some patients treated with drugs acting directly at the CNS such as the serotonin antagonist cyproheptadine and the γ-aminobutyric acid (GABA)-ergic sodium valproate [2,136].

All these lines of evidence can be seriously challenged. Many are simply attributable to the hypercortisolic state; altered EEG patterns, abnormal GH, PRL, gonadotropin and TSH secretory patterns all return to normal when the source of hormone excess is removed [2,158,159,161]. The beneficial effect of CNS-directed drugs is debated particularly because it was based on uncontrolled studies; subsequent elegant studies have shown that many with Cushing's disease have spontaneous fluctuations with long-lasting periods of apparent total remission – whether or not the patients are treated with CNS-directed or dopaminergic drugs [280].

Corticotroph cell hyperplasia has been reported in pituitaries of patients with Cushing's disease [153–155,281,282]. Because CRH exerts a growth-stimulatory action on corticotroph cells in animals [215,216] and because corticotroph cell hyperplasia has been observed in pituitaries obtained from patients with Cushing's syndrome resulting from chronic CRH oversecretion by hypothalamic [283] or ectopic [284,285] tumors, this histologic finding is generally taken as a strong argument for CRH involvement [286]. Establishing this histologic diagnosis is of utmost difficulty [14]. It should not be accepted when obtained on limited surgical materials. Some adenomas may escape surgical exploration because of an ectopic location, and the difficult histologic diagnosis of corticotroph hyperplasia certainly requires that the whole gland be thoroughly examined since the corticotroph cells are not scattered randomly in the gland, but rather show clusters of densely aggregated cells [147,287]. If this histologic diagnosis can be demonstrated under the necessary scrutiny in a patient with the clinical and biologic features of Cushing's disease, then it probably offers the best evidence of CRH dependence. Yet it would still need to be proven that CRH is of hypothalamic origin, and not from an occult ectopic source, and if so, that it is not merely a functional and transient hypothalamic CRH dysfunction associated with disorders like depression, chronic stress and general resistance to glucocorticoids.

Even the finding of corticotroph cell hyperplasia is not definitive proof that it is CRH-mediated. Evidence has been provided for the existence of primary multinodular corticotroph hyperplasia [288]. Thus the ultimate proof still requires the unambiguous demonstration that hypothalamic CRH is indeed overproduced. Plasma CRH is normal or low in patients with Cushing's disease, although the significance of these peripheral plasma values may not be absolutely relevant [289,290]. CRH rather appears to be low in the cerebrospinal fluid (CSF) of patients with Cushing's disease [291], in contrast with depressed patients [292,293]. Although CRH analogues that exert an antagonist activity have been used in the rat [294], such a molecule remains to be constructed for human studies. It certainly would constitute a unique heuristic tool and the sole way to definitively establish a pathophysiologic role for CRH in Cushing's disease.

DOES CORTICOTROPH CELL HYPERPLASIA PRECEDE ADENOMA FORMATION?

That hyperplasia often precedes the formation of a clonal tumor has long been recognized in animal models and in humans, and brilliantly demonstrated by the recent use of powerful transgenic animal models [295]. Site-directed expression of the SV40T antigen in the mouse pancreatic β-cell first induces hyperplasia of the endocrine cells [296]. As a result of a second and spontaneous event, an occasional clonal β-cell tumor develops. It is thought that this experimental model somehow reproduces the long-proposed two-step theory of Knudson for spontaneous oncogenesis [297]. In humans the familial form of medullary thyroid cancer (Sipple syndrome) provides the best example of a naturally occurring endocrine cancer where tumoral transformation is preceded by a state of general hyperplasia of C cells [298]. The molecular mechanisms responsible for the different steps have been unravelled in privileged situations in humans, such as the retinoblastoma. In most other cases they are still unknown. The local expression of angiogenic compounds may be the tumor-promoting factor [299]. On these grounds it is interesting to remember that a recently characterized angiogenic factor, vascular endothelial growth factor or vasculotropin, was isolated from pituitary folliculostellate cells [300,301] and the mouse corticotroph cell line AtT-20 [302].

Increasingly, the pituitary is becoming the target of site-directed oncogenesis in various transgenic animals. Transgenic mice expressing the human GHRH gene develop selective hyperplasia of the GH cells [303,304]. It will be of major interest to observe if authentic tumors eventually develop with time. Various genes have been targeted to pituitary corticotroph cells in transgenic mice using transgenes placed under the promoter of the rat POMC gene [305,306]. Expression of SV40T antigen provoked marked development of both anterior pituitary corticotrophs and intermediate-lobe melanotrophs [307]; whether true clonal tumors secondarily develop is not yet known. Other approaches have been used recently that create experimental models of Cushing's disease in transgenic animals [308]. ACTH-producing pituitary tumors were generated with the polyoma early region promoter linked to a cDNA encoding the polyoma large T antigen [309]. Chronic ACTH and corticosteroid overproduction was induced by targeting the expression of an antisense message to the glucocorticoid receptor type II [310], and in transgenic mice over-expressing CRH [311]. In this latter experimental model pituitary corticotroph hyperplasia was observed. It will be crucial to determine if adenomatous lesions ultimately develop.

In humans, the evidence that hyperplasia precedes the formation of a pituitary adenoma is still scant; although pregnancy is a condition with PRL cell hyperplasia, no association is clearly found to suggest that it is a risk factor for subsequent development of a PRL-secreting tumor. The ectopic GHRH syndrome is almost always associated with GH cell hyperplasia when pituitary examination is performed [312]. Similarly, pituitary enlargement occurring in states of long-lasting peripheral hormone deprivation (hypothyroidism, hypogonadism) is, as a rule, associated with hyperplasia and reverses with adequate treatment. Whether true tumors have really developed under such conditions remains to be established unequivocally.

The evidence that primary CRH hyperactivity may be responsible for corticotroph cell hyperplasia secondarily initiating the formation of an adenoma is based on theoretical, histologic and clinical grounds: (1) CRH exerts a growth-stimulatory action on corticotroph cells; (2) associations of a corricotroph adenoma and corticotroph hyperplasia have been found [149–152]; and (3) an increased number of stressful events have been found in patients with Cushing's disease [313,314]. It suggested that prolonged CRH overactivity eventually led to the formation of the adenoma. Clinical experience does not indicate that depressed patients are particularly at risk for Cushing's disease. More interesting are the patients whose disease recurs after "successful" removal of a pituitary adenoma [129,315]. It is speculated that the original hypothalamic CRH overactivity had been transiently silenced by the hypercortisolism, and recovers its activity after removal of the pituitary adenoma. In fact, there is simply no way to be sure that the recurrence is not due to the regrowth of a small amount of tumoral cells that had escaped the surgeon's skill and which can be removed by a second pituitary surgery [316,317].

Thus, although such a mechanism remains a possibility (Figure 16.11), there is certainly at the present time no definitive proof that corticotroph cell

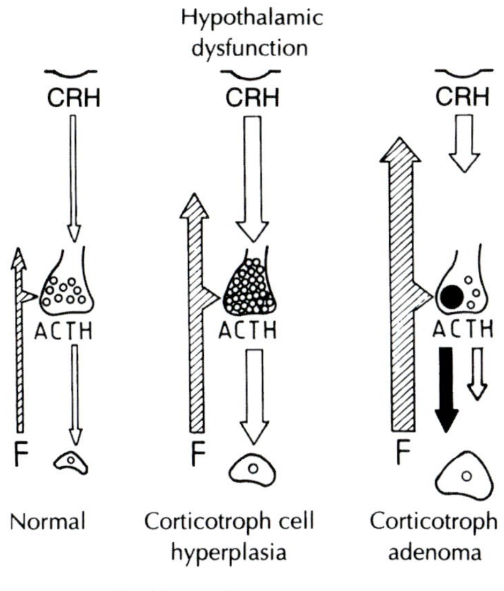

FIGURE 16.11 Pathogenesis of Cushing's disease. Schematic view of a tentative hypothalamic hypothesis. ACTH, adrenocorticotropic hormone; CRH, corticotropin-releasing hormone; F, cortisol.

hyperplasia is a prerequisite condition leading to the formation of a pituitary adenoma. Progress in this field might come from new experimental approaches generating chronic pituitary stimulation by CRH in animals [311,318] and whenever an anti-CRH analogue will be available for clinical studies.

EFFECTS OF CHRONIC ACTH AND POMC PEPTIDE OVERSECRETION

Effects on the Adrenal

Effects of ACTH on Corticosteroid Secretion

Steroidogenesis in the zona fasciculata and the zona reticularis of the adrenal cortex is regulated predominantly, if not exclusively, by ACTH. Binding of the pituitary peptide to its specific membrane receptor induces an immediate secretion of glucocorticoids, androgens and mineralocorticoids [319,320]. The primary mediator of ACTH action is cAMP and cAMP-dependent protein kinase; protein kinase C does not directly mediate the actions of ACTH although interactions between the two kinase systems have been described [321].

Because little steroid is stored in the gland, increased secretion is the reflection of increased synthesis [320]. ACTH primarily acts to increase the rate-limiting step of steroid synthesis (the conversion of cholesterol to pregnenolone) by enhancing the accessibility of cholesterol to the substrate-binding site of cytochrome P450. This action requires a rapid protein synthesis and a labile protein called steroidogenesis activator polypeptide (SAP) has recently been characterized [322]. In the long term, ACTH action also involves a stimulatory effect on the expression of various key enzymes of steroidogenesis, most likely at the transcriptional level [323,324].

In contrast with some other endocrine functions in humans, chronic adrenocortical stimulation by ACTH does not induce a desensitization state. Indeed the opposite occurs; the adrenocortical response is amplified [325]. This long-recognized phenomenon had been attributed to a "trophic" effect of ACTH though recent knowledge has shed a molecular explanation. Adrenocortical cells exposed to ACTH in vitro acquire an increased number of ACTH receptors and an increased rate of protein G_s expression [326–329]. Thus the binding of ACTH and the transducing apparatus are both amplified, explaining the higher sensitivity and the greater response potential of chronically stimulated cells.

Fascinating results have recently unmasked an autocrine network that operates on adrenocortical cells. In response to ACTH various growth factors are secreted. Insulin-like growth factor-I (IGF-I) is secreted [330,331] and acts on its own receptors to stimulate the differentiated functions of adrenocortical cells [332,333]. In contrast, transforming growth factor-β (TGF-β) exerts inhibitory effects, its receptors being also regulated by ACTH. Moreover, ACTH favors the release of angiogenic factors such as fibroblast growth factor (bFGF) and IGF-II, thus stimulating the growth of the adrenals and of their vascular system as well [321].

Although much work remains to be done to unravel the physiologic relevance of each individual system and their integrated implications in the final adrenocortical response, these autocrine factors stress the importance of the adrenal glands as potential amplifiers of corticotroph activity. In comparison with normal cells, hyperplastic adrenocortical cells of Cushing's disease have particular qualities: (1) they are more sensitive to low doses of ACTH; and (2) their response to ACTH stimulation is higher and longer [325,334]. If Cushing's disease is defined as a set-point defect at the pituitary level, it is conceivable that increased responsiveness of chronically stimulated adrenal glands may lower the amount of ACTH needed to maintain the same degree of cortisol oversecretion. Diminished ACTH secretion would thus occur in parallel with adrenal hyper-responsiveness, sometimes to the point where plasma immunoreactive ACTH reaches the lower limit of sensitivity of a given RIA. This reciprocal interaction between the adrenals and the pituitary adenoma may explain why no good correlation is found between plasma ACTH levels and the level of cortisol overproduction in patients with Cushing's disease [335].

The mechanisms of adrenal androgen secretion grossly parallel those of cortisol [320]. Thus dehydroepiandrosterone (DHEA), DHEA sulfate (DHEAS) and Δ-4-androstenedione are elevated in Cushing's disease [336]. Their peripheral transformation to testosterone and dihydrotestosterone may lead to a moderate state of androgen excess in females [337]. Dissociation between cortisol and adrenal androgens is observed, however, in the particular situation of patients resuming normal corticotroph function after successful pituitary surgery. DHEAS remains suppressed for months or years after plasma cortisol has normalized [336].

The action of ACTH on adrenal mineralocorticoids is more complex. In the zona glomerulosa ACTH acutely stimulates aldosterone release [338]. Yet this action is only transient, since increased concentrations of cortisol in the adrenal cortex inactivate cytochrome P450 11-β-corticosterone methyl oxidase. In contrast, in the zona fasciculata and reticularis the stimulatory action of ACTH is permanent. Thus 11-deoxycorticosterone (DOC), corticosterone (B), and often 18-OH-DOC, are elevated whereas aldosterone and 18-OH-B are normal or slightly suppressed in parallel with low plasma renin activity. The concentration of plasma zona fasciculata mineralocorticoids (DOC) is directly correlated to that of ACTH and participates as one determinant in the mechanism of high blood pressure [338,339].

Various physiologic agents have recently gained a new interest as possible regulators of ACTH action at the adrenal level or even as regulators themselves. Angiotensin II, serotonin [340], interleukins and as yet unidentified monocyte products [341] have shown some apparent stimulatory actions. Atrial natriuretic factor inhibits the action of ACTH both on the zona glomerulosa and the zona fasciculata [342]. Peptides with anti-ACTH action (corticostatins) have been isolated from rabbit lung and peritoneal neutrophils which are unrelated to POMC [343]. Although the pathophysiologic relevance of these observations remains elusive they may offer some speculative thoughts on new therapeutic approaches.

Effects of Non-ACTH POMC Peptides on Corticosteroid Secretions

N-terminal fragment, γ3-MSH, β- and γ-LPH, β-MSH, α-MSH and β-endorphin have all been shown to exert some effect on adrenal secretions [344–350]. In comparison with ACTH much higher concentrations were required, raising some doubt about their real significance and possible minor contamination (less than 0.1%) of purified preparations [344]. An aldosterone-stimulating activity of the N-terminal fragment [35,349], β-LPH [346], β-endorphin [348], β-MSH [347], α-MSH [345] and γ3-MSH [350] has been reported. Specific receptors to Lys-γ3-MSH have been described in the rat adrenal [351] where it would act essentially as a synergic molecule with ACTH. The clinical relevance of these results remains somewhat uncertain, primarily because of the weak intrinsic action of the peptides, and also because peptides like γ3-MSH and β-MSH are not normally found within normal or tumoral human pituitaries [168,352].

Besides, in patients with Cushing's disease, increased plasma immunoreactive Lys-γ3-MSH has been occasionally reported in some patients with idiopathic hyperaldosteronism [353], a finding which could not be confirmed by others in the same type of patients nor in other patients with dexamethasone-suppressible hyperaldosteronism. As to the somewhat elusive pituitary aldosterone-stimulating factor (ASF), it appears to be unrelated to POMC [354].

Although often suggested, the definite demonstration that some abnormal fragments of POMC processing, preferentially generated in nonpituitary tumors responsible for the ectopic ACTH syndrome, somehow enhance the secretion of mineralocorticoids by the adrenals still remains to be made. Similarly, that cortical adrenal androgen-stimulating hormone (CASH) – or joining peptide 1–12 – is a specific regulator of adrenocortical androgens has not been confirmed [355]. ACTH 7–38 or corticotrophin-inhibiting peptide (CIP) exerts an anti-ACTH action [356]. Although occasionally described in some pituitary extracts it is not a significant product of POMC in the human normal or tumoral pituitary.

Effects of ACTH on Adrenocortical Growth

Hypophysectomy results in adrenal cortex atrophy that is restored by the sole administration ofACTH [320]. Thus, in vivo, ACTH is the predominant if not the exclusive trophic factor for the adrenals. Prolonged in vivo stimulation with chronic ACTH administration or oversecretion eventually leads to an increase in total adrenal protein and RNA synthesis. Cell proliferation is indicated by an increase in total DNA [320]; the resulting adrenocortical hyperplasia participates in the amplified response of the chronically stimulated gland, and the weight of each gland can be greatly increased.

The exact mechanism whereby ACTH promotes adrenocortical growth still remains somewhat mysterious, since in vitro studies show a paradoxical negative effect of ACTH on adrenocortical cell proliferation [321]. As already mentioned, the growth-stimulatory effect of ACTH in vivo most likely proceeds through the activation of a local and complex network of autocrine growth factors and their own receptors which appear to trigger the expression of early cellular protooncogenes such as *c-fos* [357]. Although a number of other substances, including POMC-peptides such as γ3-MSH [358], have been shown to exert some adrenocortical growth effect they do not appear to be sufficiently potent to exert a direct effect in vivo.

Extra-adrenal Effects of ACTH and POMC Peptides

ACTH, β- and γ-LPH all contain a common heptapeptide (Met-Glu-His-Phe-Arg-Trp-Gly) which bears the melanocyte-stimulating activity present within POMC [28]. As measured in the frog skin bioassay the three molecules have essentially the same intrinsic bioactivity [359]. The more potent peptides (x100) α-MSH and β-MSH_{5-22} are not formed in normal and tumoral anterior pituitaries in humans. They may be generated in some nonpituitary tumors responsible for ectopic ACTH syndrome [352]. Thus in Cushing's disease and in Nelson's syndrome high plasma levels of ACTH, β-LPH and γ-LPH all participate, for essentially the same part, in the hyperpigmentation.

The same core heptapeptide is responsible for the lipolytic activity of the LPHs and ACTH. This effect is species-specific and observed predominantly in the rabbit. Human (and rat) adipocytes are essentially not responsive.

Because a small, but definite, amount of β-endorphin is formed in the anterior pituitary the question has arisen of the potential effect of this highly powerful analgesic. Very high levels of authentic nonacetylated, presumably fully bioactive, β-endorphin have been measured and chemically identified in the plasma of some patients with Nelson's syndrome. These patients showed no evidence of analgesia and had no response after naloxone administration [360]. This observation emphasizes the total lack of analgesic action of circulating β-endorphin which cannot cross the blood–brain barrier to act on its CNS receptors. CSF β-endorphin levels were low or normal in patients with Cushing's disease and even in Nelson's patients with highly elevated plasma levels [361].

PATHOLOGY OF THE ADRENAL IN CUSHING'S DISEASE

Simple Diffuse Hyperplasia

The most common adrenocortical lesion of Cushing's disease is bilateral simple diffuse hyperplasia [4]. The two glands are symmetrically (and generally moderately) enlarged, weighing between 5 and 12 g each at operation. The glands are yellow or brown and the cortex appears regularly widened on section. On light microscope examination a wide inner zone of compact zona reticularis cells separated from an outer zone of clear cells is observed. The zona glomerulosa is not changed. The cells themselves usually appear normal. Already in this form of hyperplasia small nodular lesions are found which emphasize the essential continuity of this condition with the nodular hyperplastic form with large, macroscopic nodules [362].

Multinodular Hyperplasia

Although this definition is somewhat arbitrary, it is generally used whenever one or several macroscopic (visible to the naked eye) yellow nodules are present [4,6].

Such glands, in general, have a greater weight than in simple diffuse hyperplasia. The size of the nodules displays an extremely wide range of variation, from a few millimeters to several centimeters. Although as a rule they occur in both glands, marked asymmetry is occasionally seen, which may falsely indicate an autonomous adenoma-like lesion. In contrast to the autonomous adenomas, a constant feature that must be thoroughly examined, is that the attached cortex which lies in between the nodules is always hyperplastic [4]. With the light microscope, nodular cells show features not dissimilar to those of the hyperplastic regions with alternate collections of compact and clear cells.

Controversy still exists on the mechanism leading to nodular formation, its possible implication as a transient state leading to the formation of autonomous adenomas, and even adrenal carcinomas [337–342]. A large body of evidence suggests that in most cases multinodular hyperplasia is an anatomical variant that has kept its normal ACTH dependency: (1) unilateral adrenalectomy of a highly predominant and asymmetrical gland fails to cure the hypercortisolism [369]; (2) in many cases a fine hormonal evaluation is consistent with a pituitary source of ACTH as the responsible drive of cortisol oversecretion [367]; and (3) finally the finding and removal of a pituitary microadenoma has convincingly been shown to cure such patients [370]. It is assumed that multinodular hyperplasia results from long-standing ACTH stimulation of the adrenal cortex [371].

In other cases the situation is less clear, particularly because the ACTH dependency of the hypercortisolism is in question [372–374]; plasma ACTH is undetectable, the 17-hydroxycorticosteroids not stimulated by the metyrapone test, and cortisol secretion poorly or not at all suppressed by the classic high-dose dexamethasone test. None of these data are alone sufficient to prove that ACTH secretion is suppressed. A nondetectable plasma ACTH level simply may be under the lower limit of the assay and still be present in sufficient amounts to stimulate a large mass of adrenal cells [375,376] that have been shown to be even more sensitive to ACTH than simple hyperplastic cells [377]. Some patients who did not respond to the classic high-dose (8 mg/day) dexamethasone suppression test subsequently responded to a higher dose of 16 or 32 mg [378]. It thus appears that the "autonomy" of cortisol secretion may be only apparent and not actual in many cases; and hormonal tests must be interpreted with the view that a large mass of highly ACTH-sensitive adrenocortical cells may somehow modify the classic limits of their responses [375,376,378].

Yet there remain some cases of authentic multinodular hyperplasia where the most thorough investigations have failed to detect the slightest indication of basal or stimulated (CRH) ACTH activity, including inferior petrosal sinus [379] or after bilateral adrenalectomy [380]. In these cases an ACTH-independent bilateral macronodular adrenal hyperplasia must be diagnosed [380]. The cause of this syndrome remains elusive. Privileged observations have suggested that "transition from pituitary-dependent to adrenal-dependent Cushing's syndrome" [368,381,382] may occur, providing a tentative explanation if not a definite proof. An alternate hypothesis is that some as yet unidentified non-ACTH factors exert a stimulatory action on normal – or more likely adenomatous – adrenocortical cells [379,380].

Cushing's Disease and Adrenocortical Carcinoma

The development of an adrenocortical carcinoma has been reported in exceptional patients with long-lasting Cushing's disease and multinodular hyperplasia [366,383]. In one case the patient had evidence of a 5-mm pituitary cystic basophil adenoma found at autopsy [384]. Similar, and exceptional, observations of occasional malignant adrenocortical lesions have been made in patients with poorly controlled congenital adrenal hyperplasia [383]. They raise the question of the possible role of ACTH on the generation or, more likely, the growth promotion of a concurrent adrenocortical adenoma. Convincing evidence that chronic ACTH stimulation may eventually generate an autonomous adrenocortical lesion is still lacking.

Adrenal Rests

Accessory adrenocortical tissue is often found in ectopic sites [383]. Classically it contains only the cortical component of the gland. The most usual sites include the celiac plexus, the kidney, the gonads, the broad ligaments, the epididymis and the spermatic cord. They may also occur beneath the liver capsule.

Capsular extrusions are collections of adrenocortical cells just outside the capsule of the adrenal glands. They are thus distinct from adrenal nodules. Histologically they appear to contain only zona fasciculata cells. They are ACTH-sensitive and may develop concomitantly with diffuse adrenocortical hyperplasia.

These accessory adrenocortical tissues probably explain why persistent cortisol secretion is not exceptional after an apparent total bilateral adrenalectomy [385]. They may be reactivated by the chronic stimulatory effect of highly elevated ACTH plasma levels and even become the source of excess steroid secretion in Nelson's syndrome.

OTHER CAUSES OF CUSHING'S SYNDROME

Understanding the pathophysiologic mechanisms of these conditions is essential to the principles of the differential diagnosis of Cushing's syndrome.

ACTH-dependent Spontaneous Cushing's Syndromes

CRH-secreting Tumors

CRH-secreting tumors have recently been recognized as a cause of chronic pituitary ACTH oversecretion, and hence Cushing's syndrome [285].

Rare hypothalamic tumors have been described such as gangliocytomas [283]. More patients have presented with ectopic CRH syndrome. The most frequent nonhypothalamic tumors responsible for CRH secretion have been the prostate, small-cell lung cancers, colon carcinomas, nephroblastoma, thyroid medullar carcinomas and bronchial carcinoids [285,386]. Pituitary tissue obtained in such patients exhibited the expected corticotroph cell hyperplasia [283–285]. In general the patients presented with mild clinical features of hypercortisolism.

Although, theoretically, chronic CRH hypersecretion by a nonhypothalamic tumor might induce pituitary ACTH oversecretion, some pathophysiologic aspects of the syndrome remain ambiguous. First, CRH is only a weak ACTH stimulator [387], CRH infusion in normal volunteers for three consecutive days induced only a slight ACTH and cortisol rise, although plasma CRH values were extraordinarily high, up to 10 000 pg/ml [388]. Moreover, the placenta, which is a "physiologic" source of ectopic CRH, induces very high plasma CRH values (up to 1000 pg/ml) during the last trimester of pregnancy [290], yet plasma free cortisol again is only slightly elevated [389,390]. The poor stimulatory action of circulating CRH on ACTH secretion in these two conditions is tentatively explained by two reasons: (1) the down-regulation of CRH receptors at the pituitary level by glucocorticoids [391–393]; and (2) the buffering effect of large amounts of circulating CRH-binding protein is similar in males and females, and independent of estrogen action [394,395]. Second, most patients with

Cushing's syndrome due to ectopic CRH production had much lower plasma CRH values [285,290,396,397] than those observed in pregnant women. Third, when the CRH-secreting tumors could be examined in most cases they were found to contain ACTH and/or other POMC products as well [386,397,398].

Thus, except for a single case where a metastasis located at the median eminence [285] might have been the source of excess CRH acting directly at the pituitary level (surprisingly, in this patient, cortisol was not suppressed by dexamethasone), skipping the buffering effect of the CRH-binding protein [395], there is still some question as to whether moderately elevated plasma CRH levels originating from an ectopic source can ultimately induce a state of chronic ACTH oversecretion. The definitive proof should be accepted when removal of a tumor harboring only CRH (and not ACTH) eliminates Cushing's syndrome.

Probably because of the limited number of reported cases and the pending questions regarding its pathophysiologic mechanism, ectopic CRH syndrome has not been ascribed a clear basal or dynamic specific hormonal pattern.

Besides CRH, ectopic secretion of bombesin has been claimed to induce pituitary ACTH oversecretion leading to another cause of ectopic Cushing's syndrome with a somewhat analogous mechanism [399]. This proposal remains to be confirmed.

Ectopic ACTH Syndrome

Probably first reported by Brown in 1928 [400], the existence of ectopic ACTH syndrome was definitively established by Liddle's group in the 1960s [401]. Since that time a number of reviews have documented its prevalence as a cause of Cushing's syndrome, its various clinical presentations and its specific hormonal pattern [402–404].

Recent advances in the molecular aspects of ACTH biosynthesis and POMC gene expression have shed new light on its pathophysiologic mechanism [405]. POMC gene expression is a ubiquitous phenomenon which normally occurs in many nonpituitary tissues [52–59]; a highly dominant mode of POMC gene expression proceeds through a transcription initiation starting at the 5′ end of the third exon generating a short, truncated, POMC RNA that contains the coding region for ACTH but lacks that for a signal peptide of the precursor and which therefore is nonfunctional [55,57,58]. For a nonpituitary tissue, or tumor, to produce ectopic ACTH syndrome several essential qualitative and quantitative conditions must be met.

1. A shift in POMC gene transcription initiation must occur which directs the generation of a pituitary-like POMC mRNA, the translation product of which may enter the secretory pathway.
2. A maturation process must occur which releases at least some $ACTH_{1-39}$.
3. Ultimately, if some genuine $ACTH_{1-39}$ happens to be properly formed it must be secreted in excess, a quantitative aspect which depends on the rate of gene transcription on the one hand, and the amount of functional tumor mass on the other.

The molecular mechanisms of ACTH oversecretion in pituitary and nonpituitary tumors are schematically shown in Figure 16.12. In pituitary tumors the overall process of POMC gene expression appears qualitatively unaltered, yet exaggerated; in nonpituitary tumors

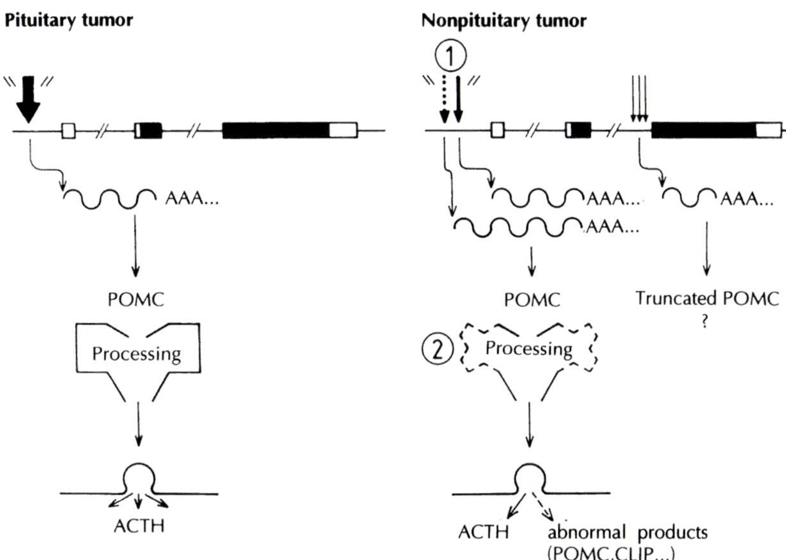

FIGURE 16.12 Schematic presentation of the molecular mechanisms of proopiomelanocortin (POMC) gene expression and adrenocorticotropic hormone (ACTH) oversecretion in a pituitary tumor (left panel) and a nonpituitary tumor (right panel).

various types of POMC transcripts are formed and different maturation processes operate that are appropriate for the resident hormone precursor of the given tissue (e.g., procalcitonin in a medullary thyroid carcinoma, progastrin-releasing peptide in a bronchial tumor) and more or less efficient for the ectopic POMC. Hence an abnormal maturation pattern of POMC is a classic, although inconstant, feature of ectopic ACTH syndrome. POMC may be poorly processed [62,406,407] or abnormal fragments such as CLIP and hβ-$MSHSH_{5-22}$ may be generated [61,352,408,409]. These processing abnormalities diminish the tissue's ability to secrete authentic ACTH – the sole bioactive peptide in terms of steroidogenesis – and somehow protect the patients from the consequences of the tumor production. They also provide the investigator with subtle molecular clues that an ACTH-dependent Cushing's syndrome may originate from a nonpituitary source. The V3 vasopressin receptor is abundantly expressed on carcinoid tumors also producing ACTH [85], in contrast to small-cell lung carcinomas. In these latter tumors with ectopic ACTH secretion, aberrant transcription of POMC may be directly related to the neoplastic phenotype [413].

Another hallmark of ectopic ACTH syndrome is its production being totally unresponsive to glucocorticoid feedback, providing the basis for hormonal investigation. Apparently this lack of glucocorticoid sensitivity is not due to a lack of glucocorticoid receptor within the tumor [410]. Apart from exceptional cases [396,411,412], these tumors are also unresponsive to CRH. Because the long-standing hypercortisolic state has appropriately suppressed the pituitary ACTH, the patients do not respond to the CRH test in vivo, in contrast to patients with Cushing's disease [218].

Although the classic sources of ectopic ACTH syndrome are tumors derived from endocrine tissues [403] recent observations imply mononuclear cells as possible alternate sources. These data should be analyzed in view of the recent report that POMC gene expression and ACTH production occur normally in some circulating mononuclear cells [59,414].

Cortisol Hyper-reactive Syndrome

The case was recently described of a patient who exhibited some clinical features of Cushing's syndrome but had low levels of plasma and urinary cortisol [415]. Cellular studies revealed that his tissues were abnormally sensitive to the action of glucocorticoids; higher affinity and higher response of aromatase to glucocorticoids were found in isolated adipocytes. Although ACTH was low and poorly reactive to the CRH test it is not clear whether the small amount of secreted cortisol is still under the control of inappropriately secreted pituitary ACTH.

ACTH-independent Spontaneous Cushing's syndrome

Primary Adrenocortical Tumors

Primary adrenocortical tumors cause approximately 20% of the cases of spontaneous Cushing's syndrome in adults [2]. Benign adenomas and adrenocortical carcinomas distribute evenly. As for Cushing's disease, a female preponderance is noted (Table 16.2). Chronic glucocorticoid excess induces an appropriate suppression of pituitary ACTH. The contralateral and the nontumorous ipsilateral adrenals are both atrophic [4,383]. Cortisol secretion is autonomous and unresponsive to either glucocorticoid deprivation or administration. Most benign adrenocortical adenomas respond to exogenously administered ACTH, and most adrenocortical carcinomas do not [16]. Whereas benign tumors are usually small and secrete exclusively cortisol, malignant tumors are much larger, and secrete a whole array of steroid precursors and androgens. Removal of a benign adrenal adenoma induces an immediate and definitive cure with often transient, sometimes long-lasting, hypocorticotropism. Malignant adrenocortical tumors are highly aggressive; in most series the survival rate is only 20% 5 years after diagnosis [16,17].

Other Adrenocortical Disorders

PRIMARY PIGMENTED NODULAR ADRENAL DISEASE (PPNAD)

This rare condition occurs primarily in childhood [416]. Cortisol oversecretion is autonomous with hormone dynamics essentially similar to those encountered in cases of adrenocortical adenomas. Pituitary ACTH is suppressed, unresponsive to the CRH test or to cortisol deprivation (metyrapone test), and cortisol secretion is unresponsive to the dexamethasone suppression tests. However, this primary adrenal disorder is driven by bilateral adrenocortical lesions; the two glands harbor numerous nodular lesions that appear typically brown or black. The adrenal's size is classically not increased. Histologically, the nodules consist of typical compact adrenocortical cells with eosinophilic cytoplasm containing brown pigment. The adrenocortical tissue which lies in between the nodules has been variously described as normal or more often atrophic; the latter aspect separates this condition from the more usual and ACTH-dependent multinodular hyperplasia. Other features add to the concept that adrenocortical nodular dysplasia is a separate entity. It may be part of a more complex clinical spectrum called the Carney complex which associates myxomas of the heart, skin, or breast, pigmented skin lesions, endocrine tumors and peripheral nerve tumors (schwannomas), and which is often a hereditary condition transmitted as a Mendelian autosomal dominant trait [417,418]. It was recently shown that germline mutations of the regulatory subunit R1-α of the protein kinase A (PKA) were present in a majority of such patients [419,420].

ACTH-INDEPENDENT BILATERAL MACRONODULAR ADRENAL HYPERPLASIA

Already mentioned, this condition suggests that non-ACTH factors may induce cortisol hypersecretion by nodular and hyperplastic adrenocortical glands [379,380]. Exceptional familial cases have been reported [421]. A recent report convincingly demonstrates that such adrenocortical lesions had acquired an inappropriate sensitivity to gastric inhibitory polypeptide that stimulated cortisol release in vivo and in vitro, also explaining why the patient had high plasma cortisol increases after meals [422,423]. This led to the concept of various "illegitimate" receptor expressions on some adrenal tumors: β-adrenergic-, vasopressin-, LH-receptors inducing variable clinical phenotypes and pharmacologic responses [423a].

In McCune-Albright syndrome, nodular hyperfunction may occur in different endocrine tissues including the adrenal glands where it can lead to hypercortisolism. It has been demonstrated that this syndrome is caused by a somatic mutation of the α-subunit of the G-protein, which activates adenylyl cyclase [424]; thus cAMP production is constitutively activated and cortisol overproduction is genuinely autonomous in the affected areas of the gland.

Gonadal Tumors

Exceptional cases of cortisol-secreting testicular and ovarian tumors have been described [425,426]. Whether these originated from ectopic adrenocortical cells is of speculative interest.

Iatrogenic Cushing's Syndromes

Exogenous Glucocorticoids

By far the most frequent cause of Cushing's syndrome is iatrogenic [427]. Patients given high doses of glucocorticoids invariably develop the clinical features of Cushing's syndrome, the severity of which depends on many variables, including the intrinsic glucocorticoid activity of the given drug, its in vivo bioavailability, the dose and duration of treatment, the mode of administration and the personal sensitivity of each individual [428]. Drug administration may be facticious [429,430] and raise serious difficulties in the differential diagnosis, particularly with the recently described cortisol hyper-reactive syndrome [415]. The syndrome may also result from large-dose administration of progestins, which possess a glucocorticoid action [431] or from ritonavir (a protease inhibitor that inhibits P4503A4, and is used to "boost" levels of other protease inhibitors) coadministration with glucocorticoids in HIV-infected patients [432]. In all these situations pituitary ACTH is suppressed and the adrenals are atrophic.

Exogenous Cortrosyn

Cortrosyn may be administered chronically in patients as an antiinflammatory or antiedematous agent. It will invariably induce the clinical features of Cushing's syndrome with highly elevated cortisol, adrenal androgens and DOC. In a way similar to that which occurs in ectopic ACTH syndrome, pituitary ACTH (and other POMC-peptides) will be suppressed.

CLINICAL FEATURES

On a historical note, it has been proposed that the first published case of Cushing's disease was "a near miss" mistakenly described by Osler in 1899 as having "an acute myxoedematous condition ..." [433,434]. The unequivocal description of this condition is attributed to the pioneering work of his most famous student Harvey Cushing, who published the case of Minnie G. first in 1912 [435]; and later again in his classical monograph of 1932 [106] with 11 more cases. Minnie G. was

> a young (16y) woman ... of most extraordinary appearance. Her round face was dusky and cyanosed, and there was an abnormal growth of hair, particularly noticeable on the sides of the forehead, upper lip, and chin. The mucous membranes were of bright colour despite her history of frequent bleeding. Her abdominous body had the appearance of a full-term pregnancy ... numerous purplish striae were present over the stretched skin of the lower abdomen ... the peculiar tense and painful adiposity affecting face, neck and trunk was in marked contrast to her comparatively spare extremities ... (the) ... most striking feature was the rapidly acquired adiposity of peculiar distribution in an amenorrheic young woman ...

DESCRIPTION OF THE CONDITION

Centripetal fat deposition is the most common manifestation of glucocorticoid excess and often the initial symptom of the patient [2,3,436]. Although weight gain is classic it may be minimal and the peculiar distribution of adipose tissue readily distinguishes it from simple obesity. Fat accumulates in the face and the supraclavicular and dorsocervical fat pads, leading to the typical moon faces and buffalo-hump, most often accompanied by facial plethora. It may exhibit inflammatory features with hot and reddish skin and may be slightly painful [106]. This acquired habitus change is best evidenced by comparison with anterior photographs. Fat also accumulates over the thorax and the abdomen, which becomes protuberant. Development of lipomatosis in various situations has been occasionally described and may induce a reversible widening of the mediastinum on chest X-ray [437]. Abnormal fat distribution is of variable degrees; it is probably the most sensitive symptom of Cushing's disease, being exceptionally absent [438,439]. It disappears rapidly and totally after cortisol hypersecretion is reduced. The fine pathophysiologic mechanism that determines fat redistribution probably lies in the differential sensitivity of central and peripheral adipocytes to the opposite lipolytic and lipogenic actions of cortisol excess on the one hand, and secondary hyperinsulinism on the other [2].

Less frequent, but certainly crucial, are the clinical features that pertain to the protein-wasting effect of cortisol. Absent in simple obesity they have a high diagnostic value and must be thoroughly searched for at examination.

1. Skin thinning due to the atrophy of the epidermis and the underlying connective tissue may be mild and is best appreciated by rubbing the skin gently over the tibial crest. In some patients the skin is so fragile that it can be scratched simply by removing a strip of adhesive tape. Skin thinning and tension over accumulated fat both account for the plethoric appearance of the face and the purple aspect of striae due to the streaks of capillaries, which almost become visible. Striae are indeed present in many patients and are most commonly located on the abdomen and flanks, but also on the breasts, hips and axillae. In contrast with the usually whitish and small striae often seen after pregnancy or rapid weight gain, the striae of Cushing's disease are typically purple to red, and wide (>1 cm). Almost 62% of patients complain of easy bruisability, whereas it is relatively uncommon in simple obesity [439]. The minimal trauma generate multiple ecchymotic lesions or purpura especially on the forearm; blood collection often results in large ecchymotic lesions. Minor wounds heal slowly and are the source of postoperative complications at the incision site. The most superficial wounds, especially frequent on the lower extremities, may lead to indolent infection and ulceration that take months to disappear. Lower-limb edema is frequent and does not always result from congestive heart failure but rather from increased capillary permeability. Protein wasting is responsible for a generalized tissue fragility. Surgeons usually find the tissues tear easily. Spontaneous ruptures occur, mainly of tendons.
2. Muscle wasting is frequent and characteristically proximal leading to fatiguability, muscle atrophy occurring mostly in the lower limbs [440]. It is found on formal testing in about 60% of patients [439]. Disappearance of muscle mass may become apparent and measurable; it contrasts with the truncal obesity. The weakness may be so severe as to prevent the patient from getting up from a chair without help.
3. Bone wasting results in general osteoporosis. Cushing's disease is associated with bone loss and an increased risk of fractures. The prevalence of osteoporosis (T score −2.5 SD or lower) assessed by bone mineral density using dual-energy X-ray absorptiometry is about 40% [441]. Patients have a low Z score in the lumbar spine (with a mean of −1.59 SD when taking into account the most important studies) and in the femoral site (−1.1 SD) [441−449]. Particularly vulnerable is the vertebral body; loss of bone density is almost invariably present when searched by sophisticated means such as dual-photon-absorptiometry. Compression fractures of the spine are evident on plain X-rays in about 20% of the patients and almost half of the patients complain of backache [439]. Neurologic complications almost never happen. In contrast, kyphosis and loss of height, sometimes dramatic (up to 20 cm), are frequent. Pathologic fractures can occur elsewhere, particularly in the ribs and pelvis [441]. Demineralization is readily visible on skull X-rays and shading of the dorsum sellae is quite common, indicating cortisol action, rather than an expanding pituitary adenoma. Renal stones, as a consequence of hypercalciuria, are present in 15% of cases [439]. In children, Cushing's disease almost invariably provokes growth retardation, if not growth arrest. Without treatment, the final adult height is reduced and peak bone mass lowered.
4. The patient with chronic hypercortisolism has impaired defense mechanisms against infections. There is no recent study on Cushing's disaese dealing with this subject, but in the 1950s [3], severe infectious complications were reported in 42% of untreated patients. Banal bronchopulmonary infections may take a most aggressive, life-threatening course. Superficial mucocutaneous infections are extremely frequent, such as tinea versicolor and ungueal mycosis, which will only subside with control of the hypercortisolism.
5. A majority of patients have high blood pressure [372,450−452]. It may occasionally be severe, inducing cardiac hypertrophy and eventually congestive heart failure. The pathophysiologic mechanism of hypertension in Cushing's disease is complex and multifactorial due to both the glucocorticoid effect of cortisol [453,454] and to the mineralocorticoid effect of cortisol and DOC [455].

Well-defined carotid wall plaques are detected in one-third of patients with active or cured Cushing's disease [456]. Increased susceptibility to both arterial and venous thrombosis is also present due to lipid [457] and coagulation [458,459,460] disturbances. A systematic review on 15 studies in 476 patients with Cushing's syndrome, including 398 patients with Cushing's disease [460], reported a risk of 1.9 and 2.5% thromboembolic complications not provoked by surgery, mostly occurring during persistent hypercortisolism or relapse. Hypercoagulability was suggested by high levels of factor VIII, factor IX and von Willebrand factor, and by evidence of enhanced thrombin generation but the overall effect on fibrinolysis remains unclear [460]. Cardiovascular complications are the major threats of the disease and contribute greatly to its morbidity and mortality rate [3,18,19,461,462]. Successful removal of the pituitary microadenoma reduces high blood pressure [463].

6. Hirsutism due to a slight excess of adrenocortical androgens is extremely frequent in women. Moderate hair growth is visible on the face (upper lips, chin, sideburns), and less often on the chest, breasts, abdomen and upper thighs. A dorsal lanugo is often observed; some degree of acne and seborrhea are frequent. Frank virilism (temporal hair loss, coarsening of the voice, clitoral hypertrophy) occasionally occurs and would rather point to another cause of Cushing's syndrome, especially an adrenocortical carcinoma. Excess adrenal androgens and cortisol both suppress gonadotroph function, resulting in an array of gonadal dysfunctions. Most female patients have oligomenorrhea or amenorrhea, and infertility is frequent. Rare patients may also have concomitant hyperprolactinemia [464,465]. In male patients the curtailed gonadotroph function [466] induces a dramatic fall in testosterone which is not compensated by the increased adrenocortical androgens. It results in loss of libido and diminished sexual performance. Loss of sexual hair and reduced testis size are observed. Gynecomastia does not usually develop.
7. Psychic disturbances are extremely common. They are highly variable both in their expression and severity and do not correlate with the intensity of the hypercortisolism. They are most often mild, limited to anxiety, increased emotional lability and irritability of unwarranted euphoria. Sleep disorders are also frequent. Severe psychotic symptoms may occur such as depression, manic disorders, delusions and/or hallucinations, and may ultimately lead to suicide. No clean link is found between the premorbid psychologic status and the type of morbid psychologic manifestations [467]. In many cases controlling the hypercortisolism results in dramatic improvement with complete disappearance of the psychic manifestations. Impairment in short-term memory and cognition is common [20,468–470]. The quality of life is reduced in patients with Cushing's disease using the generic short form 36 (SF-36) autoquestionnaire, an integrated measure of physical and psychological well-being or other questionnaire [19,471–475]. The quality of life score improves partially after treatment [471,473–476]. A score of Cushing symptoms was inversely related to SF-36 [473]. Other identified factors for worse quality of life among various studies are active hypercortisolism, female gender, young age at diagnosis, recent hospitalization, adrenal insufficiency, hypopituitarism, anxiety and depression.

The skin, as already mentioned, is often plethoric, especially on the face. Hyperpigmentation is almost never observed in the usual, uncomplicated forms of Cushing's disease, where ACTH and LPH plasma levels are only moderately elevated. In contrast it is a frequent symptom of patients whose treatment is directed primarily at the adrenals, especially after total bilateral adrenalectomy.

Miscellaneous clinical features have been claimed to be associated with Cushing's disease and reported as classic manifestations, although they now appear rare and not obviously related to glucocorticoid excess. These include thirst and polyuria in the absence of glycosuria or severe hypokalemia, and a tendency to exophthalmos, which might result from orbital fat accumulation. Cataract is rarely present unless as a secondary consequence of diabetes mellitus [439]. Although exceptional, symptoms related to the mass effect of a pituitary tumor (headache, visual defect, pituitary insufficiency) should be looked for systematically.

DIAGNOSIS OF CUSHING'S DISEASE

Routine Laboratory Tests

Routine laboratory tests may provide some clue to the diagnosis, their major interest being to measure the severity of the disease which is not only related to the rate of cortisol secretion but also, for each individual, to their personal sensitivity to glucocorticoids. They will be most useful for the follow-up of treated patients.

Altered counts of circulating leukocytes are frequent, showing increased neutrophils and decreased lymphocytes and eosinophils [436]. Significantly increased hemoglobin, although classically reported, is actually rare. Serum electrolytes are usually normal. In severe cases hypokalemia, alkalosis and hypernatremia develop in response to high levels of cortisol and DOC.

Impairment of glucose tolerance is frequent, between 39 and 94% depending on the studies which include all causes of Cushing's syndrome [450]. Reduced glucose tolerance (defined as blood glucose levels 7.8–11.1 mmol/L 2 h after an oral glucose tolerance test) is reported in 21–64% of patients with Cushing's syndrome; diabetes mellitus (defined by fasting blood glucose levels at or above 7.0 mmol/L or 11.1 mmol/L or greater 2 h after an oral glucose tolerance test) is reported in 20–47% of patients with Cushing's syndrome [439,477,478]. Rarely, patients develop ketosis and may require transient insulin treatment. The mechanisms of the diabetogenic effect of cortisol are well known and increased insulin plasma levels reflect the state of insulin resistance.

Plasma calcium and phosphate are usually normal and a mild hypercalciuria is reported in up to 40% of cases [436]. Lipid abnormalities are encountered in 37.5–52% of patients with Cushing's syndrome [3,457,478]. These are most often mild, showing a slight increase in triglycerides or combined hyperlipoproteinemia, especially in patients with impaired glucose tolerance.

Chest X-ray and electrocardiogram are normal except in cases of rib fractures and cardiac enlargement due to high blood pressure. Kidney function and liver tests are normal. Serum immunoglobulin G (IgG) has been reported to be slightly depressed. Bone mass is reduced in most patients, as are biochemical markers of bone formation like osteocalcin [443–447,479].

TABLE 16.3 Prevalences of Clinical Features of Cushing's Syndrome among 211 Patients in whom the Syndrome was Suspected.

Clinical Feature	Patients with Cushing's Syndrome	Patients without Cushing's Syndrome
Osteoporosis*	0.64	0.03
Central obesity*	0.90	0.29
Generalized obesity*	0.03	0.62
Weakness*	0.65	0.07
Plethora*	0.82	0.31
WBC ≥11 000/mm^{3*}	0.58	0.30
Acen*	0.52	0.24
Striae (red or purple)*	0.46	0.22
Diastolic blood pressure ≥105mmHg*	0.39	0.17
Edema (pitting)*	0.38	0.17
Hirsutism*	0.50	0.29
Ecchymoses*	0.53	0.06
Serum K^+ ≤3.6 mEq/L*	0.25	0.04
Oligomenorrhea	0.72	0.51
Headaches	0.41	0.37
VPRC ≥49	0.37	0.32
Females	0.65	0.77
Abnormal GTT	0.88	0.77
Age ≤35 years	0.55	0.52

* *Prevalences differed significantly (p <0.05) in the two groups.*
WBC, white blood cells; VPRC, volume of packed red cells; GTT, glucose tolerance test.
From Nugent et al. [438].

Clues to Clinical Diagnosis of Chronic Hypercortisolism

The clinical features of hypercortisolism cover a wide spectrum of symptoms and signs. Many, such as obesity, high blood pressure and psychologic disturbances, are extremely common and yet Cushing's disease is rarely their cause. Thus several authors have attempted to characterize each sign and/or symptom according to its sensitivity and specificity by comparing its prevalence in patients and in suspected (obese) subjects [436,438,439], the sensitivity of a sign or symptom being the percentage of patients with Cushing's syndrome who present it; the specificity of a sign or symptom being the percentage of subjects without Cushing's syndrome who do not present it. As shown in Table 16.3 [438] abnormal fat distribution (central obesity) is the most sensitive sign, and evidence of protein wasting (osteoporosis, myopathy) is highly specific. In the absence of fat redistribution, the likelihood of Cushing's disease is slim; in the presence of protein wasting, weight gain is highly suggestive of Cushing's syndrome. This scheme provides a most useful guide that will prove highly fruitful for the clinical approach to many suspected cases.

Particular Clinical Presentations

Difficulties for Diagnosis

Many patients with Cushing's disease present with a highly suggestive combination of symptoms and signs, as just described, while in other cases, the clinical picture is less clear and often misleading for several reasons.

1. In some patients, the clinical features are less complete and sometimes one symptom may predominate. An occasional patient has been misdirected for months or even years to rheumatologic, cardiologic, or psychiatric clinics before it is realized Cushing's syndrome is

responsible for the symptomatology. Some patients exhibit the syndrome only partially, and one symptom can dominate the whole picture. Mild forms may be mistaken for all sorts of ill-defined conditions, such as polycystic ovary syndrome, idiopathic hirsutism, idiopathic cyclic edema and essential hypertension. The reported prevalence of Cushing's syndrome is between 1 and 9.5% in screening studies of patients with type 2 diabetes [21,24,25], between 0.5 and 1% in patients with hypertension [480,481] and as high as 10.8% in patients with osteoporosis [26].

2. At both extremes, the intensity of the disease generates diagnostic difficulties. Mild forms may be mistaken for many ill-defined conditions, including polycystic ovary syndrome, essential hypertension, idiopathic cyclic edema [87] and idiopathic hirsutism. Alternatively, a rare case of authentic Cushing's disease may present with symptoms so severe (including profound myopathy and hypokalemia) that they will irresistibly suggest the ectopic ACTH syndrome.
3. Most patients with Cushing's disease exhibit some fluctuation of cortisol secretion, others display a truly cyclic pattern (Figure 16.13) [280,483–488]. Episodes of active hypercortisolism are separated by periods of normal pituitary–adrenal activity of varying lengths. Some exhibit a fairly regular pattern of episodic hypercortisolism and complain of "swelling" from time to time [489]. A slight delay in obtaining the necessary blood, salivary, or urine samples to establish the hypercortisolism may allow the diagnosis to be missed. The simplest way to make this diagnosis is to educate the patient to collect a 24-hour or overnight [280] urine sample or bedtime [490,491] saliva sample at the time when they feel that symptoms have recurred.
4. In the mild forms of Cushing's disease, the diagnosis is often less apparent in men than in women. It is claimed that some persistent testicular androgens offer a better protection against the protein-wasting effect of cortisol.
5. In rare instances the first presenting symptoms will be those of a pituitary tumor. Careful evaluation of a macroadenoma might clearly indicate a state of ACTH hypersecretion in a patient who had no evident feature of chronic hypercortisolism. These findings may even be secondarily encountered during the careful monitoring of what was primarily diagnosed as a nonfunctional pituitary adenoma, stressing the need for prolonged follow-up of such patients [252–254].
6. Quite exceptionally, Cushing's disease may be recognized in the systematic work-up of a patient with MEN I or during family screening of familial isolated pituitary adenoma due to AIP mutation (see above).

Cushing's Disease in Children

In children, Cushing's disease almost invariably provokes growth retardation, if not growth arrest [8,9,492]. A decrease in growth rate may be the sole symptom in mild forms of the disease where the final diagnosis is often delayed. However, weight gain with centripetal obesity, like in adults, is present in most cases. Hormonal and imaging data have no particular aspect at this age. The occurrence of highly aggressive pituitary tumors has been reported [493,494]. The most usual treatment is selective adenomectomy by the

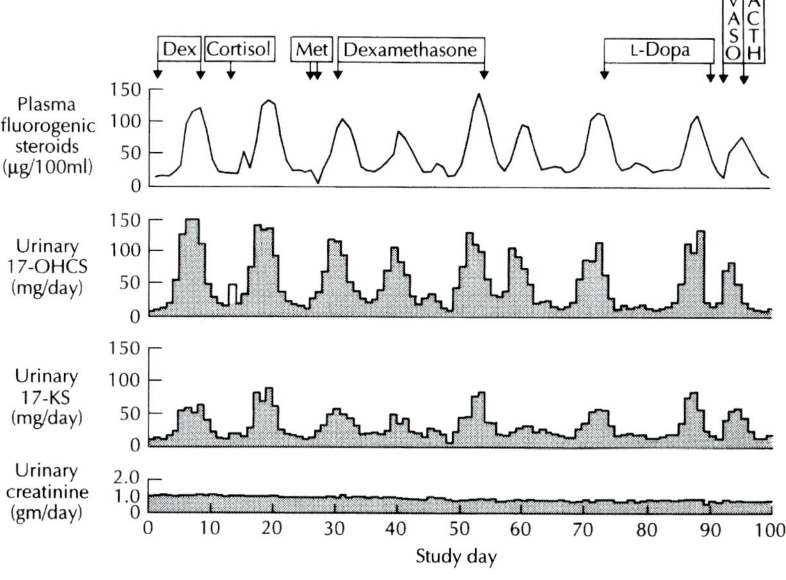

FIGURE 16.13 A case of cyclic Cushing's disease. Summary of the patient's daily morning plasma cortisol levels and daily 24-h urinary excretion of 17-hydroxycorticosteroids (17-OHCS) and 17-ketogenic steroid (17-KS) over a 100-day study period. *From Brown et al. [483].*

transsphenoidal route with a success rate of about 45–85% [495,496].

Cushing's Disease in Pregnant Women

Pregnancy occurs rarely in a hypercortisolic woman because of the hypofertility associated with this condition. To date less than 100 well-documented cases have been reported with Cushing's syndrome of all causes [497–500]. It should be outlined that an abnormal preponderance of adrenocortical tumors is found in most series during pregnancy.

In mild cases of Cushing's disease the clinical diagnosis may be obscured by features frequently present in pregnancy such as weight gain, high blood pressure, abdominal striae and impaired glucose tolerance. However, the presence of exaggerated morphological changes, virilism and especially catabolic features and hypokalemia, should raise suspicion.

The physiologic modifications of pituitary–adrenal homeostasis in normal pregnancy also hamper the biologic diagnosis. The normal and slight hypercortisolic state of late pregnancy may be difficult to distinguish from that of genuine Cushing's disease. Probably the best indicators would be the indices of free plasma cortisol (24-hour urinary cortisol excretion and salivary cortisol) showing a definite increase – in comparison with standard values at the same stage of pregnancy – and a lack of circadian rhythm [389,501,502]. Increased free testosterone may also be of help. Advancing normal gestation is associated with increasing loss of suppressibility after dexamethasone. No studies have developed a diagnostic threshold for interpretation of dexamethasone tests. Pregnant patients with ACTH-independent Cushing's syndrome do not consistently have low (<10 pg/ml; 2.2 pmol/L) or suppressed (<5 pg/ml; 1.1 pmol/L) plasma ACTH values. The ACTH values must be interpreted with caution. When in doubt between ACTH-dependent Cushing's syndrome and adrenal Cushing's syndrome, the 8 mg overnight dexamethasone suppression test may be useful [499]. The efficacy of the CRH stimulation test for differential diagnosis between Cushing's disease and adrenal Cushing's syndrome, and between Cushing's disease and ectopic ACTH secretion is unknown due to the limited number of reported cases. However, the responsiveness to CRH in pregnant women with Cushing's disease appears to be conserved, particularly in the first months of pregnancy. Its safety, its criteria and its diagnostic value have not been established [499]. The benefit of magnetic resonance imaging (MRI) during the first trimester must be carefully weighed because of its potential teratogenicity. Moreover, MRI should be performed without contrast agent (gadolinium) given the uncertainty about its safety, which limits considerably its sensitivity for detecting microadenomas. Macroadenomas appear more frequent than in nonpregnant patients. A typical image of pituitary adenoma (greater than 6 mm) with concordant biological tests makes the diagnosis of Cushing's disease highly likely.

Hypercortisolism during the course of pregnancy is associated with a high rate of maternal and fetal complications. Maternal complications occur in more than two-thirds of cases. The two main ones are hypertension and impaired glucose tolerance, reported respectively in 68% and 25% of cases. A pre-eclampsia or eclampsia is seen in 10% of cases. The cardiovascular, psychiatric and bone complications are rare, about 5% each. Of 136 observations collected in the review of the literature by Lindsay et al. [499], two maternal deaths were reported. Fetal complications are frequent, especially prematurity and intrauterine growth retardation (approximately 45% and 20%, respectively). Miscarriages and stillbirths were reported in 5% and 6% of cases, respectively, and at least three deaths of newborns. Adrenal insufficiency and fetal virilization are rare. Malformations do not seem more frequent. There is no Cushing's syndrome in newborns, confirming the protective effect of placental 11-beta hydroxysteroid dehydrogenase type 2. Symptomatic treatment of diabetes and high blood pressure is always necessary. Among the 40 cases of pregnant women with Cushing's disease compiled by Lindsay [499], only 20% underwent transsphenoidal pituitary surgery and 17% had an adrenalectomy during pregnancy, mainly in the second trimester (the period during which the fetal risk is lower and laparoscopy for adrenal surgery is still feasible). Metyrapone and ketoconazole, two inhibitors of cortisol synthesis, are theoretically contraindicated, but isolated observations or small series have been reported. Under metyrapone, an improvement of hypercortisolism was observed in ten patients, but the stimulation of precursors with mineralocorticoid activity may be responsible for hypertension, and it may provoke fetal hypoadrenalism [503].

Most anticortisolic drugs are contraindicated: metyrapone has been rarely used [503]. Transsphenoidal surgery should be a relatively safe procedure during pregnancy but until now it has only been reported once [504]. Few cases of spontaneous resolution after delivery have been reported [505].

Course of Cushing's Disease

Until recently Cushing's disease was a most severe condition with high morbidity and mortality rates. In older series, Cushing's disease ultimately led to death in a majority of untreated patients. Cardiovascular complications [3] were the predominant causes followed by infections and suicide [18,19,461,462]. In an epidemiological study during the period from 1975 through 1992 in Spain in 49 patients affected by Cushing's disease, among which disease remission was obtained in around 80% of cases during these years, a four-fold higher mortality was demonstrated, mainly due to cardiovascular diseases, and associated with age, persistence of hypertension and impaired glucose tolerance [18]. More recent studies are much more optimistic in cured patients after transsphenoidal surgery with a long-term mortality not significantly different from that in the general population [19,461,462]. In an investigation during the period from 1985 through 1995 in Denmark in 45 patients with Cushing's disease who had been cured through transsphenoidal neurosurgery, only one had died. The standard mortality ratio was not significantly different from that in the control population [19]. However, in the same study, in 20 patients with persistent hypercortisolism after initial neurosurgery, six had died which represents a five-times higher mortality rate than normal population [19]. The ultimate prognosis of Cushing's disease depends upon the severity of the hypercortisolic state and the aggressiveness of the pituitary tumor.

Several factors determine the severity of the hypercortisolic state in a given patient: the level of cortisol overproduction, the duration of hypercortisolism, and above all, some intrinsic and so far not fully identified factors that establish a different set-point of peripheral glucocorticoid sensitivity for each individual, and in the same individual in different target tissues. This explains the variable clinical features that are observed in patients with similar indices of hypercortisolism, and that in the same individual a defined target tissue seems to suffer more than the others. Because most, if not all, patients can now be cured of their disease (or at least hypercortisolism may be controlled) the practical question has become whether the clinical manifestations of Cushing's disease are reversible after successful treatment. Some patients truly are rejuvenated. As a rule younger patients obtain more benefit from a cure than older patients. In the latter group skin changes, muscle wasting and osteoporosis improve less obviously. Only recently have studies with dual-photon absorptiometry shown that suppression of hypercortisolism seemed to induce a rise in bone mass [506]. Therefore, because some effects of chronic hypercortisolism, especially in older adults, induce changes that are not easily reversible, not only should these patients be treated aggressively, they should also be treated rapidly.

The growth potential of the pituitary tumor may be another determinant of the final prognosis. Rare cases of spontaneous cure of Cushing's disease have been reported. They are thought to result from infarction and/or calcification of a pituitary adenoma [507,508]. In a minority of patients tumor growth seems to be boosted by bilateral total adrenalectomy, eventually leading to Nelson's syndrome. This rare occurrence is unpredictable. It is another argument that pinpoints the pituitary as the more logical and first target of therapeutic strategies.

DIAGNOSTIC PROCEDURES

Two steps should be used in the diagnostic approach. First, establish that chronic hypercortisolism or Cushing's syndrome is present; second, identify its cause with its specific prognostic and therapeutic implications.

It is essential that the investigative work-up be done in a coordinated, and somewhat compulsive, fashion with the clear assumption that a diagnostic certainty is the best assurance of an appropriate treatment.

The greatest difficulties are encountered when therapeutic procedures have been prematurely initiated in patients who subsequently turn out to have been misdiagnosed. Assessment of the pituitary–adrenal axis at that time may present insurmountable obstacles. Only then is it regretted that sufficient time had not been allocated to perform the initial work-up. This approach requires a skilled nursing staff, well trained to perform basal and dynamic hormonal evaluations, as well as indisputable steroid and peptide assays. Sophisticated imaging techniques must also be capable of identifying inconspicuous anatomic lesions that can be as small as a few millimeters in diameter.

HORMONAL EVALUATION

Establishing the Hypercortisolic State

The numerous and nonspecific clinical features of chronic hypercortisolism explain why Cushing's syndrome is often considered; the low incidence of this syndrome explains why it is exceptionally confirmed. It was thus essential to develop the means to assess the cortisolic state and to identify, for a given individual, whether it is inappropriately high. An ideal parameter would be that which shows no overlap between normal subjects, including obese, and patients with a hypercortisolic state, whatever the cause.

Baseline Measurements

LATE NIGHT SERUM CORTISOL

Serum cortisol is easily measured by competitive protein-binding assay or currently, by more specific immunoassays [509]. As a group, patients with Cushing's syndrome have higher morning serum cortisol values [510], yet around 50% fall within the normal

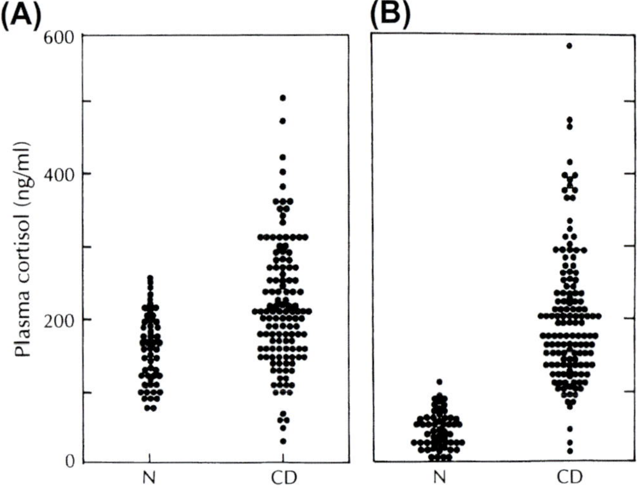

FIGURE 16.14 Plasma cortisol of the same 125 patients with Cushing's disease (CD) were obtained at 8:00 a.m. (A) and 8:00 p.m. (B) They are compared with those of normal subjects (N) at the same times.

range [450,511,512]. Because patients with Cushing's syndrome typically lack a normal circadian rhythm this overlap progressively disappears during the day (Figure 16.14). Studies obtained from multiple series showed that normal values were found in 17% of 182 patients between 4:00 and 9:00 p.m. but in only 3.4% of 147 patients at 11:00 p.m. [509]. A single sleeping midnight serum cortisol of <50 nmol/L (1.8 μg/dl) effectively excludes Cushing's syndrome; an awake midnight serum cortisol of >207 nmol/L (7.5 μg/dl) is highly suggestive of Cushing's syndrome [25,513–517] Late evening serum cortisol has a good sensitivity but suffers from two drawbacks: (1) normal subjects show frequent fluctuations of serum cortisol and so do patients with Cushing's syndrome [118–120,517,518]; thus a trough value in a patient may overlap with an occasional burst of cortisol in a normal subject, including in the evening; and (2) serum cortisol measures the total (free + bound) circulating hormone; it will therefore be altered whenever corticosteroid-binding globulin (CBG) concentration varies [517,518].

Repeat serum cortisol measurements are used to assess the lack of circadian rhythm in patients with Cushing's syndrome. Various sampling frequencies – at least six per day – and mathematical paradigms have been proposed to define a normal, and an abnormal, circadian pattern [512,519]. They do not help so much to establish the diagnosis as to appreciate the ultimate quality of a therapeutic regimen. In theory, an ideal treatment should not only control the hypercortisolism but also restore a qualitatively normal pituitary–adrenal homeostasis, including a normal circadian rhythm. Plasma cortisol may be used as the end point of the various suppression tests (see below); it is inescapable in patients with chronic renal failure [520].

Some authors have used continuous blood withdrawal with a peristaltic pump to measure the integrated concentration of plasma cortisol over different lengths of time. It was found that the 24-hour integrative plasma cortisol reliably separated normal subjects from patients with Cushing's syndrome [115,116]; then a shortened collecting period over 6 hours proved equally efficient, provided that it was performed between 8:00 p.m. and 2:00 a.m. [521]. This approach is probably more interesting as a research tool than as a routine laboratory procedure; further curtailing the time of withdrawal would ultimately end up at an equally efficient and certainly less cumbersome single blood collection at 11:00 p.m.

Blood free cortisol is the best indicator of the cortisolic state. Not only is it biologically relevant, but it is also a highly sensitive parameter. Since plasma CBG is not totally saturated at normal plasma cortisol values a further elevation increases the ratio of free/bound cortisol. Whenever cortisol production increases, variations of free plasma cortisol are amplified in comparison with those of total plasma cortisol [522,523]. Measurement of blood free cortisol requires sophisticated techniques which cannot be easily performed.

LATE NIGHT SALIVARY CORTISOL

Salivary cortisol concentration is a reliable indicator of blood free cortisol [524]. It offers a convenient, nonstressful way of sample collection, even in outpatients (Figure 16.15) and a special device has been developed to measure its integrated concentration over time [525]. Many studies would suggest that it can readily substitute for serum cortisol with an at least equal performance [490,502,514,517,518,526–528].

24-HOUR URINARY CORTISOL EXCRETION (URINARY CORTISOL)

Basal urinary collections have long provided the sole index of adrenocortical activity of a given individual. The 17-hydroxycorticosteroids measured by the Porter and Silber reaction and/or the 17-ketogenic steroids secondarily measured by the Zimmerman reaction have been extensively used. They suffer from several limitations. First, as many as 25% of obese subjects overlap with patients with Cushing's syndrome [509]. This overlap is reduced when the excretion of 17-hydroxycorticosteroids is expressed in mg/day and mg/g of urinary creatinine [511]. Second, situations of increased (obesity, hyperthyroidism) or decreased (hypothyroidism) cortisol metabolism induce parallel variations in urinary 17-hydroxycorticosteroids which do not correspond to a hyper- or hypocortisolic state but simply to adaptive changes in cortisol production rate

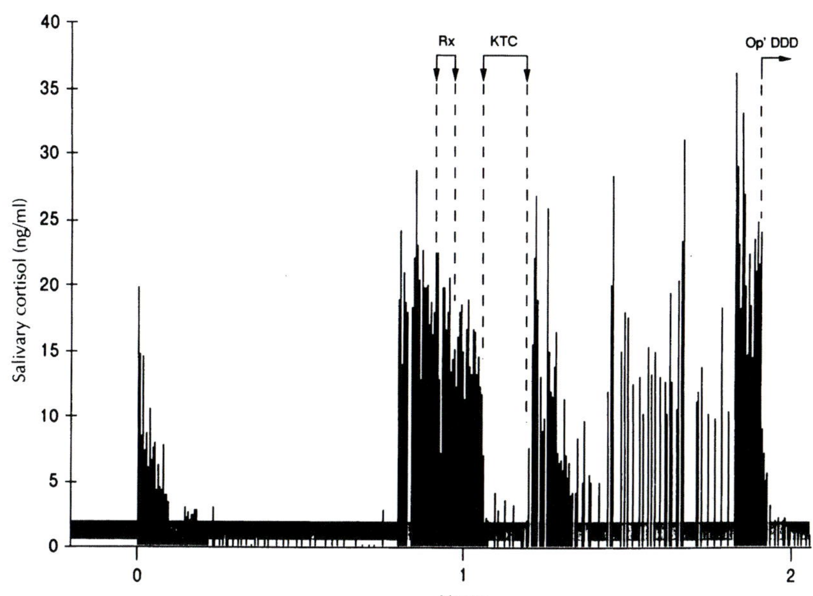

FIGURE 16.15 Two-year follow-up of 10:00 p.m. salivary cortisol in a patient with Cushing's disease. Spontaneous fluctuations of the disease and the response to various therapeutic regimens are observed. R_x, pituitary radiotherapy; KTC, ketoconazole. The horizontal black bar indicates the normal range of 10:00 p.m. salivary cortisol.

[529–531]. Drugs that accelerate or derive cortisol metabolism in the liver (phenyl-hydantoin, barbiturates, 1,1-dichloro-2–(o-chlorophenyl)-2-(*p*-chlorophenyl)-ethane (*op*'DDD)) alter the measured urinary 17-hydroxycorticosteroids without (or before for *op*'DDD) altering the production rate and the plasma levels of cortisol [518,532,533]. For these reasons the baseline urinary 17-hydroxycorticosteroids should no longer be used to diagnose Cushing's syndrome.

In contrast with cortisol metabolites, 24-hour urinary cortisol excretion is an almost ideal marker of the corticolic state. Urinary cortisol is measured by competitive protein-binding assay after extraction, or by immunoassay. Because it is correlated with the levels of blood free cortisol, urinary cortisol excretion has several invaluable qualities: (1) it is biologically relevant, being a reflection of how much biologically active, i.e., free, cortisol has been circulating over the last 24-hour period [534]; (2) it is a highly sensitive marker, since whenever the cortisol production rate increases two-fold, urinary cortisol excretion increases four-fold, whereas the 17-hydroxycorticosteroids and plasma cortisol increase only two-fold (Figure 16.16); and (3) it is not altered in obese patients, in estrogen-treated females, or by drugs or conditions that modify cortisol metabolism [511,535]. A number of studies have verified that the theoretical advantages of urinary cortisol excretion actually offer a practical gain for the diagnosis of Cushing's syndrome [509]. An almost perfect distinction is obtained between patients with Cushing's syndrome and normal subjects, provided that the urine collection is well done, and that the laboratory has validated its normal values in a large population of normal subjects

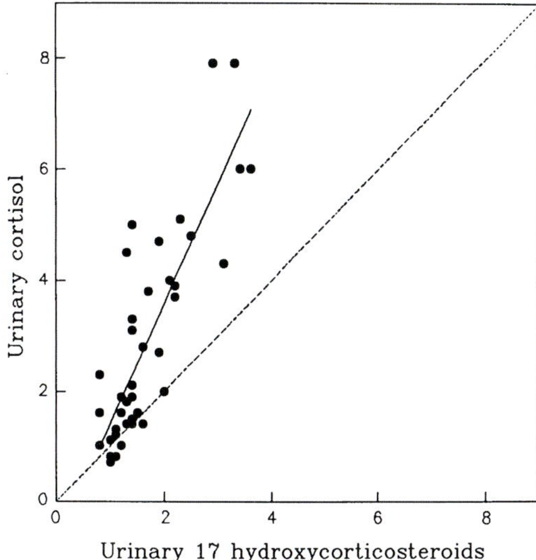

FIGURE 16.16 Correlation between the relative variations of urinary cortisol and 17-hydroxycorticosteroids in response to the stimulatory action of RU 486 in patients with Cushing's disease.

(Figure 16.17). This single basal measurement has a diagnostic accuracy comparable to the reference low-dose dexamethasone suppression tests [512,536,537]. Variations on the theme have been developed that measure urinary cortisol excretion over short (and different) periods of time to obtain a circadian pattern. Unsurprisingly, urinary cortisol excretion shows the same variations as plasma cortisol [538]. Vesperal (20–24-hour) [539] or overnight [280] urinary cortisol excretion have proved excellent diagnostic tools; they offer an obvious gain in convenience for the work-up or the follow-up of outpatients.

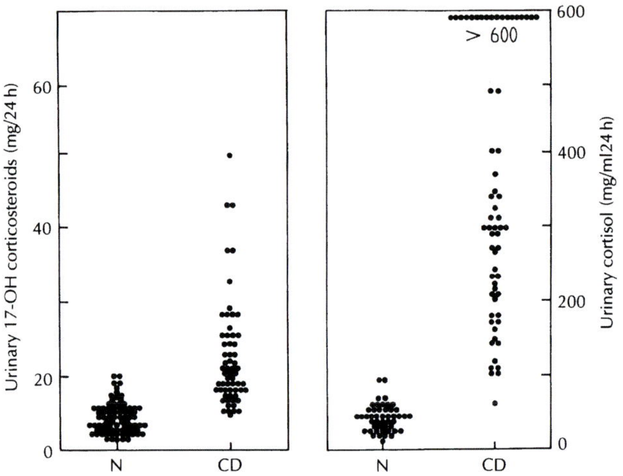

FIGURE 16.17 Baseline urinary 17-hydroxycorticosteroids and cortisol in the same 61 patients with Cushing's disease (CD) are compared with the values obtained in normal subjects (N).

CORTISOL PRODUCTION RATE

Daily cortisol production rate has an excellent sensitivity, since all patients with Cushing's syndrome have, as expected, increased cortisol production rates [509]. It has several disadvantages: (1) it is a difficult and cumbersome procedure requiring the administration of labeled isotopes; and (2) it has a poor specificity since cortisol production rate appropriately rises whenever cortisol metabolism is increased [511]. This adaptive reaction simply maintains the eucortisolic state. The recent development of a more practical analytic procedure using a stable isotope may renew this approach [540].

Suppression Tests

These tests were established in the late 1950s and early 1960s at a time when the sole measurement of baseline urinary 17-hydroxycorticosteroids offered a poor predictive value to separate normal subjects from patients with Cushing's syndrome.

THE CLASSIC LOW-DOSE DEXAMETHASONE SUPPRESSION TEST

The scientific knowledge on pituitary adrenal regulation had led Liddle to surmise that "... the fact that in Cushing's syndrome cortisol secretion is manifestly excessive implies that the normal restraint on pituitary or adrenal function is not operating properly ... " To test this hypothesis it was "... desirable that the steroid selected for the purpose of suppressing ACTH be one which did not itself contribute appreciably to the level of 17-hydroxycorticoids in the urine ... " [123]. Thus synthetic steroid analogues were selected because of their high glucocorticoid potency. It was anticipated that they would suppress ACTH when given in minute amounts as compared to the daily amount of normally secreted cortisol. It was established that 0.5 mg dexamethasone, given every 6 hours for eight doses (2 mg/day) induced almost complete suppression of urinary 17-hydroxycorticosteroid excretion on the second day of administration in normal subjects (<2.5 mg/g urinary creatinine). In contrast, almost all patients with Cushing's syndrome, whatever the etiology, maintained relatively high levels (>2.5 mg/g urinary creatinine), indicating that their feedback mechanism indeed was " ... not operating properly ... " Thus this low dose of dexamethasone allowed a convenient and efficient means to separate patients with, and subjects without, Cushing's syndrome [123,509,511,531].

In adults or in pediatric patients weighing more than 40 kg, dexamethasone is given in doses of 0.5 mg for 48 h, at 6 h intervals, beginning at 09:00 h on day 1 (i.e., at 09:00, 15:00, 21:00 and 03:00 h) and obtaining serum cortisol at 09:00 h, 6 h after the last dose of dexamethasone or beginning at 12:00 h (i.e., at 12:00, 18:00, 00:00 and 06:00 h) and obtaining serum cortisol at 08:00 h, 2 h after the last dexamethasone dose [541]. For pediatric patients weighing less than 40 kg, the dose is adjusted to 30 μg/kg/d (in divided doses) [9].

Initially appreciated through measurement of the urinary 17-hydroxycorticosteroids, the suppressive effect of the low-dose dexamethasone test has been subsequently evaluated by measuring urinary cortisol excretion (normal response: less than 27 nmol/24 h; 10 μg by 24 hours) or morning serum (normal response: less than 50 nmoles/L; or 1.8 μg/dl) or salivary cortisol collected precisely 2 hours after the last oral dose of dexamethasone, with an equal diagnostic accuracy [518,537,542,543].

Analysis of multiseries gathering several hundred cases showed that less than 5% of patients with Cushing's syndrome had normal suppression, but as many as 30% of subjects (and only an exceptional subject) without the syndrome failed to suppress normally. Furthermore, drugs that accelerate dexamethasone metabolism by induction of CYP3A4 may falsely elevate serum and urinary cortisol (false-positive responses); conversely, drugs that impair dexamethasone metabolism by inhibition of CYP3A4 may falsely decrease serum and urinary cortisol (false-negative responses).

Some authors have proposed improvement the test by tailoring the dose of dexamethasone according to body weight and administering 20 μg/kg each day rather than a fixed dose of 2 mg/day [511]. In children, it is certainly essential to adjust the dexamethasone dose [544], usually to body surface area at 2 mg/day per 1.73 m^2 for the classic low-dose dexamethasone suppression test. Since it was designed, the classic low-dose dexamethasone suppression test has been considered the most reliable means to confirm or rule out the diagnosis of Cushing's syndrome[509].

THE OVERNIGHT 1 MG DEXAMETHASONE SUPPRESSION TEST

Based on the same theoretical grounds, numerous alternate suppression tests have been proposed which attempted to offer some practical advantage over the classic approach. Probably the most popular is the overnight 1 mg dexamethasone suppression test [545]. Dexamethasone (1 mg) is administered orally between 11:00 and 12:00 p.m. and serum cortisol is measured the next morning between 8:00 and 9:00 a.m. This test is simple in outpatients. In normal subjects plasma cortisol values will be suppressed below a definite limit (established by each laboratory, and depending on the assay method). The recommended cutoff is 50 nmoles/L (or 1.8 μg/dl or 18 ng/ml), which achieves high sensitivity rates and specificity rates of 80% [517,518]. Drugs that modify dexamethasone metabolism are the same as those seen for the classic low-dose dexamethasone suppression test. A number of series have established the high sensitivity of the test, since only an exceptional patient with Cushing's syndrome will suppress normally [509].

Unfortunately the test's specificity is not good, since it has been found positive (lack of normal suppression) in as many as 13% of obese subjects and in 23% of hospitalized or chronically ill patients [509]. It may also be falsely positive in women taking estrogen. Thus, although it does not show the same diagnostic accuracy as the classic low-dose dexamethasone test it is still highly useful, and convenient, to eliminate diagnosis of Cushing's syndrome in outpatients.

As an alternative to blood collection, salivary cortisol has been used to assess the suppressive effect of the overnight 1 mg dexamethasone test with essentially similar results [490]. Further studies are needed to establish whether it will improve the specificity of the test.

Different authors have used different criteria to establish the cutoff point for normal suppression; it may be chosen as the upper limit of the normal range, the mean plus 1, 2, or 3 standard deviations, or even arbitrarily. These manipulations have implications, since raising the cutoff point increases the test specificity (less false-positive), but at the same time decreases the sensitivity (more false-negative). A sound philosophy [546] is probably to use stringent cutoff points that tend to lower the specificity since it is more acceptable to restudy a subject with suspected Cushing's syndrome than to miss the diagnosis. These limitations apply to the interpretation of other tests. A reasonable approach to diagnosis sometimes necessitates repeating tests, which must always be correlated with the clinical observation.

OTHER SUPPRESSION TESTS

Some have proposed suppression of cortisol by intravenous dexamethasone infusion in order to avoid (hypothetical) variations due to interindividual differences in the rate of dexamethasone absorption. Various dosages and times of administration have been used that all successfully achieved the desired separation between patients with Cushing's syndrome and normal (or obese) subjects [547–549].

In the field of dexamethasone suppression the ingenuity of many investigators has led to the development of many different tests. The result is extraordinarily reassuring since, even if some tests are better, all work essentially in the same manner and therefore offer an effective confirmation to the hypothesis that initiated this approach. The trick really is to use a potent glucocorticoid agonist and to titrate its dosage of administration so that it will be sufficient to totally suppress cortisol production of all normal subjects (including obese), yet insufficient to totally suppress cortisol production in all patients with Cushing's disease and, of course, in those with other causes of Cushing's syndrome.

Establishing the ACTH-driven Hypercortisolic State

When the diagnosis of Cushing's syndrome has been unequivocally obtained, its etiological investigation relies, above all, upon the appreciation of the corticotroph function.

Plasma ACTH

The first successful approach was that of Liddle's group in 1961 [108] who used the Lipscomb and Nelson [107] ACTH bioassay "... in search of a definitive answer to the question of whether the pituitary secretes abnormal quantities of corticotropin (ACTH) in Cushing's disease ... " The answer was positive, and was rapidly confirmed by others.

A few years later Berson and Yalow chose the ACTH assay as one of their first RIAs developed in humans and immediately applied this new method to the investigation of the pituitary–adrenal axis [64]. Until recently ACTH RIA has been the method of choice to assess corticotroph function because of its sensitivity and specificity [550].

ACTH is rapidly destroyed in blood by enzymes. Special care is necessary to obtain adequate plasma samples for RIA. The RIA itself presents difficulties that pertain to the low plasma concentrations, the strong affinity of ACTH for absorption to glassware, a tendency for the labeled tracer to undergo incubation damage and interference of plasma with a given antiserum. There is therefore an absolute need that both blood collection and ACTH RIA be performed expertly. The diagnostic implications of plasma ACTH determination are too important to allow uncertainty of sampling and testing.

Because various antisera will be directed against various epitopes of the molecule, some discrepancies have been observed between different RIAs, and between a given RIA and the bioassay [550,551]. Over the years many reliable RIAs have been developed using either extracted or unextracted plasma [550].

Other means to measure plasma ACTH have been developed. Radioreceptor assays [552] and the cytochemical or redox bioassay [553] have the advantage of measuring bioactive ACTH. The redox bioassay offers extraordinary sensitivity that is at least 100 times better than that of most RIAs. However, these two theoretical advantages are not really needed for diagnostic investigation of Cushing's syndrome and thus cannot compete with the ease of RIAs.

IRMAs, in contrast, offer theoretical and practical advantages as well over classical RIAs [171,554,555]; the sensitivity is somewhat better than that of most RIAs, although in the same order of magnitude (0.2 pmole/L or 1 pg/ml at best). The specificity is improved by definition since only intact $ACTH_{1-39}$ is measured. Although ACTH fragments are not measured by IRMAs they may interfere with the assay system at high concentrations by saturating the first antibody. Failure to recognize this may lead to erroneous interpretation [556]. Most important is the convenience of the IRMAs, which can be performed on unextracted plasma, with results obtained rapidly – within 24 hours – on a wide range of plasma values. Blood manipulations require fewer precautions than with RIAs since the "sandwich" effect protects the ACTH molecule during the incubation. Recent studies have largely confirmed the validity and efficacy of ACTH IRMAs which yield results which correlate almost perfectly with those obtained by the best RIAs in the same plasma samples [555]. Thus, because of their unique practical convenience it is anticipated that ACTH IRMAs are the method of choice for evaluating plasma ACTH.

In normal subjects, morning plasma ACTH constantly ranges between <2.2 and 17.6 pmol/L (<10 and 80 pg/ml) in most laboratories. Numerous series have shown that patients with Cushing's disease have morning plasma ACTH levels that tend to be slightly elevated; ACTH is almost always measurable, between half and two-thirds of the patients have values within the normal range, and the values of the others usually do not exceed 40 pmol/L (or 180 pg/ml) (Figure 16.18) [112,113,509]. Thus, morning plasma ACTH does not fully separate patients with Cushing's disease from normal, just like morning plasma cortisol. This overlap disappears when ACTH is measured later in the day [557]. At this stage of the diagnostic procedure this overlap really is not troublesome since the goal is to separate the different causes of Cushing's syndrome. In that prospect the information is invaluable; that ACTH plasma level is merely measurable is totally inappropriate and unquestionably indicates that the hypercortisolic state is ACTH-driven. It eliminates the patients whose Cushing's syndrome is secondary to an autonomously secreting adrenocortical tumor. In this latter situation pituitary ACTH secretion is appropriately suppressed and ACTH plasma levels are invariably undetectable [509], that is, under the lower sensitivity limit of the RIAs. It does not eliminate the patient with ectopic ACTH syndrome. If at least one of the two ACTH measurements is greater than 15–20 pg/ml (3.3–4.4 pmol/L) during the hypercortisolism phase, it is very likely that the Cushing's syndrome is ACTH-dependent. If there is any doubt, it is advisable to carry out a CRH test or even a high-dose dexamethasone suppression test and a CT scan of the adrenal glands [25,518].

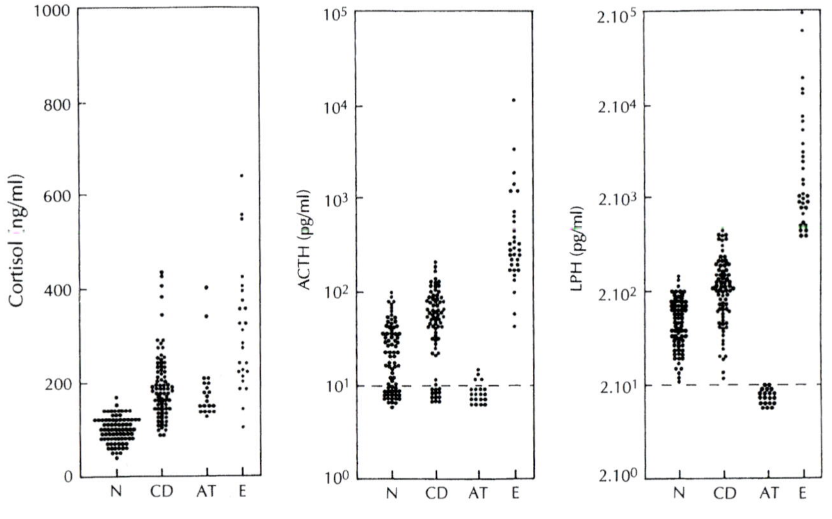

FIGURE 16.18 Morning plasma values for cortisol, adrenocorticotropic hormone (ACTH) and lipotropin (LPH) in the same blood sample obtained from normal subjects (N), patients with Cushing's disease (CD), patients with a cortisol-secreting adrenocortical tumor (AT) and patients with ectopic ACTH syndrome (E).

Plasma Non-ACTH POMC Peptides

Almost all natural POMC peptides have been measured in human blood: the N-terminal fragment [168,558,559], joining peptide [38,560], β-LPH and γ-LPH [113,561–563] and β-endorphin [564,565]. Since they are secreted concomitantly with ACTH by the pituitary corticotrophs the plasma levels of any of them constantly show almost perfect correlations with all the others (Figure 16.19). The molar plasma ratio of two POMC fragments is usually close to one, with slight differences related to different metabolic clearance rates. Thus it is not surprising that plasma determination of any non-ACTH POMC fragment provides the investigator with essentially the same diagnostic accuracy as that of ACTH itself (see Figure 16.18).

On a practical basis LPH RIAs have been the most popular non-ACTH POMC fragments studied. They were the first available but also offer several practical advantages. In contrast with ACTH, both β-LPH and γ-LPH are extremely stable in blood; immunoreactive plasma LPH values will remain unchanged in blood kept at room temperature for 24 hours [117], so that handling of blood collection is much less troublesome. Because there are large species differences in the common amino terminal region of the β- and γ-LPHs, these molecules are highly antigenic and antibodies with high affinity may be easily raised. Hence direct LPH RIA in a small volume (50 μl) of unextracted plasma is readily feasible [117]. Like ACTH, plasma immunoreactive LPH tends to be slightly elevated in Cushing's disease, and its value completely discriminates patients with Cushing's disease and patients with autonomous cortisol-secreting adrenocortical tumors who always have undetectable plasma values

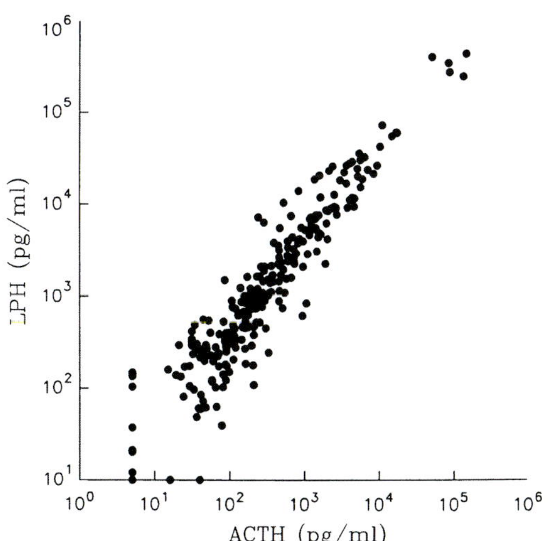

FIGURE 16.19 Correlation between plasma immunoreactive lipotropin (LPH) and adrenocorticotropic hormone (ACTH) baseline values in patients with Cushing's disease and Nelson's syndrome.

[113]. Other reports have shown essentially identical results using the N-terminal fragment, the joining peptide, or the β-endorphin RIAs.

Plasma Adrenocortical Androgens

The pattern of adrenocortical steroid secretion provides some clues in the etiologic work-up [2]. Because ACTH also regulates adrenocortical androgen secretion the latter tend to be elevated in Cushing's disease (and ectopic ACTH syndrome), whereas they are decreased in benign adrenocortical adenoma since this tumor typically produces only glucocorticoids that suppress pituitary ACTH secretion [336,337,566]. These notions are most helpful for the diagnosis of female patients: low plasma testosterone, DHEAS and Δ-4-androstenedione will be suggestive of a benign adrenocortical adenoma. Slightly elevated androgens will point to Cushing's disease but will not rule out ectopic ACTH syndrome. Highly increased androgens will suggest an adrenocortical carcinoma [16].

Establishing the Pituitary Origin of the ACTH-driven Hypercortisolic State

At this point it becomes necessary to discriminate between patients whose ACTH oversecretion is of pituitary (Cushing's disease) or nonpituitary (ectopic ACTH syndrome) origin.

Over the years various approaches have been developed to find the source of ACTH oversecretion in Cushing's syndrome. Essential clues are provided by sophisticated measurement of corticotroph function that, besides the quantitative and qualitative assessment of its baseline levels, will also require dynamic manipulations and sometimes invasive tracking investigations. Because many of these procedures were primarily set to eliminate an adrenocortical tumor as well, this aspect will also be discussed briefly.

Baseline Corticotroph Function

PLASMA ACTH LEVELS

The ACTH plasma level by itself provides a first clue to the source of ACTH oversecretion. Patients with ectopic ACTH syndrome tend to have higher levels than patients with Cushing's disease. Yet the overlap between the two groups is wide, notably in corticotroph macrodenomas, ACTH values may be high [63,113,509] and further investigations are needed for a clear separation (Figure 16.18).

PLASMA NON-ACTH POMC PEPTIDES

Altered POMC maturation is common in nonpituitary tumors, and decidedly unusual in pituitary corticotroph adenomas [60,62]. This subtle mechanism may be useful in detecting abnormal POMC fragments in blood that would pinpoint, although not identify, a nonpituitary origin of the ACTH oversecretion.

Partial degradation of ACTH into CLIP is fairly common in nonpituitary tumors (see Figure 16.8) [61]. CLIP escapes detection by most (sufficiently specific) ACTH RIAs as well as by ACTH IRMAs. Since the LPHs are unaffected by the altered POMC processing the plasma LPH/ACTH ratio is increased [113].

Gel filtration chromatography and/or high-pressure liquid chromatography (HPLC) of plasma samples or extracts will also detect abnormal molecular forms of ACTH, or unusual molecules like β-MSH_{5-22} [352]. Elegant multitargeted IRMA systems have been developed that can recognize by simple direct plasma assays the occurrence of an abnormal POMC processing at a given location on the precursor molecule [567,568].

These approaches have their limitations, however. Besides being only available to highly specialized laboratories, their sensitivity is low and their specificity also is not perfect. Rare cases of pituitary macroadenoma have been described which convincingly did not process POMC normally [63,172,173].

TUMOR MARKERS

Some tumours that cause ectopic ACTH secretion have powerful tumor markers, which must be measured if there is any doubt, such as pheochromocytomas (urinary and plasma-free normetanephrine and normetanephrine), medullary thyroid carcinoma (calcitonin) and gastrinomas (gastrin). Chromogranin A had a positive predictive value of 83% and a negative predictive value of 70% for the diagnosis of EAS in an NIH study on six patients with occult ectopic ACTH secretion diagnosed by central venous catheterization, 11 patients with histologically proven ectopic ACTH secretion and 25 patients with Cushing's disease [569]. Other tumor markers may be measured: calcitonin and its derivatives (for other neuroendocrine tumors than medullary carcinoma), urinary 5-hydroxyindoleacetic acid, glycoprotein alpha-subunit, free hCG beta-subunit, carcinoembryonic antigen, neuron-specific enolase, vasoactive intestinal peptide, glucagon, etc., have less diagnosic accuracy.

Dynamics of the Corticotroph Function

THE CLASSIC HIGH-DOSE DEXAMETHASONE SUPPRESSION TEST

The purpose here is to test the pituitary-dependency of the hypercortisolic state. In the classic [123] test dexamethasone is given orally at the dose of 2 mg every 6 hours (8 mg/day) for 2 days. Urinary corticosteroids are measured on the second day of dexamethasone administration and compared with their pretreatment (control) value. In the original paper of Liddle, all patients with Cushing's disease decreased their urinary 17-hydroxycorticosteroid to less then 50% of control values, whereas all those with adrenocortical tumors failed to reach this level of suppression [123]. Since this report it has been stated by many authors that all patients with Cushing's disease should suppress to less than 50% of their control values on the high-dose dexamethasone suppression test. Actually "... the degree of suppression is not crucial, as long as it is beyond the day-to-day fluctuations observed during control periods. In response to large doses of dexamethasone ... most (patients with Cushing's disease) exhibit decreases to less than 50% of their control values. A few, however, have been known merely to exhibit decreases to 70 to 80% of their control values" [531].

Numerous series have confirmed that whereas some 60–85% of patients with Cushing's disease suppress to less than 50% of their control values on the high-dose dexamethasone test, no rigid cutoff level should be given that rules out the diagnosis of Cushing's disease [25,509]. The specificity can be improved using a cutoff of cortisol suppression greater than 90%, although a specificity of 100% can never be attained [25,518,570]. In some patients with authentic Cushing's disease this level of suppression (50–60% of baseline) could be obtained only by administering much higher doses of dexamethasone, sometimes up to 32 mg/day [378,509]. Some data suggest that these patients have a more severe disease as judged by baseline plasma and urinary cortisol [571].

If this test has a great specificity to eliminate autonomous secreting adrenocortical tumors, it is somewhat less powerful to eliminate ectopic ACTH syndrome where an apparent suppression is not rarely observed [412,509,572].

Comparing previous and current dexamethasone urinary corticosteroid values does not only evaluate the effect of dexamethasone, but also the effect of time. Many tumors have spontaneously cycling or fluctuating activities that may induce large variations over a 2 day period. Thus an ACTH-secreting nonpituitary tumor that would spontaneously decrease its activity at the time when the test is performed could be erroneously interpreted as being suppressed by dexamethasone [573]. Alternatively a paradoxical increase in cortisol secretion has been occasionally observed in patients with authentic Cushing's disease, a phenomenon best explained by spontaneous fluctuations of the disease [483,484,574]. The only way to avoid this flaw for a single individual would be to obtain repeated urinary values to establish the degree of spontaneous variations, and/or to repeat the test itself to evaluate whether it is reproducible.

The high-dose dexamethasone test often confirms information already available from the classic low-dose dexamethasone test. Many patients with Cushing's disease who, by definition, fail to completely suppress on the low-dose test, however exhibit a definite decrease in their urinary corticosteroids. Thus, at the same time these patients exhibit an abnormal degree of resistance to the suppressive effect of glucocorticoids, which is the hallmark of Cushing's disease.

Some variations have been brought to the classic test which measure urinary cortisol instead of 17-hydroxycorticosteroid [570] or morning plasma cortisol before and after the 2 days of dexamethasone administration, with essentially the same diagnostic accuracy.

THE OVERNIGHT 8 MG DEXAMETHASONE SUPPRESSION TEST

In this test 8 mg of dexamethasone is given orally as a single dose at 23:00 or 24:00 h and the 08:00 h or 09:00 h serum cortisol the next morning is compared with that of the previous (control) day. The proposed cutoff point for a positive response (suppressibility) is a serum cortisol decrease to 50% or less of its control value [575]. With this arbitrary criterion, two studies gathering 73 patients with Cushing's disease, eight with adrenocortical tumors and 12 with ectopic ACTH syndrome, compared this overnight test directly with the classic high-dose dexamethasone suppression test performed in the same patients. This test appeared at least as efficient if not better, with 89% sensitivity and 100% specificity for the diagnosis of Cushing's disease [576]. That this overnight suppression test reaches higher diagnostic accuracy than the classic test may be explained by the simple fact that it is a stronger one since the 8 mg dose is given as a single administration. In the same manner as for the classic test, there is no theoretical reason to fix a rigid cutoff at a 50% decrease.

Others have studied the acute variations of plasma cortisol during dexamethasone infusion [577] to discriminate pituitary-dependent Cushing's disease.

THE METYRAPONE TEST

The purpose of this test is not dissimilar to that of the high-dose dexamethasone suppression test since it also evaluates the pituitary-dependency of the adrenocortical hyperfunction. The approach is just the inverse, i.e., to observe the corticotroph response to cortisol deprivation.

In the classic test [578] 750 mg of metyrapone is given every 4 hours for six doses. Urinary (24-hour) 17-hydroxycorticosteroids are measured the day before, the day of and the day after metyrapone administration. Normal subjects usually show at least a two-fold rise in urinary 17-hydroxycorticosteroids on the treatment day or on the day after, compared with the day before, reaching values above 10 mg/day [578,579]. Results obtained from more than 100 patients with Cushing's disease from different studies showed that virtually all patients responded to metyrapone with an increase in urinary 17-hydroxycorticosteroids. The sensitivity of the test reaches almost 98% [509]. In many patients an explosive response is obtained (up to 100 mg/24 h). Thus, failure to respond to metyrapone essentially excludes the diagnosis of Cushing's disease.

If this test has a great specificity to eliminate adrenocortical tumors it is less powerful to eliminate ectopic ACTH syndrome [572]. When the diagnostic accuracies of the metyrapone and the classic high-dose dexamethasone suppression tests are compared, similar figures are obtained, indicating that they merely address the same question as to whether the pituitary is involved.

Alternate methods have been proposed including the use of single-dose metyrapone tests [448,580]. Measuring plasma 11-deoxycortisol to assess the response to metyrapone in Cushing's syndrome requires special precautions. In Cushing's disease spontaneous and short fluctuations in ACTH activity may blunt the plasma 11-deoxycortisol increase. Whatever the cause of Cushing's syndrome, blockade of the 11-β-hydroxylase will automatically, and inevitably, increase plasma 11-deoxycortisol whether or not an ACTH rise is triggered. In the case of an adrenocortical tumor, the plasma 11-deoxycortisol increase will remain much lower than that observed in Cushing's disease. However, in patients with ectopic ACTH syndrome, especially if ACTH plasma levels are high, plasma 11-deoxycortisol will rise to levels identical with those reached in Cushing's disease, even though the ACTH levels do not change [581]. These flaws are avoided in the classic metyrapone test evaluated on the urinary 17-hydroxycorticosteroids, because they are the sum of cortisol and 11-deoxycortisol metabolites they will only rise if ACTH secretion increases. Thus it is highly recommended that the metyrapone test be performed in its classic setting with the total urinary 17-hydroxycorticosteroids as the best parameter.

The LPH plasma levels rise in response to metyrapone in patients with Cushing's disease and could help to discriminate them from those with ectopic ACTH syndrome where no response is observed [581]. The true diagnostic value of this approach is not well established.

DIRECT ASSESSMENT OF PITUITARY ACTH RESERVE

Several secretagogues that act specifically on the corticotroph cell in the normal subject have been used in Cushing's syndrome with the assumption that they would only trigger further ACTH secretion if the latter were of pituitary origin.

THE LVP TEST LVP is a synthetic peptide analogue of AVP that exhibits the same agonistic activity on the pituitary V_1 receptors. It is administered as a bolus intramuscular injection of 10 IU. Plasma cortisol and ACTH are measured before, and up to 60 minutes after, injection [111]. LVP has long been the sole ACTH secretagogue with a direct pituitary action. Its use has been limited because of its low stimulatory activity in comparison with its effects on smooth muscle V_1 receptors which generate gastrointestinal symptoms, general pallor and high blood pressure. These unwanted effects contraindicate its use in older subjects or patients at risk for coronary heart disease or glaucoma. In the diagnostic work-up its major interest is to achieve a complete separation between patients with adrenocortical tumors, where ACTH levels remain undetectable, and the rare patients with Cushing's disease who have low-to-undetectable baseline ACTH and in whom LVP invariably restores measurable plasma ACTH [113]. The use of LVP to discriminate between Cushing's disease and ectopic ACTH syndrome has not been established. The LVP test is abandoned in clinical practice because of the high incidence of side effects, and the substitute use of the desmopressin test.

THE DESMOPRESSIN TEST More recently the desmopressin (1-deamino-8D-arginine vasopressin) (which is a V2 and V3 agonist) has been used as a more potent ACTH secretagogue in Cushing's disease, with less side effects. Response is assessed by measuring ACTH, serum cortisol and possibly salivary cortisol, at various intervals − 30 minutes before, basally, 15, 30, 45 and 60 minutes after intravenous administration of 10 μg of desmopressin with serial blood samples obtained from an indwelling catheter inserted in a forearm vein. Patients have to restrict fluid intake for the remainder of the day to avoid water overload. Adverse effects are limited to a short-lived flushing sensation, a transient tachycardia, mild and transient decrease in blood pressure, headache, abdominal pain, or weight increase. There are several criteria for interpretation in the literature (parameter: ACTH or cortisol; threshold: a relative increase of more than 35−50% in ACTH or of more than 20−36% in cortisol) [25]. The desmopressin test induces a positive ACTH response in ca. 85% of patients with Cushing's disease [582−584]. Yet, since the V3 receptor is expressed in as many as 30% of ectopic tumors secreting ACTH [87,584], the usefulness of the desmopressin test is limited in the differential diagnosis of ACTH-dependent Cushing's syndrome. It might be more interesting in the postoperative assessment to predict recurrence after pituitary surgery as normal subjects rarely respond to the test [25,585,586].

THE CRH TEST A major breakthrough was achieved with the isolation, characterization and synthesis of ovine CRH in 1981 [71]. This discovery opened up new avenues to investigators of corticotroph function in humans [290,586,587]. Thorough studies in normal subjects rapidly showed that the ovine peptide was active in humans, eliciting an ACTH response that was definitively higher than that elicited by LVP, but still lower than that obtained after insulin-induced hypoglycemia [387,588]. Dose−response studies indicated that administration of 10 μg/kg body weight maximally stimulated cortisol release, while larger amounts could induce still higher ACTH responses [387, 589]. Synthetic ovine CRH (in many countries including the United States of America) or synthetic human CRH (in Europe) is administered intravenously at a dose of 100 μg in adults or 1 μg/kg body weight in children. Response is assessed by measuring ACTH, serum cortisol and possibly salivary cortisol 30 minutes before, baseline, 15, 30, 45 and 60 minutes after administration of CRH with serial blood samples obtained from an indwelling catheter inserted in a forearm vein. The test is well tolerated; the few side effects are mild facial flushing and neck tightness. In contrast with normal subjects, the time of day when the test is performed has no particular implication in Cushing's syndrome, but for convenience it may be performed in the morning. Data comparing the ovine and human CRH peptides in the same patients confirm that the former has a higher potency and provides a better diagnostic accuracy, largely outweighing the theoretical advantage of using a homologous peptide, at least for a single-dose testing [590].

The theoretical promise of the CRH test relies on it being a potent and specific stimulator of pituitary ACTH, thus allowing a better separation between patients with Cushing's disease, adrenocortical tumors, and, especially, ectopic ACTH syndrome (Figure 16.20) [218].

As with many tests confusion arises with the various ways different authors not only administer CRH but also appreciate an "exaggerated" or a "flat" response [586]. Criteria for a positive or negative response are seldom defined. In a survey of ten published series [218,591−599], Kaye and Crapo [576] developed their own criteria from these combined data: a positive response would be a relative increase of more than 50% in ACTH or of more than 20% in cortisol; a negative response would be a relative increase of less than 50% in ACTH or of less than 20% in cortisol. With these criteria, the sensitivity and specificity of the CRH test for the diagnosis of Cushing's disease would be 80 and 95% using the ACTH response, and 91 and 95% using the cortisol response. There is a general agreement that the test has a high diagnostic accuracy which compares favorably with that of the classic high-dose dexamethasone suppression test [600]. In evaluating 100 patients with Cushing's disease and 16 patients with ectopic ACTH secretion, a single a.m. CRH stimulation was

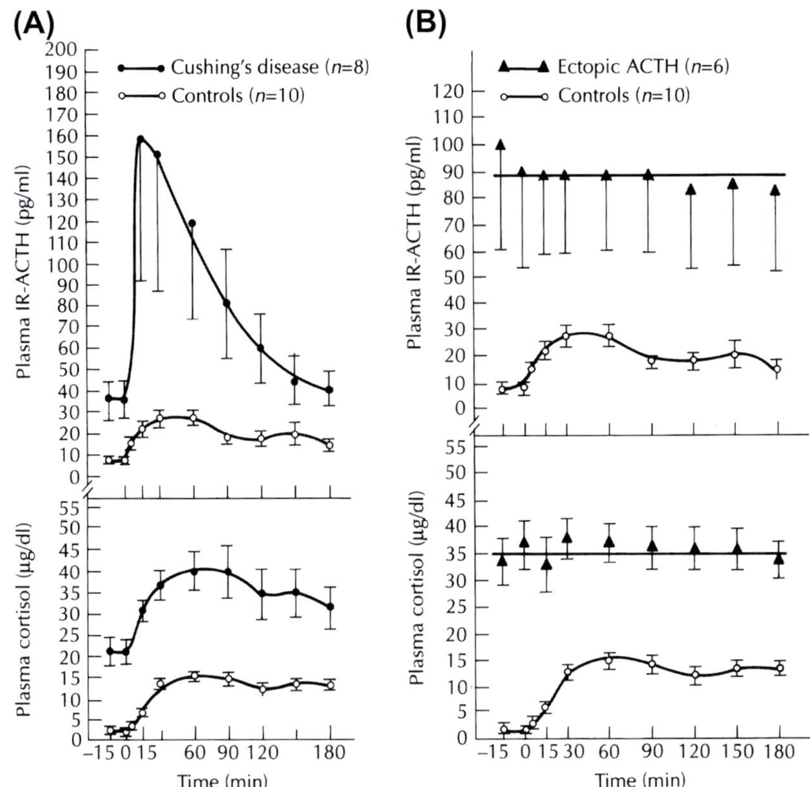

FIGURE 16.20 Responses of plasma immunoreactive (IR) adrenocorticotropic hormone (ACTH) and cortisol to corticotropin-releasing hormone (means ± SEM) in eight untreated patients with Cushing's disease. (A) six patients with Cushing's syndrome due to ectopic ACTH secretion; (B) and ten controls. *From Chrousos et al. [196].*

performed. Seven percent of patients with ACTH-dependent Cushing's did not respond, while no patient with ectopic ACTH secretion responded to CRH [601]. A positive response is highly suggestive of Cushing's disease, and the stronger the response the higher the probability. In another study with 101 patients with Cushing's disease and 14 patients with ectopic ACTH secretion, the sensitivity and specificity of the human CRH test for the diagnosis of Cushing's disease was 70 and 100% using a relative increase of more than 105% in ACTH, and 85 and 100% using a relative increase of more than 14% in cortisol response [602].

There is a general agreement that the test has a high diagnostic accuracy which compares favorably with that of the classic high-dose dexamethasone suppression test [600]. In the series where both tests were applied to the same patients, similar diagnostic accuracies were found [592,595,603–606]. In some cases however, the two tests did not agree, leading some authors to advocate a combined-test strategy to achieve the correct diagnosis. Authentic cases of Cushing's disease that did not respond to CRH have been reported by several authors and account for the 86% sensitivity of the test [576]. The stimulatory action of CRH can be strengthened by the synergistic effect of AVP or its V_1 analogues [607]. Data obtained with a combined CRH/AVP test showed that all patients with Cushing's disease responded positively [608]. A desmopressin-CRH test may be more discriminatory, with a specificity of 80–100% [609,610].

Occasional patients with ectopic ACTH syndrome exhibited an apparent positive response [412,592]. In some cases it may be questioned whether the ACTH increase originated from the tumor or the normal pituitary. Diagnostic difficulty is particularly important in the exceptional cases of bronchial carcinoid tumors that also respond to the high-dose dexamethasone suppression test and metyrapone [412]. Whether these responses are apparent or real is not proved, although in vitro studies tend to indicate that an occasional non-pituitary tumor may be authentically CRH-responsive [396]. These rare cases may lead to unwarranted pituitary surgery for a mistakenly proposed diagnosis of Cushing's disease. They are the ones which would justify systematic bilateral inferior petrosal sinus sampling.

That the pituitary tumor responsible for Cushing's disease further increases its ACTH secretion in response to CRH is further evidence of its intrinsic relative resistance to glucocorticoids. Indeed, the state of chronic hypercortisolism should normally suppress CRH action on the corticotrophs. Thus it is not surprising to observe that the CRH and the high-dose dexamethasone suppression tests each provide essentially the same diagnostic accuracy [600], since both assess the relative insensitivity to glucocorticoids of the pituitary tumor.

Tracking the ACTH Source: Bilateral Inferior Petrosal Sinus Sampling

The availability of reliable plasma ACTH RIAs – and more recently IRMAs – has prompted the development of invasive sampling procedures aimed at collecting blood draining immediately from the pituitary gland. The goal of this approach is two-fold: first to establish whether ACTH oversecretion is of pituitary or nonpituitary origin; and second, and in the case of Cushing's disease, to lateralize the pituitary location of a microadenoma.

A reliable technique requires that blood sampling be done close enough to the pituitary, that is, within the inferior petrosal sinus. Because a pituitary adenoma will lateralize its secretion in the ipsilateral inferior petrosal sinus it is essential that both sinuses be catheterized. Both sinuses and peripheral blood must be sampled simultaneously [586].

A central-to-peripheral ACTH gradient is calculated by the ratio of ACTH plasma levels in the inferior petrosal sinus with the highest level over ACTH in the peripheral blood. In patients with Cushing's disease this gradient is almost always over 2, with a mean of 15. In patients with ectopic ACTH syndrome this gradient is almost always lower than 1.7. Some have reported that the test can be improved by simultaneous CRH stimulation which increases the gradient [611–613]. A basal central:peripheral ratio of >2:1 or a CRH stimulated ratio of >3:1 is indicative of Cushing's disease. Analysis of different series and individual case reports all confirm the great diagnostic power of the procedure to discriminate between Cushing's disease and ectopic ACTH syndrome with a sensitivity and a specificity of 94% [611–617,619–626].

The main causes of false-negatives are inferior petrosal sinus sampling that is not sufficiently selective, plexiform vascularization in at least one sinus, abnormal venous drainage of an adenoma which is intrasphenoidal but not strictly intrasellar and intermittent ACTH secretion in a case of Cushing's disease. Most of these causes may be avoided by refering to an experienced neuroradiologist [627], checking catheter position with a venous angiogram and measuring prolactin, along with ACTH [628,629]. The main causes of false-positives are investigation done during a period of normal cortisol levels in the presence of a tumor causing ectopic but intermittent ACTH secretion [629], and ectopic tumor secretion of CRH [629,630]. Some false positives may be avoided by checking the consistency of hypercortisolism during the days before the procedure and preceding the catheterism by careful investigations for an endocrine tumor.

Although somewhat invasive, particularly considering the general vascular fragility of patients with Cushing's syndrome, there are few serious side effects reported. Venous thromboembolism, sixth nerve palsy, veinous subarachnoid hemmorhage, brain stem infarction [616,631,633–635]. The slight discomfort of the technique [632] is largely overcome by its diagnostic accuracy. This investigation should only be considered and performed in centers where there is a great deal of experience in the matter.

Some propose cavernous sinuses [636] or jugular venous sampling [637–639] and some substitute CRH by desmopressin, without major adverse effects during or after the procedure [640,641].

In the case of Cushing's disease this procedure also helps to localize the pituitary microadenoma by evaluating the sinus-to-sinus ACTH gradient [620,621,642]. A gradient over 1.5 lateralizes the adenoma to the pituitary half draining in the ipsilateral sinus with the highest ACTH level. Some have reported that the test can be improved by simultaneous CRH stimulation which increases the gradient [611–613]. Variable efficacy of this approach has been reported, often with a high success rate [576]. In fact this technique is not diagnosis-directed; its goal is to help the neurosurgeon remove a pituitary microadenoma that would not be readily picked up by imaging techniques and possibly not seen at surgery. Successful blind hemihypophysectomies directed by sampling lateralization have been claimed [611,621]. Obvious difficulties are anticipated in previously operated patients, and with macroadenomas and microadenomas situated centrally. Incorrect lateralizations have been reported [615,616,642] in patients with Cushing's disease. Several authors have recently reported that other pituitary hormones (PRL, GH, α-subunit) colateralize with ACTH on the ipsilateral sinus draining the microadenoma [620,643–645]. Since these non-ACTH peptides were not detected by immunohistologic studies in the removed adenomas they raise the question of a nonspecific effect of the adenoma on pituitary blood flow, or of an as yet undemonstrated local, and general, paracrine effect of the tumor. An incorrect position of the catheter might explain a colateralization of ACTH and prolactin.

IMAGING TECHNIQUES

The Pituitary

Skull X-ray and Tomograms

Because most pituitary corticotroph adenomas are small, gross deformation of the pituitary sella is rarely encountered [646] in untreated Cushing's disease. They may be demonstrated in patients who develop Nelson's syndrome, and in the rare patients with an initial macroadenoma. Skull X-rays will often show evidence of osteopenia of the dorsum sellae, and provide the neurosurgeon with useful indications on the bone landmarks and state of pneumatization of the sphenoidal sinus.

CT Scanning

With the development of pituitary surgery as the treatment of choice for Cushing's disease, preoperative localization of a pituitary adenoma is more important. CT has been for a long time the only imaging technique for the pituitary gland. With coronal images and an adequate method of injection, CT can achieve a sensitivity no higher than 50% [130,134,576,647–649]. The microadenoma will appear as a hypodense round lesion; a mass effect on the pituitary stalk and diaphragma will depend on the size of the lesion. The specificity of CT is not perfect since abnormal images are not infrequent and may provide false-positive results in patients with other causes of Cushing's syndrome [650,651]. CT scanning also easily recognizes the exceptional initial macroadenoma (Figure 16.21).

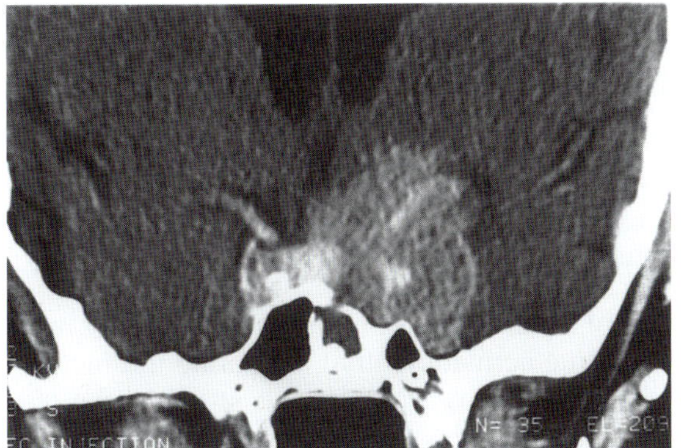

FIGURE 16.21 A huge corticotroph macroadenoma detected by computed tomography scan in a patient with mild clinical features of Cushing's disease and a cyclic evolution.

MRI

This technique has significantly improved our ability to detect pituitary microadenomas in Cushing's disease. Several studies have shown that many patients with a negative CT have a positive MRI [652–654]. Pituitary MRI should be performed in all patients with ACTH-dependent Cushing's syndrome.

Pituitary MRI consists of sagittal and coronal T_1-weighted images, coronal T_2-weighted spin echo MRI images in thin sections before gadolinium, followed by a dynamic coronal T_1 sequence beginning simultaneously with the contrast injection, and, as required, a T_1-weighted 3D gradient echo sequence (ED3D). Typical of a microadenoma is a hypointense signal better delimited after enhancement (Figure 16.22). It is often easier to detect (and sometimes visible only) after gadolinium injection on dynamic sequences or in ED3D sequence. Although this is very rare, corticotropic adenoma should be sought outside the intrasellar region (in the cavernous sinuses, sphenoidal sinuses, nasopharyngeal area) if the pituitary has no focal signal abnormality that is suggestive of adenoma. MRI may reveal pituitary adenoma in no more than 36–78% of cases in adult series [576,625,626,652,653,655–657]. Furthermore, false-positives occur where there is pituitary incidentaloma and artefact [625,658]. In addition, MRI determines the size of the adenoma, how it relates to the cavernous sinuses and whether or not it is invasive. The imaging will guide the surgeon, avoiding the need for overly aggressive surgery and the accompanying complications. The imaging will provide a picture of air distribution in the sphenoid sinus, will identify sphenoid

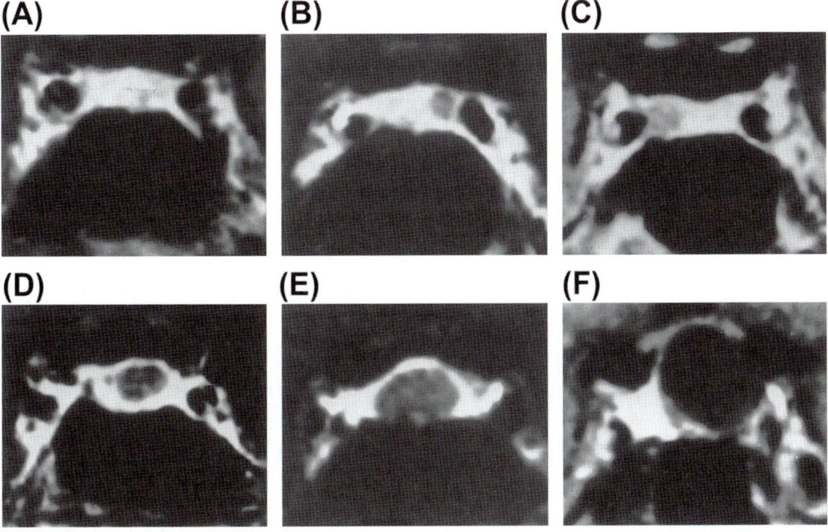

FIGURE 16.22 Pituitary magnetic resonance image in Cushing's disease. T_1-weighted images obtained in the coronal plane with gadolinium enhancement. Adenomas of increasing size are depicted from (A) to (F).

sinusitis, empty sella syndrome, carotid ectasia, etc., which will all influence surgical strategy.

The Adrenals

The main, and crucial, goal of adrenal imaging in Cushing's syndrome is to rule out an adrenal tumor. Adrenal imaging may be indicated if doubt persist between ACTH-dependent and ACTH-independent Cushing's syndrome in cases of sometimes low ACTH levels, with a CRH test and a high-dose dexamethasone suppression test. It is advisable to carry out an adrenal imaging before bilateral adrenalectomy [25,450,518].

Standard X-ray, tomography, ultrasonography and retroperitoneal pneumography have all been outrated by the highly effective and noninvasive techniques using MRI and especially CT scanning.

As a result of chronic stimulation by excess ACTH the two adrenal glands develop hyperplasia exhibiting CT features that will be essentially the same in Cushing's disease and ectopic ACTH syndrome. As a rule both glands are moderately enlarged; there is no reliable measure of the adrenals but a loss of normal concavity of their borders is considered pathologic. Occasional nodules may be present, probably more frequently in Cushing's disease than in ectopic ACTH syndrome. Macronodular hyperplasia develops in up to 15% of patients with Cushing's disease [369]. In cases where it is highly asymmetrical with a predominant macronodule on one side, an erroneous diagnosis of adrenocortical adenoma may be made that possibly leads to an unwarranted and unsuccessful unilateral adrenalectomy. Great care should be exerted to analyze the contralateral gland which, in contrast with a benign adrenocortical adenoma, will not show the characteristic features of adrenal atrophy [369]. This is also the rare situation where adrenal scintigraphy with iodocholesterol [659] will be of help in definitively proving the bilateral, although asymmetrical, functional lesions in the case of macronodular hyperplasia, in contrast with the strictly unilateral isotope uptake by a benign adrenocortical adenoma [660,661].

No adrenocortical tumor large enough to cause Cushing's syndrome, i.e., >1.5 cm, should escape detection by CT. A benign adrenocortical adenoma is readily visible in the fat-filled perirenal area of these patients and it is essential to appreciate the atrophic aspect of the contralateral gland by comparing its thickness with that of the diaphragma crus [379]. Adrenocortical carcinomas, as a rule, are characteristically large and partly necrotic tumors. They may contain calcifications or hemorrhagic areas. At this stage MRI can be used as the most sensitive method in the preoperative assessment of vascular patency of the inferior vena cava and of locoregional invasion (liver, kidney and pancreas) using sagittal and coronal planes.

PITFALLS IN DIAGNOSIS

Drug Interactions

A more extensive description of drug interactions is provided in Chapter 9.

Inducers of High CBG Plasma Levels

High estrogen states, as encountered in pregnancy and in oral contraceptive treatment, induce increased plasma CBG levels. This modification is accompanied by a parallel increase in plasma cortisol [662]. Persistence of a normal pituitary–adrenal axis is easily demonstrated by other indices; free plasma cortisol and salivary cortisol are normal and have normal circadian variations, while 24-hour urinary cortisol excretion is normal. Although false-positive responses to the overnight 1 mg dexamethasone suppression test are occasionally observed, the classic low-dose dexamethasone test is normal [509,511]. In late pregnancy the situation is more complex due to additional factors that profoundly modify the pituitary–adrenal homeostasis (see below).

op′DDD and/or some of its metabolites have been shown to have estrogen-like actions [663]. In some individuals highly elevated plasma CBG levels may obscure a proper evaluation of the drug's action on cortisol production. Urinary and/or salivary measurements bypass this potential pitfall.

Liver Enzyme Inducers

Several drugs have the common property of inducing liver enzyme activations that accelerate the metabolism of endogenous and/or exogenous steroids and of some pharmacologic agents [429].

op′DDD [533], rifampicin [664], phenytoin [665] and barbiturates [666] divert cortisol metabolism toward 6β-hydroxycortisol. This highly polar compound escapes the extraction usually performed on urine samples, artifactually lowering the result of the Porter and Silber assay. This explains why the urinary 17-hydroxycorticosteroids drop within a few days after the onset of *op*′DDD treatment, whereas plasma cortisol remains unchanged until the delayed adrenolytic action of the drug begins its effect, generally only after a few weeks.

Anticonvulsants like phenytoin and barbiturates also accelerate dexamethasone metabolism [532]. Patients on these drugs have false-positive low-dose dexamethasone suppression tests [509]. In some patients with suspected Cushing's syndrome it may be difficult to interrupt their anticonvulsant treatment. It has been proposed to monitor the test with concomitant measurement of plasma dexamethasone [667]; alternatively, because cortisol metabolism is less accelerated a suppression test has been calibrated where plasma corticosterone suppressibility is assessed after oral administration of 50 mg cortisol at midnight [668]. In such patients, however, basal urinary cortisol excretion is normal.

Antiglucocorticoids (RU 486)

Although this newly developed drug is used primarily as an antiprogesterone it also exerts an antiglucocorticoid action that is readily observed within a few hours after a single oral administration [669,670]. As expected, plasma and urinary cortisol are elevated and suppressibility by dexamethasone is altered. Because of the long duration of action of the drug, this state of general glucocorticoid resistance is still noticeable up to 3 days after single-dose administration [671]. Pilot studies have been performed where patients received long-term therapy with RU 486 (200–400 mg/day) up to several months, for breast cancer. A two- to three-fold plasma cortisol increase was observed after 2 weeks of treatment which plateaued thereafter and was not modified by the 1 mg overnight dexamethasone suppression test [672].

This increased pituitary–adrenocortical activity is an adaptive, and appropriate, response to the state of drug-induced glucocorticoid resistance. As expected, no clinical feature of hypercortisolism is observed.

Glucocorticoids

A rare patient may present with clinical features of glucocorticoid excess while on glucocorticoid treatment for an inflammatory disease, and also have an endogenous cause of Cushing's syndrome. The diagnosis may be easily made in the case of an autonomously secreting adrenocortical tumor. It is theoretically much more difficult in the rare case where Cushing's disease is suspected, since the abnormal pituitary ACTH secretion may have been somewhat sensitive to the suppressive effect of exogenous steroids.

Glycyrrhetinic Acid

Glycyrrhetinic acid, a hydrolytic product of glycyrrhizic acid, has long been recognized as a causative agent of a pseudohyperaldosteronism syndrome. Its mechanism of action has been unraveled [673]. The compound inhibits the enzyme 11-β-hydroxysteroid dehydrogenase which mainly converts cortisol to the inactive cortisone. Because this enzyme activity is present in the kidney, its inhibition induces a local excess of cortisol which will act, in a spill-over mechanism, on the kidney mineralocorticoid (or glucocorticoid type I) receptor and exert a mineralocorticoid-like effect [674]. As a consequence of the blockade of cortisol metabolism in the kidney urinary cortisol is increased; plasma cortisol is unchanged. Thus urinary cortisol is a false indicator of the cortisolic state in subjects under liquorice abuse [675].

Intercurrent Pathologic States

Simple obesity has long been a major diagnostic problem when urinary 17-hydroxycorticosteroids were the usual markers of adrenocortical activity [526]. Obesity per se induces an increased metabolic clearance rate of cortisol [529,530]. As an adaptive and appropriate response the cortisol production rate is increased with increased urinary cortisol metabolites. It has now been clearly demonstrated that the more appropriate parameters of baseline cortisol homeostasis (plasma and salivary cortisol, circadian rhythm and urinary cortisol excretion), and the classic low-dose dexamethasone suppression test are all normal in simple obesity [509].

Hyperthyroidism also accelerates cortisol metabolism with the same consequences as simple obesity, with urinary 17-hydroxycorticosteroids being elevated. Other parameters of cortisol homeostasis remain normal. Hypothyroidism induces the opposite abnormalities, i.e., low urinary 17-hydroxycorticosteroids [572].

Chronic renal failure has been mistakenly associated with abnormal glucocorticoid regulation, including diminished suppressibility by dexamethasone [677]. Because urinary measurements are evidently useless special caution must be applied to the sole possible plasma measurements. Polar metabolites of cortisol accumulate in blood to such high levels that they may significantly interfere in some cortisol assays that are not sufficiently specific. With the necessary precautions, including plasma extraction or highly specific immunoassay, plasma cortisol is normal and normally suppressible by the classic low-dose dexamethasone test [520,676,679]. Correct assessment of the pituitary–adrenal axis may be further hampered by the finding of increased plasma LPH levels [175,520], especially in hemodialysis patients, due solely to a decreased plasma clearance of LPH [680]. Plasma ACTH remains normal [520]. Patients with HIV infection, especially if treated with protease inhibitors, may exhibit features of pseudo-Cushing's syndrome, including fat pads and central obesity. Appropriate ACTH/cortisol suppression after dexamethasone excludes the diagnosis of Cushing's disease [678].

An exceptional patient has been reported who had both Addison's and Cushing's diseases [681]. The diagnosis was achieved by demonstrating the lack of normal circadian ACTH rhythm (which is normally preserved in Addison's disease) under precise conditions of cortisol administration.

Hypercortisolic States without Cushing's Syndrome

Various pathologic or physiologic conditions may be associated with biochemical, and sometimes clinical,

TABLE 16.4 Hypercortisolic States without Cushing's Syndrome

Functional hypothalamic CRH oversecretion
Depression
Anorexia nervosa
Alcoholism
Chronic stress
Strenuous exercice
Nonhypothalamic CRH oversecretion
Pregnancy
General insensitivity of glucocorticoids
Familial resistance to glucocorticoids
Pregnancy
RU 486

CRH, corticotropin-releasing hormone.

evidences of endogenous glucocorticoid excess (Table 16.4). In these situations, increased cortisol production is thought to be driven by pituitary ACTH oversecretion secondary to CNS disorder or to an appropriate adaptive reaction. This functional hypercortisolic state (sometimes called "pseudo-Cushing") is usually mild and transient and regresses with its cause. Hence it is not classically regarded as a cause of genuine Cushing's syndrome, but has long been recognized and best studied in depressed patients.

Depression

Patients with severe endogenous depression often exhibit biochemical stigmata of hypercortisolism [291]. Plasma cortisol and urinary steroids excretion are increased, and are not suppressed normally on the classic low-dose dexamethasone test. Activation of the pituitary–adrenal axis is fairly specific of depression among other conditions of primary affective disorders and may be observed in as many as 40–60% of patients in some series [290]. These observations eventually led to the routine use of differently designed and debated dexamethasone suppression tests as a biologic means for both the diagnosis and the follow-up of such patients.

Normal or slightly increased plasma ACTH levels indicate that the disorder is pituitary driven. A fine evaluation of the hypothalamic–pituitary–adrenal axis of depressed patients has recently shed new light on the pathophysiologic mechanism leading to the hypercortisolic state of this disorder [682]. Depressed patients have an attenuated plasma ACTH response to CRH in comparison with normal controls, yet their basal plasma cortisol levels are elevated, and respond normally to CRH. These results indicate that the pituitary corticotroph is intrinsically normal, the attenuated ACTH response to CRH showing that they are sensitive to the negative feedback of increased cortisol levels (just the reverse happens in Cushing's disease). The normal cortisol response to CRH, in spite of blunted ACTH rise, is compatible with hyperplasia and hyper-responsiveness of the adrenal cortex, as has been independently reported by others in depressed patients [683]. The dynamics of ACTH are similar to those observed in normal subjects administered long-term CRH infusion [388] and therefore point to the hypothalamus or suprahypothalamic regions as the primary cause of ACTH oversecretion. Although the source and significance of CSF CRH is debated [290], the finding that depressed patients have increased CSF CRH levels [292], which eventually appear to correlate positively with the degree of pituitary–adrenocortical overactivity [293], has been taken as a further indication that this condition is due to a hypothalamic dysfunction with CRH overproduction.

Whatever the exact pathophysiologic mechanism, the hypercortisolic state that accompanies depression often creates a serious diagnostic problem. A depressed patient may present with obesity, mild hirsutism, slight hypertension and moderate glucose intolerance. Although none of these is by itself absolutely conclusive, several features may more or less distinguish between transient functional hypercortisolism and true Cushing's syndrome with secondary depression. Classically in depression:

1. The hypercortisolic state is clinically and biologically mild. Urinary cortisol excretion almost never exceeds three times the upper limit of normal [684];
2. The circadian pattern of plasma cortisol levels is less disrupted and sometimes a phase-shift phenomenon is merely observed [685,686];
3. Cortisol response to insulin-induced hypoglycemia is present in depressed patients in contrast to patients with Cushing's syndrome of any cause, including Cushing's disease [121,122,509];
4. ACTH response to CRH is attenuated in contrast to the exaggerated response of Cushing's disease, a wide overlap, nevertheless is observed [682]; (see also further Tests to distinguish between "pseudo-Cushing" and Cushing's syndrome)
5. Finally, imaging investigations should find no evidence of adrenocortical or pituitary tumor.

Cases have been reported where depression preceded the occurrence of true Cushing's disease, raising the question of possible pathophysiologic role for CRH, and further complicating the diagnostic issue.

Anorexia Nervosa

Anorexia nervosa is associated with an array of neuroendocrine disorders among which sustained hypercortisolism is frequent (see Chapter 18) [291]. Increased urinary cortisol and lack of normal suppression by the classic low-dose dexamethasone test may be found. Clinical features of hypercortisolism are absent probably because of the mild hypercortisolic state and the lack of sufficient substrates, more likely than because of a hypothetic down-regulation of glucocorticoid receptors. The fine evaluation of ACTH and cortisol response to CRH in underweight patients with anorexia nervosa reveals patterns very similar to those observed in depressed patients [687]. Together with the finding of an increased CSF CRH level in anorexia nervosa [688,689] these data point to a hypothalamic or suprahypothalamic origin of pituitary–adrenocortical overactivity in anorexia nervosa. An exceptional case has been reported where authentic Cushing's disease with a pituitary adenoma found at surgery occurred 2 years after the onset of anorexia nervosa [690]. In contrast with depressed patients there is generally no clinical hesitation for the diagnosis. Abnormal corticotroph dynamics are corrected with weight restoration, and they might simply represent a nonspecific manifestation of inanition [691].

Alcoholism

Patients with chronic alcoholism may present with clinical and biochemical features of glucocorticoid excess creating a pseudo-Cushing's syndrome [692–694]. General fatigue, diminished muscle strength, plethoric facies, truncal obesity and abdominal striae may be encountered, which all mimic the typical clinical features of Cushing's syndrome [372]. A diagnosis which is further supported by the finding of increased plasma cortisol and urinary steroid excretion, a disrupted circadian rhythm and lack of normal response to the classic low-dose dexamethasone suppression test.

Alterations of the hypothalamic–pituitary–adrenal axis consistent with a hypothalamic origin are found in patients under chronic alcohol abuse, yet they are mild and present only in a minority of patients. Thus, it remains to be determined whether these functional abnormalities are associated with the propensity for alcohol abuse, are caused by ethanol intake possibly through a decrease of 11-β-hydroxysteroid dehydrogenase activity [695,696], or simply related to a common CNS disorder also responsible for depression.

Whatever the mechanism involved, alcoholic pseudo-Cushing's syndrome is a real diagnostic challenge. The simplest and most effective way to avoid a false diagnosis is to think of alcoholism and to observe the nice parallel decrease and normalization of cortisol indices and liver function tests during alcohol withdrawal in hospitalized patients [692–694,697].

Stress

Transient states of glucocorticoid excess without clinical stigmata commonly accompany an array of stressful conditions. They are thought to represent normal adaptive activation of the hypothalamic–pituitary–adrenal axis. Many such situations are encountered, including surgery, test-taking, various acute and chronic illnesses, terminal illnesses, extended burns and diabetes mellitus [509,698,699]. The simple stress of hospitalization has been claimed to increase glucocorticoid secretion. These observations emphasize the absolute need to await the resolution of any stressful intercurrent condition before initiating a proper diagnostic evaluation.

Strenuous Exercise

Slight alterations of the pituitary–adrenal axis may be encountered in response to physical exercise [700]. In a recent study, moderate elevation in baseline plasma cortisol and a blunted ACTH and cortisol response to CRH were observed in normal men running more than 45 miles per week [586].

Pregnancy

Normal pregnancy is associated with a profound hormonal turmoil that significantly alters glucocorticoid homeostasis (see also Chapter 17).

In the first months of pregnancy increased estrogens induce a two- to three-fold rise in plasma CBG that reaches a maximum at about 3 months and plateaus thereafter [662]. This generates a parallel rise in plasma cortisol but, in a similar manner to that observed in women on estrogen contraception, it does not induce a true hypercortisolic state since plasma free cortisol, and salivary and urinary cortisol remain within the normal range.

With time more significant alterations develop that culminate in the last trimester when unequivocal features of a hypercortisolic state are found, at least from a biochemical viewpoint. Mean unbound and salivary cortisol and urinary cortisol excretion show a two- to three-fold increase [389,390,501]. Thirty percent of women have 24-hour urinary cortisol excretion above the upper limit of normal, nonpregnant women, and most have an abnormal response to the classic low-dose dexamethasone suppression test [701].

The mechanism and consequences of this slight state of authentic hypercortisolism are not totally understood. However, major advances have been made in recent years which illuminate this intriguing problem.

The normal placenta has been identified as a large and physiologic site for CRH gene expression [702], depositing enormous quantities of the peptide into the maternal blood flow. Plasma CRH levels in late pregnancy may attain peaks of several thousand picograms per milliliter in comparison with the picograms per milliliter range in normal, nonpregnant women [394]. Although a large proportion of circulating CRH is bound to a carrier protein [703,704], strikingly elevated levels of free and bioactive CRH circulate at this time. Under such conditions and because plasma ACTH levels in pregnant women show a moderate but significant rise of about two- to three-fold [701], it first seemed logical to charge placental CRH as a natural culprit. The situation, however, is not as clear; no correlation has been found between plasma CRH and pituitary–adrenal parameters [389]. Conservation of a perfectly normal, although slightly shifted upward, circadian rhythm of salivary cortisol is in sharp contrast with the steady-state of high plasma CRH levels [389]. It points to an unrestrained hypothalamic drive that continues to operate and which overcomes both peripheral CRH and the expected negative feedback of increased plasma free cortisol. Whether it is related to a direct action of hypothalamic CRH at the pituitary, to AVP, or to an as yet unidentified factor, is unknown.

Progesterone exerts an antiglucocorticoid action on rat pituitary corticotroph cells [705]; it has been hypothesized that prolonged and highly elevated progesterone levels induce a state of relative and general glucocorticoid resistance [389]. This would explain the slight shift in plasma free cortisol with conserved normal circadian rhythm, the abnormal dexamethasone suppressibility, and also the absence of peripheral clinical features of hypercortisolism. This hypothesis is reinforced by the recent finding that the change in salivary cortisol after delivery correlated with the increase in serum progesterone concentration in late prenancy [389].

Some have suggested that increased plasma ACTH in pregnancy might result from placental secretion [701] and/or a reviviscent intermediate lobe of the pituitary [706,707].

Familial Resistance to Glucocorticoids

This newly recognized syndrome was first identified in a patient with hypertension and hypokalemia [708]. Fine hormonal evaluation showed no evidence of aldosterone oversecretion or adrenocortical enzyme blockade. Instead evidence of glucocorticoid excess was found; plasma cortisol and urinary cortisol were elevated. Suppression of plasma cortisol by increasing doses of dexamethasone was abnormal with a shift to the right of the dose–response curve demonstrating the relative resistance of the pituitary to the negative glucocorticoid feedback in a manner similar to that observed in Cushing's disease [709]. Two features were different; there was a normal circadian rhythm of plasma cortisol, and a total absence of clinical features of hypercortisolism. These observations suggested that the state of glucocorticoid resistance was not restricted to the pituitary, but was general. This hypothesis was reinforced by the finding of decreased glucocorticoid binding affinity of the patient's fibroblasts [709], and recently established by the cloning of the glucocorticoid receptor in an affected patient. A single base substitution (A→T) at position 2054 changed Asp_{641} to Val within a highly conserved and hitherto supposedly functional region of the ligand-binding domain of the receptor, explaining the loss of affinity [189]. This rare familial syndrome has now been identified in several families, amounting to about 20 such patients. The clinical and biochemical features severely affect the patients with homozygous defects. Increased activity of the pituitary–adrenal axis is an adaptive, and thus appropriate, reaction. The hypertension and hypokalemia are explained by the increased mineralocorticoid activity due to excess DOC and cortisol acting on the normally sensitive mineralocorticoid receptor.

Tests to Distinguish between "Pseudo-Cushing" and Cushing's Syndrome

These tests have been developed primarily to distinguish between the functional hypercortisolism of depression and genuine Cushing's syndrome.

THE COMBINED DEXAMETHASONE–CRH TEST

The hypothesis is that patients with pseudo-Cushing's syndrome are under chronic CRH stimulation due to their stressful situation and show a blunted response to exogenous CRH after dexamethasone administration. The initial protocol consisted of giving dexamethaone in doses of 0.5 mg for 48 h, at 6 h intervals, beginning at 12:00 h (i.e., at 12:00, 18:00, 00:00 and 06:00 h) and obtaining serum cortisol at 08:00 h, and then administering ovine-sequence CRH (1 μg/kg) i.v. at 08:00 h, 2 h after the last dexamethasone dose. The plasma cortisol value 15 min after CRH is expected to be greater than 38 nmol/liter (or 1.4 μg/dl or 14 ng/ml) in patients with Cushing's syndrome, but to remain suppressed in normal subjects and in patients with pseudo-Cushing's syndrome. Recent studies [710–713] reported lower specificity of the Dex-CRH test than the initial publication by the National Institutes of Health (NIH) group [714] such that this test gave no better results than the repeated assessment of the other screening tests. The cutoff proposed with ovine CRH cannot be extended to human CRH, widely used in Europe, which stimulates ACTH and cortisol secretion less than the ovine CRH. Furthermore, the interval between dexamethasone and CRH is longer than in the NIH protocol if the dexamethasone dose starts at 10:00 h instead of 12:00 h. Lastly, human CRH is expensive, just as is the 48 h hospitalization often needed to strictly respect the dexamethasone test protocol. A better diagnostic accuracy was obtained with a cortisol threshold of 70 nmol/L (25 ng/ml or 2.5 μg/dl) or with an ACTH threshold of 5.9 pmol/L (27 pg/ml) 15 min after ovine CRH (1 μg/kg, maximum 100 μg) at 08:00 h, 2 h after the last dose of dexamethasone [711].

THE CRH TEST

A recent Italian study [715], attempted to rehabilitate the CRH test in the differential diagnosis between ACTH-dependent Cushing's syndrome and pseudo-Cushing, first described by the NIH group [682]. Using a combination of two hCRH test parameters they showed that ACTH-dependent Cushing's syndrome can be diagnosed with specificity and sensitivity both over 90% [715].

THE DESMOPRESSIN TEST

In two publications of Italian groups (Milan and Naples), the desmopressin test has a good diagnosis accuracy (94%) with a threshold of ACTH of 6 pmol/L (27 pg/ml) [710,716], that was comparable to that of the dexamethasone-CRH test, even in patients with only mild hypercortisolism. Besides, desmopressin is cheaper than CRH and the desmopressin test is more convenient than dexamethasone-CRH which required 2 days' hospitalization. Furthermore, the desmopressin test may be useful in the differential diagnosis of ACTH-dependent Cushing's syndrome, and above all in the post-transsphenoidal survey of Cushing's disease. Like the dexamethasone-CRH test and perhaps the CRH test, the desmopressin test may prove useful for patients with mild hypercortisolism and normal ACTH levels, in whom the differential diagnosis has narrowed to Cushing's disease or pseudo-Cushing. Unlike the CRH test, dexamethasone-CRH and desmopressin tests cannot be applied in patients with ACTH-independent Cushing's syndrome.

Normal Suppression with the Classic Low-dose Dexamethasone Test in Authentic Cushing's Disease

It has been estimated that a minority of patients (5%) with authentic Cushing's disease suppress normally with the classic low-dose dexamethasone test, and thus are false-negatives [509]. Returning to the original data provides a simple explanation [123]. The first trials to titrate the daily amount of synthetic glucocorticoid necessary to suppress urinary 17-hydroxycorticosteroids used two different molecules with different potencies, namely Δ^1-9α-fluorocortisol and Δ^1-16α-methyl-9α-fluorocortisol (or dexamethasone). Titration curves readily show that complete suppression requires 2 mg/day of the first compound, but only $\leq$1 mg/day of dexamethasone. Curiously, in the original paper both drugs are used under the same generic name "ΔFF" leading the author to anticipate that "... although these two compounds were used interchangeably in the present study, it is possible that smaller doses of dexamethasone would be appropriate, in view of the apparent greater potency of this agent" [123].

In occasional patients with Cushing's disease, normal suppressibility by the classic low-dose dexamethasone test has been attributed to a decreased metabolic clearance rate for dexamethasone [717,718]. Simultaneous measurements of plasma endogenous cortisol and dexamethasone provide a means to evaluate suppressibility in comparison with the dose–response curve obtained in normal patients [668,718].

Other causes of apparently normal suppression in Cushing's disease are encountered in the rare patients with true cyclical episodes of hypercortisolism whenever the test is performed during a quiescent phase.

Etiologic Pitfalls

Cushing's Disease Mimicking an Autonomous Adrenocortical Tumor

The classic situation is that of a patient with Cushing's syndrome with apparent autonomous cortisol oversecretion [372]: urinary 17-hydroxycorticosteroids fail to suppress with the classic high-dose dexamethasone test, basal ACTH is low or undetectable and adrenal imaging reveals a unilateral adrenal mass. When a unilateral adrenalectomy is performed, although transiently ameliorated, the hypercortisolism inevitably recurs, allowing a correct and a posteriori diagnosis of Cushing's disease in its macronodular hyperplastic form. This situation is not uncommon and the diagnosis would be correctly established if strict criteria were used.

1. Establishing autonomous cortisol production requires indisputable proof. It has previously been noted how the high-dose dexamethasone test should be interpreted with more subtlety and how it must be sometimes strengthened [378]. The ACTH RIA may be insensitive and undetectable basal plasma ACTH levels may become detectable with a better assay or after LVP or CRH stimulation [113]. A metyrapone test may also be of help showing a rise in urinary 17-hydroxycorticosteroids. Thus, in many cases what appears as an autonomous adrenocortical activity does not resist a closer, and stronger, examination.
2. The second aspect that needs thorough evaluation is adrenal imaging. Although it may be highly asymmetrical to the point of mimicking a unilateral adrenocortical tumor, the macronodular hyperplasia of Cushing's disease is not accompanied by contralateral atrophy, as is the case in a true autonomous adrenocortical adenoma [369]. Thus careful examination of the contralateral gland on CT scan almost invariably confirms the diagnosis. It may be in this rare situation where iodocholesterol scanning may be helpful, showing asymmetrical but bilateral isotope uptake [660,661].

Severe Cushing's Disease Mimicking Classic Ectopic ACTH Syndrome

The clinical presentation of genuine Cushing's disease may be severe enough to mimic the classic form of ectopic ACTH syndrome, with rapid onset, profound myopathy, severe hypokalemia and definite hyperpigmentation [174,719]. Although the dynamic exploration of the corticotroph function may be concordant with Cushing's disease, in some cases the correct diagnosis is obscured by some unexpected responses, such as a lack of suppressibility on the classic high-dose dexamethasone tests and sometimes lack of response to the CRH test [576]. In most cases, however, pituitary imaging will point to the source of ACTH often showing a large macroadenoma on CT scan or MRI. If necessary, and if possible, bilateral inferior petrosal sinus sampling should ultimately provide the unequivocal solution.

Mild Ectopic ACTH Syndrome Mimicking Classic Cushing's Disease

It has become increasingly recognized that some non-pituitary tumors provoke a Cushing's syndrome with both clinical and biochemical features similar to those of classic Cushing's disease [572]. Mild and slowly progressive symptoms are found together with dynamic tests strictly compatible with a nonautonomous, glucocorticoid responsive, cortisol overproduction [372].

In a minority of such cases a positive response to the CRH test is another pitfall for diagnosis [396,412,592]. Because most of these patients have had small and rather indolent bronchial carcinoid tumors [720] that until recently had escaped the usual means of detection by standard X-ray, many have undergone unsuccessful pituitary surgery [721]. In some patients the correct diagnosis was made up to 10 years later [372].

The rare but classic occult carcinoid tumor which can be suspected because of the detection of abnormal circulating POMC fragments and successfully detected by chest CT scan or MRI should always be borne in mind. The clear evidence of a pituitary microadenoma on MRI helps to eliminate this possibility. If it is not detectable, the slight risk of an unwarranted pituitary surgery should be weighed against the mild risk and discomfort of bilateral inferior petrosal sinus sampling which, at this stage, offers the sole and highly efficient means to separate the two conditions.

STRATEGY

Because there are different causes of Cushing's syndrome and many different tests to distinguish between them, the final diagnosis can theoretically be obtained by many different paths. Thus a general strategy is needed, the aim of which is to obtain a certain diagnosis with the minimum risk and discomfort for the patient at the maximum cost–benefit ratio. It should always be guided by the clinical features of the given patient and proceed in a stepwise fashion.

A Clinically Driven Strategy

Which Patients to Screen for Cushing's Syndrome?

Classically, the diagnosis of Cushing's syndrome requires a clinical presentation compatible with that originally described by Harvey Cushing [106]. Indeed, it may be wise to recall that in its absence no such investigation should be undertaken.

Recently, however, some emphasis has been put on the frequent occurrence of "occult" or "subclinical" Cushing's syndrome, probably more often associated with adrenal cortical adenomas than with corticotroph adenomas. For these reasons an Endocrine Society Clinical Practice Guideline also suggests that " Patients with unusual features for age (e.g., osteoporosis, hypertension) ..." be also screened for hypercortisolism [518].

When to Screen for Cushing's Syndrome?

In patients with severe stressful conditions or pathological situations known to be accompanied by functional hypercortisolism (anorexia nervosa, alcoholism), the fine exploration of glucocorticoid homeostasis should cautiously await the disappearance of the primary disorder. A patient with authentic Cushing's syndrome may have such severe complications of disease that some tests which could further compromise the condition may be contraindicated. Thus, the diagnostic approach may be modulated by some particular clinical presentations. There may be cases where it is important to delay testing, and others where it is urgent to treat and bypass tests. In the vast majority of cases, however, a defined and coordinated procedure can be applied.

A Stepwise Strategy

A two-step diagnostic approach should first establish the hypercortisolic state and subsequently its cause.

The Hypercortisolic State

Recent studies and consensus conferences have aimed at establishing a hierarchy between the various diagnostic approaches whereby one can distinguish the more usual and easy tests that are sufficient in the vast majority of cases ("first-line" tests), and those that can be necessary to confirm a difficult case ("second-line" tests) [25,450,518].

THE FIRST-LINE TESTS

They are expected to be highly sensitive, simple to perform, possible in outpatients and not costly. Late night salivary cortisol, 24 h urine cortisol, 1 mg and 2 mg 48 h dexamethasone suppression tests and combined strategies based on these tests have similar accuracies [517]. The use of one of the first-line tests is recommended: at least two measurements of 24 h urine cortisol [518]; two measurements of late night salivary cortisol (at bedtime or between 23:00–24:00 h) [518]; 1 mg overnight dexamethasone suppression test [518] or, in certain populations, 2 mg 48 h dexamethasone suppression test [518]. For some centers, the 2 mg 48 h dexamethasone suppression test is considered as a second-line test rather that a first-line test because it is not simple to carry out in an outpatient even if adequate written instructions are provided. In special populations, some tests are preferred: urine cortisol in pregnant women [518]; urine cortisol and late night salivary cortisol in patients receiving drugs that modify dexamethasone clearance [518]; 1 mg overnight dexamethasone suppression test in patients with severe renal failure (consensus); urine cortisol and late night salivary cortisol in suspected cyclic Cushing's syndrome [518]; 1 mg overnight dexamethasone suppression test or late night cortisol [518] in the case of an adrenal incidentaloma. Intermittent Cushing's syndrome should be considered if the clinical impression contrasts with normal laboratory tests or even transient cortisol deficiency [518].

SECOND-LINE TESTS

When the hypercortisolism is severe, the diagnosis is easily confirmed by repeating first-line tests. The specific second-line tests are useful if doubts persist between Cushing's syndrome and a functional hypercortisolic state, the pseudo-Cushing state, as in patients suffering from depression and chronic alcoholism. The specific second-line tests are the following: midnight serum cortisol, serum and salivary cortisol cycle, dexamethasone-CRH test, desmopressin test, CRH test [518].

The Cause of the Hypercortisolic State

The first step to identify the cause of Cushing's syndrome is to measure plasma ACTH.

An ACTH level that is less than 5–10 pg/ml (1.1–2.2 pmol/L) on two separate occasions confirms that the Cushing's syndrome is ACTH-independent. If at least one of the two ACTH measurements is greater than 15–20 pg/ml (3.3–4.4 pmol/L) during the hypercortisolism phase, it is very likely that the Cushing's syndrome is ACTH-dependent. If there is any doubt, it is advisable to carry out a CRH test or even a high-dose dexamethasone suppression test and a CT scan of the adrenal glands [25,450,518].

The final diagnosis of Cushing's syndrome will invariably rely on the combination of several diagnostic procedures using both hormonal and imaging tests that are summarized in Figure 16.23.

Diagnosis of Cushing's disease is based on a combination of several types of investigation including dynamic tests (high-dose dexamethasone suppression test; CRH; for some teams, desmopressin stimulation test), tumor markers, pituitary MRI, thoraco–abdomino–pelvic CT scan (if necessary, somatostatin receptor scintigraphy), and bilateral inferior petrosal sinus sampling for ACTH.

Bilateral inferior petrosal sinus sampling is being increasingly performed with a high diagnostic accuracy to separate pituitary and nonpituitary sources of ACTH. It has led some groups to propose its systematic use as the main if not sole diagnostic procedure for the etiologic work-up. However, because it represents an invasive technique, particularly considering the vascular fragility of these patients, and because its performance may rely above all on the skill of one particular investigator, others are reluctant to consider this test as a primary, systematic and routine diagnostic procedure for etiology.

A reasonable strategy therefore establishes the diagnosis of Cushing's disease on the basis of concordant dynamic testing of the pituitary corticotroph function and the simultaneous presence of a pituitary microadenoma by MRI. In the case of a negative pituitary imaging a thorough and systematic search for a nonpituitary tumor should be undertaken. Bilateral inferior petrosal sinus sampling may be considered with the expectation that it will avoid unwarranted transsphenoidal surgery in the rare case of an occult ectopic ACTH syndrome mimicking Cushing's disease, and that it will provide useful information on the lateralization of the pituitary microadenoma for the surgeon in cases where the disease is confirmed [25,450].

TREATMENT

In identifying the goals of treatment for Cushing's disease, the morbidity and mortality of untreated chronic hypercortisolism dictate that the condition be treated rapidly and actively in most patients.

Such goals are to correct adrenocortical oversecretion, ablate or destroy the primary tumoral lesion, respect anterior pituitary functions possibly restoring a normal pituitary–adrenal axis, and eventually reverse the peripheral manifestations of steroid excess.

These ideal goals cannot always be achieved and in many cases the treatment will only permit a patient to be controlled but not cured. Correction of adrenocortical oversecretion may be accompanied by persistent abnormality of the circadian rhythm (on *op*′DDD),

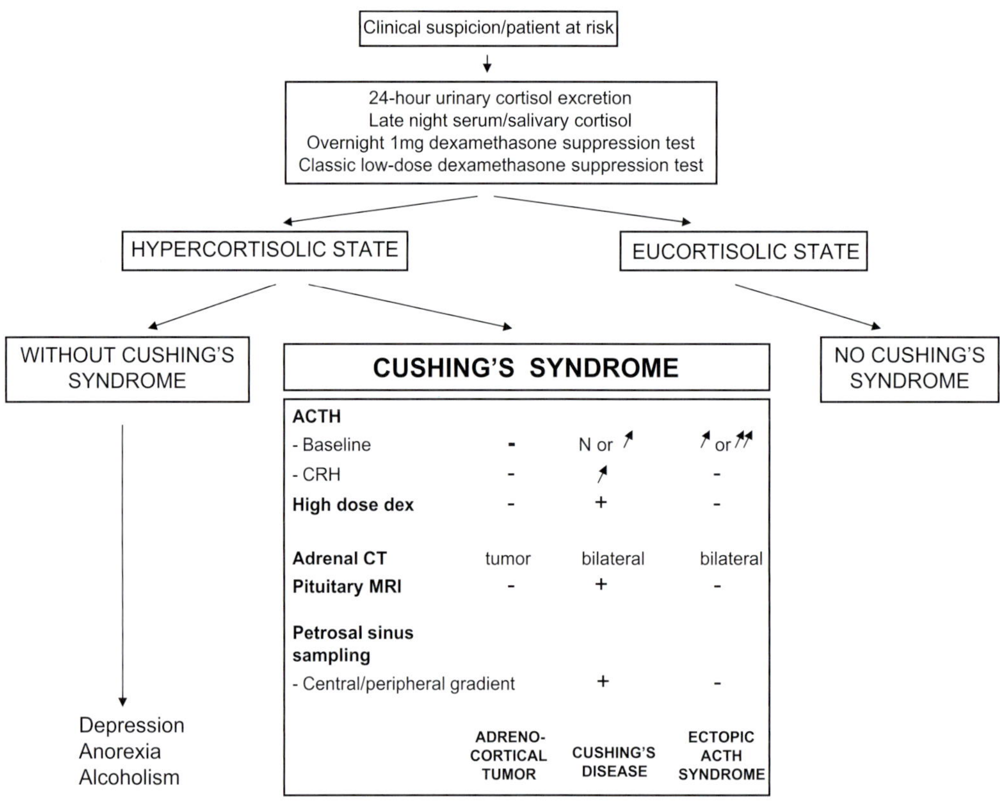

FIGURE 16.23 Pathways to the diagnosis of Cushing's syndrome. ACTH, adrenocorticotroptic hormone; CRH, corticotropin-releasing hormone; CT, computed tomography; MRI, magnetic resonance imaging.

a need for life-long (bilateral adrenal surgery) or transient (selective pituitary adenomectomy) steroid coverage, or progressive development of pituitary insufficiency (radiotherapy).

Over the years various strategies have been developed directed at either the adrenals or the pituitary and using surgical, radiation and pharmacologic approaches either alone or in various combinations. Several recent reviews address the overall treatment options and strategies [450,722–724].

Today, surgical removal of a pituitary microadenoma by the transsphenoidal route appears as the only therapeutic means capable of curing a patient. Yet, it is not always feasible nor always successful. And long-term follow-up of "cured" patients does not always restore a perfect quality of life [473,725].

PITUITARY-DIRECTED THERAPIES

Surgery

Pituitary surgery emerged as a major therapeutic approach in the late 1970s. Two groups [127,128] who performed it systematically in patients who had no evidence of sellar enlargement on skull X-ray demonstrated that most patients harbored a microadenoma in their pituitary and were cured by its selective removal. The rationale that guided this systematic approach was based on the prevalence of such microadenomas at autopsy [3,106], the reported successes in occasional patients who had been operated on [726–728], and the convenience and safety of a novel neurosurgical procedure, namely the transsphenoidal route [727,729]. Over the last 10 years transsphenoidal pituitary exploration has become widespread in many centers and more than a thousand operated patients have been reported in published series.

Prior to surgery, patients should be prepared so that severe hypertension and hyperglycemia are controlled and infected areas eradicated. Depending on the severity of the hypercortisolic state some patients may need a course of anticortisolic treatment for several months before surgery. In all cases patients should receive glucocorticoid coverage during surgery and the operation should be performed only by experienced neurosurgeons, preferably in referral centers. Under these strict conditions the transsphenoidal approach is considered a safe procedure [616]. Mortality is exceptionally reported as a consequence of meningitis [129], bleeding [730], or delayed myocardial infarction [651], accounting for five operation-related deaths in about

550 published patients [731]. CSF leak occurs in 3–8% of cases. Mild and transient complications such as diabetes insipidus and facial and periorbital hematomas are more frequent.

A successful surgical outcome of a selective adenomectomy characteristically induces a state of usually transient, although sometimes lasting up to several years, corticotroph deficiency during which steroid coverage is necessary. In most patients a progressive return to a completely normal pituitary–adrenal axis is observed. All baseline measurements, all dynamic tests and the circadian rhythm of cortisol are normal (Figure 16.24) [129,134,158–160,163,188]. Late night salivary cortisol is also validated to assess the outcome of pituitary surgery [732]. Thus pituitary surgery has the potential to cure patients.

Estimating the cure rate of pituitary surgery is difficult when comparing the results of different series. There are variable criteria for cure [733–737], variable durations of follow-up after surgery, and even variable surgical techniques and strategies. If an immediate success (or initial cure) is defined as the patient with a normal or a low cortisolic state in the first 1–3 months after surgery, there is a general agreement for a high early success rate. Screening the results of more than 800 operated patients reported in 14 series from 14 different centers published between 1979 and 1989 shows that the early success rates varied between 66 and 88% [738]. In the seven largest series which report between 60 and 216 cases, this number varies between 70 and 92% [129–135]. These figures are confirmed by more recent series [739,740], and similar success rates are reported whether the patients were operated by the classical sublabial transseptal approach or the newer transnasal combined endoscopic microsurgery [741]; with the latter approach, there was less blood loss, and both the time of anesthesia and the hospital stay were shorter.

These encouraging figures must be tempered by the fact that some patients who were early successes by the best criteria [315] eventually relapse. The rate of recurrence is difficult to analyze in the various series for lack of uniformity and because the valid figure, i.e., relapse rate (patients x years of follow-up) is only rarely reported. It has been estimated at about 8% [731], although it can be as high as 15% [129,738] in some series. With longer time of follow-up, recent series have reported recurrence rates of 25% at 5 years [742], or a final success rate at 10 years of only 56% [743]. The postoperative work-up shows that, as a group, patients who ultimately recur have higher cortisol responses to CRH and higher baseline urinary cortisol excretion than other early cured patients who will not recur [129,738]. Also, the ACTH response to desmopressin, in the postoperative period, has been more and more recognized as a good predictor of later recurrence in a number of series [744–749]; because, in contrast with CRH, desmopressin response is rather specific to the

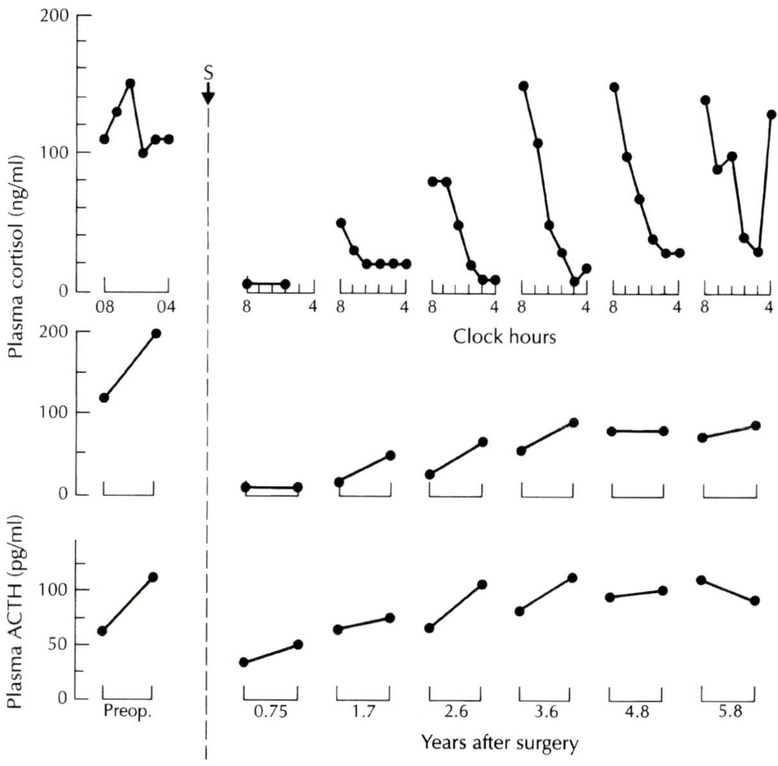

FIGURE 16.24 Long-term follow-up of pituitary–adrenal function after successful pituitary surgery (S). (A) Circadian variation of plasma cortisol. (B, C) Plasma cortisol and adrenocorticotropic hormone (ACTH) responses to the lysine vasopressin (LVP) test. *From Guilhaume et al. [129].*

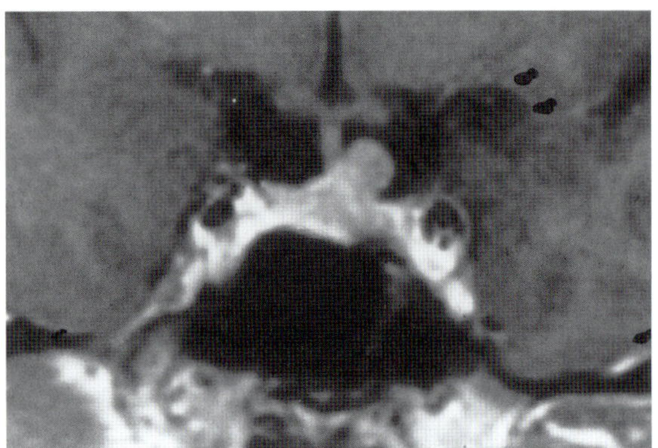

FIGURE 16.25 Pituitary magnetic resonance image exhibiting a corticotroph adenoma situated above the sella turcica.

sole tumoral corticotroph cells, this test is both sensitive and specific. Since true recurrences may occur as late as 10 years, or even more, postoperatively, it is recommended that all initially cured patients be regularly – and indefinitely – followed. The reason for relapses remains obscure. It has been interpreted by some as the manifestation of a persistent hypothalamic drive that would have been primarily responsible for the development of a pituitary adenoma; alternatively a partial adenomectomy could spare a small population of tumoral cells that subsequently regrow [316,317].

A crucial question is to understand the reasons for the early surgical failures. Some circumstances provide an obvious explanation: (1) profuse local bleeding, often due to dural venous sinus, may prevent exposure of the gland [130]; (2) a pituitary adenoma may be located above the sella (Figure 16.25) or even in the sphenoid sinus [138,139]; or (3) a patient with an occult ectopic ACTH syndrome may have been misdiagnosed [572,721].

Excluding these causes there are still patients who are unexpected surgical failures, either because the exploration cannot detect the adenoma or because removal of an apparent adenoma does not control the hypercortisolism. A thorough search for an indicator that would predict a favorable or unfavorable surgical outcome has not clearly distinguished a convincing predictive biochemical parameter [129]. It has been proposed that the cure rate was lower in patients with large macroadenomas [130] with paradoxical responses to TRH and/or LHRH [738], with circulating autoantibodies against pituitary ACTH-producing cells [750], and in those with evidence of intermediate lobe involvement [270]. These suggestions remain controversial [731]. A positive pituitary MRI imaging is positively [740] – or not [751] – associated with a higher likelihood of surgical success.

Better correlations have emerged from studies systematically comparing the surgical outcome and histologic characteristics of the removed pituitary fragments [129,130,731,752]. One study reported that tumoral cells in the excised tissue were more prevalent in early successes (72%) than in surgical failures (24%, $p < 0.01$) [129]. The fact that adenomatous cells were not identified in most surgical failures suggested that either a pituitary adenoma was present which had been missed, or that there was no adenoma in the pituitary. The latter, which would favor a hypothalamic hypothesis for some Cushing's disease [152], actually is hardly tenable since no evidence of corticotroph cell hyperplasia was found histologically in this same study [129,752]. A much more likely explanation is that most of the time surgical failure occurs because a microadenoma was indeed present but missed. The fact that pre- and postoperative urinary cortisol excretion and plasma ACTH remained absolutely unchanged in patients who failed surgery despite removal of a significant portion (ca. 50%) of their anterior pituitary can be taken as an indication that only suppressed corticotroph cells had been removed, leaving the adenoma in situ [129]. Some patients have finally been cured when a microadenoma was found at a second operation [135,317]. There is no theoretical reason why it should be easy to explore a solid organ and discover inconspicuous lesions a few millimeters in size under a microscopic view that is often blurred by hemorrhages, and at the same time ignore the lures of small microcystic structures lying close to the posterior lobe. Thus, technical difficulties should not be minimized as an evident cause of surgical failure.

The surgical outcome does not always correlate with the histological data when some patients are cured after a mere exploration of the pituitary [130] or when no adenomatous cells were apparently removed [129,752], and others being surgical failures although such cells were found [129]. In a large series reporting 216 cases the primary predictor of failure of surgery was the existence of lateral extrasellar extension of the tumor [130]. Some groups have advocated that total hypophysectomy be performed systematically in order to diminish the risk of failure [753]. Others find no improved early success with this strategy [731]. Although total hypophysectomy appears to lower the risk of relapses it certainly augments the risks of hypopituitarism, and many recommend it in particular patients – usually postmenopausal women – and only if the surgeon fails to identify the adenoma [130].

In an attempt to improve the efficacy of pituitary surgery several groups have tried to develop new approaches to help the neurosurgeon find the microadenoma, or at least locate the pituitary half which harbors the lesion. Perioperative histologic examinations and ACTH determinations in peripituitary blood [754] have been claimed to be of help. But the most popular approach has been bilateral inferior petrosal sinus sampling. A ratio of the ACTH level on one side to the other greater than 1.5 indicates that the adenoma lies in that same half of the pituitary gland [611,621]. Because some patients have been cured by hemihypophysectomy guided on the sole results of this test it may be indicated in the patients with no MRI evidence of microadenoma. It might avoid the total hypophysectomy, with its life-long hormone replacement, proposed by some if the surgical exploration were negative. Yet this technique should probably be reserved for experienced teams and its real diagnostic accuracy is variably appreciated [615,642].

Pituitary surgery has re-emerged as a most fruitful treatment of Cushing's disease. It essentially provides a rapid and easily assessable result with a high rate of success in expert hands. It has been successfully performed in a patient with an empty sella [755]. Its major causes of failure are anatomic due to the lateral extension, the small size, or the inaccessibility of the tumor. It is the sole treatment that results in a complete restitution ad integrum of the pituitary–adrenal axis. After successful pituitary surgery in 161 patients treated for Cushing's disease, long-term (mean of 8.7 years) survival was similar to that expected from an age- and sex-matched control population [461]. In the case of failure of a selective adenomectomy or partial hypophysectomy all other therapeutic strategies remain open, including a second attempt at transsphenoidal exploration, although usually with a lower success rate compared to first surgery [756–758]. It is ideally performed and evaluated by an integrated team with an endocrinologist, a radiologist, a neurosurgeon and a histologist. Transsphenoidal pituitary surgery for ACTH-secreting pituitary tumors is associated with a higher complication rate than that observed after similar surgery for other pituitary tumor cell types. About 13% of patients undergoing tumor resection in an experienced center develop complications, especially deep vein thrombosis [616].

Radiation

Conventional Radiotherapy

Probably the first patient to receive pituitary irradiation for Cushing's disease was patient E. G. F. (or case 11 of Cushing's monograph) who was almost dying from his condition when:

> "… he was given … four X-ray treatments. During their course, he felt particularly miserable, but, his downward progression for the preceding month was unmistakably checked. The improvement in his general condition was so striking it must have been something more than coincidence …" [106].

Subsequently conventional megavoltage pituitary irradiation has been proposed as a first-line treatment of Cushing's disease. Success rates vary between groups depending on the proposed criteria to define cure. Because this treatment usually does not restore a normal circadian rhythm or a normal response to the classic low-dose dexamethasone suppression test, the criteria for "cured" or "improved" patients are most often set arbitrarily according to some plasma cortisol or urinary steroid values. In a series of 51 irradiated patients, out of 44 who had been followed-up for more than 1 year, ten were judged cured (urinary 17-hydroxycorticosteroids <7 mg/g creatinine) for periods up to 14 years, and 13 others were judged improved (urinary 17-hydroxycorticosteroids <10 mg/g creatinine) [759]. Subsequent re-evaluation of this group showed that the success rate was especially high in the children (<20 years old) with 80% being cured, and it was suggested that only about 15% of adults would be cured with an additional 30% improved [760]. Other groups have reported success rates somewhat higher, in the 50% range [761,762]. Most groups have delivered between 35 and 52 Gy with a daily fractional dose of ca. 200 cGy. Lower doses (20 Gy) have a high relapse rate [763].

The response to radiotherapy is slow, taking months or years for a full effect. Significant complications of modern radiotherapy are rare provided that the total and fractional doses remain within established limits. The most frequent is the late occurrence of hypopituitarism [763,764]. Serious complications such as injury to optic nerve or chiasma, radiation-induced carcinogenesis and brain necrosis have also been reported in occasional patients with Cushing's disease. However, they are truly exceptional for total doses of less than 50 Gy [765].

Because of its limitations as the sole treatment of Cushing's disease, pituitary radiotherapy has been combined with various other therapeutic regimens [766]. Its combination with unilateral adrenalectomy does not seem justified in view of the poor success rate [767]. More logically and more efficiently, pituitary irradiation is associated with transient adrenocortical-directed medical treatment such as metyrapone, *op*′DDD, or ketoconazole [768–771] until it has achieved its full effect. Twenty-five of 30 patients with persistent or recurrent Cushing's disease after pituitary surgery who underwent radiation were in remission for a median follow-up of 42 months under combined ketoconazole treatment [768]. No recurrences occurred, and most patients were controlled within 2 years, especially when receiving concomitant ketoconazole therapy. Pituitary irradiation is probably undisputed in large macroadenomas that are either inoperable or only partially removed by surgery because of local extension [762]. Some controversy still exists on its prophylactic action for Nelson's syndrome in patients subjected to bilateral adrenalectomy.

Stereotactic Radiosurgery with the γ-Knife

An original device called a γ-knife has been developed and efficiently used for the last 20 years at the Karolinska Institute of Stockholm. A hemispheric instrument (collimator helmet) allows a cerebral target to be placed at a constant and exact intersection of 201 beams of ^{60}Co radiation that simultaneously crossfire to the lesion. This technique achieves high precision and can deliver a fixed dose of radiation to areas ranging in size from 4 cm to a few millimeters without major side effects. The complete treatment is achieved in a single painless session of 5–30 minutes. The γ-knife has been widely used to destroy pituitary adenomas with a high success rate, reaching 76% in Cushing's disease with no relapses [771]. These impressive figures were not confirmed in more recent series from other centers where only 44–54% of the patients were in remission, and with some recurrences [772,773]. It would be desirable that this radiation procedure be extended to several other centers, allowing a wider and more significant evaluation of what appears as a highly promising therapeutic means for its convenience and, hopefully, its high success rate.

Heavy-particle Radiotherapy

The use of heavy particles (α-particle irradiation or proton-beam therapy) allows the delivery of a higher dose of radiation on a smaller-volume target. Reported success rates appear somewhat higher than with conventional radiotherapy, between 65 and 80% [774,775]. This gain in efficacy is offset by an increased incidence of side effects such as optic nerve alteration, oculomotor palsies and hypopituitarism. These methods are not applicable to large tumors with suprasellar or sinus extension, and they are only available in a limited number of specialized centers with a cyclotron.

Radioactive Implants

Direct implantation of radioactive seeds within the sella has been claimed a safe and efficient treatment in the limited centers that perform this specialized stereotactic approach [776,777]. Local interstitial irradiation is delivered by ^{198}Au or ^{90}Y. In the largest recently reported series of 86 patients, 77% had achieved remission after 1 year [778]. The authors emphasize the lack of recurrence of their cured patients as a major advantage over pituitary surgery. Yet interstitial irradiation is associated with a 50% incidence of hypopituitarism which compares quite unfavorably with conventional radiotherapy, and especially with surgery.

Medical Treatments

Various drugs have been tentatively used to try to suppress oversecretion of ACTH in Cushing's disease. Whatever the promises of the initial studies it is fair to say that in the long range none has gained a level of credibility that could favorably compare with that of the other therapeutic means [779].

Cyproheptadine

In the mid-1970s the first cases of cyproheptadine-induced remissions were reported in three patients with Cushing's disease [780]. Clinical and laboratory improvement manifested after 2–3 months of treatment at a dose of 24 mg/day. The drug subsequently proved also to be efficient in cases with Nelson's syndrome [781]. The course of treated patients soon appeared highly variable. Some remained in remission long after (up to 3 years) the drug was discontinued, a majority relapsed either immediately after drug cessation or even while still under therapy [136].

Cyproheptadine possesses an array of pharmacologic actions since it is simultaneously antiserotonergic, antihistaminergic, anticholinergic and antidopaminergic [136]. It is usually claimed that cyproheptadine blocks ACTH secretion in humans at the hypothalamic level through its antiserotonin action and its supposed beneficial therapeutic effect in Cushing's disease has been taken as an indication that an intrinsic hypothalamic abnormality was at the origin of the disease [136]. Yet in vitro studies have also shown a direct inhibitory effect of cyproheptadine on ACTH release from cultured human pituitary adenoma cells [203].

Cyproheptadine administration constantly induces undesirable side effects, such as hyperphagia, weight gain and sedation. Today it seems quite clear that antiserotonin drugs have a questionable therapeutic efficacy, through an unclear mechanism of action and at the price of constant undesirable side effects.

Sodium Valproate

Sodium valproate, another CNS-directed drug, has been reported to induce clinical remissions in some patients with Cushing's disease or Nelson's syndrome [782,783]. This indirect GABAergic drug, which acts by inhibiting GABA transaminase, could theoretically lower CRH production [136]. The promises of its action have not been confirmed by long-term studies [784,785].

Bromocriptine and Dopamine Agonists

The dopaminergic agent bromocriptine has initially been reported to cause an acute suppression of ACTH in a subset of patients with Cushing's disease or Nelson's syndrome [786–788]. Long-term remissions have been subsequently reported in occasional patients with Cushing's disease. It has been suggested that bromocriptine-responsive patients harbored a distinctive type of pituitary adenoma that would originate from intermediate-lobe remnants [270]. This hypothesis has been debated [271,276]. A single controlled study established that bromocriptine was no more effective than placebo to acutely lower cortisol in most, if not all, patients with Cushing's disease [270]. It remains possible, however, that an occasional tumor acquires some unexpected sensitivity to the dopaminergic drug, yet it remains exceptional [274,788].

The development of new D2 dopamine agonists such as cabergoline, and the fine analysis of the D2 dopamine receptor expression, both at the mRNA and the protein levels, in human pituitary corticotroph adenomas has reopened the field. Two teams from Italy and the Netherlands have convincingly shown that this signaling pathway was present and functional in a definite number of these adenomas [277]. Subsequent clinical trials have shown that some patients with Cushing's disease could normalize their urinary cortisol excretion under cabergoline treatment [789]. Yet this trial was uncontrolled, and only a minority of patients (ca. one-third) were normalized, and some actually recurred after a few months of treatment. Some have proposed to combine cabergoline with ketoconazole [790], also with limited success.

Somatostatin and its Analogues

Since the initial report showing that somatostatin infusion induced a partial decrease of plasma ACTH in five patients with Nelson's syndrome [791] there have been a few studies of its action in Cushing's disease and Nelson's syndrome using the analogue SMS 201-995 (octreotide). The clearest conclusion of these various anecdotal reports is that the somatostatin analogue is ineffective in treating Cushing's disease [792], in contrast to what is observed in some, but not all, patients with ectopic ACTH syndrome [793].

New interest was recently gained in the field with recent somatostatin analogues with broader specificities. SOM 230 has high affinity for the somatostatin receptor subtype 5 also. This latter receptor is more expressed in corticotroph adenomas than the type 2 which is actually suppressed under excess cortisol; on these theoretical grounds it was hypothesized that SOM 230 might suppress ACTH oversecretion of corticotroph adenomas [794–796]. A first multicenter, phase II trial with pasireotide (SOM 230) was undertaken in 29 patients with Cushing's disease: on a short-term period of 15 days, five patients (17%) had normalized their urinary cortisol excretion [797].

Other Drug Treatments

On the basis of experimental studies showing the involvement of PPAR gamma and/or retinoic acid on the regulation of proopiomelanocortin gene expression [104,105], tentative – uncontrolled – therapeutic studies have been performed: PPAR agonists (rosiglitazone or pioglitazone) showed no convincing effects on a small series of patients with either Cushing's disease or Nelson's syndrome [798–803]; retinoic acid had some effect on animal models [804,805].

CRH does not induce a state of pituitary corticotroph desensitization on tumor cells in vitro [180]. There is no theoretical reason to believe that chronic administration of a powerful CRH analogue would inhibit ACTH secretion by a pituitary tumor.

Although various peptides (corticostatins) and ACTH analogues [356] with anti-ACTH activity have been described, none has been used for pharmacologic or therapeutic trials in humans not adapted to treatment of Cushing's disease.

At the present time there is no effective means to pharmacologically control ACTH secretion or counteract its peripheral action in Cushing's disease. The promises of the first trials with various CNS-directed compounds have not been confirmed in the long term. The proven efficacy of a drug should be unequivocally established only on the basis of well-designed and well-controlled trials [274,806]. Elegant studies have shown that many patients with Cushing's disease have spontaneous fluctuations of their disease activity. It was nicely demonstrated that various CNS-directed drugs had a variable efficacy in the same patient that simply correlated with phases of spontaneous remissions [280]. These considerations are not trivial. It is not exceptional that a patient is referred to a specialized center after several months, or years, of a totally inefficient treatment trustfully administered on the basis of its alleged but not proven benefit.

ADRENAL-DIRECTED THERAPIES

Surgery

Total Bilateral Adrenalectomy

The recognition that adrenocortical overactivity was the common denominator of all spontaneous Cushing's syndromes and the availability of steroid replacement therapy both boosted the indication of total bilateral adrenalectomy as a radical treatment of Cushing's disease in the early 1950s [807,808]. The obvious and major advantage of this surgical option is its unequaled efficacy to control the hypercortisolic state that is constant and immediate.

The first series reported a high operative mortality rate in the range of 5–10% [808]. A high incidence of postoperative complications was also a major concern in those fragile patients. Wound infections, poor healing, pancreatic injury, acute cholecystitis, pulmonary infections and thromboembolism were the most frequent causes of a high morbidity rate. Some teams have advocated the posterior approach to the adrenals simultaneously by two surgical teams to expedite the procedure and minimize the postoperative morbidity of the more classic transabdominal approach [807].

In reality, the important dogma is to operate on patients who have been prepared, that is after a significant period of eucortisolic state, most often obtained by pharmacologic means. Although it remains a difficult surgical procedure, its mortality is now almost negligible and morbidity is greatly reduced with these precautions, provided that it is performed by a skilled and experienced surgical team, usually now by a laparoscopic approach. The most recent series stress the safety of the procedure and the excellent long-term benefit, if not perfect [475,476].

Adrenalectomized patients will require life-long steroid coverage by gluco- and mineralocorticoids with its unavoidable constraints, need for adaptation, education and the risk of acute adrenal insufficiency.

Unexpectedly, some patients resume endogenous cortisol secretion that may even lead to recurrence of their hypercortisolism, years after a total bilateral adrenalectomy. This occurrence is not exceptional, being reported in as many as 10% of cases [233,385,809]. It is due to the presence of some adrenal rests that have escaped the surgeon's knife or to accessory glands located in various sites and which have regrown under the stimulatory action of chronically and highly elevated ACTH plasma levels.

In some patients, the drastic cortisol deprivation induced by adrenal surgery seems to trigger a definite boost in the growth and secretory activity of the pituitary tumor which was at the origin of the disease. Sellar deformations and clinical hyperpigmentation occur, with increased plasma ACTH levels, defining Nelson's syndrome [810,811]. These tumors often grow aggressively, which may bear a significant morbidity and even mortality [233].

Thus the high efficacy of adrenal surgery is counterbalanced by several disadvantages [812]. It is reasonable to propose such an approach only when pituitary-directed treatments have failed or are contraindicated.

Other Surgical Approaches

Subtotal resection of the adrenals had been initially proposed as the theoretically ideal surgical option. Retrospective analysis of various series shows that it actually fails in its object of restoring normal adrenocortical function in almost 90% of patients; most become adrenal-insufficient requiring steroid coverage, and almost 20–25% relapse [233].

Others have proposed total bilateral adrenalectomy and adrenal autotransplantation, either by inserting slices of the gland within and under the rectus muscle [813], or by transplanting one-third of a gland by vascular connection between the adrenal and the saphenous veins [814,815]. It seems that an occasional success may occur where the transplanted tissue remains active, eventually visualized by iodocholesterol scanning, and capable of delivering a reasonable amount of endogenous steroids up to 11 years after surgery [814]. The fine-tuning of cortisol homeostasis in such conditions is hardly predictable. Long-term follow-up of eight adrenal autotransplants gave rather unfavorable results [816].

Medical Treatments

op′DDD: An Adrenolytic Drug

In the late 1940s it was found by serendipity that the insecticide DDD provoked a selective necrosis of the dog adrenal cortex that predominated in the zona fasciculata and reticularis [817]. A contaminant of the crude DDD preparation exhibited the effective adrenolytic action: 1,1-dichloro-2-(o-chlorophenyl)-2-(*p*-chlorophenyl)-ethane or *op′*DDD. This compound was first used in humans for the chemotherapy of adrenocortical carcinomas where it exhibited a clear adrenolytic action [819]. Its therapeutic use was soon extended to the treatment of Cushing's disease [770,819–821].

*op′*DDD is a highly lipophilic compound with particular kinetics. Its absorption rate is very variable depending on the vehicle [822]. Compared with the commercially available tablets it is better absorbed when given in milk or chocolate, and poorly absorbed when micronized with the gastroresistant cellulose acetylphthalate. In this case much higher doses must be given (up to 12 g/day), in comparison with a usual dose of 3 g/day in its tablet form, but gastrointestinal side effects are minimized. The drug is stored in the adrenals and in the fat [823] and has been detected in the blood as long as 20 months after treatment cessation [824].

The most common side effects of *op′*DDD are digestive and neurologic [770]. Nausea and anorexia have been recorded in about 30% of patients; dizziness, apathy and general weakness are often encountered transiently. All these side effects are generally minor; they disappear spontaneously or after lowering the dose. It is quite exceptional that they require more than a few days of drug interruption. More severe neurologic symptoms such as ataxia and tremor are extremely rare.

Similar symptoms may result from adrenal insufficiency and before attributing them to a toxic effect of the drug vigorous glucocorticoid administration should be attempted. Adrenal insufficiency may occur in hydrocortisone-supplemented patients because through its effect on liver enzymes the drug accelerates the metabolism of exogenously administered steroids

[533]. In some cases much higher doses of hydrocortisone are needed than usually required to supplement an Addisonian patient [825,826].

op′DDD almost constantly provokes a series of biochemical alterations that reflect its being a major inducer of liver microsomal enzymes [825]. Plasma γ-glutamyl transferase and alkaline phosphatase are increased but hepatitis never occurs. Blood cholesterol also invariably rises to a mean value of 3.6 g/L [770]. Caution should be exerted to adjust any intercurrent treatment involving liver metabolism (such as antivitamin K), and estrogen-containing birth control pills may be inefficient. Many patients on *op*′DDD treatment show features of an estrogen-like effect: gynecomastia occurs in as many as 50% of male patients [770], and large increases in plasma CBG, sex-binding globulin and thyroxine-binding globulin (up to six times baseline) have been reported. These actions are to be related to that of chlorinated insecticides such as *op*′DDD [673]. Although not demonstrated directly for *op*′DDD it is conceivable that the compound or one of its metabolites is also a potent estrogen-like agent. These effects, coupled with the rise in plasma cholesterol, obviously raise serious questions about a possible deleterious vascular effect, yet curiously there has been no systematic study of the general effect of *op*′DDD on vascular risk and on coagulation homeostasis. No renal or hematologic toxicity (apart from rare leucopenia) has been described. Allergic reactions (skin rash) are rare and transient. Diminished total and free T_4 has been reported and may be related to a competition between *op*′DDD and T_4 on thyroxine-binding globulin [827]. Interestingly the gonads are not a target of *op*′DDD action, which does not interfere with gonadal steroidogenesis [828]. Because of its presumed teratogenic effect contraception should be ensured in treated females and pregnancy only allowed after at least 2 years of interruption of the treatment; babies born from such patients have shown no abnormalities.

Patients with Cushing's disease almost invariably reduce their cortisol production on *op*′DDD [770]. As already mentioned the response should not be assessed only on plasma cortisol or on urinary 17-hydroxycorticosteroids, which may be artifactually altered. Direct indicators of plasma free cortisol such as salivary or urinary cortisol are the best parameters. Decreased cortisol production is a slow phenomenon that is manifest after 1 or 2 months of treatment. Because the action of the drug is somewhat predominant on the zona fasciculata and reticularis the mineralocorticoid secretion has been claimed to be more preserved [820]. In many cases, however, it can also be fully suppressed [770].

op′DDD provokes mitochondrial degeneration in adrenal cortical cells [820] and evidence for an altered activity of 11-β-hydroxylase has been observed in patients with Cushing's disease with a slight increase in plasma DOC and 11-deoxycortisol levels and in the ratios of DOC/corticosterone and 11-deoxycortisol/cortisol [829]. Yet the particular and invaluable property of *op*′DDD is that it is not merely an enzyme inhibitor, but truly an adrenolytic drug. The decreased cortisol production results from a loss of adrenocortical cells. This mechanism of action is different from that of the classic enzyme inhibitors which only block, more or less completely, the steroidogenesis pathway; hence the enormous advantage of *op*′DDD. In contrast with the pure enzyme inhibitors its efficacy is not compromised by an escape phenomenon. It is nicely corroborated by the rise in ACTH and LPH which is invariably triggered in response to the relative cortisol deprivation (Figure 16.26). Because the treatment with *op*′DDD had been so efficient many patients refused adrenal surgery that had initially been planned after a medical preparation with the drug! Thus, it became possible to observe the long-term effect of *op*′DDD as the sole treatment of Cushing's disease [770]. Whereas about 80% of patients responded to treatment, it appeared that hypercortisolism recurred in most after cessation of the drug; 60% relapses were observed within 2–69 months.

Although *op*′DDD is a highly effective adrenolytic drug with unique properties, its use as sole therapy in

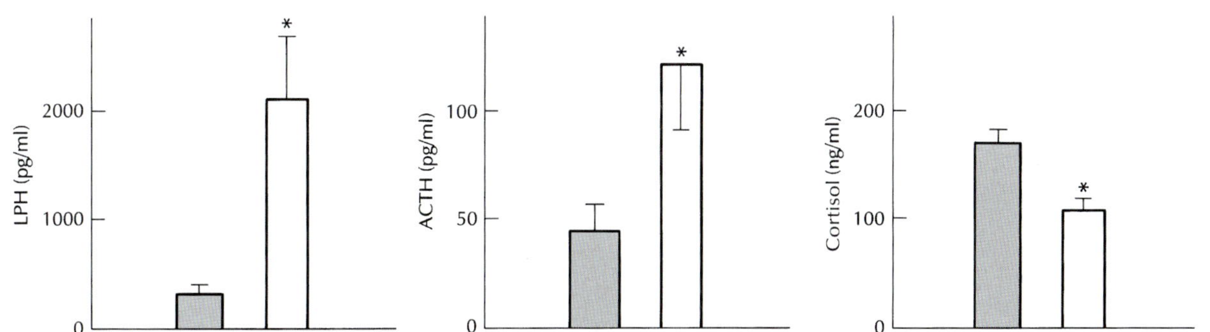

FIGURE 16.26 Values (mean + SEM) of morning plasma lipotropin (LPH), adrenocorticotropic hormone (ACTH), and cortisol in patients with Cushing's disease before therapy (stippled bars) and on *op*′*DDD* (clear bars). *From Kuhn et al. [130]*

Cushing's disease has several limitations. Because of its numerous and serious side effects, its particular kinetics and its highly variable bioavailability, it necessitates close and repeated monitoring. The drug cannot pretend to cure a patient, but merely to control the hypercortisolism to a variable extent, and this has to be regularly evaluated. Many patients will develop adrenal insufficiency. Although its efficacy may last for years in a given patient, its effect is most often only transient.

A better indication of *op*′DDD is probably when transient control of hypercortisolism is needed, for example, waiting for the full effect of pituitary irradiation to become manifest [769,770], or to prepare a severely ill patient for pituitary or adrenal surgery. In the latter situation, the close observation of ACTH variations under prolonged reduction of plasma cortisol may be a predictive value of the aggressiveness of the pituitary tumor.

Inhibitors of Cortisol Synthesis

Various pharmacologic agents that inhibit cortisol synthesis have been tentatively proposed for the treatment of Cushing's disease.

METYRAPONE

Metyrapone inhibits 11-β-hydroxylase activity, blocking the last step of adrenal steroid biosynthesis, the conversion of the biologically inactive 11-deoxycortisol to cortisol. As expected, patients with Cushing's disease respond to the cortisol-lowering effect of metyrapone by an overshoot of ACTH secretion that is anticipated to override the partial enzyme blockade [581]. Few reports describe its effectiveness in occasional patients [830,831]. A single group has systematically studied its long-term (up to 66 months) effect in patients with Cushing's disease. Although ACTH did rise in response to the drug (750–4000 mg/day) it apparently was not sufficient to overcome the metyrapone blockade [832]. As noted elsewhere the patients of this study had also received pituitary radiotherapy, which may explain why the anticipated escape phenomenon was not reported in these very patients [833]. Furthermore, metyrapone often results in some general side effects including nausea and dizziness; it increases the secretion of adrenocortical androgens and may result in intolerable worsening of hirsutism in female patients [832]. Thus, the beneficial effect of metyrapone as sole treatment of Cushing's disease appears far from evident. It may be useful as an adjunct treatment while awaiting the full effect of pituitary irradiation. It may gain in power if administered concomitantly with other cortisol-lowering drugs [834,835] and may be useful for its rapid onset of action.

AMINOGLUTETHIMIDE

Aminoglutethimide blocks the first step in adrenal steroid biosynthesis. Its use in patients with Cushing's disease has provided inconsistent results that are outweighed by its frequent side effects [836], which include somnolence, dizziness and skin rash. Its use has been proposed in association with metyrapone [835].

Imidazole Derivatives: Ketoconazole and Etomidate

The anticortisolic drug of the imidazole family, ketoconazole, inhibits various steps of adrenal and testicular steroidogenesis [837]. Cortisol synthesis is inhibited at the levels of the 20–22 desmolase and 11-β-hydroxylase. Several studies initiated in the late 1980s have shown its rapid cortisol-lowering action in patients with Cushing's disease [838,839] and its prolonged beneficial effect as the sole treatment in some series [840–842]. The ACTH response to long-term ketoconazole administration is somewhat variable, although it was increased in some patients, with an exaggerated response to CRH [843]. The successful action of long-term ketoconazole administration may be restricted, as for metyrapone, to patients who were concomitantly subjected to pituitary irradiation [840]. Around 50% of patients with Cushing's disease appear to be controlled in the long term [844]. Patients have been reported who progressively escaped from the beneficial effect of ketoconazole [845]. Thus the real efficacy of the drug as the sole treatment of Cushing's disease should await further evaluation. It has few side effects besides the rare toxic hepatitis.

Another imidazole derivative, the anesthetic drug etomidate, also inhibits cortisol synthesis. It was recently shown that it can be safely administered intravenously at a nonhypnotic dose with a dramatic and immediate cortisol-lowering effect [846]. It is proposed as an alternative for the rapid control of severe hypercortisolic states.

RU 486: Hopes and Limitations

The potent antiglucocorticoid action of RU 486 in humans raised the hope of a potential new pharmacologic approach in the treatment of patients with chronic hypercortisolism. The first reported case indeed showed a dramatic beneficial effect of the drug in a patient with ectopic ACTH syndrome [847].

The situation in Cushing's disease is completely different. Based on the known pathophysiologic mechanism of the disease it was anticipated that RU 486 would antagonize cortisol action not only at the periphery but also at the pituitary, and immediately trigger a brisk ACTH and cortisol rise. A study performed in five patients with Cushing's disease given the drug (400 mg/day) for 3 consecutive days confirmed this fear [848]. All indices of corticotroph and adrenocortical activities showed a major rise (Figure 16.27). Urinary

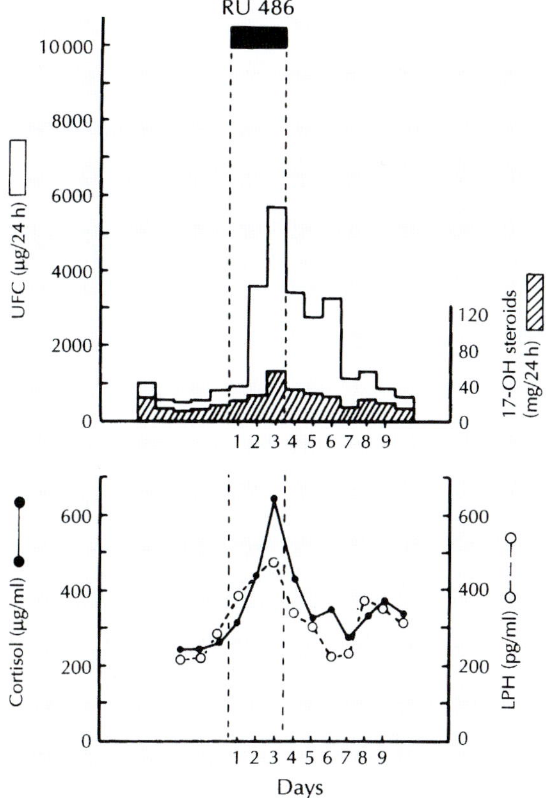

FIGURE 16.27 Pituitary–adrenal response to RU 486 (400 mg/day for 3 days) in a patient with Cushing's disease. LPH, lipotropin; 17-OH, 17-hydroxycorticosteroids; UFC, urinary free cortisol.

free cortisol increased ten-fold in some patients! Thus this short-term study demonstrated that RU 486 administration in Cushing's disease will inevitably provoke an immediate pituitary retort. What will be the final balance at the peripheral target organ between the action of RU 486 and the increased endogenous cortisol is unknown. At the present time a sensitive and convenient way of evaluating this peripheral balance that would allow the drug to be administered safely is lacking, especially in view of its long duration of action. Although it is possible that RU 486 may help to control hypercortisolism in some urgent situations [849], it should not be considered as a routine alternative for treating patients with Cushing's disease. The "merits and pitfalls" of RU 486 (mifepristone) in Cushing's syndrome have been reviewed recently [850].

NELSON'S SYNDROME

Classically

Don H. Nelson reported in 1958 the case of "*... a patient who, three years after bilateral adrenalectomy for hyper-adrenocorticisim, was found to have a chromophobe tumor of the pituitary gland that was secreting large quantities of ACTH*" [810]. At that time the fine pathophysiologic mechanism of "*Cushing's syndrome due to bilateral adrenal hyperplasia*" was undecided and even the role of the pituitary was debated, essentially because the lack of a sensitive ACTH assay did not allow measurement of the hormone in such patients. There was something prophetic in Nelson's paper where he described the first ten patients bearing his syndrome: "*Ten patients, previously adrenalectomized for Cushing's syndrome, who have subsequently developed evidence of a disturbance of the pituitary gland, have been studied.*" The recognition of this new entity was indeed illuminating; it pointed at the pituitary as the genuine cause of Cushing's syndrome due to bilateral adrenal hyperplasia [811]. The evidence of "a disturbance of the pituitary gland" relied on an array of variously associated and more or less sensitive indicators such as hyperpigmentation, enlarged pituitary gland by roentgenologic examination or visual field defect, and increased plasma ACTH [231,811].

Precisely because the definition of Nelson's syndrome is variously appreciated, its incidence after adrenal surgery has been variably estimated as ranging from 5 to 78% in some series [2]. Judged on plasma ACTH increase as well as on hyperpigmentation, evidence of pituitary disease progress after adrenal surgery is almost constant [113,812]. The diagnosis of Nelson's syndrome was based upon classic criteria, i.e., the occurrence of both hyperpigmentation and roentgenographic evidence of sellar enlargement. Although poorly sensitive, these criteria have two major advantages: (1) they have always been available allowing retrospective studies on large series of patients; and (2) the occurrence of a sellar enlargement most often corresponds to a pituitary tumor the size of which is relevant for a significant morbidity.

On the basis of these criteria, the prevalence of Nelson's syndrome is lower, but still highly variable ranging from 8–38% [2,231,851–853]. Some authors report that pituitary tumors may occur as late as 16 years after surgery [852,853] although it is not known whether the patients were all regularly followed. The ACTH rise within the year after adrenal surgery discriminates between the patients who will subsequently develop Nelson's syndrome and those who will not [854,855]. Children seem to be more prone to develop Nelson's syndrome [856]. No parameter has been found that could predict the behavior of the pituitary adenoma in response to the adrenal surgery. Recent data suggest that the ACTH rise in response to *op'*DDD-induced cortisol long-term deprivation discriminated between patients at risk and the others, the former showing a definitely higher ACTH retort. Whether pituitary irradiation offers a prophylactic means against Nelson's syndrome has been debated [759,852–854]. In our own series, none of 18 patients who received pituitary irradiation before or within 3 years after adrenal surgery developed Nelson's syndrome.

Corticotroph tumors of Nelson's syndrome occasionally behaved in an aggressive manner [857]. True pituitary cancers with extracranial metastases have been described [229,231,852]. Plasma ACTH is usually above 1000 pg/ml and can reach the very high values of 100,000 pg/ml. Hyperpigmentation is invariably present. Stimulation of adrenal rests may lead to recurrent hypercortisolism with concomitant androgen and DOC oversecretion [385,858,859]. Treatment of such tumors is of utmost difficulty; surgery is almost always incomplete and irradiation therapy has limited efficacy [113,761]. An occasional tumor may spontaneously infarct [507]. These tumors may ultimately cause the death of a patient whose hypercortisolism is perfectly controlled [233].

Nelson's Syndrome or Corticotroph Tumor Progression?

Today we know that the corticotroph adenoma is indeed the cause of Cushing's disease, and we can use highly sensitive imaging and biological means to visualize it and assess its function through pituitary MRI and ACTH measurements with immunoassays. These modern approaches are now routinely used for the follow-up of patients with Cushing's disease.

Rather than "wait" for the occurrence of Nelson syndrome, as "defined" originally (Figure 16.28, upper), we can now "detect," early and precisely, the possible occurrence of corticotroph tumor progression, long before the "classical" features of Nelson's syndrome (Figure 16.28, lower)!

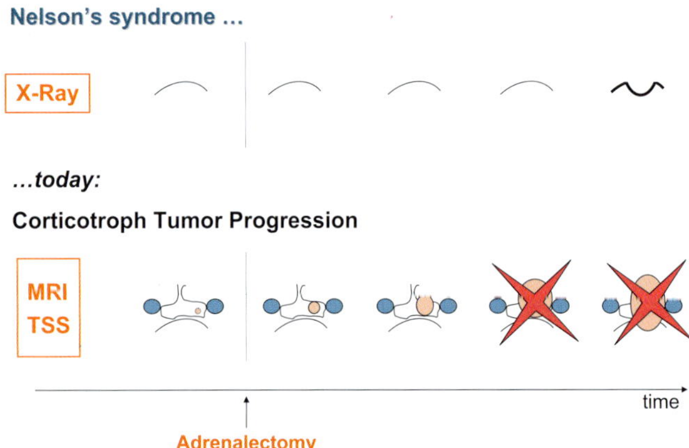

FIGURE 16.28 Nelson's syndrome ... or corticotroph tumor progression? Late diagnosis of Nelson's syndrome, originally, when the diagnosis means lacked sensitivity (upper part). Close follow-up of possible corticotroph tumor progression, with modern tools such as pituitary MRI (lower part).

We recently studied [860] the rate of occurrence of corticotroph tumor progression in a cohort of 53 patients with Cushing's disease who were carefully followed in a single center after bilateral adrenalectomy, using repeat MRI, for a median duration of follow-up after adrenalectomy of 4.6 years (range 0.5–13.5). None had received pituitary radiotherapy. CTP was defined either by the occurrence of an adenoma at MRI, or the growth of a pre-existing adenoma on pituitary MRI.

Three years after adrenalectomy, the proportion of patients showing evidence of corticotroph tumor progression reached 39%; this number tended to plateau at 47% after 7 years. Thus ca. 50% of the patients showed no evidence of corticotroph tumor progression after this time period. Corticotroph tumor progression can indeed be easily detected by repeat pituitary MRI [861]. It is recommended that it be performed before and 6 months after adrenalectomy, then every year, at least for the next 5–6 years. In the absence of corticotroph tumor progression it seems reasonable to increase the time intervals of MRI surveillance thereafter.

The historical cases of Nelson's syndrome were characterized by large invasive pituitary macroadenomas presenting a major therapeutic challenge. Today with pituitary MRI the tumor could have been detected much earlier at a smaller size, and the surgical procedures have improved, as well as the radiotherapeutic protocol.

After adrenalectomy, the goal is not to cure the pituitary adenoma, but rather to manage corticotroph tumor progression so that no complication related to the tumor burden occurs. Indeed, a microadenoma appeared on MRI after adrenalectomy may not be removed as long as it does not grow, especially in patients with high-risk pituitary surgery. Alternatively, if necessary corticotroph tumor progression can be treated by surgery and/or radiotherapy [861–864].

Pathophysiological Hypotheses

A suggested mechanism is that total bilateral adrenalectomy provokes a dramatic cortisol deprivation state that triggers not only an overshoot of ACTH secretion but also a burst of tumor growth. Adrenalectomized patients receive steroid coverage in a total dosage that may surpass the physiologic substitution. However, on a daily basis the pituitary tumor is totally deprived of cortisol for several hours during the night. This is probably the major difference with the patient who still has two adrenals and a permanent production of cortisol during 24 hours. Although it has been amply demonstrated and finely explained how cortisol deprivation stimulates ACTH production it still remains to be shown if, and how, cortisol also acts on the growth of corticotroph cells. As already suggested, restored hypothalamic CRH activity may participate in the pathophysiologic mechanism of the tumor growth. So far there has been no means to evaluate the growth potential of a pituitary corticotroph adenoma. Because it remains an unpredictable event which somehow appears to be triggered by cortisol lowering it adds another reason why all efforts should be made to choose as a first-line treatment the therapeutic means which at the same time ablates this threat.

STRATEGY

Pituitary Surgery as the First-line Treatment

The Transsphenoidal Approach

Pituitary surgery offers the success rate, and the quality of cure that undoubtedly designate it as the best therapeutic option. A systematic approach by the transsphenoidal route is indicated whenever the dynamic hormonal tests are all concordant with the diagnosis of Cushing's disease, if the evidence for a pituitary adenoma has been obtained by MRI or by bilateral inferior petrosal sinus sampling if there is no obvious extrasellar lateral extension. It can be chosen as a first-line treatment in the moderately severe patient who does not require a prior preparation with anticortisolic drugs.

If a microadenoma is found at exploration it is selectively removed by partial hypophysectomy. Most patients will be immediately cured. Long-term follow-up is necessary since late recurrences may occur.

If the surgical exploration fails to identify an adenomatous lesion some have advocated immediate total hypophysectomy. It seems fair, however, to suggest only a partial hypophysectomy at a first operation. In some cases a small microadenoma will be excised and the patient will be cured. With the hope of increasing the odds of a successful blind partial hypophysectomy in the case of a negative transsphenoidal exploration some groups perform a systematic bilateral inferior petrosal sinus sampling procedure prior to surgery. If a clear lateralization of ACTH is found it pinpoints the side of the gland which should be removed, since it presumably harbors the inconspicuous corticotroph adenoma too small to be seen by the surgeon. It may be fair however to restrict this invasive procedure only to the patients who have no visible lesion on pituitary MRI.

Failure of Pituitary Surgery

In case of initial surgical failure the partial hypophysectomy option has three advantages: (1) the overall pituitary function is not compromised; (2) histologic examination of the obtained pituitary tissue provides information to explain the failure; and (3) all therapeutic options remain open, including a second surgical attempt at the pituitary [735,736].

The excised pituitary tissue may show no tumoral tissue but only "normal" pituitary fragments with few corticotroph cells, some of them exhibiting Crooke's hyaline features. The first consideration should be that of a diagnostic error, especially a missed occult ectopic ACTH syndrome. A complete re-evaluation of the patient should be undertaken. If Cushing's disease is ultimately confirmed the surgical failure may be best explained by the fact that a microadenoma does exist, but was missed.

Alternatively, histologic examination of the removed tissue may reveal the presence of tumoral cells within fragments of normal pituitary. In that situation it is highly likely that only part of an adenoma has been excised.

A Second Trial of Pituitary Surgery?

This option can be envisaged only after the diagnosis of Cushing's disease has been thoroughly reassessed, and the presence of a pituitary microadenoma clearly demonstrated either by bilateral inferior petrosal sinus sampling or after repeat MRI in the patient treated by anticortisolic drugs. It should not be performed if evidence of extrasellar lateral extension has been obtained. Secondary successes are reported in about 73% of patients [317]. In selected patients a total hypophysectomy may be planned in the prospect of increasing the odds of definitive success. Whatever the option the risk of compromising the overall pituitary function is maximized [317].

This strategy applies also to patients in whom the disease recurs.

When Pituitary Surgery is Questionable as a First-line Treatment

Some situations raise serious doubt on the probability that first-line pituitary surgery will be successful and may command a different strategy.

The classic situation is when the diagnosis between Cushing's disease and ectopic ACTH syndrome is unclear. The hormonal dynamics are consistent with Cushing's disease but the pituitary MRI is negative, or the hormonal dynamics are not strictly concordant with Cushing's disease. Bilateral inferior petrosal sinus sampling offers the theoretical means to resolve this ambiguity and has proved its efficacy in some groups. However, it is not a widely accepted procedure because of its invasiveness, the need for an experienced radiologic team and its diagnostic limitations [461]. A safe and practical alternative is to administer adrenal-directed therapy with drugs such as *op*′DDD or ketoconazole [844]. At the same time the hypercortisolism will be treated and close surveillance of the corticotroph function, of pituitary MRI and other potential sources of nonpituitary ACTH should be conducted. Although this approach precludes the further use of dynamic hormonal testing it is a strategy that often provides time to secondarily detect an emerging small pituitary adenoma or sometimes a small bronchial carcinoid tumor. It is acceptable in view of the usually low agressiveness of these tumors and allows subsequent surgical treatment of these lesions in well-prepared patients.

Rare pituitary tumors presenting with evidence of lateral extrasellar extension in the cavernous sinus are better detected by MRI. These potentially aggressive tumors should best be treated with combined radiotherapy and *op′*DDD.

The severity of the hypercortisolism may be enough to preclude immediate pituitary surgery. The patient may be prepared for surgery by a course of anticortisolic treatment for several months.

Alternatively, a mild or cyclic form of Cushing's disease may first require further close surveillance and repeat hormonal evaluation before a radical treatment option is undertaken.

After Pituitary Surgery has Failed

At that time there is no ideal or easy treatment!

It is most often necessary to control the hypercortisolism with an adrenal-directed treatment. It is our experience that *op′*DDD has the highest long-term efficacy. Others would favor the less toxic ketoconazole. Depending on the aggressiveness of the pituitary tumor simultaneous radiotherapy is often indicated and anticortisolic drugs may be discontinued later.

In rare cases of failure, total bilateral adrenalectomy may eventually be necessary, provided that the corticotroph tumor progression is closely monitored.

The role of dopamine or somatostatin analogues remains to be fully established.

PERSPECTIVES

Great promise has arisen from the early successes of pituitary surgery. These patients should be followed regularly and for a long time. The recurrence rates that will be observed in the years to come will permit a sound judgment on the long-term efficacy of this therapeutic approach.

In some cases, a small adenoma lying deep in a small pituitary gland remains a challenge for the therapist. It may not be totally unrealistic to envisage the development of more sensitive techniques that will detect and destroy these inconspicuous lesions. CRH analogues may be designed to target the appropriate isotopes or drugs specifically on the tumor cells eventually providing a convenient, elegant, and, hopefully, efficient new therapeutic approach.

What is also needed is a practical and sensitive biochemical marker of the peripheral action of glucocorticoids. It would be a most useful aid to evaluate the real efficacy of all therapeutic means. It would also help to better evaluate those frequent patients who look somewhat hypercortisolic but have "normal" hormonal investigations. There may well be a large fringe of ill-defined pathologic states that potentially result from a slight disruption of cortisol homeostasis and cannot be detected by present modes of investigation uniformly directed toward the sole assessment of cortisol production rather than toward its action.

Acknowledgments

The authors are greatly indebted to Professor P. Thomopoulos and Dr H. Escourolle for their comments and participation in obtaining hormonal data; to Professor L. Olivier and Dr E. Vila-Porcile for fruitful discussions and for the histologic illustrations; to Dr J. P. Abecassis and Professor A. Bonnin for their comments and the imaging illustrations; to MM J. F. Massias and F. Lenne for their contribution to the artwork. They express their deep gratitude to Dr C. Bertagna for her benevolent and tolerant review of the text. This work would not have been possible without the invaluable secretarial expertise of Mrs M. Le Scouarnec.

References

[1] T.A. Huff, Clinical syndromes related to disorders of adrenocorticotrophic hormone, in: M.B. Allen, V.B. Makesh (Eds.), The Pituitary: A Current Review, Academic Press, New York, 1977, pp. 153–168.

[2] J.D. Baxter, J.B. Tyrrell, The adrenal cortex, in: P. Felig, J.D. Baxter, A.E. Broadus, L.A. Frohman (Eds.), Endocrinology and Metabolism, McGraw-Hill, New York, 1981, pp. 385–510.

[3] C.M. Plotz, A.L. Knowlton, C. Ragan, The natural history of Cushing's syndrome, Am J Med 13 (1952) 597–614.

[4] A.M. Neville, M.J. O'Hare, Aspects of structure, function and pathology, in: V.H.T. James (Ed.), The Adrenal Gland, Raven Press, New York, 1979, pp. 1–66.

[5] R.G. McArthur, M.D. Cloutier, A.B. Hayles, R.G. Sprague, Cushing's disease in children, Mayo Clin Proc 47 (1972) 318–326.

[6] A.M. Neville, T. Symington, Bilateral adrenocortical hyperplasia in children with Cushing's syndrome, J Pathol 107 (1972) 95–106.

[7] A.L. Hartley, J.M. Birsh, H.B. Mardsen, H. Reid, M. Harris, V. Blair, Adrenocortical tumors: Epidemiological and familial aspects, Arch Dis Child 62 (1987) 683–689.

[8] M.O. Savage, L.F. Chan, A.B. Grossman, H.L. Storr, Work-up and management of paediatric Cushing's syndrome, Curr Opin Endocrinol Diabetes Obes 15 (4) (2008) 346–351.

[9] M.A. Magiakou, G. Mastorakos, E.H. Oldfield, M.T. Gomez, J.L. Doppman, G.B. Cutler Jr, et al., Cushing's syndrome in children and adolescents. Presentation, diagnosis, and therapy, N Engl J Med 331 (10) (1994) 629–636.

[10] L. Alexander, D. Appleton, R. Hall, W.M. Ross, R. Wilkinson, Epidemiology of acromegaly in the Newcastle region, Clin Endocrinol 12 (1980) 71–79.

[11] E.B. Gold, Epidemiology of pituitary adenomas, Epidemiol Rev 3 (1981) 163–183.

[12] Biometrics Branch, National Cancer Institute, S.J. Cutler, J.L. Young (Eds.), Third National Cancer Survey: Incidence data, 41, Government Printing Office: National Cancer Institute Monograph, Washington, 1975, pp. 75–78.

[13] N.S. Ross, D.C. Aron, Hormonal evaluation of the patient with an incidentally discovered adrenal mass, N Engl J Med 323 (1990) 1401–1405.

[14] K. Kovacs, E. Horvath, Pathology of pituitary tumors, Endocrinol Metab Clin North Am 16 (1987) 529–551.

[15] A.M. Hutter, D.E. Kayhoe, Adrenal cortical carcinoma. Clinical features of 138 patients, Am J Med 41 (1966) 572–580.

[16] C. Bertagna, D.N. Orth, Clinical and laboratory findings and results of therapy in 58 patients with adrenocortical tumors admitted to a single medical center (1951 to 1978), Am J Med 71 (1981) 855–875.

[17] J.P. Luton, S. Cerdas, L. Billaud, et al., Clinical features of adrenocortical carcinoma, prognostic factors, and the effect of mitotane therapy, N Engl J Med 322 (1990) 1195–1201.

[18] J. Etxabe, J.A. Vazquez, Morbidity and mortality in Cushing's disease: An epidemiological approach, Clin Endocrinol (Oxf) 40 (4) (1994) 479–484.

[19] J. Lindholm, S. Juul, J.O. Jørgensen, J. Astrup, P. Bjerre, U. Feldt-Rasmussen, et al., Incidence and late prognosis of Cushing's syndrome: A population-based study, J Clin Endocrinol Metab 86 (1) (2001) 117–123.

[20] C.G. Patil, S.P. Lad, G.R. Harsh, E.R. Laws Jr., M. Boakye, National trends, complications, and outcomes following transsphenoidal surgery for Cushing's disease from 1993 to 2002, Neurosurg Focus 23 (2007) E7.

[21] B. Catargi, V. Rigalleau, A. Poussin, N. Ronci-Chaix, V. Bex, V. Vergnot, et al., Occult Cushing's syndrome in type-2 diabetes, J Clin Endocrinol Metab 88 (2003) 5808–5813.

[22] L.N. Contreras, E. Cardoso, M.P. Lozano, J. Pozzo, P. Pagano, H. Claus-Hermbeg, [Detection of preclinical Cushing's syndrome in overweight type 2 diabetic patients], Medicina (B Aires) 60 (2000) 326–330.

[23] M.S. Caetano, C. Silva Rdo, C.E. Kater, Increased diagnostic probability of subclinical Cushing's syndrome in a population sample of overweight adult patients with type 2 diabetes mellitus, Arq Bras Endocrinol Metabol 51 (2007) 1118–1127.

[24] G. Reimondo, A. Pia, B. Allasino, F. Tassone, S. Bovio, G. Borretta, et al., Screening of Cushing's syndrome in adult patients with newly diagnosed diabetes mellitus, Clin Endocrinol (Oxf) 67 (2007) 225–229.

[25] G. Arnaldi, A. Angeli, A.B. Atkinson, X. Bertagna, F. Cavagnini, G.P. Chrousos, et al., Diagnosis and complications of Cushing's syndrome: A consensus statement, J Clin Endocrinol Metab 88 (2003) 5593–5602.

[26] I. Chiodini, M.L. Mascia, S. Muscarella, C. Battista, S. Minisola, M. Arosio, et al., Subclinical hypercortisolism among outpatients referred for osteoporosis, Ann Intern Med 147 (2007) 541–548.

[27] B.A. Eipper, R.E. Mains, Structure and biosynthesis of pro-adrenocorticotropin/endorphin and related peptides, Endocr Rev 1 (1980) 1–27.

[28] S. Nakanishi, A. Anoue, T. Kita, et al., Nucleotide sequence of cloned cDNA for bovine corticotropin-β-lipotropin precursor, Nature 278 (1979) 423–427.

[29] A.C.Y. Chang, M. Cochet, S.N. Cohen, Structural organisation of human genomic DNA encoding the proopiomelanocortin peptide, Proc Nat Acad Sci USA 77 (1980) 4890–4894.

[30] P. Whitfeld, P. Seeburg, J. Shine, The human proopiomelanocortin gene: Organization, sequence and interspersion with repetitive DNA, DNA 1 (1982) 133–143.

[31] H. Takahashi, Y. Hakamata, Y. Watanabe, R. Kikuno, T. Miyata, S. Numa, Complete nucleotide sequence of the human corticotropin-β-lipotropin precursor gene, Nucleic Acids Res 11 (1983) 6847–6858.

[32] B.U. Zabel, S.L. Naylor, A.Y. Sakaguchi, et al., High resolution chromosal localization of human genes for amylase, proopiomelanocortin and a DNA fragment (D3 S1) by in situ hybridization, Proc Nat Acad Sci USA 80 (1983) 6932–6936.

[33] J. Feder, F. Migone, A.C.Y. Chang, et al., A DNA polymorphism in close physical linkage with the proopiomelanocortin gene, Am J Hum Genet 35 (1983) 1090–1096.

[34] A.I. Smith, J.W. Funder, Proopiomelanocortin processing in the pituitary, central nervous system and peripheral tissues, Endocr Rev 9 (1988) 159–179.

[35] N. Seidah, J. Rochemont, J. Hamelin, M. Lis, M. Chretien, Primary structure of the major human pituitary proopiomelanocortin NH_2-terminal glycopeptide. Evidence for an aldosterone-stimulating activity, J Biol Chem 256 (1981) 7977–7984.

[36] E. Estivariz, J. Hope, C. McLean, P.J. Lowry, Purification and characterization of a gamma-melanotropin precursor from frozen human pituitary glands, Biochem J 191 (1980) 125–132.

[37] N.G. Seidah, J. Rochemont, J. Hamelin, S. Benjannet, M. Chretien, The missing fragment of the pro-sequence of human proopiomelanocortin: Sequence and evidence for C-terminal amidation, Biochem Biophys Res Commun 102 (1981) 710–716.

[38] X. Bertagna, F. Camus, F. Lenne, F. Girard, J.P. Luton, Human joining peptide: A proopiomelanocortin product secreted as a homodimer, Mol Endocrinol 2 (1988) 1108–1114.

[39] M. Fenger, H.A. Johnsen, Alpha-amidated peptides derived from proopiomelanocortin in normal human pituitary, Biochem J 250 (1988) 781–788.

[40] A.P. Scott, P.J. Lowry, Adrenocorticotrophic and melanocyte stimulating peptides in the human pituitary, Biochem J 139 (1974) 593–602.

[41] N. Tanaka, K. Abe, S. Miyakawa, S. Ohnami, M. Tanaka, T. Takeuchi, Analysis of human pituitary and tumor adrenocorticotropin using isoelectric focusing, J Clin Endocrinol Metab 48 (1979) 559–565.

[42] R.G. Allen, E. Orwoll, J.W. Kendall, E. Herbert, The distribution of forms of adrenocorticotropin and β-endorphin in normal, tumorous and autopsy human anterior pituitary tissues; virtual absence of 13K adrenocorticotropin, J Clin Endocrinol Metab 51 (1980) 376–380.

[43] K. Tanaka, W.E. Nicholson, D.N. Orth, The nature of immunoreactive lipotropins in human plasma and tissue extracts, J Clin Invest 62 (1978) 94–104.

[44] D.N. Orth, W.E. Nicholson, High molecular weight forms of human ACTH are glycoproteins, J Clin Endocrinol Metab 44 (1977) 214–217.

[45] A.F. Bradbury, M.D.A. Finnie, D.G. Smyth, Mechanism of C-terminal amide formation by pituitary enzymes, Nature 298 (1982) 686–688.

[46] B.A. Eipper, L. Park, H.T. Keutmann, R. Mains, Amidation of joining peptide, a major Pro-ACTH/Endorphin derived product peptide, J Biol Chem 261 (1986) 8686–8694.

[47] H.P. Bennent, C.A. Browne, S. Solomon, Biosynthesis of phosphorylated forms of corticotropin related peptides, Proc Nat Acad Sci USA 78 (1981) 4713–4717.

[48] B.A. Eipper, R.E. Mains, Phosphorylation of proadrenocorticotropin/endorphin derived peptides, J Biol Chem 257 (1982) 4907–4915.

[49] A.P. Scott, P.J. Lowry, J.G. Ratcliffe, L.H. Rees, J. Landon, Corticotropin-like peptides in the rat pituitary, J Endocrinol 61 (1974) 355–367.

[50] D.T. Krieger, The multiple faces of proopiomelanocortin, a prototype precursor molecule, Clin Res 31 (1983) 342–353.

[51] R.E. Silman, T. Chard, P.J. Lowry, I. Smith, I.M. Young, Human foetal pituitary peptides and parturition, Nature 260 (1976) 716–718.

[52] C.L. Chen, J.P. Mather, P.L. Morris, C.W. Bardin, Expression of proopiomelanocortin-like gene in the testis and epididymis, Proc Nat Acad Sci USA 81 (1984) 5672–5675.

[53] J.E. Pintar, B.S. Shacter, A.B. Herman, S. Durgerian, D.T. Krieger, Characterization and localization of proopiomelanocortin messenger RNA in the adult rat testis, Science 225 (1984) 632–634.

[54] L. Jeannotte, J.P.H. Burbach, J. Drouin, Unusual proopiomelanocortin ribonucleic acids in extrapituitary tissues; intronless transcripts in testes and long poly (A)+ tails in hypothalamus, Mol Endocrinol 1 (1987) 749–757.

[55] T. Lacaze-Masmonteil, Y. de Keyzer, J.P. Luton, A. Kahn, X. Bertagna, Characterization of proopiomelanocortin transcripts in human non-pituitary tissues, Proc Nat Acad Sci USA 84 (1987) 7261–7265.

[56] H. Jingami, S. Nakanishi, H. Imura, S. Numa, Tissue distribution of messenger RNAs coding for opioid peptide precursors and related RNA, Eur J Biochem 142 (1984) 441–447.

[57] C.R. De Bold, W.E. Nicholson, D.N. Orth, Immunoreactive proopiomelanocortin (POMC) peptides and POMC-like messenger ribonucleic acid are present in many rat nonpituitary tissues, Endocrinology 122 (1988) 2648–2657.

[58] A.J.L. Clark, P.M. Lavender, P. Coates, M.R. Johnson, L.H. Rees, In vitro and in vivo analysis of the processing and fate of the peptide products of the short proopiomelanocortin mRNA, Mol Endocrinol 4 (1990) 1737–1743.

[59] R. Buzetti, L. Mc Loughlin, P.M. Lavender, A.J.L. Clark, L.H. Rees, Expression of proopiomelanocortin gene and quantification of adrenocorticotrophic hormone-like immunoreactivity in human normal peripheral mononuclear cells and lymphoid and myeloid malignancies, J Clin Invest 83 (1989) 733–737.

[60] Y. De Keyzer, X. Bertagna, F. Lenne, F. Girard, J.P. Luton, A. Kahn, Altered proopiomelanocortin gene expression in ACTH producing nonpituitary tumors, J Clin Invest 76 (1985) 1892–1898.

[61] D. Vieau, J.F. Massias, F. Girard, J.P. Luton, X. Bertagna, Corticotrophin-like intermediary lobe peptide as a marker of alternate proopiomelanocortin processing in ACTH-producing nonpituitary tumours, Clin Endocrinol 31 (1989) 691–700.

[62] S.J. Ratter, G. Gillies, H. Hope, et al., Pro-opiocortin related peptides in human pituitary and ectopic ACTH secreting tumors, Clin Endocrinol 18 (1983) 211–218.

[63] M.L. Raffin-Sanson, J.F. Massias, C. Dumont, M.C. Raux-Demay, M.F. Proeschel, J.P. Luton, et al., High plasma proopiomelanocortin in aggressive adrenocorticotropin-secreting tumors, J Clin Endocrinol Metab 81 (12) (1996) 4272–4277.

[64] S.A. Berson, R.S. Yalow, Radioimmunoassay of ACTH in plasma, J Clin Invest 47 (1968) 2725–2751.

[65] D.T. Krieger, W. Allen, Relationship of bioassayable and immunoassayable plasma ACTH and cortisol concentrations in normal subjects and in patients with Cushing's disease, J Clin Endocrinol Metab 10 (1975) 675–687.

[66] J.H. Liu, R.R. Kazer, D.D. Rasmussen, Characterization of the twenty-four hour secretion patterns of adrenocorticotropin and cortisol in normal women and patients with Cushing's disease, J Clin Endocrinol Metab 64 (1987) 1027–1035.

[67] J.D. Veldhuis, A. Iranmanesh, M.K. Johnson, G. Lizarralde, Amplitude, but not frequency, modulation of adrenocorticotropin secretory bursts gives rise to the nyctohemeral rhythm of the corticotropic axis in man, J Clin Endocrinol Metab 71 (1990) 452–463.

[68] A. Iranmanesh, G. Lizarralde, D. Short, J.D. Veldhuis, Intensive venous sampling paradigms disclose high frequency adrenocorticotropin release episodes in normal men, J Clin Endocrinol Metab 71 (1990) 1276–1283.

[69] D.T. Krieger, W. Allen, F. Rizzo, H.P. Krieger, Characterization of the normal temporal pattern of plasma corticosteroids levels. Circadian adrenal periodicity, J Clin Endocrinol Metab 32 (1971) 266–284.

[70] C. Rivier, J. Rivier, W. Vale, Inhibition of adrenocorticotropic hormone secretion in the rat by immunoneutralization of corticotropin-releasing factor, Science 218 (1982) 377–379.

[71] W. Vale, J. Spiess, C. Rivier, J. Rivier, Characterization of a 41-residue ovine hypothalamic peptide that stimulates secretion of corticotropin and β-endorphin, Science 213 (1981) 1394–1397.

[72] F. Labrie, R. Veilleux, G. Lefevre, D.H. Coy, J. Sueiras-Diaz, A.V. Schally, Corticotropin-releasing factor stimulates accumulation of adenosine 3′,5′ monophosphate in rat pituitary corticotrophs, Science 216 (1982) 1007–1008.

[73] G. Aguilera, J.P. Harwood, J.X. Wilson, J. Morell, J.H. Brown, K.J. Catt, Mechanisms of action of corticotropin-releasing factor and other regulators of corticotropin release in the rat pituitary cells, J Biol Chem 258 (1983) 8039–8045.

[74] P. Carvalho, G. Aguilera, Protein kinase C mediates the effect of vasopressin in pituitary corticotrophs, Mol Endocrinol 3 (1989) 1935–1943.

[75] G.E. Gillies, E.A. Linton, P.J. Lowry, Corticotropin releasing activity of the new CRF is potentiated several times by vasopressin, Nature 299 (1982) 355–357.

[76] A.B. Abou-Samra, J.P. Harwood, V.C. Manganiello, K.J. Catt, G. Aguilera, Phorbol 12-myristate 13-acetate and vasopressin potentiate the effect of corticotropin-releasing factor on cyclic AMP production in rat anterior pituitary cells, J Biol Chem 262 (1987) 1129–1136.

[77] Y. Oki, W.E. Nicholson, D.N. Orth, Role of protein kinase-C in the adrenocorticotropin secretory response to arginine vasopressin (AVP) and the synergistic response to AVP and corticotropin-releasing factor by perifused rat anterior pituitary cells, Endocrinology 127 (1990) 350–357.

[78] V. Giguere, F. Labrie, Vasopressin potentiates cyclic AMP accumulation and ACTH release induced by corticotropin-releasing factor (CRF) in rat anterior pituitary cells in culture, Endocrinology 111 (1982) 1752–1754.

[79] H.U. Affolter, T. Reisine, Corticotropin releasing factor increases proopiomelanocortin messenger RNA in mouse anterior pituitary tumor cells, J Biol Chem 260 (1985) 15477–15481.

[80] J.P. Gagner, J. Drouin, Opposite regulation of pro-opiomelanocortin gene transcription by glucocorticoids and CRH, Mol Cell Endocrinol 40 (1985) 25–32.

[81] T.O. Bruhn, R.E. Sutton, C. Rivier, W. Vale, Corticotropin releasing factor regulates proopiomelanocortin messenger RNA levels in vivo, Neuroendocrinology 39 (1984) 170–175.

[82] C.R. De Bold, W.R. Sheldon, G.S. De Cherney, et al., Arginine vasopressin potentiates adrenocorticotropin release induced by ovine corticotropin releasing factor, J Clin Invest 73 (1984) 533–538.

[83] S.W.J. Lamberts, T. Verleun, R. Oosterom, F. de Jong, W.H.L. Hackeng, Corticotropin releasing factor (ovine) and vasopressin exert a synergistic effect on adrenocorticotropin release in man, J Clin Endocrinol Metab 58 (1984) 298–303.

[84] J.H. Liu, K. Muse, P. Contrepas, et al., Augmentation of ACTH-releasing activity of synthetic corticotropin releasing factor by vasopressin in women, J Clin Endocrinol Metab 57 (1983) 1087–1089.

[85] Y. de Keyzer, F. Lenne, C. Auzan, et al., The pituitary V3 vasopressin receptor and the corticotroph phenotype in ectopic ACTH syndrome, J Clin Invest 97 (1996) 1311–1318.

[86] Y. de Keyzer, C. Auzan, F. Lenne, C. Beldjord, M. Thibonnier, X. Bertagna, et al., Cloning and characterization of the human V3 pituitary vasopressin receptor, FEBS Lett 356 (2–3) (1994) 215–220.

[87] P. René, Y. de Keyzer, The vasopressin receptor of corticotroph pituitary cells, Prog Brain Res 139 (2002) 345–357.

[88] G.W. Liddle, D. Osland, C.K. Meador, Normal and abnormal regulation of corticotropin secretion in man, Recent Prog Horm Res 18 (1962) 125–166.

[89] H. Jingami, S. Matsukura, S. Numa, H. Imura, Effects of adrenalectomy and dexamethasone administration on the level of preprocorticotropin-releasing factor messenger ribonucleic acid (mRNA) in the hypothalamus and adrenocorticotropin/beta-lipotropin precursor mRNA in the pituitary in rats, Endocrinology 117 (1985) 1314–1320.

[90] W. Vale, J. Vaughan, M. Smith, G. Yamamoto, J. Rivier, C. Rivier, Effects of synthetic ovine corticotropin-releasing factor, glucocorticoids, catecholamines, neuro-hypophysial peptides, and other substances on cultured corticotropic cells, Endocrinology 113 (1983) 1121–1131.

[91] L.M. Bilezikjian, W.W. Vale, Glucocorticoids inhibit corticotropin-releasing factor-induced production of adenosine 3′,5′-monophosphate in cultured anterior pituitary cells, Endocrinology 113 (1983) 657–662.

[92] J.L. Roberts, C.L.C. Chen, J.H. Eberwine, et al., Glucocorticoid regulation of proopiomelanocortin gene expression in rodent pituitary, Recent Prog Horm Res 38 (1982) 227–256.

[93] J.H. Eberwine, J.L. Roberts, Glucocorticoid regulation of proopiomelanocortin gene transcription in the rat pituitary, J Biol Chem 259 (1984) 2166–2170.

[94] A. Bateman, A. Singh, T. Kral, S. Solomon, The immune-hypothalamic—pituitary—adrenal axis, Endocr Rev 10 (1989) 92–112.

[95] F. Berkenbosch, J. Van Oers, A. Del Rey, F. Tilders, H. Besedovsky, Corticotropin releasing factor producing neurons in the rat activated by interleukin 1, Science 238 (1987) 524–526.

[96] Y. Naitoh, J. Fukata, T. Tominaga, et al., Interleukin-6 stimulates the secretion of adrenocorticotropic hormone in conscious freely moving rats, Biochem Biophys Res Commun 155 (1988) 1459–1463.

[97] B.L. Spangelo, A.M. Judd, P.C. Isakson, R.M. MacLeod, Interleukin-6 stimulates anterior pituitary hormone release in vitro, Endocrinology 125 (1989) 575–577.

[98] J.I. Koenig, K. Snow, B.D. Clark, et al., Intrinsic pituitary interleukin-1 β is induced by bacterial lipopolysaccharide, Endocrinology 126 (1990) 3053–3058.

[99] H. Vankelecom, P. Carmeliet, J. Van Damme, A. Billiau, C. Denef, Production of interleukin-6 by folliculo-stellate cells in the anterior pituitary gland in a hystiotypic cell aggregate culture system, Neuroendocrinology 49 (1989) 102–106.

[100]. S. Melmed, gp130-Related cytokines and their receptors in the pituitary, Trends Endocrinol Metab 8 (10) (1997) 391–397.

[101] H. Houben, C. Denef, Regulatory peptides produced in the anterior pituitary, Trends Endocrinol Metab 1 (1990) 398–402.

[102] W.B. Malarkey, B.J. Zvara, Interleukin-1 beta and other cytokines stimulate adrenocorticotropin release from cultured pituitary cells of patients with Cushing's disease, J Clin Endocrinol Metab 69 (1989) 196–199.

[103] E. Arzt, G. Stelzer, U. Renner, M. Lange, O.A. Muller, G.K. Stalla, Interleukin-2 and interleukin-2 receptor expression in human corticotrophic adenoma and murine pituitary cultures, J Clin Invest 90 (1992) 1944–1951.

[104] A.P. Heaney, M. Fernando, W.H. Yong, S. Melmed, Functional PPAR-gamma receptor is a novel therapeutic target for ACTH-secreting pituitary adenomas, Nat Med 8 (11) (2002) 1281–1287.

[105] M. Páez-Pereda, D. Kovalovsky, U. Hopfner, M. Theodoropoulou, U. Pagotto, E. Uhl, et al., Retinoic acid prevents experimental Cushing syndrome, J Clin Invest 108 (8) (2001) 1123–1131.

[106] H. Cushing, The basophil adenomas of the pituitary body and their clinical manifestations, Bull Johns Hopkins Hosp 50 (1932) 137–195.

[107] H.S. Lipscomb, D.H. Nelson, A sensitive biologic assay for ACTH, Endocrinology 71 (1962) 13–23.

[108] W.C. Williams, D. Island, R.A.A. Oldfield, W. Grant, Blood corticotropin (ACTH) levels in Cushing's disease, J Clin Endocrinol Metab 21 (1961) 426–432.

[109] D.H. Nelson, J.G. Sprunt, R.B. Mims, Plasma ACTH determinations in 58 patients before or after adrenalectomy for Cushing's syndrome, J Clin Endocrinol Metab 26 (1966) 722–728.

[110] R. Ney, N. Shimizu, W.E. Nicholson, D.P. Island, G.W. Liddle, Correlation of plasma ACTH concentration with adrenocortical response in normal human subjects, surgical patients, and patients with Cushing's disease, J Clin Invest 42 (1963) 1669–1677.

[111] M.C. Raux, M. Binoux, J.P. Luton, M.T. Pham Huu Trung, F. Girard, Studies of ACTH secretion control in 116 cases of Cushing's syndrome, J Clin Endocrinol Metab 40 (1975) 186–197.

[112] G.M. Besser, J. Landon, Plasma levels of immunoreactive corticotrophin in patients with Cushing's syndrome, Br Med J 4 (1968) 552–554.

[113] J.M. Kuhn, M.F. Proeschel, D. Seurin, X. Bertagna, J.P. Luton, F. Girard, Comparative assessment of ACTH and lipotropin plasma levels in the diagnosis and follow-up of patients with Cushing's syndrome: A study of 210 cases, Am J Med 86 (1989) 678–684.

[114] D.M. Cook, J.W. Kendall, J.P. Allen, Nyctohemeral variation and suppressibility of plasma ACTH in various stages of Cushing's disease, Clin Endocrinol 5 (1976) 303–312.

[115] K. Pirich, J. Vierhapper, 24-hour serum concentration profile of cortisol in patients with Cushing's disease, Exp Clin Endocrinol 92 (1988) 275–279.

[116] Z. Zadik, L. De Lacerda, A.A.H. De Carmargo, B.P. Hamilton, C.J. Migeon, A.A. Kowarski, A comparative study of urinary 17-hydroxy-corticosteroids, urinary free cortisol, and the integrated concentration of plasma cortisol, J Clin Endocrinol Metab 51 (1980) 1099–1101.

[117] J.M. Kuhn, D. Seurin, X. Bertagna, R. Hadjiat, P. Thieblot, F. Girard, Les lipotropines (β- et γ-LPH) marqueurs fiables de la fonction corticotrope, Ann Endocrinol 45 (1984) 369–374.

[118] H. Vetter, R. Strass, J.M. Bayer, Short-term fluctuations in plasma cortisol in Cushing's syndrome, Clin Endocrinol 6 (1977) 1–4.

[119] L. Hellman, E.D. Weitzman, H. Roffwarg, D.K. Fukishima, K. Yoshida, T.F. Gallagher, Cortisol is secreted episodically in Cushing's syndrome, J Clin Endocrinol Metab 30 (1970) 686–689.

[120] P. Sederberg-Olsen, C. Binder, H. Kehlet, A.M. Neville, L.M. Nielsen, Episodic variation in plasma corticosteroids in subjects with Cushing's syndrome of differing etiology, J Clin Endocrinol Metab 36 (1973) 906–910.
[121] K. Von Werder, R.P. Smilo, S. Hane, P.H. Forsham, Pituitary response to stress in Cushing's disease, Acta Endocrinol 67 (1971) 127–140.
[122] G.M. Besser, C.R.W. Edwards, Cushing's syndrome, in: A.S. Mason (Ed.), Clinics in Endocrinology and Metabolism, WB Saunders, London, 1972, pp. 451–490.
[123] G.W. Liddle, Tests of pituitary—adrenal suppressibility in the diagnosis of Cushing's syndrome, J Clin Endocrinol Metab 20 (1960) 1539–1560.
[124] D.N. Orth, C.R. De Bold, G.S. De Cherney, et al., Pituitary microadenomas causing Cushing's disease respond to corticotrophin-releasing factor, J Clin Endocrinol Metab 55 (1982) 1017–1019.
[125] G.F.F.M. Pieters, A.R.M.M. Hermus, A.G.H. Smals, A.K.M. Bartelink, T.J. Benraad, P.W.C. Kloppenborg, Responsiveness of the hypophyseal—adrenocortical axis to corticotropin releasing factor in pituitary-dependent Cushing's disease, J Clin Endocrinol Metab 57 (1983) 513–516.
[126] H. Bricaire, J.P. Luton, La physiopathologie du syndrome de Cushing, Acta Clin Belgica 24 (1969) 131–148.
[127] J.B. Tyrrell, R.M. Brooks, P.A. Fitzgeral, P.B. Cofoid, P.H. Forsham, C.W. Wilson, Cushing's disease: Selective transsphenoidal resection of pituitary adenomas, N Engl J Med 298 (1978) 753–758.
[128] R.M. Salassa, E.R. Laws, P.C. Carpenter, R.C. Northcutt, Transsphenoidal removal of pituitary microadenoma in Cushing's disease, Mayo Clin Proc 53 (1978) 24–28.
[129] B. Guilhaume, X. Bertagna, M. Thomsen, et al., Transsphenoidal pituitary surgery for the treatment of Cushing's disease: Results in 64 patients and long term follow-up studies, J Clin Endocrinol Metab 66 (1988) 1056–1064.
[130] T.J. Mampalam, J.B. Tyrrell, C.B. Wilson, Transsphenoidal microsurgery for Cushing's disease: A report of 216 cases, Ann Intern Med 109 (1988) 487–493.
[131] P.C. Carpenter, Cushing's syndrome: Update of diagnosis and management, Mayo Clin Proc 61 (1986) 49–58.
[132] D.K. Ludecke, Present status of surgical treatment of ACTH-secreting pituitary adenomas in Cushing's disease, in: S.W.J. Lamberts, F.J.H. Tilders, E.A. Van DerVeen, J. Assies (Eds.), Trends in Diagnosis and Treatment of Pituitary Adenomas, Free University Press, Amsterdam, 1984, pp. 315–323.
[133] J. Hardy, Cushing's disease — 50 years later, Can J Neurol Sci 9 (1982) 375–381.
[134] R. Fahlbusch, M. Bushfelder, O.A. Muller, Transsphenoidal surgery for Cushing's disease, J R Soc Med 79 (1986) 262–269.
[135] T. Nakane, A. Kuwayama, M. Watanabe, et al., Long term results of transsphenoidal adenomectomy in patients with Cushing's disease, Neurosurgery 21 (1987) 218–222.
[136]. D.T. Krieger, Physiopathology of Cushing's disease, Endocr Rev 4 (1983) 22–43.
[137] F. Robert, G. Pelletier, J. Hardy, Pituitary adenomas in Cushing's disease, Arch Pathol Lab Med 102 (1978) 448–455.
[138] D.E. Schteingart, W.F. Chandler, R.V. Lloyd, G. Ibarra-Perez, Cushing's syndrome caused by an ectopic pituitary adenoma, Neurosurgery 21 (1987) 223–227.
[139] J. Kammer, R. George, Cushing's disease in a patient with an ectopic pituitary adenoma, JAMA 246 (1981) 2722–2724.
[140] J. Duoskova, Z. Putz, An intracranial tumor in an unusual location associated with Cushing's syndrome, Cesk Patol 21 (1985) 113–117.
[141] W.M. Burch, R.S. Kramer, P.D. Kenan, C.B. Hammond, Cushing's disease caused by an ectopic pituitary adenoma within the sphenoid sinus, N Engl J Med 312 (1985) 587–588.
[142] C.A. Axiotis, H.A. Lippes, M.J. Merino, N.C. DeLanerolle, A.F. Stewart, B. Kinder, Corticotroph cell pituitary adenoma within an ovarian teratoma. A new cause of Cushing's syndrome, Am J Surg Pathol 11 (1987) 218–224.
[143] L. Olivier, E. Vila-Porcile, M.P. Dubois, J. Racadot, F. Peillon, Histological and cytological aspects of pituitary adenomas in Cushing's disease, in: P.J. Derome, C.P. Jedynak, F. Peillon (Eds.), Pituitary Adenomas, Biology, Physiopathology and Treatment, Asclepios Publishers, France, 1980, pp. 19–32.
[144] L. Olivier, E. Vila-Porcile, F. Peillon, J. Racadot, Etude en microscopie electronique des grains de secrétion basophiles dans les cellules hypophysaires tumorales de la maladie de Cushing, C R Soc Biol 166 (1972) 1591–1600.
[145] A.C. Crooke, A change in the basophil cells of the pituitary gland common to conditions which exhibit the syndrome attributed to basophil adenoma, J Path Bact 41 (1935) 339–349.
[146] E. Porcile, J. Racadot, Ultrastructure des cellules de Crooke observées dans l'hypophyse humaine au cours de la maladie de Cushing, C R Acad Sci 263 (1966) 948–951.
[147] R.F. Phifer, S.S. Spicer, D.N. Orth, Specific demonstrations of the human hypophyseal cells which produce adrenocorticotrophic hormone, J Clin Endocrinol Metab 31 (1970) 347–361.
[148] J. Trouillas, C. Girod, G. Sassolas, et al., A human β-endorphin pituitary adenoma, J Clin Endocrinol Metab 58 (1984) 242–249.
[149] S.W.J. Lamberts, S.Z. Stefanko, S. De Lange, et al., Failure of clinical remission after transsphenoidal removal of a microadenoma in a patient with Cushing's disease; multiple hyperplastic and adenomatous cell nests in surrounding pituitary tissue, J Clin Endocrinol Metab 50 (1980) 793–798.
[150] D. Ludecke, R. Kautzky, W. Saeger, D. Schrader, Selective removal of hypersecreting pituitary adenomas, Acta Neurochir 35 (1976) 27–42.
[151] W. Saeger, D.L. Ludecke, F. Geisler, The anterior lobe in Cushing's disease/syndrome, in: D.L. Ludecke, G.P. Chrousos, G. Tolis (Eds.), ACTH, Cushing's Syndrome, and Other Hypercortisolemic States., Raven Press, New York, 1990, pp. 147–156.
[152] D.M. Cook, P.J. McCarthy, Failure of hypophysectomy to correct pituitary-dependent Cushing's disease in two patients, Arch Intern Med 148 (1988) 2497–2500.
[153] W. Saeger, D.K. Ludecke, Pituitary hyperplasia. Definition, light and electron microscopical structures and significance in surgical specimens, Virchows Arch 399 (1983) 277–287.
[154] R. Martin, Y. Cetin, G.L. Fehm, R. Fahlbusch, K.H. Voigt, Multiple cellular forms of corticotrophs in surgically removed pituitary adenomas and periadenomatous tissue in Cushing's disease, Am J Pathol 106 (1982) 332–341.
[155] M.E. Molitch, Pathogenesis of pituitary tumors, Endocrinol Metab Clin North Am 16 (1987) 503–527.
[156] T. Suda, H. Demura, R. Demura, K. Jibiki, F. Tozawa, K. Shizume, Anterior pituitary hormones in plasma and pituitaries from patients with Cushing's disease, J Clin Endocrinol Metab 51 (1980) 1048–1053.
[157] T. Suda, Y. Abe, H. Demura, et al., ACTH, β LPH and β endorphin in pituitary adenomas of the patients with Cushing's disease: activation of β-LPH conversion to β-endorphin, J Clin Endocrinol Metab 49 (1979) 475–477.
[158] P.A. Fitzgerald, D.C. Aron, J.W. Findling, et al., Cushing's disease: Transient secondary adrenal insufficiency after selective removal of pituitary microadenomas: Evidence for a pituitary origin, J Clin Endocrinol Metab 54 (1982) 413–422.

[159] A.M. Schnall, J.S. Brodkey, B. Kaufman, O.H. Pearson, Pituitary function after removal of pituitary microadenomas in Cushing's disease, J Clin Endocrinol Metab 47 (1978) 410–417.

[160] P.C. Avgerinos, G.P. Chrousos, L.K. Nieman, E.H. Oldfield, D.L. Loriaux, G.B. Cutler Jr., The corticotropin releasing hormone test in the post-operative evaluation of patients with Cushing's syndrome, J Clin Endocrinol Metab 65 (1987) 906–913.

[161] A. Kuwayama, N. Kageyama, T. Nakane, M. Watanabe, N. Kanie, Anterior pituitary function after transsphenoidal selective adenomectomy in patients with Cushing's disease, J Clin Endocrinol Metab 53 (1981) 163–172.

[162] S.W.J. Lamberts, J.G.M. Klijn, F.H. de Jong, The recovery of the hypothalamo—pituitary—adrenal axis after transsphenoidal operation in three patients with Cushing's disease, Acta Endocrinol 98 (1981) 580–585.

[163] R.M. Boyer, M. Witkin, A. Carruth, J. Ramsey, Circadian cortisol rhythms in Cushing's disease, J Clin Endocrinol Metab 48 (1979) 760–765.

[164] T. Suda, F. Tozawa, M. Yamada, et al., Effects of corticotropin-releasing hormone and dexamethasone on proopiomelanocortin messenger RNA level in human corticotroph adenoma cells in vitro, J Clin Invest 82 (1988) 110–114.

[165] A.J.L. Clark, P.M. Lavender, G.M. Besser, L.H. Rees, Pro-opiomelanocortin mRNA size heterogeneity in ACTH-dependent Cushing's syndrome, J Mol Endocrinol 2 (1988) 3–9.

[166] T. Nayaya, H. Seo, A. Kuwayama, et al., Pro-opiomelanocortin gene expression in silent corticotroph-cell adenoma and Cushing's disease, J Neurosurg 72 (1990) 262–267.

[167] Y. De Keyzer, X. Bertagna, J.P. Luton, A. Kahn, Variable modes of proopiomelanocortin gene transcription in human tumors, Mol Endocrinol 3 (1989) 215–223.

[168] X. Bertagna, D. Seurin, L. Pique, J.P. Luton, H. Bricaire, F. Girard, Peptides related to the NH_2 terminal end of proopiocortin in man, J Clin Endocrinol Metab 56 (1983) 489–495.

[169] T. Shibasaki, H. Masui, G. Sato, N. Ling, R. Guillemin, Secretion pattern of pro-opiomelanocortin-derived peptides by a pituitary adenoma from a patient with Cushing's disease, J Clin Endocrinol Metab 52 (1981) 350–353.

[170] X. Bertagna, J.P. Luton, M. Binoux, H. Bricaire, F. Girard, Characterization of lipotropin-, corticotropin-, and β-endorphin-immunoreactive materials secreted in vitro by a human pituitary adenoma responsible for a case of Nelson's syndrome, J Clin Endocrinol Metab 49 (1979) 527–532.

[171] H. Raff, J.W. Findling, A new immunoradiometric assay for corticotropin evaluated in normal subjects and patients with Cushing's syndrome, Clin Chem 35 (1989) 596–600.

[172] P.J. Fuller, A.T.W. Lim, J.W. Barlow, et al., A pituitary tumor producing high molecular weight adrenocorticotropin-related peptides: Clinical and cell culture studies, J Clin Endocrinol Metab 58 (1984) 134–142.

[173] M. Reincke, B. Allolio, W. Saeger, D. Kaulen, W. Winkelmann, A pituitary adenoma secreting high molecular weight adrenocorticotropin without evidence of Cushing's disease, J Clin Endocrinol Metab 65 (1987) 1296–1300.

[174] A.C. Hale, J.B. Millar, S.J. Ratter, J.D. Pickard, I. Doniach, L.H. Rees, A case of pituitary dependent Cushing's disease with clinical and biochemical features of the ectopic ACTH syndrome, Clin Endocrinol 22 (1985) 479–488.

[175] X. Bertagna, W.J. Stone, W.E. Nicholson, C.D. Mount, D.N. Orth, Simultaneous assay of immunoreactive β-lipotropin, gamma-lipotropin, and β-endorphin in plasma of normal human subjects, patients with ACTH/LPH hypersecretory syndromes, and patients undergoing chronic hemodialysis, J Clin Invest 67 (1981) 124–133.

[176] E.M. Brown, M.S. Le Boff, M. Detting, J.T. Posillico, C. Chen, Secretory control in normal and abnormal parathyroid tissue, Recent Prog Horm Res 43 (1987) 337–382.

[177] A.R. Wolfsen, W.D. Odell, The dose-response relationship of ACTH and cortisol in Cushing's disease, Clin Endocrinol 12 (1980) 557–568.

[178] E.M. Pardes, J.W. de Yampey, R.J. Soto, D.F. Moses, A.F. De Nicola, A correlative study between glucocorticoid receptor levels in human mononuclear leukocytes and biochemical data in Cushing's disease, Acta Endocrinol 120 (1989) 55–61.

[179] K. Kontula, R. Pelkonen, L. Andersson, A. Sivula, Glucocorticoid receptors in adrenocorticoid disorders, J Clin Endocrinol Metab 51 (1980) 654–657.

[180] M. Grino, F. Boudouresque, B. Conte-Devolx, et al., In vitro corticotropin-releasing hormone (CRH) stimulation of adrenocorticotropin release from corticotroph adenoma cells: Effect of prolonged exposure to CRH and its interaction with cortisol, J Clin Endocrinol Metab 66 (1988) 770–775.

[181] R. Oosterom, T. Verleun, P. Vitterlinden, et al., ACTH and β-endorphin secretion by three corticotropic adenomas in culture. Effect of culture time, dexamethasone, vasopressin and synthetic corticotropin-releasing factor, Acta Endocrinol 106 (1984) 21–29.

[182] T. Suda, N. Tomori, F. Tozawa, H. Demura, K. Shizume, Effects of corticotropin-releasing factor and other materials on adrenocorticotropin secretion from pituitary glands of patients with Cushing's disease in vitro, J Clin Endocrinol Metab 59 (1984) 840–845.

[183] M.C. White, E.F. Adams, M. Loizou, K. Mashiter, R. Fahlbush, Ovine corticotropin-releasing factor stimulates ACTH release from human corticotrophinoma cells in culture: Interaction with hydrocortisone and arginine vasopressin, Clin Endocrinol 23 (1985) 295–302.

[184] K. Mashiter, E.F. Adams, G. Gillies, S. Van Noorden, S. Ratter, Adrenocorticotropin and lipotropin secretion by dispersed cell cultures of a human corticotropic adenoma: Effect of hypothalamic extract, arginine vasopressin, hydrocortisone and serotonin, J Clin Endocrinol Metab 51 (1980) 566–572.

[185] G. Gillies, S. Ratter, A. Grossman, et al., Secretion of ACTH, LPH, and β-endorphin from human pituitary tumors in vitro, Clin Endocrinol 13 (1980) 197–205.

[186] S.W.J. Lamberts, E.G. Bons, P. Vitterlinden, Studies on the glucocorticoid-receptor blocking action of RU 38486 in cultured ACTH-secreting human pituitary tumour cells and normal rat pituitary cells, Acta Endocrinol 109 (1985) 64–69.

[187] L. Lane, E. Oldfield, D. Brandon, Normal human glucocorticoid receptor gene in pituitary adenomas. The Endocrine Society, 71st Annual Meeting, Seattle, 1989 366, Abstract 1374.

[188] N.A. Huizenga, P. de Lange, J.W. Koper, R.N. Clayton, W.E. Farrell, A.J. van der Lely, et al., Human adrenocorticotropin-secreting pituitary adenomas show frequent loss of heterozygosity at the glucocorticoid receptor gene locus, J Clin Endocrinol Metab 83 (3) (1998) 917–921.

[189] D.M. Hurley, D. Accili, C.A. Stratakis, et al., Point mutation causing a single aminoacid substitution in the hormone binding domain of the glucocorticoid receptor in familial glucocorticoid resistance, J Clin Invest 87 (1991) 680–686.

[190] M. Qi, B.J. Hamilton, D. DeFranco, v-Mos oncoproteins affect the nuclear retention and reutilization of glucocorticoid receptors, Mol Endocrinol 3 (1989) 1279–1288.

[191] R. Jaggi, B. Salmons, D. Muellener, B. Groner, The v-Mos and Ha-ras oncogene expression represses glucocorticoid hormone-dependent transcription from the mouse mammary tumour virus LTR, EMBO J 5 (1986) 2609–2616.

[192] A. Kahn, Effets antiprolifératif et anti-inflammatoire des glucocorticoides par inhibition des complexes Jun-Fos, Medecine/Sciences 6 (1990) 1003–1005.

[193] H.F. Yan-Yen, J.C. Chambard, Y.L. Sun, et al., Transcriptional interference between c-Jun and glucocorticoid receptor: Mutual inhibition of DNA binding due to direct protein—protein interaction, Cell 62 (1990) 1205–1215.

[194] L.M. Bilezikjian, A.L. Blount, W.W. Vale, The cellular actions of vasopressin on corticotrophs of the anterior pituitary: Resistance to glucocorticoid action, Mol Endocrinol 1 (1987) 451–458.

[195] K.E. Sheppard, J.L. Roberts, M. Blum, Down regulation of glucocorticoid receptor by CRF in AtT20 cells is via an adenylate cyclase dependent mechanism. The Endocrine Society, 72nd Annual Meeting, Atlanta, 1990 222, Abstract 790.

[196] L. Vallar, A. Spada, G. Giannattasio, Altered G and adenylate cyclase activity in human GH-secreting pituitary adenomas, Nature 330 (1987) 566–568.

[197] C.A. Landis, S.B. Masters, A. Spada, A.M. Pace, H.R. Bourne, L. Vallar, GTPase inhibiting mutations activate the alpha chain of G and stimulate adenylyl cyclase in human pituitary tumours, Nature 340 (1989) 692–696.

[198] J. Lyons, C.A. Landis, G. Harsh, Two G protein oncogenes in human endocrine tumors, Science 249 (1990) 655–659.

[199] J. Bertherat, A. Horvath, L. Groussin, S. Grabar, S. Boikos, L. Cazabat, et al., Mutations in regulatory subunit type 1A of cyclic adenosine 5′-monophosphate-dependent protein kinase (PRKAR1A): Phenotype analysis in 353 patients and 80 different genotypes, J Clin Endocrinol Metab 94 (6) (2009) 2085–2091.

[200] G.F.F.M. Pieters, A.G.H. Smals, T.J. Benraad, P.W.C. Kloppenborg, Plasma cortisol response to thyrotropin-releasing hormone and luteinizing hormone-releasing hormone in Cushing's disease, J Clin Endocrinol Metab 48 (1979) 874–876.

[201] D.T. Krieger, M. Luria, Plasma ACTH and cortisol responses to TRF, vasopressin or hypoglycemia in Cushing's disease and Nelson's syndrome, J Clin Endocrinol Metab 44 (1977) 361–368.

[202] G.F.F.M. Pieters, A.G.H. Smals, H.J.M. Goverde, G.J. Pesman, E. Meyer, P.W.C. Kloppenborg, Adrenocorticotropin and cortisol responsiveness to thyrotropin-releasing hormone discloses two subsets of patients with Cushing's disease, J Clin Endocrinol Metab 55 (1982) 1188–1197.

[203] M. Ishibashi, T. Yamahi, Direct effects of thyrotropin-releasing hormone, cyproheptadine, and dopamine on adrenocorticotropin secretion from human corticotroph adenoma cells in vitro, J Clin Invest 68 (1981) 1018–1027.

[204] S. Oki, Y. Nakai, K. Nakao, H. Imura, Plasma β-endorphin responses to somatostatin, thyrotropin-releasing hormone, or vasopressin in Nelson's syndrome, J Clin Endocrinol Metab 50 (1980) 194–197.

[205] G. Vlotides, T. Eigler, S. Melmed, Pituitary tumor-transforming gene: Physiology and implications for tumorigenesis, Endocr Rev 28 (2) (2007) 165–186.

[206] T. Tateno, H. Izumiyama, M. Doi, T. Yoshimoto, M. Shichiri, N. Inoshita, et al., Differential gene expression in ACTH-secreting and non-functioning pituitary tumors, Eur J Endocrinol 157 (6) (2007) 717–724.

[207] B.W. Scheithauer, K. Kovacs, R.V. Randall, The pituitary gland in untreated Addison's disease: A histological and immunocytologic study of 18 adenohypophyses, Arch Pathol Lab Med 107 (1983) 484–487.

[208] R. Clayton, V. Schrieber, A.C. Burden, Secondary pituitary hyperplasia in Addison's disease, Lancet (1977) 954–956.

[209] B. Krautli, J. Muller, A.M. Landolt, F. Von Schulthess, ACTH producing pituitary adenoma in Addison's disease: Two cases treated by transsphenoidal microsurgery, Acta Endocrinol 99 (1982) 357–363.

[210] Y. Toshihiko, S. Kensaku, A. Masaaki, N. Hajime, K. Ken Ichi, I. Hiroschi, Probable ACTH secreting pituitary tumor in association with Addison's disease, Acta Endocrinol 110 (1985) 36–41.

[211] K.N. Westlund, G. Aguilera, G.V. Childs, Quantification of morphological changes in pituitary corticotropes produced by in vivo corticotropin-releasing factor stimulation and adrenalectomy, Endocrinology 116 (1985) 439–445.

[212] E.R. Siperstein, K.G. Miller, Hypertrophy of the ACTH-producing cell following adrenalectomy: A quantitative electron microscopic study, Endocrinology 93 (1973) 1257–1268.

[213] J. Resetic, Z. Reiner, D. Lüdecke, V. Riznar-Resetic, M. Sekso, The effects of cortisol, 11-epicortisol, and lysine vasopressin on DNA and RNA synthesis in isolated human adrenocorticotropic hormone-secreting pituitary tumor cells, Steroids 55 (1990) 98–100.

[214] N. Billestrup, R.L. Mitchell, W. Vale, I. Verma, Growth hormone-releasing factor induces c-fos expression in cultured primary pituitary cells, Mol Endocrinol 1 (1987) 300–305.

[215] B.J. Gertz, L.N. Contreras, D.J. McComb, K. Kovacs, J.B. Tyrrell, M.F. Dallman, Chronic administration of corticotropin releasing factor increases pituitary corticotroph number, Endocrinology 120 (1987) 381–388.

[216] M.J. Horacek, G.T. Campbell, C.A. Blake, Effects of corticotrophin-releasing hormone on corticotrophs in anterior pituitary gland allografts in hypophysectomized, orchidectomized hamsters, Cell Tissue Res 258 (1989) 65–68.

[217] O.A. Muller, H.G. Dorr, B. Hagen, G.K. Stalla, K. Von Werder, Corticotropin releasing factor stimulation test in normal controls and patients with disturbances of the hypothalamo—pituitary—adrenal axis, Klin Wochenschr 60 (1982) 1485–1491.

[218] G.P. Chrousos, J.M. Schulte, E.H. Oldfield, P.W. Gold, G.B. Cutler Jr., D.L. Loriaux, The corticotropin-releasing factor stimulation test. An aid in the evaluation of patients with Cushing's syndrome, N Engl J Med 310 (1984) 622–626.

[219] M. Binoux, M. Gourmelen-Combourieu, J.P. Luton, M.T. Pham Huu Trung, F. Girard, Etude de l'ACTH plasmatique au cours de 100 épreuves à la lysine vasopressme chez l'homme, Acta Endocrinol 68 (1971) 1–30.

[220] T. Suda, F. Tozawa, T. Mouri, et al., Effect of cyproheptadine, reserpine and synthetic corticotropin-releasing factor on pituitary glands from patients with Cushing's disease, J Clin Endocrinol Metab 56 (1983) 1094–1099.

[221] A. Spada, F. Reza-Elahi, A. Lania, M. Bassetti, E. Atti, Inhibition of basal and corticotropin-releasing hormone-stimulated adenylate cyclase activity and cytosolic Ca^{2+} levels by somatostatin in human corticotropin-secreting pituitary adenomas, J Clin Endocrinol Metab 70 (1990) 1262–1268.

[222] P. Mollard, P. Vacher, J. Guerin, M.A. Rogawski, B. Dufy, Electrical properties of cultured human adrenocorticotropin-secreting adenoma cells: Effects of high K^{+}, corticotropin-releasing factor and angiotensin II. Endocrinology 121 (1987) 395 405.

[223] P.L.M. Dahia, A.B. Grossman, The molecular pathogenesis of carticotroph tumors, Endoc Rev 20 (1999) 136–155.

[224] J.M. Alexander, B.M.K. Biller, H. Bikkal, A. Arnold, A. Klibanski, Clinically non-functioning pituitary tumors are monoclonal in origin, J Clin Invest 86 (1990) 336–340.

[225] V. Herman, J. Fagin, R. Gonsky, K. Kovacs, S. Melmed, Clonal origin of pituitary adenomas, J Clin Endocrinol Metab 71 (1990) 1427–1433.

[226] H.M. Schulte, E.H. Oldfield, B. Allolio, D.A. Katz, R.A. Berkman, I.U. Ali, Clonal composition of pituitary adenomas in patients with Cushing's disease: Determination by X-chromosome inactivation analysis, J Clin Endocrinol Metab 73 (1991) 1302–1308.

[227] C. Gicquel, Y. Le Bouc, J.P. Luton, F. Girard, X. Bertagna, Monoclonality of corticotroph macroadenomas in Cushing's disease, J Clin Endocrinol Metab 75 (1992) 472–475.

[228] B.M.K. Biller, J.M. Alexander, N.T. Zervas, E.T. Hedley-Whilte, A. Arnold, A. Klibanski, Clonal origins of adrenocorticotropin-secreting pituitary tissue in Cushing's disease, J Clin Endocrinol Metab 75 (1992) 1303–1309.

[229] J.L. Gabrilove, P.J. Anderson, N.S. Halmi, Pituitary proopiomelanocortin-cell carcinoma occurring in conjunction with a gliobastoma in a patient with Cushing's disease and subsequent Nelson's syndrome, Clin Endocrinol 25 (1986) 117–126.

[230] W. Forbes, Carcinoma of the pituitary gland with metastases to the liver in a case of Cushing's syndrome, J Path Bact 59 (1947) 137–144.

[231] R.M. Salassa, T.P. Kearns, J.W. Kernohan, R.G. Sprague, C.S. MacCarty, Pituitary tumors in patients with Cushing's syndrome, J Clin Endocrinol Metab 19 (1959) 1523–1529.

[232] T. Masuda, Y. Akasaka, Y. Ishikawa, et al., An ACTH-producing pituitary carcinoma developing Cushing's disease, Pathol Res Pract 195 (1999) 183–187.

[233] R.B. Welbourn, Survival and causes of death after adrenalectomy for Cushing's disease, Surgery 97 (1985) 16–20.

[234] S.H. Sherry, A.T. Guay, A.K. Lee, et al., Concurrent production of adrenocorticotropin and prolactin from two distinct cell lines in a single pituitary adenoma: A detailed immunohistochemical analysis, J Clin Endocrinol Metab 55 (1982) 947–955.

[235] G. Giannattasio, M. Bassetti, Human pituitary adenomas. Recent advances in morphological studies, J Endocrinol Invest 13 (1990) 435–454.

[236] J.F. Rehfeld, J. Lindholm, B.N. Anderson, et al., Pituitary tumors containing cholecystokinin, N Engl J Med 316 (1987) 1244–1247.

[237] J.H. Steel, S. Van Noorden, J. Ballesta, et al., Localization of 7B2, Neuromedin B and Neuromedin U in specific cell types of rat, mouse, and human pituitary in rat hypothalamus, and in 30 human pituitary and extrapituitary tumors, Endocrinology 122 (1988) 270–282.

[238] M.E. Vrontakis, T. Sano, K. Kovacs, H.G. Friesen, Presence of galanin-like immunoreactivity in nontumorous corticotrophs and corticotroph adenomas of the human pituitary, J Clin Endocrinol Metab 70 (1990) 747–751.

[239] L.J. Deftos, D.T. O'Connor, C.B. Wilson, P.A. Fitzgerald, Human pituitary tumors secrete chromogranin-A, J Clin Endocrinol Metab 68 (1989) 869–872.

[240] K. Sekiya, M.A. Ghatei, M.J. Salahuddin, et al., Production of GAWK (chromogranin B 420–493) like immunoreactivity by endocrine tumors and its possible diagnostic value, J Clin Invest 83 (1989) 1834–1842.

[241] D. Vieau, F. Lenne, J.P. Luton, X. Bertagna, Marqueurs de différenciation endocrine et secrétions ectopiques d'ACTH, Ann Endocrinol 50 (1989) 310 (Abstract).

[242] K. Tatemoto, S. Efendic, V. Mutt, G. Makk, G. Feistner, J. Barchas, Pancreastatin, a novel pancreatic peptide that inhibits insulin secretion, Nature 324 (1986) 476–478.

[243] B.H. Fasciotto, S.U. Gorr, D.J. DeFranco, M.A. Levine, D.V. Cohn, Pancreastatin, a presumed product of chromogranin-A (secretory protein-I) processing, inhibits secretion from porcine parathyroid cells in culture, Endocrinology 125 (1989) 1617–1622.

[244] G.S. Wand, D.T. O'Connor, M. Takiyynddin, M.A. Levine, A proposed role for chromogranin A as a glucocorticoid-responsive autocrine inhibitor of ACTH secretion, The Endocrine Society, 72nd Annual Meeting, Atlanta, 1990 789222 (Abstract).

[245] S.L. Asa, J. Henderson, D. Goltzman, D.J. Drucker, Parathyroid hormone-like peptide in normal and neoplastic human endocrine tissues, J Clin Endocrinol Metab 71 (1989) 1112–1118.

[246] J. Price, A.C. Nieuwenhuyzen Kruseman, I. Doniach, T.A. Howlett, G.M. Besser, L.H. Rees, Bombesin like peptides in human endocrine tumors: Quantitation, biochemical characterization, and secretion, J Clin Endocrinol Metab 60 (1985) 1097–1103.

[247] G. Tramu, J.C. Beauvillain, M. Mazzuca, P. Fossati, A. Martin-Linquette, J.L. Christiaens, Dissociation des résultats obtenus en immunofluoresce avec des antiserums anti-ACTH dans trois cas d'adénomes "chromophobe" sans hypercorticisme, Ann Endocrinol 37 (1976) 55–56.

[248] K. Kovacs, E. Horvath, T.A. Bayley, S.T. Hassaram, C. Ezrin, Silent corticotroph cell adenoma with lysosomal accumulation and crinophagy. A distinct clinicopathologic entity, Am J Med 64 (1978) 492–499.

[249] J. Hassoun, C. Charpin, P. Jaquet, J.C. Lissitzky, F. Grisoli, M. Toga, Corticolipotropin immunoreactivity in silent chromophobe adenomas: A light and electron microscopic study, Arch Pathol Lab Med 106 (1982) 25–30.

[250] E. Horvath, K. Kovacs, D.W. Killinger, H.S. Smyth, M.E. Platts, W. Singer, Silent corticotropic adenomas of the human pituitary gland: A histologic, immunocytologic and ultrastructural study, Am J Pathol 98 (1980) 617–638.

[251] E. Horvath, K. Kovacs, H.S. Smyth, et al., A novel type of pituitary adenoma: Morphological features and clinical correlations, J Clin Endocrinol Metab 66 (1988) 1111–1118.

[252] E.L. Gogel, P.R. Salber, J.B. Tyrrell, M.L. Rosenblum, J.W. Findling, Cushing's disease in a patient with a "non-functioning" pituitary tumor. Spontaneous development and remission, Arch Intern Med 143 (1983) 1040–1042.

[253] N.J.A. Vaughan, C.M. Laroche, I. Goodman, M.J. Davies, J.S. Jenkins, Pituitary Cushing's disease arising from a previously non-functional corticotrophin chromophobe adenoma, Clin Endocrinol 22 (1985) 147–153.

[254] M.E. Cooper, R.M.L. Murray, R. Kalnins, J. Woodward, G. Jerums, The development of Cushing's syndrome from a previously silent pituitary tumour, Aust NZ J Med 17 (1987) 249–251.

[255] P. Werner, Endocrine adenomatosis and peptic ulcer in a large kindred, Am J Med 35 (1963) 205–212.

[256] M.L. Brandi, S.J. Marx, G.D. Aurbach, L.A. Fitzpatrick, Familial multiple endocrine neoplasia type I: A new look at pathophysiology, Endocr Rev 8 (1987) 391–405.

[257] H.S. Ballard, B. Frame, R.J. Harstock, Familial multiple endocrine adenoma—peptide ulcer complex, Medicine 43 (1964) 481–516.

[258] P.N. Maton, J.D. Gardner, R.T. Jensen, Cushing's syndrome in patients with the Zollinger-Ellison syndrome, N Engl J Med 315 (1986) 1–5.

[259] D. Gaitan, P.T. Loosen, D.N. Orth, Two patients with Cushing's disease in a kindred with multiple endocrine neoplasia type I, J Clin Endocrinol Metab 76 (1993) 1580–1582.

[260] C. Larsson, B. Skogseid, K. Oberg, Y. Nakamura, M. Nordenshjold. Multiple endocrine neoplasia type I gene maps to chromosome 11 and is lost in insulinoma. Nature 198; 332: 85–87.

[261] C. Bystrom, C. Larsson, C. Blomberg, et al., Localization of the MEN 1 gene to a small region within chromosome 11q13 by deletion mapping in tumors, Proc Nat Acad Sci USA 87 (1990) 1968–1972.

[262] O. Vierimaa, M. Georgitsi, R. Lehtonen, P. Vahteristo, A. Kokko, A. Raitila, et al., Pituitary adenoma predisposition caused by germline mutations in the AIP gene, Science 312 (5777) (2006) 1228–1230.

[263] A.F. Daly, J.F. Vanbellinghen, S.K. Khoo, M.L. Jaffrain-Rea, L.A. Naves, M.A. Guitelman, et al., Aryl hydrocarbon receptor-interacting protein gene mutations in familial isolated pituitary adenomas: Analysis in 73 families, J Clin Endocrinol Metab 92 (5) (2007) 1891–1896.

[264] M.S. Elston, K.L. McDonald, R.J. Clifton-Bligh, B.G. Robinson, Familial pituitary tumor syndromes, Nat Rev Endocrinol 5 (8) (2009) 453–461.

[265] M.R. Celio, A. Pasi, E. Burgisser, G. Buetti, V. Hollt, C.H. Gramsch, Proopiocortin fragments in normal adult pituitary: Distribution and ultrastructural characterisation of immunoreactive cells, Acta Endocrinol 95 (1980) 27–40.

[266] M.E. Peterson, D.T. Krieger, W.D. Durcker, N.S. Halmi, Immunocytochemical study of the hypophysis in 25 dogs with pituitary-dependent hyperadrenocorticism, Acta Endocrinol 101 (1982) 15–24.

[267] J.N. Moore, J. Steiss, W.E. Nicholson, D.N. Orth, A case of pituitary adrenocorticotropin-dependent Cushing's syndrome in the horse, Endocrinology 104 (1979) 576–582.

[268] D.N. Orth, M.A. Holscher, M.G. Wilson, W.E. Nicholson, R.E. Plue, C.D. Mount, Equine Cushing's disease: Plasma immunoreactive proopiomelanocortin peptide and cortisol levels basally and in response to diagnostic tests, Endocrinology 110 (1982) 1430.

[269] M.G. Wilson, W.E. Nicholson, M.A. Holscher, B.J. Scherrer, C.D. Mount, D.N. Orth, Proopiomelanocortin peptides in normal pituitary, pituitary tumor, and plasma of normal and Cushing's horses, Endocrinology 110 (1982) 941–954.

[270] S.W.J. Lamberts, S.A. De Lange, S.Z. Stefanko, Adrenocorticotropin-secreting pituitary adenomas originate from the anterior or the intermediate lobe in Cushing's disease: Differences in the regulation of hormone secretion, J Clin Endocrinol Metab 54 (1982) 286–291.

[271] A.M. McNicol, G.M. Teasdale, G.H. Beastall, A study of corticotroph adenomas in Cushing's disease: No evidence of intermediate lobe origin, Clin Endocrinol 24 (1986) 715–722.

[272] C. Raffel, J.E. Boggan, L.F. Eng, R.L. Davis, C.B. Wilson, Pituitary adenomas in Cushing's disease: Do they arise from the intermediate lobe? Surg Neurol 30 (1988) 125–130.

[273] H. Nakashima, Y. Hirata, M. Uchihashi, M. Tomita, T. Fujita, Effect of ovine corticotrophin releasing factor, bromocriptine, and dopamine on release of ACTH and beta-endorphin in a patient with Cushing's disease, Acta Endocrinol 109 (1985) 7–12.

[274] A.C. Hale, P.J. Coates, I. Doniach, et al., A bromocriptine-responsive corticotroph adenoma secreting alpha-MSH in a patient with Cushing's disease, Clin Endocrinol 28 (1988) 215–223.

[275] T.A. Howlett, J.A.H. Wass, L.H. Rees, G.M. Besser, Plasma cortisol response to dopamine agonists in Cushing's disease: The importance of background variability, J Endocrinol Invest 10 (1987) 53.

[276] R.J.M. Croughs, H.P.F. Koppeschaar, J.W. Van't Verlaat, A.M. McNicol, Bromocriptine-responsive Cushing's disease associated with anterior pituitary corticotroph hyperplasia or normal pituitary gland, J Clin Endocrinol Metab 68 (1989) 495–498.

[277] R. Pivonello, D. Ferone, W.W. de Herder, J.M. Kros, M.L. De Caro, M. Arvigo, et al., Dopamine receptor expression and function in corticotroph pituitary tumors, J Clin Endocrinol Metab 89 (5) (2004) 2452–2462.

[278] D.T. Krieger, S.M. Glick, Sleep EEG stages and plasma growth hormone concentration in states of endogenous and exogenous hypercortisolemia or ACTH elevation, J Clin Endocrinol Metab 39 (1974) 986–1000.

[279] E. Van Cauter, S. Refetoff, Evidence for two subtypes of Cushing's disease based on the analysis of episodic cortisol secretion, N Engl J Med 312 (1985) 1343–1349.

[280] A.B. Atkinson, A.L. Kennedy, D.J. Carson, D.R. Hadden, J.A. Weaver, B. Sheridan, Five cases of cyclical Cushing's syndrome, Br Med J 291 (1985) 1453–1457.

[281] A.M. Schnall, K. Kovacs, J.S. Brodkey, O.H. Pearson, Pituitary Cushing's disease without adenoma, Acta Endocrinol 94 (1980) 297–303.

[282] P.E. McKeever, M.C. Koppelman, D. Metcalf, E. Quindlen, P.L. Kourblith, C.A. Stroot, Refractory Cushing's disease caused by multinodular ACTH cell hyperplasia, J Neuropathol Exp Neurol 41 (1982) 490–499.

[283] S.L. Asa, K. Kovacs, G.T. Tindall, D.L. Barrow, E. Howath, P. Versei, Cushing's disease associated with an intrasellar gangliocytoma producing corticotrophin-releasing factor, Ann Intern Med 101 (1984) 789–793.

[284] J.L. Belsky, B. Cuello, L.W. Swanson, D.M. Simmons, R.M. Sarrett, F. Braza, Cushing's syndrome due to ectopic production of corticotropin-releasing factor, J Clin Endocrinol Metab 60 (1985) 496–500.

[285] R. Carey, S. Varma, C. Drake, et al., Ectopic secretion of corticotropin-releasing factor as a cause of Cushing's syndrome, N Engl J Med 311 (1984) 13–20.

[286] A.M. McNicol, Current topics in neuropathology. Cushing's disease, Neuropathol Appl Neurobiol 11 (1985) 485–494.

[287] R.F. Phifer, D.N. Orth, S.S. Spicer, Specific demonstration of the human hypophyseal adrenocorticomelanotropic (ACTH/MSH) cell, J Clin Endocrinol Metab 39 (1974) 684–692.

[288] W.F. Young, B.W. Scheithauer, H. Gharib, E.R. Laws Jr., P.C. Carpenter, Cushing's syndrome due to primary multinodular corticotrope hyperplasia, Mayo Clin Proc 63 (1988) 256–262.

[289] T. Suda, N. Tomori, F. Yajima, et al., Immunoreactive corticotropin-releasing factor in human plasma, J Clin Invest 76 (1985) 2026–2029.

[290] E.A. Linton, P.J. Lowry, Corticotrophin releasing factor in man and its measurements: A review, Clin Endocrinol 31 (1989) 225–249.

[291] M. Altemus, P.W. Gold, Neuroendocrinology and psychiatric illness, Front Neuroendocrinol 11 (1990) 32–38.

[292] C.B. Nemeroff, E. Widerlov, G. Bissette, et al., Elevated concentrations of corticotropin-releasing-factor like immunoreactivity in depressed patients, Science 226 (1984) 1342–1344.

[293] A. Roy, D. Pickar, S. Paul, A. Doran, G.P. Chrousos, P.W. Gold, CSF corticotropin releasing hormone in depressed patients and normal control subjects, Am J Psychiatry 144 (1987) 641–644.

[294] C. Rivier, J. Rivier, W. Vale, Synthetic competitive antagonists of corticotropin-releasing factor: Effect on ACTH secretion in the rat, Science 224 (1984) 889–891.

[295] D. Hanahan, Dissecting multistep tumorigenesis in transgenic mice, Annu Rev Genet 22 (1988) 479–519.

[296] D. Hanahan, Heritable formation of pancreatic β-cell tumors in transgenic mice expressing recombinant insulin/simian virus 40 oncogenes, Nature 315 (1985) 115–122.

[297] A.G. Knudson, Genetics of human cancer, Annu Rev Genet 20 (1986) 231–251.

[298] H.J. Wolfe, K.E.W. Melvin, S.J. Cervio-Skinner, et al., C-Cell hyperplasia preceding medullary thyroid carcinoma, N Engl J Med 289 (1973) 437–441.

[299] J. Folkman, K. Watson, D. Ingber, D. Hanahan, Induction of angiogenesis during the transition from hyperplasia to neoplasia, Nature 339 (1989) 58–61.

[300] D. Gospodarowicz, J.A. Abraham, J. Schilling, Isolation and characterization of a vascular endothelial cell mitogen produced by pituitary-derived folliculo stellate cells, Biochem J 86 (1989) 7311–7315.

[301] N. Ferrara, W.J. Henzel, Pituitary follicular cells secrete a novel heparin-binding growth factor specific for vascular endothelial cells, Biochem Biophys Res Commun 161 (1989) 851–856.

[302] J. Plouet, J. Schilling, D. Gospodarowicz, Isolation and characterization of a newly identified endothelial cell mitogene produced by pituitary AtT-20 cells, EMBO J 8 (1989) 3801–3806.

[303] K.E. Mayo, R.L. Hammer, L.W. Swanson, R.L. Brinster, M.G. Rosenfeld, R.M. Evans, Dramatic pituitary hyperplasia in transgenic mice expressing a human growth hormone-releasing factor gene, Mol Endocrinol 2 (1988) 606–612.

[304] L. Stefaneanu, K. Kovacs, E. Korvath, et al., Adenohypophysial changes in mice transgenic for human growth hormone-releasing factor: A histological, immunocytochemical, and electron microscopic investigation, Endocrinology 125 (1989) 2710–2718.

[305] G.D. Hammer, V. Fairchild-Huntress, M.J. Low, Pituitary-specific and hormonally regulated gene expression directed by the rat proopiomelanocortin promoter in transgenic mice, Mol Endocrinol 4 (1990) 1689–1697.

[306] Y. Tremblay, I. Tretjakoff, A. Pterson, T. Antakly, C. Xian Zhang, J. Drouin, Pituitary-specific expression and glucocorticoid regulation of a proopiomelanocortin fusion gene in transgenic mice, Proc Nat Acad Sci USA 85 (1988) 8890–8894.

[307] G.D. Hammer, V. Fairchild-Huntress, M.J. Low, A POMC-SV 40 T antigen fusion gene induces differentiated pituitary tumors and thymic hyperplasia in transgenic mice. The Endocrine Society, 72nd Annual Meeting, Atlanta, 1990 221, Abstract 787.

[308] T.A. Stewart, Models of human endocrine disorders in transgenic rodents, TEM 4 (1993) 136–141.

[309] A. Helseth, G.P. Siegal, E. Hang, V.L. Bautch, Transgenic mice that develop pituitary tumors — a model for Cushing's disease, Am J Pathol 140 (1992) 1071–1080.

[310] M.C. Pepin, F. Pothier, N. Barden, Impaired type II glucocorticoid-receptor function in mice bearing antisense RNA transgene, Nature 355 (1992) 725–728.

[311] M.P. Stenzel-Poore, V.A. Cameron, J. Vaughan, P.E. Sawchenko, W. Vale, Development of Cushing's syndrome in corticotropin-releasing factor transgenic mice, Endocrinology 130 (1992) 3378–3386.

[312] T. Sano, S.L. Asa, K. Kovacs, Growth hormone-releasing hormone-producing tumors: Clinical, biochemical, and morphological manifestations, Endocr Rev 9 (1988) 357–373.

[313] N. Sonino, G.A. Fava, S. Grandi, F. Mantero, M. Boscaro, Stressful life events in the pathogenesis of Cushing's syndrome, Clin Endocrinol 29 (1988) 617–623.

[314] N. Sonino, G.A. Fava, M. Boscaro, A role for life events in the pathogenesis of Cushing's disease, Clin Endocrinol 3 (1993) 261–264.

[315] S.W.J. Lamberts, J.G.M. Klijn, F.H. de Jong, The definition of true recurrence of pituitary-dependent Cushing's syndrome after transsphenoidal operation, Clin Endocrinol 26 (1987) 707–712.

[316] A. Kuwayama, Long-term results of pituitary surgery in Cushing's disease, in: D.L. Ludecke, G.P. Chrousos, G. Tolis (Eds.), ACTH, Cushing's Syndrome, and other Hypercortisolemic States., Raven Press, New York, 1990, pp. 289–295.

[317] R.B. Friedman, E.H. Oldfield, L.K. Nieman, et al., Repeat transsphenoidal surgery for Cushing's disease, J Neurosurg 71 (1989) 520–527.

[318] G.D. Hammer, G. Mueller, B. Lin, J.S. Petrides, B.A. Roos, M.J. Low, Ectopic corticotropin-releasing hormone produced by a transfected cell line chronically activates the pituitary-adrenal axis in transkaryotic rats, Endocrinology 130 (1992) 1975–1985.

[319] M.T. Jones, Control of adrenocortical hormone secretion, in: V.H.T. James (Ed.), The Adrenal Gland, Raven Press, New York, 1979, pp. 93–130.

[320] G.N. Gill, ACTH regulation of the adrenal cortex, in: G.N. Gill (Ed.), Pharmacology of Adrenal Cortical Hormones, Pergamon, New York, 1979, pp. 35–66.

[321] P.J. Hornsby, The mechanism of action of ACTH in the adrenal cortex, in: B.A. Cooke, R.J.B. King, H.J. Van Der Molen (Eds.), Hormones and their Actions, Part II. Elsevier Science Publishers BV, Biomedical Division, 1988, pp. 193–210.

[322] L.M. Mertz, R.C. Pedersen, The kinetics of steroidogenesis activator polypeptide in the rat adrenal cortex. Effects of adrenocorticotropin, cyclic adenosine 3′:5′ monophosphate cycloheximide and circadian rhythm, J Biol Chem 264 (1989) 15274–15279.

[323] M.R. Waterman, E.R. Simpson, Regulation of the biosynthesis of cytochromes P-450 involved in steroid hormone synthesis, Mol Cell Endocrinol 39 (1985) 81–89.

[324] M.E. John, M.C. John, V. Boggaram, E.R. Simpson, M.R. Waterman, Transcriptional regulation of steroid hydroxylase genes by corticotropin, Proc Nat Acad Sci USA 83 (1986) 4715–4719.

[325] G.W. Liddle, Regulation of adrenocortical function in man, in: N.P. Christy (Ed.), The Human Adrenal Cortex, Harper and Row, New York, 1971, pp. 41–68.

[326] A. Penhoat, C. Jailiard, J.M. Saez, Corticotropin positively regulates its own receptors and cAMP response in cultured bovine adrenal cells, Proc Nat Acad Sci USA 86 (1989) 4978–4981.

[327] M. Begeot, D. Langlois, A. Penhoat, J.M. Saez, Variations in guanine-binding proteins (Gs, Gi) in cultured bovine adrenal cells. Consequences on the effects of phorbol and cholera-toxin-induced cAMP production, Eur J Biochem 174 (1988) 317–321.

[328] K.G. Mountjoy, L.S. Robbins, M.T. Mortrud, R.D. Cone, The cloning of a family of genes that encode the melanocortin receptors, Science 257 (1992) 1248–1251.

[329] M.C. Lebrethon, A. Penhoat, D. Naville, C. Jaillard, J.M. Saez, Regulation of ACTH-receptor mRNA level by ACTH and angiotensin II in human (HAC) and bovine (BAC) cultured fasciculata-reticularis cells. 75th meeting of the American Endo Soc, Las Vegas (June 1993) abstract 1680.

[330] A. Penhoat, D. Naville, C. Jaillard, P.G. Chatelain, J.M. Saez, Hormonal regulation of insulin-like growth factor I secretion by bovine adrenal cells, J Biol Chem 264 (1989) 6858–6862.

[331] I. Louveau, A. Penhoat, J.M. Saez, Regulation of IGF-1 receptors by corticotropin and angiotensin-II in cultured bovine adrenocortical cells, Biochem Biophys Res Commun 163 (1989) 32–36.

[332] A. Penhoat, P.G. Chatelain, C. Jaillard, J.M. Saez, Characterization of somatomedin-C/insulin-like growth factor I and insulin receptors on cultured bovine adrenal fasciculata cells. Role of these peptides on adrenal cell function, Endocrinology 122 (1988) 2518–2526.

[333] W.E. Rainey, I. Viard, J.I. Mason, C. Cochet, E.M. Chambaz, J.M. Saez, Effects of transforming growth factor beta on ovine adrenocortical cells, Mol Cell Endocrinol 60 (1988) 189–198.

[334] J. Kolanowski, J. Crabbe, Le mécanisme de l'hyperreactivité corticosurrénale à la corticotropine (ACTH) dans la maladie de Cushing, Horm Res 13 (1980) 337 (Abstract).

[335] C.D. West, L.I. Dolman, Plasma ACTH radioimmunoassays in the diagnosis of pituitary—adrenal dysfunction, Ann NY Acad Sci 297 (1977) 205–219.

[336] T. Yamaji, M. Ishibashik, H. Sekihara, A. Itabashi, T. Yanaihara, Serum dehydroepiandrosterone sulfate in Cushing's syndrome, J Clin Endocrinol Metab (1984) 1164–1168.

[337] A.G.H. Smals, P.W.C. Kloppenborg, T.J. Benraad, Plasma testosterone profiles in Cushing's syndrome, J Clin Endocrinol Metab 45 (1977) 240–245.

[338] C.E. Kater, E.G. Biglieri, N. Brust, B. Chang, J. Hirai, I. Irony, Stimulation and suppression of the mineralocorticoid hormones in normal subjects and adrenocortical disorders, Endocr Rev 10 (1989) 149–164.

[339] M. Schambelan, P.E. Slaton Jr., E.G. Biglieri, Mineralocorticoid production in hyperadrenocorticism, Am J Med 51 (1971) 299–303.

[340] H. Lefebvre, S. Idres, C. Delarue, et al., Effect de la serotonine (-5-HT) sur la secretion du cortisol par le cortex surrénalien humain in vitro. Role paracrine possible de la 5-HT medullo surrénalienne sur la secrétion des glucocorticoides, Ann Endocrinol 50 (1989) 307 (Abstract).

[341] R.X. Whitcomb, W.M. Linehan, L.M. Wahl, R.A. Knazek, Monocytes stimulate cortisol production by cultured human adrenocortical cells, J Clin Endocrinol Metab 66 (1988) 33–38.

[342] M. Naruse, K. Obana, K. Naruse, et al., Atrial natriuretic polypeptide inhibits cortisol secretion as well as aldosterone secretion in vitro from human adrenal tissue, J Clin Endocrinol Metab 64 (1987) 10–16.

[343] Q. Zhu, S. Solomon, Isolation and mode of action of rabbit corticostatic peptides, Endocrinology 130 (1992) 1413–1423.

[344] M.T. Pham Huu Trung, N. De Smitter, A. Boggio, X. Bertagna, E. Girard, Responses of isolated guinea-pig adrenal cells to ACTH and pro-opiocortin derived peptides, Endocrinology 100 (1982) 1819–1821.

[345] G.P. Vinson, B.J. Whitehouse, A. Dell, T. Etienne, H.R. Morris, Characterization of an adrenal zona glomerulosa-stimulating component of posterior pituitary extracts as alpha-MSH, Nature 284 (1980) 464–467.

[346] H. Matsuoka, P.J. Mulrow, C.H. Li, β-lipotropin: A new aldosterone-stimulating factor, Science 209 (1980) 307–308.

[347] H. Matsuoka, P.J. Mulrow, R. Franco-Saenz, C.H. Li, Stimulation of aldosterone production by β-melanotropin, Nature 291 (1981) 155–156.

[348] H.G. Gullner, J.R. Gill, β-endorphin selectively stimulates aldosterone secretion in hypophysectomized, nephrectomized dogs, J Clin Invest 71 (1983) 124–128.

[349] P. Lis, P. Hamet, J. Gutokowska, et al., Effect of N-terminal portion of proopiomelanocortin on aldosterone release by human adrenal adenoma in vitro, J Clin Endocrinol Metab 52 (1981) 1053–1056.

[350] R.C. Pedersen, A.C. Brownie, N. Ling, Pro-adrenocorticotropin/endorphin-derived peptides: Coordinate action on adrenal steroidogenesis, Science 208 (1980) 1044–1045.

[351] R.C. Pedersen, A.C. Brownie, Lys-Gamma3-melanotropin binds with high affinity to the rat adrenal cortex, Endocrinology 112 (1983) 1279–1287.

[352] X. Bertagna, F. Lenne, D. Comar, et al., Human beta-melanocyte stimulating hormone revisited, Proc Nat Acad Sci USA 83 (1986) 9719–9723.

[353] G.Y. Griffing, B. Berelowitz, M. Hudson, et al., Plasma immunoreactive gamma melanotropin in patients with idiopathic hyperaldosteronism, aldosterone-producing adenomas, and essential hypertension, J Clin Invest 76 (1985) 163–169.

[354] R.M. Carey, S. Sen, Recent progress in the control of aldosterone secretion, Recent Prog Horm Res 42 (1986) 251–296.

[355] A. Penhoat, P. Sanchez, C. Jaillard, D. Langlois, M. Begeot, J.M. Saez, Human proopiomelanocortin (79–76), a proposed cortical-androgen stimulating hormone does not affect steroidogenesis in cultured human adult adrenal cells, J Clin Endocrinol Metab 72 (1991) 23–26.

[356] C.H. Li, D. Chung, D. Yamashiro, C.Y. Lee, Isolation, characterization, and synthesis of a corticotropin-inhibiting peptide from human pituitary glands, Biochemistry 75 (1978) 4306–4309.

[357] J. Koistinaho, R. Roivanen, G. Yang, Circadian rhythm in c-fos protein expression in the rat adrenal cortex, Mol Cell Endocrinol 71 (1990) R1–R6.

[358] P.J. Lowry, L. Silas, C. McLean, E.A. Linton, F.E. Estivary, Pro-gamma-melanocyte-stimulating hormone cleavage in adrenal gland undergoing compensatory growth, Nature 306 (1983) 70–73.

[359] D.N. Orth, K. Tanaka, W.G. Nicholson, Melanocyte stimulating hormones (MSH's) and lipotropic hormones (LPH's), in: B.M. Jaffe, H.R. Behrman (Eds.), Methods of Hormone Radioimmunoassay, Academic Press, New York, 1979, pp. 285–313.

[360] J.C. Willer, L. Sheng-Shu, X. Bertagna, F. Girard, Pituitary β-endorphin not involved in pain control in some pathophysiological conditions, Lancet (1984) 295–296.

[361] K. Nakao, S. Oki, I. Tanaka, et al., Immunoreactive-β-endorphin and adrenocorticotropin in human cerebrospinal fluid, J Clin Invest 66 (1980) 1383–1390.

[362] A.M. Neville, M.J. O'Hare, Histopathology of the human adrenal cortex, Clin Endocrinol Metab 14 (1985) 791–820.

[363] H. Bricaire, J.P. Luton, M. Ghozland, M. Forest, La polymicroadénomatose de la cortico-surrénale dans le syndrome de Cushing. A propos de 15 observations, Ann Med Interne 121 (1970) 755–777.

[364] P. Cuginin, P. Battisti, L. Di Palma, et al., "GIANT" macronodular adrenal hyperplasia causing Cushing's syndrome: Case report and review of the literature on a clinical distinction of adrenocortical nodular pathology associated with hypercortisolism, Endocrinol Jpn 36 (1989) 101–116.

[365] S.W.J. Lamberts, J. Zuiderwijk, P. Uitterlinden, J.J. Blijd, H.A. Bruining, F.H. de Jong, Characterization of adrenal autonomy in Cushing's syndrome: A comparison between in vivo and in vitro responsiveness of the adrenal gland, J Clin Endocrinol Metab 70 (1990) 192–199.

[366] J.P. Luton, A. Krivitzky, Ph Thieblot, M. Forest, H. Bricaire, Hyperplasie polyadénomateuse maligne bilatérale des surrénales partiellement hormono-dépendantes, Ann Endocrinol 39 (1978) 1–14.

[367] S. Leiba, B. Shindel, I. Weinberger, et al., Cushing's disease coexisting with a single macronodule simulating adenoma of the adrenal cortex, Acta Endocrinol 112 (1986) 323–328.

[368] A.R. Hermus, G.F. Pieters, A.G. Smals, et al., Transition from pituitary-dependent to adrenal-dependent Cushing's syndrome, N Engl J Med 318 (1988) 966–970.

[369] J.L. Doppman, D.L. Miller, A.J. Dwyer, et al., Macronodular adrenal hyperplasia in Cushing's disease, Radiology 166 (1988) 347–352.

[370] D.C. Aron, J.W. Findling, P.A. Fitzgerald, et al., Pituitary ACTH dependency of nodular adrenal hyperplasia in Cushing's syndrome. Report of two cases and review of the literature, Am J Med 71 (1981) 302–306.

[371] A.G.H. Smals, G.F.F.M. Pieters, U.J.C. Van Haelst, P.W.C. Kloppenborg, Macronodular adrenocortical hyperplasia in long-standing Cushing's disease, J Clin Endocrinol Metab 58 (1984) 25–31.

[372] J. Newell-Price, P. Trainer, M. Besser, A. Grossman, The diagnosis and differential diagnosis of Cushing's syndrome and pseudo-Cushing's states, Endo Rev 19 (1998) 647–672.

[373] J.P. Luton, La poly-micro-adénomatose dans les syndromes de Cushing, Editorial, Presse Med 78 (1970) 43.

[374] J.L. De Gennes, J.P. Luton, H. Bricaire, Réponses négatives à la Métopirone dans le syndrome de Cushing à adénome ou adénomatose cortico-surrénale, Ann Endocrinol 32 (1971) 601–607.

[375] K. Hashimoto, Y. Kawada, K. Murakami, et al., Cortisol responsiveness to insulin-induced hypoglycemia in Cushing's syndrome with huge nodular adrenocortical hyperplasia, Endocrinol Jpn 33 (1986) 479–487.

[376] S. Makino, K. Hashimoto, M. Sugiyama, et al., Cushing's syndrome due to huge nodular adrenocortical hyperplasia with fluctuation of urinary 17-OHCS excretion, Endocrinol Jpn 36 (1989) 655–663.

[377] S.W.J. Lamberts, E.G. Bons, H.A. Bruining, Different sensitivity to adrenocorticotropin of dispersed adrenocortical cells from patients with Cushing's disease with macronodular and diffuse adrenal hyperplasia, J Clin Endocrinol Metab 58 (1984) 1106–1110.

[378] H.R. Fish, D.O. Sobel, C.A. Miegel, Macronodular adrenal hyperplasia with hypothalamic—pituitary—adrenal suppression by ultrahigh-dose dexamethasone: regression following hypophysectomy, Clin Neuropharmacol 9 (1986) 303–308.

[379] R.A. Cheitlin, M. Westphal, C.M. Cabrea, D.K. Fujii, J. Snyder, P.A. Fitzgerald, Cushing's syndrome due to bilateral adrenal macronodular hyperplasia with undetectable ACTH: Cell culture of adenoma cells on extracellular matrix, Horm Res 29 (1988) 162–167.

[380] C.D. Malchoff, J. Rosa, C.R. DeBold, et al., Adrenocorticotropin-independent bilateral macronodular adrenal hyperplasia: An unusual cause of Cushing's syndrome, J Clin Endocrinol Metab 68 (1989) 855–860.

[381] H. Watanobe, T. Kawagishi, Y. Hirai, T. Sato, M. Tsutsui, Cushing's syndrome presenting the coexistence of a pituitary corticotrophic cell hyperplasia and a unilateral functional adrenal adenoma, Acta Endocrinol 110 (1985) 302–307.

[382] B. Hocher, V. Bähr, S. Dorfmüller, W. Oelkers, Hypercortisolism with non-pigmented micronodular adrenal hyperplasia: Transition from pituitary-dependent to adrenal dependent Cushing's syndrome, Acta Endocrinol 128 (1993) 120–125.

[383] D.L. Page, R.A. DeLellis, A.J. Hough, Tumors of the Adrenal. Atlas of Tumor Pathology, fascicle 23, second series, Armed Forces Institute of Pathology, Washington, 1985.

[384] D.C. Anderson, D.F. Child, C.H. Sutcliffe, C.H. Buckley, D. Davies, D. Longson, Cushing's syndrome, nodular adrenal hyperplasia and virilizing carcinoma, Clin Endocrinol 9 (1978) 1–14.

[385] R.A. Chalmers, L. Mashiter, G.F. Joplin, Residual adrenocortical function after bilateral "total" adrenalectomy for Cushing's disease, Lancet (1981) 1196–1199.

[386] S. Melmed, R.J. Rushakoff, Ectopic pituitary and hypothalamic hormone syndromes, Endocrinol Metab Clin North Am 16 (1987) 805–821.

[387] D.N. Orth, R.V. Jackson, G.S. De Cherney, et al., Effect of synthetic ovine corticotropin-releasing factor, J Clin Invest 71 (1983) 587–595.

[388] H.M. Schulte, G.P. Chrousos, P.W. Gold, et al., Continuous administration of synthetic ovine CRF in man, J Clin Invest 75 (1985) 1781–1785.

[389] B. Allolio, J. Hoffmann, E.A. Linton, W. Winkelmann, M. Kusche, H.M. Schulte, Diurnal salivary cortisol patterns during pregnancy and after delivery: Relationship to plasma corticotrophin-releasing-hormone, Clin Endocrinol 33 (1990) 279–289.

[390] A.B. Abou-Samra, M. Pugeat, H. Dechaud, et al., Increased plasma concentration of N-terminal lipotrophin and unbound cortisol during pregnancy, Clin Endocrinol 20 (1984) 221–228.

[391] J. Schwartz, N. Billestrup, M. Perrin, J. Rivier, W. Vale, Identification of corticotropin-releasing factor (CRF) target cells and effects of dexamethasone on binding in anterior pituitary using a fluorescent analog of CRF, Endocrinology 119 (1986) 2376–2382.

[392] G.V. Childs, J.L. Moreil, A. Niendorf, G. Aguilera, Cytochemical studies of corticotropin-releasing factor (CRF) receptors in anterior lobe corticotropes: Binding, glucocorticoid regulation, and endocytosis of (Biotiny1-Ser1) CRF, Endocrinology 119 (1986) 2129–2142.

[393] R.L. Huager, M.A. Millan, K.J. Catt, G. Aguilera, Differential regulation of brain and pituitary corticotropin-releasing factor receptors by corticosterone, Endocrinology 120 (1987) 1527–1533.

[394] E.A. Linton, C.D.A. Wolfe, D.P. Behan, P.J. Lowry, A specific carrier substance for human corticotrophin releasing factor in late gestational maternal plasma which could mask the ACTH-releasing activity, Clin Endocrinol 28 (1988) 315–324.

[395] E.A. Linton, D.P. Behan, P.W. Saphier, P.J. Lowry, Corticotropin-releasing hormone (CRH)-binding protein: Reduction in the adrenocorticotropin-releasing activity of placental but not hypothalamic CRF, J Clin Endocrinol Metab 70 (1990) 1574–1580.

[396] T. Suda, M. Kondo, R. Totani, et al., Ectopic ACTH syndrome caused by lung cancer that responded to corticotropin-releasing hormone, J Clin Endocrinol Metab 63 (1986) 1047–1051.

[397] M.C. Ràux-Demay, M.F. Proeschel, Y. de Keyzer, X. Bertagna, J.P. Luton, F. Girard, Characterization of human corticotrophin releasing hormone and proopiomelanocortin related peptides in a thymic carcinoid tumor responsible for Cushing's syndrome, Clin Endocrinol 29 (1988) 649–657.

[398] G.V. Upton, T.T. Amatruda, Evidence for the presence of tumor peptides with corticotropin-releasing factor like activity in the ectopic ACTH syndrome, N Engl J Med 285 (1971) 419–424.

[399] T.A. Hewlett, J. Price, A.C. Hale, et al., Pituitary ACTH dependent Cushing's syndrome due to ectopic production of a bombesin-like peptide by a medullary carcinoma of the thyroid, Clin Endocrinol 22 (1985) 91–101.

[400] W.H. Brown, A case of plunglandular syndrome: Diabetes of bearded women, Lancet (1928) 1022–1023.

[401] C.K. Meador, G.W. Liddle, D.P. Island, et al., Cause of Cushing's syndrome in patients with tumors arising from "nonendocrine" tissue, J Clin Endocrinol Metab 22 (1962) 693–703.

[402] G.W. Liddle, W.E. Nicholson, D.P. Island, D.N. Orth, L. Abe, S.C. Lowder, Clinical and laboratory studies of ectopic humoral syndromes, Recent Prog Horm Res 25 (1969) 283–314.

[403] D.N. Orth, Ectopic hormone production, in: P. Felig, J.D. Baxter, A.E. Broadus, L.A. Frohman (Eds.), Endocrinology and Metabolism, McGraw-Hill, New York, 1981, pp. 191–217.

[404] L.H. Rees, J.G. Ratcliffe, Ectopic hormone production by non-endocrine tumours, Clin Endocrinol 3 (1974) 263–299.

[405] A. White, A.J.L. Clark, The cellular and molecular basis of the ectopic ACTH syndrome, Clin Endocrinol 39 (1993) 131–142.

[406] R.S. Yalow, S.A. Berson, Size heterogeneity of immunoreactive human ACTH in plasma and in extracts of pituitary glands and ACTH-producing thymoma, Biochem Biophys Res Commun 44 (1971) 439–445.

[407] X.Y. Bertagna, W.E. Nicholson, G.D. Sorenson, O.S. Pettengill, C.D. Mount, D.N. Orth, Corticotropin, lipotropin, and β-endorphin production by a human nonpituitary tumor in tissue culture: evidence for a common precursor, Proc Nat Acad Sci USA 75 (1978) 5160–5164.

[408] D.N. Orth, W.E. Nicholson, W.M. Mitchell, D.P. Island, G.W. Liddle, Biologic and immunologic characterization and physical separation of ACTH and ACTH fragments in the ectopic ACTH syndrome, J Clin Invest 52 (1973) 1756–1769.

[409] J.G. Ratcliffe, A.P. Scott, H.P.J. Bennett, et al., Production of a corticotrophin-like intermediate lobe peptide and of corticotrophin by a bronchial carcinoid tumour, Clin Endocrinol 2 (1973) 51–55.

[410] A.J.L. Clark, M.F. Stewart, P.M. Lavender, et al., Defective glucocorticoid regulation of proopiomelanocortin gene expression and peptide secretion in a small cell lung cancer cell line, J Clin Endocrinol Metab 70 (1990) 485–490.

[411] R. Oosterom, T. Verleun, H.A. Bruining, W.H.L. Hackeng, S.W.J. Lamberts, Secretion of adrenocorticotropin, β-endorphin and calcitonin by cultured medullary thyroid carcinoma cells. Effects of synthetic corticotropin-releasing factor and lysine vasopressin, Acta Endocrinol 113 (1986) 65–72.

[412] C.D. Malchoff, D.N. Orth, C. Abboud, J.A. Carney, P.C. Pairolero, R.M. Carey, Ectopic ACTH syndrome caused by a bronchial carcinoid tumor responsive to dexamethasone, metyrapone, and corticotropin-releasing factor, Am J Med 84 (1988) 760–764.

[413] M.L. Raffin-Sanson, Y. de Keyzer, X. Bertagna, Syndromes of ectopic ACTH secretion: Recent pathophysiological progresses and their clinical implications, The Endocrinologist 10 (2000) 97–106.

[414] W.J. Meyer III, E.M. Smith, G.E. Richards, A. Cavallo, A.C. Morrill, J.E. Blalock, In vivo immunoreactive adrenocorticotropin (ACTH) production by human mononuclear leukocytes from normal and ACTH-deficient individuals, J Clin Endocrinol Metab 64 (1987) 98–105.

[415] S. Iida, Y. Nakamura, H. Fujii, et al., A patient with hypocortisolism and Cushing's syndrome-like manifestations: Cortisol hyperreactive syndrome, J Clin Endocrinol Metab 70 (1990) 729–737.

[416] C.K. Meador, B. Bowdoin, W.C. Owen, T.A. Farmer, Primary adrenocortical nodular dysplasia: A rare cause of Cushing's syndrome, J Clin Endocrinol Metab 27 (1967) 1255–1263.

[417] J.A. Carney, L.S. Hruska, G.D. Beauchamp, H. Gordon, Dominant inheritance of the complex of myxomas, spotty pigmentation, and endocrine overactivity, Mayo Clin Proc 61 (1986) 165–172.

[418] W.F. Young, J.A. Carney, B.U. Musa, N.M. Wulffraat, J.W. Lens, H.A. Drexhage, Familial Cushing's syndrome due to primary pigmented nodular adrenocortical disease, N Engl J Med 321 (1989) 1659–1664.

[419] L.S. Kirschner, F. Sandrini, J. Monbo, J.P. Lin, J.A. Carney, C.A. Stratakis, Genetic heterogeneity and spectrum of mutations of the PRKAR1A gene in patients with the Carney complex, Hum Mol Genet 9 (2000) 3037–3046.

[420] M. Casey, C.J. Vaughan, J. He, et al., Mutations in the protein kinase A R 1alpha regulatory subunit cause familial cardiac myxomas and Carney complex, J Clin Invest 107 (2001) 235.

[421] J.L. Findlay, L.R. Sheeler, W.C. Engeland, D.C. Aron, Familial adrenocorticotropin-independent Cushing's syndrome with bilateral macronodular adrenal hyperplasia, J Clin Endocrinol Metab 76 (1993) 189–191.

[422] A. Lacroix, E. Bolte, J. Tremblay, et al., Gastric inhibitory polypeptide-dependent cortisol hypersecretion — a new cause of Cushing's syndrome, N Engl J Med 327 (1992) 974–980.

[423] Y. Reznik, V. Allali-Zerah, J.A. Chayvialle, et al., Food dependent Cushing's syndrome mediated by aberrant adrenal sensitivity to gastric inhibitory polypeptide, N Engl J Med 327 (1992) 981–986.

[423a] A. Lacroix, N. Ndiaye, J. Tremblay, P. Hamet, Ectopic and abnormal hormone receptors in adrenal Cushing's syndrome, Endocr Rev 22 (2001) 75–110.

[424] L.S. Weinstein, A. Shenker, P.V. Gejman, M.J. Merino, E. Friedman, A.M. Spiegel, Activating mutations of the stimulatory G protein in the McCune-Albright syndrome, N Engl J Med 325 (1991) 1688–1695.

[425] K. Knyrim, M. Higi, D.L. Hossfeld, S. Seeber, C.G. Schmidt, Autonomous cortisol secretion by a metastatic Leydig cell carcinoma associated with Klinefelter's syndrome, J Cancer Res Clin Oncol 100 (1981) 85–93.

[426] N.J. Marieb, S. Splangler, M. Kashgarian, A. Heimann, M.L. Schwartz, P.E. Schwartz, Cushing's syndrome secondary to ectopic cortisol production by ovarian carcinoma, J Clin Endocrinol Metab 57 (1983) 737–740.

[427] N.P. Christy, Iatrogenic Cushing's syndrome, in: N.P. Christy (Ed.), The Human Adrenal Cortex, Harper and Row, New York, 1971, pp. 395–425.

[428] J.B. Tyrrell, J.D. Baxter, Endocrinology and metabolism, in: P. Felig, J.D. Baxter, A.E. Broadus, A.L. Frohman (Eds.), Glucocorticoid Therapy, McGraw-Hill, New York, 1981, pp. 599–623.

[429] J.P. O'Hare, J.A. Vale, S. Wood, R.J. Corrall, Factitious Cushing's syndrome, Acta Endocrinol 111 (1986) 165–167.

[430] D.M. Cook, A.W. Meikle, Factitious Cushing's syndrome, J Clin Endocrinol Metab 61 (1985) 385–387.

[431] K. Siminioski, P. Goss, D.J. Drucker, The Cushing's syndrome induced by medroxyprogesterone acetate, Ann Intern Med 111 (1989) 758–760.

[432] K. Samaras, S. Pett, A. Gowers, M. McMurchie, D.A. Cooper, Iatrogenic Cushing's syndrome with osteoporosis and secondary adrenal failure in human immunodeficiency virus-infected patients receiving inhaled corticosteroids and ritonavir-boosted protease inhibitors: six cases, J Clin Endocrinol Metab 90 (7) (2005) 4394–4398.

[433] M.D. Altschule, A near miss. Osler's early description of Cushing's syndrome with, regrettably, no post-mortem examination, N Engl J Med 302 (1980) 1153–1155.

[434] W. Osler, An actue myxoedematous condition, with tachycardia, glycosuria, melaena, mania, and death, J Nerv Ment Dis 26 (1899) 65–71.

[435] H. Cushing, The Pituitary Body and its Disorders, Lippincott, Philadelphia, 1912.

[436] E.J. Ross, P. Marshall-Jones, M. Friedman, Cushing's syndrome: Diagnostic criteria, Q J Med 35 (1966) 149–192.

[437] L.C. Santini, J.L. Williams, Mediastinal widening (presumable lipomatosis) in Cushing's syndrome, N Engl J Med 284 (1971) 1357–1359.

[438] C.A. Nugent, H.R. Warner, J.T. Dunn, F.H. Tyler, Probability theory in the diagnosis of Cushing's syndrome, J Clin Endocrinol Metab 24 (1964) 621–627.

[439] E.J. Ross, D.C. Linch, Cushing's syndrome-killing disease: Discriminatory value of signs and symptoms aiding early diagnosis, Lancet (1982) 646–649.

[440] J.P. Luton, J.C. Valcke, G. Turpin, M. Forest, H. Bricaire, Muscle et syndrome de Cushing, Ann Endocrinol 31 (1970) 157–169.

[441] N. Ohmori, K. Nomura, K. Ohmori, Y. Kato, T. Itoh, K. Takano, Osteoporosis is more prevalent in adrenal than in pituitary Cushing's syndrome, Endocr J 50 (2003) 1–7.

[442] P.J. Manning, M.C. Evans, I.R. Reid, Normal bone mineral density following cure of Cushing's syndrome, Clin Endocrinol (Oxf) 36 (1992) 229–234.

[443] A.R. Hermus, A.G. Smals, L.M. Swinkels, D.A. Huysmans, G.F. Pieters, C.F. Sweep, et al., Bone mineral density and bone turnover before and after surgical cure of Cushing's syndrome, J Clin Endocrinol Metab 80 (1995) 2859–2865.

[444] I. Chiodini, V. Carnevale, M. Torlontano, S. Fusilli, G. Guglielmi, M. Pileri, et al., Alterations of bone turnover and bone mass at different skeletal sites due to pure glucocorticoid excess: Study in eumenorrheic patients with Cushing's syndrome, J Clin Endocrinol Metab 83 (1998) 1863–1867.

[445] K. Godang, T. Ueland, J. Bollerslev, Decreased bone area, bone mineral content, formative markers, and increased bone resorptive markers in endogenous Cushing's syndrome, Eur J Endocrinol 141 (1999) 126–131.

[446] C. Kristo, K. Godang, T. Ueland, E. Lien, P. Aukrust, S.S. Froland, et al., Raised serum levels of interleukin-8 and interleukin-18 in relation to bone metabolism in endogenous Cushing's syndrome, Eur J Endocrinol 146 (2002) 389–395.

[447] C. Kristo, R. Jemtland, T. Ueland, K. Godang, J. Bollerslev, Restoration of the coupling process and normalization of bone mass following successful treatment of endogenous Cushing's syndrome: A prospective, long-term study, Eur J Endocrinol 154 (2006) 109–118.

[448] C.M. Francucci, P. Pantanetti, G.G. Garrapa, F. Massi, G. Arnaldi, F. Mantero, Bone metabolism and mass in women with Cushing's syndrome and adrenal incidentaloma, Clin Endocrinol (Oxf) 57 (2002) 587–593.

[449] C. Di Somma, R. Pivonello, S. Loche, A. Faggiano, M. Klain, M. Salvatore, et al., Effect of 2 years of cortisol normalization on the impaired bone mass and turnover in adolescent and adult patients with Cushing's disease: A prospective study, Clin Endocrinol (Oxf) 58 (2003) 302–308.

[450] J. Newell-Price, X. Bertagna, A.B. Grossman, L.K. Nieman, Cushing's syndrome, Lancet 367 (9522) (2006) 1605–1617.

[451] M.L. Muiesan, M. Lupia, M. Salvetti, C. Grigoletto, N. Sonino, M. Boscaro, et al., Left ventricular structural and functional characteristics in Cushing's syndrome, J Am Coll Cardiol 41 (2003) 2275–2279.

[452] F. Fallo, P. Maffei, A. Dalla Pozza, M. Carli, P. Della Mea, M. Lupia, et al., Cardiovascular autonomic function in Cushing's syndrome, J Endocrinol Invest 32 (2009) 41–45.

[453] H. Bricaire, M. Thibonnier, M. Hautecouverture, P. Corvol, J.P. Luton, Variations du système rénine angiotensine aldostérone dans la maladie de Cushing, Nouv Presse Med 9 (1980) 1007–1009.

[454] C.M. Ritchie, B. Sheridan, R. Fraser, et al., Studies on the pathogenesis of hypertension in Cushing's disease and acromegaly, Q J Med 280 (1990) 855–867.

[455] T. Saruta, H. Suzuki, M. Handa, Y. Igarash, K. Kondo, S. Senba, Multiple factors contribute to the pathogenesis of hypertension in Cushing's syndrome, J Clin Endocrinol Metab 62 (1986) 275–279.

[456] A. Faggiano, R. Pivonello, S. Spiezia, M.C. De Martino, M. Filippella, C. Di Somma, et al., Cardiovascular risk factors and common carotid artery caliber and stiffness in patients with Cushing's disease during active disease and 1 year after disease remission, J Clin Endocrinol Metab 88 (2003) 2527–2533.

[457] J.P. Luton, C.H. Richard, M.H. Laudat, J.C. Pinon, H. Bricaire, Manifestations cardiovasculaires et anomalies lipidiques au cours du syndrome de Cushing, Nouv Presse Med 11 (1982) 2693–2698.

[458] G.M. Patrassi, R. Dal Bo Zanon, M. Boscaro, S. Martinelli, A. Girolami, Further studies on the hypercoagulable state of patients with Cushing's syndrome, Thromb Haemost (1985) 518–520.

[459] M. Boscaro, N. Sonino, A. Scarda, L. Barzon, F. Fallo, M.T. Sartori, et al., Anticoagulant prophylaxis markedly reduces thromboembolic complications in Cushing's syndrome, J Clin Endocrinol Metab 87 (2002) 3662–3666.

[460] B. Van Zaane, E. Nur, A. Squizzato, O.M. Dekkers, M.T. Twickler, E. Fliers, et al., Hypercoagulable state in Cushing's syndrome: A systematic review, J Clin Endocrinol Metab 94 (8) (2009) 2743–2750.

[461] B. Swearingen, B.M.K. Biller, F.G. Barker II, et al., Long-term mortality after transsphenoidal surgery for Cushing disease, Ann Int Med 130 (1999) 821–824.

[462] L. Pikkarainen, T. Sane, A. Reunanen, The survival and well-being of patients treated for Cushing's syndrome, J Intern Med 245 (1999) 463–468.

[463] D.K. Ludecke, G. Niedworok, Results of microsurgery in Cushing's disease and effect on hypertension, Cardiology 72 (1985) 91–94.

[464] T.H. Jurney, H. De Ruyter, R.A. Vigersky, Cushing's disease presenting as amenorrhoea with hyperprolactinaemia: Report of two cases, Clin Endocrinol 14 (1981) 539–545.

[465] T. Yamaji, M. Ishibashi, A. Teramoto, T. Fukushima, Hyperprolactinemia in Cushing's disease and Nelson's syndrome, J Clin Endocrinol Metab 58 (1984) 790–795.

[466] J.P. Luton, P. Thieblot, J.C. Valcke, J. Mahoudeau, H. Bricaire, Reversible gonadotropin deficiency in male Cushing's disease, J Clin Endocrinol Metab 45 (1977) 488–495.

[467] P.H. Mazet, D. Simon, J.P. Luton, H. Bricaire, Syndrome de Cushing: Symptomatologie psychique et personnalité de 50 malades, Nouv Presse Med 10 (1981) 2565–2570.

[468] N. Sonino, G.A. Fava, Psychiatric disorders associated with Cushing's syndrome. Epidemiology, pathophysiology and treatment, CNS Drugs 15 (5) (2001) 361–373.

[469] H. Forget, A. Lacroix, H. Cohen, Persistent cognitive impairment following surgical treatment of Cushing's syndrome, Psychoneuroendocrinology 27 (3) (2002) 367–383.

[470] I. Bourdeau, C. Bard, H. Forget, Y. Boulanger, H. Cohen, A. Lacroix, Cognitive function and cerebral assessment in patients who have Cushing's syndrome, Endocrinol Metab Clin North Am 34 (2) (2005) 357–369.

[471] M.T. Hawn, D. Cook, C. Deveney, B.C. Sheppard, Quality of life after laparoscopic bilateral adrenalectomy for Cushing's disease, Surgery 132 (6) (2002) 1064–1068.

[472] N. Sonino, S. Bonnini, F. Fallo, M. Boscaro, G.A. Fava, Personality characteristics and quality of life in patients treated for Cushing's syndrome, Clin Endocrinol (Oxf) 64 (3) (2006) 314–318.

[473] J.R. Lindsay, T. Nansel, S. Baid, J. Gumowski, L.K. Nieman, Long-term impaired quality of life in Cushing's syndrome despite initial improvement after surgical remission, J Clin Endocrinol Metab 91 (2) (2006) 447–453.

[474] S.M. Webb, X. Badia, M.J. Barahona, A. Colao, C.J. Strasburger, A. Tabarin, et al., Evaluation of health-related quality of life in patients with Cushing's syndrome with a new questionnaire, Eur J Endocrinol 158 (5) (2008) 623–630.

[475] P.W. Smith, K.C. Turza, C.O. Carter, M.L. Vance, E.R. Laws, J.B. Hanks, Bilateral adrenalectomy for refractory Cushing disease: A safe and definitive therapy, J Am Coll Surg 208 (6) (2009) 1059–1064.

[476] S.K. Thompson, A.V. Hayman, W.H. Ludlam, C.W. Deveney, D.L. Loriaux, B.C. Sheppard, Improved quality of life after bilateral laparoscopic adrenalectomy for Cushing's disease: A 10-year experience, Ann Surg 245 (5) (2007) 790–794.

[477] J.P. Luton, G. Strauch, D. Salmon, M. Linard, H. Bricaire, Etude de la glycorégulation au cours des syndromes de Cushing avant et après thérapeutique. Journées endocrinologiques de Langue Française, Paris. La Revue Française d'Endocrinologie Clinique, Nutrition et Métabolisme 1973; 4: 315–320.

[478] T. Mancini, B. Kola, F. Mantero, M. Boscaro, G. Arnaldi, High cardiovascular risk in patients with Cushing's syndrome according to 1999 WHO/ISH guidelines, Clin Endocrinol (Oxf) 61 (6) (2004) 768–777.

[479] A. Sartorio, B. Ambrosi, P. Colombo, F. Morabito, G. Faglia, Osteocalcin levels in Cushing's disease before and after treatment, Horm Metab Res 20 (1998) 70.

[480] G.H. Anderson Jr, N. Blakeman, D.H. Streeten, The effect of age on prevalence of secondary forms of hypertension in 4429 consecutively referred patients, J Hypertens 12 (5) (1994) 609–615.

[481] M. Omura, J. Saito, K. Yamaguchi, Y. Kakuta, T. Nishikawa, Prospective study on the prevalence of secondary hypertension among hypertensive patients visiting a general outpatient clinic in Japan, Hypertens Res 27 (3) (2004) 193–202.

[482] R.D. Brown, G.R. Van Loon, D.N. Orth, G.W. Liddle, Cushing's disease with periodic hormonogenesis: One explanation for paradoxical response to dexamethasone, J Clin Endocrinol Metab 36 (1973) 445–451.

[483] B. Liberman, B.L. Wajchenberg, M.A. Tambascia, C.H. Mesquita, Periodic remission in Cushing's disease with paradoxical dexamethasone response: An expression of periodic hormonogenesis, J Clin Endocrinol Metab 43 (1976) 913–918.

[484] D.E. Schteingart, A.L. McKenzie, Twelve-hour cycles of adrenocorticotropin and cortisol secretion in Cushing's disease, J Clin Endocrinol Metab 51 (1980) 1195–1198.

[485] A.H. Vagnucci, E. Evans, Cushing's disease with intermittent hypercortisolism, Am J Med 80 (1986) 83–88.

[486] H.U. Schweikert, H.L. Fehm, R. Fahlbusch, et al., Cyclic Cushing's syndrome combined with cortisol suppressible, dexamethasone non-suppressible ACTH secretion: A new variant of Cushing's syndrome, Acta Endocrinol 110 (1985) 289–295.

[487] K.I. Alexandraki, G.A. Kaltsas, A.M. Isidori, S.A. Akker, W.M. Drake, S.L. Chew, et al., The prevalence and characteristic features of cyclicity and variability in Cushing's disease, Eur J Endocrinol 160 (6) (2009) 1011–1018.

[488] O. Kuchel, E. Bolte, M. Chretien, et al., Cyclical edema and hypokalemia due to occult episodic hypercorticism, J Clin Endocrinol Metab 64 (1987) 170–174.

[489] M.H. Laudat, S. Cerdas, C. Fournier, D. Guiban, B. Guilhaume, J.P. Luton, Salivary cortisol measurement: A practical approach to assess pituitary–adrenal function, J Clin Endocrinol Metab 66 (1988) 343–348.

[490] A.R. Hermus, G.F. Pieters, G.F. Borm, et al., Unpredictable hypersecretion of cortisol in Cushing's disease: Detection by daily salivary cortisol measurements, Acta Endocrinol 5 (1993) 428–432.

[491] M.C. Raux-Demay, F. Girard, Hyperfonctionnement corticosurrénalien, in: J. Bertrand, R. Rappaport, P.C. Sizonenko (Eds.), Endocrinologie Pediatrique, Payot, Lausanne, 1982, pp. 471–481.

[492] W.L. Miller, J.J. Townsend, M.M. Grumbach, A.L. Kaplan, An infant with Cushing's disease due to an adrenocorticotropin-producing pituitary adenoma, J Clin Endocrinol Metab 48 (1979) 1017–1025.

[493] H. Stegner, D.K. Ludecke, M. Kadrnka-Lovrencie, N. Stahnke, R.P. Willig, Cushing's disease due to an unusually large adenoma of the pituitary gland in infancy, Eur J Pediatr 143 (1985) 221–223.

[494] D.M. Styne, M.M. Grumbach, S.L. Kaplan, C.B. Wilson, F.A. Conte, Treatment of Cushing's disease in childhood and adolescence by transsphenoidal micoradenomectomy, N Engl J Med 310 (1984) 889–893.

[495] D. Batista, M. Gennari, J. Riar, R. Chang, M.F. Keil, E.H. Oldfield, et al., An assessment of petrosal sinus sampling for localization of pituitary microadenomas in children with Cushing disease, J Clin Endocrinol Metab 91 (1) (2006) 221–224.

[496] D.C. Aron, A.M. Schnall, L.R. Sheeler, Cushing's syndrome and pregnancy, Am J Obstet Gynecol 162 (1990) 244–252.

[497] J. Pickart, A.L. Jochen, C.N. Sadur, F.D. Hofeldt, Cushing's syndrome in pregnancy, Obstet Gynecol Surv 45 (1990) 87–93.

[498] J.R. Lindsay, L.K. Nieman, The hypothalamic–pituitary–adrenal axis in pregnancy: Challenges in disease detection and treatment, Endocr Rev 26 (6) (2005) 775–799.

[499] J.R. Lindsay, J. Jonklaas, E.H. Oldfield, L.K. Nieman, Cushing's syndrome during pregnancy: Personal experience and review of the literature, J Clin Endocrinol Metab 90 (5) (2005) 3077–3083.

[500] M.H. Laudat, B. Guilhaume, P. Blot, C. Fournier, J.P. Giauque, J.P. Luton, Etat hormonal de la grossess: Modification du cortisol et de la testostérone, Ann Endocrinol 48 (1987) 334–338.

[501] A. Viardot, P. Huber, J.J. Puder, H. Zulewski, U. Keller, B. Müller, Reproducibility of nighttime salivary cortisol and its use in the diagnosis of hypercortisolism compared with urinary free cortisol and overnight dexamethasone suppression test, J Clin Endocrinol Metab 90 (10) (2005) 5730–5736.

[502] M.J.J. Gormley, D.R. Haden, T.L. Kennedy, D.A.D. Montgomery, G.A. Murnaghan, B. Sheridan, Cushing's syndrome in pregnancy treatment with metyrapone, Clin Endocrinol (1982) 283–293.

[503] I.F. Casson, J.C. Davis, R.V. Jeffreys, J.H. Silas, J. Williams, P.E. Bekchetz, Successful management of Cushing's disease during pregnancy by transsphenoidal adenectomy, Clin Endocrinol 27 (1987) 423–428.

[504] D.C. Aron, A.M. Schnall, L.R. Sheeler, Spontaneous resolution of Cushing's syndrome after pregnancy, Am J Obstet Gynecol 162 (1990) 472–474.

[505] N.A. Pocock, J.A. Eisman, C.R. Dunstan, R.A. Evans, D.J. Thomas, N.L. Huq, Recovery from steroid-induced osteoporosis, Ann Intern Med 107 (1987) 319–323.

[506] J.W. Findling, J.B. Tyrrell, D.C. Aron, P.A. Fitzgerald, C.B. Wilson, P.H. Forsham, Silent pituitary apoplexy: Subclinical infarction of an adrenocorticotropin-producing pituitary adenoma, J Clin Endocrinol Metab 52 (1981) 95–97.

[507] K.A. La Civita, S. McDonald, Cyclic Cushing's disease in association with a pituitary stone, South Med J 82 (1989) 1174–1176.

[508] L. Crapo, Cushing's syndrome: A review of diagnostic tests, Metabolism 28 (1979) 955–977.

[509] M. Klose, M. Lange, A.K. Rasmussen, N.E. Skakkebaek, L. Hilsted, E. Haug, et al., Factors influencing the adrenocorticotropin test: Role of contemporary cortisol assays, body composition, and oral contraceptive agents, J Clin Endocrinol Metab 92 (4) (2007) 1326–1333.

[510] D.H.P. Streeten, C.T. Stevenson, T.G. Dalakos, J.J. Nicholas, L.G. Dennick, H. Fellerman, The diagnosis of hypercortisolism. Biochemical criteria differentiating patients from lean and obese normal subjects and from females on oral contraceptives, J Clin Endocrinol Metab 29 (1969) 1191–1211.

[511] R.L. Eddy, A.L. Jones, P.F. Gilliland, J.D. Ibarra Jr., J.Q. Thompson, J.F. McMurry, Cushing's syndrome: A prospective study of diagnostic methods, Am J Med 55 (1973) 621–630.

[512] D.A. Papanicolaou, J.A. Yahovski, G.B. Cutler, G.P. Chrousos, L.K. Nieman, A single midnight serum cortisol measurement distinguishes Cushing's syndrome from pseudo-Cushing states, J Clin Endocrinol Metab 83 (1998) 1163–1167.

[513] P. Putignano, P. Toja, A. Dubini, F. Pecori Giraldi, S.M. Corsello, F. Cavagnini, Midnight salivary cortisol versus urinary free and midnight serum cortisol as screening tests for Cushing's syndrome, J Clin Endocrinol Metab 88 (2003) 4153–4157.

[514] G. Reimondo, B. Allasino, S. Bovio, P. Paccotti, A. Angeli, M. Terzolo, Evaluation of the effectiveness of midnight serum cortisol in the diagnostic procedures for Cushing's syndrome, Eur J Endocrinol 153 (2005) 803–809.

[515] F. Pecori Giraldi, A.G. Ambrogio, M. De Martin, L.M. Fatti, M. Scacchi, F. Cavagnini, Specificity of first-line tests for the diagnosis of Cushing's syndrome: Assessment in a large series, J Clin Endocrinol Metab 92 (2007) 4123–4129.

[516] M.B. Elamin, M.H. Murad, R. Mullan, D. Erickson, K. Harris, S. Nadeem, et al., Accuracy of diagnostic tests for Cushing's syndrome: A systematic review and metaanalyses, J Clin Endocrinol Metab 93 (2008) 1553–1562.

[517] L.K. Nieman, B.M. Biller, J.W. Findling, J. Newell-Price, M.O. Savage, P.M. Stewart, et al., The diagnosis of Cushing's syndrome: An Endocrine Society Clinical Practice Guideline, J Clin Endocrinol Metab 93 (5) (2008) 1526–1540.

[518] T. Nichols, C.A. Nugent, F.H. Tyler, Steroid laboratory tests in the diagnosis of Cushing's syndrome, Am J Med 45 (1968) 116–128.

[519] X. Bertagna, M. Donnadieu, M. Binoux, F. Girard, Dynamics and characterization of immunoreactive β-MSH in hemodialysis patients. Its relationship to ACTH, J Clin Endocrinol Metab 45 (1977) 1179–1186.

[520] Z. Zadik, L. De Lacerda, A.A. Kowarski, Evaluation of the 6-hour integrated concentration of cortisol as a diagnostic procedure for Cushing's syndrome, J Clin Endocrinol Metab 54 (1982) 1072–1074.

[521] M. Follenius, G. Brandenberger, Plasma free cortisol during secretory episodes, J Clin Endocrinol Metab 62 (1986) 609–612.

[522] P. Robin, J. Predine, E. Milgrom, Assay of unbound cortisol in plasma, J Clin Endocrinol Metab 46 (1978) 277–283.

[523] T. Umeda, R. Hiramatsu, T. Iwaoka, T. Shimadda, F. Miura, T. Sato, Use of saliva for monitoring unbound free cortisol levels in serum, Clin Chim Acta 110 (1981) 245–253.

[524] J.E. Shipley, N.E. Alessi, S.E. Wade, A.D. Haegele, B. Helmbold, Utility of an oral diffusion sink (ODS) device for quantification of saliva corticosteroids in human subjects, J Clin Endocrinol Metab 74 (1992) 698–700.

[525] R.F. Vining, R.A. McGinley, J.J. Maksvytis, K. Yho, Salivary cortisol: A better measure of adrenal cortical function than serum cortisol, Ann Clin Biochem 20 (1983) 329–335.

[526] M. Yaneva, H. Mosnier-Pudar, M.A. Dugué, S. Grabar, Y. Fulla, X. Bertagna, Midnight salivary cortisol for the initial diagnosis of Cushing's syndrome of various causes, J Clin Endocrinol Metab 89 (7) (2004) 3345–3351.

[527] H. Raff, J.L. Raff, J.W. Findling, Late-night salivary cortisol as a screening test for Cushing's syndrome, J Clin Endocrinol Metab 83 (8) (1998) 2681–2686.

[528] C.J. Migeon, O.C. Green, J.P. Eckert, Study of adrenocortical function in obesity, Metabolism 12 (1963) 718–739.

[529] J.A. Prezio, G. Carreon, E. Clerkin, C.R. Meloni, L.H. Kyle, J.J. Canary, Influence of body composition on adrenal function in obesity, J Clin Endocrinol Metab 24 (1964) 481–485.

[530] G.W. Liddle, K.L. Melmon, The adrenals, in: R.H. Williams (Ed.), Textbook of Endocrinology, fifth edn., WB Saunders, Philadelphia, 1974, pp. 233–322.

[531] A.N. Elias, G. Gwinup, Effects of some clinically encountered drugs on steroid synthesis and degradation, Metabolism 29 (1980) 582–595.

[532] T. Bledsoe, D.P. Island, R.L. Ney, G.W. Liddle, An effect of op'DDD on the extra-adrenal metabolism of cortisol in man, J Clin Endocrinol Metab 24 (1964) 1303–1311.

[533] J. Lindholm, Studies on some parameters of adrenocortical function, Acta Endocrinol 72 (1973) 1–155.

[534] C.G. Beardwell, C.W. Burke, C.L. Cope, Urinary free cortisol measured by competitive protein binding, J Endocrinol 43 (1968) 79–89.

[535] B.E.P. Murphy, Clinical evaluation of urinary cortisol determinations by competitive protein-binding radioassay, J Clin Endocrinol Metab 28 (1968) 343–348.

[536] G. Vidal-Trecan, M.H. Laudat, P. Thornopoulos, J.P. Luton, H. Bricaire, Urinary free corticoids: An evaluation of their usefulness in the diagnosis of Cushing's syndrome, Acta Endocrinol 103 (1983) 110–115.

[537] J. Kobberling, A. Von Zur Muhlen, The circadian rhythm of free cortisol determined by urine sampling at two-hour intervals in normal subjects and in patients with severe obesity or Cushing's syndrome, J Clin Endocrinol Metab 38 (1973) 313–319.

[538] M.H. Laudat, L. Billaud, P. Thomopoulos, O. Vera, A. Yllia, J.P. Luton, Evening urinary free corticoids: A screening test in Cushing's syndrome and incidentally discovered adrenal tumours, Acta Endocrinol 119 (1988) 459–464.

[539] N.V. Esteban, T. Loughlin, A.L. Yergey, et al., Daily cortisol production rate in man determined by stable isotope dilution/mass spectrometry, J Clin Endocrinol Metab 71 (1991) 39–45.

[540] J.A. Yanovski, G.B. Cutler Jr, G.P. Chrousos, L.K. Nieman, Corticotropin-releasing hormone stimulation following low-dose dexamethasone administration. A new test to distinguish Cushing's syndrome from pseudo-Cushing's states, JAMA 269 (17) (1993) 2232–2238.

[541] L. Kennedy, A.B. Atkinson, H. Johnston, B. Sheridan, D.R. Hadden, Serum cortisol concentrations during low dose dexamethasone suppression test to screen for Cushing's syndrome, Br Med J 289 (1984) 1188–1191.

[542] W.W. Luthold, J.A. Marcondes, B.L. Wajchenberg, Salivary cortisol for the evaluation of Cushing's syndrome, Clin Chim Acta 151 (1985) 33–39.

[543] P.C. Hindmarsh, C.G. Brook, Single dose dexamethasone suppression test in children: Dose relationship to body size, Clin Endocrinol 23 (1985) 67–70.

[544] C.A. Nugent, T. Nichols, F.H. Tyler, Diagnosis of Cushing's syndrome — single dose dexamethasone suppression test, Arch Intern Med 116 (1965) 172–176.

[545] C. Cronin, D. Igoe, M.J. Duffy, S.K. Cunningham, T.J. McKenna, The overnight dexamethasone test is a worthwhile screening procedure, Clin Endocrinol 33 (1990) 27–33.

[546] V.H.T. James, J. Landon, V. Wynn, Oral and intravenous suppression tests in the diagnosis of Cushing's syndrome, J Endocrinol 33 (1965) 515–524.

[547] A.B. Abou-Samra, H. Dechaud, B. Estom, et al., β-Lipotropin and cortisol responses to an intravenous infusion of dexamethasone suppression test in Cushing's syndrome and obesity, J Clin Endocrinol Metab 61 (1985) 116–119.

[548] A.B. Atkinson, E.J. McAteer, D.R. Hadden, L. Kennedy, B. Sheridan, A.I. Traub, A weight-related intravenous dexamethasone suppression test distinguishes obese controls from patients with Cushing's syndrome, Acta Endocrinol 120 (1989) 753–759.

[549] D.N. Orth, Adrenocortictropic hormone (ACTH), in: B.M. Jaffe, H.R. Behrman (Eds.), Methods of Hormone Radioimmunoassay, Academic Press, New York, 1979, pp. 245–284.

[550] G.M. Besser, D.N. Orth, W.E. Nicholson, R.L. Bynny, K. Abe, J.P. Woodham, Dissociation of disappearance of bioactive and radioimmunoreactive ACTH from plasma in man, J Clin Endocrinol Metab 32 (1971) 595–603.

[551] R.J. Lefkowtiz, J. Roth, I. Pastan, Radio-receptor assay of adrenocorticotropic hormone: New approach to assay of polypeptide hormone in plasma, Science 170 (1970) 633–635.

[552] J. Chayen, N. Loveridge, J.R. Daly, A sensitive bioassay for adrenocorticotrophic hormone in human plasma, Clin Endocrinol 1 (1972) 219–233.

[553] S.C. Hodgkinson, B. Allolio, J. Landon, P.J. Lowry, Development of a non-extracted "two-site" immunoradiometric assay for corticotropin utilizing extreme amino- and carboxy-terminally directed antibodies, Biochem J 218 (1984) 703–711.

[554] J.W. Findling, W.C. Engeland, H. Raff, The use of immunoradiometricassay for the measurement of ACTH in human plasma, Trends Endocrinol Metab 1 (1990) 283–287.

[555] H. Raff, J.W. Findling, J. Wong, Short loop adrenocorticotropin feedback after ACTH 1–24 in injection in man is an artifact of the immunoradiometric assay, J Clin Endocrinol Metab 69 (1989) 678–680.

[556] P.M. Horrock, D.R. London, Diagnostic value of 9 am plasma adrenocorticotrophic hormone concentrations in Cushing's disease, Br Med J 285 (1982) 1302–1303.

[557] J. Hope, S.J. Ratter, F.E. Estivariz, L. McLoughlin, P.J. Lowry, Development of a radioimmunoassay for an amino-terminal peptide of pro-opiocortin containing the gamma-MSH region: Measurement and characterization in human plasma, Clin Endocrinol 15 (1981) 221–227.

[558] J.S.D. Chan, N.G. Seidah, M. Chretien, Measurement of N-terminal (1–76) of human proopiomelanocortin in human plasma: Correlation with adrenocorticotropin, J Clin Endocrinol Metab 56 (1983) 791–796.

[559] M. Phlipponneau, F. Lenne, M.F. Proeschel, F. Girard, J.P. Luton, X. Bertagna, Plasma immunoreactive joining peptide in man: A new marker of proopiomelanocortin processing and corticotroph function, J Clin Endocrinol Metab 76 (1993) 325–329.

[560] J.J.H. Gilkes, L.H. Rees, G.M. Besser, Plasma immunoreactive corticotrophin and lipotrophin in Cushing's syndrome and Addison's disease, Br Med J 1 (1977) 996–998.

[561] E. Wiedemann, T. Saito, J.A. Linfoot, C.H. Li, Radio-immunoassay for human β-lipotropin in unextracted plasma, J Clin Endocrinol Metab 45 (1977) 1108–1111.

[562] D.T. Krieger, A.S. Liotta, T. Suda, A. Goodgold, E. London, Human plasma immunoreactive lipotropin and adrenocorticotropin in normal subjects and in patients with pituitary—adrenal disease, J Clin Endocrinol Metab 48 (1979) 566–571.

[563] E. Wiedemann, T. Saito, J.A. Linfoot, C.H. Li, Specific radioimmunoassay of human β-endorphin in unextracted plasma, J Clin Endocrinol Metab 49 (1979) 478–480.

[564] R. Smith, A. Grossman, R. Gaillard, et al., Studies on circulating metenkephalin and β-endorphin: Normal subjects and patients with renal and adrenal disease, Clin Endocrinol 15 (1981) 291–300.

[565] D.M. Halpin, J.M. Burrin, G.F. Joplin, Serum testosterone levels in women with Cushing's disease, Acta Endocrinol 122 (1990) 71–75.

[566] S.R. Crosby, M.F. Stewart, J.G. Ratcliffe, A. White, Direct measurement of the precursors of adrenocorticotropin in human plasma by two-site immunoradiometric assay, J Clin Endocrinol Metab 67 (1988) 1272–1277.

[567] P.J. Lowry, E.A. Linton, S.C. Hodgkinson, Analysis of peptide hormones of the hypothalamic–pituitary–adrenal axis using "two-site" immunoradiometric assays, Horm Res 32 (1989) 25–29.

[568] M.S. Zemskova, E.S. Nylen, N.J. Patronas, E.H. Oldfield, K.L. Becker, L.K. Nieman, Diagnostic accuracy of chromogranin A and calcitonin precursors measurements for the discrimination of ectopic ACTH secretion from Cushing's disease, J Clin Endocrinol Metab 94 (8) (2009) 2962–2965.

[569] M.R. Flack, E.H. Oldfield, G.B. Cutler Jr., M.H. Zweig, J.D. Malley, G.P. Chrousos, et al., Urine free cortisol in the high-dose dexamethasone suppression test for the differential diagnosis of the Cushing syndrome, Ann Intern Med 116 (3) (1992) 211–217.

[570] E. Odagiri, R. Demura, H. Demura, et al., The changes in plasma cortisol and urinary free cortisol by an overnight dexamethasone suppression test in patients with Cushing's disease, Endocrinol Jpn 35 (1988) 795–802.

[571] T.A. Howlett, P.L. Drury, L. Perry, I. Doniach, L.H. Ress, G.M. Besser, Diagnosis and management of ACTH-dependent Cushing's syndrome: Comparison of the features in ectopic and pituitary ACTH production, Clin Endocrinol 24 (1986) 699–713.

[572] R.E. Bailey, Periodic hormonogenesis — a new phenomenon. Periodicity in function of a hormone-producing tumor in man, J Clin Endocrinol Metab 32 (1971) 317–327.

[573] B. Liberman, B.L. Wajchenberg, M.A. Tambascia, C.H. Mesquita, Periodic remission in Cushing's disease with paradoxical dexamethasone response: An expression of periodic hormonogenesis, J Clin Endocrinol Metab 43 (1976) 913–918.

[574] J.B. Tyrrell, J.W. Findling, D.C. Aron, P.A. Fitzgerald, P.H. Forsham, An overnight high-dose dexamethasone suppression test for rapid differential diagnosis of Cushing's syndrome, Ann Intern Med 104 (1986) 180–186.

[575] T.B. Kaye, L. Crapo, The Cushing syndrome: An update on diagnostic tests, Ann Intern Med 112 (1990) 434–444.

[576] R.J.M. Croughs, R. Docter, F.H. DeJong, Comparison of oral and intravenous dexamethasone suppression tests in the differential diagnosis of Cushing's syndrome, Acta Endocrinol 72 (1973) 54–62.

[577] G.W. Liddle, H.L. Estet, J.W. Kendall, W.C. Williams, A.W. Townes, Clinical application of a new test of pituitary reserve, J Clin Endocrinol Metab 19 (1959) 875–894.

[578] D.H.P. Streeten, G.H. Anderson, T.G. Dalakos, et al., Normal and abnormal function of the hypothalamic—pituitary—adrenocortical system in man, Endocr Rev 5 (1984) 371–394.

[579] M. Spiger, W. Jubiz, A.W. Meikle, C.D. West, F.H. Tyler, Single-dose metyrapone test: Review of a four-year experience, Arch Intern Med 135 (1975) 698–700.

[580] A.B. Abou-Samra, M. Fevre-Montange, M. Pugeat, et al., The value of β-lipotrophin measurement during the short metyrapone test in patients with pituitary diseases and in Cushing's syndrome, Acta Endocrinol 105 (1984) 441–448.

[581] D.A. Malerbi, B.B. Mendonca, B. Liberman, S.P. Toledo, M.C. Corradini, M.B. Cunha-Neto, et al., The desmopressin stimulation test in the differential diagnosis of Cushing's syndrome, Clin Endocrinol (Oxf) 38 (1993) 463–472.

[582] M. Moro, P. Putignano, M. Losa, C. Invitti, C. Maraschini, F. Cavagnini, The desmopressin test in the differential diagnosis between Cushing's disease and pseudo-Cushing states, J Clin Endocrinol Metab 85 (2000) 3569–3574.

[583] P.L. Dahia, A.B. Grossman, The molecular pathogenesis of corticotroph tumors, Endocr Rev. 20 (2) (1999) 136–155.

[584] M. Losa, P. Mortini, S. Dylgjeri, R. Barzaghi, A. Franzin, C. Mandelli, et al., Desmopressin stimulation test before and after pituitary surgery in patients with Cushing's disease, Clin Endocrinol (Oxf) 55 (2001) 61–68.

[585] P. Colombo, C. Dall'Asta, L. Barbetta, et al., Usefulness of the desmopressin test in the post-operative evaluation of patients with Cushing's disease, Eur J Endocrinol 143 (2000) 227–234.

[586] D.N. Orth, Corticotropin-releasing hormone in humans, Endocr Rev 13 (1992) 164–191.

[587] A. Grossman, A.C. Nieuwenhuyzen Kruseman, L. Perry, et al., New hypothalamic hormone, corticotropin releasing factor, specifically stimulates the release of adrenocorticotrophic hormone and cortisol in men, Lancet (1982) 921–922.

[588] S.J. Watson, J.F. Lopez, E.A. Young, W. Vale, J. Rivier, R.A. Knazek, Effects of low dose oCRH in humans: Endocrine relationships and beta-endorphin-beta lipotropin responses, J Clin Endocrinol Metab 66 (1988) 10–15.

[589] L.K. Nieman, G.B. Cutler, E.H. Oldfield, D.L. Loriaux, G.P. Chrousos, The ovine corticotropin-releasing hormone (CRH) stimulation test is superior to the human CRF stimulation test for the diagnosis of Cushing's disease, J Clin Endocrinol Metab 69 (1989) 165–169.

[590] G.P. Chrousos, L. Nieman, B. Nisula, et al., Corticotropin-releasing factor stimulation test, N Engl J Med 311 (1984) 471–473.

[591] L.K. Nieman, G.P. Chrousos, E.H. Oldfield, P.C. Avgerinos, G.B. Cutler, D.L. Loraux, The ovine corticotropin-releasing hormone stimulation test and the dexamethasone suppression test in the differential diagnosis of Cushing's syndrome, Ann Intern Med 105 (1986) 862–867.

[592] J. Newell-Price, A. Grossman, Diagnosis and management of Cushing's syndrome, Lancet 353 (1999) 2087–2088.

[593] M. Boscaro, A. Rampazzo, N. Sonino, G. Merola, M. Scanarini, F. Mantero, Corticotropin releasing hormone stimulation test: Diagnostic aspects in Cushing's syndrome, J Endocrinol Invest 10 (1987) 297–302.

[594] A.R. Hermus, G.F. Pieters, G.J. Pesman, A.G. Smals, T.J. Benraad, P.W. Kloppenborg, The corticotropin-releasing-hormone test versus the high dose dexamethasone test in the differential diagnosis of Cushing's syndrome, Lancet (1986) 540–544.

[595] H. Jorgensen, S. Skare, H. Frey, K.F. Hanssen, N. Norman, Effects of synthetic corticotropin-releasing factor in normal individuals and in patients with hypothalamic—pituitary—adrenocortical disorders, Acta Med Scand 218 (1985) 79–84.

[596] O.A. Muller, G.K. Stalla, K. Von Werder, Corticotropin-releasing-factor: A new tool for the differential diagnosis of Cushing's syndrome, J Clin Endocrinol Metab 57 (1983) 227–229.

[597] V. Schrell, R. Fahlbusch, M. Bushfelder, S. Riedi, G.K. Stall, O.A. Muller, Corticotropin-releasing hormone stimulation test before and after transsphenoidal selective micro-adenomectomy in 30 patients with Cushing's disease, J Clin Endocrinol Metab 64 (1987) 1150–1159.

[598] O.A. Muller, G.K. Stalla, K. Von Werder, CRH in Cushing's syndrome, Horm Metab Res 16 (1987) 51–58.

[599] D.N. Orth, Cushing's syndrome, N Engl J Med 332 (1995) 791–803.

[600] L.K. Nieman, E.H. Oldfield, R. Wesley, et al., A simplified morning ovine corticotropin-releasing hormone stimulation test for the differential diagnosis of ACTH-dependent Cushing's syndrome, J Clin Endocrinol Metab 77 (1993) 308–312.

[601] J. Newell-Price, D.G. Morris, W.M. Drake, M. Korbonits, J.P. Monson, G.M. Besser, et al., Optimal response criteria for the human CRH test in the differential diagnosis of ACTH-dependent Cushing's syndrome, J Clin Endocrinol Metab 87 (4) (2002) 1640–1645.

[602] A.B. Grossman, T.A. Howlett, L. Perry, et al., CRF in the differential diagnosis of Cushing's syndrome: A comparison with the dexamethasone suppression test, Clin Endocrinol 29 (1988) 167–178.

[603] M.I. Wiggam, A.P. Heaney, E.M. McIlrath, D.R. McCance, B. Sheridan, D.R. Hadden, et al., Bilateral inferior petrosal sinus sampling in the differential diagnosis of adrenocorticotropin-dependent Cushing's syndrome: A comparison with other diagnostic tests, J Clin Endocrinol Metab 85 (4) (2000) 1525–1532.

[604] I. Ilias, D.J. Torpy, K. Pacak, N. Mullen, R.A. Wesley, L.K. Nieman, Cushing's syndrome due to ectopic corticotropin secretion: Twenty years' experience at the National Institutes of Health, J Clin Endocrinol Metab 90 (8) (2005) 4955–4962.

[605] A.M. Isidori, G.A. Kaltsas, C. Pozza, V. Frajese, J. Newell-Price, R.H. Reznek, et al., The ectopic adrenocorticotropin syndrome: Clinical features, diagnosis, management, and long-term follow-up, J Clin Endocrinol Metab 91 (2) (2006) 371–377.

[606] C. Favrod-Coune, M.C. Raux-Demay, M.F. Proeschel, X. Bertagna, F. Girard, J.P. Luton, Potentiation of the classic ovine corticotrophin-releasing hormone stimulation test by the combined administration of small doses of lysine vasopressin, Clin Endocrinol 28 (1993) 405–410.

[607] G. Dickstein, C.R. DeBold, D. Gaitan, et al., Plasma ACTH and cortisol responses to ovine corticotropin-releasing hormone (CRF), arginine vasopressin (AVP), CRH plus AVP, and CRH plus metyrapone in patients with Cushing's disease, J Clin Endocrinol Metab 81 (1996) 2934–2941.

[608] J. Newell-Price, L. Perry, S. Medbak, J. Monson, M. Savage, M. Besser, et al., A combined test using desmopressin and corticotropin-releasing hormone in the differential diagnosis of Cushing's syndrome, J Clin Endocrinol Metab 82 (1) (1997) 176–181.

[609] S. Tsagarakis, C. Tsigos, V. Vasiliou, P. Tsiotra, J. Kaskarelis, C. Sotiropoulou, et al., The desmopressin and combined CRH-desmopressin tests in the differential diagnosis of ACTH-dependent Cushing's syndrome: Constraints imposed by the expression of V2 vasopressin receptors in tumors with ectopic ACTH secretion, J Clin Endocrinol Metab 87 (4) (2002) 1646–1653.

[610] H.M. Schulte, B. Allolio, R.W. Gunther, et al., Bilateral and simultaneous sinus petrosus inferior catheterization in patients with Cushing's syndrome: Plasma-immunoreactive-ACTH-concentrations before and after administration of CRF, Horm Metab Res 16 (1987) 66–67.

[611] E.H. Oldfield, J.L. Doppman, L.K. Nieman, et al., Petrosal sinus sampling with and without corticotrophin-releasing hormone for the differential diagnosis of Cushing's syndrome, N Engl J Med 325 (1991) 897–905.

[612] F. Vignati, M.E. Berselli, G. Scialfa, E. Boccardi, P. Loli, Bilateral and simultaneous venous sampling of inferior petrosal sinuses for ACTH and PRL determination: Preoperative localization of ACTH-secreting microadenomas, J Endocrinol Invest 12 (1989) 235–238.

[613] A.M. Landolt, A. Valavanis, J. Girard, A.N. Eberle, Corticotrophin-releasing factor-test used with bilateral, simultaneous inferior petrosal sinus blood-sampling for the diagnosis of pituitary-dependent Cushing's disease, Clin Endocrinol 25 (1986) 687–696.

[614] F.S. Bonelli, J. Huston III, P.C. Carpenter, et al., Adrenocorticotropic hormone-dependent Cushing's syndrome: Sensitivity and specificity of inferior petrosal sinus sampling, Am J Neuroradiol 21 (2000) 690–696.

[615] P.L. Semple, E.R. Laws, Complications in a contemporary series of patients who underwent transsphenoidal surgery for Cushing's disease, J Neurosurg 91 (1999) 175–179.

[616] J.W. Findling, M.E. Kehoe, J.L. Shaker, H. Raff, Routine inferior petrosal sinus sampling in the differential diagnosis of adrenocorticotropin (ACTH)-dependent Cushing's syndrome: Early recognition of the occult ectopic ACTH syndrome, J Clin Endocrinol Metab 73 (1991) 408–413.

[617] L. Bessac, I. Bachelot, A. Vasdev, et al., Le cathétérisme des sinus pétreux inférieurs. Sa place dans le diagnostic du syndrome de Cushing. Expérience de 23 explorations, Ann Endocrinol 53 (1992) 16–27.

[618] A. Tabarin, J.F. Greselle, F. San-Galli, et al., Usefulness of the corticotropin-releasing hormone test during bilateral inferior petrosal sinus sampling for the diagnosis of Cushing's disease, J Clin Endocrinol Metab 75 (1991) 53–59.

[619] M.I. Wiggam, A.P. Heaney, E.M. McIlrath, et al., Bilateral inferior petrosal sinus sampling in the differential diagnosis of adrenocorticotropin-dependent Cushing's syndrome: A comparison with other diagnostic tests, J Clin Endocrinol Metab 85 (2000) 1525–1532.

[620] E.H. Oldfield, G.P. Chrousos, H.M. Schulte, et al., Preoperative lateralization of ACTH-secreting pituitary microadenomas by bilateral and simultaneous inferior petrosal venous sinus sampling, N Engl J Med 312 (1985) 100–103.

[621] H.C. Taylor, M.E. Velasco, J.S. Brodkey, Remission of pituitary-dependent Cushing's disease after removal of nonneoplastic pituitary gland, Arch Intern Med 140 (1980) 1366–1368.

[622] A. Colao, A. Faggiano, R. Pivonello, F. Pecori Giraldi, F. Cavagnini, G. Lombardi, Study Group of the Italian Endocrinology Society on the Pathophsiology of the Hypothalamic–Pituitary–Adrenal Axis. Inferior petrosal sinus sampling in the differential diagnosis of Cushing's syndrome: results of an Italian multicenter study, Eur J Endocrinol 144 (5) (2001) 499–507.

[623] B. Swearingen, L. Katznelson, K. Miller, S. Grinspoon, A. Waltman, D.J. Dorer, et al., Diagnostic errors after inferior petrosal sinus sampling, J Clin Endocrinol Metab 89 (8) (2004) 3752–3763.

[624] R.M. Testa, N. Albiger, G. Occhi, F. Sanguin, M. Scanarini, S. Berlucchi, et al., The usefulness of combined biochemical tests in the diagnosis of Cushing's disease with negative pituitary magnetic resonance imaging, Eur J Endocrinol 156 (2) (2007) 241–248.

[625] S. Jehle, J.E. Walsh, P.U. Freda, K.D. Post, Selective use of bilateral inferior petrosal sinus sampling in patients with adrenocorticotropin-dependent Cushing's syndrome prior to transsphenoidal surgery, J Clin Endocrinol Metab 93 (12) (2008) 4624–4632.

[626] G.A. Kaltsas, M.G. Giannulis, J.D. Newell-Price, J.E. Dacie, C. Thakkar, F. Afshar, et al., A critical analysis of the value of simultaneous inferior petrosal sinus sampling in Cushing's disease and the occult ectopic adrenocorticotropin syndrome, J Clin Endocrinol Metab 84 (2) (1999) 487–492.

[627] J.W. Findling, M.E. Kehoe, H. Raff, Identification of patients with Cushing's disease with negative pituitary adrenocorticotropin gradients during inferior petrosal sinus sampling: Prolactin as an index of pituitary venous effluent, J Clin Endocrinol Metab 89 (12) (2004) 6005–6009.

[628] V. Lefournier, M. Martinie, A. Vasdev, P. Bessou, J.G. Passagia, F. Labat-Moleur, et al., Accuracy of bilateral inferior petrosal or cavernous sinuses sampling in predicting the lateralization of Cushing's disease pituitary microadenoma: Influence of catheter position and anatomy of venous drainage, J Clin Endocrinol Metab 88 (1) (2003) 196–203.

[629] J. Young, C. Deneux, M. Grino, C. Oliver, P. Chanson, G. Schaison, Pitfall of petrosal sinus sampling in a Cushing's syndrome secondary to ectopic adrenocorticotropin-corticotropin releasing hormone (ACTH-CRH) secretion, J Clin Endocrinol Metab 83 (2) (1998) 305–308.

[630] D.L. Miller, J.L. Doppman, S.B. Peterman, L.K. Nieman, E.H. Oldfield, R. Chang, Neurologic complications of petrosal sinus sampling, Radiology 185 (1) (1992) 143–147.

[631] D.C. Aron, J.W. Findling, J.B. Tyrrell, Cushing's disease, Endocrinol Metab Clin North Am 16 (1987) 705–730.

[632] V. Lefournier, B. Gatta, M. Martinie, A. Vasdev, A. Tabarin, P. Bessou, et al., One transient neurological complication (sixth nerve palsy) in 166 consecutive inferior petrosal sinus samplings for the etiological diagnosis of Cushing's syndrome, J Clin Endocrinol Metab 84 (9) (1999) 3401–3402.

[633] C.D. Gandhi, S.A. Meyer, A.B. Patel, D.M. Johnson, K.D. Post, Neurologic complications of inferior petrosal sinus sampling, Am J Neuroradiol 29 (4) (2008) 760–765.

[634] F.S. Bonelli, J. Huston 3rd, F.B. Meyer, P.C. Carpenter, Venous subarachnoid hemorrhage after inferior petrosal sinus sampling for adrenocorticotropic hormone, Am J Neuroradiol 20 (2) (1999) 306–307.

[635] A. Teramoto, S. Nemoto, K. Takakura, Y. Sasaki, T. Machida, Selective venous sampling directly from cavernous sinus in Cushing's syndrome, J Clin Endocrinol Metab 76 (1993) 637–641.

[636] J.L. Doppman, E.H. Oldfield, L.K. Nieman, Bilateral sampling of the internal jugular vein to distinguish between mechanisms of adrenocorticotropic hormone-dependent Cushing syndrome, Ann Intern Med 128 (1) (1998) 33–36.

[637] D. Erickson, J. Huston 3rd, W.F. Young Jr., P.C. Carpenter, R.A. Wermers, F.S. Bonelli, et al., Internal jugular vein sampling in adrenocorticotropic hormone-dependent Cushing's syndrome: A comparison with inferior petrosal sinus sampling, Clin Endocrinol (Oxf) 60 (4) (2004) 413–419.

[638] I. Ilias, R. Chang, K. Pacak, E.H. Oldfield, R. Wesley, J. Doppman, et al., Jugular venous sampling: An alternative to petrosal sinus sampling for the diagnostic evaluation of adrenocorticotropic hormone-dependent Cushing's syndrome, J Clin Endocrinol Metab 89 (8) (2004) 3795–3800.

[639] M.C. Machado, S.V. de Sa, S. Domenice, M.C. Fragoso, P. Puglia Jr., M.A. Pereira, et al., The role of desmopressin in bilateral and simultaneous inferior petrosal sinus sampling for differential diagnosis of ACTH-dependent Cushing's syndrome, Clin Endocrinol (Oxf) 66 (1) (2007) 136–142.

[640] F. Castinetti, I. Morange, H. Dufour, P. Jaquet, B. Conte-Devolx, N. Girard, et al., Desmopressin test during petrosal sinus sampling: A valuable tool to discriminate pituitary or ectopic ACTH-dependent Cushing's syndrome, Eur J Endocrinol 157 (3) (2007) 271–277.

[641] G.P. Chrousos, T.H. Schuermeyer, J. Doppman, et al., NIH conference. Clinical applications of corticotropin-releasing factor, Ann Intern Med 102 (1985) 344–358.

[642] L.S. Jackson, E.R. Savolaine, R. Franco-Saenz, False lateralization of a pituitary microadenoma, Ann Intern Med 108 (1988) 767–768.
[643] H.M. Schulte, B. Allolio, R.W. Gunther, et al., Selective bilateral and simultaneous catheterization of the inferior petrosal sinus: CRF stimulates prolactin secretion from ACTH-producing microadenomas in Cushing's disease, Clin Endocrinol 28 (1988) 289–295.
[644] B. Allolio, R.W. Gunther, G. Benker, D. Reinwein, W. Winkelmann, H.M. Schulte, A multihormonal response to corticotropin-releasing hormone in inferior petrosal sinus blood of patients with Cushing's disease, J Clin Endocrinol Metab 71 (1990) 1195–1203.
[645] P.A. Crock, R.G. Pestell, A.J. Calenti, et al., Multiple pituitary hormone gradients from inferior petrosal sinus sampling in Cushing's disease, Acta Endocrinol 119 (1988) 75–80.
[646] D.P. MacErlean, F.H. Doyle, The pituitary fossa in Cushing's syndrome. A retrospective analysis of 93 patients, Br J Radiol 49 (1976) 820–826.
[647] S.C. Saris, N.J. Patronas, J.L. Doppman, et al., Cushing's syndrome: Pituitary CT scanning, Radiology 162 (1987) 775–777.
[648] S. Marcovitz, R. Wee, J. Chan, J. Hardy, The diagnostic accuracy of preoperative CT scanning in the evaluation of pituitary ACTH-secreting adenomas, Am J Roentgenol 149 (1987) 803–806.
[649] W.F. Chandler, D.E. Schteingart, R.V. LLoyd, P.E. McKeever, G. Ibarra-Perez, Surgical treatment of Cushing's disease, J Neurosurg 66 (1987) 204–212.
[650] J.W. Findling, J.B. Tyrrell, Occult ectopic secretion of corticotropin, Arch Intern Med 146 (1986) 929–933.
[651] J.E. Boggan, J.B. Tyrrell, C.B. Wilson, Transsphenoidal microsurgical management of Cushing's disease, J Neurosurg 59 (1983) 195–200.
[652] A.J. Dwyer, J.A. Frank, J.L. Doppman, et al., Pituitary adenomas in patients with Cushing disease: Initial experience with Gd-DTPA-enhanced MR imaging, Radiology 163 (1987) 421–426.
[653] W.W. Peck, W.P. Dillon, D. Norman, T.H. Newton, C.B. Wilson, MR high-resolution, imaging of pituitary microadenomas at 1.5 T: Experience with Cushing's disease, Am J Roentgenol 152 (1989) 145–151.
[654] J.L. Doppman, J.A. Frank, A.J. Dwyer, et al., Gadolinium DTPA enhanced MR imaging of ACTH-secreting microadenomas of the pituitary gland, J Comput Assist Tomogr 12 (1988) 728–735.
[655] M. Buchfelder, R. Nistor, R. Fahlbusch, W.J. Huk, The accuracy of CT and MR evaluation of the sella turcica for detection of adrenocorticotropic hormone-secreting adenomas in Cushing disease, Am J Neuroradiol 14 (5) (1993) 1183–1190.
[656] C. Invitti, F. Pecori Giraldi, M. de Martin, F. Cavagnini, Diagnosis and management of Cushing's syndrome: Results of an Italian multicentre study. Study Group of the Italian Society of Endocrinology on the pathophysiology of the hypothalamic–pituitary–adrenal axis, J Clin Endocrinol Metab 84 (2) (1999) 440–448.
[657] A. Tabarin, F. Laurent, B. Catargi, F. Olivier-Puel, R. Lescene, J. Berge, et al., Comparative evaluation of conventional and dynamic magnetic resonance imaging of the pituitary gland for the diagnosis of Cushing's disease, Clin Endocrinol (Oxf) 49 (3) (1998) 293–300.
[658] W.A. Hall, M.G. Luciano, J.L. Doppman, N.J. Patronas, E.H. Oldfield, Pituitary magnetic resonance imaging in normal human volunteers: Occult adenomas in the general population, Ann Intern Med 120 (10) (1994) 817–820.
[659] A. Venot, J.P. Luton, P.H. Bouchard, J.C. Roucayrol, H. Bricaire, Original scintigraphic patterns with radiocholesterol and post Op'DDD results in hypercortisolic patients (Communication). World Federation of Nuclear Medicine and Biology, Second International Congress, Washington, 1978.
[660] F. Bui, C. Macri, L. Varotto, M. Boscaro, F. Mantero, Adrenal scintigraphy in the morphological and functional evaluation of Cushing's syndrome, Cardiology 72 (1985) 76–83.
[661] N.E. Watson Jr., R.J. Cowan, H.M. Chilton, The utility of adrenal scintigraphy in Cushing's syndrome and hyperaldosteronism, Clin Nucl Med 10 (1985) 539–542.
[662] E. Demey-Ponsart, J.M. Foidart, J. Sulon, J.C. Sodoyez, CBG serum, free and total cortisol and circadian patterns of adrenal function in normal pregnancy, J Seteroid Biochem 16 (1982) 165–169.
[663] R.J. Gellert, W. Meroy Heinrichs, R.S. Swerdloff, DDT homologues: Estrogen-like effects on the vagina, uterus and pituitary of the rat, Endocrinology 91 (1972) 1095–1100.
[664] S. Tamada, I. Kazayoshi, Induction of hepatic cortisol 6β-hydroxylase by rifampicine, Lancet i (1976) 366–367.
[665] H. Gharib, J.M. Munoz, Endocrine manifestations of diphenylhydantoin therapy, Metabolism 23 (1974) 515–524.
[666] S. Burstein, H.L. Kimball, E.L. Klaibe, et al., Metabolism of 2 and 6β-hydroxycortisol in man. Determination of production rates of 6β-hydroxycortisol with and without phenobarbital administration, J Clin Endocrinol Metab 27 (1967) 491–499.
[667] A.W. Meikle, Dexamethasone suppression tests: Usefulness of simultaneous measurement of plasma cortisol and dexamethasone, Clin Endocrinol 16 (1982) 401–408.
[668] A.W. Meikle, J.B. Stanchfield, C.D. West, F.H. Tyler, Hydrocortisone suppression test for Cushing's syndrome, Arch Intern Med 134 (1974) 1068–1071.
[669] R.C. Gaillard, A. Riondel, M.F. Muller, W. Hermann, E.E. Baulieu, RU 486: A steroid with antiglucocorticoid activity that only disinhibits the human pituitary—adrenal system at a specific time of the day, Proc Nat Acad Sci USA 81 (1984) 3879–3882.
[670] X. Bertagna, C. Bertagna, J.P. Luton, J.M. Husson, F. Girard, The new steroid analog RU 486 inhibits glucocorticoid action in man, J Clin Endocrinol Metab 59 (1984) 25–28.
[671] M.C. Raux-Demay, T. Pierret, M. Bouvier d'Yvoire, X. Bertagna, F. Girard, Transient inhibition of RU 486 antiglucocorticoid action by dexamethasone, J Clin Endocrinol Metab 70 (1990) 230–233.
[672] J.G.M. Klijn, F.H. de Jong, G.H. Bakker, S.W.J. Lamberts, C.J. Rodenburg, J. Alexieva-Figush, Antiprogestins, a new form of endocrine therapy for human breast cancer, Cancer Res 49 (1989) 2851–2856.
[673] P.M. Stewart, A.M. Wallace, R. Valentino, D. Burt, C.H.L. Shackleton, C.R.W. Edwards, Mineralocorticoid activity of liquorice: 11β-hydroxysteroid dehydrogenase deficiency comes of age, Lancet (1987) 821–824.
[674] P.M. Stewart, J.E.T. Corrie, C.H.L. Shackleton, C.R.W. Edwards, Syndrome of apparent mineralocorticoid excess: A defect in the cortisol—cortisone shuttle, J Clin Invest 82 (1988) 340–349.
[675] M.A. MacKenzie, W.H.L. Hoefnagels, R.W.M.M. Jansen, T.J. Benraad, P.W.C. Kloppenborg, The influence of glycyrrhetinic acid on plasma cortisol and cortisone in healthy young volunteers, J Clin Endocrinol Metab 70 (1990) 1637–1643.
[676] K.L. Cohen, Metabolic, endocrine, and drug induced interference with pituitary function tests: A review, Metabolism 26 (1977) 1165–1177.

[677] E.Z. Wallace, P. Rosman, N. Toshav, A. Sacerdote, A. Balthazar, Pituitary—adrenocortical function in chronic renal failure: Studies of episodic secretion of cortisol and dexamethasone suppressibility, J Clin Endocrinol Metab 50 (1979) 46–51.

[678] K.K. Miller, P.A. Dally, D. Sentochnik, et al., Pseudo-Cushing's syndrome in human immunodeficiency virus-infected patients, Clin Infec Diseases 27 (1998) 68–72.

[679] R.J. Workman, W.K. Vaughn, W.J. Stone, Dexamethasone suppression testing in chronic renal failure: Pharmacokinetics of dexamethasone and demonstration of a normal hypothalamic—pituitary—adrenal axis, J Clin Endocrinol Metab 63 (1986) 741–746.

[680] N. Aronin, A.S. Liotta, B. Shickmanter, G.C. Schussler, D.T. Krieger, Impaired clearance of β-lipotropin in uremia, J Clin Endocrinol Metab 53 (1981) 797–800.

[681] R.N. Dexter, D.N. Orth, K. Abe, W.E. Nicholson, G.W. Liddle, Cushing's disease without hypercortisolism, J Clin Endocrinol Metab 30 (1970) 573–579.

[682] P.W. Gold, L. Loriaux, A. Roy, et al., Responses to corticotropin-releasing hormone in the hypercortisolism of depression and Cushing's disease, N Engl J Med 314 (1986) 1329–1335.

[683] J.D. Amsterdam, A. Winocur, E. Abelman, I. Lucki, K. Rickels, Cosyntropin (ACTH 1–24) stimulation test in depressed patients and healthy subjects, Am J Psychiatry 140 (1983) 907–909.

[684] B.J. Carroll, G.C. Curtis, B.M. Davies, J. Mendels, A.A. Sugarman, Urinary free cortisol excretion in depression, Psychol Med 6 (1976) 43–50.

[685] E.J. Sachar, L. Hellman, H.P. Roffwarg, F.S. Halpern, D.K. Fukushima, T.F. Gallagher, Disrupted 24-hr patterns of cortisol secretion in psychotic depression, Arch Gen Psychiatry 28 (1973) 19–26.

[686] J.A. Schlechte, B. Sherman, B. Pfohl, A comparison of adrenal cortical function in patients with depressive illness and Cushing's disease, Horm Res 23 (1986) 1–8.

[687] P.W. Gold, H. Gwirtsman, P.C. Avgerinos, et al., Abnormal hypothalamic—pituitary—adrenal function in anorexia nervosa, N Engl J Med 314 (1986) 1335–1342.

[688] M. Hotta, T. Shibasaki, A. Masuda, et al., The responses of plasma adrenocorticotropin and cortisol to corticotropin-releasing hormone (CRH) and cerebrospinal fluid immunoreactive CRH in anorexia nervosa patients, J Clin Endocrinol Metab 62 (1986) 319–324.

[689] W.H. Kaye, J. Gwirtsman, D.T. George, et al., Elevated cerebrospinal fluid levels of immunoreactive corticotropin releasing hormone in anorexia nervosa: Relationship to state of nutrition, adrenal function, and intensity of depression, J Clin Endocrinol Metab 64 (1987) 203–208.

[690] J.L. Katz, J. Weiner, J. Kream, B. Zumoff, Cushing's disease in a young woman with anorexia nervosa: Pathophysiological implications, Can J Psychiatry 31 (1986) 861–864.

[691] M.M. Fichter, K.M. Pirke, F. Holsboer, Weight loss causes neuroendocrine distrubances: Experimental study in healthy starving subjects, Psychiatry Res 17 (1986) 61–72.

[692] A.G. Smals, P.W. Kloppenborg, K.T. Njo, J.M. Knoben, C.M. Ruland, Alcohol-induced Cushingoid syndrome, Br Med J 2 (1976) 1298.

[693] L.H. Rees, G.M. Besser, W.J. Jeffcoate, D.J. Goldie, W. Marks, Alcohol-induced pseudo-Cushing's syndrome, Lancet (1977) 726–728.

[694] S. Kirkman, D.H. Nelson, Alcohol-induced pseudo-Cushing's disease: A study of prevalence with review of the literature, Metabolism 37 (1988) 390–394.

[695] J.D. Berman, D.M. Cook, M. Buchman, L.D. Keith, Diminished adrenocorticotropin response to insulin-induced hypoglycemia in nondepressed, actively drinking male alcoholics, J Clin Endocrinol Metab 71 (1990) 712–717.

[696] P.M. Stewart, P. Burra, C.H.L. Shackleton, M.C. Sheppard, E. Elias, 11 Beta-hydroxysteroid dehydrogenase deficiency and glucocorticoid status in patients with alcoholic and non alcoholic chronic liver disease, J Clin Endocrinol Metab 76 (1993) 748–751.

[697] S.W.J. Lamberts, J.G.M. Klijn, F.H. de Jong, J.C. Birkenhager, Hormone secretion in alcohol-induced pseudo-Cushing's syndrome, JAMA 242 (1979) 1640–1643.

[698] C.T. Sawin, Measurement of plasma cortisol in the diagnosis of Cushing's syndrome, Ann Intern Med 68 (1968) 624–631.

[699] E.M. Gold, The Cushing syndromes: Changing views of diagnosis and treatment, Ann Intern Med 90 (1979) 829–844.

[700] F. Petraglia, C. Barletta, F. Facchinetti, et al., Response of circulating adrenocorticotropin beta-endorphin, beta-lipotropin and cortisol to athletic competition, Acta Endocrinol 118 (1988) 332–336.

[701] L.H. Rees, C.W. Burke, T. Chard, S.W. Evans, A.T. Letchworth, Possible placental origin of ACTH in normal human pregnancy, Nature 234 (1975) 620–622.

[702] M. Grino, G.P. Chrousos, A.N. Margioris, The corticotropin releasing hormone gene is expressed in human placenta, Biochem Biophys Res Commun 148 (1987) 1208–1214.

[703] D.N. Orth, C.D. Mount, Specific high affinity binding protein for human corticotrophin releasing hormone in normal human plasma, Biochem Biophys Res Commun 143 (1987) 411–417.

[704] E.A. Linton, P.J. Lowry, A large molecular weight carrier substance for CRF-41 in human plasma, J Endocrinol 111 (1986) 150.

[705] A.B. Abou Samra, B. Loras, M. Pugeat, J. Tourniaire, J. Bertrand, Demonstration of an antiglucocorticoid action of progesterone on the corticosterone inhibition of β-endorphin release by rat anterior pituitary in primary culture, Endocrinology 115 (1984) 1471–1475.

[706] A.B. Abou Samra, M. Pugeat, H. Dechaux, L. Nachury, J. Tourniaire, Acute dopaminergic blockade by sulpiride stimulates β-endorphin secretion in pregnant women, Clin Endocrinol 21 (1984) 583–588.

[707] G.F.F.M. Pieters, A.G.H. Smals, H.J.M. Goverde, P.W.C. Kloppenborg, Paradoxical responsiveness of adrenocorticotropin and cortisol to thyrotropin releasing hormone (TRH) in pregnant women. Evidence for intermediate lobe activity? J Clin Endocrinol Metab 55 (1981) 387–389.

[708] A.C.M. Vingerhoeds, J.H.H. Thijssen, F. Schwarz, Spontaneous hypercortisolism without Cushing's syndrome, J Clin Endocrinol Metab 43 (1975) 1128–1133.

[709] G.P. Chrousos, A. Vingerhoeds, D. Brandon, et al., Primary cortisol resistance in man. A glucocorticoid receptor-mediated disease, J Clin Invest 69 (1982) 1261–1269.

[710] F. Pecori Giraldi, R. Pivonello, A.G. Ambrogio, M.C. De Martino, M. De Martin, M. Scacchi, et al., The dexamethasone-suppressed corticotropin-releasing hormone stimulation test and the desmopressin test to distinguish Cushing's syndrome from pseudo-Cushing's states, Clin Endocrinol (Oxf) 66 (2007) 251–257.

[711] D. Erickson, N. Natt, T. Nippoldt, W.F. Young Jr., P.C. Carpenter, T. Petterson, et al., Dexamethasone-suppressed corticotropin-releasing hormone stimulation test for diagnosis of mild hypercortisolism, J Clin Endocrinol Metab 92 (2007) 2972–2976.

[712] B. Gatta, O. Chabre, C. Cortet, M. Martinie, J.B. Corcuff, P. Roger, et al., Reevaluation of the combined dexamethasone suppression-corticotropin-releasing hormone test for differentiation of mild Cushing's disease from pseudo-Cushing's syndrome, J Clin Endocrinol Metab 92 (11) (2007) 4290–4293.

[713] N.M. Martin, W.S. Dhillo, A. Banerjee, A. Abdulali, C.N. Jayasena, M. Donaldson, et al., Comparison of the dexamethasone-suppressed corticotropin-releasing hormone test and low-dose dexamethasone suppression test in the diagnosis of Cushing's syndrome, J Clin Endocrinol Metab 91 (7) (2006) 2582–2586.

[714] J.A. Yanovski, G.B. Cutler Jr., G.P. Chrousos, L.K. Nieman, Corticotropin-releasing hormone stimulation following low-dose dexamethasone administration. A new test to distinguish Cushing's syndrome from pseudo-Cushing's states, JAMA 269 (17) (1993) 2232–2238.

[715] G. Arnaldi, G. Tirabassi, R. Papa, G. Furlani, L. Trementino, M. Cardinaletti, et al., Human corticotropin releasing hormone test performance in the differential diagnosis between Cushing's disease and pseudo-Cushing state is enhanced by combined ACTH and cortisol analysis, Eur J Endocrinol 160 (6) (2009) 891–898.

[716] M. Moro, P. Putignano, M. Losa, C. Invitti, C. Maraschini, F. Cavagnini, The desmopressin test in the differential diagnosis between Cushing's disease and pseudo-Cushing states, J Clin Endocrinol Metab 85 (2000) 3569–3574.

[717] J.F. Caro, A.W. Meikle, J.H. Check, S.N. Cohen, Normal suppression to dexamethasone in Cushing's disease: An expression of decreased metabolic clearance for dexamethasone, J Clin Endocrinol Metab 47 (1978) 667–670.

[718] A.W. Meikle, L.G. Lagerquist, F.H. Tyler, Apparently normal pituitary—adrenal suppressibility in Cushing's syndrome: Dexamethasone metabolism and plasma levels, J Lab Clin Med 86 (1975) 472–478.

[719] J.D. Fachnie, M.S. Zafar, R.C. Melinger, J.L. Chason, D.M. Kahkonen, Pituitary carcinoma mimics the ectopic adrenocorticotropin syndrome, J Clin Endocrinol Metab 50 (1980) 1062–1065.

[720] A.M.S. Mason, J.G. Ratcliffe, R.M. Buckle, A.S. Mason, ACTH secretion by bronchial carcinoid tumours, Clin Endocrinol 1 (1972) 3–25.

[721] D.F. Federman, E.J. Mark, Persistance of Cushing's syndrome after hypophysectomy, N Engl J Med 305 (1981) 1637–1643.

[722] P.M. Stewart, S. Petersenn, Rationale for treatment and therapeutic options in Cushing's disease, Best Pract Res Clin Endocrinol Metab 23 (Suppl 1) (2009) S15–S22.

[723] X. Bertagna, L. Guignat, L. Groussin, J. Bertherat, Cushing's disease, Best Pract Res Clin Endocrinol Metab 23 (5) (2009) 607–623.

[724] B.M. Biller, A.B. Grossman, P.M. Stewart, S. Melmed, X. Bertagna, J. Bertherat, et al., Treatment of adrenocorticotropin-dependent Cushing's syndrome: A consensus statement, J Clin Endocrinol Metab 93 (7) (2008) 2454–2462.

[725] A.H. Heald, S. Ghosh, S. Bray, C. Gibson, S.G. Anderson, H. Buckler, et al., Long-term negative impact on quality of life in patients with successfully treated Cushing's disease, Clin Endocrinol (Oxf) 61 (4) (2004) 458–465.

[726] L.G. Lagerquist, A.W. Meikle, C.D. West, F.H. Tyler, Cushing's disease with cure by resection of a pituitary adenoma: Evidence against a primary hypothalamic defect, Am J Med 57 (1974) 826–830.

[727] J. Hardy, Transsphenoidal microsurgery of the normal and pathological pituitary, Clin Neurosurg 16 (1969) 185–217.

[728] S.T. Bigos, F. Robert, G. Pelletier, J. Hardy, Cure of Cushing's disease by trans-sphenoidal removal of a microadenoma from a pituitary gland despite a radiographically normal sella turcica, J Clin Endocrinol Metab 45 (1977) 1251–1260.

[729] G. Guiot, J. Bouche, A. Opriou, Les indications de 1'abord sphenoidal dans les adénomes hypophysaires, Nouv Presse Med 75 (1967) 1563–1568.

[730] S.T. Bigos, M. Somma, E. Rasio, et al., Cushing's disease: Management by transsphenoidal pituitary microsurgery, J Clin Endocrinol Metab 50 (1980) 348–354.

[731] C.A. Carrasco, J. Coste, L. Guignat, L. Groussin, M.A. Dugué, S. Gaillard, et al., Midnight salivary cortisol determination for assessing the outcome of transsphenoidal surgery in Cushing's disease, J Clin Endocrinol Metab 93 (12) (2008) 4728–4734.

[732] C.E. Burke, C.B.T. Adams, M.M. Esiri, C. Morris, J.S. Bevan, Transsphenoidal surgery for Cushing's disease: Does what is removed determine the endocrine outcome? Clin Endocrinol 33 (1990) 525–537.

[733] D.R. McCance, D.S. Gordon, T.F. Fannin, et al., Assessment of endocrine function after transsphenoidal surgery for Cushing's disease, Clin Endocrinol 38 (1993) 79–86.

[734] P.J. Trainer, H.S. Lawrie, J. Verhelst, et al., Transsphenoidal resection in Cushing's disease: Undetectable serum cortisol as the definition of successful treatment, Clin Endocrinol 38 (1983) 73–78.

[735] D. Bochicchio, M. Losa, M. Buchfelder, Factors influencing the intermediate and late outcome of Cushing's disease treated by transsphenoidal surgery: A retrospective study by the European Cushing's disease survey group, J Clin Endocrinol Metab 80 (1995) 3114–3120.

[736] D.R. McCane, M. Besser, A.B. Atkinson, Assessment of cure after transsphenoidal surgery for Cushing's disease, Clin Endocrinol 44 (1996) 1–6.

[737] L.S. Blevins Jr., J.H. Christy, Cushing's disease due to ACTH-secreting macroadenomas: Management issues, The Endocrinologist 9 (1999) 257–262.

[738] G.D. Hammer, J.B. Tyrrell, K.R. Lamborn, C.B. Applebury, E.T. Hannegan, S. Bell, et al., Transsphenoidal microsurgery for Cushing's disease: Initial outcome and long-term results, J Clin Endocrinol Metab 89 (12) (2004) 6348–6357.

[739] B.M. Hofmann, M. Hlavac, R. Martinez, M. Buchfelder, O.A. Müller, R.T. Fahlbusch, Long-term results after microsurgery for Cushing disease: Experience with 426 primary operations over 35 years, J Neurosurg 108 (1) (2008) 9–18.

[740] J.L. Atkinson, W.F. Young Jr, F.B. Meyer, D.H. Davis, T.B. Nippoldt, D. Erickson, et al., Sublabial transseptal vs transnasal combined endoscopic microsurgery in patients with Cushing disease and MRI-depicted microadenomas, Mayo Clin Proc 83 (5) (2008) 550–553.

[741] C.G. Patil, D.M. Prevedello, S.P. Lad, M.L. Vance, M.O. Thorner, L. Katznelson, et al., Late recurrences of Cushing's disease after initial successful transsphenoidal surgery, J Clin Endocrinol Metab 93 (2) (2008) 358–362.

[742] A.B. Atkinson, A. Kennedy, M.I. Wiggam, D.R. McCance, B. Sheridan, Long-term remission rates after pituitary surgery for Cushing's disease: The need for long-term surveillance, Clin Endocrinol (Oxf) 63 (5) (2005) 549–559.

[743] R.A. Alwani, W.W. de Herder, M.O. van Aken, J.H. van den Berge, E.J. Delwel, A.H. Dallenga, et al., Biochemical predictors of outcome of pituitary surgery for Cushing's disease, Neuroendocrinology 91 (2) (2010) 169–178.

[744] M. Losa, R. Bianchi, R. Barzaghi, M. Giovanelli, P. Mortini, Persistent drenocorticotropin response to desmopressin in the early postoperative period predicts recurrence of Cushing's disease, J Clin Endocrinol Metab 94 (9) (2009) 3322–3328.

[745] F. Castinetti, M. Martinie, I. Morange, H. Dufour, N. Sturm, J.G. Passagia, et al., A combined dexamethasone desmopressin test as an early marker of postsurgical recurrence in Cushing's disease, J Clin Endocrinol Metab 94 (6) (2009) 1897–1903.

[746] B. Ambrosi, A.E. Malavazos, E. Passeri, C. Dall'Asta, Desmopressin test may predict the risk of recurrence in Cushing's disease, Clin Endocrinol (Oxf) 70 (5) (2009) 811.

[747] D.J. Romanholi, M.C. Machado, C.C. Pereira, D.S. Danilovic, M.A. Pereira, V.A. Cescato, et al., Role for postoperative cortisol response to desmopressin in predicting the risk for recurrent Cushing's disease, Clin Endocrinol (Oxf) 69 (1) (2008) 117–122.

[748] C. Dall'asta, L. Barbetta, L. Bonavina, P. Beck-Peccoz, B. Ambrosi, Recurrence of Cushing's disease preceded by the reappearance of ACTH and cortisol responses to desmopressin test, Pituitary 7 (3) (2004) 183–188.

[749] G.F.F.M. Pieters, A.R.M.M. Hermus, E. Meijer, A.G.H. Smals, P.W.C. Kloppenborg, Predictive factors for initial cure and relapse rate after pituitary surgery for Cushing's disease, J Clin Endocrinol Metab 69 (1989) 1122–1126.

[750] S. Salenave, B. Gatta, S. Pecheur, F. San-Galli, A. Visot, P. Lasjaunias, et al., Pituitary magnetic resonance imaging findings do not influence surgical outcome in adrenocorticotropin-secreting microadenomas, J Clin Endocrinol Metab 89 (7) (2004) 3371–3376.

[751] W.A. Scherbaum, U. Schrell, M. Gluck, R. Fahlbusch, E.F. Pfeiffer, Autoantibodies to pituitary corticotropin-producing cells: Possible marker for unfavourable outcome after pituitary microsurgery for Cushing's disease, Lancet (1987) 1394–1396.

[752] L. Olivier, E. Vali-Porcile, Pituitary pathology in Cushing's disease. Histology and morphometry of pituitary tissues removed through microsurgery, Pathol Res Pract 183 (1988) 587–591.

[753] J.P. Thomas, S.H. Richards, Long term results of radical hypophysectomy for Cushing's disease, Clin Endocrinol 19 (1983) 629–636.

[754] D.K. Ludecke, Intraoperative measurement of adrenocorticotropic hormone in peripituitary blood in Cushing's disease, Neurosurgery 24 (1989) 201–205.

[755] A. Ganguly, J.B. Stanchfield, T.S. Roberts, C.D. West, F.H. Tyler, Cushing's syndrome in a patient with an empty selle turcica and a microadenoma of the adenohypophysis, Am J Med 60 (1976) 306–309.

[756] J.L. Doppman, R. Chang, E.H. Oldfield, G. Chrousos, C.A. Stratakis, L.K. Nieman, The hypoplastic inferior petrosal sinus: A potential source of false-negative results in petrosal sampling for Cushing's disease, J Clin Endocrinol Metab 84 (2) (1999) 533–540.

[757] C.G. Patil, A. Veeravagu, D.M. Prevedello, L. Katznelson, M.L. Vance, E.R. Laws Jr., Outcomes after repeat transsphenoidal surgery for recurrent Cushing's disease, Neurosurgery 63 (2) (2008) 266–270, discussion 270–271.

[758] M.A. Wagenmakers, R.T. Netea-Maier, E.J. van Lindert, H.J. Timmers, J.A. Grotenhuis, A.R. Hermus, Repeated transsphenoidal pituitary surgery (TS) via the endoscopic technique: A good therapeutic option for recurrent or persistent Cushing's disease (CD), Clin Endocrinol (Oxf) 70 (2) (2009) 274–280.

[759] D.N. Orth, G.W. Liddle, Results of treatment in 108 patients with Cushing's syndrome, N Engl J Med 285 (1971) 243–247.

[760] A.S. Jennings, G.W. Liddle, D.N. Orth, Results of treating childhood Cushing's disease with pituitary irradiation, N Engl J Med 297 (1977) 957–962.

[761] T.A. Howlett, P.N. Plowman, J.A.H. Wass, L.H. Rees, A.E. Jones, G.M. Besser, Megavoltage pituitary irradiation in the management of Cushing's disease and Nelson's syndrome: Long-term follow-up, Clin Endocrinol 31 (1989) 309–323.

[762] F.E. Helberg, G.E. Sheline, Radiotherapy of pituitary tumors, Endocrinol Metab Clin North Am (1987) 667–684.

[763] M.D. Littley, S.M. Shalet, C.G. Beardwell, S.R. Ahmed, M.L. Sutton, Long-term follow-up of low-dose external pituitary irradiation for Cushing's disease, Clin Endocrinol 33 (1990) 445–455.

[764] G.F. Sharpe, P. Kendall-Taylor, R.W.G. Prescott, et al., Pituitary function following megavoltage therapy for Cushing's disease: Long term follow up, Clin Endocrinol 22 (1985) 169–177.

[765] S. Aristizabal, W.L. Caldwell, J. Avila, E.G. Mayer, Relationship of time dose factors to tumour control and complications in the treatment of Cushing's disease, Int J Radiat Oncol Biol Phys 2 (1977) 47–54.

[766] M. Murayama, K. Yasuda, Y. Minamori, L. Mercado-Asis, N. Yamakita, K. Miura, Long-term follow-up of Cushing's disease treated with reserpine and pituitary irradiation, J Clin Endocrinol Metab 75 (1992) 935–942.

[767] S.W.J. Lamberts, F.H. de Jong, J.C. Birkenhager, Evaluation of a therapeutic regimen in Cushing's disease. The predictability of the result of unilateral adrenalectomy followed by external pituitary irradiation, Acta Endocrinol 86 (1977) 146–155.

[768] J. Estrada, M. Boronat, M. Mielgo, et al., The long-term outcome of pituitary irradiation after unsuccessful transsphenoidal surgery in Cushing's disease, N Engl J Med 336 (1997) 172–177.

[769] D.E. Schteingart, H.S. Tsao, C.I. Taylor, A. McKenzie, R. Victoria, B.A. Therrien, Sustained remission of Cushing's disease with mitotane and pituitary irradiation, Ann Intern Med 5 (1980) 613–619.

[770] J.P. Luton, J.A. Mahoudeau, P.H. Bouchard, et al., Treatment of Cushing's disease by op'DDD. Survey of 62 cases, N Engl J Med 300 (1979) 459–464.

[771] M. Degerblad, T. Rahn, G. Bergstrand, M. Thoren, Long-term results of stereotactic radiosurgery to the pituitary gland in Cushing's disease, Acta Endocrinol 112 (1986) 310–314.

[772] J. Jagannathan, J.P. Sheehan, N. Pouratian, E.R. Laws, L. Steiner, M.L. Vance, Gamma knife surgery for Cushing's disease, J Neurosurg 106 (6) (2007) 980–987.

[773] F. Castinetti, M. Nagai, H. Dufour, J.M. Kuhn, I. Morange, P. Jaquet, et al., Gamma knife radiosurgery is a successful adjunctive treatment in Cushing's disease, Eur J Endocrinol 156 (1) (2007) 91–98.

[774] J.A. Linfoot, Heavy ion therapy: Alpha particle therapy of pituitary tumors, in: J.A. Linfoot (Ed.), Recent Advances in the Diagnosis and Treatment of Pituitary Tumors, Raven Press, New York, 1979, pp. 245–267.

[775] R.N. Kjelberg, B. Kliman, Lifetime effectiveness — a system of therapy for pituitary adenomas, emphasizing Bragg peak proton hypophysectomy, in: J.A. Linfoot (Ed.), Recent Advances in the Diagnosis and Treatment of Pituitary Tumors, Raven Press, New York, 1979, pp. 269–288.

[776] C.W. Burke, F.H. Doyle, G.F. Joplin, R.N. Arnot, D.P. MacErlean, T. Russel Fraser, Cushing's disease: Treatment by pituitary implantation of radioactive gold or yttrium seeds, Q J Med 168 (1973) 693–714.

[777] J. Cassar, F.H. Doyle, P.D. Lewis, K. Mashiter, S.V. Van Noorden, G.F. Joplin, Treatment of Nelson's syndrome by pituitary implantation of yttrium-90 or gold-198, Br Med J 2 (1976) 269–272.

[778] L.M. Sandler, N.T. Richards, D.H. Carr, K. Mashiter, G.F. Joplin, Long term follow-up of patients with Cushing's disease treated by interstitial irradiation, J Clin Endocrinol Metab 65 (1987) 441–447.

[779] J.W. Miller, L. Crapo, The medical treatment of Cushing's syndrome, Endocr Rev 14 (1993) 443–458.

[780] D.T. Krieger, L. Amorosa, F. Linick, Cyproheptadine-induced remission of Cushing's disease, N Engl J Med 293 (1975) 893–896.

[781] N. Aronin, D.T. Krieger, Persistent remission of Nelson's syndrome following discontinuance of cyproheptadine treatment, N Engl J Med 302 (1980) 453.

[782] A.N. Elias, G. Gwinup, L.J. Valenta, Effects of valproic acid, naloxone and hydrocortisone in Nelson's syndrome and Cushing's disease, Clin Endocrinol 15 (1981) 151–154.

[783] M.T. Jones, B. Gillham, U. Beckford, et al., Effect of treatment with sodium valproate and diazepam on plasma corticotropin in Nelson's syndrome, Lancet (1981) 1179–1181. i.

[784] W. Kelly, J.E. Adams, I. Laing, D. Longson, D. Davies, Long-term treatment of Nelson's syndrome with sodium valproate, Clin Endocrinol 28 (1988) 195–204.

[785] B. Allolio, W. Winkelmann, D. Kaulen, F. Hipp, R. Mies, Valproate in Cushing's disease, Lancet. i (1982) 171.

[786] S.W.J. Lamberts, J.G.M. Klijin, M. De Quijada, et al., The mechanism of the suppressive action of bromocriptine on adrenocorticotropin secretion in patients with Cushing's disease and Nelson's syndrome, J Clin Endocrinol Metab 51 (1980) 307–311.

[787] A.L. Kennedy, B. Sheridan, D.A.D. Montgomery, ACTH and cortisol response to bromocriptine, and results of long-term therapy in Cushing's disease, Acta Endocrinol 89 (1978) 461–468.

[788] A.B. Atkinson, A.L. Kennedy, B. Sheridon, Six year remission of ACTH-dependent Cushing's syndrome using bromocriptine, Postgrad Med J 61 (1985) 239–242.

[789] R. Pivonello, M.C. De Martino, P. Cappabianca, M. De Leo, A. Faggiano, G. Lombardi, et al., The medical treatment of Cushing's disease: Effectiveness of chronic treatment with the dopamine agonist cabergoline in patients unsuccessfully treated by surgery, J Clin Endocrinol Metab 94 (1) (2009) 223–230.

[790] L. Vilar, L.A. Naves, M.F. Azevedo, M.J. Arruda, C.M. Arahata, E. Moura, L. Silva, et al., Effectiveness of cabergoline in monotherapy and combined with ketoconazole in the management of Cushing's disease, Pituitary 13 (2) (2010) 123–129.

[791] J.B. Tyrrell, M. Lorenzi, J.E. Gerich, P.H. Forsham, Inhibition by somatostatin of ACTH secretion in Nelson's syndrome, J Clin Endocrinol Metab 40 (1975) 1125–1127.

[792] S.W.J. Lamberts, The role of somatostatin in the regulation of anterior pituitary hormone secretion and the use of its analogs in the treatment of human pituitary tumors, Endocr Rev 9 (1988) 417–436.

[793] X. Bertagna, C. Favrod-Coune, H. Escourolle, et al., Suppression of ectopic ACTH secretion by the long-acting somatostatin analog SMS 201–995, J Clin Endocrinol Metab 68 (1989) 988–991.

[794] C. de Bruin, R.A. Feelders, A.M. Waaijers, P.M. van Koetsveld, D.M. Sprij-Mooij, S.W. Lamberts, et al., Differential regulation of human dopamine D2 and somatostatin receptor subtype expression by glucocorticoids in vitro, J Mol Endocrinol 42 (1) (2009) 47–56.

[795] C. de Bruin, A.M. Pereira, R.A. Feelders, J.A. Romijn, F. Roelfsema, D.M. Sprij-Mooij, et al., Coexpression of dopamine and somatostatin receptor subtypes in corticotroph adenomas, J Clin Endocrinol Metab 94 (4) (2009) 1118–1124.

[796] L.J. Hofland, J. van der Hoek, R. Feelders, M.O. van Aken, P.M. van Koetsveld, M. Waaijers, et al., The multi-ligand somatostatin analogue SOM230 inhibits ACTH secretion by cultured human corticotroph adenomas via somatostatin receptor type 5, Eur J Endocrinol 152 (4) (2005) 645–654.

[797] M. Boscaro, W.H. Ludlam, B. Atkinson, J.E. Glusman, S. Petersenn, M. Reincke, et al., Treatment of pituitary-dependent Cushing's disease with the multireceptor ligand somatostatin analog pasireotide (SOM230): A multicenter, phase II trial, J Clin Endocrinol Metab 94 (1) (2009) 115–122.

[798] J. Kreutzer, I. Jeske, B. Hofmann, I. Blumcke, R. Fahlbusch, M. Buchfelder, et al., No effect of the PPAR-gamma agonist rosiglitazone on ACTH or cortisol secretion in Nelson's syndrome and Cushing's disease in vitro and in vivo, Clin Neuropathol 28 (6) (2009) 430–439.

[799] D. Suri, R.E. Weiss, Effect of pioglitazone on adrenocorticotropic hormone and cortisol secretion in Cushing's disease, J Clin Endocrinol Metab 90 (3) (2005) 1340–1346.

[800] B. Ambrosi, C. Dall'Asta, S. Cannavo, R. Libe, T. Vigo, P. Epaminonda, et al., Effects of chronic administration of PPAR-gamma ligand rosiglitazone in Cushing's disease, Eur J Endocrinol 151 (2) (2004) 173–178.

[801] A. Munir, F. Song, P. Ince, S.J. Walters, R. Ross, J. Newell-Price, Ineffectiveness of rosiglitazone therapy in Nelson's syndrome, J Clin Endocrinol Metab 92 (5) (2007) 1758–1763.

[802] K.R. Mullan, H. Leslie, D.R. McCance, B. Sheridan, A.B. Atkinson, The PPAR-gamma activator rosiglitazone fails to lower plasma ACTH levels in patients with Nelson's syndrome, Clin Endocrinol (Oxf) 64 (5) (2006) 519–522.

[803] F. Pecori Giraldi, C. Scaroni, E. Arvat, M. Martin, R. Giordano, N. Albiger, et al., Effect of protracted treatment with rosiglitazone, a PPARgamma agonist, in patients with Cushing's disease, Clin Endocrinol (Oxf) 64 (2) (2006) 219–224.

[804] M. Labeur, M. Paez-Pereda, E. Arzt, G.K. Stalla, Potential of retinoic acid derivatives for the treatment of corticotroph pituitary adenomas, Rev Endocr Metab Disord 10 (2) (2009) 103–109.

[805] V. Castillo, D. Giacomini, M. Páez-Pereda, J. Stalla, M. Labeur, M. Theodoropoulou, et al., Retinoic acid as a novel medical therapy for Cushing's disease in dogs, Endocrinology 147 (9) (2006) 4438–4444.

[806] H.P. Kopperschaar, R.J. Croughs, J.H. Thijssen, F. Schwarz, Response to neurotransmitter modulating drugs in patients with Cushing's disease, Clin Endocrinol 25 (1986) 661–667.

[807] H.W. Scott, G.W. Liddle, J.L. Mulherin, T.J. McKenna, S.L. Stroup, R.K. Rhamy, Surgical experience with Cushing's disease, Ann Surg 185 (1977) 524–534.

[808] R.B. Welbourn, D.A.D. Montgomery, T.L. Kennedy, The natural history of treated Cushing's syndrome, Br J Surg 58 (1971) 1–17.

[809] L. Kemink, A. Hermus, G. Pieters, T.H. Benraad, A. Smals, P. Kloppenborg, Residual adrenocortical function after bilateral adrenalectomy for pituitary-dependent Cushing's syndrome, J Clin Endocrinol Metab 75 (1992) 1211–1214.

[810] D.H. Nelson, J.W. Meakin, J.B. Dealy, D.D. Matson, K. Emerson, G.W. Thorn, ACTH-producing tumor of the pituitary gland, N Engl J Med 259 (1958) 161–164.

[811] D.H. Nelson, J.W. Meakin, G.W. Thorn, ACTH-producing pituitary tumors following adrenalectomy for Cushing's syndrome, Ann Intern Med 52 (1960) 560–569.

[812] W.F. Kelly, I.A. MacFarlane, D. Longson, D. Davis, H. Sutcliffe, Cushing's disease treated by total adrenalectomy: Long term observation in 43 patients, Q J Med 52 (1983) 224–231.

[813] M.D. Urban, P.A. Lee, R.K. Danisk, C.J. Migeon, Treatment of Cushing's disease with bilateral adrenalectomy and autotransplantation, Horm Res 13 (1980) 81–89.

[814] D. Barzilai, G. Dickstein, Y. Kanter, Y. Plavnick, A. Schramek, Complete remission of Cushing's disease by total bilateral adrenalectomy and adrenal autotransplantation, J Clin Endocrinol Metab 50 (1980) 853–856.

[815] Y.M. Xu, Y. Qiao, P. Wu, Z.D. Chen, N.T. Jin, Adrenal autotransplantation with attached blood vessels for treatment of Cushing's disease, J Urol 141 (1989) 6–8.

[816] J.D. Hardy, D.O. Moore, H.G. Langford, Cushing's disease today. Late follow-up of 17 adrenalectomy patients with emphasis on eight with adrenal autotransplants, Ann Surg 201 (1985) 595–603.

[817] A.A. Nelson, G. Woodard, Severe adrenal cortical atrophy (cytotoxic) and hepatic damage produced in dogs by feeding 2,2 bis (parachorophenyl)-1,1 dichloroethane (DDD or TDE), Arch Path 48 (1949) 387–394.

[818] D.M. Bergenstal, M.B. Lipsett, R.H. Moy, R. Hertz, Regression of adrenal cancer and suppression of adrenal function in man by *op*'DDD, Trans Assoc Am Physicians 72 (1959) 341–350.

[819] A.L. Southren, S. Tochimoto, L. Strom, A. Ratuschni, H. Ross, G. Gordon, Remission in Cushing's syndrome with *op*'DDD, J Clin Endocrinol Metab 26 (1966) 268–278.

[820] T.E. Temple, D.J. Jones, G.W. Liddle, R.N. Dexter, Treatment of Cushing's disease. Correction of hypercortisolism by *op*'DDD without induction of aldosterone deficiency, N Engl J Med 281 (1969) 801–805.

[821] H. Bricaire, J.P. Luton, Douze ans de traitement médical de la maladie de Cushing: Usage prolongé de 1'*op*'DDD dans quarante six cas, Nouv Presse Med 5 (1976) 325–329.

[822] A.J. Moolenaar, H. Van Slooten, A.P. Van Seters, D. Smeenk, Blood levels of *op*'DDD following administration in various vehicles after a single dose and during long-term treatment, Cancer Chemother Pharmacol 7 (1981) 51–54.

[823] Y. Touitou, A.J. Moolenaar, A. Bogdan, A. Auzeby, J.P. Luton, *op*'DDD (mitotane) treatment for Cushing's syndrome: Adrenal drug concentration and inhibition in vitro of steroid synthesis, Eur J Clin Pharmacol 29 (1985) 483–487.

[824] S. Leiba, R. Weinstein, B. Shindel, et al., The protracted effect of *op*'DDD in Cushing's disease and its impact on adrenal morphogenesis of young human embryo, Ann Endocrinol 50 (1989) 49–53.

[825] R.V. Hague, W. May, D.R. Cullen, Hepatic microsomal enzyme induction and adrenal crisis due to *op*'DDD therapy for metastatic adrenocortical carcinoma, Clin Endocrinol 31 (1989) 51–57.

[826] G.B. Robinson, I.B. Hales, A.J. Henniker, et al., The effect of *op*'DDD on adrenal steroid replacement therapy requirements, Clin Endocrinol 27 (1987) 437–444.

[827] J.S. Marshall, L.S. Tomkins, Effect of *op*'DDD and similar compounds on thyroxine binding globulin, J Clin Endocrinol Metab 28 (1968) 386–392.

[828] M. Ojima, S. Hashimoto, N. Itoh, et al., Effects of *op*'DDD on pituitary–gonadal function in patients with Cushing's disease, Nippon Naibunpi Gakkai Zasshi 64 (1988) 451–462.

[829] R.D. Brown, W.E. Nicholson, W.T. Chick, C.A. Stroott, Effect of *op*'DDD on human adrenal steroid 11β-hydroxylation activity, J Clin Endocrinol Metab 36 (1973) 730–733.

[830] J. Donckier, J.M. Burrin, I.D. Ramsay, G.F. Joplin, Successful control of Cushing's disease in the elderly with long term metyrapone, Postgrad Med J 62 (1986) 727–730.

[831] G. Dickstein, M. Lahav, Z. Shen-Orr, Y. Edoute, D. Barzilai, Primary therapy for Cushing's disease with metyrapone, JAMA 255 (1986) 1167–1169.

[832] W.J. Jeffcoate, L.H. Rees, S. Tomlin, A.E. Jones, C.R.W. Edwards, G.M. Besser, Metyrapone in long-term management of Cushing's disease, Br Med J 2 (1977) 215–217.

[833] D.N. Orth, Metyrapone is useful only as adjunctive therapy in Cushing's disease, Ann Intern Med 89 (1978) 128–130.

[834] D.F. Child, C.W. Burke, D.M. Burley, L.H. Rees, T.R. Fraser, Drug control of Cushing's syndrome. Combined aminoglutethimide and metyrapone therapy, Acta Endocrinol 82 (1976) 330–341.

[835] M. Thoren, U. Adamson, H.E. Sjöberg, Ammoglutethimide and metyrapone in the management of Cushing's syndrome, Acta Endocrinol 109 (1985) 451–457.

[836] D.E. Schteingart, J.W. Conn, Effects of aminoglutethimide upon adrenal function and cortisol metabolism in Cushing's syndrome, J Clin Endocrinol Metab 27 (1967) 1657–1666.

[837] N. Sonino, The use of ketoconazole as an inhibitor of steroid production, N Engl J Med 317 (1987) 812–818.

[838] S. Cerdas, L. Billaud, B. Guilhaume, M.H. Laudat, X. Bertagna, J.P. Luton, Effets à court terme du ketoconazole dans les syndromes de Cushing, Ann Endocrinol 50 (1989) 489–496.

[839] D.R. McCance, D.R. Hadden, L. Kennedy, B. Sheridan, A.B. Atkinson, Clinical experience with ketoconazole as a therapy for patients with Cushing's syndrome, Clin Endocrinol 27 (1987) 593–599.

[840] P. Loli, M.E. Berselli, M. Tagliafferri, The use of ketoconazole in the treatment of Cushing's syndrome, J Clin Endocrinol Metab 63 (1986) 1365–1371.

[841] M. Sonino, M. Boscaro, G. Merola, F. Mantero, Prolonged treatment of Cushing's disease by ketoconazole, J Clin Endocrinol Metab 61 (1985) 718–722.

[842] A. Angeli, R. Frairia, Ketoconazole therapy in Cushing's disease, Lancet (1985) 821.

[843] M. Boscaro, N. Sonino, A. Rampazzo, F. Mantero, Response of pituitary–adrenal axis to corticotrophin releasing hormone in patients with Cushing's disease before and after ketoconazole treatment, Clin Endocrinol 27 (1987) 461–467.

[844] F. Castinetti, I. Morange, P. Jaquet, B. Conte-Devolx, T. Brue, Ketoconazole revisited: A preoperative or postoperative treatment in Cushing's disease, Eur J Endocrinol 158 (1) (2008) 91–99.

[845] C. Tsigos, D.A. Papanicolaou, G.P. Chrousos, Advances in the diagnosis and treatment of Cushing's syndrome, Bailliere's, Clin Endocrinol and Metab 9 (1995) 315–336.

[846] H.M. Schulte, G. Benker, D. Reinwein, W.G. Sippell, B. Allolio, Infusion of low dose etomidate: Correction of hypercortisolemia in patients with Cushing's syndrome and dose-response relationship in normal subjects, J Clin Endocrinol Metab 70 (1990) 1426–1430.

[847] L.K. Nieman, G.P. Chrousos, C. Kellner, et al., Successful treatment of Cushing's syndrome with the glucocorticoid antagonist RU 486, J Clin Endocrinol Metab 61 (1985) 536–540.

[848] X. Bertagna, C. Bertagna, M.H. Laudat, J.M. Husson, F. Girard, J.P. Luton, Pituitary–adrenal response to the antigulcocorticoid action of RU 486 in Cushing's syndrome, J Clin Endocrinol Metab 63 (1986) 639–643.

[849] A.J. Van der Lely, K. Fockin, R.C. Van der Mast, S.W.J. Lamberts, Rapid reversal of acute psychosis in the Cushing's syndrome with the cortisol receptor antagonist mifepristone (RU 486), Ann Int Med 114 (1991) 143–144.

[850] F. Castinetti, M. Fassnacht, S. Johanssen, M. Terzolo, P. Bouchard, P. Chanson, et al., Merits and pitfalls of mifepristone in Cushing's syndrome, Eur J Endocrinol 160 (6) (2009) 1003–1010.

[851] A.A. Kasperlik-Zaluska, J. Nielubowicz, J. Wislawski, et al., Nelson's syndrome: Incidence and prognosis, Clin Endocrinol 19 (1983) 693–698.

[852] S.A.G. Kemink, A.G.H. Smals, A.R.M.M. Hermus, et al., Nelson's syndrome: A review, The Endocrinologist 7 (1997) 5–9.

[853] K.L. Cohen, R.H. Noth, T. Pechinski, Incidence of pituitary tumors following adrenalectomy, Arch Intern Med 138 (1978) 575–579.

[854] A.H. Barnett, J.H. Livesey, K. Friday, R.A. Donald, E.A. Espiner, Comparison of preoperative and postoperative ACTH concentrations after bilateral adrenalectomy in Cushing's disease, Clin Endocrinol 18 (1983) 301–305.

[855] A.C. Moreira, M. Castro, H.R. Machado, Longitudinal evaluation of adrenocorticotrophin and beta-lipotrophin plasma levels following bilateral adrenalectomy in patients with Cushing's syndrome, Clin Endocrinol 39 (1993) 91–96.

[856] N.J. Hopwood, F.M. Kenny, Incidence of Nelson's syndrome after adrenalectomy for Cushing's disease in children, Am J Dis Child 131 (1977) 1353–1356.

[857] R.A. Bonner, K. Mukai, J.H. Oppenheimer, Two unusual variants of Nelson's syndrome, J Clin Endocrinol Metab 49 (1979) 23–29.

[858] C. Verdonk, C. Guerin, E. Lufkin, S.F. Hodgson, Activation of virilizing adrenal rest tissues by excessive ACTH production, Am J Med 73 (1982) 455–459.

[859] N.G. Baranetsky, R.D. Zipser, U. Goebelmann, et al., Adrenocorticotropin-dependent virilizing paraovarian tumors in Nelson's syndrome, J Clin Endocrinol Metab 49 (1979) 381–386.

[860] G. Assié, H. Bahurel, J. Coste, S. Silvera, M. Kujas, M.A. Dugué, et al., Corticotroph tumor progression after adrenalectomy in Cushing's disease: A reappraisal of Nelson's syndrome, J Clin Endocrinol Metab 92 (1) (2007) 172–179.

[861] H. Bahurel-Barrera, G. Assie, S. Silvera, X. Bertagna, J. Coste, P. Legmann, Inter- and intra-observer variability in detection and progression assessment with MRI of microadenoma in Cushing's disease patients followed up after bilateral adrenalectomy, Pituitary 11 (3) (2008) 263–269.

[862] G. Assié, H. Bahurel, J. Bertherat, M. Kujas, P. Legmann, X. Bertagna, The Nelson's syndrome ... revisited, Pituitary 7 (4) (2004) 209–215.

[863] P.A. Kelly, G. Samandouras, A.B. Grossman, F. Afshar, G.M. Besser, P.J. Jenkins, Neurosurgical treatment of Nelson's syndrome, J Clin Endocrinol Metab 87 (12) (2002) 5465–5469.

[864] M. Hornyak, M.H. Weiss, D.H. Nelson, W.T. Couldwell, Nelson syndrome: Historical perspectives and current concepts, Neurosurg Focus 23 (3) (2007) E12.

CHAPTER

17

Thyrotropin-Secreting Pituitary Tumors

Vanessa Rouach [1], *Yona Greenman* [1,2]

[1] Institute of Endocrinology, Metabolism and Hypertension, Tel Aviv-Sourasky Medical Center, Tel Aviv, Israel
[2] Sackler School of Medicine, Tel Aviv University, Tel Aviv, Israel

The coexistence of hyperthyroidism, a pituitary mass and excessive thyrotropin production demonstrated using a thyroid-stimulating hormone (TSH) bioassay, was first described in 1960 [1]. The diagnosis of thyrotropin-secreting adenomas (TSPA) is based on the demonstration of elevated serum thyroid hormones in the presence of elevated or normal TSH levels. The possibility of making this diagnosis was compromised at first by the inability of early radioimmunoassays to distinguish between normal and suppressed TSH levels. In patients with primary thyroid disease, which is by far the most common cause of hyperthyroidism, TSH levels are suppressed by the elevated peripheral thyroid hormones, and are thus undetectable in serum. When TSH itself is responsible for thyroid hyperstimulation, it is readily detected, being either inappropriately in the normal range or actually elevated. Because of the past laboratory limitations, patients were often misdiagnosed as having primary hyperthyroidism, leading to erroneous therapeutic decisions. The introduction of sensitive TSH immunoassays led to an improvement in the detection rate of these pituitary tumors. Nevertheless, they remain a rare disorder, being the least prevalent among all pituitary adenomas. In a large pathological series, TSPA represented 0.6% of the adenomas found in postmortem pituitaries [2], whereas in surgical series 0.9–1.5% of pituitary adenomas [3,4] were thyrotropinomas. A relatively higher rate of 2.8% was reported by Beck Peccoz et al. in a detailed review from 1996 [5].

This chapter reviews the pathophysiology, clinical characteristics, diagnosis and therapeutic approach to TSH-secreting adenomas.

PATHOGENESIS

The role of disordered hypothalamic or peripheral endocrine function vs. the presence of intrinsic lesions in the pituitary cell in the pathogenesis of pituitary adenomas has been the focus of intense investigations. TSH-secreting tumors, as other types of pituitary adenomas, were found to be monoclonal in origin [6,7]. Nevertheless, the precise mechanisms involved in pituitary cell transformation remain undefined. A number of etiologic factors are proposed, including mutations in pituitary tumor-susceptibility genes, overactivation of proliferative cell-signaling pathways, under-expression of tumor suppressor genes, mostly those involved in cell cycle regulation, and alterations in hormone-regulatory pathways [8]. It is probable that many of these factors interact to initiate transformation and promote tumor cell proliferation. Data on alterations that may be central or more specific to the development of TSPA are scarce, due to the relative rarity of these tumors, and are discussed below.

Hormone Regulatory Pathways

The secretion of TSH, a glycoprotein hormone composed of α- and β-subunits, is controlled by the integrated thyrotroph response to humoral and central signals. Thyrotropin-releasing hormone (TRH) secreted by neurons in the paraventricular nucleus of the hypothalamus is the major stimulator of TSH secretion [9]. TRH also controls post-translational glycosylation of TSH, which is important for its biologic activity [10]. Thyroid hormones mediate the negative feedback regulation of the TSH and TRH genes. Thyroxine (T_4) is converted to triiodothyronine (T_3) by a type II 5′-deiodinase (D2). It then binds to thyroid hormone nuclear receptors (TR) that interact with thyroid-hormone-responsive elements on the promoter regions of TRH and TSH subunit genes, inhibiting their transcription rate [11].

The Pituitary, Third Edition, DOI: 10.1016/B978-0-12-380926-1.10017-3

Pituitary Hyperplasia in Long-standing Hypothyroidism

Loss of thyroid hormone feedback inhibition leads not only to TRH and TSH hypersecretion, but also to proliferation of TSH-secreting cells with frank compensatory hyperplasia. Thyrotroph hyperplasia may be associated with prolactin cell hyperplasia and hyperprolactinemia, probably as a result of sustained TRH stimulation [12]. Histology reveals the preserved anterior pituitary acinar pattern surrounded by a reticulin-fiber network, but individual acini are larger, and contain many "thyroidectomy cells." These are large pale cells with eccentric nuclei and abundant vacuolated cytoplasm characteristically present in the pituitaries of experimentally induced hypothyroid rats, as well as in patients with untreated protracted hypothyroidism. The hyperplasic cells probably originate from division of pre-existing thyrotrophs and differentiation of stem cells into mature TSH-secreting cells. In addition, growth hormone (GH) and TSH bihormonal cells or "thyrosomatotrophs" have been identified in the pituitary of patients with protracted primary hypothyroidism, supporting the notion of transdifferentiation of somatotrophs to thyrotrophs contributing to the generation of thyroid cell hyperplasia [13]. Enlargement of the pituitary gland due to long-standing hypothyroidism is a well-recognized disorder. Pituitary enlargement is sometimes prominent, with growth into the suprasellar space, mimicking a neoplastic process. Recognition of this entity has important clinical implications, as thyroxine replacement therapy fully resolves these "pseudotumors" of the pituitary, avoiding inadvertent surgery [12]. In rare cases, hyperplasia to adenoma transition may occur, and monoclonal TSPA arising in the background of hyperplasia have been reported in a few patients with long-standing untreated hypothyroidism [7,14]. However, most TSPA are primary pituitary lesions unassociated with thyroid failure and without underlying thyrotroph hyperplasia, suggesting that TRH stimulation does not play a central role in tumorigenesis, although it may act as a growth promoter of transformed cells.

Impaired Thyroid Hormone Negative Feedback

Defective negative feedback of thyroid hormones on TRH or TSH secretion could also be involved in the pathogenesis of TSH-secreting tumors. In most patients harboring TSPA, TSH levels do not suppress after administration of thyroid hormones. One possible explanation could be alterations in expression or activity of deiodinase enzymes, leading to decreased T_3 concentration in the tumoral tissue. Indeed, type 3 deiodinase (D3), that catalyzes the inactivation of biologically active T_3 to diiodothyronine and T_4 to inactive reverse T_3 (rT_3), has been found to have a 6.5-fold increased expression in pituitary tumors, in comparison to normal pituitary tissue. In particular, the TSH-secreting tumor examined in that series expressed a 13.1-fold excess of D3 mRNA and reduced D2 mRNA (0.1-fold of normal pituitaries), suggesting that this pattern of deiodinase expression may contribute to the tumor resistance to thyroid hormone feedback [15]. Another mechanism for impaired thyroid hormone feedback could involve alterations in thyroid hormone receptors (TR). There are two major classes of TR, TRα and TRβ, each of which undergoes alternative splicing to generated α1 and α2 or β1 and β2 isoforms [16]. TRα2 is unable to bind ligand and has a dominant-negative effect on TR-mediated transcription. TRα1, TRβ1 and TRβ2 are T_3-binding isoforms and are expressed in the thyrotroph and the TRH neurons. However, TRβ2 is the most abundantly expressed isoform in the hypothalamic–pituitary system. A few studies on the expression and structure of TR have been reported in TSPA. Sequencing of TRα1 and TRβ1 from six tumors has been reported as normal [5], whereas no TRα1, TRα2 and TRβ1 mRNA expression was detected in one tumor [17]. In another study, normal expression levels of TRα and TRβ mRNA were detected in two TSH-secreting tumors, but the nuclear proteins were undetectable, suggesting a post-transcriptional defect in RNA processing [18]. Abnormal TRβ has been found in two TSH-secreting adenomas. In the first case, alternative splicing caused a 135 bp deletion within the ligand-binding domain of TRβ2 [19]. In the second case, a somatic mutation was identified in the ligand-binding domain of TRβ, that caused a His to Tyr substitution at codon 435 of TRβ1 corresponding to codon 450 of TRβ2 [20]. Both TRβ variants had impaired thyroid hormone binding, impaired T_3-dependent negative regulation of TSHβ and glycoprotein α-subunit genes, and showed dominant negative activity on the wild-type TRβ, accounting for the defective negative regulation of TSH in these tumors. Interestingly, the mutation found in the second case occurred in the same codon in which mutations causing the syndrome of resistance to thyroid hormone (RTH) have been previously identified. Nevertheless, TSH-secreting tumors have been rarely reported [21] in the several hundred patients diagnosed with RTH, suggesting that mutations in TRβ are not sufficient to induce tumor formation.

Altered Hypothalamic Signaling

Increased hypothalamic hormone stimulation or, alternatively, defective action of inhibitory hypothalamic hormones could be involved in increased thyrotroph proliferation and TSH secretion.

TRH

As already mentioned, TRH is the major stimulatory factor in TSH secretion. Mutations leading to constitutive activation of the TRH receptor or components of its signal transduction pathway could also be potentially involved in TSPA pathogenesis. Nevertheless, no mutations on the TRH receptor, Gαq, Gα11, or Gαs were detected in the tumors screened [22,23].

DOPAMINE

Dopamine (DA) and its agonists inhibit TSH secretion, while DA-receptor-blocking agents such as metoclopramide and domperidone increase TSH concentration both in euthyroid and hypothyroid subjects. The description of TSH-secreting tumors in two patients receiving long-term phenothiazine treatment raised the possibility of a facilitatory effect of this DA receptor-blocking drug in the development of these tumors [24]. It should be noted, however, that long-term phenothiazine treatment does not enhance plasma TSH levels. Although impaired DA receptor function could potentially be associated with TSH-secreting tumors, no mutations on the dopamine type 2 receptor gene were detected in three TSPA tested [25].

SOMATOSTATIN

Somatostatin lowers serum TSH concentrations in normal and hypothyroid patients, and also reduces the serum TSH response to TRH. TSH-secreting tumors express somatostatin receptors, evidenced by the presence of specific somatostatin-binding sites, measured either on membrane preparations or on frozen tumor sections by autoradiography [26,27]. Recently, somatostatin receptor (SSTR) subtype expression was examined in four TSH-secreting tumors. SSTR2 mRNA was detected in all tumors and the expression was significantly higher than that in normal pituitary. All other receptor subtypes except for SSTR4 were expressed in the tumors, albeit at lower levels [28]. Loss of heterozygosity at the SSTR5 locus has been described in one TSH-secreting adenoma that was associated with unusual tumor aggressiveness and resistance to treatment with somatostatin analogues [29]. An inactivating mutation in the SSTR5 gene has been described in one case of GH-secreting tumor [30], but not in TSPA. Hence, the somatostatin inhibitory pathway seems to be intact and not involved in the pathogenesis of these tumors.

Alterations in Pituitary Transcription Factors

The β-TSH gene is under transcriptional control of Pit-1, a transcription factor restricted to the anterior pituitary gland, and specifically expressed in thyrotrophs, lactotrophs and somatotrophs. Since Pit-1 is critical for the survival and proliferation of these cells, its possible role in pituitary tumorigenesis has been investigated. Collectively, the data suggest that pituitary tumorigenesis is not associated with altered expression of this gene. Pit-1 transcripts of normal size and sequence were found in GH-, PRL- and TSH-secreting tumors [31].

Familial/Genetic Syndromes

Pituitary tumors may develop as a consequence of germline mutations causing familial syndromes. The multiple endocrine neoplasia type 1 syndrome (MEN1) is an autosomal dominant disorder caused by mutations in the MEN1 gene, which acts as a tumor suppressor gene. Forty percent of patients with the MEN1 syndrome develop pituitary adenomas, with a predominance of macroprolactinomas [32]. TSPA associated with the MEN1 syndrome has been reported in very few cases [33–35]. The McCune-Albright syndrome is caused by mosaicism for an activating mutation of GNAS, the gene encoding Gs-α. Pituitary hormone hypersecretion in this syndrome is usually secondary to somatotroph hyperplasia or GH-secreting tumors, but one patient with a plurihormonal tumor secreting GH, TSH and prolactin has been reported [36]. Finally, thyrotropinomas represent 1% of pituitary tumors in the familial isolated pituitary adenoma syndrome, which is caused by mutations in the aryl hydrocarbon receptor interacting protein gene [37].

Oncogenes, Tumor Suppressor Genes and Growth Factors

Molecular studies have shown that amplified, mutated or over-expressed oncogenes, or inactivated tumor suppressor genes prevalent in other neoplasms are rarely involved in the development of pituitary tumors. Loss of heterozygosity on 11q13 was found in three of 13 TSPA, but none of them had mutations on the menin gene located in this region [38]. The gsp oncogene detected in 40% of GH-secreting tumors is not expressed in thyrotropinomas [23]. Basic fibroblast growth factor (bFGF) has been found to be over-expressed in TSH-secreting adenomas, suggesting that it may play a role in cell proliferation and the development of fibrosis in these tumors [39]. The pituitary tumor transforming gene (PTTG) is over-expressed in pituitary tumors and its level of expression seems to correlate with the degree of invasiveness in secretory adenomas [40]. The number of TSPA studied in these series was small, not allowing for a precise assessment of the degree of PTTG mRNA expression in these tumors. PTTG was found to be positively correlated with bFGF [41] and VEGF expression [42], suggesting that PTTG may induce angiogenic growth and progression of pituitary tumors. PTTG-targeted over-expression using the α-glycoprotein subunit promoter was associated with the development of plurihormonal hyperplasia and microadenomas, secreting TSH, LH and GH [43] in a transgenic mouse model.

Abnormal Cell Signaling Pathways

The PI3K/AKT/mTOR pathway is altered in pituitary tumors. AKT was found to be over-expressed as well as overactivated by phosphorylation in all types of pituitary adenomas [44]. In a mouse model of TSH-secreting tumors, in which a knockin mutation in the TRβ gene causes complete loss of thyroid hormone binding and transcription activity of the receptor, AKT and its downstream effectors mTOR and $p70^{S6K}$ were found to be activated in the mouse pituitaries, causing increased cell proliferation and decreased apoptosis [45]. Furthermore, the tumors had over-expression of cyclin D1 and hyperphosphorylation of RB, contributing to aberrant pituitary growth [46].

PATHOLOGY

Thyrotrophs represent approximately 5% of adenohypophyseal cells. They derive from precursors that express the transcription factor Pit-1, and require additional expression of thyrotroph embryonic factor (TEF) and Gata2 for differentiation [47].

Thyrotroph cell adenomas are composed of chromophobic cells that immunostain positively for TSHβ, α-subunit and Pit-1. On electron microscopy, thyrotroph cell adenomas consist of elongated angular cells with long cytoplasmic processes containing small sparse, spherical secretory granules (50–200 nm), usually lining up along the cell membrane [48]. An interesting feature of TSH-secreting tumors is that many are plurihormonal, producing α-subunits, PRL, GH, LH and FSH, in different combinations, in addition to TSH [4]. Most frequently GH and PRL are cosecreted with TSH, in line with the common transcription regulation by Pit-1 shared by these hormones. TSPA may be monomorphous, consisting of one morphologically distinct cell type that produces two or more hormones, or plurimorphous, being composed of two or more morphologically distinct cell types each producing different hormones, sometimes in the same secretory granule [49–51]. Despite positive immunostaining in the cell cytoplasm, hormone production may not always be manifest clinically, or by increased serum TSH levels. This discrepancy could be due to synthesis of TSH molecules that are either not being secreted or are not detected by routine assay methods. Secretion of uncombined α- and β-subunits that are biologically inactive could explain the lack of clinical expression of these tumors.

TSH-secreting tumors are usually invasive macroadenomas that tend to have a very fibrous consistency, possibly due to increased expression of bFGF [39]. In a recent series, three of ten TSH-secreting tumors were classified as atypical adenomas according to the World Health Organization criteria (invasive growth, increased mitotic activity, and positive staining for p53 and Ki67 in greater than 3% of cells) [52]. Nevertheless, these three tumors did not recur or metastasize, indicating a lack of relationship between the morphological features and the biological behavior in these cases.

Thus far, two TSH-secreting carcinoma cases have been described [53,54]. Besides being locally invasive, there was also evidence of tumor metastasis to lung, liver, bone and the abdominal cavity in one case [53], and in brain tissue in the other [54].

CLINICAL FEATURES

The mean age at diagnosis is approximately 45 years, ranging from 8 to 84, with a female to male ratio of 1:1.18 (Table 17.1). The clinical presentation is related to the pattern of hormone hypersecretion by the adenoma, as well as to the presence of compression of neighboring structures by the tumor, depending on its size.

Hyperthyroidism

Most patients with TSH-secreting tumors present with classic symptoms and signs of hyperthyroidism of variable severity, indistinguishable from those caused by primary thyroid disease. Unlike Graves' disease, however, ophthalmopathy, pretibial myxedema and acropachy are absent, and the female preponderance characteristic of autoimmune thyroid disease is not apparent. The history of thyroid dysfunction is often long, with a diagnosis delay that may reach several years, mainly if patients are misdiagnosed as having Graves' disease, which may lead to inappropriate thyroidectomy or radio-iodine thyroid ablation in about 30% of them [5]. The mean delay between documentation of hyperthyroidism and diagnosis of a TSH adenoma was 6 ± 2 years in patients with intact thyroid, as opposed to 12 ± 3 years in those with previously treated thyroids [55]. Some patients were misdiagnosed for over 20 years [55–57]. Nevertheless, more recent series report a significantly shorter latency time between onset of symptoms and diagnosis. Cardiovascular symptoms related to thyrotoxicosis such as tachycardia, atrial fibrillation and heart failure are not frequently described, and episodes of periodic paralysis have been rarely reported [58–61]. Unilateral exophthalmos due to orbital invasion by the pituitary tumor has been reported in three patients with TSPA [62–64], whereas

TABLE 17.1 Clinical Characteristics of Patients with TSH-Secreting Pituitary Tumors

		Ref	n.	Mean Age(years)	F/M Ratio	Goiter	Visual Impairment	Acromegaly	Hyperprolactinemia	Macrodenomas
E Macchia et al.	2009	[76]	26	45	15/11	21/26	3/26	1/26	0/26	11/26
G Marucci et al.	2009	[52]	10	46.5	5/5	1/10		1/10		10/10
MS Elston et al.	2009	[150]	6	43	3/3	6/6	2/6	1/6		5/6
MJ Clarke et al.	2008	[65]	21	46	6/15		8/21	1/21		16/21
F Roelfsema et al.	2008	[104]	5		1/4	5/5				4/5
A Yoshihara et al.	2007	[82]	8		1/7					
T keinitz et al.	2007	[56]	5	58.6	5/0	4/5			1/5	3/5
R Ness-Abramof et al.	2007	[81]	11	44.8	5/6		6/11	2/11		10/11
F Boqazzi et al.	2006	[94]	8	45	6/2					
D Mannavola et al.	2005	[123]	8		5/3					5/8
A Teramoto et al.	2004	[57]	20	41.2	16/4	16/20		3/20	3/20	18/20
HV Socin et al.	2003	[66]	43	44	20/23			8/43	9/43	34/41
YY Wu et al.	2003	[80]	7	48	6/1			1/7		6/7
NJ Sarlis et al.	2003	[105]	21							20/21
P Caron et al.	2001	[147]	11	43	6/5				1/11	9/11
JM Kuhn et al.	2000	[95]	18		9/9	5/18	2/18			11/16
F Brucker-Davis et al.	1999	[55]	25	44	17/8	20/25	9/25	1/25	3/25	23/25
M Losa et al.	1999	[133]	24	40.1	11/13			5/24	2/24	18/24
M Losa et al.	1997	[108]	5		3/2					4/5
L Persani et al.	1997	[125]	10							
P Beck-Peccoz et al.	1996	[5]	280	41	140/115	166/177	53/126		9/30	172/243
Total			572	45	1.18	(244/292) 84%	(83/233) 36%	(24/183) 13%	(28/184) 15%	(379/505) 75%

bilateral exophthalmos was present in a few patients who subsequently developed autoimmune thyroiditis [5]. The prevalence of antithyroid antibodies in patients with TSH-secreting tumors is low, similar to that encountered in the general population. However, the diagnosis of TSPA may be delayed by the association with Hashimoto's thyroiditis [65–67], because of the absence of hyperthyroidism in these patients [7,68,69]. In situations such as these, the inadequate suppression of TSH during L-thyroxine replacement therapy should suggest the presence of autonomous TSH hypersecretion from a pituitary tumor.

Goiter

The thyroid gland is enlarged as assessed by physical examination in about 90% of patients. Thyroid nodules are frequently reported, but differentiated thyroid carcinomas were documented in only a few cases [70–73]. It is unusual for the thyroid mass to be the presenting symptom of TSPA, although a patient with a rapidly growing goiter causing dyspnea and stridor, with tracheal compression leading to tracheomalacia, has been reported [74].

Goiters are frequent even in patients who had previously undergone thyroidectomy, since the thyroid remnant may enlarge as a consequence of persistent TSH stimulation. In fact, regrowth of the thyroid gland after thyroidectomy in patients inappropriately treated for primary thyroid disease may alert the physician to the presence of excess TSH production.

Pituitary Tumor Mass Effect

TSH-secreting tumors are usually large, with a 75% rate of macroadenomas at the time of diagnosis (Table 17.1). Consequently, signs and symptoms secondary to compression of surrounding anatomic structures are common. Visual field defects and impaired vision are reported in approximately 35% of patients and complaints of headaches are not uncommon. Studies of anterior pituitary hormone function are not reported in detail in most case series, therefore the prevalence of hypopituitarism cannot be accurately assessed. Symptoms indicative of hypogonadism such as amenorrhea, impotence and decrease libido are reported in 15–20% of cases, but they may often be secondary to coexistent hyperprolactinemia. The high frequency of invasive macroadenomas in this tumor subtype has often been attributed to the delay in diagnosis that was common before the era of sensitive TSH immunoassays. An increased incidence of invasive macroadenomas in patients who have previously undergone thyroid ablation has been reported, in comparison to intrasellar tumors that were more frequent in patients with untreated thyroid [5,75]. The invasiveness of the tumors in patients with a history of previous thyroid ablation has been paralleled to that described in patients developing Nelson's syndrome after bilateral adrenalectomy for Cushing's disease.

With the considerable evolution of the diagnosis of TSPA in the last two decades due to the widespread availability of ultrasensitive methods for TSH measurement, and the improvement in pituitary imaging, it could be anticipated that tumors would be diagnosed at an earlier stage. Indeed, there are reports of an increase in the relative incidence of microadenoma [66]. In contrast, according to a recent series, the high ratio between macro- and microadenomas has remained stable over time. Moreover, the latency in diagnosis was significantly shorter over time in macroadenomas, implying that TSPA tend to be large and invasive in nature, and not as a consequence of diagnosis delay [76].

Hormone Cosecretion

Cosecretion of GH occurs commonly, being reported in approximately 15% of patients (Table 17.1). In some patients with acromegaly, signs and symptoms of hyperthyroidism may be clinically missed, as the clinical picture related to GH hypersecretion may predominate. Hyperprolactinemia has been reported in almost 20% of patients, mostly manifesting with amenorrhea, galactorrhea, impotence, or decreased libido in addition to TSH-induced hyperthyroidism (Table 17.1). Although cosecretion of prolactin by the tumor itself is common, in some of the patients hyperprolactinemia may be secondary to stalk compression by the large TSPA. Cosecretion of FSH and/or LH is uncommon, being found in about 1% of cases. LH hypersecretion may rarely manifest with elevated androgen levels [77].

Immunohistochemical studies report a larger incidence of hormonal co-expression, suggesting that these hormones may not be secreted in large enough quantities to lead to clinical disease [65,78,79]. Positive immunostaining for ACTH has been reported in eight cases, with no clinical evidence of hypercortisolism [65,77,80,81].

TSH-secreting tumors occurring in the context of multiple endocrine neoplasia syndrome type 1 [33–35] and in McCune-Albright syndrome [36] have also been described.

DIAGNOSIS

Laboratory Studies

The presence of elevated, inappropriately normal, or just detectable TSH levels, measured by a reliable and sensitive assay, concurrently with elevated peripheral

TABLE 17.2 Laboratory Characteristics of Patients with TSH-Secreting Pituitary Tumors

		Ref	n.	Thyrotoxicosis	TSH Range (mU/l)	Elevated α-SU	α-SU/TSH Molar Ratio >1
E Macchia et al.	2009	[76]	26	18/26	1.4–9	18/26	25/26
G Marucci et al.	2009	[52]	10	8/10			
MS Elston et al.	2009	[150]	6	6/6		3/6	3/6
MJ Clarke et al.	2008	[65]	21	10/21			
F Roelfsema et al.	2008	[104]	5	5/5	1.4–5.8	3/5	
A Yoshihara et al.	2007	[82]	8	8/8	0.4–8.2		
T keinitz et al.	2007	[56]	5	5/5	2–126	3/5	3/5
R Ness-Abramof et al.	2007	[81]	11	6/11			
F Boqazzi et al.	2006	[94]	8			7/8	7/8
D Mannavola et al.	2005	[123]	8			1/5	1/5
A Teramoto et al.	2004	[57]	20		0.46–55	15/19	19/19
HV Socin et al.	2003	[66]	43	32/43	0.1–12	13/43	
YY Wu et al.	2003	[80]	7			1/3	3/3
NJ Sarlis et al.	2003	[105]	21				
P Caron et al.	2001	[147]	11				
JM Kuhn et al.	2000	[95]	18	18/18			
F Brucker-Davis et al.	1999	[55]	25	22/25	1.1–393	8/14	12/14
M Losa et al.	1999	[133]	24	20/24			
M Losa et al.	1997	[108]	5		1.1–7.8		
L Persani et al.	1997	[125]	10	2/10			
P Beck-Peccoz et al.	1996	[5]	280			93/142	108/135
Total			572	(160/212)75%	0.46–393	(195/428) 46%	(181/221) 82%

thyroid hormones is essential for the diagnosis of a TSH-secreting tumor. Nevertheless, many patients initially misdiagnosed and treated for primary hyperthyroidism were rendered euthyroid or hypothyroid by thyroid ablation and were no longer hyperthyroid at the time of diagnosis. Currently available sensitive TSH immunometric assays clearly distinguish the markedly suppressed TSH levels found in primary hyperthyroidism from conditions in which the thyrotroph is not suppressed to such a degree. The importance of early diagnosis should be emphasized, as it may increase the chances of identifying smaller tumors with a more favorable outcome [5,66]. TSH levels vary widely, ranging from 0.4 [57,82] to 393 mU/L [55,56] in recent series. Mean TSH levels are several-fold higher in patients previously treated with thyroid ablation, despite peripheral thyroid hormone levels still in the hyperthyroid range [5,55]. Serum TSH levels do not appear to correlate with the severity of clinical hyperthyroidism, suggesting the existence of TSH molecules with variable biologic activity [83]. TSH molecules secreted by these tumors are immunologically identical to native TSH [50,84] but the biologic/immunologic (B/I) ratio of serum or tumor-derived TSH from patients with thyrotropinomas is usually increased [85–88]. Variant or aberrant glycosylation of the TSH glycoprotein may explain the altered B/I ratio found in the molecule secreted by TSPA [84,89].

In earlier series α-subunit levels were elevated in the majority of patients with TSH-secreting tumors, being as such an important diagnostic tool. Nevertheless, in more recent series, normal α-subunits levels were observed in 35% [5,69] to 60% of cases (Table 17.2) [66]. Normal α-subunit levels seem to be found more frequently in microadenomas than in macroadenomas [66,69]. Furthermore, caution should be exercised when evaluating α-subunit levels in menopausal women or in men with primary hypogonadism, as the elevated gonadotropins could contribute to the observed elevated α-subunit level, which is common to the glycoprotein hormones. In these patients, different normal criteria have been suggested [90].

An α-subunit/TSH molar ratio greater than 1 is found in about 80% of patients with documented TSPA (Table 17.2) [5,51,55,66]. This ratio is helpful in the differential diagnosis between thyrotropinomas and nontumorous TSH hypersecretion, where the ratio is usually less than unity.

Dynamic Tests

Dynamic testing is important mainly in patients in whom imaging does not reveal a defined pituitary mass or when only a microadenoma is apparent. In these cases, the association of resistance to thyroid hormone with a pituitary incidentaloma may be difficult to discern from a TSH-secreting tumor [91]. As mentioned above, a normal α-subunit level or a normal α-subunit/TSH molar ratio in this situation would not rule out a small thyrotropinoma. The combined use of the T_3 suppression test and the TRH test have increased specificity and sensitivity for the diagnosis work-up in these situations [92].

TRH Test

Absence of a TSH response to exogenous TRH stimulation was initially believed to be a universal finding in patients with TSPA, implying autonomous TSH hypersecretion by the tumor. Although this is true for most patients, over 20% do in fact respond normally to TRH, with a poststimulatory doubling of basal TSH levels [55,66,93]. Thus, a blunt TSH response to TRH stimulation supports the presence of a TSPA, but a normal test by no means excludes the diagnosis. The α-subunit and the TSH responses to TRH are usually parallel, but in some instances a TRH-induced rise in α-subunit values occurred despite an absent TSH response. In patients with hyperthyroidism, discrepancies between TSH and α-subunit responses to TRH are pathognomonic of TSPA cosecreting other pituitary hormones [51]. According to Brucker-Davis et al., in patients with intact thyroid, the most sensitive test to identify a TSH-secreting adenoma was an elevated α-subunit/TSH ratio (83%), followed by an elevated α-subunit level (75%), a flat or decreased response to TRH (71%) and an elevated baseline TSH (43%). A flat or decreased response to TRH was the most specific test for the diagnosis of TSPA (96%), followed by elevated α-subunit (90%), elevated baseline TSH (88%) and elevated α-subunit/TSH ratio (65%). The TSH response to TRH had the best positive and negative predictive value. In patients with prior thyroid treatment, the TRH test was less sensitive (64%), but was highly specific (100%) [55].

T_3 Suppression Test

Patients harboring TSH-secreting tumors do not suppress TSH levels normally after exogenous administration of T_3 or T_4. In two series of TSPA, only about 20% of tested patients responded by a slight reduction of TSH levels after T_3 administration for 10 days [93,94]. A complete inhibition of TSH secretion after T_3 suppression test (80–100 μg per day for 8–10 days) has never been recorded in patients with TSPA [5,55,66]. In this latter condition, T_3 suppression seems to be the most sensitive and specific test in assessing the presence of a TSPA. However, this test is contraindicated in elderly patients or in those with coronary heart disease. Reduction of circulating T_4 or T_3 by antithyroid drugs results in elevation of TSH levels in the majority of patients. This suggests that endogenous elevated thyroid hormone levels have some inhibitory effect on tumor thyrotroph function.

Octreotide Test

Somatostatin inhibits TSH secretion in physiological conditions and in most TSPA since they express somatostatin receptors and retain the sensitivity to native somatostatin and its analogues (octreotide and lanreotide) [26,95]. Somatostatin infusion or acute octreotide administration reduced TSH levels in most patients tested [5,57]. TSH levels decreased by more than 50% of baseline after the acute subcutaneous (s.c.) administration of 50–100 μg of octreotide in 95% of patients [96]. Nevertheless, patients with resistance to thyroid hormone have been shown to respond with a similar degree of TSH reduction after s.c. injection of 100 μg of octreotide. However, continued treatment with octreotide-LAR for 2 months did not change TSH and peripheral thyroid hormone levels in patients with RTH. Free thyroid hormones normalized or significantly decreased in 7/8 patients with TSPA, although TSH levels remained unchanged [83]. Thus, a 2-month clinical trial with somatostatin analogues, but not the acute octreotide test, may assist in the differential diagnosis of difficult cases of central hyperthyroidism.

Circadian Secretion of TSH

In other hormone-secreting pituitary adenomas, e.g., Cushing's disease and prolactinoma, hormone secretion is characterized by diminished or absent diurnal amplitude, increased basal secretion, increased pulse frequency and diminished secretory regularity [97–99]. Similarly, circadian and pulsatile TSH secretion was absent in most patients with TSH-secreting tumors [100,101]. TSH pulsatility was detected in three patients [51,102,103], but the physiologic circadian TSH variation was absent. In a recent study by Roelfsema et al. the TSH secretion pattern studied in five patients was characterized by increased pulse frequency, delayed diurnal rhythm, enhanced basal secretion, spikiness and disorderliness [104].

Pituitary Imaging

Most reported thyrotropinomas are large macroadenomas which frequently invade surrounding structures such as the cavernous and sphenoid sinuses; they also extend suprasellarly, and may compress the optic chiasm. Delayed diagnosis and previous inadvertent ablative therapy to the thyroid gland, thereby reducing endogenous negative feedback on the thyrotroph, have been implicated as possible causes for this relatively aggressive tumor proliferation [5,85]. On the other hand, it is possible that the tumors display an inherently more invasive growth behavior irrespective of diagnosis delay [76].

CT and MRI imaging are currently used for the evaluation of pituitary and parasellar abnormalities and masses, but MRI has the additional advantage of better delineating the relationship of pituitary tumors to surrounding structures. In 80% of patients thyrotropinomas were hypoenhancing with respect to the normal pituitary after gadolinium administration [105].

According to recent series, about 20% of cases are microadenomas, which are mainly diagnosed by CT and/or MRI, although in isolated cases explorative transsphenoidal surgery [85] or inferior petrosal sinus sampling [106] were necessary for tumor localization. About one-quarter of patients harboring macroadenomas had minimal or no suprasellar extension, while the remainder had either marked suprasellar extension or invasion of sphenoidal and cavernous sinuses. Collectively, about 30% of the patients harbored either microadenomas or small enclosed macroadenomas with better clinical prognosis, whereas in 70% of them larger tumors were evident. Some of these tumors were highly invasive, extending to the hypothalamus, brain stem, or orbit [63]. Curiously, two cases of highly calcified tumors ("pituitary stones") have been reported [107].

Thyrotropinomas have been successfully imaged by means of indium-111 pentetreotide single-photon emission tomography, thus further confirming the presence of somatostatin receptors in these tumors in vivo [108]. There was a trend for a direct correlation between the degree of TSH inhibition after acute octreotide administration and the degree of radioisotope uptake by the tumor, but larger series are necessary to confirm these findings. This imaging modality may also play a role in the identification of ectopic tumors, although so far only two cases of ectopic TSPA have been reported in the nasopharynx [109,110]. The presence of tumoral dopamine receptors has been demonstrated in vivo by iodine-123 iodobenzamine scanning in one patient [111,112].

DIFFERENTIAL DIAGNOSIS

Faced with a patient with elevated thyroid hormone levels and detectable circulating TSH, two important clinical diagnoses should be considered. These include inappropriate TSH secretion and euthyroid hyperthyroxinemia. The syndrome of inappropriate TSH secretion comprises two entities: (1) neoplastic TSH secretion; and (2) nonneoplastic pituitary hypersecretion of TSH due to thyroid hormone resistance.

Resistance to Thyroid Hormones (RTH)

The syndrome of resistance to thyroid hormone (RTH) is a rare inherited autosomal dominant disease [113], most commonly caused by heterozygous point mutations in the TRβ gene [114,115]. Thyroid hormone receptors are ligand-gated transcription factors [116], and most RTH mutations affect the C-terminal ligand-binding domain, reducing TRβ affinity for T_3 or impairing the interaction with the corepressors or coactivators involved in thyroid hormone action. The defective TRβ exerts a dominant negative effect on the normal allele by engaging it in homodimerization.

The clinical manifestations of RTH are variable, and patients may be metabolically hypo-, hyper-, or euthyroid. In addition to altered thyroid function, patients often present with goiter. Interestingly, there appear to be two distinct forms of the disease; generalized resistance affects all tissues, whereas patients with isolated pituitary resistance exhibit specific central defects in feedback inhibition of thyroid hormone, with normal peripheral responses [117]. In generalized RTH, patients are often asymptomatic due to elevated thyroid hormones compensating for the reduced affinity of the mutant TRβ for T_3. Patients with more severe mutations may have symptoms of hypothyroidism. One exception is that patients with generalized RTH can display tachycardia, a classic symptom of hyperthyroidism, because heart rate is predominantly controlled by the TRα isoform, which is unaffected by RTH mutations. On the other hand, patients with central RTH generally display symptoms of hyperthyroidism along with elevated TSH levels [118,119]. The separate existence of two forms of RTH is controversial, since the same mutations have been found in both types of disorders. Investigators have often suggested that generalized and central RTH represent opposite poles of the same continuum of disease symptoms [118,120]. In a recent study, Wondisford and colleagues introduced a naturally occurring mutation (R429Q) into the germline of mice at the TRβ locus. The mice developed typical characteristics of central RTH. The group showed that the mutation, which impairs TR homodimerization and corepressor binding, is associated with selective impairment of thyroid hormone-mediated gene repression, not affecting actions mediated by hormone binding with coactivators and positive gene regulation [121]. They propose that this is the key feature that distinguishes central RTH mutations from generalized RTH mutations [122]. Interestingly, in 15% of patients with RTH no mutations in the TRβ gene have been identified, raising the possibility that deficiency/mutations in cofactors may be involved in the etiology of these cases.

Biochemically, no differences in basal values of TSH and free thyroid hormone levels are seen in patients with TSPA compared to those with RTH, but the latter have normal α-subunit levels and α-subunit/TSH molar ratios are less than 1 [89]. When dynamically tested, they usually display an exaggerated TSH stimulation by TRH, and often TSH levels are suppressible by thyroid hormones, in contrast to patients harboring thyrotropinomas. The response to long-acting somatostatin analogues may also be useful in this differential diagnosis as patients with TSPA usually display a marked decrease in thyroid hormone levels, while patients with RTH do not respond [89,123].

Peripheral markers of thyroid hormone action may also assist in the differential diagnosis of these two entities. Circulating sex-hormone-binding globulin (SHBG) is elevated in over 90% of TSPA patients, reflecting clinical hyperthyroidism, whereas levels are usually normal in generalized thyroid hormone resistance [124]. Similarly, markers of bone turnover such as carboxyterminal cross-linked telopeptide of type I collagen (ICTP) are elevated in the hyperthyroid state caused by TSH-secreting tumors and are in the normal range in thyroid resistance syndrome [125]. An occasional patient with a TSH-secreting microadenoma not demonstrable by imaging techniques may be difficult to distinguish from patients with selective pituitary resistance to thyroid hormones. In these cases screening family members for thyroid function abnormalities may be helpful. Alternatively, direct screening for TRβ mutations may be required.

Recently, thyroid color flow Doppler sonography (CFDS) has been suggested as an adjunctive tool for differentiating patients with TSPA versus RTH. Baseline CFDS pattern and peak systolic velocity were elevated in both conditions at baseline, but after the T_3 suppression test these parameters normalized in most patients with RTH, but not in those with TSPA [94].

Recent discoveries of genetic defects that alter cell membrane transport of thyroid hormone and its metabolism broadened the definition of RTH to include all defects that could reduce the biological activity of thyroid hormones. A defect in the active transport of T_3 into cells was first described in 2004 [126]. It is caused by mutations in the monocarboxylate transporter 8 (MT8) gene located on the X chromosome. Affected males present with severe psychomotor disorders and an unusual combination of low levels of T_4, high concentrations of T_3, and low levels of reverse T_3. Another cause of impaired biological activity of thyroid hormone is decreased generation of deiodinase 2. Inherited partial deficiency of selenoprotein enzymes, including deiodinases that generate T_3, was identified in two families in 2005 [127]. It is caused by mutations in the selenocysteine insertion sequence-binding protein 2 gene (*SECISBP2*), thus producing a variable decrease in several selenoproteins. The characteristic laboratory findings in subjects with SBP2 mutations are high T_4, low T_3, high rT_3, and slightly elevated levels of TSH.

Euthyroid Hyperthyroxinemia

Several disorders cause euthyroid hyperthyroxinemia [128]. They are not uncommon and should be ruled out before considering an extensive work-up for inappropriate TSH secretion.

1. Artifactual high thyroxine levels can be caused by thyroxine-binding antibodies, although the interference is uncommon with current assays [129].
2. TSH levels may be spuriously elevated in some assays due to the presence of anti-TSH antibodies or heterophile antibodies, the most common of which are the human antimouse immunoglobulins [130].
3. Abnormalities in circulating thyroid-binding proteins may also cause elevated total thyroxine levels with normal TSH levels. Increased TBG levels, either congenital or secondary to estrogen, drugs, or liver disease, are not uncommon. In these patients the free thyroid hormone levels are also normal. Similarly, increased binding to prealbumin or albumin, as occurs in familial dysalbuminemic hyperthyroxinemia, or to transthyretin [131] may cause a similar biochemical profile.
4. Situations in which there is inhibition of T_4 to T_3 conversion, including drugs that inhibit 5′-deiodinase activity, 5′-deiodinase deficiency, or the sick-euthyroid syndrome, can lead to elevated thyroxine levels. T_3 levels may be normal or low and rT_3 levels are elevated in these patients.

Clinically, when exogenous thyroxine treatment is given, there is a period of approximately 6 weeks for TSH to be effectively lowered and achieve steady-state levels. In this "disequilibrium" situation, that also occurs physiologically during the neonatal period, elevated thyroxine levels may occur in the presence of detectable TSH levels [132].

The conditions to be considered when evaluating a patient for a TSH-secreting tumor are summarized in Table 17.3.

TABLE 17.3 Differential Diagnosis of Inappropriate TSH Secretion

	Total T_4	Free T_4	T_3	TSH
TSH-secreting tumor	↑	↑	↑	↑or N
Reduced thyroid hormone sensitivity				
GRTH	↑	↑	↑	↑or N
PRTH	↑	↑	↑	↑or N
MCT8 mutation	↓	↓	↑	↑or N
SBP2 mutation	↑	↑	↓	↑or N
Euthyroid hyperthyroxinemia				
Alterations in thyroid binding proteins	↑	N	↑	N
Interference of antibodies in thyroid hormone and TSH assays	↑ or N	↑ or N	↑ or N	↑ or N
Inhibition of T_4 to T_3 conversion	↑	↑	↓	N
Acute non-thyroidal illness	↑ or N	↑ or N	↓↓	N or ↑

N, normal; ↑, increased; ↓, decreased; GRTH, generalized resistance to thyroid hormone; PRTH, pituitary resistance to thyroid hormone; MCT8, monocarboxylate transporter 8; SBP2, selenocysteine insertion sequence binding protein 2.

TREATMENT

Surgery

The goal of therapy in patients with TSH-secreting adenomas is to restore euthyroidism in hyperthyroid patients and eliminate the symptoms of mass effect in patients with large tumors. Therefore, selective transsphenoidal pituitary surgery is the preferred initial therapy for these patients as it provides the possibility of complete removal of neoplastic tissue and definitive cure, thus controlling hyperthyroidism, while preserving anterior pituitary function [133]. The major obstacles to analysis of surgical results are the lack of universally accepted criteria of cure and the fact that series are usually small due to the rarity of the disease. Surgical "cure," defined as normalization of thyroid hormone and TSH levels, and absence of residual mass on pituitary imaging, has been documented in about 40% of patients after surgery [5]. This number has remained stable in most series from the past 10 years [55,66,133], although three recent series have reported long-term remission in approximately 50% [57,65,76] or even 80% of cases [52].

Not surprisingly, most patients cured by surgery alone had either microadenomas or macroadenomas with minimal or no extrasellar expansion. An additional third had normalization of thyroid function despite the presence of residual tumor on imaging studies. The value of pituitary surgery in patients with larger tumors where total excision is not feasible should be underscored. Debulking of tumor mass often provides improvement in visual field defects, CNS symptoms and hyperthyroidism.

Radiotherapy

Radiation therapy has been used as an adjuvant to surgery in patients not in remission after surgery. In some patients, tumor growth was stabilized and patients became euthyroid, despite persistently elevated TSH levels. The actual cure rate for radiotherapy is probably underestimated due to lack of long-term follow-up studies. Taking into consideration the well-known late side effects of radiotherapy, it is now prescribed less frequently. The risk of complications is potentially lower when techniques such as stereotactic radiosurgery are used, as radiation is delivered to the region of interest with less exposure of surrounding brain tissue. However, long-term follow-up studies in general are few, and specifically the small number of TSPA treated with these techniques precludes accurate evaluation of efficacy and complication rates. The use of radiotherapy should be carefully weighted in light of the current availability of efficacious medical treatment such as somatostatin analogues. This treatment modality should probably be reserved for patients with residual tumors unresponsive to medical treatment.

Medical Treatment

Therapy directed at the thyroid gland level was previously used in a large number of patients either because they were initially diagnosed as having primary thyroid disease, or as an attempt to control hyperthyroidism until the pituitary tumor could be targeted. Antithyroid drugs reduced thyroid hormone levels, at least temporarily, in most patients. About one-third of patients underwent partial or total thyroidectomy, or radioactive iodine ablation, sometimes on multiple occasions [134,135] because of recurrence of goiter and hyperthyroidism. In some instances, ablative thyroid therapy was used after unsuccessful pituitary surgery in an attempt to control the hyperthyroidism [50,63]. Importantly, all therapies directed to the thyroid gland result in increased TSH secretion by the pituitary gland, and in the long term carry the potential risk of causing tumor expansion [5,136]. As such, direct antithyroid treatment should be avoided, reserving the use of antithyroid drugs for short-term preparation for pituitary surgery. β-Adrenergic blocking agents such as propranolol provide temporary symptomatic relief and could be used as adjunct therapy.

Dopamine Agonists

Dopamine agonists are seldom effective for the treatment of TSH-secreting adenomas. In two small series, the administration of bromocriptine reduced TSH levels in only 20% of patients tested [57,86]. In a few patients, the DA agonist may in fact reduce α-subunit levels, without altering TSH levels [100,101,137]. Tumor shrinkage has been reported only in those with combined excess of TSH and PRL [57,66,138,139]. However, Kienitz et al. recently reported that euthyroidism was restored and that tumor size remained stable in three out of four patients who received dopamine agonist therapy [56]. Two of them had microadenomas and two had macroadenomas. The fourth patient developed tachycardia and a paradoxical elevation of TSH that led to discontinuation of cabergoline. A similar case of a paradoxical rise of TSH to bromocriptine has been previously reported [140], but the mechanism remains unclear. Two additional cases of normalization of thyroid function with cabergoline have been reported, one of which has been resistant to therapy with somatostatin analogues [81,141].

Somatostatin Analogues

Treatment with long-acting somatostatin analogues is the main medical modality available for TSH-secreting tumors [142]. Autoradiograpy and binding studies have demonstrated the expression of somatostatin receptors (SSTR) in TSH-secreting adenomas. Expression analysis of somatostatin receptor subtypes has been conducted in very few tumors; in one case analyzed by qualitative RT-PCR the tumor expressed predominantly SSTR2, but all SSTR types except for SSTR1 mRNA were also expressed (Figure 17.1) [143]. In four additional cases analyzed by quantitative RT-PCR, SSTR2, SSTR1 and SSTR5 were the most abundantly expressed subtypes [28]. The presence of SSTR2 in all tumors tested explains the good clinical response of these tumors to treatment with the currently available somatostatin analogues, which preferentially bind to this SSTR subtype. The clinical response sometimes can be dramatic, with marked tumor shrinkage occurring after just a few weeks of treatment (Figure 17.2). During short-term treatment (up to 2 weeks) octreotide induced a mean 74% decrease in TSH level in 90% of patients, with normalization of thyroid hormone levels in 73% [96]. A parallel decrease in α-subunits was reported in 78% of them. With treatment extension, the percentage of cases in which there was thyroid function normalization increased to 84–95%, tumor shrinkage was reported in 40–50%, improvement in visual fields occurred in 75% of patients and goiter size reduction was reported in 20% of them [5,96]. An impressive improvement in visual field defects occurring just

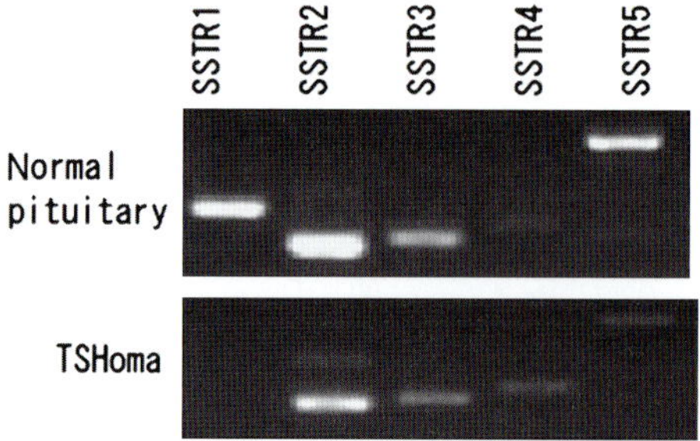

FIGURE 17.1 Expression of somatostatin receptor subtypes in a TSH-secreting tumor in comparison to the expression in normal pituitary. *From Usui et al. [143].*

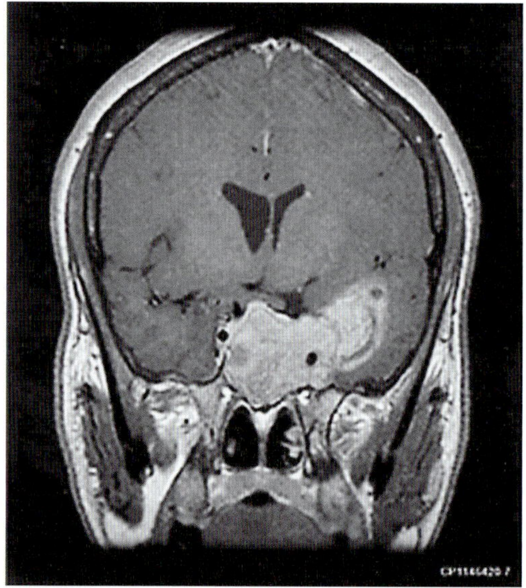

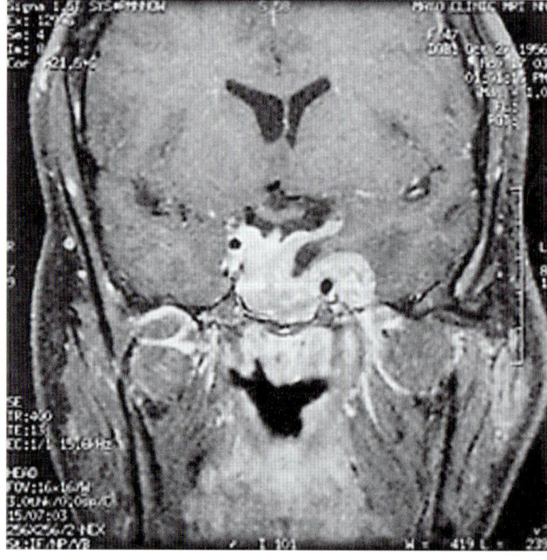

FIGURE 17.2 Marked tumor volume reduction of a mixed TSH/GH-secreting tumor after 1 week of therapy with s.c. octreotide 50 μg t.i.d and one I.M. injection of Octreotide-LAR 20 mg. (A) Baseline; (B) 2 months after treatment. *From Atkinson et al. [151].*

3 hours after initiation of treatment has been reported [144]. In about 20% of patients on octreotide an escape of TSH hypersecretion without increased thyroid hormone levels was observed. The tachyphylaxis was successfully reversed by increasing the dose of octreotide. True escape from therapy occurred in 10–12% of patients, with complete resistance in 4% of cases. The dose of octreotide in patients with TSH-secreting adenomas to achieve TSH normalization was reported to be lower than that needed to suppress GH in GH-secreting adenomas [5,60,69,96,144,145].

Slow-release depot preparations of octreotide (Sandostatin-LAR) and somatuline (Lanreotide) have been shown to be equally effective in the treatment of TSH-secreting tumors, with the added advantage of increased tolerability and acceptance by patients [95,146,147].

Primary medical therapy with somatostatin analogues has been reported by a few investigators [66,147]. Reduction in TSH levels, thyroid hormone normalization and tumor shrinkage rates were similar in the 26 patients reported by Socin et al. to those reported when medical treatment was given postoperatively. Nevertheless, surgical outcome did not improve in the 19 patients who received presurgical octreotide therapy. In a recent large series Macchia and colleagues reported 15 patients treated preoperatively by somatostatin analogues with an apparent, although not statistically significant, increase in success rate in micro- but not in macroadenomas [76]. Chronic medical treatment was given in eight patients because of poor general condition, absence of a visible adenoma on MRI or patient preference [66,81]. This treatment was rendered successfully. Hence, although the number of reported patients is small, it seems that primary treatment with somatostatin analogues may be recommended under specific circumstances.

Of interest are the findings of octreotide treatment in pregnant women. This treatment was effective in restoring euthyroidism in the mother and had no side effects on development and thyroid function of the fetuses [148,149].

CRITERIA OF CURE AND FOLLOW-UP

No single criterion is sufficient to define cure of thyrotropinoma patients. Normalization of thyroid hormone and TSH levels, albeit a clinical goal, does not necessarily reflect cure, as it may occur despite the presence of significant residual tumor mass. Undetectable TSH levels in the early postoperative period in patients who were hyperthyroid before surgery are highly predictive of complete tumor removal as all these patients were reported to have a normal postoperative MRI and normal TSH suppression after T_3 administration [69]. Nevertheless, recurrence may also occur after apparent complete tumor surgical excision, especially in patients in whom dynamic stimulatory and suppressive tests of TSH secretion remain abnormal.

Because of the relative rarity of these tumors and the lack of homogeneous large treatment series, recurrence and follow-up data are still missing. Thus, careful long-term monitoring of these patients is indicated.

CONCLUSIONS

With improvement in diagnostic techniques and increased awareness of the disease, TSH-secreting tumors are being more readily detected. It appears that diagnosis of the disease at an earlier stage of tumor growth may improve prognosis. As there are essentially few unique aspects of the clinical presentation of these hyperthyroid patients, their initial distinction from patients with primary thyroid disease is difficult, justifying the recommendation of routine TSH measurements in the basal evaluation of hyperthyroid patients. Pituitary microsurgery is the cornerstone of treatment, providing a good chance of remission for small tumors, or improvement of symptoms by debulking larger tumors. Somatostatin analogues are recommended as second-line treatment after unsuccessful surgery, in view of their high effectiveness in controlling tumoral hypersecretion and tumor growth. Radiotherapy should be reserved for the rare patients unresponsive to treatment with somatostatin analogues. With the availability of improved diagnostic and therapeutic tools the aggressive behavior usually associated with these rare pituitary tumors may be successfully controlled in most patients.

References

[1] J.W. Jailer, D.A. Holub, Remission of Grave's disease following radiotherapy of a pituitary neoplasm, Am J Med 28 (1960) 497–500.

[2] H. Buurman, W. Saeger, Subclinical adenomas in postmortem pituitaries: Classification and correlations to clinical data, Eur J Endocrinol 154 (2006) 753–758.

[3] J.R.E. Davis, W.E. Farrel, R.N. Clayton, Pituitary tumors, Reproduction 121 (2001) 363–371.

[4] W. Saeger, D.K. Lüdecke, M. Buchfelder, R. Fahlbusch, H.J. Quabbe, S. Petersenn, Pathohistological classification of pituitary tumors: 10 years of experience with the German Pituitary Tumor Registry, Eur J Endocrinol 156 (2007) 203–216.

[5] P. Beck-Peccoz, F. Brucker-Davis, L. Persani, R.C. Smallridge, B.D. Weintraub, Thyrotropin-secreting pituitary tumors, Endocr Rev 17 (1996) 610–638.

[6] S. Mantovani, P. Beck-Peccoz, K. Saccomanno, A. Spada, G. Faglia, F. Barbetti, TSH-secreting pituitary adenomas are monoclonal in origin, Proceedings of the 77th Annual Meeting of the Endocrine Society, Washington DC, 1995, p. 412 (abstract P2-485).

[7] W. Ma, H. Ikeda, N. Watabe, M. Kanno, T. Yoshimoto, A plurihormonal TSH-producing pituitary tumor of monoclonal origin in a patient with hypothyroidism, Horm Res 59 (2003) 257–261.
[8] D. Dworakowska, A. Grossman, The pathophysiology of pituitary adenomas, Best Prac Res Clin Endocrinol Metab 23 (2009) 525–541.
[9] M.I. Chiamolera, F.E. Wondisford, Minireview: Thyrotropin-releasing hormone and the thyroid hormone feedback mechanism, Endocrinology 150 (2009) 1091–1096.
[10] L. Persani, Hypothalamic thyrotropin-releasing hormone and thyrotropin biological activity, Thyroid 10 (1998) 941–946.
[11] E.D. Abel, R.S. Ahima, M.E. Boers, J.K. Elmquist, F.E. Wondisford, Critical role for thyroid hormone receptor β2 in the regulation of paraventricular thyrotropin-releasing hormone neurons, J Clin Invest 107 (2001) 1017–1023.
[12] E. Horvath, K. Kovacs, B.W. Scheithauer, Pituitary hyperplasia, Pituitary 1 (1999) 169–180.
[13] S. Vidal, E. Horvath, K. Kovacs, S.M. Cohen, R.V. Lloyd, B.W. Scheithauer, Transdifferentiation of somatotrophs to thyrotrophs in the pituitary of patients with protracted primary hypothyroidism, Virchows Arch 436 (2000) 43–51.
[14] N.H. Ghannam, M.M. Hammami, Z. Muttair, S.M. Bakheet, Primary hypothyroidism-associated TSH-secreting pituitary adenoma/hyperplasia presenting as a bleeding nasal mass and extremely elevated TSH level, J Endocrinol Invest 22 (1999) 419–423.
[15] L.A. Tannahill, T.J. Visser, C.J. McCabe, S. Kachilele, K. Boelaert, M.C. Sheppard, et al., Dysregulation of iodothyronine deiodinase enzyme expression and function in human pituitary tumours, Clin Endocrinol 56 (2002) 735–743.
[16] A. Aranda, O. Martinez-Iglesias, L. Ruiz-Llorente, V. Garcia-Carpizo, A. Zambrano, Thyroid receptor: Roles in cancer, Trends Endocrinol Metab 20 (2009) 318–324.
[17] C.J. Wang, S.L. Howng, K.H. Lin, Expression of thyroid hormone receptors in human pituitary tumor cells, Cancer Lett 91 (1995) 79–83.
[18] N.J. Gittoes, C.J. McCabe, J. Verhaeg, M.C. Sheppard, J.A. Franklin, An abnormality of thyroid hormone receptor expression may explain abnormal thyrotropin production in thyrotropin-secreting pituitary tumors, Thyroid 8 (1998) 9–14.
[19] S. Ando, N.J. Sarlis, J. Krishnan, X. Feng, S. Refetoff, M.Q. Zhang, et al., Aberrant splicing of thyroid hormone receptor in a TSH-secreting pituitary tumor is a mechanism for hormone resistance, Mol Endocrinol 15 (2001) 1529–1538.
[20] S. Ando, N.J. Sarlis, E.H. Oldfield, P.M. Yen, Somatic mutation of TRβ can cause a defect in negative regulation of TSH in a TSH-secreting pituitary tumor, J Clin Endocrinol Metab 86 (2001) 5572–5576.
[21] K. Watanabe, T. Kameya, A. Yamauchi, et al., Thyrotropin-producing microadenoma associated with pituitary resistance to thyroid hormone, J Clin Endocrinol Metab 76 (1993) 1025–1030.
[22] E. Faccenda, S. Melmed, J.S. Bevan, K.A. Eidne, Structure of the thyrotropin-releasing hormone receptor in human pituitary adenomas, Clin Endocrinol 44 (1996) 341–347.
[23] Q. Dong, F. Brucker-Davis, B.D. Weintraub, et al., Screening of candidate oncogenes in human thyrotroph tumors: Absence of activating mutations of the G alpha q, G alpha 11, G alpha s, or thyrothropin-releasing hormone receptor genes, J Clin Endocrinol Metab 81 1134-1140
[24] F.P.M. Dunne, M.P. Feely, J.B. Ferriss, C. Keohane, D. Murphy, I. Perry, Hyperthyroidism, inappropriate plasma TSH and pituitary adenoma in three patients, two receiving long-term phenothiazine therapy, Q J Med 75 (1990) 345–354.
[25] E. Friedman, E.F. Adams, A. Hoog, et al., Normal structural dopamine type 2 receptor gene in prolactin-secreting and other pituitary tumors, J Clin Endocrinol Metab 78 (1994) 568–574.
[26] J. Bertherat, T. Brue, A. Engalbert, et al., Somatostatin receptors on thyrotropin-secreting pituitary adenomas: Comparison with the inhibitory effects of octreotide upon in vivo and in vitro hormonal secretions, J Clin Endocrinol Metab 75 (1992) 540–546.
[27] M. Polak, J. Bertherat, J.Y. Li, et al., A human TSH-secreting adenoma: Endocrine, biochemical and morphological studies. Evidence of somatostatin receptors by using quantitative autoradiography. Clinical and biological improvement by SMS 201-995 treatment, Acta Endocrinol (Copenh) 124 (1991) 479–486.
[28] K. Horiguchi, M. Yamada, R. Umezawa, T. Satoh, K. Hashimoto, M. Tosaka, et al., Somatostatin receptor subtypes mRNA in TSH secreting pituitary adenomas: A case showing a dramatic reduction in tumor size during short octreotide treatment, Endocrine J 54 (2007) 371–378.
[29] M. Filopanti, E. Ballare, G. Lania, et al., Loss of heterozygosity at the SS receptor type % locus in human GH and TSH-secreting pituitary adenomas, J Endocrinol Invest 10 (2004) 937–942.
[30] A. Lania, G. Mantovani, A. Spada, Genetic abnormalities of somatostatin receptors in pituitary tumors, Mol Cell Endocrinol 1–2 (2008) 180–186.
[31] I. Pellegrini-Bouiller, I. Morange-Ramos, A. Barlier, G. Gunz, A. Enjalbert, P. Jaquet, Pit-1 gene expression in human pituitary tumors, Horm Res 47 (1997) 251–258.
[32] B. Verges, F. Boureille, P. Goudet, et al., Pituitary disease in MEN type 1 (MEN1): Data from the France–Belgium MEN1 multicenter study, J Clin Endocrinol Metab 87 (2002) 457–465.
[33] A.G. Wynne, I.T. Gharib, B. Scheithauer, D.H. Davis, S.L. Freeman, E. Horvath, Hyperthyroidism due to inappropriate secretion of thyrotropin in 10 patients, Am J Med 92 (1992) 15–24.
[34] J.R. Burgess, J.J. Shepherd, T.M. Greenaway, Thyrotropinomas in multiple endocrine neoplasia type 1 (MEN-1), Aust NZ J Med 24 (1994) 740–741.
[35] T.J. Taylor, S.S. Donlon, A.E. Bale, R.C. Smallridge, T.B. Francis, R.S. Christensen, et al., Treatment of a thyrotropinoma with octreotide-LAR in a patient with multiple endocrine neoplasia-1, Thyroid 10 (2000) 1001–1007.
[36] A. Gessl, M. Freissmuth, T. Czech, et al., Growth hormone-prolactin-thyrotropin-secreting pituitary adenoma in atypical McCune-Albright syndrome with functionally normal Gs alpha protein, J Clin Endocrinol Metab 79 (1994) 1128–1134.
[37] M.A. Tichomirowa, A.F. Daly, A. Beckers, Familial pituitary adenomas, J Intern Med 266 (2009) 5–18.
[38] C. Asteria, M. Anagni, L. Persani, et al., Loss of heterozygosity of the MEN1 gene in a large series of TSH-secreting pituitary adenomas, J Endocrinol Invest 24 (2001) 796–801.
[39] S. Ezzat, E. Horvath, K. Kovacs, H.S. Smyth, W. Singer, S.L. Asa, Basic fibroblast growth factor expression in two prolactin and thyrotropin-producing pituitary adenomas, Endocr Pathol 6 (1995) 125–134.
[40] F. Salehi, K. Kovacs, B.W. Scheithauer, R.V. Lloyd, M. Cusimano, Pituitary tumor-transforming gene in endocrine and other neoplasms: A review and update, Endocrine-related Cancer 15 (2008) 721–742.
[41] A.P. Heaney, G.A. Horwitz, Z. Wang, R. Singson, S. Melmed, Early involvement of estrogen-induced pituitary tumor transforming gene and fibroblast growth factor expression in prolactinoma pathogenesis, Nat Med 5 (1999) 1317–1321.

[42] C.J. McCabe, K. Boelaert, L.A. Tannahill, et al., Vascular endothelial growth factor, its receptor KDR/Flk-1, and pituitary transforming gene in pituitary tumors, J Clin Endocrinol Metabol 87 (2002) 4238–4244.

[43] R.A. Abbud, I. Takumi, E.M. Barker, S.G. Ren, D.Y. Chen, K. Wawrowsky, et al., Early multipotential pituitary focal hyperplasia in the alpha-subunit of glycoprotein hormone-driven pituitary tumor-transforming gene transgenic mice, Mol Endocrinol 19 (2005) 1383–1391.

[44] M. Musat, M. Korbonits, B. Kola, et al., Enhanced protein kinase B/AKT signaling in pituitary tumours, Endocrine-related Cancer 12 (2005) 423–433.

[45] C. Lu, M.C. Willingham, F. Furuya, S. Cheng, Activation of phospatidylinositol 3-kinase signaling promotes aberrant pituitary growth in a mouse model of thyroid-stimulating hormone-secreting pituitary tumors, Endocrinology 149 (2008) 3339–3345.

[46] H. Furumoto, H. Ying, G.V.R. Chandramouli, et al., An unliganded thyroid hormone β receptor activates the cyclin D1/cyclin-dependent kinase/retinoblastoma/E2F pathway and induces pituitary tumorigenesis, Mol Cell Biol 25 (2005) 124–135.

[47] M. Al-Shraim, S.L. Asa, The 2004 world health organization classification of pituitary tumors: What is new? Acta Neuropathol 111 (2006) 1–7.

[48] R.Y. Osamura, H. Kajiya, M. Takei, N. Egashira, M. Tobita, S. Takekoshi, et al., Pathology of the human pituitary adenomas, Histochem Cell Biol 130 (2008) 495–507.

[49] W.B. Malarkey, K. Kovacs, T.M. O'Dorisio, Response of a GH and TSH-secreting pituitary adenoma to a somatostatin analogue (SMS 201-995): Evidence that GH and TSH coexist in the same cell and secretory granules, Neuroendocrinology 49 (1989) 267–274.

[50] M. Kuzuya, K. Inoue, M. Ishibashi, et al., Endocrine and immunohistochemical studies on thyrotropin (TSH)-secreting pituitary adenomas: Responses of TSH, α-subunit and growth hormone to hypothalamic releasing hormones and their distribution in adenoma cells, J Clin Endocrinol Metab 71 (1990) 1103–1111.

[51] M. Terzolo, F. Orlandi, M. Basseti, et al., Hyperthyroidism due to a pituitary adenoma composed of two different cell types, one secreting alpha-subunit alone and another cosecreting alpha-subunit and thyrotropin, J Clin Endocrinol Metab 72 (1991) 415–421.

[52] G. Marucci, M. Faustini-Fustini, A. Righi, E. Pasquini, G. Frank, R. Agati, et al., Thyrotropin secreting pituitary tumors: Significance of "atypical adenomas" in a series of 10 patients and association with Hashimoto thyroiditis as a cause of delay in diagnosis, J Clin Pathol 62 (2009) 455–459.

[53] A.J. Mixson, T.C. Friedman, D.A. Katz, et al., Thyrotropin-secreting pituitary carcinoma, J Clin Endocrinol Metab 76 (1993) 529–533.

[54] R.L. Brown, T. Muzzafar, R. Wollman, R.E. Weiss, A pituitary carcinoma secreting TSH and prolactin: A non-secreting adenoma gone awry, Eur J Endocrinol 154 (2006) 639–643.

[55] F. Brucker-Davis, E.H. Oldfield, M.C. Skarulis, J.L. Doppman, B.D. Weintraub, Thyrotropin-secreting pituitary tumors: Diagnostic criteria, thyroid hormone sensitivity, and treatment outcome in 25 patients followed at the National Institutes of Health, J Clin Endocrinol Metab 84 (1999) 476–486.

[56] T. Kienitz, M. Quinkler, C.J. Strasburger, M. Ventz, Long-term management in five cases of TSH-secreting pituitary adenomas: A single center study and review of the literature, Eur J Endocrinol 157 (2007) 39–46.

[57] A. Teramoto, N. Sanno, S. Tahara, Y.R. Osamura, Pathological study of thyrotropin-secreting pituitary adenoma: Plurihormonality and medical treatment, Acta Neuropathol 108 (2004) 147–153.

[58] J.T. George, J.C. Thow, B. Matthews, M.P. Pye, V. Jayagopal, Atrial fibrillation associated with a thyroid stimulating hormone-secreting adenoma of the pituitary gland leading to a presentation of acute cardiac decompensation: A case report, J Med Case Reports 28 (2008) 67.

[59] F.S. Hsu, W.S. Tsai, T. Chau, H.H. Chen, Y.C. Chen, S.H. Lin, Thyrotropin-secreting pituitary adenoma presenting as hypokalemic periodic paralysis, Am J Med Sci 325 (2003) 48–50.

[60] M.P. Fischler, W.H. Reinhart, TSH-secreting pituitary macroadenoma: Rapid tumor shrinkage and recovery from hyperthyroidism with octreotide, J Endocrinol Invest 22 (1999) 64–65.

[61] S. Zuniga, V. Mendoza, I.F. Espinoza, A. Zarate, M. Mason, M. Mercado, A plurihormonal TSH-secreting pituitary microadenoma: Report of a case with an atypical clinical presentation and transient response to bromocriptine therapy, Endocr Pathol 8 (1997) 81–86.

[62] S. Suntarnlohanakul, L. MoSuwan, P. Vasiknanont, N. Phuenpathom, N. Chongchitnant, TSH secreting pituitary adenoma in children: A case report, J Med Assoc Thai 73 (1990) 175–179.

[63] J.G. Yovos, J.M. Falko, T.M. O'Dorisio, W.B. Malarkey, S. Cataland, C.C. Capen, Thyrotoxicosis and a thyrotropin-secreting pituitary tumor causing unilateral exophthalmos, J Clin Endocrinol Metab 53 (1981) 338–343.

[64] S.A. Hill, J.M. Falko, C.B. Wilson, W.E. Hunt, Thyrotrophin-producing pituitary adenomas, J Neurosurg 57 (1982) 515–519.

[65] M.J. Clarke, D. Erickson, M.R. Castro, J.L. Atkinson, Thyroid-stimulating hormone pituitary adenomas, J Neurosurg 109 (2008) 17–22.

[66] H.V. Socin, P. Chanson, B. Delemer, A. Tabarin, V. Rohmer, J. Mockel, et al., The changing spectrum of TSH-secreting pituitary adenomas: Diagnosis and management in 43 patients, Eur J Endocrinol 148 (2003) 433–442.

[67] S.B. Iskandar, E. Supit, R.M. Jordan, A.N. Peiris, Thyrotropin-secreting pituitary tumor and Hashimoto's disease: A novel association, South Med J 96 (2003) 933–936.

[68] M.F. Langlois, J.B. Lamarche, D. Bellabarba, Long-standing goiter and hypothyroidism: An unusual presentation of a TSH-secreting adenoma, Thyroid 6 (1996) 329–335.

[69] M. Losa, M. Giovanelli, L. Persani, P. Mortini, G. Faglia, P. Beck-Peccoz, Criteria of cure and follow-up of central hyperthyroidism due to thyrotropin-secreting pituitary adenomas, J Clin Endocrinol Metab 81 (1996) 3084–3090.

[70] M. Poggi, S. Monti, C. Pascucci, V. Toscano, A rare case of follicular thyroid carcinoma in a patient with thyrotropin-secreting pituitary adenoma, Am J Med Sci 337 (2009) 462–465.

[71] S. Ohta, S. Nishizawa, Y. Oki, H. Namba, Coexistence of thyrotropin-producing pituitary adenoma with papillary adenocarcinoma of the thyroid – a case report and surgical strategy, Pituitary 4 (2001) 271–274.

[72] A.L. Calle-Pascual, E. Yuste, P. Martin, et al., Association of a thyrotropin-secreting pituitary adenoma and a thyroid follicular carcinoma, J Endocrinol Invest 14 (1991) 499–502.

[73] P. Gasparoni, D. Rubello, L. Persani, P. Beck-Peccoz, Unusual association between a thyrotropin-secreting pituitary adenoma and a papillary thyroid carcinoma, Thyroid 8 (1998) 181–183.

[74] K. Horn, F. Erhardt, R. Fahlbusch, C.R. Pickardt, K. Werder, P.C. Scriba, Recurrent goiter, hyperthyroidism, galactorrhea and amenorrhea due to a thyrotropin and prolactin-producing pituitary tumor, J Clin Endocrinol Metab 43 (1976) 137–143.

[75] P. Beck-Peccoz, L. Persani, S. Mantovani, D. Cortelazzi, C. Asteria, Thyrotropin-secreting pituitary adenomas, Metabolism 45 (8 Suppl 1) (1996) 75–79.

[76] E. Macchia, M. Gasperi, M. Lombardi, L. Morselli, A. Pinchera, G. Acerbi, G. Rossi, E. Martino, Clinical aspects and therapeutic outcome in thyrotropin-secreting pituitary adenomas: A single center experience, J Endocrinol Invest 32 (2009) 773–779.

[77] W. Saeger, D.K. Lüdecke, Pituitary adenomas with hyperfunction of TSH. Frequency, histological classification, immunocytochemistry and ultrastructure, Virchows Arch A Pathol Anat Histol 394 (1982) 255–267.

[78] F. Roelfsema, S. Kok, P. Kok, A.M. Pereira, N.R. Biermasz, J.W. Smit, et al., Pituitary-hormone secretion by thyrotropinomas, Pituitary 12 (2009) 200–210.

[79] N. Sanno, A. Teramoto, A. Matsuno, S. Takekoshi, R.Y. Osamura, GH and PRL gene expression by nonradioisotopic in situ hybridization in TSH-secreting pituitary adenomas, J Clin Endocrinol Metab 80 (1995) 2518–2522.

[80] Y.Y. Wu, H.Y. Chang, J.D. Lin, K.W. Chen, Y.Y. Huang, S.M. Jung, Clinical characteristics of patients with thyrotropin-secreting pituitary adenoma, J Formos Med Assoc 102 (2003) 164–171.

[81] R. Ness-Abramof, A. Ishay, G. Harel, N. Sylvetzky, E. Baron, Y. Greenman, et al., TSH-secreting pituitary adenomas: Follow-up of 11 cases and review of the literature, Pituitary 10 (2007) 307–310.

[82] A. Yoshihara, O. Isozaki, N. Hizuka, Y. Nozoe, C. Harada, M. Ono, et al., Expression of type 5 somatostatin receptor in TSH-secreting pituitary adenomas: A possible marker for predicting long-term response to octreotide therapy, Endocr J 54 (2007) 133–138.

[83] P. Beck-Peccoz, L. Persani, Variable biological activity of thyroid-stimulating hormone, Eur J Endocrinol 131 (1994) 331–340.

[84] P. Beck-Peccoz, G. Piscitelli, S. Amr, et al., Endocrine, biochemical, and morphological studies of a pituitary adenoma secreting growth hormone, thyrotropin (TSH), and alpha-subunit: Evidence for secretion of TSH with increased bioactivity, J Clin Endocrinol Metab 62 (1986) 704–710.

[85] N. Gesundheit, P.A. Petrick, M. Nissim, et al., Thyrotropin-secreting pituitary adenomas: Clinical and biochemical heterogeneity, Ann Intern Med 111 (1989) 827–835.

[86] J.S. Bevan, C.W. Burke, M.M. Esiri, et al., Studies of two thyrotrophin-secreting pituitary adenomas: Evidence for dopamine receptor deficiency, Clin Endocrinol 31 (1989) 59–70.

[87] S. Savastano, G. Lombardi, B. Merola, et al., Hyperthyroidism due to a thyroid-stimulating hormone (TSH)-secreting pituitary adenoma associated with functional hyperprolactinemia, Acta Endocrinol 116 (1987) 452–458.

[88] S. Filetti, B. Rapoport, D.C. Aron, E.C. Greenspan, C.B. Wilson, W. Fraser, TSH and TSH subunit production by human thyrotrophic tumor cells in monolayer culture, Acta Endocrinol 99 (1982) 224–231.

[89] J.A. Magner, A. Klibanski, H. Fein, et al., Ricin and lentil lectin affinity chromatography reveals oligosaccharide heterogeneity of thyrotropin secreted by 12 human pituitary tumors, Metabolism 41 (1992) 1009–1015.

[90] P. Beck-Peccoz, L. Persani, G. Faglia, Glycoprotein hormone α-subunit in pituitary adenomas, Trends Endocrinol Metab 3 (1992) 41–45.

[91] J.D. Safer, S.D. Colan, L.M. Fraser, F.E. Wondisford, A pituitary tumor in a patient with thyroid hormone resistance: A diagnostic dilemma, Thyroid 11 (2001) 281–291.

[92] P. Beck-Peccoz, L. Persani, D. Mannavola, I. Campi, Pituitary tumours: TSH-secreting adenomas, Best Pract Res Clin Endocrinol Metab 23 (2009) 597–606.

[93] Y. Greenman, S. Melmed, Thyrotropin-secreting pituitary tumors, in: S. Melmed (Ed.), The Pituitary, first ed., Blackwell Science, Cambridge, 1995, pp. 546–558.

[94] F. Bogazzi, L. Manetti, L. Tomisti, G. Rossi, C. Cosci, C. Sardella, et al., Thyroid color flow Doppler sonography: An adjunctive tool for differentiating patients with inappropriate thyrotropin (TSH) secretion due to TSH-secreting pituitary adenoma or resistance to thyroid hormone, Thyroid 16 (2006) 989–995.

[95] J.M. Kuhn, S. Arlot, H. Lefebvre, P. Caron, C. Cortet-Rudelli, F. Archambaud, et al., Evaluation of the treatment of thyrotropin-secreting pituitary adenomas with a slow release formulation of the somatostatin analog lanreotide, J Clin Endocrinol Metab 85 (2000) 1487–1491.

[96] P. Chanson, B. Weintraub, A.G. Harris, Octreotide therapy for thyroid-stimulating hormone-secreting pituitary adenomas, Ann Intern Med 119 (1993) 236–240.

[97] M.O. van Aken, A.M. Pereira, G. van den Berg, J.A. Romijn, J.D. Veldhuis, F. Roelfsema, Profound amplification of secretory-burst mass and anomalous regularity of ACTH secretory process in patients with Nelson's syndrome compared with Cushing's disease, Clin Endocrinol (Oxf) 60 (2004) 765–772.

[98] R. Groote Veldman, G. van den Berg, S.M. Pincus, M. Frölich, J.D. Veldhuis, F. Roelfsema, Increased episodic release and disorderliness of prolactin secretion in both micro- and macroprolactinomas, Eur J Endocrinol 140 (1999) 192–200.

[99] G. van den Berg, M. Frölich, J.D. Veldhuis, F. Roelfsema, Growth hormone secretion in recently operated acromegalic patients, J Clin Endocrinol Metab 79 (1994) 1706–1715.

[100] A. Beckers, R. Abs, C. Mahler, et al., Thyrotropin-secreting pituitary adenomas: Report of seven cases, J Clin Endocrinol Metab 72 (1991) 477–483.

[101] M.H. Samuels, W.M. Wood, D.E. Gordon, et al., Clinical and molecular studies of a thyrotropin secreting pituitary adenoma, J Clin Endocrinol Metab 68 (1989) 1211–1215.

[102] G. Brabant, K. Prank, U. Ranft, et al., Circadian and pulsatile TSH secretion under physiological and pathophysiological conditions, Horm Metab Res 23 (suppl) (1990) 12–17.

[103] R. Adriaanse, G. Brabant, E. Endert, F.J. Bemelman, W.M. Wiersinga, Pulsatile thyrotropin and prolactin secretion in a patient with a mixed thyrotropin- and prolactin-secreting pituitary adenoma, Eur J Endocrinol 130 (1994) 113–120.

[104] F. Roelfsema, A.M. Pereira, D.M. Keenan, J.D. Veldhuis, J.A. Romijn, Thyrotropin secretion by thyrotropinomas is characterized by increased pulse frequency, delayed diurnal rhythm, enhanced basal secretion, spikiness, and disorderliness, J Clin Endocrinol Metab 93 (2008) 4052–4057.

[105] N.J. Sarlis, L. Gourgiotis, C.A. Koch, M.C. Skarulis, F. Brucker-Davis, J.L. Doppman, et al., MR imaging features of thyrotropin-secreting pituitary adenomas at initial presentation, Am J Roentgenol 181 (2003) 577–582.

[106] S.I. Frank, N. Gesundheit, J.L. Doppman, et al., Preoperative lateralization of pituitary microadenomas by petrosal sinus sampling: Utility in two patients with non-ACTH-secreting tumors, Am J Med 87 (1989) 679–682.

[107] J. Webster, J.R. Peters, R. John, et al., Pituitary stone: Two cases of densely calcified thyrotropin-secreting pituitary adenomas, Clin Endocrinol 40 (1994) 137–143.

[108] M. Losa, P. Magnani, P. Mortini, et al., Indium-111 pentetreotide single-photon emission tomography in patients with TSH-secreting pituitary adenomas: Correlation with the effect of a single administration of octreotide on serum TSL levels, Eur J Nucl Med 24 (1997) 728–731.

[109] D.S. Cooper, B.M. Wening, Hyperthyroidism caused by an ectopic TSH-secreting pituitary tumor, Thyroid 6 (1996) 337–343.

[110] E. Pasquini, M. Faustini-Fustini, V. Sciarretta, D. Saggese, F. Roncaroli, D. Serra, et al., Ectopic TSH-secreting pituitary adenoma of the vomerosphenoidal junction, Eur J Endocrinol 148 (2003) 253–257.

[111] N.P. Verhoeff, F.J. Bemelman, W.M. Wiersinga, E.A. van-Royen, Imaging of dopamine D2 and somatostatin receptors in vivo using single-photon emission tomography in a patient with a TSH/PRL-producing pituitary macroadenoma, Eur J Nucl Med 20 (1993) 555–561.

[112] W.W. deHerder, A.E. Reijs, D.J. Kwekkeboom, et al., In vivo imaging of pituitary tumors using a radiolabelled dopamine D2 receptor radioligand, Clin Endocrinol 45 (1996) 755–767.

[113] S. Refetoff, R.E. Weiss, S.J. Usala, The syndromes of resistance to thyroid hormone, Endocr Rev 14 (1993) 348–399.

[114] P.M. Yen, Molecular basis of resistance to thyroid hormone, Trends Endocrinol Metab 14 (2003) 327–333.

[115] V.K. Chatterjee, Resistance to thyroid hormone and peroxisome-proliferator-activated receptor resistance, Biochem Soc Trans 29 (2001) 227–231.

[116] P.M. Yen, Physiological and molecular basis of thyroid hormone action, Physiol Rev 81 (2001) 1097–1142.

[117] M.T. McDermott, E.C. Ridgway, Central hyperthyroidism, Endocrinol Metabol Clinics North America 27 (1998) 187–203.

[118] P. Beck-Peccoz, V.K. Chatterjee, The variable clinical phenotype in thyroid hormone resistance syndrome, Thyroid 4 (1994) 225–232.

[119] F. Brucker-Davis, M.C. Skarulis, M.B. Grace, J. Benichou, P. Hauser, E. Wiggs, et al., Genetic and clinical features of 42 kindreds with resistance to thyroid hormone. The National Institutes of Health Prospective Study, Ann Int Med 123 (1995) 572–583.

[120] R.E. Weiss, S. Refetoff, Resistance to thyroid hormone, Rev Endocrine Metabolic Disorders 1 (2000) 97–108.

[121] D.S. Machado, A. Sabet, L.A. Santiago, A.R. Sidhaye, M.I. Chiamolera, T.M. Ortiga-Carvalho, et al., A thyroid hormone receptor mutation that dissociates thyroid hormone regulation of gene expression in vivo, Proc Nat Acad Sci USA 106 (2009) 9441–9446.

[122] P. Webb, Another story of mice and men: The types of RTH, Proc Nat Acad Sci USA 106 (2009) 9129–9130.

[123] D. Mannavola, L. Persani, G. Vannucchi, M. Zanardelli, L. Fugazzola, U. Verga, et al., Different responses to chronic somatostatin analogues in patients with central hyperthyroidism, Clin Endocrinol (Oxf) 62 (2005) 176–181.

[124] P. Beck Peccoz, R. Roncoroni, S. Mariotti, et al., Sex hormone-binding globulin measurement in patients with inappropriate secretion of thyrotropin (IST): Evidence against selective pituitary thyroid hormone resistance in nonneoplastic IST, J Clin Endocrinol Metab 71 (1990) 19–25.

[125]. L. Persani, D. Preziati, C.H. Matthews, A. Sartorio, V.K. Chatterjee, P. Beck-Peccoz, Serum levels of carboxy-terminal cross-linked telopeptide of type I collagen (ICTP) in the differential diagnosis of the syndrome of inappropriate secretion of TSH, Clin Endocrinol 47 (1997) 207–214.

[126] E.C. Friesema, A. Grueters, H. Biebermann, H. Krude, A. von Moers, M. Reeser, et al., Association between mutations in a thyroid hormone transporter and severe X-linked psychomotor retardation, Lancet 364 (2004) 1435–1437.

[127] A.M. Dumitrescu, X.H. Liao, M.S. Abdullah, J. Lado-Abeal, F.A. Majed, L.C. Moeller, et al., Mutations in SECISBP2 result in abnormal thyroid hormone metabolism, Nat Genet 37 (2005) 1247–1252.

[128] G.C. Borst, C. Eil, K.D. Burman, Euthyroid hyperthyroxinemia, Ann Intern Med 98 (1983) 366–378.

[129] P. Glendenning, D. Siriwardhana, K. Hoad, A. Musk, Thyroxine autoantibody interference is an uncommon cause of inappropriate TSH secretion using the Immulite 2000 assay, Clin Chim Acta 403 (2009) 136–138.

[130] M.J. Tan, F. Tan, R. Hawkins, W.K. Cheah, J.J. Mukherjee, A hyperthyroid patient with measurable thyroid-stimulating hormone concentration – a trap for the unwary, Ann Acad Med Singapore 35 (2006) 500–503.

[131] D. Cartwright, P. O'Shea, O. Rajanayagam, M. Agostini, P. Barker, C. Moran, et al., Familial dysalbuminemic hyperthyroxinemia: A persistent diagnostic challenge, Clin Chem 55 (2009) 1044–1046.

[132] N. Gesundheit, Thyrotropin induced hyperthyroidism, in: L.E. Braverman, R.D. Utiger (Eds.), Werner and Ingbar's The Thyroid, a Fundamental and Clinical Text, sixth ed., JB Lippincott, Philadelphia, 1991, pp. 682–691.

[133] M. Losa, P. Mortini, A. Franzin, R. Barzaghi, C. Mandelli, M. Giovanelli, Surgical management of thyrotropin-secreting pituitary adenomas, Pituitary 2 (1999) 127–131.

[134] M. Simard, C.J. Mirrell, A.E. Pekary, J. Drexler, K. Kovacs, J.M. Hershman, Hormonal control of thyrotropin and growth hormone secretion in a human thyrotrope pituitary adenoma studied in vitro, Acta Endocrinol 119 (1988) 283–290.

[135] F. Grisoli, T. Leclercg, J.P. Winteler, et al., Thyroid-stimulating hormone pituitary adenomas and hyperthyroidism, Surg Neurol 25 (1986) 361–368.

[136] I.E. McCutcheon, B.D. Weintraub, E.H. Oldfield, Surgical treatment of thyrotropin-secreting pituitary adenomas, J Neurosurg 73 (1990) 674–683.

137. P. Beck-Peccoz, G. Piscitelli, S. Amr, et al., Endocrine, biochemical, and morphological studies of a pituitary adenoma secreting growth hormone, thyrotropin (TSH), and alpha-subunit: Evidence for secretion of TSH with increased bioactivity, J Clin Endocrinol Metab 62 (1986) 704–710.

[138] A. Colao, R. Pivonello, C. Di Somma, S. Savastano, L.F. Grasso, G. Lombardi, Medical therapy of pituitary adenomas: Effects on tumor shrinkage, Rev Endocr Metab Disord 10 (2009) 111–123.

[139] J.R. Mulinda, S. Hasinski, L.I. Rose, Successful therapy for a mixed thyrotropin- and prolactin-secreting pituitary macroadenoma with cabergoline, Endocr Pract 5 (1999) 76–79.

[140] P. Chanson, J. Orgiazzi, P.J. Derome, D. Bression, C.P. Jedynak, J. Trouillas, et al., Paradoxical response of thyrotropin to L-dopa and presence of dopaminergic receptors in a thyrotropin-secreting pituitary adenoma, J Clin Endocrinol Metab 59 (1984) 542–546.

[141] F. Mouton, F. Faivre-Defrance, C. Cortet-Rudelli, R. Assaker, G. Soto-Ares, S. Defoort-Dhellemmes, et al., TSH-secreting adenoma improved with cabergoline, Ann Endocrinol (Paris) 69 (2008) 244–248.

[142] P. Chanson, A. Warnet, Treatment of thyroid-stimulating hormone secreting adenomas with octreotide, Metabolism 41 (suppl.2) (1992) 62–65.

[143] T. Usui, S. Izawa, T. Sano, T. Tagami, D. Nagata, A. Shimatsu, et al., Clinical and molecular features of a TSH-secreting pituitary microadenoma, Pituitary 8 (2005) 127–134.

[144] A. Warnet, E. Lajeunie, F. Gelbert, et al., Shrinkage of a primary thyrotropin-secreting pituitary adenoma treated with the long-acting somatostatin analogue octreotide (SMS 201-995), Acta Endocrinol 124 (1991) 487–491.

[145] A. Colao, M. Filippella, C. Di Somma, S. Manzi, F. Rota, R. Pivonello, et al., Somatostatin analogs in treatment of non-growth hormone-secreting pituitary adenomas, Endocrine 20 (2003) 279–283.

[146] A. Gancel, P. Vuillermet, A. Legrand, F. Catus, F. Thomas, J.M. Kuhn, Effects of a slow-release formulation of the new somatostatin analogue lanreotide in TSH-secreting pituitary adenomas, Clin Endocrinol (Oxf) 40 (1994) 421–428.

[147] P. Caron, S. Arlot, C. Bauters, P. Chanson, J.M. Kuhn, M. Pugeat, et al., Efficacy of the long-acting octreotide formulation (octreotide-LAR) in patients with thyrotropin-secreting pituitary adenomas, J Clin Endocrinol Metab 86 (2001) 2849–2853.

[148] P. Caron, C. Gerbeau, L. Pradayrol, C. Simonetta, F. Bayard, Successful pregnancy in an infertile woman with a thyrotropin-secreting macroadenoma treated with somatostatin analog (octreotide), J Clin Endocrinol Metab 81 (1996) 1164–1168.

[149] G. Blackhurst, M.W. Strachan, D. Collie, A. Gregor, P.F. Statham, J.E. Seckl, The treatment of a thyrotropin-secreting pituitary macroadenoma with octreotide in twin pregnancy, Clin Endocrinol (Oxf) 57 (2002) 401–404.

[150] M.S. Elston, J.V. Conaglen, Clinical and biochemical characteristics of patients with TSH-secreting pituitary adenomas from one New Zealand centre, Intern Med J 40(3) (2009) 214–219.

[151] J.L. Atkinson, C.F. Abboud, J.I. Lane, Dramatic volume reduction of a large GH/TSH secreting pituitary tumor with short term octreotide therapy, Pituitary 8 (2005) 89–91.

CHAPTER

18

Gonadotroph Adenomas

Peter J. Snyder

University of Pennsylvania, Philadelphia, Pennsylvania, USA

Adenomas that arise from the gonadotroph cells are among the most common adenomas of the pituitary gland, but they are the most difficult to recognize because they secrete inefficiently and the secreted products – intact gonadotropins and their subunits – often do not produce a readily recognizable clinical syndrome. Consequently, these adenomas are often not recognized until they become so large as to cause neurologic symptoms. A minority, however, do cause recognizable clinical syndromes.

PATHOPHYSIOLOGY

Gonadotroph adenomas usually synthesize and secrete the products of the normal gonadotroph cell, intact gonadotropins – follicle-stimulating hormone (FSH) and luteinizing hormone (LH) – and their subunits – α, FSHβ and LHβ – but the secretion usually differs from that of other pituitary adenomas in two ways. First, gonadotroph adenomas secrete inefficiently compared to many other pituitary adenomas. Macroadenomas that arise from lactotroph cells, for example, typically produce serum prolactin concentrations 100–1000 times normal. Macroadenomas that arise from gonadotroph cells, in contrast, may produce serum concentrations of its secretory products up to ten times normal, but often not above normal at all; in those cases the secretory nature of the adenomas can be recognized only by their response to stimulation and/or by their secretory behavior in vitro. Second, gonadotroph adenomas usually do not secrete intact gonadotropins and their subunits in the same proportions as do normal gonadotroph cells.

Secretion in Vivo

Basal Secretion

INTACT FSH AND LH

Gonadotroph adenomas often produce supranormal basal serum concentrations of intact FSH but less commonly of intact LH [1]. The degree of FSH elevation is minimal to ten times normal. Some gonadotroph adenomas, however, can be recognized only in vitro and not in vivo, as described below.

The FSH secreted by gonadotroph adenomas is apparently normal, or nearly normal, qualitatively. The size of the FSH appears similar to that of intact FSH, not of the FSH subunits, α and FSHβ [2], and the pattern of charge on the FSH secreted also appears to be normal [3]. In addition, FSH from patients with gonadotroph adenomas is biologically active in vitro; in fact, the ratio of biologic to immunologic activity in the sera of men with gonadotroph adenomas is even greater than that of age-matched normal men [4,5]. In vivo biologic activity, however, has not been tested and would not necessarily parallel the in vitro activity, since in vivo activity depends on the clearance of FSH as well as its intrinsic activity.

The basal serum concentration of intact LH may be slightly supranormal but is rarely substantially supranormal in patients who have gonadotroph adenomas. When it is elevated in a male, the serum testosterone concentration, as one would predict, is also supranormal [6–9]. In most men with gonadotroph adenomas the serum LH concentration is within the normal range or slightly elevated and the testosterone concentration is normal or subnormal [10]. When the testosterone is subnormal, it increases rapidly to normal in response to administration of exogenous human chorionic gonadotropin, suggesting a secondary cause of the hypogonadism, presumably due to compression of the normal gonadotroph cells by the large but inefficient gonadotroph adenoma.

GONADOTROPIN SUBUNITS: α, FSHβ AND LHβ

Gonadotroph adenomas may produce supranormal basal serum concentrations of α, FSHβ and LHβ subunits. When gonadotroph adenomas are identified

The Pituitary, Third Edition, DOI: 10.1016/B978-0-12-380926-1.10018-5

by a supranormal basal serum FSH concentration, many [1,2,11–13], perhaps one-third [1], of the patients also exhibit a supranormal serum α-subunit concentration. The degree of elevation of the α-subunit concentration can be more or less than that of the FSH concentration. Those few gonadotroph adenomas recognized by their supranormal serum concentration of intact LH also may exhibit a supranormal serum α concentration [7,8]. Some pituitary adenomas produce supranormal serum concentrations of α-subunit but not of intact FSH or LH [14,15]; many of these are probably also gonadotroph adenomas, because they may secrete intact FSH, as well as α-subunit, in culture [16]. Gonadotroph adenomas identified by supranormal basal serum FSH concentrations generally produce supranormal basal concentrations of serum FSHβ as well [10].

The α, LHβ and FSHβ genes in gonadotroph adenomas appear to be the same as those in the normal pituitary. The transcriptional start sites of the α- and LHβ-subunit genes in gonadotroph adenomas have been shown to be identical to those in the normal pituitary by S-1 nuclease mapping [17].

OTHER SECRETORY PRODUCTS

Documented or presumed gonadotroph adenomas have occasionally been shown to secrete products other than gonadotropins and their subunits. One patient was found to have an adenoma that produced supranormal serum concentrations of FSH and TSH [18]. About one-third of patients with acromegaly have supranormal serum concentrations of α-subunit [19], but both in vivo [20] and in vitro [21,22] evidence suggests that the α-subunit in these patients is secreted by the adenomatous somatotroph cells.

Stimulated Secretion

Administration of thyrotropin-releasing hormone (TRH) to patients who have gonadotroph adenomas often produces an increase in their serum concentration of LHβ-subunit, and less often intact FSH and LH. These responses are characteristic of gonadotroph adenomas, because normal men and women show no response of intact FSH and FSHβ, and no more than a 33% increase in intact LH and LHß [10,23,24]. In a study of 16 women who had pituitary macroadenomas that were clinically nonfunctioning, 11 could be identified as being of gonadotroph origin by their LHβ-subunit responses to TRH; four had responses of intact LH and three of intact FSH (Figure 18.1) [23]. Of 38 men who had pituitary macroadenomas that were clinically nonfunctioning, 14 had responses of LHß, five of intact LH and four intact FSH (Figure 18.2) [10].

Administration of GnRH to patients who have gonadotroph adenomas results in widely variable FSH and LH responses, from subnormal to supranormal. It is not possible to determine if the increase in FSH or LH is secreted by adenomatous or normal gonadotroph cells.

Synthesis and Secretion in Vitro

Basal Secretion

When gonadotroph adenomas that are recognized in vivo by supranormal basal or stimulated serum concentrations of gonadotropins and/or their subunits are excised and studied in vitro, they usually synthesize and secrete large amounts of the same intact hormones and subunits they had in vivo, confirming the gonadotroph nature of the adenomas. These adenomas often synthesize and secrete large amounts of other

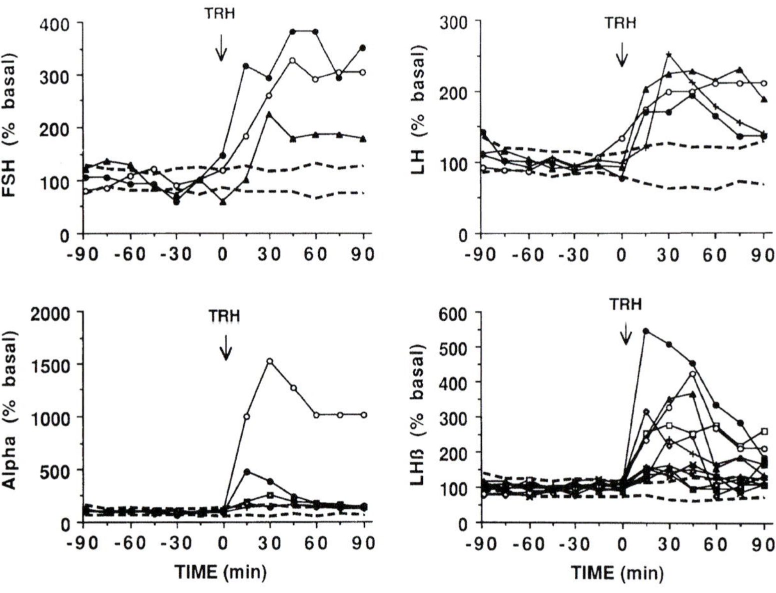

FIGURE 18.1 Increases in the serum concentrations of intact FSH, LH, alpha subunit, and, mostly, LHβ subunit to TRH in 16 women with adenomas that had been thought to be "nonsecreting" on the basis of basal serum hormone concentrations. The dashed lines show the ranges of serum concentrations in 16 age-matched healthy women. Eleven women with "nonsecreting" adenomas exhibited significant responses to TRH of LHβ subunit, four of intact LH and α-subunit, and three of FSH. *From Daneshdoost et al. [23].*

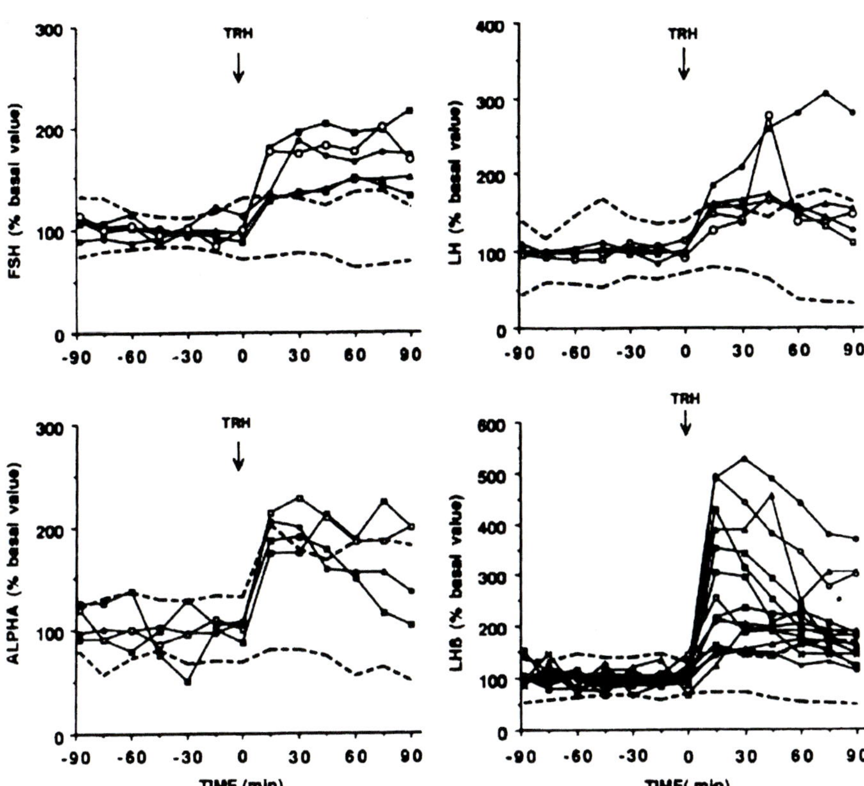

FIGURE 18.2 Increases in the serum concentrations of intact FSH, LH, α-subunit, and, mostly, LHβ subunit to TRH in 38 men with adenomas that had been thought to be "nonsecreting" on the basis of basal serum hormone concentrations. The dashed lines show the ranges of serum concentrations in age-matched healthy men. *From Daneshdoost et al. [10].*

gonadotroph cell products as well. For example, when adenomas that produce supranormal serum FSH concentrations in vivo are excised and established in dispersed cell culture, they usually secrete large amounts of FSH, but they often also secrete intact LH [16]. Similarly, adenomas that produce a supranormal serum concentration of α-subunit but not of intact FSH may secrete as much FSH in culture as adenomas that produced supranormal serum FSH concentrations [16]. Not surprisingly, adenomas that produce supranormal serum FSH concentrations stain immunospecifically for FSH and LH [25].

When pituitary adenomas that are not associated in vivo with supranormal serum concentrations of any pituitary hormones, i.e., so called "nonsecreting" or "nonfunctional" adenomas, are studied in vitro, a majority have been shown to synthesize and secrete intact gonadotropins and/or their subunits in vitro, demonstrating that they are also gonadotroph adenomas. The results are similar whatever the in vitro technique: dispersed cell culture and assay of the culture medium [26–28], immunospecific staining of fixed adenoma tissue [26–29], or extraction of mRNA (Table 18.1) [17]. Using these techniques 70–100% of "nonsecreting adenomas" have been found to synthesize and/or secrete some combination of intact FSH and LH and α-, FSHβ- and LHβ-subunits. Up to 25% of these adenomas demonstrate intact TSH, TSHβ, or α, but only sporadic adenomas show evidence of prolactin, growth hormone, or ACTH.

Stimulated Secretion

Gonadotroph adenomas, whether initially identified in vivo or only in vitro, may respond in culture to stimulation with both GnRH and TRH. In one study gonadotropin-releasing hormone (GnRH) stimulated the secretion of LH in two of five adenomas and FSH in two of six [30]. Unlike the responses of gonadotropins to GnRH in vivo, which cannot be ascribed with certainty to normal or adenomatous gonadotroph cells, the locus of the responses of adenoma cell culture to GnRH seems clear. TRH stimulated the secretion of LH in three of five and FSH in two of six adenomas [30].

PATHOLOGY

Gonadotroph adenomas are not usually recognized until they become very large, but they differ little, if any, from other pituitary macroadenomas in gross pathologic appearance or by light or electron microscopy. Gonadotroph adenomas can be reliably distinguished pathologically from other pituitary adenomas only by detecting the expression of the FSHβ, LHβ, or α-subunit genes by immunospecific staining for the subunits in adenoma tissue, extracting their mRNAs from adenoma

TABLE 18.1 Synthesis and Secretion *in Vitro* of Pituitary Hormones by "Nonsecreting" Pituitary Adenomas

	Immunostaining (%)	Hormone Secretion in Culture (%)	mRNA (%)
Authors	Black et al. [29]	Asa et al. [26]	Jameson et al. [17]
No. of patients	36	12	13
FSHβ, LHβ, α	66.7	100	69.3
TSHβ, α	33.3	25	7.7
Prolactin	16.7	0	0
Growth hormone	2.8	0	0
ACTH	8.5	0	7.7

In each study the authors examined by an in vitro technique (immunospecific staining, hormone secretion in culture, or mRNA expression) surgically excised pituitary adenoma tissue that had been judged to be "nonsecreting" by basal serum hormone concentrations in vivo.

tissue, or by secretion of intact gonadotropins or the subunits by cultured adenoma cells.

Gross Pathology

Because excessive secretion of gonadotropins and their subunits does not often cause a recognizable clinical syndrome, gonadotroph adenomas are generally not recognized until they become so large that they cause neurological symptoms. Gonadotroph adenomas, however, do not differ in their gross pathologic characteristics from other pituitary adenomas of similar size. Like other pituitary macroadenomas, they may extend outside of the sella turcica in any direction. Superior extension may elevate and compress the optic chiasm and even compress the hypothalamus and third ventricle; lateral extension into the cavernous sinuses may encase the internal carotid arteries and compress the oculomotor nerves; inferior extension into the sphenoid sinus may cause CSF rhinorrhea. Focal areas of hemorrhage are often found within gonadotroph adenomas, but most are not associated with the clinical syndrome of pituitary apoplexy.

Light Microscopy

By light microscopy gonadotroph adenomas often differ little from other pituitary adenomas when stained with hematoxylin and eosin. As in other pituitary adenomas, the cells are not arranged in the normal pituitary glandular pattern but instead are in cords [25,31], sometimes interspersed with varying amounts of fibrous tissue. In any one adenoma the cells are usually similar in size, but vary considerably among adenomas. The cytoplasm stains neither with hematoxylin nor eosin, so for many years gonadotroph adenomas were called "chromophobe adenomas." This term, which implied that the cells were hormonally inactive, contributed to the erroneous impression that the adenomas were nonsecreting.

By immunospecific staining, gonadotroph adenomas can often be recognized when stained specifically for gonadotropin subunits. Not only do adenomas associated with elevated serum gonadotropin concentrations stain for gonadotropin subunits (Figure 18.3) [25,31], so do more than 70% of adenomas that are associated with no supranormal serum concentration of any pituitary hormone [26,27,29]. The percentage of cells that stain immunospecifically for gonadotropin subunits, however, is smaller than the percentage of somatotroph or lactotroph adenoma cells that stain for growth hormone of prolactin. The intensity of staining of gonadotroph adenomas is also less than that of somatotroph

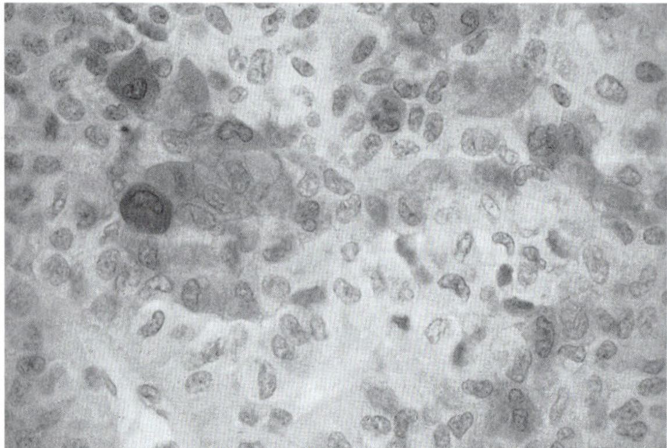

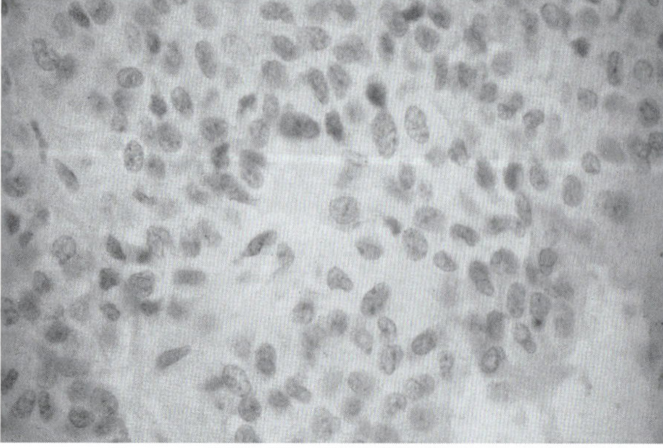

FIGURE 18.3 Demonstration of FSH and LH in gonadotroph adenoma cells by immunoperoxidase staining. The left panel shows positive cytoplasmic staining (brown color) in several cells for FSH; staining for LH was similarly positive. The right panel shows no cytoplasmic staining for prolactin; staining for growth hormone was similarly negative.

and lactotroph adenomas. Some gonadotroph adenomas, however, cannot be recognized at all by immunospecific staining. Many adenomas that do not stain immunospecifically for any pituitary hormone and are called "null cell" or "oncocytic" (because of densely packed mitochondria) secrete intact gonadotropins and/or their subunits in cell culture [26].

Electron Microscopy

The electron microscopic appearance of gonadotroph adenomas is variable. Some adenomatous gonadotroph cells have numerous secretory granules of varying sizes and cytoplasmic organelles, and others have sparse secretory granules and few organelles [25]. Yet others have numerous mitochondria ("oncocytes") and few secretory granules [27].

ETIOLOGY

Gonadotroph adenomas appear to be true neoplasms, arising from a somatic mutation of a single progenitor cell that divides repetitively. The evidence for this view comes from studies that show that virtually all pituitary adenomas, including gonadotroph adenomas, are monoclonal, that is, arise from a somatic mutation of a single cell. In one study of five women whose pituitary macroadenomas expressed some combination of FSHβ, LHβ and a subunit, and whose peripheral leukocytes were heterozygous for HPRT, the adenomas had predominantly one allele or the other (Figure 18.4) [32]. This study suggests that gonadotroph adenomas arise from a somatic mutation of a single progenitor cell that then proliferates, but what mutation and what causes the transformation remains unknown.

Specific mutations have been identified in patients who have hereditary pituitary adenomas, e.g., in multiple endocrine neoplasia type I (MEN I), the Carney complex and familial isolated acromegaly. In MEN I, a mutation of the MENI gene results in decreased expression of the tumor suppressor protein menin, which results in the development of adenomas of the pituitary, parathyroids and pancreas [33]. All types of pituitary adenomas can occur in MEN I, most commonly lactotroph and somatotroph adenomas, but including, less often, gonadotroph adenomas [34,35] and adenomas identified as nonfunctioning [36–38].

Less is known about mutations responsible for the development of sporadic pituitary adenomas. About 40% of somatotroph adenomas are associated with mutations of the gene encoding the α-subunit of the G stimulatory protein (Gsα), as consequence constitutively activating adenylyl cyclase and increasing cAMP, which is mitogenic to somatotroph cells, thereby causing somatotroph adenomas [39].

Mutations that cause other pituitary adenomas, including gonadotroph adenomas, are not known. Investigators have searched, directly or indirectly, for many other mutations that might be causally related to the development of other pituitary adenomas, including genes that express c-Myc, c-fos, c-myb [40], ras [41,42], retinoblastoma suppresser [43–45], IL-6 [46], pituitary adenylate cyclase activating peptides [47], protein kinase C [48], epidermal growth factor [49], transforming growth factor β [50], gonadotropin-releasing hormone [51], gonadotropin-releasing hormone receptor [52], activin [53] and follistatin [54], but none has been clearly

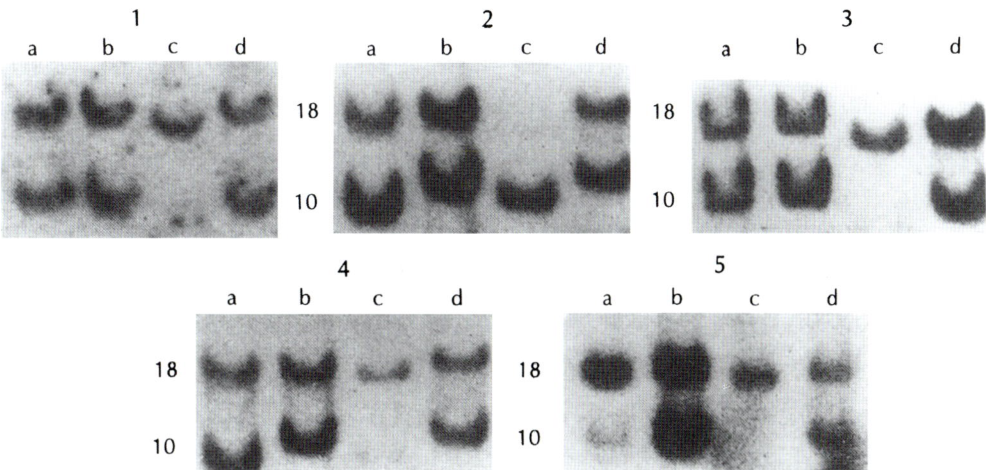

FIGURE 18.4 Demonstration of the apparent monoclonality of five pituitary adenomas. The bands represent DNA fragments of the HPRT gene from the peripheral leukocytes (lanes a and b) and pituitary adenoma cells (lanes c and d) of five women. The leukocytes of each patient show both alleles of the gene (lane b), but the adenoma cells show only one allele (lane c), supporting the hypothesis that these adenomas arose from clonal expansion of a single cell. *From Alexander et al. [32].*

associated with the pathogenesis of any human pituitary adenomas.

Three genes have been identified that might be related to the pathogenesis of pituitary adenomas. One is the pituitary tumor transforming gene (PTTG), which was cloned from GH4 cells, a rat pituitary tumor cell line [55]. It is over-expressed in the majority of human pituitary adenomas of all cell types compared with nonadenomatous pituitary tissue [56]. Another is a truncated form of the fibroblast growth factor receptor-4, which has been identified in all types of human pituitary adenomas [57]. A third is the MEG3 tumor suppressor gene, expression of which is selectively lost in nonfunctioning adenomas by hypermethylation [58].

External hormonal stimulation from the hypothalamus seems unlikely to be a primary cause of gonadotroph adenomas, but might have a secondary effect on adenoma growth and probably has an effect on adenoma secretion. The possibility that gonadotroph adenomas could arise from stimulation of the gonadotroph cells as a consequence of testosterone deficiency in long-standing primary hypogonadism was raised because of the observation that patients who have long-standing primary hypogonadism do develop some degree of pituitary enlargement [59]. However, the historical, clinical and hormonal characteristics of patients with gonadotroph adenomas are quite distinct from those of patients with primary hypogonadism, as discussed under differential diagnosis. And yet, hormonal secretion by gonadotroph adenomas does seem to be dependent on endogenous GnRH, since administration of the GnRH antagonist Nal-Glu GnRH to patients with gonadotroph adenomas and supranormal serum FSH concentrations lowers the FSH to normal [60].

Histologic evidence also supports the view that gonadotroph adenomas are true neoplasms. Gonadotroph adenomas are composed of sheets of similar pituitary cells, rather than a mixture of various kinds of pituitary cells arranged in a sinusoidal pattern, as occurs in the normal pituitary. In Klinefelter's syndrome and other kinds of primary hypogonadism, the pituitary shows, instead, gonadotroph cell hyperplasia, although one patient has been reported to have both Klinefelter's syndrome and a gonadotroph adenoma [61].

CLINICAL PRESENTATION

Gonadotroph adenomas usually come to clinical attention when they become so large as to cause neurologic symptoms, most commonly impaired vision (Table 18.2). The large size may also cause deficient hormonal secretion from the nonadenomatous pituitary; these deficiencies may even be recognizable at the time of presentation, but they are usually not the impetus for the patient seeking medical attention. Gonadotroph adenomas are probably not recognized when they are microadenomas because these adenomas are usually so inefficient hormonally that when they are of "micro" size (less than 1 cm) they probably do not produce elevated serum gonadotropin or subunit concentrations. Some gonadotroph adenomas are first recognized as an incidental finding when an MRI of the head is performed for an unrelated reason. Increasingly, these adenomas are recognized because of a clinical syndrome related to gonadotropin hypersecretion.

TABLE 18.2 Clinical Presentations of Gonadotroph Adenomas

NEUROLOGIC SYMPTOMS
Visual impairment
Headache
Other (diplopia, seizures, CSF rhinorrhea, etc.)
INCIDENTAL FINDING
When magnetic resonance imaging is performed because of an unrelated symptom
CLINICAL SYNDROMES SPECIFIC TO GONADOTROPH ADENOMAS
Ovarian hyperstimulation due to secretion of intact FSH in a premenopausal woman
Premature puberty due to secretion of intact LH in a boy
Large testicular size due to secretion of intact LH in a man
Pituitary apoplexy following GnRH or GnRH analogue administration
Acute GnRH administration
GnRH analogue treatment for prostate cancer

Neurologic Symptoms

Impaired vision is the symptom that most commonly leads a patient with a gonadotroph adenoma to seek medical attention. Visual impairment is caused by suprasellar extension of the adenoma that compresses the optic chiasm. If the extension is in the midline, the greatest compression occurs in the middle of the chiasm, the site of the fibers that cross and serve the nasal retinae and therefore receive visual signals from the temporal fields. Vision from the temporal fields is thus compromised first, beginning with the superior quadrants. Suprasellar extension may also occur asymmetrically; if laterally, it could impair vision in one nasal field; if anteriorly, it could impair vision in all of one eye but not the other. When compression becomes more severe, central visual acuity is also affected. Some patients recognize the localized beginnings of their visual deficit, but others notice only that they cannot see what they once could. The onset of the deficit is usually so gradual that patients often do not seek ophthalmological consultation for months or even years. Even then the reason for the deficit may not be recognized unless a visual field examination is performed, and the diagnosis may be delayed further.

Other neurologic symptoms that may cause a patient with a gonadotroph adenoma to seek medical attention are headaches, caused presumably by expansion of the sella; diplopia, caused by oculomotor nerve compression due to lateral extension of the adenoma; CSF rhinorrhea, caused by inferior extension of the adenoma; and the excruciating headache and the diplopia caused by pituitary apoplexy, sudden hemorrhage into the adenoma.

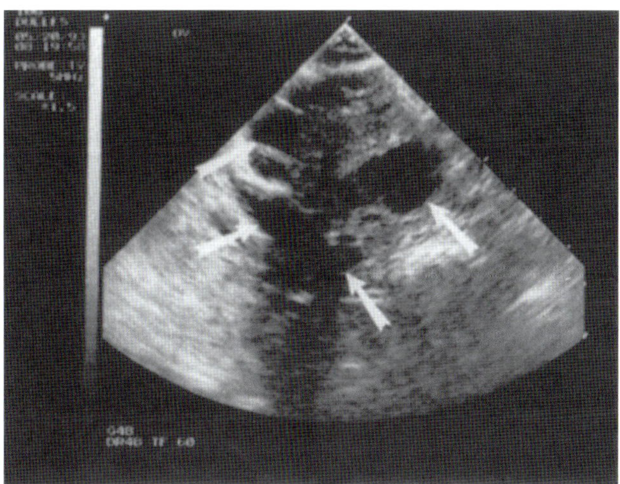

FIGURE 18.5 Multiple ovarian cysts as seen by ultrasonography in a premenopausal woman who had a gonadotroph adenoma hypersecreting FSH and causing ovarian hyperstimulation syndrome. Arrows point to the cysts. *From Djerassi et al. [62].*

Incidental Finding on MRI

Sellar masses are increasingly recognized as incidental findings when an MRI is performed for an unrelated reason, such as head trauma in a motor vehicle accident (Table 18.2). If the lesion is >1 cm, evaluation may reveal evidence of a gonadotroph adenoma or of any other pituitary adenoma (see Diagnosis, below). If the lesion is clinically nonfunctioning, it still may well be a gonadotroph adenoma.

Clinical Syndromes Specific to Gonadotroph Adenomas

Gonadotroph adenomas sometimes result in recognizable clinical syndromes (Table 18.2). One syndrome is ovarian hyperstimulation when a gonadotroph adenoma secretes intact FSH in a premenopausal woman. Since the first case was described [62], many more have been reported [63–70]. Continuous secretion of FSH by the adenoma, in contrast to cyclical secretion by normal gonadotroph cells, results in very large ovaries with oligomenorrhea and multiple, large cysts and widened endometrial stripe, which can be detected by pelvic ultrasound (Figure 18.5). This clinical picture can be mistaken for polycystic ovarian syndrome, but administration of a superactive GnRH analogue to a patient with a gonadotroph adenoma results in increased, rather than decreased, FSH secretion, as well as increased serum estradiol and ovarian size [63]. The serum FSH concentration in these patients typically is elevated, the LH concentration is suppressed, and the concentrations of α-subunit and estradiol are elevated. The estradiol concentration is often higher than 500 pg/ml and sometimes as high as 2000 pg/ml. In some patients the serum FSH concentration is within the normal range but the LH concentration is suppressed. Excision of the gonadotroph adenoma can lead to restoration of normal gonadotropin secretion and ovarian function, and pregnancy can occur [63,66,69].

In a man, a clinical presentation of a gonadotroph adenoma with elevated serum FSH concentration is large testicular size in spite of hypogonadism [71]. In contrast, men who have secondary hypogonadism of other causes usually have testes that are normal to slightly small.

A rare clinical presentation is premature puberty in a boy caused by a gonadotroph adenoma hypersecreting intact LH, resulting in increased serum testosterone [72,73]. Secretion of intact LH by gonadotroph adenomas is also rare in men. When it does occur, the result is supranormal serum testosterone concentration [6–8,74], but that condition is usually not associated with any clinical manifestations.

Another clinical presentation, although not due to hormonal hypersecretion, is pituitary apoplexy following the bolus administration of GnRH or the administration of a GnRH analogue to patients with a gonadotroph adenoma. Recent reports describe the discovery of previously unrecognized gonadotroph adenomas when GnRH superactive analogues were administered to treat prostate cancer [75–78]. Enlargement of a gonadotroph adenoma, without apoplexy, was also been reported when a superactive GnRH analogue was administered for prostate cancer [79].

Symptoms of Pituitary Hormonal Deficiencies

At the time of initial presentation due to a neurologic symptom, many patients with gonadotroph adenomas, when questioned, admit to symptoms of pituitary hormonal deficiencies. Ironically, the most common pituitary hormonal deficiency is of LH, as a result of compression of the normal gonadotroph cells by the adenoma and lack of secretion of a substantial amount of intact LH by the adenomatous gonadotroph cells. The result in men is a subnormal serum testosterone concentration, which produces symptoms of decreased energy and libido. The result in premenopausal women is amenorrhea. Secondary hypothyroidism (low serum thyroxine but TSH not elevated) and secondary hypoadrenalism (low early morning cortisol but ACTH not elevated) may also occur.

DIAGNOSIS

The process of making the diagnosis of a gonadotroph adenoma usually proceeds first from recognizing that a patient's visual abnormality or other symptom could represent a sellar mass, then to confirming the presence of a sellar mass by magnetic resonance imaging (MRI), and finally to finding secretory abnormalities of gonadotropins and their subunits characteristic of gonadotroph adenomas. Sometimes the sellar mass is found serendipitously when an MRI of the head is performed because of an unrelated symptom.

Visual and Other Abnormalities

The visual abnormality most characteristic of a sellar mass is diminished vision in the temporal fields. Either or both eyes may be affected, and to variable degrees. Diminished visual acuity occurs when the optic chiasm is more severely compressed. Depending on the direction of suprasellar extension of the adenoma, other patterns of visual loss may also occur, so a sellar lesion should be suspected when any pattern of visual loss is unexplained.

Other neurologic abnormalities that should raise the suspicion of a sellar mass are headaches, oculomotor nerve palsies and CSF rhinorrhea. The quality of the headaches is not specific. Amenorrhea should also raise the suspicion of a sellar mass.

Imaging of the Pituitary

MRI is sufficiently sensitive to demonstrate any pituitary adenoma that has become so large as to impair vision or cause any other neurologic symptom. Because gonadotroph adenomas are generally hormonally inefficient, by the time a gonadotroph adenoma produces supranormal serum concentrations of intact gonadotropins or their subunits, it is sufficiently large to be seen by MRI.

MRI will not distinguish a gonadotroph adenoma from other pituitary macroadenomas or from other large sellar lesions. However, a clear distinction between an intrasellar mass lesion and the normal pituitary is evidence that the lesion is not a pituitary adenoma.

Hormonal Abnormalities

Intrasellar mass lesions detected by MRI should be evaluated further by measurement of serum concentrations of pituitary hormones to determine if the lesion is of pituitary or nonpituitary origin, and if pituitary, the cell of origin. A pituitary adenoma of gonadotroph or thyrotroph cell origin should be suspected if the serum prolactin concentration is less than 100 ng/ml, the patient does not appear acromegalic, the serum IGF-1 concentration is not supranormal, the patient does not have Cushing's syndrome and does not have supranormal urine cortisol excretion. A lesion of nonpituitary origin could also account for these findings. Preoperative recognition that an intrasellar mass lesion is of gonadotroph origin depends on finding specific combinations of the serum concentrations of gonadotropins and their subunits (see Table 18.4). The combinations differ somewhat in men and women.

Men

A supranormal serum FSH concentration in a man who has a sellar mass >1 cm usually indicates that the lesion is a gonadotroph adenoma (Table 18.3). The diagnosis is strengthened if he also has other characteristic features of a gonadotroph adenoma, such as a supranormal basal serum concentration of α-subunit or responses of intact FSH and LH or of LHβ to TRH (Table 18.3). A supranormal serum LH accompanied by a supranormal serum testosterone, whether or not accompanied by a supranormal FSH, is strong evidence that the lesion is one of the unusual gonadotroph adenomas that secrete intact LH (Table 18.3). A supranormal serum

TABLE 18.3 In Vivo Hormonal Criteria for the Diagnosis of Gonadotroph Adenomas* (any one or any combination of the following)

Men	Women
SUPRANORMAL BASAL SERUM CONCENTRATIONS OF	
FSH†	FSH, but not LH
α-subunit	α-subunit relative to FSH and LH
LH and testosterone	
SUPRANORMAL RESPONSE TO TRH OF	
FSH	FSH
LH	LH
LHβ (most common)	LHβ (most common)

* *Assuming the patient has a pituitary macroadenoma.*
† *Assuming the patient does not have a history of primary hypogonadism.*

α-subunit as the sole basal serum abnormality indicates that the intrasellar lesion is of gonadotroph or thyrotroph origin. TRH stimulation of intact FSH or LH or of LHβ subunit would confirm a gonadotroph origin. If the basal serum concentrations of FSH, LH and α-subunit are all supranormal, TRH stimulation of FSH, LH, or LHβ subunit would also suggest that the adenoma is of gonadotroph origin (Table 18.3).

Women

Recognizing the gonadotroph origin of an intrasellar mass on the basis of basal serum hormone concentrations of intact FSH and LH is more difficult in women than in men. In a woman over 50 years old who has an intrasellar mass and elevated gonadotropins, distinguishing between the adenoma and normal postmenopausal gonadotroph cells as the source is usually not possible on the basis of the basal gonadotropins alone. Similarly, in a woman under 50 years old who has an intrasellar mass and elevated serum gonadotropins, distinguishing between the adenoma and premature ovarian failure as the source of the gonadotropins is also not usually possible on the basis of the FSH and LH values alone. A few combinations of basal FSH, LH and α-subunit values, however, do suggest strongly that an intrasellar mass is a gonadotroph adenoma. A markedly supranormal FSH associated with a subnormal LH, for example, most likely indicates a gonadotroph adenoma, rather than the postmenopausal state or premature ovarian failure (Table 18.4). A serum α-subunit concentration that is supranormal when intact FSH and LH are not, or is supranormal out of proportion to FSH and LH, also suggests a gonadotroph adenoma (Table 18.4). More commonly, an intrasellar mass in a woman may be recognized as a gonadotroph adenoma by an increase in the FSH or LH, or even more frequently, the LHβ-subunit, in response to TRH (Figure 18.1). (Note: Synthetic TRH for diagnostic use is available in many countries, but not in the United States. Commercial assays are widely available for α-subunit, but not for LHβ or FSHβ.)

TABLE 18.4 Gonadotroph Adenoma Presenting as Ovarian Hyperstimulation in a Premenopausal Woman. Basal Serum Hormone Concentrations in a 39-year-old Woman who Presented with Oligomenorrhea

Hormone	Patient's Value	Normal Range
FSH (mIU/ml)	17.8	5.4–12.4
LH (mIU/ml)	0.7	1.7–7.7
α-subunit (ng/ml)	23.3	0.1–1.0
Estradiol (pg/ml)	588	30–100

Ultrasound images of the ovaries and uterus are shown in Figure 18.5.
From Djerassi et al.[62]

Distinguishing a Gonadotroph Adenoma from Primary Hypogonadism

The question of distinguishing a gonadotroph adenoma from primary hypogonadism may be raised, because in both conditions serum concentrations of intact gonadotropins and their subunits may be supranormal and gonadal steroids may be subnormal. Furthermore, long-standing primary hypogonadism may cause some enlargement of the pituitary as a consequence of gonadotroph hyperplasia [59]. In practice, however, making this distinction is usually quite easy, because each exhibits a different clinical presentation and each a different set of hormonal secretory characteristics (Table 18.5). The major clinical distinction results from the observation that pituitary enlargement due to primary hypogonadism usually does not occur unless the hypogonadism is severe, untreated and of many years duration. Consequently, such patients, both men and women, usually appear severely hypogonadal clinically. In contrast, men and women who have gonadotroph adenomas may be hypogonadal, but the hypogonadism is usually not severe or of long duration. Consequently, they do not appear hypogonadal clinically. The major difference in basal hormonal concentrations is the elevation of both FSH and LH in patients who have primary hypogonadism and the elevation of FSH but usually not LH, and sometimes by a greater elevation of α-subunit, in patients who have gonadotroph adenomas.

TABLE 18.5 Comparison of Characteristics of Gonadotroph Adenomas and Primary Hypogonadism in Men

	Gonadotroph Adenoma	Primary Hypogonadism
Puberty	Normal	Often incomplete
Fertility history	Normal	Subnormal
Testicular size	Normal	Small
Serum testosterone	Low to high	Low to normal
Testosterone response to hCG (when basal value is subnormal)	Marked, to well within normal range	Subnormal
Serum FSH	High	High
Serum LH	Usually normal or slightly high	High if testosterone is low
α-subunit	High to very high	High
FSH response to TRH	Common	Absent
LHβ response to TRH	Very common	Absent

The major difference in hormonal responses to TRH is that patients who have gonadotroph adenomas often exhibit responses of FSH, LH and, more commonly, LHβ-subunit [10,23], but patients who have primary hypogonadism do not [24]. Another clear difference is that men who have a subnormal serum testosterone on the basis of a gonadotroph adenoma exhibit an increase to well within the normal range when treated with hCG for 4 days [80], but men with primary hypogonadism do not.

Abnormal Secretion of other Pituitary Hormones

Pituitary adenomas that secrete intact gonadotropins and/or their subunits usually do not secrete other pituitary hormones as well, but concomitant secretion of TSH and prolactin has been reported rarely. A serum prolactin concentration that is elevated but under 100 ng/ml, however, suggests not concomitant secretion by the adenoma but increased secretion by normal lactotroph cells that are less than normally inhibited because of stalk compression by the adenoma.

Deficient secretion of other pituitary hormones often occurs due to the mass effect of the typically large gonadotroph adenomas and should always be investigated. Measurement of basal serum concentrations of thyroxine, cortisol and testosterone in men and estradiol in women, and of ACTH reserve is usually necessary.

TABLE 18.6 Comparison of Treatments for Gonadotroph Adenomas

Treatment	Indications	Complications
Transsphenoidal surgery	Intrasellar mass with suprasellar extension and visual impairment	Worsening of vision, ocular palsy, hematoma, CSF rhinorrhea, meningitis, diabetes insipidus, hypopituitarism
Transcranial surgery	Large, residual symptomatic extrasellar tissue following transsphenoidal surgery	Same as above, but more likely
Radiation	Primary treatment: intrasellar mass with only mild suprasellar extension	Transient: fatigue, nausea, hair loss, loss of taste and smell
	Adjuvant treatment: substantial residual adenoma tissue after surgery	Permanent: hypopituitarism, blindness
Observation	Vision intact	Visual impairment
Medications (dopamine agonists, somatostatin analogues)		Often ineffective

TREATMENT

When gonadotroph adenomas are not detected until they become so large that they cause significant visual impairment, treatment must be directed at reducing adenoma mass and restoring vision as soon as possible. Surgery, usually transsphenoidal, is the only treatment that meets this criterion (Table 18.6). Gonadotroph adenomas are usually sensitive to radiation, which may be used to prevent regrowth if substantial adenoma tissue remains after surgery or to treat primarily if an adenoma is detected before it becomes so large as to cause neurologic symptoms. Several pharmacologic treatments have been tried, but none reduce adenoma size reliably.

Surgery

Surgical Approaches

Transsphenoidal surgery using the operating microscope replaced transcranial surgery in the 1970s as the preferred treatment for sellar masses thought to be below the diaphragm sella, because that approach allowed excision of more of the mass with fewer serious complications. In the past decade an increasing number of neurosurgeons have been using endoscopic surgery [81–83] instead of, or in addition to, the operating microscope, and now several series each report experience with more than 100 patients who have undergone a procedure involving endoscopy. Some surgeons employ the endoscope exclusively [84–86]. Others use transsphenoidal surgery with the operative microscope for primary resection and then use an endoscope to extend surgery within and beyond the sella [87]. Another technique for guiding surgery is intraoperative MRI, to determine the extent of sellar mass remaining after initial debulking [88], especially for very large adenomas that extend far outside the sella [89]. Similarly, intraoperative Doppler also allows operating near and within the cavernous sinuses without damaging the internal carotid arteries [90] and thus allows a larger amount of the adenoma to be excised. Neurosurgeons are using these and other techniques to extend the reach of surgery in and around the sella to include the cavernous sinuses and suprasellar regions. Some neurosurgeons are now operating on suprasellar lesions, such as craniopharyngiomas, via a transsphenoidal approach [91–93].

Efficacy of Surgery

Transsphenoidal surgery almost always results in a decrease in adenoma size (Figure 18.6) [94] and concomitantly an improvement in vision (Figure 18.7) and decrease in hormone hypersecretion (Figure 18.8) [94]. Seventy to eighty percent of patients who have abnormal visual fields due to a gonadotroph adenoma in one series experienced improvement following transsphenoidal surgery [94]. This improvement is similar to that of all macroadenomas. In one series of 230 patients whose visual fields were abnormal before transsphenoidal surgery, the fields improved in 73%, remained the same in 23% and worsened in 4% (Table 18.7) [95]. In another series of 113 pituitary adenomas that extended beyond the sella, 81% of those with visual field defects before surgery experienced improvement in fields after surgery, 19% remained the same and none worsened [96]. Few reports of endoscopic surgery describe the degree of mass removal or change in postoperative vision.

Complications of Surgery

Serious complications of transsphenoidal surgery are uncommon, but appear to be greater when the adenoma is very large and the surgeon has performed fewer transsphenoidal procedures. In a survey in which

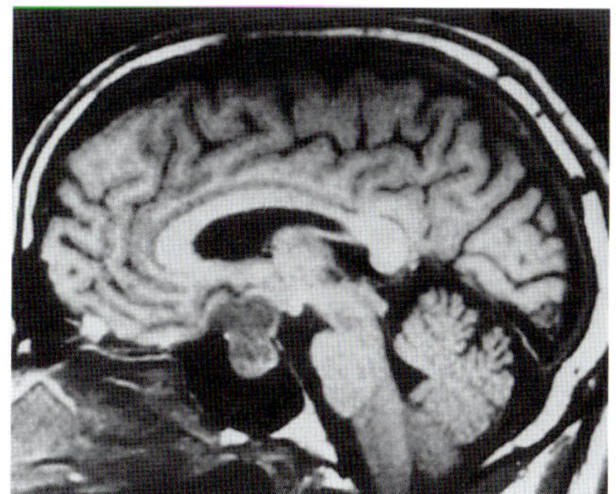

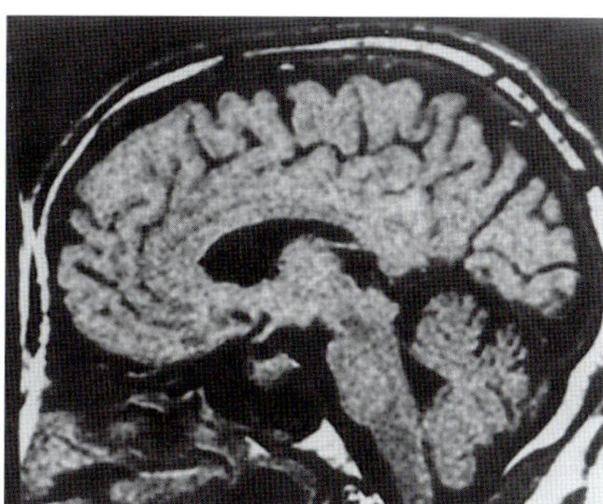

FIGURE 18.6 Reduction in gonadotroph adenoma size by transsphenoidal surgery as seen by magnetic resonance imaging in sagittal views. The left panel shows the large figure-eight-shaped adenoma extending far above the sella and elevating the optic chiasm. The right panel shows that most of the adenoma has been excised and that the optic chiasm has been restored to its customary position. Improvement in his vision is shown in Figure 18.7.

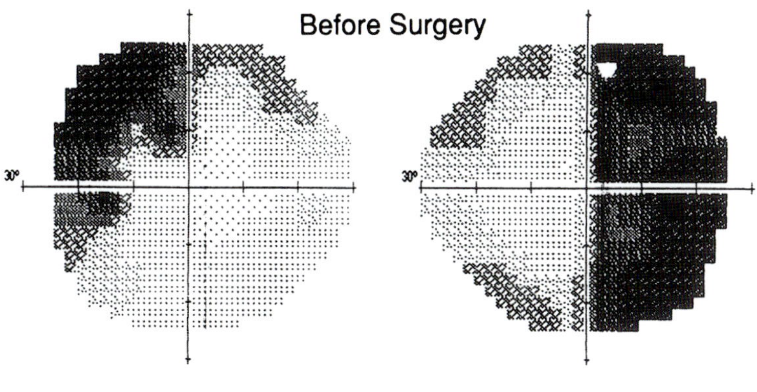

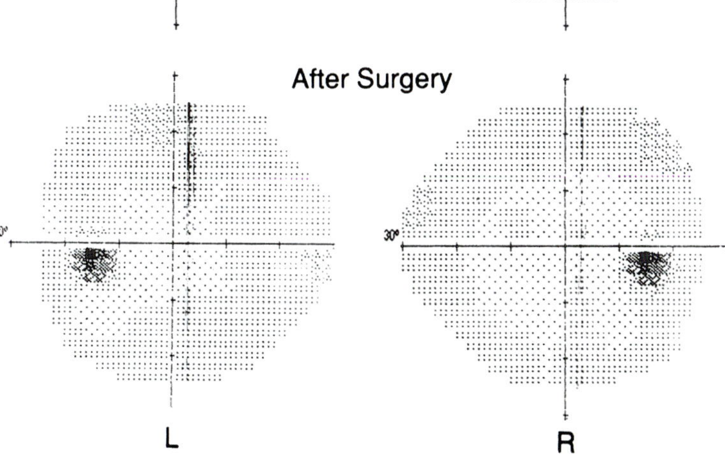

FIGURE 18.7 Visual fields performed on an automated Humphrey instrument in a 42-year-old man with a gonadotroph adenoma before (upper pair) and 4 weeks after (lower pair) transsphenoidal excision of much of the adenoma. Before surgery he had a complete right temporal defect and a left superior temporal defect; afterwards visual fields were normal. Magnetic resonance imaging of his adenoma before and after surgery is shown in Figure 18.6. *Courtesy of Dr Peter J. Savino.*

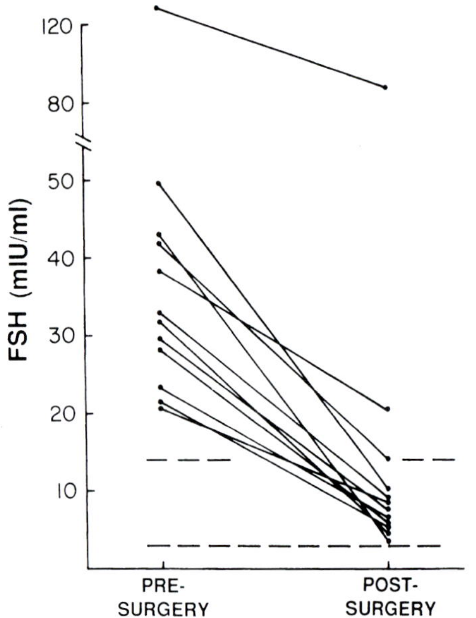

FIGURE 18.8 Serum FSH concentrations in 12 men with gonadotroph adenomas before and 4–6 weeks after transsphenoidal surgery. The decreases in FSH correlated with the decrease in size as determined by imaging. *From Harris et al. [94].*

TABLE 18.7 Efficacy of Transsphenoidal Surgery for Restoring Vision in Patients who have Pituitary Macroadenomas

	Number of Patients (%) Whose Vision was:			
Visual Parameter	**Number of Patients**	**Better**	**Unchanged**	**Worse**
ACUITY				
Normal before surgery	181	NA	99	1
Abnormal before surgery	104	50	49	1
FIELDS				
Normal before surgery	71	NA	99	1
Abnormal before surgery	214	76	20	4

Adapted from[95].

neurosurgeons were asked to report their own experience (Table 18.8), serious complications reported by the 958 respondents included carotid artery injury (1.1%), central nervous system injury (1.3%), loss of vision (1.8%), ophthalmoplegia (1.4%), hemorrhage or swelling of the residual tumor (2.9%), cerebrospinal fluid leak (3.9%), meningitis (1.5%) and death (0.9%) [97]. The chances of anterior pituitary insufficiencies (19.4%) and diabetes insipidus (17.8%) were higher. The incidence of each complication was higher among neurosurgeons who were less experienced. Among neurosurgeons who reported performing fewer than 200 transsphenoidal procedures, 1.2% of the procedures resulted in death, but among neurosurgeons who reported performing more than 500 procedures, only 0.2% resulted in death. Although these results are based on retrospective self-reporting via questionnaire, they provide a broader assessment of complications of transsphenoidal surgery than that provided by the most experienced pituitary surgeons [98–100], whose complication rates are closer to those of the most experienced group above [97].

An even broader assessment is provided by a study using the Nationwide Inpatient Sample, 1996–2000, of 5497 operations at 538 hospitals by 825 surgeons, which also demonstrated that surgeons who performed more transsphenoidal operations had fewer complications than those who performed fewer [101]. Odds ratio for one or more complications of surgery or perioperative care was 0.76 for a five-fold larger case load per surgeon (95% confidence interval 0.65–0.89; $p = 0.005$). The lowest quartile of surgeons in this survey performed only one transsphenoidal procedure a year and the highest only eight or more per year, illustrating dramatically that this survey represented a much broader sampling than that of the primarily pituitary neurosurgeons above.

Complication rates are also greater in patients who have had prior pituitary surgery than in those who never had, and even greater in those whose prior

TABLE 18.8 Complications of Transsphenoidal Surgery in Relationship to the Experience of the Surgeon

	Percent of Operations Resulting in Complication		
	Number of Previous Operations		
Complication	**<200**	**20–500**	**>500**
Carotid artery injury	1.4	0.6	0.4
Central nervous system injury	1.6	0.9	0.6
Hemorrhage into tumor bed	2.8	4.0	0.8
Loss of vision	2.4	0.8	0.5
Ophthalmoplegia	1.9	0.8	0.4
Cerebrospinal fluid leak	4.2	2.8	0.5
Meningitis	1.9	0.8	0.5
Nasal septum perforation	7.6	4.6	3.3
Anterior pituitary insufficiency	20.6	14.9	7.2
Diabetes insipidus	19.0	NA	7.6
Death	1.2	0.6	0.2

Data were collected from participating surgeons by questionnaire. Adapted from [97].

surgery was via craniotomy than in those whose prior surgery was transsphenoidal [102].

Evaluation of the Results of Surgery

The results of surgery should initially be evaluated 4–6 weeks afterwards. Residual adenoma tissue should be evaluated by MRI and by measurement of whatever hormones or subunits had been elevated before surgery. The functions of the nonadenomatous anterior pituitary should also be re-evaluated postoperatively, as should vasopressin secretion. Neuroophthalmologic function should likewise be re-evaluated.

Radiation

Techniques of Radiation

Radiation therapy has been used to treat pituitary adenomas for decades. The standard technique during the latter half of the 20th century employed a supervoltage source to deliver a total of 45–50 Gy in daily 2 Gy doses via three external portals. Much of our information about the long-term effects of radiation on pituitary adenomas and surrounding tissues is based on patients treated by this technique. This technique, however, has now been supplanted by techniques in which the radiation is delivered stereotactically, to attempt to minimize the amount of radiation to which the brain and other surrounding structures are exposed. Current techniques employ radiation from one of several sources: protons from a cyclotron ("proton beam"), high-energy X-rays from a linear accelerator ("LINAC"), or gamma radiation from a ^{60}Co source ("gamma knife") (Table 18.9). Radiation from a linear accelerator or a cyclotron can be administered either in a single dose or in multiple fractions over several weeks, whereas radiation from a ^{60}Co source can be administered only as a single dose. Single-dose techniques are often referred to as "radiosurgery," although no surgery is involved. All of the techniques use computer-generated models, so that the radiation conforms to the boundaries of the lesion. Proton beam treatment has an additional theoretical advantage with regard to delivering radiation differentially to the lesion, in that the beam of protons exhibits a peak, delivered to the tumor, followed by a rapid decrease in energy just after the peak, so that the normal tissue adjacent to the tumor is exposed to much less energy. Single-dose techniques are reserved for lesions that are a certain minimal distance, e.g., 3–5 mm, from the optic chiasm and optic nerves, because the dose of radiation delivered is highly likely to damage those structures and cause blindness.

Efficacy of Radiation

Studies of prestereotactic radiation administered following surgery for a pituitary macroadenoma generally showed efficacy in preventing regrowth of the adenoma [103–105]. In one study of men who had prestereotactic radiation therapy following surgery for clinically nonfunctioning pituitary macroadenomas, only 7% of the 63 patients who received radiation following surgery developed new visual impairment requiring additional treatment during the subsequent 15 years, but 66% of the 63 who did not receive radiation developed new visual impairment [103].

Several series have been reported in recent years describing the efficacy of stereotactic methods of radiation in preventing recurrence of pituitary adenomas and other sellar tumors. In series of patients treated with fractionated radiotherapy using a linear accelerator [106–109] or proton beam [110] observed for a median of 40 months or more, adenoma size was reduced or stable in 90–100%. In a review of 25 studies involving 1621 patients, of whom 452 had clinically nonfunctioning pituitary adenomas and who were treated with single-dose radiation from a linear accelerator, gamma source, or proton beam, adenoma size was controlled in about 90% during a follow-up that was more than 40 months in half the patients [111]. In a report from a single center at which 100 clinically nonfunctioning adenomas were treated with single-dose radiation from a gamma source, followed for a median of 45 months, adenoma volume decreased or remained stable in 92% of patients [112].

Complications of Radiation

The long-term side effects after prestereotactic radiation include hypopituitarism and neurologic deficits. Hypopituitarism, in several studies, began about a year or more after radiation, and by 10 years afterwards about 50% of patients had a deficiency of

TABLE 18.9 Comparison of Options for Radiation Therapy for Pituitary Adenomas

Radiation Source	Type of Radiation	Common Name	Availability of Fractionated Doses	Availability of Single Dose
Linear accelerator	X-radiation	LINAC	Yes	Yes
^{60}Cobalt	Gamma radiation	Gamma knife	No	Yes
Cyclotron	Protons	Proton beam	Yes	Yes

ACTH, TSH, or LH [113–115]. Neurological side effects occurred less commonly. Blindness due to optic neuritis [116], brain tumors and cerebrovascular accidents attributed to accelerated local atherosclerosis were reported as case reports and in some series [117,118], but other series reported no neurologic sequelae [119]. Although decreased cognitive function has been reported anecdotally after radiation, one systematic study did not confirm this effect [120].

Although current radiotherapy techniques offer the theoretical advantage of targeting the tumor by stereotactic means, pituitary deficiencies and neurological complications also occur with these techniques. In the series of 100 patients with clinically nonfunctioning adenomas treated with single-dose gamma radiation and followed for a median of 45 months, 20% developed new hypopituitarism [112]. In the review of 35 studies involving 1621 patients, optic neuropathy occurred in about 1%, other cranial neuropathies in 1.3% and parenchymal brain damage in about 0.8% [111].

Management of Patients after Radiation

Hormonal evaluation, both for excessive secretion of whichever intact gonadotropins and their subunits were secreted excessively by the adenoma prior to treatment, and for deficient secretion by the nonadenomatous pituitary, should be performed 6 and 12 months after radiation and once a year thereafter. Evaluation of size by MRI should be performed 1 year after radiation and, if the mass is smaller, less frequently thereafter. Neuroophthalmologic evaluation should be repeated after radiation if it had been abnormal before.

Pharmacologic Treatment

Several drugs have been administered in attempts to treat gonadotroph adenomas, but so far none has been found that reduces their size consistently and substantially.

Although dopamine does not decrease gonadotropin secretion to an appreciable degree in normal subjects, bromocriptine has been reported to reduce the secretion of intact gonadotropins and α-subunit in a few patients and even to improve vision in one, but not to reduce adenoma size [121,122]. CV 205-504 has also been reported to reduce secretion and adenoma size in occasional patients [123]. Cabergoline has been reported to reduce α-subunit concentration in a single patient with a gonadotroph adenoma [124] and to decrease adenoma volume by 10–18% in seven of 13 other patients with gonadotroph adenomas [125].

The somatostatin analogue, octreotide, has been used to treat gonadotroph adenomas because of the demonstration that somatostatin itself may decrease secretion by gonadotroph adenomas in vitro. Although there have been occasional reports of dramatic decreases in the size of gonadotroph adenomas associated with octreotide administration [126,127] and some improvement in vision, the majority of patients have little if any improvement in adenoma size or vision [126–128].

Several agonist analogues of GnRH have been administered to patients with gonadotroph adenomas, based on the rationale that chronic administration of these agonists causes down-regulation of GnRH receptors on, and decreased secretion of FSH and LH from, normal gonadotroph cells. Administration of GnRH agonist analogues to patients with gonadotroph adenomas, however, generally produces either an agonist effect or no effect on secretion and no effect on adenoma size [129,130].

Potent antagonist analogues of GnRH have also been tried. Administration for 1 week of the GnRH antagonist, Nal-Glu GnRH, to men with gonadotroph adenomas reduced their elevated FSH concentrations to normal [60]. However, when Nal-Glu administration was continued for 6 months, although FSH remained suppressed, adenoma size did not decrease [131].

Observation

Observation alone is a reasonable course for a patient who has a sellar mass, even if it extends outside of the sella and elevates the optic chiasm, as long as the mass is not associated with neurologic symptoms, especially for patients whose surgical risk is high or who prefer not to have surgery until necessary. In a series of 40 patients with clinically nonfunctioning sellar masses, 24 "macro" and 16 "micro," who were followed for a mean of 42 months, the 48-month probability of enlargement was 19% for the micro lesions and 44% for the macros [132]. New or worse visual field defects were observed in 67% of the macro lesions that increased in size. In a series of 28 patients with clinically nonfunctioning sellar masses, all "macro," followed for an average of 84 months, 14 increased in size in an average of 118 months, six requiring surgery for worsening visual field; eight decreased in size [133].

References

[1] P.J. Snyder, Gonadotroph cell adenomas of the pituitary, Endocr Rev 6 (1985) 552–563.

[2] P.J. Snyder, J. Johnson, R. Muzyka, Abnormal secretion of glycoprotein α-subunit and follicle-stimulating hormone (FSH) β-subunit in men with pituitary adenomas and FSH hypersecretion, J Clin Endocrinol Metab 51 (1980) 579–584.

[3] S.C. Chappel, H.M. Bashey, P.J. Snyder, Similar isoelectric profiles of FSH from gonadotroph cell adenomas and non-adenomatous pituitaries, Acta Endocrinol (Copenh) 113 (3) (1986) 311–316.

[4] A.B. Galway, J.W. Hsueh, L. Daneshdoost, M.H. Zhou, S.N. Pavlou, P.J. Snyder, Gonadotroph adenomas in men produce biologically active follicle-stimulating hormone, J Clin Endocrinol Metab 71 (1990) 907–912.

[5] S. Borgato, L. Persani, R. Romoli, D. Cortelazzi, A. Spada, P. Beck-Peccoz, Serum FSH bioactivity and inhibin levels in patients with gonadotropin secreting and nonfunctioning pituitary adenomas, J Endocrinol Invest 21 (1998) 372–379.

[6] P.J. Snyder, F.H. Sterling, Hypersecretion of LH and FSH by a pituitary adenoma, J Clin Endocrinol Metab 42 (1976) 544–550.

[7] A. Klibanski, P.J. Deutsch, J.L. Jameson, et al., Luteinizing hormone-secreting pituitary tumor: Biosynthetic characterization and clinical studies, J Clin Endocrinol Metab 64 (1987) 536–542.

[8] R.D. Peterson, I.A. Kourides, M. Horwith, E.D. Vaughn, B.B. Saxena, R.A.R. Fraser, Luteinizing hormone and α-subunit-secreting Pituitary tumor: Positive feedback of estrogen, J Clin Endocrinol Metab 51 (1981) 692–698.

[9] M.D. Whitaker, J.C. Prior, B. Scheithauer, L. Dolman, F. Durity, M.R. Pudek, Gonadotrophin-secreting pituitary tumour: Report and review, Clin Endocrinol 22 (1985) 43–48.

[10] L. Daneshdoost, T.A. Gennarelli, H.M. Bashey, P.J. Savino, R.C. Sergott, T.M. Bosley, et al., Identification of gonadotroph adenomas in men with clinically nonfunctioning adenomas by the LHβ subunit response to TRH, J Clin Endocrinol Metab 77 (1993) 1352–1355.

[11] J.L. Borges, E.C. Ridgway, K. Kovacs, A.D. Rogol, M.O. Thorner, Follicle-stimulating hormone-secreting pituitary tumor with concomitant elevation of serum α-subunit levels, J Clin Endocrinol Metab 58 (1984) 937–941.

[12] A.J. Chapman, A. MacFarlane, S.M. Shalet, C.G. Beardwell, J. Dutton, M.L. Sutton, Discordant serum α-subunit and FSH concentrations in a woman with a pituitary tumour, Clin Endocrinol 21 (1984) 123–129.

[13] R. Demura, K. Jibiki, O. Kubo, et al., The significance of α-subunit as a tumor marker for gonadotropin-producing pituitary adenomas, J Clin Endocrinol Metab 63 (1986) 564–569.

[14] A. Klibanski, E.C. Ridgway, N.T. Zervas, Pure alpha subunit-secreting pituitary tumors, J Neurosurg 59 (1983) 585–589.

[15] E.C. Ridgway, A. Klibanski, P.W. Ladenson, et al., Pure alpha-secreting pituitary adenomas, N Engl J Med 304 (1981) 1254–1259.

[16] P.J. Snyder, H.M. Bashey, J.L. Phillips, T.A. Gennarelli, Comparison of hormonal secretory behavior of gonadotroph cell adenomas in vivo and in culture, J Clin Endocrinol Metab 61 (6) (1985 Dec) 1061–1065.

[17] J.L. Jameson, A. Klibanski, P.M. Black, et al., Glycoprotein hormone genes are expressed in clinically nonfunctioning pituitary adenomas, J Clin Invest 80 (1987) 1472–1478.

[18] Y. Konde, N. Kugal, S. Kimura, et al., A case of pituitary adenoma with possible simultaneous secretion of thyrotropin and follicle-stimulating hormone, J Clin Endocrinol Metab 54 (1982) 397–403.

[19] D.S. Oppenheim, A.R. Kana, J.S. Sangha, A. Klibanski, A prevalence of alpha subunit hypersecretion in patients with pituitary tumors clinically nonfunctioning and somatotroph adenomas, J Clin Endocrinol Metab 70 (1990) 859–864.

[20] P. Beck-Peccoz, M. Bassetti, A. Spada, et al., Glycoprotein hormone alpha subunit response to growth hormone (GH)-releasing hormone in patients with active acromegaly. Evidence for alpha subunit and GH co-existence in the same tumor cell, J Clin Endocrinol Metab 61 (1985) 541–546.

[21] L.J. Hofland, P.M. Van Koetsveld, T.M. Verleun, S.W.J. Lamberts, Glycoprotein hormone alpha-subunit and prolactin release by cultured pituitary adenoma cells from acromegalic patients correlation with GH release, Clin Endocrinol 30 (1989) 601–611.

[22] M.C. White, P. Newland, M. Daniels, et al., Growth hormone secreting pituitary adenomas are heterogeneous in cell culture and commonly secrete glycoprotein hormone alpha subunit, Clin Endocrinol 25 (1986) 173–179.

[23] L. Daneshdoost, T.A. Gennarelli, H.M. Bashey, P.J. Savino, R.C. Sergott, T.M. Bosley, et al., Recognition of gonadotroph adenomas in women, N Engl J Med 324 (9) (1991) 589–594.

[24] P.J. Snyder, R. Muzyka, J. Johnson, R.D. Utiger, Thyrotropin-releasing hormone provokes abnormal follicle-stimulating hormone (FSH) and luteinizing hormone responses in men who have pituitary adenomas and FSH hypersecretion, J Clin Endocrinol Metab 51 (1980) 744–748.

[25] J. Trouillas, C. Girod, G. Sassolas, B. Claustrat, The human gonadotropic adenoma pathologic diagnosis and hormonal correlations in 26 tumors, Semin Diagnost Pathol 3 (1986) 42–57.

[26] S.L. Asa, B.M. Gerne, W. Singer, E. Horvath, K. Kovacs, H.S. Smyth, Gonadotropin secretion in vitro by human pituitary null cell adenomas and oncocytomas, J Clin Endocrinol Metab 62 (1986) 1011–1019.

[27] K. Mashiter, E. Adams, S. Van Noorden, Secretion of LH, FSH and PRL shown by cell culture and immunocytochemistry of human functionless pituitary adenomas, Clin Endocrinol 15 (1981) 103–112.

[28] S. Yamada, S.L. Asa, K. Kovacs, P. Muller, H.S. Smyth, Analysis of hormone secretion by clinically nonfunctioning human pituitary adenomas using the reverse hemolytic plaque assay, J Clin Endocrinol Metab 68 (1) (1989) 73–80.

[29] P.M. Black, D.W. Hsu, A. Klibanski, B. Kliman, J.L. Jameson, E.C. Ridgway, et al., Hormone production in clinically nonfunctioning pituitary adenoma, J Neurosurg 66 (1987) 244–250.

[30] D.J. Kwekkeboom, F.H. de Jong, S.W. Lamberts, Gonadotropin release by clinically nonfunctioning and gonadotroph pituitary adenomas in vivo and in vitro: Relation to sex and effects of thyrotropin-releasing hormone, gonadotropin-releasing hormone, and bromocriptine, J Clin Endocrinol Metab 68 (6) (1989) 1128–1135.

[31] E. Horvath, K. Kovacs, Gonadotroph adenomas of the human pituitary: Sex-related fine-structural dichotomy. A histologic, immunocytochemical, and electron-microscopic study of 30 tumors, Am J Pathol 117 (3) (1984) 429–440.

[32] J.M. Alexander, B.M.K. Biller, H. Bikkal, N.T. Zervas, A. Arnold, A. Klibanski, Clinically nonfunctioning pituitary tumors are monoclonal in orgin, J Clin Invest 86 (1990) 336–340.

[33] S.C. Chandrasekhapappa, S.C. Guru, P. Manickam, S.E. Olufemi, F.S. Collins, M.R. Emmert-Buck, et al., Positional cloning of the gene for multiple endocrine neoplasia-type 1, Science 276 (1997) 404–407.

[34] M. Benito, S.L. Asa, V.A. Livolsi, V.A. West, P.J. Snyder, Gonadotroph tumor associated with multiple endocrine neoplasia type 1, J Clin Endocrinol Metab 90 (1) (2005) 570–574.

[35] S. Sztal-Mazer, D.J. Topliss, R.W. Simpson, P.S. Hamblin, J.V. Rosenfeld, C.A. McLean, Gonadotroph adenoma in multiple endocrine neoplasia type 1, Endocr Pract 14 (5) (2008) 592–594.

[36] J.H. Bassett, S.A. Forbes, A.A. Pannett, S.E. Lloyd, P.T. Christie, C. Wooding, et al., Characterization of mutations in patients with multiple endocrine neoplasia type 1, Am J Hum Genet 62 (2) (1998) 232–244.

[37] A. Cebrian, S. Ruiz-Llorente, A. Cascon, M. Pollan, J.J. Diez, A. Pico, et al., Mutational and gross deletion study of the MEN1 gene and correlation with clinical features in Spanish patients, J Med Genet 40 (5) (2003) e72.

[38] B. Verges, F. Boureille, P. Goudet, A. Murat, A. Beckers, G. Sassolas, et al., Pituitary disease in MEN type 1 (MEN1): Data from the France–Belgium MEN1 multicenter study, J Clin Endocrinol Metab 87 (2) (2002) 457–465.

[39] C.A. Landis, S.B. Masters, A. Spada, A.M. Pace, H.R. Bourne, L. Vallar, GTPase inhibiting mutations activate the α chain of G_s and stimulate adenylate cyclase in human pituitary tumors, Nature 340 (1989) 692–696.

[40] M. Woloschak, J.L. Roberts, K. Post, c-Myc, c-fos, and c-myb gene expression in human pituitary adenomas, J Clin Endocrinol Metab 79 (1994) 253–257.

[41] W.Y. Cai, J.M. Alexander, E.T. Hedley-Whyte, B.W. Scheithauer, J.L. Jameson, N.T. Zervas, et al., Ras mutations in human prolactinomas and pituitary carcinomas, J Clin Endocrinol Metab 78 (1994) 89–93.

[42] L. Pei, S. Melmed, B. Scheithauer, K. Kovacs, D. Prager, H-ras mutations in human pituitary carcinoma metastases, J Clin Endocrinol Metab 78 (1994) 842–846.

[43] V.L. Cryns, J.M. Alexander, A. Klibanski, A. Arnold, The retinoblastoma gene in human pituitary tumors, J Clin Endocrinol Metab 77 (1993) 644–646.

[44] H. Ikeda, R.L. Beauchamp, T. Yoshimoto, D.W. Yandell, Detection of heterozygous mutation in the retinoblastoma gene in a human pituitary adenoma using pcr-sscp analysis and direct sequencing, Endo Path 6 (1995) 189–196.

[45] J. Zhu, S.P. Leon, A.H. Beggs, L. Busque, D.G. Gilliland, P.M. Black, Human pituitary adenomas show no loss of heterozygosity at the retinoblastoma gene locus, J Clin Endocrinol Metab 78 (1994) 922–927.

[46] T.H. Jones, S. Justice, A. Price, K. Chapman, Interleukin-6 secreting human pituitary adenomas in vitro, J Clin Endocrinol Metab 73 (1991) 207–209.

[47] P. Robberecht, P. Vertongen, B. Velkeniers, P. DeNeef, P. Vergani, C. Raftopoulos, et al., Receptors for pituitary adenylate cyclase activating peptides in human pituitary adenomas, J Clin Endocrinol Metab 77 (1993) 1235–1239.

[48] V. Alvaro, L. Levy, C. Dubray, A. Roche, F. Peillon, B. Querat, et al., Invasive human pituitary tumors express a point-mutated alpha-protein kinase-C, J Clin Endocrinol Metab 77 (1993) 1125–1129.

[49] V. LeRiche, S.L. Asa, S. Ezzat, Epidermal growth factor and its receptor (EGF-R) in human pituitary adenomas: EGF-R correlates with tumor aggressiveness, J Clin Endocrinol Metab 81 (1996) 656–662.

[50] S. Ezzat, I.A. Walpola, L. Ramyar, H.S. Smythe, S.L. Asa, Membrane-anchored expression of transforming growth factor alpha in human pituitary adenoma cells, J Clin Endocrinol Metab 80 (1995) 534–539.

[51] G.M. Miller, J.M. Alexander, A. Klibanski, Gonadotropin-releasing hormone messenger RNA expression in gonadotroph tumors and normal human pituitary, J Clin Endocrinol Metab 81 (1996) 80–83.

[52] J.M. Alexander, A. Klibanski, Gonadotropin-releasing hormone receptor mRNA expression by human pituitary tumors in vitro, J Clin Invest 93 (1994) 2332–2339.

[53] G. Haddad, J.L. Penabad, H.M. Bashey, S.L. Asa, T.A. Gennarelli, R. Cirullo, et al., Expression of activin/inhibin subunit messenger ribonucleic acids by gonadotroph adenomas, J Clin Endocrinol Metab 79 (1994) 1399–1403.

[54] J.L. Penabad, H.M. Bashey, S.L. Asa, G. Haddad, K.D. Davis, A.B. Herbst, et al., Decreased follistatin gene expression in gonadotroph adenomas, J Clin Endocrinol Metab 81 (1996) 3397–3403.

[55] L. Pei, S. Melmed, Isolation and characterization of a pituitary tumor-transforming gene (PTTG), Mol Endocrinol 11 (4) (1997) 433–441.

[56] X. Zhang, G.A. Horwitz, T.R. Prezant, A. Valentini, M. Nakashima, M.D. Bronstein, et al., Structure, expression, and function of human pituitary tumor-transforming gene (PTTG), Mol Endocrinol 13 (1) (1999) 156–166.

[57] S. Ezzat, L. Zheng, X.F. Zhu, G.E. Wu, S.L. Asa, Targeted expression of a human pituitary tumor-derived isoform of FGF receptor-4 recapitulates pituitary tumorigenesis, J Clin Invest 109 (1) (2002) 69–78.

[58] R. Gejman, D.L. Batista, Y. Zhong, Y. Zhou, X. Zhang, B. Swearingen, et al., Selective loss of MEG3 expression and intergenic differentially methylated region hypermethylation in the MEG3/DLK1 locus in human clinically nonfunctioning pituitary adenomas, J Clin Endocrinol Metab 93 (10) (2008) 4119–4125.

[59] N.A. Samaan, A.V. Stephans, J. Danziger, J. Trujillo, Reactive pituitary abnormalities in patients with Klinefelter's and Turner's syndromes, Arch Intern Med 139 (1979) 198–201.

[60] L. Daneshdoost, S. Pavlou, M.E. Molitch, Inhibition of follicle-stimulating hormone secretion from gonadotroph adenomas by repetitive administration of a gonadotropin-releasing hormone antagonist, J Clin Endocrinol Metab 71 (1990) 92–97.

[61] B.W. Scheithauer, M. Moschopulos, K. Kovacs, B.S. Jhaveri, T. Percek, R.V. Lloyd, The pituitary in Klinefelter syndrome, Endocr Pathol 16 (2) (2005) 133–138.

[62] A. Djerassi, C. Coutifaris, V.A. West, S.L. Asa, S.C. Kapoor, S.N. Pavlou, et al., Gonadotroph adenoma in a premenopausal woman secreting follicle-stimulating hormone and causing ovarian hyperstimulation, J Clin Endocrinol Metab 80 (2) (1995) 591–594.

[63] A.J. Castelbaum, H. Bigdeli, K.D. Post, M.F. Freedman, P.J. Snyder, Exacerbation of ovarian hyperstimulation by leuprolide reveals a gonadotroph adenoma, Fertil Steril 78 (6) (2002) 1311–1313.

[64] S. Christin-Maitre, C. Rongieres-Bertrand, M.L. Kottler, N. Lahlou, R. Frydman, P. Touraine, et al., A spontaneous and severe hyperstimulation of the ovaries revealing a gonadotroph adenoma, J Clin Endocrinol Metab 83 (10) (1998) 3450–3453.

[65] O. Cooper, J.L. Geller, S. Melmed, Ovarian hyperstimulation syndrome caused by an FSH-secreting pituitary adenoma, Nat Clin Pract Endocrinol Metab 4 (4) (2008) 234–238.

[66] M. Ghayuri, J.H. Liu, Ovarian hyperstimulation syndrome caused by pituitary gonadotroph adenoma secreting follicle-stimulating hormone, Obstet Gynecol 109 (2 Pt2) (2007) 547–549.

[67] E. Mor, I.A. Rodi, A. Bayrak, R.J. Paulson, R.Z. Sokol, Diagnosis of pituitary gonadotroph adenomas in reproductive-aged women, Fertil Steril 84 (3) (2005) 757.

[68] V. Sicilia, J. Earle, S.G. Mezitis, Multiple ovarian cysts and oligomenorrhea as the initial manifestations of a gonadotropin-secreting pituitary macroadenoma, Endocr Pract 12 (4) (2006) 417–421.

[69] T. Sugita, K. Seki, Y. Nagai, N. Saeki, A. Yamaura, S. Ohigashi, et al., Successful pregnancy and delivery after removal of gonadotrope adenoma secreting follicle-stimulating hormone in a 29-year-old amenorrheic woman, Gynecol Obstet Invest 59 (3) (2005) 138–143.

[70] M.J. Valimaki, A. Tiitinen, H. Alfthan, A. Paetau, A. Poranen, T. Sane, et al., Ovarian hyperstimulation caused by gonadotroph adenoma secreting follicle-stimulating hormone in a 28-year-old woman, J Clin Endocrinol Metab 84 (11) (1999) 4204–4208.

[71] D. Heseltine, M.C. White, P. Kendall-Taylor, D.M. De Kretser, W. Kelly, Testicular enlargement and elevated serum inhibin concentrations occur in patients with pituitary macroadenomas secreting follicle stimulating hormone, Clin Endocrinol (Oxf) 31 (4) (1989) 411–423.
[72] B. Ambrosi, M. Basstti, R. Ferrario, G. Medri, G. Giannattsio, G. Faglia, Precocious puberty in a boy with a PRL, LH- and FSH-secreting pituitary tumour: Hormonal and immunocytochemical studies, Acta Endocrinol 122 (1990) 569–576.
[73] M. Faggiano, T. Criscuolo, I. Perrone, C. Quarto, A.A. Sinisi, Sexual prococity in a boy due to hypersecretion of LH and prolactin by a pituitary adenoma, Acta Endocrinol 102 (1983) 167–172.
[74] R. Demura, O. Kubo, H. Demura, K. Shizume, FSH and LH secreting pituitary adenoma, J Clin Endocrinol Metab 45 (1977) 653–657.
[75] P. Chanson, G. Schaison, Pituitary apoplexy caused by GnRH-agonist treatment revealing gonadotroph adenoma, J Clin Endocrinol Metab 1995 (80) (1995) 2267–2268.
[76] A. Davis, S. Goel, M. Picolos, M. Wang, V. Lavis, Pituitary apoplexy after leuprolide, Pituitary 9 (3) (2006) 263–265.
[77] Y. Reznik, F. Chapon, N. Lahlou, N. Deboucher, J. Mahoudeau, Pituitary apoplexy of a gonadotroph adenoma following gonadotrophin releasing hormone agonist therapy for prostatic cancer, J Endocrinol Invest 20 (9) (1997) 566–568.
[78] R. Sahli, E. Christ, D. Kuhlen, O. Giger, I. Vajtai, Sellar collision tumor involving pituitary gonadotroph adenoma and chondroma: A potential clinical diagnosis, Pituitary (2009). Sep 17.
[79] W. Massoud, P. Paparel, J.G. Lopez, P. Perrin, M. Daumont, A. Ruffion, Discovery of a pituitary adenoma following treatment with a gonadotropin-releasing hormone agonist in a patient with prostate cancer, Int J Urol 13 (1) (2006) 87–88.
[80] P.J. Snyder, H. Bigdeli, D.F. Gardner, et al., Gonadal function in fifty men with untreated pituitary adenomas, J Clin Endocrinol Metab 48 (1979) 309–314.
[81] P. Cappabianca, L.M. Cavallo, A. Colao, M. Del Basso De Caro, F. Esposito, S. Cirillo, et al., Endoscopic endonasal transsphenoidal approach: Outcome analysis of 100 consecutive procedures, Minim Invasive Neurosurg 45 (4) (2002) 193–200.
[82] H.D. Jho, Endoscopic transsphenoidal surgery, J Neurooncol 54 (2) (2001) 187–195.
[83] T. Kawamata, H. Iseki, R. Ishizaki, T. Hori, Minimally invasive endoscope-assisted endonasal trans-sphenoidal microsurgery for pituitary tumors: Experience with 215 cases comparing with sublabial trans-sphenoidal approach, Neurol Res 24 (3) (2002) 259–265.
[84] A.R. Dehdashti, A. Ganna, K. Karabatsou, F. Gentili, Pure endoscopic endonasal approach for pituitary adenomas: Early surgical results in 200 patients and comparison with previous microsurgical series, Neurosurgery 62 (5) (2008) 1006–1015. discussion 15–7.
[85] G. Frank, E. Pasquini, G. Farneti, D. Mazzatenta, V. Sciarretta, V. Grasso, et al., The endoscopic versus the traditional approach in pituitary surgery, Neuroendocrinology 83 (3–4) (2006) 240–248.
[86] B.A. Senior, C.S. Ebert, K.K. Bednarski, M.K. Bassim, M. Younes, D. Sigounas, et al., Minimally invasive pituitary surgery, Laryngoscope 118 (10) (2008) 1842–1855.
[87] N. Fatemi, J.R. Dusick, M.A. de Paiva Neto, D.F. Kelly, The endonasal microscopic approach for pituitary adenomas and other parasellar tumors: A 10-year experience, Neurosurgery 63 (4 Suppl 2) (2008) 244–256, discussion 256.
[88] C. Nimsky, B. von Keller, O. Ganslandt, R. Fahlbusch, Intraoperative high-field magnetic resonance imaging in transsphenoidal surgery of hormonally inactive pituitary macroadenomas, Neurosurgery 59 (1) (2006) 105–114, discussion 114.
[89] F. Baumann, C. Schmid, R.L. Bernays, Intraoperative magnetic resonance imaging-guided transsphenoidal surgery for giant pituitary adenomas, Neurosurg Rev 33 (1) (2010) 83–90.
[90] J.R. Dusick, F. Esposito, D. Malkasian, D.F. Kelly, Avoidance of carotid artery injuries in transsphenoidal surgery with the Doppler probe and micro-hook blades, Neurosurgery 60 (4 Suppl 2) (2007) 322–328, discussion 328–329.
[91] E. de Divitiis, P. Cappabianca, L.M. Cavallo, F. Esposito, O. de Divitiis, A. Messina, Extended endoscopic transsphenoidal approach for extrasellar craniopharyngiomas, Neurosurgery 61 (5 Suppl 2) (2007) 219–227, discussion 228.
[92] P.A. Gardner, D.M. Prevedello, A.B. Kassam, C.H. Snyderman, R.L. Carrau, A.H. Mintz, The evolution of the endonasal approach for craniopharyngiomas, J Neurosurg 108 (5) (2008) 1043–1047.
[93] I. Laufer, V.K. Anand, T.H. Schwartz, Endoscopic, endonasal extended transsphenoidal, transplanum transtuberculum approach for resection of suprasellar lesions, J Neurosurg 106 (3) (2007) 400–406.
[94] R.I. Harris, N.J. Schatz, T. Gennarelli, P.J. Savino, W.H. Cobbs, P.J. Snyder, Follicle-stimulating hormone-secreting pituitary adenomas: Correlation of reduction of adenoma size with reduction of hormonal hypersecretion after transsphenoidal surgery, J Clin Endocrinol Metab 56 (6) (1983) 1288–1293.
[95] J.C. Trautmann, E.R. Laws, Visual status after transsphenoidal surgery at the Mayo Clinic, 1971–1982, Am J Ophthalmol 96 (1983) 200–208.
[96] P.M. Black, N.T. Zervas, G. Candia, Management of large pituitary adenomas by transsphenoidal surgery, Surg Neurol 29 (1988) 4434.
[97] I. Ciric, A. Ragin, C. Baumgartner, D. Pierce, Complications of transsphenoidal surgery: Results of a national survey, review of the literature, and personal experience, Neurosurg 40 (1997) 225–237.
[98] D.L. Barrow, G.T. Tindall, Loss of vision after transsphenoidal surgery, Neurosurg 27 (1990) 60–68.
[99] P.M. Black, N.T. Zervas, G.L. Candia, Incidence and management of complications of transsphenoidal operations for pituitary adenomas, Neurosurg 20 (1987) 920–924.
[100] C.B. Wilson, A decade of pituitary microsurgery, J Neurosurg 61 (1984) 814–833.
[101] F.G. Barker 2nd, A. Klibanski, B. Swearingen, Transsphenoidal surgery for pituitary tumors in the United States, 1996–2000: Mortality, morbidity, and the effects of hospital and surgeon volume, J Clin Endocrinol Metab 88 (10) (2003) 4709–4719.
[102] E.R. Laws Jr., N.C. Fode, M.J. Redmond, Transsphenoidal surgery following unsuccessful prior therapy, J Neurosurg 63 (1985) 823–829.
[103] N.J.L. Gittoes, A.S. Bates, W. Tse, B. Bullivant, M.C. Sheppard, R.N. Clayton, et al., Radiotherapy for non-functioning pituitary adenomas, Clin Endocrinol 48 (1998) 331–337.
[104] M.W. McCord, J.M. Buatti, E.M. Fennel, W.M. Mendenhall, R.M. Marcus Jr., A.L. Rhoton, et al., Radiotherapy for pituitary adenoma: Long-tem outcome and sequellae, Int J Radiation Oncology 39 (1997) 437–444.
[105] M. Zaugg, O. Adamman, R. Pescia, A.M. Landolt, External irradiation of macroinvasive pituitary adenomas with telecobalt: A retrospective study with long-term follow-up in patients irradiated with doses mostly of between 40–45 Gy, Int J Radiation Oncology Biol Phys 32 (1995) 671–680.
[106] P. Colin, N. Jovenin, B. Delemer, J. Caron, H. Grulet, A.C. Hecart, et al., Treatment of pituitary adenomas by fractionated stereotactic radiotherapy: A prospective study of 110 patients, Int J Radiat Oncol Biol Phys 62 (2) (2005) 333–341.

[107] H.B. Mackley, C.A. Reddy, S.Y. Lee, G.A. Harnisch, M.R. Mayberg, A.H. Hamrahian, et al., Intensity-modulated radiotherapy for pituitary adenomas: The preliminary report of the Cleveland Clinic experience, Int J Radiat Oncol Biol Phys 67 (1) (2007) 232–239.

[108] G. Minniti, D. Traish, S. Ashley, A. Gonsalves, M. Brada, Fractionated stereotactic conformal radiotherapy for secreting and nonsecreting pituitary adenomas, Clin Endocrinol (Oxf) 64 (5) (2006) 542–548.

[109] S.H. Paek, M.B. Downes, G. Bednarz, W.M. Keane, M. Werner-Wasik, W.J. Curran Jr., et al., Integration of surgery with fractionated stereotactic radiotherapy for treatment of nonfunctioning pituitary macroadenomas, Int J Radiat Oncol Biol Phys 61 (3) (2005) 795–808.

[110] B.B. Ronson, R.W. Schulte, K.P. Han, L.N. Loredo, J.M. Slater, J.D. Slater, Fractionated proton beam irradiation of pituitary adenomas, Int J Radiat Oncol Biol Phys 64 (2) (2006) 425–434.

[111] J.P. Sheehan, A. Niranjan, J.M. Sheehan, J.A. Jane Jr., E.R. Laws, D. Kondziolka, et al., Stereotactic radiosurgery for pituitary adenomas: An intermediate review of its safety, efficacy, and role in the neurosurgical treatment armamentarium, J Neurosurg 102 (4) (2005) 678–691.

[112] V. Mingione, C.P. Yen, M.L. Vance, M. Steiner, J. Sheehan, E.R. Laws, et al., Gamma surgery in the treatment of nonsecretory pituitary macroadenoma, J Neurosurg 104 (6) (2006) 876–883.

[113] M.D. Littley, S.M. Shalet, C.G. Beardwell, K.O. Lillehei, Hypopituitarism following external radiotherapy for pituitary tumours in adults, Quart J Med 70 (145) (1970) 160.

[114] P. Nelson, M. Goodman, J. Flickenger, D. Richardson, A. Robinson, Endocrine function in patients with large pituitary tumors treated with operative decompression and radiation therapy, Neurosurg 24 (1989) 398–400.

[115] P.J. Snyder, B.F. Fowble, N.L. Schatz, P.J. Savino, T.A. Gennarelli, Hypopituitarism following radiation therapy of pituitary adenomas, Am J Med 81 (1986) 457–462.

[116] J.L. Millar, N.A. Spry, D.S. Lamb, J. Delahunt, Blindness in patients after external beam irradiation for pituitary adenoma: Two cases occuring after small daily fractional doses, Clin Oncology 3 (1991) 291–294.

[117] M. Brada, D. Ford, S. Ashley, J.M. Bliss, S. Crowley, M. Mason, et al., Risk of second brain tumour after conservative surgery and radiotherapy for pituitary adenoma, Br Med J 304 (1993) 1343–1346.

[118] B.J. Fisher, L.E. Gaspar, B. Noone, Radiation therapy of pituitary adenoma: Delayed sequelae, Radiology 187 (1993) 843–846.

[119] R.J. Dowsett, B. Fowble, R.C. Sergott, P.J. Savino, T.M. Bosley, P.J. Snyder, et al., Results of radiotherapy in the treatment of acromegaly: Lack of ophthalmologic complications, Int J Radiation Oncology Biol Phys 19 (1990) 453–459.

[120] A.P. van Beek, A.C. van den Bergh, L.M. van den Berg, G. van den Berg, J.C. Keers, J.A. Langendijk, et al., Radiotherapy is not associated with reduced quality of life and cognitive function in patients treated for nonfunctioning pituitary adenoma, Int J Radiat Oncol Biol Phys 68 (4) (2007) 986–991.

[121] M. Berezin, D. Olchovsky, A. Pines, R. Tadmor, B. Lunenfeld, Reduction of follicle-stimulating hormone (FSH) secretion in FSH-producing pituitary adenoma by bromocriptine, J Clin Endocrinol Metab 59 (1984) 1220–1222.

[122] M.L. Vance, E.C. Ridgway, M.O. Thorner, Follicle-stimulating hormone and alpha subunit-secreting pituitary tumor treated with bromocriptine, J Clin Endocrinol Metab 61 (1985) 580–584.

[123] D.J. Kwekkeboom, S.J. Lamberts, Long-term treatment with the dopamine agonist CV 205-502 of patients with a clinically non-functioning, gonadotroph, or α-subunit secreting pituitary adenoma, Clin Endocrinol 36 (1992) 171–176.

[124] M. Giusti, L. Bocca, T. Florio, L. Foppiani, A. Corsaro, L. Auriati, et al., Cabergoline modulation of alpha-subunits and FSH secretion in a gonadotroph adenoma, J Endocrinol Invest 23 (7) (2000) 463–466.

[125] T. Lohmann, C. Trantakis, M. Biesold, S. Prothmann, S. Guenzel, R. Schober, et al., Minor tumour shrinkage in nonfunctioning pituitary adenomas by long-term treatment with the dopamine agonist cabergoline, Pituitary 4 (3) (2001) 173–178.

[126] R.A.G. Sy, R. Bernstein, K.Y. Chynn, I.A. Kourides, Reduction in size of a thyrotropin- and gonadotropin-secreting pituitary adenoma treated with octreotide acetate (somatostatin analog), J Clin Endocrinol Metab 74 (1992) 690–694.

[127] A. Warnet, A.G. Harris, E. Renard, D. Martin, A. James-Deidier, P. Chaumet-Riffaud, A prospective multicenter trial of octreotide in 24 patients with visual defects caused by nonfunctioning and gonadotropin-secreting pituitary adenomas. French Multicenter Octreotide Study Group, Neurosurgery 41 (4) (1997) 786–795, discussion 796–797.

[128] L. Katznelson, D.S. Oppenheim, F. Coughlin, B. Kliman, D.A. Schonfeld, A. Klibanski, Chronic somatostatin analog administration in patients with alpha subunit-secreting pituitary adenomas, J Clin Endocrinol Metab 75 (1992) 1318–1325.

[129] A. Klibanski, J.M. Alexander, H.A. Bikkal, D.W. Hsu, B. Swearingen, N.T. Zervas, Somatostatin regulation of glycoprotein hormone and free subunit secretion in clinically nonfunctioning and somatotroph adenomas in vitro, J Clin Endocrinol Metab 1248 (1991) 1255.

[130] S.H. Roman, M. Goldstein, I.A. Kourides, F. Comite, C.W. Bardin, D.T. Kreiger, The luteinizing hormone-releasing hormone (LHRH)agonist d-TRT^{6}-PRO^{9}-NEt]LHRH increased rather than lowered LH and alpha subunit levels in a patient with an LH-secreting pituitary tumor, J Clin Endocrinol Metab 58 (1984) 313–319.

[131] G.A. McGrath, R.J. Goncalves, J.K. Udupa, et al., New technique for quantitation of pituitary adenoma size: Use in evaluating treatment of gonadotroph adenomas with gonadotropin-releasing hormone antagonist, J Clin Endocrinol Metab 76 (1993) 1363–1368.

[132] N. Karavitaki, K. Collison, J. Halliday, J.V. Byrne, P. Price, S. Cudlip, et al., What is the natural history of nonoperated nonfunctioning pituitary adenomas? Clin Endocrinol (Oxf) 67 (6) (2007) 938–943.

[133] O.M. Dekkers, S. Hammer, R.J. de Keizer, F. Roelfsema, P.J. Schutte, J.W. Smit, et al., The natural course of non-functioning pituitary macroadenomas, Eur J Endocrinol 156 (2) (2007) 217–224.

CHAPTER

19

Nonpituitary Tumors of the Sellar Region

Olga Moshkin [1], Steffen Albrecht [2], Juan M. Bilbao [3], Kalman Kovacs [3]

[1] PRHC, Peterborough, ON, Canada [2] The Montreal's Children Hospital, McGill University Health Centre, Montreal, QC, Canada, [3] University of Toronto, Toronto, ON, Canada

The pituitary gland, sella turcica and the parasellar region can be involved by a wide variety of nonneoplastic tumor-like lesions as well as by numerous benign and malignant neoplasms (Table 19.1). Exhaustive discussion of the clinical, radiological, pathological and surgical aspects of all of these entities is obviously beyond the scope of this chapter. Detailed reviews of their pathology can be found elsewhere [1] and several extensive reviews of sellar imaging are also available [2–6]. In addition, there is a well-illustrated review of the various surgical approaches to sellar tumors [7].

ECTOPIAS

Pituitary Ectopy

An ectopic pituitary gland can mimic a suprasellar tumor [8]. Adenohypophyseal ectopy has also been associated with cerebral malformations [9] and precocious puberty [10].

Ectopy of the neurohypophysis seems to be increasingly recognized since the advent of magnetic resonance (MR) imaging: MR yields more detailed images of the pituitary–hypothalamic axis than computed tomography (CT) and furthermore, the neurohypophysis produces a typical hyperintense "bright signal" on T_1-weighted images in many (but not all) individuals [11]. Neurohypophyseal ectopy is therefore easy to recognize; the normal bright spot in the posterior aspect of the pituitary gland is missing and appears instead elsewhere, usually in the region of the median eminence. Such extrasellar ectopia of the neurohypophysis was seen in only one of 1500 cranial MRs in patients without any evidence of sellar or parasellar disease [11]; instead, it is usually part of a triad that also includes absence of the pituitary stalk and hypoplasia of the adenohypophysis [12].

Affected individuals have either severe isolated growth hormone deficiency or multiple anterior pituitary hormone insufficiencies [12]; diabetes insipidus, on the other hand, is not a feature, indicating that the ectopic posterior lobe is functioning normally. These patients have a greatly delayed and very low GH-response to GHRH infusion [13]. The triad was also seen in a pair of identical twins with a paracentric inversion of the short arm of chromosome 1; however, it is not certain whether the chromosomal alteration is causally related to the pituitary malformation [14].

Ectopia or hypoplasia/aplasia of the neurohypophysis with or without hypoplasia of the adenohypophysis can also be associated with septo-optic dysplasia (De Morsier's syndrome), which combines uni- or bilateral optic nerve hypoplasia, midline cerebral malformations and endocrine deficiencies [15–17].

Ectopic Salivary Gland Tissue

Salivary gland rests can be found in virtually all autopsy pituitaries at any age if the glands are examined by serial sections [18]. They are usually located in the posterior lobe and resemble serous acinar and duct cells of normal salivary glands [18]. In contrast to the almost universal presence of incidental salivary gland rests, symptomatic lesions are exceedingly rare, with only two reported cases [19,20]. Similarly, primary salivary gland-like tumors in the sellar region are also extremely rare: a few cases of sellar adenoid cystic carcinoma and papillary mucinous adenocarcinoma have been reported but are thought to have derived from epithelial rests within the pituitary gland, either minor salivary rests or Rathke's cleft remnants [21]; we are unaware of such tumors having occurred in the pituitary gland proper.

The Pituitary, Third Edition, DOI: 10.1016/B978-0-12-380926-1.10019-7

TABLE 19.1 Sellar Tumors and Tumor-like Lesions Other than Pituitary Adenomas

ECTOPIAS
Pituitary ectopy
Neurohypophyseal ectopy
Salivary gland rests
HAMARTOMA/CHORISTOMAS
Hypothalamic hamartoma/hamartoblastoma
CYSTS
Rathke's cleft cyst
Arachnoid cyst
Epidermoid/dermoid cyst
INFLAMMATORY LESIONS
Infection
Sarcoidosis
Lymphocytic/autoimmune hypophysitis
Granulomatous hypophysitis
Xanthomatous hypophysitis
Erdheim-Chester disease
Rosai-Dorfman disease
Others
NEOPLASMS
Granular cell tumor
Bone tumors
Chordoma
Cartilaginous tumors
Rhabdomyosarcoma
Vascular tumors
Others
Craniopharyngioma
Meningioma
Schwannoma
Glioma
Of optic pathways (pilocytic astrocytoma)
Of pituitary gland
Chordoid glioma of third ventricle
Gangliocytoma/gangliocytoma-adenoma
Germ cell tumors
Hematologic disorders
Lymphoma
Leukemia
Plasmacytoma/multiple myeloma
Langerhans cell histiocytosis
Metastases
Melanoma

HAMARTOMAS

Hypothalamic Hamartoma

Hypothalamic hamartomas are rare lesions that usually form a small pedunculated nodule attached to the floor of the third ventricle and projecting into the basal cistern; some are attached to the hypothalamus and project into the third ventricle. Histologically, they are composed of large, mature ganglion cells that resemble hypothalamic neurons; in addition, there is a highly differentiated glial stroma composed of astrocytes and oligodendrocytes. These lesions are quite "organoid" in appearance, including the presence of myelinated fiber tracts, and on a small, fragmented biopsy specimen may be difficult to distinguish histologically from normal hypothalamus without the clinical history.

Precocious puberty is one of the main manifestations of these lesions; in one large series, they accounted for 24 of 107 cases of precocious puberty of central origin [22]. They are also often associated with gelastic (laughing) seizures and behavioral problems, especially aggressive outbursts. Evidence has been presented that the hamartoma is the primary epileptogenic focus in these patients [23]. (For a more detailed discussion of the effects and therapy of hypothalamic hamartomas, the reader is referred to Chapter 8.)

The constellation of hypothalamic hamartoma, pituitary insufficiency, postaxial polydactyly, cardiac and genitourinary malformations, and imperforate anus constitutes Pallister-Hall syndrome, which can be inherited as an autosomal dominant trait [24]. In the initial reports, the hypothalamic tumors were found to be composed of immature neuronal elements and therefore called "hamartoblastomas," but in subsequent reports, lesions containing mature neurons similar to hypothalamic hamartomas were also seen [25–27], especially in older children, suggesting that the former constitute an immature stage of the latter [26,27]; this has led to the disappearance of the term "hamartoblastoma." Recently, germline mutations of the GL13 zinc finger transcription factor have been described in two affected families [24]. It remains to be seen whether sporadic hypothalamic hamartomas not associated with the syndrome carry somatic mutations of this gene.

CYSTS

Rathke's Cleft Cyst

Rathke's cleft cysts are generally believed to originate from remnants of Rathke's pouch, which is the *Anlage* of the adenohypophysis. During early embryogenesis, the anterior and posterior portions of the pouch give rise to the anterior and intermediate lobes of the pituitary gland, respectively. Later, the pouch may fail to obliterate completely, leaving behind cystic remnants at the interface between those lobes. Such cystic remnants can be found in up to one-fifth of autopsy pituitaries [28] as well as in pharyngeal pituitaries [29]. They are usually less than 5 mm in diameter [30]. Most are intrasellar with or without suprasellar extension, but some entirely suprasellar cases have been described (Figure 19.1) [31,32]. Even more rarely, they are located within the bones of the skull base [33].

Histologically, the cyst's epithelium is composed of several cell types, including ciliated columnar cells similar to respiratory epithelium, and goblet cells. There may be focal squamous metaplasia. The cyst lumen is filled with mucus but can also contain cell debris and cholesterol crystals [34]. Some pituitary adenomas are intimately admixed with cysts indistinguishable from Rathke's cleft cysts [34]. It is not clear whether these tumors represent true "transitional" neoplasms or a collision of two independent, relatively frequent lesions.

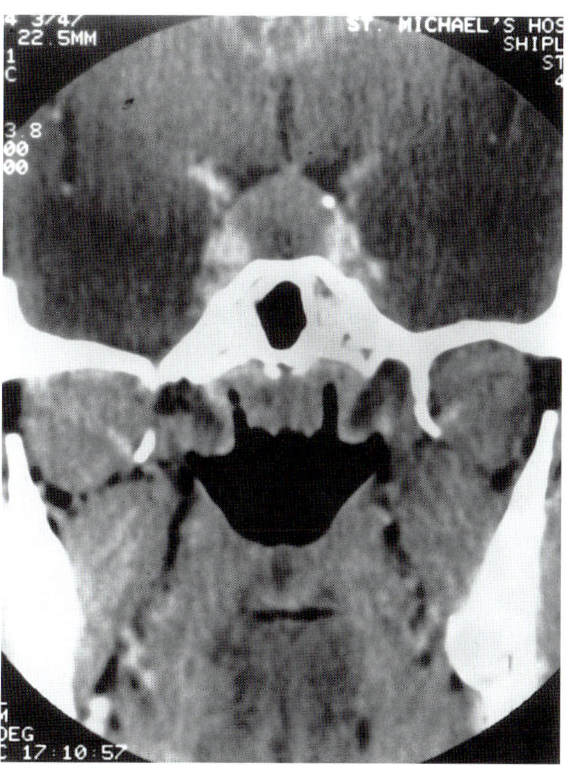

FIGURE 19.1 Cyst of Rathke's pouch cleft in a 36-year-old man who was diagnosed as having a pituitary adenoma with panhypopituitarism. Computed tomography scan revealed an isodense sellar and suprasellar mass. At operation, a thin-walled cyst was found within the expanded sella and suprasellar area. Histology revealed the collapsed cyst wall lined by a single layer of epithelial ciliated cells.

As is obvious from the prevalence of these cysts in autopsy material, most are asymptomatic. The majority of symptomatic cases occurs in adults with a 2:1 female predilection [32,35]. Most have a suprasellar extension and usually present with endocrine disturbances, visual complaints, or headache and combinations thereof [35,36]. Rarely, the patient presents acutely with a clinical picture resembling pituitary apoplexy [34]. In two such cases seen by one of the authors (S.A.), there was intense mural inflammation, possibly related to leakage of mucus. This may also explain the reports of aseptic meningitis [35] associated with Rathke's cleft cysts. Progressive enlargement of the cyst can also lead to an "empty sella" [37]. Other unusual presentations include abscess formation in the cyst [38], the Tolosa-Hunt syndrome (painful ophthalmoplegia) caused by cyst rupture with an intense inflammatory reaction in the sella and cavernous sinuses [39], hypopituitarism with granulomatous hypophysitis also associated with cyst rupture [40], hemorrhage into the cyst [34], and occurrence in identical twins [41]. By most accounts, neither the CT nor the MRI features are sufficiently distinctive to allow accurate preoperative diagnosis [32,35,36]. However, one group found that a T_2-hypointense lesion causing anterior displacement of the pituitary stalk with a posterior ledge of the diaphragma sellae was highly suggestive of a Rathke's cleft cyst [34]. Partial excision with drainage (with biopsy of the wall for histological conformation) is the treatment of choice; except for pituitary insufficiency and severe visual impairment, most deficits resolve at least partially and recurrence is unusual [32,35,36].

Epidermoid and Dermoid Cysts

Most intracranial epidermoid and dermoid cysts arise in the cerebellopontine angle, but sellar and parasellar examples also occur. Epidermoid cysts are lined by a keratinizing squamous epithelium similar to normal epidermis, hence the name. If the cyst wall also contains skin appendages, such as sebaceous glands and hair follicles, it is called a dermoid cyst. Symptoms usually arise from compression of adjacent structures [42]. Chemical meningitis secondary to spillage of keratinous debris [43] and the development of a squamous cell carcinoma in the cyst [43,44] are the two major complications. Other unusual presentations include subarachnoid hemorrhage [45], stroke [46] and rupture into the ventricular system [47]. Treatment is surgical. These cysts can coexist with arachnoid cysts [48].

Arachnoid Cysts

Arachnoid cysts account for about 1% of intracranial space-occupying lesions and about one-tenth of arachnoid cysts arise in the sellar/suprasellar region [49].

There is now general agreement that these are congenital lesions; in fact, some cases have been diagnosed prenatally [50]. The cysts arise when a split in the arachnoid fills with cerebrospinal fluid (CSF) through a unidirectional slit-valve; the pumping force is provided by arterial pulsation. This mechanism has been documented de visu by direct endoscopic observation [49].

Sellar arachnoid cysts become symptomatic by causing hydrocephalus (secondary to compression of the third ventricle), optochiasmatic and/or other neurological symptoms (such as gait disturbance) and endocrine dysfunction (pituitary insufficiency or precocious puberty) [50]. CT and MR studies show a cystic structure whose content has the same imaging characteristics as CSF. Earlier surgical approaches included cyst resection or fenestration and cystoperitoneal shunting. However, these often had significant complications and disappointing long-term outcomes. More recently, minimally invasive neuroendoscopic procedures seem to be gaining in acceptance, since they are rapid, well-tolerated and provide good long-term outcomes [50–52]. Techniques include cystocisternostomy, cystoventriculostomy and cystoventriculocisternostomy. It is noteworthy, however, that in contrast to the other symptoms, the endocrine disturbances rarely regress, probably because of permanent hypothalamic damage [50].

TUMORS

Granular Cell Tumor

This lesion is also known as choristoma, granular cell myoblastoma, granular cell pituicytoma and granular cell schwannoma. Microscopic collections of granular cells termed "tumorlets' or "tumorettes" can be found in up to 17% of unselected autopsy pituitaries [53]; they are roughly evenly distributed between the infundibulum and the posterior lobe [53,54]. Since they are not seen in patients of less than 20 years of age, they appear to be acquired rather than congenital [53,54]. The association of granular cell tumors with either pituitary adenomas [55] or multiple endocrine neoplasia, type 1 (MEN-1) [56] may be coincidental rather than a reflection of a common etiology.

Histologically, the tumors are composed of sheets and lobules of tightly packed, polyhedral cells whose key feature is their abundant, distinctly granular cytoplasm. These granules stain intensely with the periodic acid-Schiff stain and retain this property after diastase digestion. By electron microscopy, the granules appear as phagolysosomes filled with electron-dense material and membrane debris [57]. Tumors with an identical histological appearance occur in many other sites, especially the skin, tongue, breast and biliary tree. This has led to considerable controversy as to their "cell of origin," which in turn has generated a volume of literature that is completely out of proportion to the practical importance and relevance of the problem. Pending definitive settlement of this issue, their noncommittal and descriptive designation as granular cell tumors seems entirely appropriate.

These tumors only rarely become large enough to produce symptoms: Schaller et al. present one case of their own and review 42 previously reported cases [58]. Most lesions present in the fourth or fifth decade with a 2:1 female predominance. The most common presentations are visual disturbances and/or hypopituitarism. Considering their location, diabetes insipidus is surprisingly rare, with only one case having been reported [59]. Radiologically, there are sellar changes in about half the cases [60]; imaging studies show suprasellar or supra- and intrasellar lesions which enhance due to their high vascularity [58,60], but these features are not sufficiently distinctive to allow a definite radiological diagnosis [58]. Treatment is surgical [58]; consideration should be given to postoperative radiotherapy for incompletely resected lesions [58].

Gangliocytoma and Mixed Adenoma–Gangliocytoma

A gangliocytoma is a neoplasm composed of mature neurons (i.e., ganglion cells) without a glial component. About 50 such neoplasms arising in the pituitary gland or sellar region have been reported [61–63]. Roughly one-quarter are pure gangliocytomas while the remainder have a second component that is indistinguishable from a pituitary adenoma; these tumors are referred to as mixed adenoma–gangliocytomas. Tumors with both a mature neuronal and a glial component are called gangliogliomas, but these are very rare in the sella [61].

Histologically, the ganglionic component resembles hypothalamic neurons; various hypothalamic releasing hormones and other hormones such as gastrin and vasopressin [61,63] and rarely pituitary hormones [64] have been demonstrated immunohistochemically in the tumor cells. The adenomatous component may be intimately admixed or form a separate, discrete nodule.

About two-thirds of these tumors occur in women; most of the mixed tumors are associated with endocrine disturbances (usually acromegaly) [62,63] while most of the pure gangliocytomas are endocrinologically silent [63].

Three histogenetic hypotheses exist to explain the origin of the mixed adenoma–gangliocytomas: growth of the adenoma secondary to stimulation by hypothalamic releasing hormones secreted by the gangliocytoma [62]; "aberrant" neuronal differentiation in an adenoma [65]; or origin from a common neuronal–adenohypophyseal precursor cell [63].

Chordoma

Chordomas are rare, slowly growing, locally aggressive bone tumors arising in the midline. Approximately 50% involve the sacrum, 35% occur in the clivus and the remaining 15% arise in vertebrae [66]. Chordomas are thought to arise from remnants of the notochord which is the first organizer of the neuraxis during early embryogenesis and which normally disappears by the sixth week of gestation [66]. The nucleus pulposus represents its only persistent derivative; however, ectopic notochordal remnants can be found, especially at either end of the craniospinal axis [67]. In addition, incidental intradural notochordal rests called "ecchordosis physaliphora" can be seen occasionally in the region of the clivus [68] and these may give rise to the rare cases of purely intradural chordomas [69,70]. Histologically indistinguishable tumors of presumably identical histogenesis can arise in the nasopharynx [71]. Tumors of identical histological appearance arising in the soft tissues are called parachordomas.

Pathology

Grossly, the tumor can be firm to semiliquid with a lobulated, gelatinous appearance and focal calcification (Figure 19.2). Its margin can be expansile or infiltrative. The histology of chordomas is very characteristic. They are composed of lobules of large, polyhedral cells arranged in sheets and ribbons and separated by abundant mucinous ground substance. Their cytoplasm is variably vacuolated; highly vacuolated cells are called "physaliphorous" (Greek for "bubble-bearing"). In addition, there are smaller cells with nonvacuolated cytoplasm, stellate cells and intermediate forms. The cytoplasmic vacuoles contain neutral mucins while the tumor matrix is rich in acid mucopolysaccharides. By electron microscopy, the tumor cells have typical ultrastructural features of epithelial cells, including microvilli and desmosomes. Chordomas also have a typical immunohistochemical profile [72,73]: they express epithelial markers such as keratin and epithelial membrane antigen (EMA), but also S-100 protein, neural-type cadherin and the intermediate filament vimentin. This distinguishes them both from metastatic adenocarcinomas (keratin- and EMA-positive, but generally S-100 protein and vimentin-negative) and cartilaginous tumors (keratin- and EMA-negative, S-100 and vimentin-positive). They can, however, express carcinoembryonic antigen, which is also frequently expressed by adenocarcinomas.

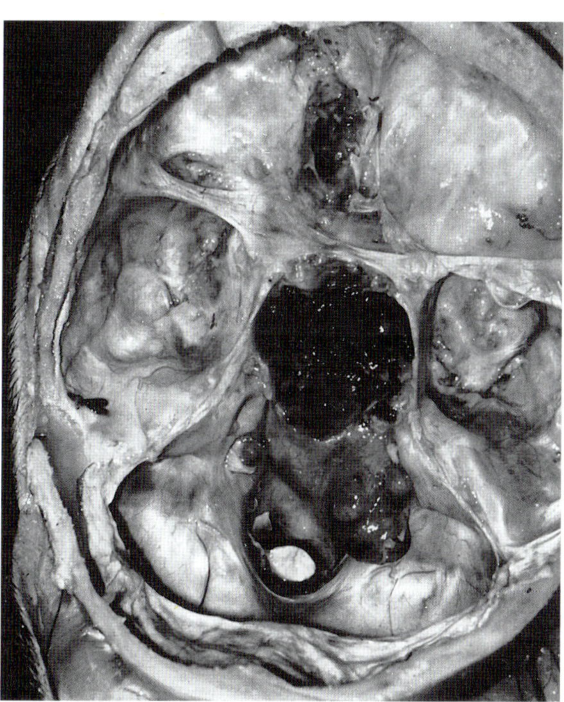

FIGURE 19.2 A 56-year-old woman died 10 years after the diagnosis of parasellar chordoma. At autopsy a large lobulated, necrotic tumor mass was found infiltrating the entire clivus, the sphenoidal sinus and the parasellar area, as well as a portion of the ethmoidal sinus. Death was due to compression and necrosis of midbrain and basal forebrain.

Clinical Aspects

Chordomas of the cranial base usually present with headache, oculomotor disturbances (especially diplopia secondary to abducens nerve paresis), other visual symptoms, intracranial hypertension, or cerebellopontine angle syndrome; endocrine disturbance is possible but uncommon. The majority of chordomas occurs in adults, most often in the fourth decade [74,75]. Patients with clival chordomas tend to be younger than those with sacral tumors. Familial chordoma with probable autosomal dominant inheritance has been described [76].

Clival chordomas are infiltrative and arise in close vicinity to vital cerebral structures (optic pathways, carotid arteries, hypothalamus/pituitary gland and brainstem). Radiological evaluation should include both CT and MR: the former is superior for determining the extent of bone involvement, while the latter is more accurate for delineation of soft tissue infiltration and the relationship of the tumor to vital cerebral structures [77]. Obviously, the optimal therapy should try to remove as much tumor as possible while causing minimal damage to these structures. Many papers have been published on the best approach to this difficult problem, sometimes with conflicting results. Multiple surgical approaches exist [78] and more than one approach may have to be used in a given patient, since the tumors are only rarely confined to a single cranial compartment [78]. A meta-analysis of the radiotherapy literature indicates that patients treated with surgery and radiotherapy do better than those treated with either modality alone [79]. There is also mounting evidence that proton-beam radiotherapy is more effective than photon-beam therapy [66,79]; unfortunately, the former is only available in a small number of specially equipped centers. Stereotactic radiosurgery can also be effective but is restricted to small tumors (greatest diameter less than 3 cm) which excludes most patients [80]; furthermore, the number of treated patients is small and follow-up is short so that these results need to be confirmed. Overall, 5-year recurrence-free survival rates of about 60–70% can be achieved [79,81]. Why female patients have a poorer prognosis in some series is not yet clear [66,74]. It is expected that advances in imaging techniques will allow more accurate radiotherapy planning, especially through three-dimensional reconstruction of the tumor and the surrounding normal structures [79], which will hopefully lead to further improvements in survival. Approximately 10% of cranial chordomas eventually metastasize [74], usually several years after diagnosis and following local recurrence. Preferred sites of metastasis are lung, liver, bone and lymph nodes [82,83].

Chordomas do rarely occur in children. As reviewed elsewhere [75,84], chordomas in children less than 5 years of age are quite aggressive, with uncontrollable local disease and early metastases often leading to death within 18 months after diagnosis; in older children, however, behavior is similar to that of adult cases.

Variants

High-grade sarcomatous areas may be present in chordomas either de novo or appear in a recurrence or a metastasis. These tumors are called "dedifferentiated chordoma" by analogy with dedifferentiated chondrosarcoma. Of the 14 cases reviewed by Belza and Urich, only two were intracranial [85]. The sarcomatous component most often has the appearance of a malignant fibrous histiocytoma, but osteosarcoma and fibrosarcoma also occur [85]. These tumors are considerably more aggressive than ordinary chordomas, with about 90% of patients developing metastases with a rapidly fatal course; there is some anecdotal evidence of partial and transient response to aggressive chemotherapy [86].

Another variant of chordoma is the so-called chondroid chordoma first described by Heffelfinger et al. in 1973 [87]. Histologically, it consists of a mixture of typical chordoma and areas that resemble cartilage. It occurs almost exclusively in the spheno-occipitial region; only rare sacrococcygeal cases have been described. Chondroid chordoma is a controversial lesion. For one thing its "true nature" is questioned. The original description was based only on routine histology and there are certainly some chordomas that contain areas that are indistinguishable from cartilage on routine stains. As reviewed elsewhere [72,73], many studies of chondroid chordoma have been published (using mostly immunohistochemistry) and the results cover the whole spectrum of possibilities, with some showing an epithelial (chordomatous) phenotype in both components, some showing a mesenchymal (cartilaginous) phenotype in both components, and yet others a truly biphasic pattern, with the authors concluding that chondroid chordoma is really a chordoma, a chondrosarcoma, or a true mixed tumor. Not only are there significant and unavoidable technical differences between these studies (choice of antibodies, etc.), but there is also no consensus on what exactly constitutes a true chondroid chordoma: what looks like a chondroid chordoma to one group [72] is considered a mixed hyaline/myxoid chondrosarcoma by another [73]. Given the lack of uniformity of diagnosis, it is not surprising that many studies have failed to confirm [74] the better prognosis for chondroid chordomas that was shown in the original description [87], those which do show a better prognosis may have included chondrosarcomas in their material, which are known to have a better prognosis than chordoma [87].

Cartilaginous Tumors

Cranial chondrosarcoma is rarer than chordoma [77], with whom it nevertheless shares a predilection for the sellar region and a similar infiltrative growth pattern. However, calcification is more frequent and abundant in the former than in the latter, and chondrosarcomas tend to arise more laterally as opposed to the midline location of chordomas [77]. As for chordomas, imaging studies should include both CT and MR for evaluation of bone and soft tissue involvement, respectively [77]. Histologically, most sellar chondrosarcomas are well differentiated and resemble hyaline cartilage; these tumors may be histologically quite bland and their malignant character only apparent because of their destructive growth pattern. Although chordomas may have some chondroid foci (see above), chondrosarcomas do not contain the typical physaliphorous cells of chordomas, and their immunohistochemical features are also different (see above). This distinction is of more than academic interest: with similar therapy, chondrosarcomas have a better prognosis than chordomas, with 5-year recurrence-free survival rates of around 90–95% [77,81].

Chondromas (also called enchondromas) are even rarer than chondrosarcomas [77]. They can occur as solitary lesions [88,89] or in the context of Ollier disease (multiple chondromas) [90] or Maffucci syndrome (multiple chondromas and hemangiomas) [91,92]; interestingly, some of the latter patients also had pituitary adenomas [92].

Craniopharyngioma

Overall, craniopharyngioma constitutes about 3% of brain tumors [93], but up to 9% in children and adolescents [94,95]; it is in fact the most frequent sellar tumor in that age group. Craniopharyngioma is classified into two histological types – adamantinomatous and papillary. The adamantinomatous craniopharyngioma occurs at all ages, from the fetal and newborn period [96,97] to late senescence [98], but is most frequent in children and adolescents [99,100]. In contrast, the papillary craniopharyngioma occurs almost exclusively in adults [99–102]. Most craniopharyngiomas are suprasellar, with or without intrasellar extension. Rare cases confined to the third ventricle or to the chiasm have been described [103–105]. In some patients, the tumor achieves giant proportions (up to 12 cm; "giant cystic craniopharyngioma"), and extends well beyond the sellar region in any direction [106]. The association of craniopharyngioma with pituitary adenoma, microadenoma, hyperplasia and other tumors has been described [107,108]. In addition, neoplasms consisting of closely intermingled pituitary adenoma and craniopharyngioma components, some containing an intermediate morphologic phenotype, were also reported [109,110].

Pathology

Craniopharyngiomas are mostly cystic or cystic-solid (Figures 19.3 and 19.4). The cysts are filled with a brownish, lipid and cholesterol-rich viscous fluid bearing more than a superficial resemblance to motor oil. Histologically, the classical craniopharyngioma

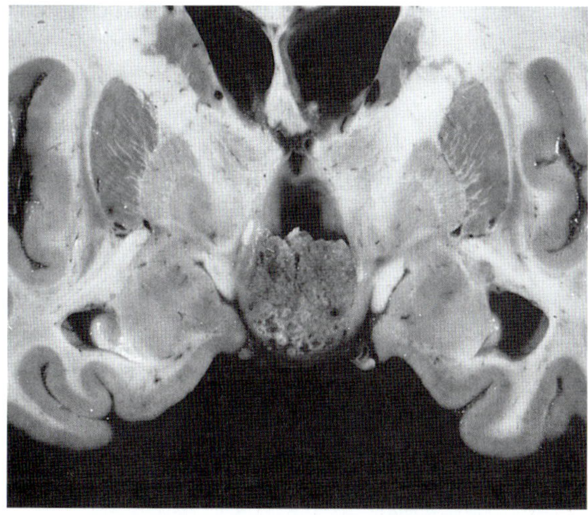

FIGURE 19.3 A 77-year-old woman presented with a 2-month history of personality changes, memory loss and shuffling gait. Computed tomography scan disclosed hydrocephalus due to ventricular compression by a suprasellar mass. The patient died in the early postoperative period of bronchopneumonia. At autopsy there was a 2.5 x 3 cm craniopharyngioma pushing upward and rostrally into the third ventricle and suprachiasmatic area.

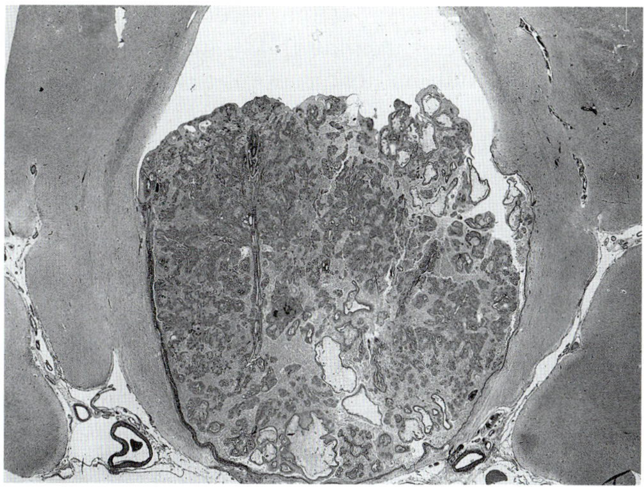

FIGURE 19.4 Low-power view of a craniopharyngioma whose growing edge occupied and expanded into the third ventricle. Note distension of infundibulum (hematoxylin and eosin staining; x5.2).

contains nests of basaloid and stellate epithelial cells that resemble the dental ameloblastic organ and are also seen in adamantinoma (a rare bone tumor with ameloblastic differentiation); consequently, this variant is called adamantinomatous. In addition, there are various amounts of squamous epithelium. Calcifications are frequent. Portions of the tumor often degenerate and the keratinous debris elicits an intense inflammatory and foreign body giant cell reaction. The papillary variant contains only squamous epithelium without any adamantinomatous component. Other features that distinguish it from the adamantinomatous variant are the presence of goblet cells [100] and the lack of calcification [99,100].

Although histologically benign, craniopharyngiomas are biologically aggressive tumors. They tend to surround and/or infiltrate vital structures such as the hypothalamus, the optic pathways and vessels of the circle of Willis. There is often intense gliosis in the brain structures adjacent to or invaded by the tumor; combined with the inflammatory reaction, this makes the tumor especially adherent to these structures and hinders attempts at complete resection. Malignant transformation has been described [111]; this appeared on the fifth recurrence after 35 years of follow-up and 8 years following radiotherapy.

Clinical Aspects

The clinical presentation of craniopharyngiomas is a direct result of their location and growth behavior. They compress the optic pathways, infiltrate the hypothalamus and can extend into the third ventricle (Figures 19.3, 19.4), thereby causing visual disturbances, hypothalamic–pituitary dysfunction and hydrocephalus, or combinations thereof [112]. The most frequent endocrine manifestations are short stature secondary to GH-deficiency and diabetes insipidus [112]; somewhat surprisingly, the syndrome of inappropriate secretion of antidiuretic hormone (SIADH) has also been reported in rare patients [112]. Another very unusual presentation is hearing loss secondary to posterior fossa involvement [113]. MR is the imaging modality of choice, especially to determine the full extent of the tumor and its relationship to adjacent brain structures [114]. Some groups find significant imaging differences between adamantinomatous and papillary craniopharyngiomas [101], while others do not [93].

The traditional therapeutic approach centered on surgical resection, with or without postoperative radiotherapy. It is generally agreed that radical resection with total removal of the tumor (confirmed by postoperative MR) is associated with the lowest rate of recurrence; only 10% of such cases in a recent series recurred [115]. However, although multiple postoperative endocrinopathies are almost universal regardless of the extent of surgery, ADH deficiency with an abnormal sense of thirst is seen only after radical surgery and constitutes a major management problem with significant morbidity and mortality [95,115]. Another complication of radical surgery is damage to arteries of the circle of Willis, leading to either hemorrhage or cerebral infarction [115]. Therefore, there is a growing consensus not to aim for radical resection at all costs in every patient, but to reserve this for tumors where complete resection can be achieved without producing additional damage to vital structures [114]. As reviewed elsewhere, subtotal excision followed by adjuvant radiotherapy produces excellent results, with 10-year recurrence-free survivals of 80–90% reported in the recent literature [115,116]. Although some groups find better outcome with papillary craniopharyngiomas than with adamantinomatous ones [99], others do not once additional parameters, such as completeness of resection, are taken into account [100,102].

Alternative therapies aimed at minimizing surgical intervention have also been developed. One promising approach is the stereotactically guided instillation of β-emitting isotopes into craniopharyngioma cysts, which has been shown to produce results similar to those of conventional therapy [94,117]; however, this method can only be applied to predominantly cystic tumors without a significant solid component. In a similar vein, intracystic administration of bleomycin was successful in a giant cystic craniopharyngioma [118]. Stereotactic radiosurgery is another option [116].

Meningioma

Meningiomas are tumors of arachnoid and meningothelial cells that account for approximately 25% of intracranial tumors in women and 13% in men [119]; this may be due to the expression of sex-steroid receptors by these tumors. They can arise anywhere in the cranial cavity; meningiomas of the sellar and parasellar regions account for about 20% of meningiomas [120]. The sphenoid ridge (Figure 19.5) and the tuberculum sellae are more frequently involved than the clivus. Sellar involvement by a meningioma is usually the result of intrasellar extension of a suprasellar meningioma; purely intrasellar menigiomas are distinctly unusual: Nozaki et al. describe one case of their own and review 17 previously reported ones [121]. Interestingly, a few patients had a synchronous pituitary adenoma and sellar meningioma [122,123]. One intrasellar meningioma occurred 8 years after radiotherapy for a pituitary adenoma [124].

Pathology

Meningiomas can display many different histological appearances, with more than ten recognized subtypes. The most frequent ones are the meningothelial, fibroblastic and transitional variants. Psammoma bodies and meningothelial whorls are helpful clues to the diagnosis. Most meningiomas are benign, slow-growing lesions and correspond to WHO grade I tumors including meningothelial, fibrous (fibroblastic), transitional (mixed), psammomatous, angiomatous, microcystic, secretory, lymphoplasmacyte-rich and metaplastic subtypes. Meningiomas with greater likelihood of recurrence and/or aggressive behavior are associated with a less-favorable clinical outcome and correspond to WHO grades II (atypical) and III (anaplastic or malignant). Grade II meningiomas include chordoid, clear cell and atypical subtypes; grade III – rhabdoid, papillary and anaplastic. The grade III meningiomas are

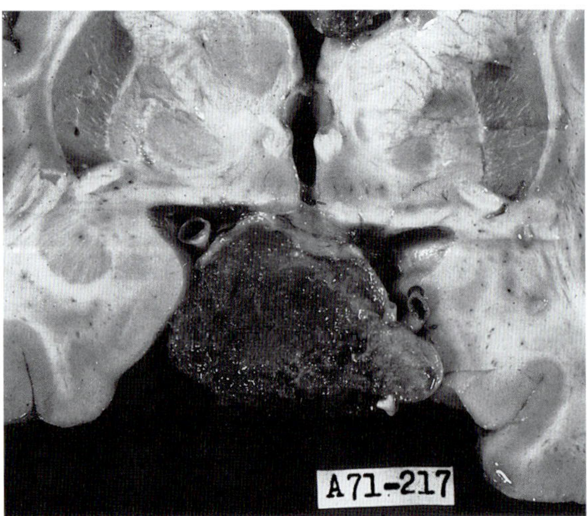

FIGURE 19.5 Meningioma of the planum sphenoidale. The well-demarcated mass in the suprasellar area compressed the anterior hypothalamus and infundibulum.

aggressive, with a propensity towards metastasis and recurrence, and are sometimes associated with prior radiation. Another aggressive variant of meningioma with a hemangiopericytic pattern is nowadays considered as a true hemangiopericytoma of the meninges rather than as a hemangiopericytic meningioma, and has been moved to mesenchymal, nonmeningothelial tumors category [125]. A positive immunoreactivity for epithelial membrane antigen (EMA), vimentin, S100, Claudin-1, Ki-67 and progesterone receptor (PR) may help in differential diagnosis. In addition, secretory meningiomas show strong positive staining for CEA in the pseudopsammomatous bodies and in the cells immediately adjacent to the lumina [125].

Clinical Aspects

Intrasellar meningiomas mimic nonfunctioning pituitary adenomas clinically, since they present with visual disturbances, partial or complete hypopituitarism, hyperprolactinemia, or combinations thereof [121]. MR is superior to CT in delineating the lesion and its relationship to adjacent intracranial structures [121], but unless a dural origin of the tumor can be clearly demonstrated, radiographic distinction from pituitary adenoma remains difficult. Resection is the treatment of choice; a purely intrasellar meningioma can be resected transsphenoidally but tumors with a suprasellar component often require a combined transsphenoidal and transcranial approach. Meningiomas are highly vascular and massive intraoperative bleeding occurred in about one-third of the reported cases [121], this can be prevented by selective preoperative endovascular embolization of the tumor's feeding vessels [121]. More recently, stereotactic radiosurgery has been proposed as an alternative therapy, both for recurrent and primary skull base meningiomas, since it produces excellent long-term tumor control with few complications [126].

Glioma

Glioma of the optic pathways is a well-documented entity that predominantly occurs in children. It has a definite association with neurofibromatosis type 1 (NF1); between one-third [127–129] and two-thirds of cases [130] occur in patients with NF1, and conversely, up to 15% of randomly screened NF1 patients have a glioma of the optic pathways, often bilaterally [131,132]. In fact, bilateral optic pathway gliomas are diagnostic of NF1. Optic pathway gliomas have also been described in a few patients with Beckwith-Wiedemann syndrome [133].

Histologically, most of these tumors are of a particular type of low-grade glioma called pilocytic astrocytoma (Figure 19.6); the term "pilocytic" refers to the elongated, "hair-like" shape of the tumor cells. Tumor cells are immunopositive for GFAP (glial fibrillary acidic protein). One of their major manifestations is obviously loss of vision; however, very young children may not complain of visual disturbances until they are nearly blind [134]. Additional manifestations depend on the tumor's location. For instance, a tumor of the optic nerve may cause proptosis, while tumors with chiasmal and/or hypothalamic involvement may be associated with hydrocephalus and endocrinopathy, such as diabetes insipidus, hypopituitarism, or precocious puberty. There is some evidence that the presentation differs between NF1 and non-NF1-associated tumors; in one series, precocious puberty was seen only with the former while intracranal hypertension and nystagmus were only seen with the latter [135].

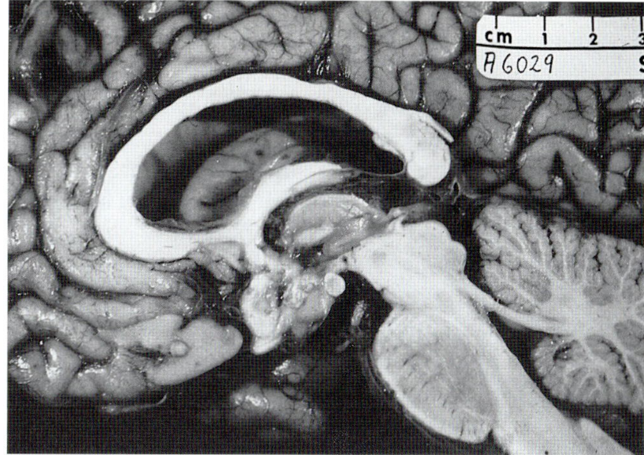

FIGURE 19.6 Pilocytic astrocytoma involving hypothalamus and walls of the third ventricle.

Therapy is controversial; the debate centers on the indication for surgery and the extent thereof, as well as the role of radiotherapy and chemotherapy. NF1-associated tumors are more indolent than non-NF1-associated cases. Most of the optic pathway gliomas discovered by routine screening in NF1 patients are asymptomatic and only a small minority progress after discovery [131,136]; in fact, even among symptomatic tumors, only about 10–20% progress [127,131]. Given the indolent nature of most NF1-associated optic pathway gliomas, therapy should be as conservative as possible; guidelines for the management of these children have been published [137]. Optic pathway gliomas not associated with NF1 have a somewhat paradoxical behavior; even though about two-thirds will eventually progress or recur, prolonged survival is still the rule, even with conservative management, with 5- and 10-year survival rates of about 90% and 75–85% being reported, respectively [127,129]. Quality of life therefore becomes a major issue against which complications of radical surgery and radiotherapy have to be weighed [127,129]. Chemotherapy is increasingly being used, especially in younger children, since it can delay the need for radiotherapy by several years [127]. It should be noted that about half of these children will have some type of treatment-requiring, persistent endocrinopathy (usually anterior and/or posterior pituitary insufficiency), related either to direct effects of the tumor, the therapy, or both [127,128].

Gliomas involving the optic pathways in adults are usually anaplastic astrocytomas or glioblastoma multiforme that are highly infiltrative (Figure 19.7). Given their location and aggressive nature, prognosis is poor; with a few exceptions [138], most patients die within a year of diagnosis [139–141].

Gliomas of the pituitary gland proper are very rare [142–144]. They can mimic nonfunctioning pituitary adenomas both radiologically [135] and endocrinologically by causing hypopituitarism and/or hyperprolactinemia [143,144], the latter presumably through stalk effect.

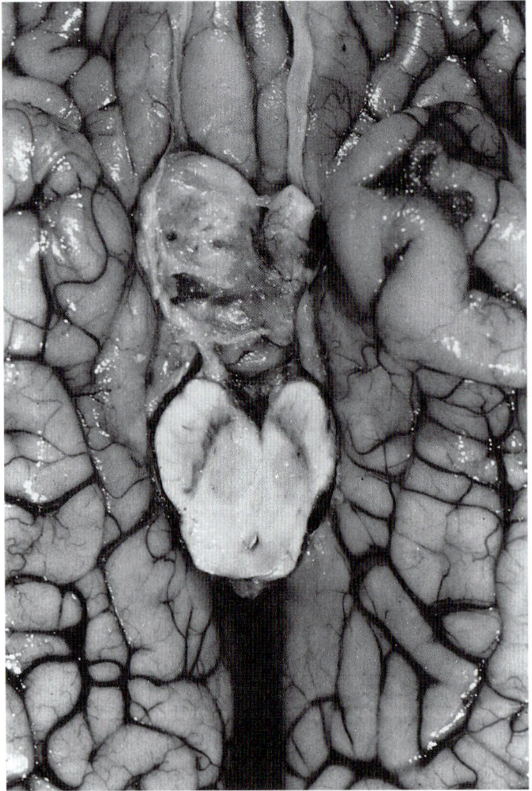

FIGURE 19.7 This 49-year-old woman presented with blurred vision and a dense left homonymous hemianopsia. X-ray studies disclosed the presence of a large hypothalamic mass with involvement of the optic chiasm and right optic nerve. At craniotomy biopsy showed a malignant astrocytoma. The tumor progressed, and the patient developed uncontrollable seizures and died 8 months after the onset of symptoms. A ventral view of the brain at autopsy revealed a massive enlargement of the optic chiasm and right optic nerve. Coronal sections of the brain showed a noncontiguous tumor mass in the right cerebral convexity, indicative of multicentric glioma.

Recently, temozolomide (TMZ), an oral alkylating agent, was introduced in the treatment of patients with malignant gliomas [145]. There were reported results of a phase II study conducted to assess the efficacy of oral TMZ in children with progressive low-grade gliomas [146]. In this study, the patients received TMZ 200 mg/m^2 by mouth for 5 days every 4 weeks. TMZ given in this schedule was successful in stabilizing disease in a significant proportion of the patients with optic pathway glioma/pilocytic astrocytoma, with manageable toxicity [146]. The tumor response to treatment was associated with 1p deletion and low expression of the DNA repair enzyme O6-methylguanine DNA methyltransferase (MGMT). It was shown that MGMT immunostaining is a good biomarker for predicting tumor chemosensitivity for temozolomide administration [147].

Recently, a very unusual type of glioma occurring in the third ventricle/suprasellar region has been described as "chordoid glioma of the third ventricle" [148]. Of the nine definite [148,149] and one probable [150] cases reported so far, all arose in adults and all but one occurred in women. Both the radiologic and histologic features are remarkably constant. The tumors were large, rounded, uniformly enhancing masses involving the suprasellar region and/or the third ventricle. They were well demarcated and not invasive. Histologically, they were composed of epithelioid cells set in an abundant myxoid matrix with a prominent lymphoplasmacytic inflammatory infiltrate. Although the histologic picture suggests a low-grade chordomatous type of epithelial neoplasm, immunohistochemical and ultrastructural studies surprisingly indicate a glial phenotype. The histogenesis and long-term prognosis of this unusual neoplasm are unclear at this point.

Germ Cell Tumors

Overall, germ cell tumors account for no more than 1% of intracranial tumors in Western countries [151]; in children, however, they constitute up to about 10% of brain tumors [151], and conversely, about 6% of pediatric germ cell tumors are intracranial [152]. Although it is reported that they constitute up to 16% of brain tumors in Japan [151], epidemiological surveys indicate a lower proportion of 1.8–3.1% [153,154]. These tumors usually arise in the midline, about two-thirds occur in the pineal region, one-third in the suprasellar area (Figure 19.8), and the remainder in the thalamus and basal ganglia. Rarely, they are centered on the pituitary fossa or limited to it [155–157]. There is a definite male predominance for pineal cases and an equally definite female predominance for suprasellar cases [158–160]; the reason for this is unknown. Intracranial germ cell tumors have been reported in association

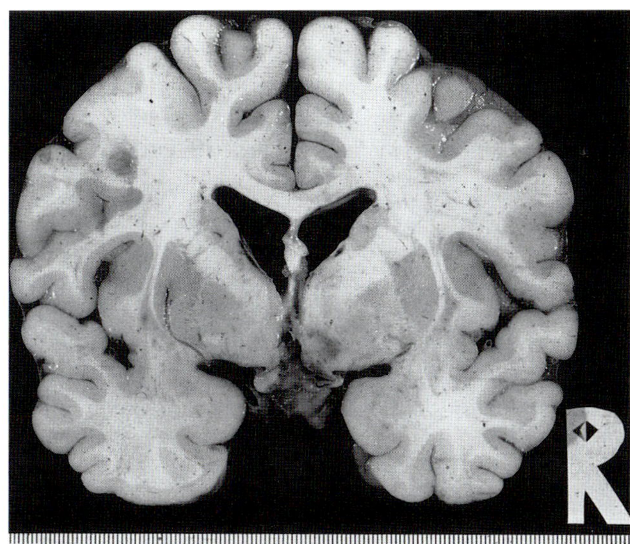

FIGURE 19.8 Germinoma infiltrated the optic tracts, infundibulum and anterior hypothalamus. The pineal gland was not involved.

with Down syndrome [161], Klinefelter syndrome [162] and Cornelia de Lange syndrome [163].

Pathology

Just like other extragonadal germ cell tumors, these tumors are presumed to arise from residual primordial germ cells that became "displaced" during their migration from the yolk sac to the genital ridges; possible mechanisms for this aberrant migration are reviewed elsewhere [164]. More recently, origin from other types of embryonal cells has been proposed [165]. Histologically, these tumors are indistinguishable from their gonadal counterparts and are classified as germinomas (called seminomas in the testis and dysgerminomas in the ovary), embryonal carcinomas, teratomas (mature or immature), endodermal sinus tumors (also called yolk-sac tumor), or choriocarcinomas. This classification is based on the stage of embryonic development that the tumor most resembles [158]: primordial germ cells (germinoma), embryonal stem cells (embryonal carcinoma), embryonic tissues (teratoma), yolk-sac endoderm (yolk-sac tumor), or trophoblast (choriocarcinoma). Detailed histological descriptions can be found elsewhere [160,166]. (Suprasellar germinomas were sometimes called "ectopic pinealomas" in the past because they bear some histologic resemblance to the fetal pineal gland. However, since they are clearly of germ cell and not of neuroepithelial origin, this term has been abandoned.) Mixed malignant germ cell tumors composed of two or more types are not uncommon. It should be noted, however, that syncytiotrophoblastic giant cells can be present in tumors other than choriocarcinoma without altering the diagnosis; choriocarcinoma is only diagnosed if both cyto- and syncytiotrophoblastic elements are present. Immunohistochemistry is useful in identifying and confirming the presence of certain elements: syncytiotrophoblastic cells are positive for β-human chorionic gonadotrophin (β-hCG), embryonal carcinoma stains for β-hCG, CD30 and α-fetoprotein (AFP), while endodermal sinus tumors usually stain only for AFP. Germinomas are usually negative for the aforementioned markers but express CD117/c-kit, OCT4 and placental alkaline phosphatase (PLAP). Documentation of expression of β-hCG and/or AFP is important for follow-up since their levels can be monitored in the patient's blood and cerebrospinal fluid for early detection of recurrence.

Clinical Aspects

The presenting symptoms of suprasellar germ cell tumors are mostly those of mass effect or precocious puberty [151,158–160]. Mass effect can produce hypopituitarism, diabetes insipidus, visual disturbances, hydrocephalus and intracranial hypertension. Symptomatic suprasellar germinomas can be tiny: in one series of children considered to have "idiopathic" central diabetes insipidus, seven only had a thickened pituitary stalk on MR; in six of these, biopsy of the stalk showed a germinoma [167]. Precocious puberty may be caused by hypothalamic destruction with release of gonadal inhibition and/or by β-hCG secretion by the tumor. Other presentations include psychosis, dementia, seizures, bulimia, or anorexia [151,158–160]. As for most lesions discussed in this chapter, MR is superior to CT in evaluating the extent of the tumor and its relationship to normal adjacent structures; however, the radiologic appearance of these tumors is not sufficiently distinctive to allow subtyping by imaging [151]. Association with a pituitary adenoma has been reported [157].

With modern microsurgical techniques and management of intracranial hypertension, pretherapy biopsy of suspected intracranial germ cell tumors has become the rule, at least in North America [151,159,168]. Since the histologic type is a major determinant of therapy and prognosis, open biopsy is preferred over stereotactic biopsy, because the latter yields considerably smaller samples that may not adequately represent the tumor, especially if it is a mixed one [151,159,168]. Furthermore, surgical debulking of tumors can achieve rapid relief of mass effect on critical structures such as the optic pathways [159].

Mature teratomas are theoretically benign and can be cured by complete surgical resection alone [151,154,166,168]. However, these tumors can be very bulky, leading to significant surgical morbidity [168]. Pure germinomas are highly radiosensitive and current radiotherapy protocols can achieve long-term survival in about 70–80% of patients [151,154]; some authors even report 10-year survival rates of more than 90%

[165]. The other types of germ cell tumors are more aggressive even when treated with a combination of surgery, radiotherapy and chemotherapy; survival rates are about half of those reported for pure germinomas [151]. Since chemotherapy has produced significant improvement of survival in patients with nongerminomatous germ cell tumors of the gonads, there are a number of trials underway assessing its role in the treatment of intracranial germ cell tumors, both as adjuvant and as neoadjuvant (pre-irradiation) therapy [151], some groups have even begun using chemotherapy and radiotherapy preoperatively [169]. In contrast to most other brain tumors, these tumors have the ability to metastasize along the CSF pathways and also outside of the central nervous system. Systemic metastases can be aided by a ventriculo-peritoneal shunt; over two dozen cases of this phenomenon have been reported, according to a recent review [170].

HEMATOLOGICAL PROLIFERATIONS

Lymphomas and Leukemias

While clinically significant involvement of the CNS by lymphomas and leukemias is mostly meningeal and extradural [171], intraparenchymal infiltrates are not uncommon at autopsy, especially with high-grade lymphomas and lymphoblastic leukemia [172]. In regard to the pituitary gland, periglandular (subcapsular) infiltration is seen in almost half the cases of adult acute lymphoblastic leukemia, but true intraparenchymal deposits are very rare [173]. Pituitary function does not appear to be affected in most cases, occasional patients suffered from the syndrome of inappropriate secretion of antidiuretic hormone [171,173]. Very rarely, the pituitary gland may be massively enlarged to the point of causing symptomatic chiasmal compression [174]. Rare cases of primary CNS lymphomas can also present because of the involvement of the hypothalamic–pituitary axis [175–177]. The pituitary gland can also be involved in systemic angiotropic lymphoma [178]. Primary pituitary lymphoma is extremely rare and recently this entity has been reported in a few papers [179–181].

Plasmacytoma

Plasmacytomas can involve the sella and simulate nonfunctioning pituitary adenomas clinically. Most of the patients reported eventually developed full-blown multiple myeloma [182–184]; only very few cases can be considered as true solitary sellar plasmacytomas [185]. Histologically, a plasmacytoma composed of relatively well-differentiated plasma cells can be mistaken for a chromophobe adenoma [186]. However, electron microscopy and immunohistochemistry will demonstrate lack of epithelial and neurosecretory features. Furthermore, clonal rearrangements of immunoglobulin genes typical of B-cell neoplasms can be demonstrated in plasmacytomas by molecular genetic studies.

Langerhans Cell Histiocytosis/Histiocytosis X

Langerhans cell histiocytosis (LCH), formerly known as histiocytosis X, can be localized, multifocal, or disseminated. Solitary lesions, especially in bone, are also referred to as eosinophilic granuloma. Histologically, lesions of LCH contain a mixed cell population composed of lymphocytes, eosinophils, foamy macrophages and Langerhans cells. The latter express S-100 protein and CD1a antigen; on ultrastructural examination, they contain peculiar cytoplasmic organelles called Birbeck granules, which are pathognomonic. Langerhans cells must be demonstrated in a lesion for a definite diagnosis of LCH.

Traditionally, LCH has been considered as a nonneoplastic, reactive histiocytic proliferation, triggered perhaps by some defect of immune regulation. However, molecular genetic clonality studies of both disseminated and localized forms have shown convincingly that all of them were clonal, and therefore neoplastic [187]. Furthermore, only the CD1a-positive cells are clonal, indicating that LCH is indeed a clonal proliferation of neoplastic Langerhans cells [187].

CNS involvement is described in a recent extensive review [188]. While not uncommon in disseminated forms of LCH (Figure 19.9), isolated lesions confined to the hypothalamic–pituitary axis are very unusual (Figure 19.10); this is sometimes referred to as Ayala's disease or Gagel's granuloma. Any part of the CNS can be involved, but the sites of predilection are the hypothalamic–pituitary axis and the pontocerebellar region. Diabetes insipidus is the most frequent manifestation, and once it is fully established, posterior pituitary function is essentially irreversibly lost, regardless of therapy [188]. Surgery and/or radiotherapy should be reserved for lesions causing mass effect [188]. Recently, debilitating progressive cerebellar degeneration in the absence of cerebellar parenchymal infiltration has been reported as a late and possibly paraneoplastic complication of LCH [189].

METASTASES

In cancer patients, metastasis to the pituitary gland is more common than pituitary adenoma; in their series of 500 autopsies, Max et al. found a prevalence of 3.6% and 1.8%, respectively [190]. Metastases are also the most

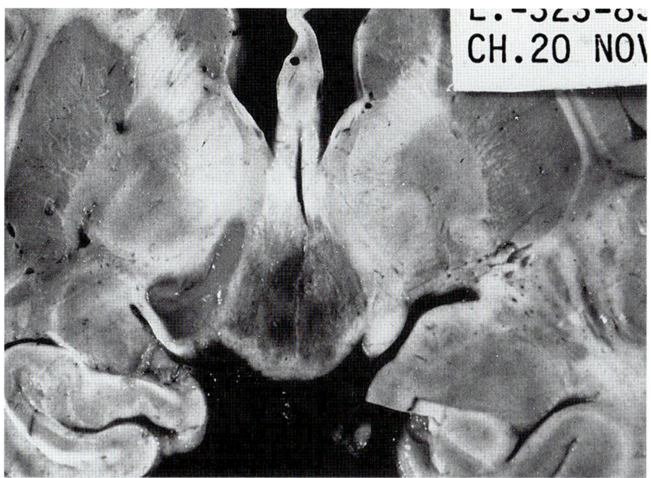

FIGURE 19.9 This patient had disseminated Langerhans cell histiocytosis. Note ill-defined infiltration of anterior hypothalamus. The lesion exhibited areas of hemorrhages, necrosis and cavitation.

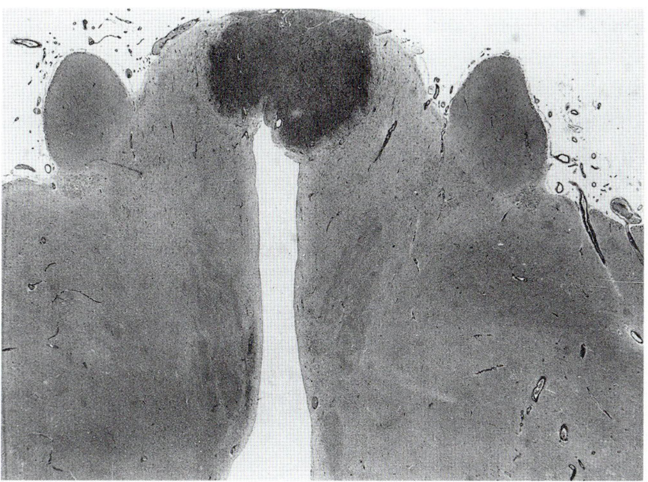

FIGURE 19.10 Incidental finding of isolated histiocytosis X of the hypothalamus (Gagel's granuloma, Ayala's disease) in a 65-year-old man. The patient had a sacral chordoma diagnosed 10 years previously and treated with several courses of radiotherapy. The tumor progressed with massive involvement of the pelvic organs. Shortly before death a computed tomography scan of the head showed a mass in the suprasellar hypothalamic area which histologically was composed of lymphocytes, histiocytes and foamy macrophages in a fibrovascular stroma.

frequent tumor of the neurohypophysis [191], which is affected about twice as often as the adenohypophysis [190]. The prevalence of pituitary metastasis in autopsy series of cancer patients ranges up to 26.7% [192] with most reports quoting around 3–5%. In an autopsy study of 739 cancer patients, one-half of the pituitary metastases constituted the only metastatic deposit in the CNS [193]. Although any tumor can metastasize to the pituitary gland, carcinomas of the breast and lung account for 50% and 20% of cases respectively, based on a review of 220 cases by McCormick et al. [194]. Conversely, 15–25% of women with metastatic breast cancer will have pituitary metastases [195,196]. Occasionally, no primary tumor can be identified [197], even at autopsy [198,199].

The mechanism of spread to the pituitary gland is most likely hematogenous; the less frequent involvement of the anterior lobe may be due to some "protective" effect of its indirect portal blood supply, as opposed to the direct systemic supply of the posterior lobe. It is of note that in patients with metastatic breast carcinoma, pituitary metastases are statistically associated with metastases in other endocrine glands and in the heart, liver and gut, suggesting that this pattern is not random [196].

The histology of the metastasis will obviously depend on the type of primary tumor, which is usually some type of adenocarcinoma. In patients without a known primary tumor, certain features may provide a clue to the origin of the lesion. For example, the presence of signet ring cells suggests a gastric carcinoma, while positive immunostaining for prostatic-specific antigen is a reliable and highly specific marker of prostatic origin.

Most pituitary metastases are asymptomatic and constitute incidental autopsy findings in patients with widely disseminated cancer. However, among patients presenting with symptomatic pituitary metastases, many have no prior history of malignancy and the primary tumor is discovered only after diagnosis of the pituitary lesion. Such was the case of nine of 14 patients in one series [197]. Presenting symptoms [186] include headache, visual field defects due to chiasmal compression [200], as well as ophthalmoplegia and ptosis secondary to involvement of the cavernous sinus and its structures [198]. Involvement of the anterior lobe can lead to hypopituitarism [197,201], which can also be caused by an isolated metastasis in the infundibulum [202]. Posterior lobe involvement may lead to diabetes insipidus; in one series of 100 consecutive cases of diabetes insipidus, 14 were caused by metastasis. The imaging appearance is usually indistinguishable from that of a pituitary adenoma [186], which is in fact the most frequent clinical misdiagnosis; the correct diagnosis can be missed even histologically [194].

Since by definition these patients suffer from metastatic disease, treatment is palliative. However, surgical decompression with or without postoperative radiotherapy can provide improvement; in one series, mean survival was 22 months [197]. Pituitary metastases from a primary prostatic carcinoma can regress with androgen blockade [203,204].

It is noteworthy that increasing numbers of carcinomas metastatic to pituitary adenomas are being reported; the primary tumors have included carcinomas of the stomach [205], lung [206,207], breast [208,209], kidney [210], prostate [211] and pancreas [211], as well as a malignant carcinoid tumor of the mediastinum [212]. Sometimes, no primary lesion could be identified [206] or the patient had more than one potential primary tumor [213]. In a patient with a known, previously "stable" pituitary adenoma, a metastasis into the adenoma can cause a rapid increase in size [205,212] or a sudden worsening of mass effect [206,207].

POSTRADIOTHERAPY TUMORS

Ionizing radiation is oncogenic and irradiation of the brain for any reason predisposes to the development of primary intracranial tumors, especially gliomas and meningiomas [214]. Even average doses as low as 1.5 Gy that were administered as therapy for tinea capitis produce a significant increase in the number of brain, as well as head and neck, tumors [214]. In one series of 334 patients with pituitary adenoma who underwent conservative surgery followed by radiotherapy, five developed a second brain tumor (two astrocytomas, two meningiomas, and one meningeal sarcoma); the cumulative risks were 1.3% and 1.9% at 10 and 20 years, respectively [215]. Gliomas have occurred following radiotherapy for various sellar tumors, including pituitary adenomas [216,217], craniopharyngiomas [216,217], optic glioma [216] and suprasellar germ cell tumors [216,218]. All patients had received radiation doses of >40 Gy; latency periods ranged from 1 to 28 years [216,217]. They may involve the suprasellar structures, but also the cerebral hemispheres, brain stem, or cerebellum. About three-quarters are malignant (anaplastic) astrocytomas or glioblastoma multiforme [216]; these are aggressive tumors and most patients die within a few months of histological diagnosis. Meningiomas also occur following sellar radiotherapy [124,219–221]; radiation doses and latency periods are similar to those of postradiotherapy gliomas. Occasionally, an unfortunate patient develops more than one postradiotherapy tumor [222].

Post-irradiation sarcoma is also a rare but well-recognized entity [223]. Kumar et al. found 29 reports of sarcomas developing after radiotherapy for pituitary adenoma; radiation doses ranged from 20 to 100 Gy and latency periods from 2.5 to 27 years [224]. As with most radiation-induced brain malignancies, prognosis was grim, with over 90% of these patients dying within 6 months of diagnosis [224].

MISCELLANEOUS LESIONS

Both intra- and parasellar schwannomas have been reported. An intrasellar schwannoma can cause hypopituitarism and mimic a nonfunctioning pituitary adenoma both clinically and radiologically [225,226]. Tumors of bone that can involve the sellar and parasellar regions include giant cell tumor [227,228], chondromyxoid fibroma [229] and brown tumor of hyperparathyroidism [230]. Even a mundane bony spur can become clinically significant when located in the sella [231]! Most uncommon are hemangioblastoma (in association with von Hippel-Lindau disease) [232], cavernous hemangioma [233], glomangioma [234], leiomyoma [235], hemangioblastoma [236], paraganglioma [237], primary melanoma [238], primary sellar thyroid follicular tumor [239] and "tumoral" extramedullary hematopoiesis [240].

Lymphocytic hypophysitis (LH) is a rare autoimmune disorder, characterized pathologically by lymphocytic infiltration of the anterior and, in some cases, of a posterior pituitary lobe and pituitary stalk (infundibulo-neurohypophysitis). Usually lymphocytes represent the dominant infiltrating cells; plasma cells may also be numerous, while other cells such as eosinophils, macrophages and neutrophils are rare. Occasional multinucleated giant cells are seen within the infiltrate in lymphocytic hypophysitis [241]. Some patients display mixed lymphocytic and granulomatous lesions, and for this reason McKeen [1984] suggested that these two forms of hypophysitis – lymphocytic and granulomatous – represent different stages of the same disease [242]. The disorder typically presents as a mass in the sellar region and mimics clinically and radiologically other nonfunctional sellar masses, more commonly pituitary adenoma. Clinical manifestations may include headache and/or visual disturbances, symptoms of hypopituitarism, polyuria and polydipsia, and rarely symptoms of hyperprolactinemia. A diagnosis of lymphocytic hypophysitis is based on histologic examination of a pituitary biopsy or on clinical, imaging and endocrinological studies when surgery is not performed. Lymphocytic hypophysitis is more common in women and shows striking association with pregnancy [241]. Recently autoimmune hypophysitis has been reported in patients with different malignant tumors treated with anticytotoxic T-lymphocyte antigen-4 (CTLA-4) [241,243].

Erdheim-Chester disease and Rosai Dorfman disease are extremely rare disorders with unique morphology which can involve the pituitary [244,245]. The etiology of these diseases is not yet known – it can be inflammatory or neoplastic. More studies are required to clarify their etiology and pathogenesis.

Last but not least, sarcoidosis, one of the great imitators, should be mentioned here as a cause of pituitary "tumor." The nervous system becomes clinically involved in about 5–10% of patients with sarcoidosis [246–248]. Most of the patients develop neurosarcoidosis during the course of systemic sarcoidosis; initial presentation because of nervous system involvement is rare. Any part of the central or peripheral nervous system can be affected, but the sites of predilection are the meninges with the base of the brain, with cranial nerve palsies being the main complaint [246–248]. With regard to the pituitary–hypothalamic axis, the hypothalamus is more frequently affected than the other components [248], with partial or complete anterior and/or posterior pituitary insufficiency being the main manifestations. Histologically, sarcoidosis is characterized by noncaseating granulomatous inflammation. However, a definitive diagnosis absolutely requires negative mircobiological cultures to exclude an infectious process. (Negative special stains for microorganisms are not sufficient, since they are considerably less sensitive than cultures.) Corticosteroids are the mainstay of therapy [248].

References

[1] B.W. Scheithauer, Pathology of the pituitary and sellar region: Exclusive of pituitary adenoma, Pathol Annu 20 (1985) 67–155.

[2] D.W. Chakeres, A. Curtin, G. Ford, Magnetic resonance imaging of pituitary and parasellar abnormalities, Radiol Clin N Am 27 (1989) 265–281.

[3] J.L. Donovan, G.M. Nesbit, Distinction of masses involving the sella and suprasellar space: Specificity of imaging features, Am J Radiol 167 (1996) 597–603.

[4] M.H. Naheedy, J.R. Haag, B. Azar-Kia, et al., MRI and CT of sellar and parasellar disorders, Radiol Clin N Am 25 (1987) 819–847.

[5] R.A. Zimmerman, Imaging of intrasellar, suprasellar and parasellar tumors, Sem Roentgenol 25 (1990) 174–197.

[6] M. Pisaneschi, G. Kapoor, Imaging the sella and parasellar region, Neuroimaging Clin N Am 15 (2005) 203–219.

[7] R.S. Isaacs, P.J. Donald, Sphenoid and sellar tumors, Otolaryngol Clin N Am 28 (1995) 1191–1229.

[8] A.R.T. Colohan, M.S. Grady, J.M. Bonnin, et al., Ectopic pituitary gland simulating a suprasellar tumor, Neurosurgery 20 (1987) 43–48.

[9] H. Ikeda, H. Niizuma, J. Suzuki, et al., A case of cebocephaly-holoprosencephaly with an aberrant adenohypophysis, Childs Nerv Syst 3 (1987) 251–254.

[10] S. Niikawa, H. Nokura, T. Uno, et al., Precocious puberty due to an ectopic pituitary gland, Neurol Med Chir 28 (1988) 681–684.

[11] B.S. Brooks, T. El Gammal, J.D. Allison, W.H. Hoffman, Frequency and variation of the pituitary bright signal on MR images, Am J Neuroradiol 10 (1989) 943–948.

[12] B.H.P. Nagel, M. Palmbach, D. Petersen, M.B. Ranke, Magnetic resonance images of 91 children with different causes of short stature: Pituitary size reflects growth hormone secretion, Eur J Pediatr 156 (1997) 758–763.

[13] M. Maghnie, A. Moretta, A. Valtorta, et al., Growth hormone response to growth-hormone-releasing hormone varies with the hypothalamic–pituitary abnormalities, Eur J Endocrinol 135 (1996) 198–204.

[14] S.F. Siegel, M. Ahdab-Barmada, S. Arslanian, T.P. Foley, Ectopic posterior pituitary tissue and paracentric inversion of the short arm of chromosome 1 in twins, Eur J Endocrinol 133 (1995) 87–92.

[15] U. Roessmann, M.E. Velasco, E.J. Small, A. Hori, Neuropathology of "septo-optic dysplasia" (de Morsier syndrome) with immunohistochemical studies of the hypothalamus and pituitary gland, J Neuropathol Exp Neurol 46 (1987) 597–608.

[16] J.A. Sorkin, P.C. Davis, L.R. Meacham, et al., Optic nerve hypoplasia: Absence of the posterior pituitary bright signal on magnetic resonance imaging correlates with diabetes insipidus, Am J Ophthalmol 122 (1996) 717–723.

[17] S. Willnow, W. Kiess, O. Butenandt, et al., Endocrine disorders in septo-optic dysplasia (de Morsier syndrome) — evaluation and follow-up of 18 patients, Eur J Pediatr 155 (1996) 179–184.

[18] S.S. Schochet, W.F. McCormick, N.S. Halmi, Salivary gland rests in the human pituitary. Light and electron microscopical study, Arch Pathol 98 (1974) 193–200.

[19] T. Kato, T. Aida, H. Abe, et al., Ectopic salivary gland within the pituitary gland, Neurol Med Chir 28 (1988) 930–933.

[20] S.B. Tatter, M.A. Edgar, A. Klibanski, B. Swearingen, Symptomatic salivary-rest cyst of the sella turcica, Acta Neurochir 135 (1995) 150–153.

[21] M.Z. Gilcrease, R. Delgado, J. Albores-Saavedra, Intrasellar adenoid cystic carcinoma and papillary mucinous adenocarcinoma: Two previously undescribed primary neoplasms at this site, Ann Diagn Pathol 3 (3) (1999) 141–147.

[22] O. Hirsch Pescovitz, F. Comite, K. Hench, et al., The NIH experience with precocious puberty: Diagnostic subgroups and response to short-term luteinizing hormone releasing hormone analogue therapy, J Pediatr 108 (1986) 47–54.

[23] R. Kuzniecky, B. Guthrie, J. Mountz, et al., Intrinsic epileptogenesis of hypothalamic hamartomas in gelastic epilepsy, Ann Neurol 42 (1997) 60–67.

[24] S. Kang, J.M. Graham, A. Haskins Olney, L.G. Biesecker, GL13 frameshift mutations cause autosomal dominant Pallister-Hall syndrome, Nat Genet 15 (1997) 266–268.

[25] P.D. Pallister, F. Hecht, J. Herrman, Three additional cases of the congenital hypothalamic "hamartoblastoma" (Pallister-Hall) syndrome, Am J Med Genet 33 (1989) 500–501.

[26] L.A. Squires, S. Constantini, D.C. Miller, J.H. Wisoff, Hypothalamic hamartoma and the Pallister-Hall syndrome, Pediatr Neurosurg 22 (1995) 303–308.

[27] K. Iafolla, J.D. Fratkin, P.K. Spiegel, et al., Case report and delineation of the congenital hypothalamic hamartoblastoma syndrome (Pallister-Hall syndrome), Am J Med Genet 33 (1989) 489–499.

[28] S. Shuangshoti, M.G. Netsky, B.S. Nashold, Epithelial cysts related to sella turcica. Proposed origin from neuroepithelium, Arch Pathol 90 (1970) 444–450.

[29] P. McGrath, Cysts of sellar and pharyngeal hypophyses, Pathology 3 (1971) 123–131.

[30] A. Keyaki, A. Hirano, J.F. Llena, Asymptomatic and symptomatic Rathke's cleft cysts, Neurol Med Chir 29 (1989) 88–93.

[31] D.L. Barrow, R.H. Spector, Y. Takei, G.T. Tindall, Symptomatic Rathke's cleft cysts located entirely in the suprasellar region: Review of diagnosis, management, and pathogenesis, Neurosurgery 16 (1985) 766–772.

[32] D.A. Ross, D. Norman, C.B. Wilson, Radiologic characteristics and results of surgical management of Rathke's cysts in 43 patients, Neurosurgery 30 (1992) 173–179.

[33] E. Hanna, J. Weissman, I.P. Janecka, Sphenoclival Rathke's cleft cysts: Embryology, clinical appearance and management, Ear Nose Throat J 77 (1998) 396–399.

[34] B.K. Kleinschmidt-DeMasters, K.O. Lillehei, J.C. Stears, The pathologic, surgical, and MR spectrum of Rathke cleft cysts, Surg Neurol 44 (1995) 19–27.

[35] J.L. Voelker, R.L. Campbell, J. Muller, Clinical, radiographic, and pathological features of symptomatic Rathke's cleft cysts, J Neurosurg 74 (1991) 535–544.

[36] W. El-Mahdy, M. Powell, Transsphenoidal management of 28 symptomatic Rathke's cleft cysts, with special reference to visual and hormonal recovery, Neurosurgery 42 (1998) 7–17.
[37] M. Baldini, L. Mosca, L. Princi, The empty sella syndrome secondary to Rathke's cleft cyst, Acta Neurochir 53 (1980) 69–78.
[38] T.G. Obenchain, D.P. Becker, Abscess formation in a Rathke's cleft cyst: Case report, J Neurosurg 36 (1972) 359–362.
[39] R.J.B. Macaulay, Ruptured Rathke's cleft cyst: A possible cause of Tolosa-Hunt syndrome, Clin Neuropathol 16 (1997) 98–102.
[40] C.H. Albini, M.H. MacGillivray, J.E. Fisher, et al., Triad of hypopituitarism, granulomatous hypophysitis, and ruptured Rathke's cleft cyst, Neurosurgery 22 (1988) 133–136.
[41] Y. Hayashi, J. Yamashita, N. Muramatsu, et al., Symptomatic Rathke's cleft cysts in identical twins: Case illustration, J Neurosurg 84 (1996) 710.
[42] K. Yamakawa, N. Shitara, S. Genka, et al., Clinical course and surgical prognosis of 33 cases of intracranial epidermoid tumors, Neurosurgery 24 (1989) 568–573.
[43] R.C. Abramson, R.B. Morawetz, M. Schlitt, Multiple complications from an intracranial epidermoid cyst: Case report and literature review, Neurosurgery (1989) 24–574.
[44] A.J. Lewis, P.W. Cooper, E.E. Kassel, M.L. Schwartz, Squamous cell carcinoma arising in a suprasellar epidermoid cyst: Case report, J Neurosurg 59 (1983) 538–541.
[45] C.W. Torbiak, R. Mazagri, S.P.K. Tchang, L.J. Clein, Parasellar epidermoid cyst presenting with subarachnoid hemorrhage, Can Assoc Radiol J 46 (1995) 392–394.
[46] T. Civit, C. Pinelli, J.P. Lescure, et al., Stroke related to a dermoid cyst: Case report, Neurosurgery 41 (1997) 1396–1399.
[47] J.E. Cohen, J.A. Abdallah, M. Garrote, Massive rupture of suprasellar dermoid cyst into ventricles, J Neurosurg 87 (1997) 963.
[48] W.H. Chang, B.S. Sharma, K. Singh, et al., A middle fossa arachnoid cyst in association with a suprasellar dermoid cyst, Indian Pediatr 26 (1989) 833–835.
[49] H.W.S. Schroeder, M.R. Gaab, Endoscopic observation of a slit-valve mechanism in a suprasellar prepontine arachnoid cyst: Case report, Neurosurgery 40 (1997) 198–200.
[50] A. Pierre-Kahn, L. Capelle, R. Brauner, et al., Presentation and management of suprasellar arachnoid cysts: Review of 20 cases, J Neurosurg 73 (1990) 355–359.
[51] H.W.S. Schroeder, M.R. Gaab, W.R. Niendorf, Neuro-endoscopic approach to arachnoid cysts, J Neurosurg 85 (1996) 293–298.
[52] P. Decq, P. Brugieres, C. Le Guerinel, et al., Percutaneous endoscopic treatment of suprasellar arachnoid cysts: Ventriculocystostomy or ventriculocystocisternostomy? Technical note, J Neurosurg 84 (1996) 696–701.
[53] W.M. Shanklin, The origin, histology, and senescence of tumorettes in the human neurohypophysis, Acta Anat 18 (1953) 1–20.
[54] S.A. Luse, J.W. Kernohan, Granular cell tumors of the stalk and posterior lobe of the pituitary gland, Cancer 8 (1955) 616–622.
[55] T. Tomita, M. Kuziez, I. Watanabe, Double tumors of anterior and posterior pituitary gland, Acta Neuropathol 54 (1981) 161 164.
[56] B.E. Tuch, J.N. Carter, G.M. Armellin, R.C. Newland, The association of a tumour of the posterior pituitary gland with multiple endocrine neoplasia type 1, Aust NZ J Med 12 (1982) 179–181.
[57] A. Landolt, Granular cell tumor of the neurohypophysis, Acta Neurochir 22 (Suppl) (1975) 120–128.
[58] B. Schaller, E. Kirsch, M. Tolnay, T. Mindermann, Symptomatic granular cell tumor of the pituitary gland: Case report and review of the literature, Neurosurgery 42 (1998) 166–171.
[59] L.B. Schlachter, G.T. Tindall, G.S. Pearl, Granular cell tumor of the pituitary gland associated with diabetes insipidus, Neurosurgery 6 (1980) 418–421.
[60] J. Vaquero, G. Leunda, J.M. Cabezudo, et al., Granular pituicytomas of the pituitary stalk, Acta Neurochir 59 (1981) 209–215.
[61] W. Saeger, D.K. Ludecke, M. Losa, Kombinierte neuronale und endokrine Tumoren der Sellaregion, Pathologe 18 (1997) 419–424.
[62] M. Morikawa, N. Tamaki, T. Kokunai, Y. Imai, Intrasellar pituitary gangliocytoadenoma presenting with acromegaly: Case report, Neurosurgery 40 (1997) 611–615.
[63] J. Towfighi, M.M. Salam, R.E. McLendon, et al., Ganglion cell-containing tumors of the pituitary gland, Arch Pathol Lab Med 120 (1996) 369–377.
[64] K.C. McCowen, J.N. Glickman, P.M. Black, et al., Gangliocytoma masquerading as a prolactinoma: Case report, J Neurosurg 91 (1999) 490–495.
[65] E. Horvath, K. Kovacs, B.W. Scheithauer, et al., Pituitary adenoma with neuronal choristoma (PANCH): Composite lesion or lineage infidelity? Ultrastruct Pathol 18 (1994) 565–574.
[66] E.C. Halperin, Why is female sex an independent predictor of shortened overall survival after proton/photon radiation therapy for skull base chordomas? Int J Rad Oncol Biol Phys 38 (1997) 225–230.
[67] T.R. Ulich, J.M. Mirra, Ecchordosis physaliphora vertebralis, Clin Orthopaed Rel Res 163 (1982) 282–289.
[68] K.L. Ho, Ecchordosis physaliphora and chordoma: A comparative ultrastructural study, Clin Neuropathol 4 (1985) 77–86.
[69] T.B. Mapstone, B. Kaufman, R.A. Ratcheson, Intradural chordoma without bone involvement: Nuclear magnetic resonance (NMR) appearance, J Neurosurg 59 (1983) 535–537.
[70] J.T. Wolfe, B.W. Scheithauer, "Intradural chordoma" or "giant ecchordosis physaliphora?" Report of two cases, Clin Neuropathol 6 (1987) 98–103.
[71] K.H. Perzin, N. Pushparaj, Nonepithelial tumors of the nasal cavity, paranasal sinuses, and nasopharynx. A clinicopathologic study. XIV: Chordomas, Cancer 57 (1986) 784–796.
[72] W.P. Walker, S.K. Landas, C.M. Bromley, M.T.M. Sturm, Immunohistochemical distinction of classical and chondroid chordomas, Mol Pathol 4 (1991) 661–666.
[73] A.E. Rosenberg, G.A. Brown, A.K. Bhan, J.M. Lee, Chondroid chordoma — a variant of chordoma. A morphologic and immunohistochemical study, Am J Clin Pathol 101 (1994) 36–41.
[74] J.X. O'Connell, L.G. Renard, N.J. Liebsch, et al., Base of skull chordoma. A correlative study of histologic and clinical features of 62 cases, Cancer 74 (1994) 2261–2267.
[75] L.A.B. Borba, O. Al-Mefty, R.E. Mrak, J. Suen, Cranial chordomas in children and adolescents, J Neurosurg 84 (1996) 584–591.
[76] J. Stepanek, S.A. Cataldo, M.J. Ebersold, et al., Familial chordoma with probable autosomal dominant inheritance, Am J Med Genet 75 (1998) 335–336.
[77] A.L. Weber, E.W. Brown, E.B. Hug, N.J. Liebsch, Cartilaginous tumors and chordomas of the cranial base, Otolaryngol Clin N Am 28 (1995) 453–471.
[78] O. Al-Mefty, L.A.B. Borba, Skull base chordomas: A management challenge, J Neurosurg 86 (1997) 182–189.
[79] P.T.H. Tai, P. Craighead, F. Bagdon, Optimization of radiotherapy for patients with cranial chordoma. A review of dose-response ratios for photon techniques, Cancer 75 (1995) 749–756.
[80] N. Muthukumar, D. Kondziolka, L.D. Lunsford, J.C. Flickinger, Stereotactic radiosurgery for chordoma and chondrosarcoma: Further experiences, Int J Rad Oncol Biol Phys 41 (1998) 387–392.

[81] E. Gay, L.N. Sekhar, E. Rubinstein, et al., Chordomas and chondrosarcomas of the cranial base: Results and follow-up of 60 patients, Neurosurgery 36 (1995) 887–897.

[82] R. Volpe, A. Mazabraud, A clinicopathologic review of 25 cases of chordoma (a pleomorphic and metastasizing neoplasm), Am J Surg Pathol 7 (1983) 161–170.

[83] P.W. Chambers, C.P. Schwinn, Chordoma, A clinicopathologic study of metastasis, Am J Clin Pathol 72 (1979) 765–776.

[84] V. Benk, N.J. Liebsch, J.E. Munzenrider, et al., Base of skull and cervical spine chordomas in children treated with high-dose irradiation, Int J Rad Oncol Biol Phys 31 (1995) 577–581.

[85] M.G. Belza, H. Urich, Chordoma and malignant fibrous histiocytoma. Evidence for transformation, Cancer 58 (1986) 1082–1087.

[86] G.F. Fleming, P.S. Heimann, J.K. Stephens, et al., Dedifferentiated chordoma. Response to aggressive chemotherapy in two cases, Cancer 72 (1993) 714–718.

[87] M.J. Heffelfinger, D.C. Dahlin, C.S. MacCarthy, J.W. Beabout, Chordomas and cartilaginous tumors at the skull base, Cancer 32 (1973) 410–420.

[88] P. Angiari, E. Torcia, R.A. Botticelli, et al., Ossifying parasellar chondroma. Case report, J Neurosurg Sci 31 (1987) 59–63.

[89] J. Dutton, Intracranial solitary chondroma. Case report, J Neurosurg 49 (1978) 460–463.

[90] H. Nakase, K. Nagata, T. Yonezawa, et al., Extensive parasellar chondroma with Ollier's disease, Acta Neurochir 140 (1998) 100–101.

[91] K.A. Bushe, M. Naumann, M. Warmuth-Metz, et al., Maffucci's syndrome with bilateral cartilaginous tumors of the cerebellopontine angle, Neurosurgery 27 (1990) 625–628.

[92] K. Miki, K. Kawamoto, Y. Kawamura, et al., A rare case of Maffucci's syndrome combined with tuberculum sellae enchondroma, pituitary adenoma and thyroid adenoma, Acta Neurochir 87 (1987) 79–85.

[93] O.P. Eldevik, M. Blaivas, T.O. Gabrielsen, et al., Craniopharyngioma: Radiologic and histologic findings and recurrence, Am J Neuroradiol 17 (1996) 1427–1439.

[94] J. Voges, V. Sturm, R. Lehrke, et al., Cystic craniopharyngioma: Long-term results after intracavitary irradiation with stereotactically applied colloidal β-emitting radioactive sources, Neurosurgery 40 (1997) 263–270.

[95] C.J. De Vile, D.B. Grant, R.D. Hayward, R. Stanhope, Growth and endocrine sequelae of craniopharyngioma, Arch Dis Child 75 (1996) 108–114.

[96] B. Azar-Kia, U.R. Krishnan, M.M. Schechter, Neonatal craniopharyngioma. Case report, J Neurosurg 42 (1975) 91–93.

[97] W. Janisch, H.G. Flegel, Kraniopahryngiom bei einem Feten, Zentralbl Allg Pathol 135 (1989) 65–69.

[98] G.S. Lederman, A. Recht, J.S. Loeffler, et al., Craniopharyngioma in an elderly patient, Cancer 60 (1987) 1077–1080.

[99] T.E. Adamson, O.D. Wiestler, P. Kleihues, M.G. Yasargil, Correlation of clinical and pathological features in surgically treated craniopharyngiomas, J Neurosurg 73 (1990) 12–17.

[100] T.B. Crotty, B.W. Scheithauer, W.F. Young, et al., Papillary craniopharyngioma: A clinicopathological study of 48 cases, J Neurosurg 83 (1995) 206–214.

[101] S. Sartoretti-Schefer, W. Wichmann, A. Aguzzi, A. Valavanis, MR differentiation of adamantinous and squamous-papillary craniopharyngiomas, Am J Neuroradiol 18 (1997) 77–87.

[102] H.L. Weiner, J.H. Wisoff, M.E. Rosenberg, et al., Craniopharyngiomas: A clinicopathological analysis of factors predictive of recurrence and functional outcome, Neurosurgery 35 (1994) 1001–1011.

[103] M.C. Brodsky, W.F. Hoyt, S.L. Barnwell, C.B. Wilson, Intrachiasmatic craniopharyngioma: A rare cause of chiasmal thickening. Case report, J Neurosurg 68 (1988) 300–302.

[104] T.A. Duff, R. Levine, Intrachiasmatic craniopharyngioma. Case report, J Neurosurg 59 (1983) 176–178.

[105] K. Kunishio, Y. Yamamoto, N. Sunami, et al., Craniopharyngioma in the third ventricle: Necropsy findings and histogenesis, J Neurol Neurosurg Psychiatry 50 (1987) 1053–1056.

[106] S.C. Young, R.A. Zimmerman, M.A. Nowell, et al., Giant cystic craniopharyngiomas, Neuroradiology 29 (1987) 468–473.

[107] N. Karavitaki, B.W. Scheithauer, J. Watt, et al., Collision lesions of the sella: Co-existence of craniopharyngioma with gonadotroph adenoma and of Rathke's cleft cyst with corticotroph adenoma, Pituitary 11 (3) (2008) 317–323.

[108] O. Moshkin, B.W. Scheithauer, L.V. Syro, et al., Collision tumors of the sella: Craniopharyngioma and silent pituitary adenoma subtype 3: Case report, Endocrine Pathology 20 (1) (2009) 50–55.

[109] M. Gokden, R. Mrak, Pituitary adenoma with craniopharyngioma component, Human Pathology 40 (8) (2009) 1189–1193.

[110] A. Yoshida, C. Sen, S. Asa, M.K. Rosenblum, Composite pituitary adenoma and craniopharyngioma? An unusual sellar neoplasm with divergent differentiation, Am J Surg Path 32 (11) (2008) 1136–1141.

[111] G.A. Nelson, O.F. Bastian, M. Schlitt, R.L. White, Malignant transformation in craniopharyngioma, Neurosurgery 22 (1988) 427–429.

[112] G. Gonzales-Portillo, T. Tomita, The syndrome of inappropriate secretion of antidiuretic hormone: An unusual presentation for childhood craniopharyngioma. Report of three cases, Neurosurgery 42 (1998) 917–922.

[113] E.S. Connolly, C.J. Winfree, P.W. Carmel, Giant posterior fossa cystic craniopharyngiomas presenting with hearing loss. Report of three cases and review of the literature, Surg Neurol 47 (1997) 291–299.

[114] R.L. Hintz, Management of craniopharyngioma, Acta Paediatr 417 (Suppl) (1996) 81–82.

[115] C.J. De Vile, D.B. Grant, B.E. Kendall, et al., Management of childhood craniopharyngioma: Can the morbidity of radical surgery be predicted? J Neurosurg 85 (1996) 73–81.

[116] D. Prasad, M. Steiner, L. Steiner, Gamma knife surgery for craniopharyngioma, Acta Neurochir 134 (1995) 167–176.

[117] B.E. Pollock, L.D. Lunsford, D. Kondziolka, et al., Phosphorus-32 intracavitary irradiation of cystic craniopharyngiomas: Current technique and long-term results, Int J Rad Oncol Biol Phys 33 (1995) 437–446.

[118] S. Cavalheiro, F.V. De Castro Sparapani, J.O.B. Franco, et al., Use of bleomycin in intratumoral chemotherapy for cystic craniopharyngioma, J Neurosurg 84 (1996) 124–126.

[119] A. Helseth, S.J. Mørk, A. Johansen, S. Tretli, Neoplasms of the central nervous system in Norway. IV. A population-based epidemiological study of meningiomas, Acta Pathol Microbiol Immunol Scand 97 (1989) 646–654.

[120] M. Rohringer, G.R. Sutherland, D.F. Louw, A.A.F. Sima, Incidence and clinicopathologic features of meningioma, J Neurosurg 71 (1989) 665–672.

[121] K. Nozaki, I. Nagata, K. Yoshida, H. Kikuchi, Intrasellar meningioma: Case report and review of the literature, Surg Neurol 47 (1997) 447–454.

[122] J. Zentner, J. Gilsbach, Pituitary adenoma and meningioma in the same patient: Report of three cases, Eur Arch Psychiatry Neurosci 238 (1989) 144–148.

[123] K. Yamada, T. Hatayama, M. Ohta, K. Sakoda, T. Uozumi, Coincidental pituitary adenoma and parasellar meningioma: Case report, Neurosurgery 19 (1986) 267–270.

[124] V. Kasantikul, S. Shuangshoti, C. Phonprasert, Intrasellar meningioma after radiotherapy for prolactinoma, J Med Assoc Thai 71 (1988) 524–527.

[125] A. Perry, D.N. Louis, B.W. Scheithauer, H. Budka, A. von Daimling, Meningiomas, in: D.N. Louis, H. Ohgaki, O.D. Wiestler, W.K. Cavenee (Eds.), WHO classification of tumours of the central nervous system, fourth ed., International Agency for Research on Cancer, Lyon, 2007, pp. 164–172.

[126] D. Kondziolka, Levy El, A. Niranjan, et al., Long-term outcomes after meningioma radiosurgery: Physician and patient perspectives, J Neurosurg 91 (1999) 44–50.

[127] A.J. Janss, R. Grundy, A. Cnaan, et al., Optic pathway and hypothalamic/chiasmatic gliomas in children younger than age 5 years with a 6-year follow-up, Cancer 75 (1995) 1051–1059.

[128] P.F. Collett-Solberg, H. Sernyak, M. Satin-Smith, et al., Endocrine outcome in long-term survivors of low-grade hypothalamic/chiasmatic glioma, Clin Endocrinol 47 (1997) 79–85.

[129] L.N. Sutton, P.T. Molloy, H. Sernyak, et al., Long-term outcome of hypothalamic/chiasmatic astrocytomas in children treated with conservative surgery, J Neurosurg 83 (1995) 583–589.

[130] R. Listernick, J. Charrow, Neurofibromatosis type 1 in childhood, J Pediatr 116 (1990) 845–853.

[131] R. Listernick, J. Charrow, M. Greenwald, M. Mets, Natural history of optic pathway tumors in children with neurofibromatosis type 1: A longitudinal study, J Pediatr 125 (1994) 63–66.

[132] J. Astrup, Natural history and clinical management of optic pathway glioma, Br J Neurosurg 17 (4) (2003) 327–335.

[133] J.M. Weinstein, M. Backonja, L.W. Houston, et al., Optic glioma associated with Beckwith-Wiedemann syndrome, Pediatr Neurol 2 (1986) 308–310.

[134] J. Suharwardy, J. Elston, The clinical presentation of children with tumours affecting the anterior visual pathways, Eye 11 (1997) 838–844.

[135] R. Listernick, C. Darling, M. Greenwald, et al., Optic pathway tumors in children: The effect of neurofibromatosis type 1 on clinical manifestations and natural history, J Pediatr 127 (1995) 718–722.

[136] I.F. Pollack, J.J. Mulvihill, Special issues in the management of gliomas in children with neurofibromatosis 1, J Neuro-Oncol 28 (1996) 257–268.

[137] R. Listernick, D.N. Louis, R.J. Packer, D.H. Gutmann, Optic pathway gliomas in children with neurofibromatosis 1: Consensus statement from the NF1 optic pathway glioma task force, Ann Neurol 41 (1997) 143–149.

[138] G.W. Albers, W.F. Hoyt, L.S. Forno, L.A. Shratter, Treatment response in malignant optic glioma of adulthood, Neurology 38 (1988) 1071–1074.

[139] W.F. Hoyt, L.G. Meshel, S. Lessell, et al., Malignant optic glioma of adulthood, Brain 96 (1973) 121–132.

[140] A. Rudd, J.E. Rees, P. Kennedy, et al., Malignant optic nerve gliomas in adults, J Clin Neuro-Ophthalmol 5 (1985) 238–243.

[141] M.J.B. Taphoorn, W.A.E.J. de Vries-Knoppert, H. Ponssen, J.G. Wolbers, Malignant optic glioma in adults. Case report, J Neurosurg 70 (1989) 277–279.

[142] M. Cynthya, Scotorne A glioma of the posterior lobe of the pituitary, J Pathol Bacteriol 69 (1) (2005) 109–112.

[143] J.B. Winer, H. Lidov, F. Scaravilli, An ependymoma involving the pituitary fossa, J Neurol Neurosurg Psychiatry 52 (1989) 1443–1444.

[144] S. Nishizawa, T. Yokoyama, K. Hinokuma, et al., Pituitary astrocytoma: Magnetic resonance and hormonal characteristics. Case illustration, J Neurosurg 87 (1997) 131.

[145] H.S. Friedman, T. Kerby, H. Calvert, Temozolomide and treatment of malignant glioma, Clin Cancer Res 6 (2000) 2585–2597.

[146] S. Gururangan, M.J. Fisher, J.C. Allen, et al., Temozolomide in children with progressive low-grade glioma, Neuro-Oncol 9 (2) (2007) 161–168.

[147] N. Levin, I. Lavon, B. Zelikovitsh, et al., Progressive low-grade oligodendrogliomas: response to temozolomide and correlation between genetic profile and O6-methylguanine DNA methyltranspherese protein expression, Cancer 106 (2006) 1759–1765.

[148] D.J. Brat, B.W. Scheithauer, S.M. Staugaitis, et al., Third ventricular chordoid glioma: A distinct clinicopathologic entity, J Neuropathol Exp Neurol 57 (1998) 283–290.

[149] I. Vajtai, Z. Varga, B.W. Scheithauer, M. Bodosi, Chordoid glioma of the third ventricle: Confirmatory report of a new entity, Hum Pathol 30 (1999) 723–726.

[150] J. Wanschitz, M. Schmidbauer, H. Maier, et al., Suprasellar meningioma with expression of glial fibrillary acidic protein: A peculiar variant, Acta Neuropathol 90 (1995) 539–544.

[151] C.S. Kretschmar, Germ cell tumors of the brain in children: A review of current literature and new advances in therapy, Cancer Invest 15 (1997) 187–198.

[152] L.P. Dehner, Gonadal and extragonadal germ cell neoplasia of childhood, Hum Pathol 14 (1983) 493–511.

[153] J.I. Kuratsu, Y. Ushio, Epidemiological study of primary intracranial tumors: A regional survey in Kumamato prefecture in the Southern part of Japan, J Neurosurg 84 (1996) 946–950.

[154] M. Matsutani, K. Sano, K. Takakura, et al., Primary intracranial germ cell tumors: A clinical analysis of 153 histologically verified cases, J Neurosurg 86 (1997) 446–455.

[155] F. Furukawa, H. Haebara, Y. Hamashima, Primary intracranial choriocarcinoma arising from the pituitary fossa. Report of an autopsy case with literature review, Acta Pathol Jpn 36 (1986) 773–781.

[156] W. Poon, H.K. Ng, K. Wong, J.R. South, Primary intrasellar germinoma presenting with cavernous sinus syndrome, Surg Neurol 30 (1988) 402–405.

[157] M. Sugiyama, I. Takumi, Y. Node, et al., Neurohypophyseal germinoma with prolactinoma. Case illustration, J Neurosurg 90 (1999) 170.

[158] M.T. Jennings, R. Gelman, F. Hochberg, Intracranial germ-cell tumors: Natural history and pathogenesis, J Neurosurg 63 (1985) 155–167.

[159] H.J. Hoffman, H. Otsubo, E.B. Hendrick, et al., Intracranial germ-cell tumors in children, J Neurosurg 74 (1991) 545–551.

[160] M.E. Rueda-Pedraza, S.A. Heifetz, I.A. Sesterhenn, G.B. Clark, Primary intracranial germ cell tumors in the first two decades of life. A clinical, light-microscopic, and immunohistochemical analysis of 54 cases, Perspect Pediatr Pathol 10 (1987) 160–207.

[161] M. Tanabe, M. Mizushima, Y. Anno, et al., Intracranial germinoma with Down's syndrome: A case report and review of the literature, Surg Neurol 47 (1997) 28–31.

[162] J.A. Prall, L. McGavran, B.S. Greffe, M.D. Partington, Intracranial malignant germ cell tumor and the Klinefelter syndrome. Case report and review of the literature, Pediatr Neurosurg 23 (1995) 219–224.

[163] A. Sato, A. Kajita, K. Sugita, et al., Cornelia de Lange syndrome with intracranial germinoma, Acta Pathol Jpn 36 (1986) 143–149.

[164] O.A. Glenn, A.J. Barkovich, Intracranial germ cell tumors: A comprehensive review of proposed embryologic derivation, Pediatr Neurosurg 24 (1996) 242–251.

[165] K. Sario, Pathogenesis of intracranial germ cell tumors revisited, J Neurosurg 90 (1999) 258–264.

[166] K.L. Salzman, A.M. Rojiani, J. Buatti, et al., Primary intracranial germ cell tumors: Clinicopathologic review of 32 cases, Pediatr Pathol Lab Med 17 (1997) 713–727.

[167] S.L. Mootha, A.J. Barkovich, M.M. Grumbach, et al., Idiopathic hypothalamic diabetes insipidus, pituitary stalk thickening, and the occult intracranial germinoma in children and adolescents, J Clin Endocrinol Metab 82 (1997) 1362–1367.

[168] S.L. Wolden, W.M. Wara, D.A. Larson, et al., Radiation therapy for primary intracranial germ-cell tumors, Int J Rad Oncol Biol Phys 32 (1995) 943–949.

[169] Y. Ushio, M. Kochi, J.I. Kuratsu, et al., Preliminary observations for a new treatment in children with primary intracranial yolk sac tumor or embryonal carcinoma. Report of five cases, J Neurosurg 90 (1999) 133–137.

[170] C.H. Rickert, M. Reznick, J. Lenelle, P. Rinaldi, Shunt-related abdominal metastasis of cerebral teratocarcinoma: Report of an unusual case and review of the literature, Neurosurgery 42 (1998) 1378–1383.

[171] T. Sheehan, R.J.G. Cuthbert, A.C. Parker, Central nervous system involvement in haematological malignancies, Clin Lab Haematol 11 (1989) 331–338.

[172] W. Janisch, H. Gerlach, D. Schreiber, et al., Isolierte neoplastische Infiltrate im Zentralnervensystem bei generalisierten Non-Hodgkin-Lymphomen. Eine prospektive pathologisch-anatomische Untersuchung, Zentralbl Pathol Anat 122 (1978) 195–203.

[173] S.R. Masse, R.W. Wolk, R.H. Conklin, Peripituitary gland involvement in acute leukemia in adults, Arch Pathol 96 (1973) 141–142.

[174] K. Nemoto, Y. Ohnishi, T. Tsukada, Chronic lymphocytic leukemia showing pituitary tumor with massive leukemic cell infiltration, and special reference to clinicopathological findings of CLL, Acta Pathol Jpn 28 (1978) 797–805.

[175] L.W. Duchen, C.S. Treip, Microgliomatosis presenting with dementia and hypopituitarism, J Pathol 98 (1969) 143–146.

[176] M. Gottfredsson, T.D. Oury, C. Bernstein, et al., Lymphoma of the pituitary gland: An unusual presentation of central nervous system lymphoma in AIDS, Am J Med 5 (1996) 563–564.

[177] F. Maiuri, Primary cerebral lymphoma presenting as steroid-responsive chiasmal syndrome, Br J Neurosurg 1 (1987) 499–502.

[178] J.H. Shanks, M. Harris, A.J. Howat, A.J. Freemont, Angiotropic lymphoma with endocrine involvement, Histopathology 31 (1997) 161–166.

[179] A. Giustina, M. Gola, M. Doga, E. Rossei, Clinical review 136. Primary lymphoma of the pituitary: An emerging clinical entity, J Clin Endocrinol Metab 86 (2002) 4567–4575.

[180] O. Moshkin, P. Muller, B.W. Scheithauer, et al., Primary pituitary lymphoma: A histological, immunohistochemical, and ultrastructural study with literature review, Endocr Pathol 20 (2009) 46–49.

[181] M. Yasuda, N. Akiyama, S. Miyamoto, et al., Primary sellar lymphoma: Intravascular large B-cell lymphoma diagnosed as a double cancer and improved with chemotherapy, and literature review of primary parasellar lymphoma, Pituitary 13 (2010) 39–47.

[182] S.J. Urbanski, J.M. Bilbao, E. Horvath, et al., Intrasellar plasmacytoma terminating in multiple myeloma: A report of a case including electron microscopical study, Surg Neurol 14 (1980) 233–236.

[183] J. Vaquero, E. Areitio, R. Martinez, Intracranial parasellar plasmacytoma, Arch Neurol 39 (1982) 738.

[184] P. Bitterman, A. Ariza, R.A. Black, et al., Multiple myeloma mimicking pituitary adenoma, Comput Radiol 10 (1986) 201–205.

[185] G.L. Mancardi, T.I. Mandybur, Solitary intracranial plasmacytoma, Cancer 51 (1983) 2226–2233.

[186] P. Juneau, W.C. Schoene, P. Black, Malignant tumors in the pituitary gland, Arch Neurol 49 (1992) 555–558.

[187] C.L. Willman, K.L. McClain, An update on clonality, cytokines, and viral etiology in Langerhans cell histiocytosis, Hematol Oncol Clin N Am 12 (1998) 407–416.

[188] N.G. Grois, B.E. Favara, G.H. Mostbeck, D. Prayer, Central nervous system disease in Langerhans cell histiocytosis, Hematol Oncol Clin N Am 12 (1998) 287–305.

[189] H. Goldberg-Stern, R. Weitz, R. Zaizov, et al., Progressive spinocerebellar degeneration "plus" associated with Langerhans cell histiocytosis: A new paraneoplastic syndrome? J Neurol Neurosurg Psychiatry 58 (1995) 180–183.

[190] M.B. Max, M.D.F. Deck, D.A. Rottenberg, Pituitary metastasis: Incidence in cancer patients and clinical differentiation from pituitary adenoma, Neurology 31 (1981) 998–1002.

[191] I.A. Felix, Pathology of the neurohypophysis, Pathol Res Pract 183 (1988) 535–537.

[192] U. Roessmann, B. Kaufman, R.L. Friede, Metastatic lesions in the sella turcica and pituitary gland, Cancer 25 (1970) 478–480.

[193] D. Schreiber, K. Bernstein, J. Schneider, Tumormetastasen im Zentralnervensystem. Eine prospektive Studie. 3. Mitteilung: Metastasen in Hypophyse, Epiphyse und Plexus chorioidei, Zentralbl Allg Pathol 126 (1986) 64–73.

[194] P.C. McCormick, K.D. Post, A.D. Kandji, A.P. Hays, Metastatic carcinoma to the pituitary gland, Br J Neurosurg 3 (1989) 71–80.

[195] K.J. Gurling, G.B.D. Scott, D.N. Baron, Metastasis in pituitary tissue removed at hypophysectomy in women with mammary carcinoma, Br J Cancer 11 (1957) 519–523.

[196] S.M. De la Monte, G.M. Hutchins, G.W. Moore, Endocrine organ metastases from breast carcinoma, Am J Pathol 114 (1984) 131–136.

[197] C.L. Branch, E.R. Laws, Metastatic tumors of the sella turcica masquerading as primary pituitary tumors, J Clin Endocrinol Metab 65 (1987) 469–474.

[198] J. Duvall, J.F. Cullen, Metastatic disease in the pituitary: Clinical features, Transact Ophthalmol Soc UK 102 (1982) 481–486.

[199] K. Kovacs, Metastatic cancer of the pituitary gland, Oncology 27 (1973) 533–542.

[200] J.C. Kattah, R.M. Silgals, H. Manz, et al., Presentation and management of parasellar and suprasellar metastatic mass lesions, J Neurol Neurosurg Psychiatry 48 (1985) 44–49.

[201] R.J. Teears, E.M. Silverman, Clinicopathologic review of 88 cases of carcinoma metastatic to the pituitary gland, Cancer 36 (1975) 216–220.

[202] E.M. Allen, S.R. Kannan, A. Powell, Infundibular metastasis and panhypopituitarism, J Natl Med Assoc 81 (1989) 325–330.

[203] U. Szuwart, H.J. Konig, H. Bennefeld, et al., Klinik der hypophysaren Metastasierungen, Onkologie 11 (1988) 66–69.

[204] M. Losa, M. Grasso, E. Giugni, et al., Metastatic prostatic adenocarcinoma presenting as a pituitary mass: Shrinkage of the lesion and clinical improvement with medical treatment, Prostate 32 (1997) 241–245.

[205] A.P. Van Seters, G.T.A.M. Bots, H. van Dulken, et al., Metastasis of an occult gastric carcinoma suggesting growth of a prolactinoma during bromocriptine therapy: A case report with a review of the literature, Neurosurgery 16 (1985) 813–817.

[206] K.D. Post, P.C. McCormick, A.P. Hays, A.G. Kandji, Metastatic carcinoma to pituitary adenoma. Report of two cases, Surg Neurol 30 (1988) 286–292.

[207] P.A. Molinatti, B.W. Scheithauer, R.V. Randall, E.R. Laws, Metastasis to pituitary adenoma, Arch Pathol Lab Med 109 (1985) 287–289.

[208] J.F. Richardson, I. Katayama, Neoplasm to neoplasm metastasis. An acidophil adenoma harbouring metastatic carcinoma: A case report, Arch Pathol 91 (1971) 135–139.

[209] E.L. Zager, E.T. Hedley-Whyte, Metastasis within a pituitary adenoma presenting with bilateral abducens palsies: Case report and review of the literature, Neurosurgery 21 (1987) 383–386.

[210] R.L. James, G. Arsenis, M. Stoler, et al., Hypophyseal metastatic renal cell carcinoma and pituitary adenoma. Case report and review of the literature, Am J Med 76 (1984) 337–340.

[211] J.A. Ramsay, K. Kovacs, B.W. Scheithauer, et al., Metastatic carcinoma to pituitary adenomas: A report of two cases, Exp Clin Endocrinol 92 (1988) 69–76.

[212] T. Abe, K. Matsumoto, M. Iida, et al., Malignant carcinoid tumor of the anterior mediastinum metastasis to a prolactin-secreting pituitary adenoma: A case report, Surg Neurol 48 (1997) 389–394.

[213] T.R. Hurley, C.M. D'Angelo, R.A. Clasen, et al., Adenocarcinoma metastatic to a growth-hormone secreting pituitary adenoma: Case report, Surg Neurol 37 (1992) 361–365.

[214] D. Hubert, M. Bertin, Tumeurs du système nerveux radio-induites chez l'homme, Bull Cancer 80 (1993) 971–983.

[215] M. Brada, D. Ford, S. Ashley, et al., Risk of second brain tumour after conservative surgery and radiotherapy for a pituitary adenoma, Br Med J 304 (1992) 1343–1346.

[216] E. Salvati, M. Artico, R. Caruso, et al., A report on radiation-induced gliomas, Cancer 67 (1991) 392–397.

[217] N.E. Simmons, E.R. Laws, Glioma occurrence after sellar irradiation: Case report and review, Neurosurgery 42 (1998) 172–178.

[218] C. Kitanaka, N. Shitara, T. Nakagomi, et al., Postradiation astrocytoma. Report of two cases, J Neurosurg 70 (1989) 469–474.

[219] S. Okamoto, H. Handa, J. Yamashita, et al., Post-irradiation brain tumors, Neurol Med Chir 25 (1985) 528–533.

[220] M. Salvati, L. Cervoni, F. Puzzilli, et al., High-dose radiation-induced meningiomas, Surg Neurol 47 (1997) 435–442.

[221] M. Bhaskara Rao, D. Rout, V.V. Radhakrishnan, Suprasellar meningioma subsequent to treatment for a pituitary adenoma: Case report, Surg Neural 47 (1997) 443–446.

[222] M.J. Alexander, A.A.F. DeSalles, U. Tomiyasu, Multiple radiation-induced intracranial lesions after treatment for pituitary adenoma. Case report, J Neurosurg 88 (1998) 111–115.

[223] W.G. Cahan, Radiation-induced sarcoma – 50 years later, Cancer 82 (1998) 6–7.

[224] P.P. Kumar, R.R. Good, F.M. Skultety, et al., Radiation-induced neoplasms of the brain, Cancer 59 (1987) 1274–1282.

[225] T. Civit, C. Pinelli, M. Klein, et al., Intrasellar schwannoma, Acta Neurochir 139 (1997) 160–161.

[226] N.F. Maartens, D.B. Ellegala, M.L. Vance, et al., Intrasellar Schwannomas: Report of two cases, Neurosurgery 52 (2003) 1200–1206.

[227] J.T. Wolfe, B.W. Scheithauer, D.C. Dahlin, Giant-cell tumor of the sphenoid bone, J Neurosurg 59 (1983) 322–327.

[228] K.K. Wu, P.M. Ross, D.C. Mitchell, H.H. Sprague, Evolution of a case of multicentric giant cell tumor over a 23-year period, Clin Orthopaed Rel Res 213 (1986) 279–288.

[229] S.B. Keel, A.K. Bhan, N.J. Liebsch, A.E. Rosenberg, Chondromyxoid fibroma of the skull base: A tumor which may be confused with chordoma and chondrosarcoma. A report of three cases and review of the literature, Am J Surg Pathol 21 (1997) 577–582.

[230] Y. Shenker, R.V. Lloyd, L. Weatherbee, et al., Ectopic prolactinoma in a patient with hyperparathyroidism and abnormal sellar radiography, J Clin Endocrinol Metab 62 (1986) 1065–1069.

[231] M. Petrus, M. Mignonat, J.C. Netter, et al., Association epine intrasellaire et hyperprolactinemie, Ann Pediatr 35 (1988) 201–203.

[232] P.D. Sawin, K.A. Follett, B.C. Wen, E.R. Laws, Symptomatic intrasellar hemangioblastoma in a child treated with subtotal resection and adjuvant radiosurgery. Case report, J Neurosurg 84 (1996) 1046–1050.

[233] M.E. Sansone, B.H. Liwnicz, T.I. Mandybur, Giant pituitary cavernous hemangioma. Case report, J Neurosurg 53 (1980) 124–126.

[234] S.L. Asa, K. Kovacs, E. Horvath, et al., Sellar glomangioma, Ultrastruct Pathol 7 (1984) 49–54.

[235] B.K. Kleinschmidt-DeMasters, G.W. Mierau, C.I. Sze, et al., Unusual dural and skull-based mesenchymal neoplasms: A report of four cases, Hum Pathol 29 (1998) 240–245.

[236] D.A. Morrison, K. Bibby, Sellar and suprasellar hemangiopericytoma mimicking pituitary adenoma, Arch Ophthalmol 115 (1997) 1201–1203.

[237] J.M. Bilbao, E. Horvath, K. Kovacs, et al., Intrasellar paraganglioma associated with hypopituitarism, Arch Pathol Lab Med 102 (1978) 95–98.

[238] M.J. Aubin, J. Hardy, R. Comtois, Primary sellar haemorrhagic melanoma: Case report and reviewof the literature, Br J Neurosurg 11 (1997) 80–83.

[239] C. Ruchti, M. Balli-Antunes, H.A. Gerber, Follicular tumor in the sellar region without primary cancer of the thyroid. Heterotopic carcinoma? Am J Clin Pathol 87 (1987) 776–780.

[240] B. Aarabi, M. Haghshenas, V. Rakeii, Visual failure caused by suprasellar extramedullary hematopoiesis in beta thalassemia: Case report, Neurosurgery 42 (1998) 922–926.

[241] P. Caturegli, I. Lupi, M. Landek-Salgado, et al., Pituitary autoimmunity: 30 years later, Autoimmun Rev 7 (2008) 631–637.

[242] D.W. McKeel, Primary hypothyroidism and hypopituitarism in a young woman: Pathological discussion, Am J Med 77 (1984) 326–329.

[243] T. Dillard, C.G. Yedinak, J. Alumkal, M. Fleseriu, Anti-CTLA-4 antibody therapy associated autoimmune hypophysitis: Serious immune related adverse events across a spectrum of cancer subtypes, Pituitary 13 (2010) 29–38.

[244] K. Kovacs, J.M. Bilbao, V. Fornasier, E. Horvath, Pituitary pathology in Erdheim-Chester disease, Endocrine Pathol 15 (2) (2004) 159–166.

[245] T. Oweity, B.W. Scheithauer, H.S. Ching, Multiple system Erdheim-Chester disease with massive hypothalamic–sellar involvement and hypopituitarism, J Neurosurg 96 (2002) 344–351.

[246] V.A. Briner, A. Muller, J.O. Gebbers, Die Neurosarkoidose, Schw Med Wochenschr 128 (1998) 799–810.

[247] N. Sato, G. Sze, J.H. Kim, Cystic pituitary mass in neurosarcoidosis, Am J Neuroradiol 18 (1997) 1182–1185.

[248] O.P. Sharma, Neurosarcoidosis, A personal perspective based on the study of 3 patients, Chest 112 (1997) 220–228.

SECTION IV

PITUITARY PROCEDURES

CHAPTER

20

Pituitary Imaging

Marcel M. Maya [1], Barry D. Pressman [2]

[1] Department of Imaging, Cedars-Sinai Medical Center, Los Angeles, CA, USA

[2] Cedars-Sinai Medical Center, Los Angeles, CA, USA

HISTORY OF PITUITARY IMAGING

Imaging of the sella turcica and of the pituitary received tremendous attention almost from the inception of radiography. It was soon recognized that changes in and around the sella turcica could reflect numerous intracranial conditions, not solely those of the pituitary itself. Further, the importance of the pituitary gland's intricate function spurred interest in the evaluation of the sella turcica as a window to the gland itself.

Plain radiography was the first and, for many decades, the only technique applicable to imaging of the sella turcica. Accordingly, there is a remarkably extensive literature pertaining to the size, shape, contour and bony density of the sella turcica and its many components. The advent of tomography and its evolution from linear, to thin-section multidirectional techniques, increased the ability to recognize and to define variations of normal and differentiate them from pathology. However, advances in surgical treatment and the effect this has had on the evaluation of the true significance of radiographic findings, indicated that even these exquisite tomographic techniques were inadequate for the ever-increasing requirement to adequately diagnose pituitary pathology. These requirements have continued to expand as a result of improvement in medical, as well as surgical, treatment.

Pneumoencephalography (PEG) and angiography were powerful diagnostic tools for pituitary evaluation. With their development it was no longer necessary to simply rely on plain film images. Rather, indirect visualization of the pituitary gland itself was available. PEG allowed for evaluation of suprasellar masses, and normal variations such as the empty sella. When supplemented with tomography, PEG was a remarkably excellent technique for imaging the sella turcica and parasellar area, but was performed with some difficulty because of the potential for complication and patient discomfort.

Angiography was, and is, also an important tool for evaluation of the pituitary gland. Originally it offered information, otherwise unavailable, concerning the status of the vital vascular structures in the parasellar area. Angiographic techniques and resolution have continued to improve and to be utilized in pituitary imaging, but conventional angiography has been largely replaced initially by CT, and then by MRI and MR angiography.

In the early 1970s the wedding of radiographic and computer technology in the form of computer-assisted tomography (CAT), now know as computed tomography (CT), resulted in a revolution in neuroimaging. At first, spatial resolution and contrast sensitivity were limited but these were rapidly improved. Accordingly, although CT initially was of limited value in the diagnosis of pituitary disease, it is now capable of fine-detail evaluation of the sella turcica, the pituitary gland itself, the suprasellar space, the cavernous sinuses and, to a greater or lesser degree, the contiguous vascular structures and the optic chiasm. The rapid progression of CT technology was remarkable, as was its impact on pituitary imaging.

As CT appeared to be reaching its limits of resolution, MRI literally exploded on the scene and relatively rapidly replaced CT for most pituitary imaging. The spatial resolution of MRI is not equivalent to that of CT, the latter having a much greater capability of defining bone detail. However, MRI has the capability of delineating glandular pathology better than CT and it far surpasses CT in definition of the parasellar and suprasellar regions. Further, there is no iodizing radiation exposure of the patient with MRI, and intravenous iodinated contrast is not required with MRI as it is with CT. However, in a large percentage of pituitary MRI studies gadolinium contrast enhancement is very useful. With the

The Pituitary, Third Edition, DOI: 10.1016/B978-0-12-380926-1.10020-3

recognition of nephrogenic systemic fibrosis as a consequence of gadolinium administration in patients with renal failure the advantage of MR over CT in this group has been reduced.

PLAIN FILMS AND TOMOGRAMS

Size and Shape of Sella

The sella turcica is best visualized on lateral views of the skull. The sellar floor can be studied on frontal radiographs angled tangentially to the plane of the floor (Caldwell view).

Numerous studies of the "normal" sella turcica size were performed and reported prior to CT and MRI. Enlargement of the sella turcica was thought to be an indicator of pituitary pathology, as were distortion of shape and contour of the sella.

A wide range of normal exists, and this has been expanded with information gained from CT and MRI. For instance, visualization of an "enlarged" empty sella in an asymptomatic patient indicates that sella turcica size alone is not a valid determinant of pituitary disease. A small sella turcica may be associated with pituitary insufficiency, but the correlation is poor [1] and most small sellas are of no significance.

According to Taveras and Wood [1], 17 mm is the upper limit of normal for the maximum anteroposterior diameter of the sella. The depth measured perpendicular to the sella floor, from a line drawn between dorsum and tuberculum, should not exceed 13 mm in most cases. The normal width varies between 10 and 15 mm. These are only guidelines, and sella turcica enlargement can only be used as a suggestion of pituitary abnormality and is certainly not sufficient for diagnosis.

Investigators have also attempted to use the area and the volume of the sella turcica to serve as better predictors of pituitary disease. The volume is the product of one-half length × width × height. An area greater than 130 square mm, and a volume greater than 1092 cubic mm, have been reported to be abnormal [2]. These techniques are limited because they do not necessarily reflect true pituitary size.

Studies of the shape of the sella turcica and the bony density of its margins are limited in their value as predictors of pituitary and/or parasellar disease. Focal erosion of the lateral margins secondary to an aneurysm, focal erosions of the floor by pituitary lesions, and selective erosion of the posteroinferior floor secondary to chronic increased intracranial pressure [3,4] are some of the more dependable findings. Thickening of the tuberculum or of the clinoid processes, and blistering of the planum sphenoidale, have frequently been reported in association with meningiomas of the sella turcica. The sellar floor may become sclerotic in some cases of craniopharyngioma and nasopharyngeal carcinoma [1].

Intrasellar, parasellar, or suprasellar fat and calcifications may be excellent indicators of pathology. Craniopharyngiomas and germ cell tumors are often associated with fat and/or calcification. Aneurysms may demonstrate eggshell or other calcification patterns. Meningiomas frequently calcify, and on rare occasions pituitary tumors calcify (pituitary stone).

Thin-section (1–2 mm), high-resolution, multidirectional tomography was initially expected to improve the sensitivity for diagnosis of pituitary lesions, particularly microadenomas. Initial enthusiasm emphasized visualization of small areas of sella floor erosion and/or depression. Unfortunately this has not stood the close scrutiny of subsequent carefully performed radiologic/pathologic/surgical studies [3,4]. In cases in which surgery showed a microadenoma, and in which tomograms were considered positive, the correlation between the actual location of the lesion and the radiographic findings was quite poor. Eventually it was recognized that tomograms added little to the diagnosis of microadenomas, although they were useful to better define such bony changes as sclerosis, bone destruction and the presence of calcification.

ANGIOGRAPHY

Angiography initially had a role in the primary diagnosis of larger pituitary lesions. Lateral displacement and medial concavity of the cavernous carotid artery are signs of an intrasellar mass. Tumor vascularity and tumor blush were also helpful but frequently difficult to detect, requiring carefully performed subtraction images. Suprasellar extension of intrasellar masses could be detected by elevation of the anterior cerebral and/or anterior communicating arteries. Hypervascularity of meningiomas and delineation of aneurysms are important capabilities of angiography.

However, angiography is of no value in the diagnosis of microadenomas. It was widely performed prior to pituitary surgery because surgeons were anxious to identify the location of the carotid arteries and to exclude an intrasellar aneurysm. Subsequently, CT and then MRI replaced the need for angiography in most cases because the position of the carotid arteries, and the possibility of an aneurysm, may be clarified by these techniques with little or no patient risk or discomfort. On occasion, additional vascular detail may be required, and can most often be obtained with MR or CT angiographic techniques.

CT

The successful application of CT to the evaluation of intrasellar pathology awaited several technical

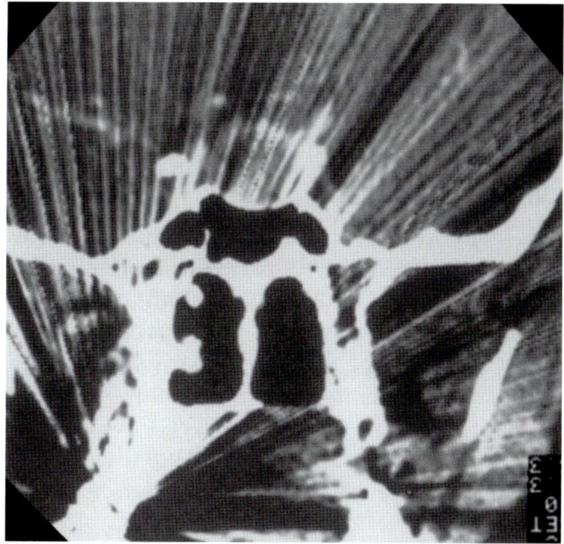

FIGURE 20.1 Artifacts from metallic dental devices obscure the pituitary tumor in this direct coronal CT image. By readjusting the angle of gantry these artifacts were avoided.

improvements. High resolution required 1–2 mm sections, a 256 × 256 matrix, and equipment with excellent signal/noise ratios without unacceptable ionizing radiation levels. Initially, axial views with coronal and sagittal computerized reformations were applied to the sella. Although this technique was useful for depiction of suprasellar and parasellar pathology, it was frequently inadequate to evaluate intrasellar disease, especially microadenomas. Direct coronal imaging was necessary, and required the patients to extend their necks maximally in the prone or supine position. Proper angling of the X-ray beam was necessary to avoid metallic streak dental artifacts (Figure 20.1). Fortunately, modern multislice high-resolution CT scanners are capable of helical acquisitions in the axial plane, allowing for high-resolution multiplanar reformation (MPR) into the crucial coronal, as well as sagittal, planes (Figure 20.2).

CT tissue contrast is limited within the pituitary without iodinated contrast administration. Although fat and calcium are well defined on noncontrast CT, these are infrequently associated with intrapituitary lesions, compared to their increased association with suprasellar and parasellar lesions. Fortunately most pituitary tumors enhance with intravenous contrast less rapidly than normal pituitary tissue, resulting in increased conspicuity of these tumors. However, there is a small but definite allergic risk attendant to the use of such agents and some patients have medical conditions that contraindicate the use of iodinated contrast agents, e.g., reduced renal function, multiple myeloma and sickle cell disease. One further drawback of CT is that it utilizes ionizing radiation, albeit with much greater soft tissue contrast than conventional radiographic techniques. The critical tissue at risk for radiation exposure is the optic lens. The lens is directly irradiated with axial CT imaging of the pituitary, receiving as much as 3–5 rads of radiation, one more factor favoring MR for pituitary imaging.

Although CT has to a great extent been replaced by MRI for pituitary evaluation, it still offers some advantages. Therefore, CT's technical factors and diagnostic considerations will be discussed.

Technical Factors

Thin slice (0.63 mm) axial helical acquisition allows for isovoxel (a cube with equality of all three dimensions) coronal and sagittal reformations. The acquisition and display matrix should be at least 256 × 256, with 512 × 512 being even more desirable for visualization of smaller microadenomas. Resolution is inadequate with coarser matrices. Intravenous iodinated contrast should be administered by rapid infusion which may

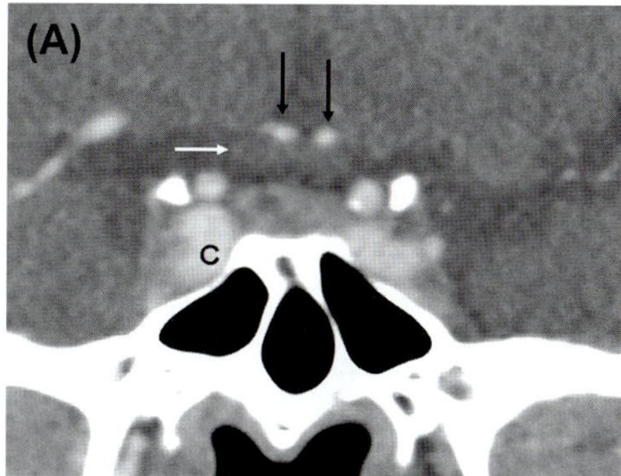

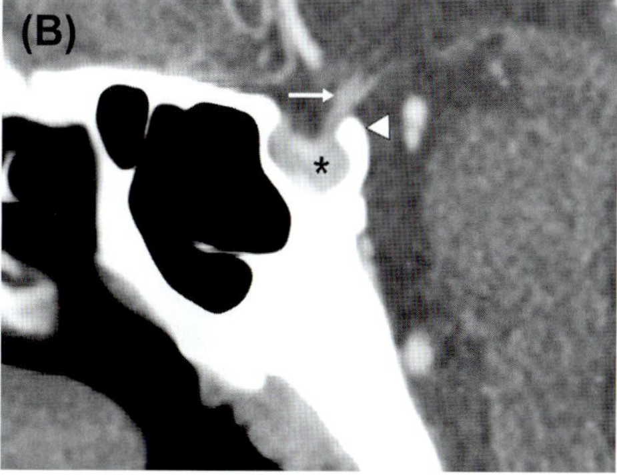

FIGURE 20.2 Coronal (A) and sagittal (B) MPRs from an axial CT. (A) Note the densely enhancing intracavernous carotid (C), and the anterior cerebral arteries (black arrows) above the faintly seen optic chiasm (white arrow). Sagittal image shows the normal anatomic relationship of the pituitary gland (*), stalk (white arrow) and bony dorsum sella (arrowhead).

be augmented by a bolus push for the initial 10–20 cc. This technique will achieve an adequate blood level and early opacification of the cavernous sinus and of the normally vascularized pituitary gland (Figure 20.2). Slower drip infusion alone may result in slow development of an adequate circulating blood level, thereby reducing the conspicuity of lesions by minimizing the difference in contrast enhancement between the normal gland and the lesion. A total dose of 40–45 g iodine has proven sufficient for most pituitary studies. Increasing the dose is unlikely to improve diagnostic accuracy but does increase the risk of morbidity, especially renal toxicity.

Normal Anatomy

The primary value of pituitary imaging by CT is not the high-resolution bone detail available but rather the direct visualization of the gland and surrounding soft tissue structures. With the use of intravenous contrast, soft tissue contrast is sufficient to define the pituitary gland, intraglandular pathology, the infundibulum, the cavernous sinuses and, to a greater or lesser extent, the suprasellar space and the optic chiasm (Figure 20.2). Pathologic fat and calcification deposits may be exquisitely defined (Figure 20.3).

The normal pituitary gland enhances with iodinated intravenous contrast because of the absence of a blood–brain barrier. It is therefore hyperdense on enhanced CT. Without iodinated contrast, gland visualization is often inadequate and pathologic conditions within the gland, the sella turcica, and the suprasellar and parasellar spaces, are frequently not demonstrated. The infundibular stalk, similar to the pituitary, also has no blood–brain barrier and enhances with contrast (Figure 20.2). Since the cavernous sinuses are mainly blood-filled, they too enhance, thereby obscuring the lateral margins of the pituitary. Carotid artery enhancement is equivalent to that of the cavernous sinuses, so that the intracavernous portions of these vessels are not delineated, but the supracavernous portions are usually well defined. The horizontal portions of the anterior and middle cerebral arteries are often well visualized. Intracavernous neural structures do not enhance and therefore may be seen as low-density structures within the enhanced sinus (Figure 20.9). Cranial nerves III and IV are superolateral in position in the cavernous sinuses, and most often are seen as a single structure. More inferiorly and laterally in the cavernous sinuses are the first and second divisions of cranial nerve V, which usually are visualized individually. The third division of the trigeminal nerve does not enter the cavernous sinus but exits the cranial cavity through the foramen ovale after leaving the trigeminal ganglion in Meckel's cave, which may be seen as a fluid density posterior to the cavernous sinus. More often than not, the abducens nerve, which is medial to cranial nerve V, is not separately defined because it is relatively small.

Medial to the cavernous sinus and caudad to the sella turcica is the sphenoid sinus, the shape of which may be quite variable Pneumatization may not be equal on the two sides, thereby resulting in asymmetrical sella turcica floor thickness. At the junction of the sphenoid septum with the sellar floor, there may be a slight depression of the floor simulating an area of pathologic erosion or remodeling, erroneously suggesting an intrasellar mass. Intrasellar and suprasellar cerebrospinal fluid (CSF) is low in density, well contrasted against the hyperdense pituitary and osseous structures. The optic nerves and chiasm are variably defined, best visualized in those patients with a greater suprasellar volume of CSF (Figure 20.2).

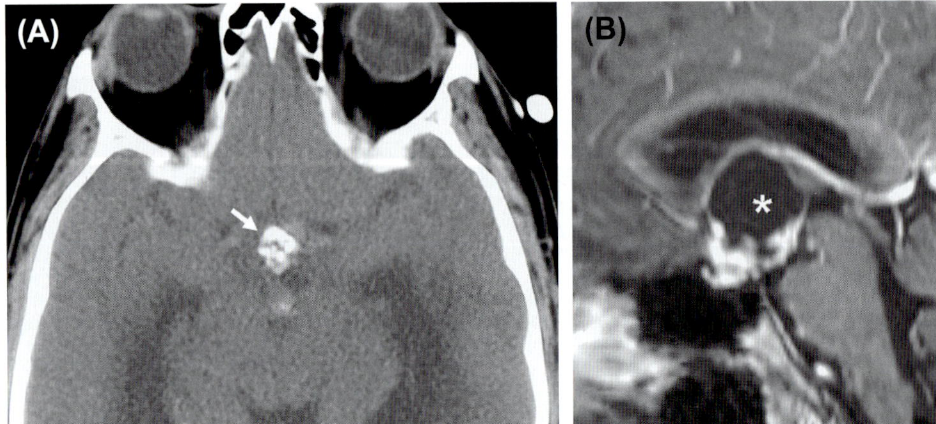

FIGURE 20.3 Axial noncontrast CT (A) and coronal MR (B) in a patient with craniopharyngioma. (A) Chunky and irregular calcification (arrow) of the suprasellar mass is quite typical of craniopharyngioma. (B) MR depicts the solid and cystic mass (*), however, is less sensitive to calcium.

The infundibulum extends to the superior margin of the pituitary from the undersurface of the hypothalamus (tuber cinereum) immediately posterior to the optic chiasm. It enhances with contrast, is relatively uniform in size, is midline in position, and its maximum diameter does not normally exceed 3 mm.

MRI: TECHNIQUE AND ANATOMY

MRI is the preferred procedure for imaging the pituitary and the parasellar regions because of its intrinsic qualities of excellent spatial resolution, multiplanar capabilities, capability for assessment of dynamic contrast enhancement and absence of ionizing radiation. MRI has therefore become the clear procedure of choice for pituitary imaging.

High-resolution MRI requires a high field-strength magnet (1.5 or 3 Tesla unit). Although the suprasellar contents may be adequately depicted on low and medium field-strength units, confidence in the diagnosis of intraglandular pathology requires the very high resolution that is obtainable only on high field-strength units. For high spatial detail, thin slices (maximum 3 mm, preferably 2 mm), a fine matrix (256 × 256 to 512 × 256), and a small field of view (16–18 cm) are needed. Since intraglandular pathology often measures no more than 1–3 mm, gaps of 1–3 mm between slices might result in missed pathology, as has been empirically discovered. Therefore, contiguous (no gap) sections are required.

High signal-to-noise ratios are required to avoid obscuring small lesions. The most widely employed pulse sequence is a conventional spin-echo T_1-weighted image (short repetition time [TR], short echo time [TE]) in the coronal plane and sagittal planes before and after gadolinium administration. Good signal-to-noise ratios can be obtained with two to four excitations. More than four excitations (averages) increase the imaging time and the likelihood of patient movement. The placement of inferior saturation bands diminish flow-related artifact, especially on postcontrast sequences. Two excitations may be used to save time for sagittal plane imaging, since experience has shown that the sagittal plane is less valuable than the coronal for defining intraglandular lesions. Although T_2-weighted imaging is usually not necessary, coronal fast spin-echo T_2-weighted sequence may be useful to improve tissue differentiation in complex cases (Figure 20.4). Coronal and sagittal images are usually sufficient. Axial imaging is reserved for those few cases with large masses in which the axial plane helps to define lateral extension (Figure 20.5). Gadolinium enhancement significantly improves tissue contrast and may show subtle lesions, particularly microadenomas that are otherwise difficult to detect on noncontrast studies [55].

Many authors advocate dynamic scanning as a technique to increase sensitivity to pituitary lesions. They suggest that with fast scanning during the early infusion of contrast, differentiation between normal and neoplastic tissue can be detected due to the differing dynamics of contrast enhancement. Several investigators compared dynamic and conventional sequences and found superior sensitivity in detection of microadenomas [5–9]. The largest and best-conducted series by Tabarin et al. [10] found that dynamic MRI had improved sensitivity, but decreased specificity compared to conventional MRIs. This study, however, was limited by using a 1.0 Tesla magnet, unlike the current state-of-the-art high-field MRs, including that used in the Friedman et al. article, which used at least a 1.5-Tesla magnet (Figure 20.6) [10,11].

The anterior pituitary generates a homogeneous or slightly heterogeneous signal, approximately isointense (of similar signal) to cortical brain on noncontrast T_1-weighted images (Figure 20.7). The signal throughout

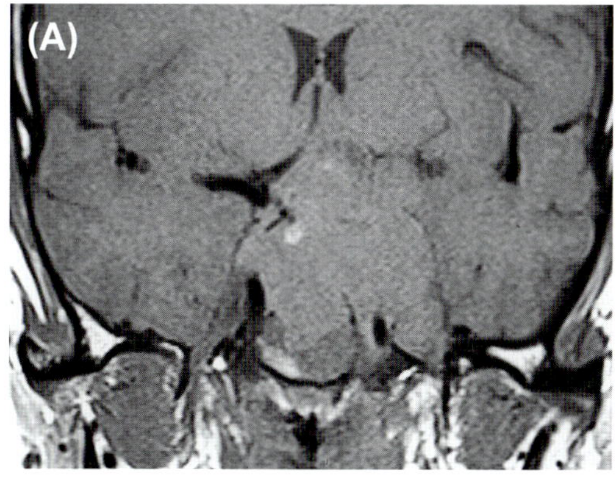

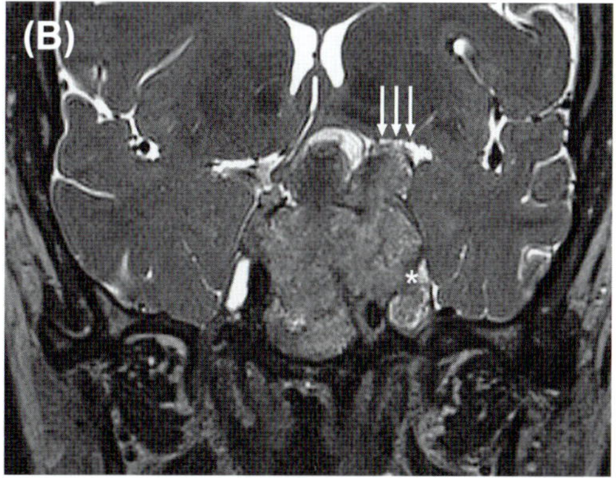

FIGURE 20.4 A 21-year-old male with a large prolactinoma. (A) Coronal precontrast T_1-weighted and (B) coronal T_2-weighted MR. Only noncontrast sequences could be obtained due to gadolinium allergy. The superior extent of the tumor and its interface with adjacent brain tissue is considerably clearer on the T_2 image (arrows). Note left-sided cavernous sinus invasion by tumor (*).

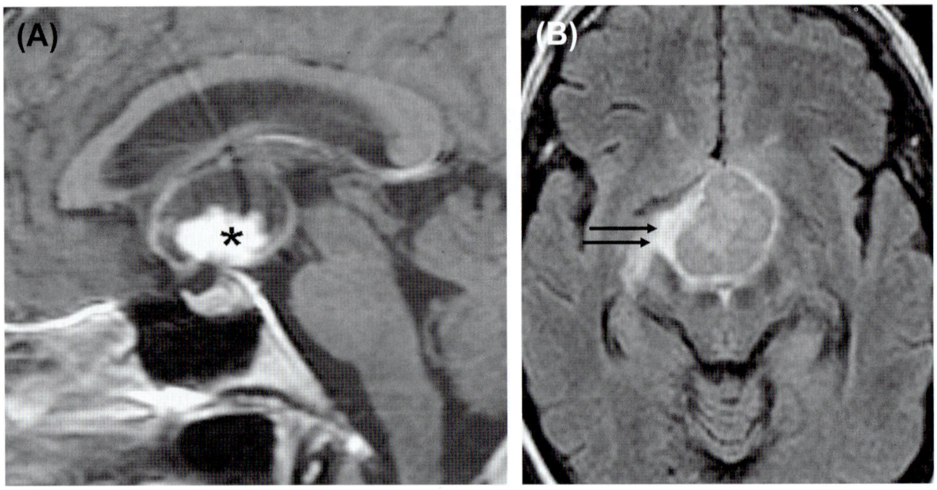

FIGURE 20.5 Craniopharyngioma. (A) Sagittal T_1-weighted MR shows a mixed solid and cystic mass (*). (B) Axial FLAIR image defines the lateral extent of the mass (arrows).

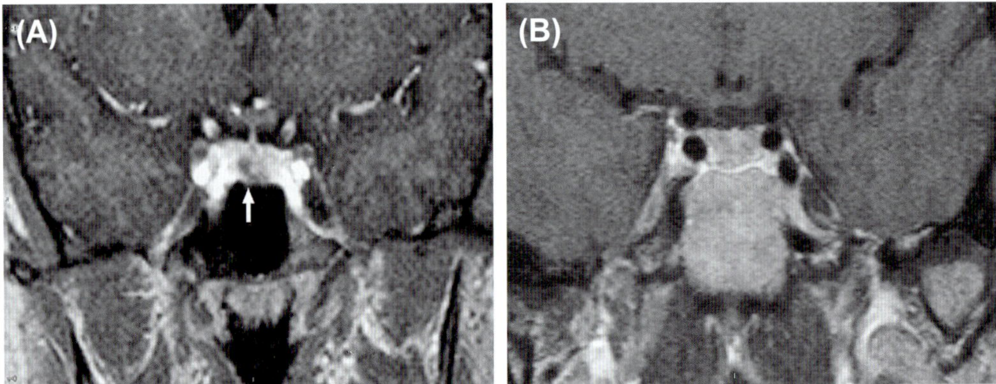

FIGURE 20.6 Dynamic MR technique. (A) Coronal dynamic image shows a hypoenhancing lesion on the right (open arrow). (B) The lesion is more difficult to discern from adjacent normal pituitary tissue on conventional postcontrast image.

the anterior pituitary is moderately to markedly increased with contrast administration. In third trimester fetuses, infants up to 2–3 months of age and pregnant females, the anterior pituitary is hyperintense in signal, thought to be secondary to hyperplasia of prolactin cells responding to placental estrogen (Figure 20.8) [12].

The cavernous sinuses are hypointense relative to the pituitary and contiguous brain and, therefore, are easily recognized. They also show enhancement with contrast. The medial dural margin of the cavernous sinus is not well seen as a separate structure whereas the lateral dural wall is usually well defined. The intracavernous neural structures are of lower intensity than the sinus itself. Rapid flow in the carotid arteries results in a signal void that clearly defines these vessels within the cavernous sinuses on noncontrast scans (Figure 20.9). Since the cavernous sinuses enhance approximately equally to the pituitary, the margin between the two is less conspicuous on contrast-enhanced scans. However, the carotid arteries and the neural structures remain visible because of the signal void (rapid flow) of the carotid arteries and the low signal (but greater than the carotid signal) of the normally nonenhancing neural structures.

In the suprasellar space the carotid, anterior and middle cerebral arteries are usually well visualized because of the signal void created by the rapid blood flow. The optic chiasm, optic nerves and infundibulum are clearly delineated on T_1-weighted images, and thereby provide excellent contrast for the vessels and neural structures. The optic chiasm and nerves do not enhance with gadolinium administration because of their blood–brain barrier, but the infundibulum enhances similarly to the pituitary (see Figure 20.12), because of the absence of a blood–brain barrier. It measures 2–3 mm in width (Figure 20.9).

The posterior pituitary is normally hyperintense (bright) on T_1-weighted images (Figure 20.10). Initially

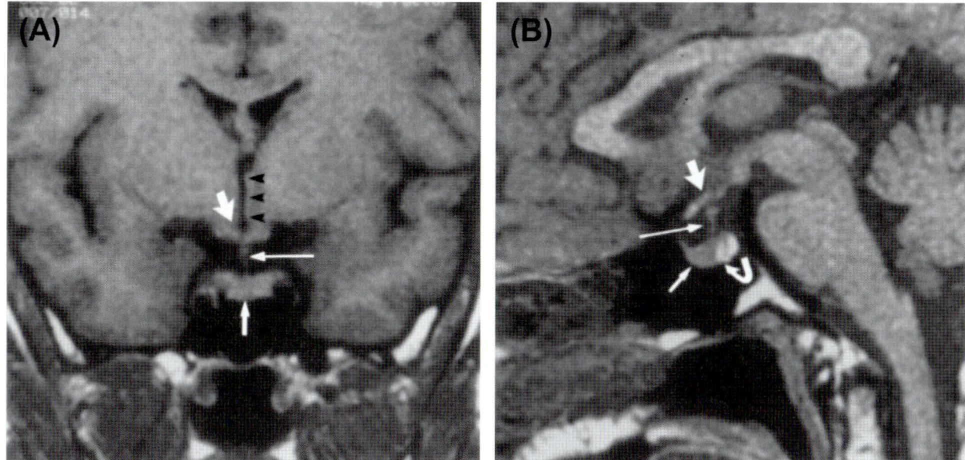

FIGURE 20.7 Normal 37-year-old woman. (A) Coronal T_1-weighted noncontrast MRI. The pituitary gland (arrow) is slightly concave superiorly. The infundibular stalk (long arrow), optic chiasm (broad arrow) and third ventricle (arrowheads) are well visualized. (B) Midline sagittal T_1-weighted noncontrast MRI. Chiasm (broad arrow), infundibular stalk (long arrow), anterior pituitary (arrow), posterior pituitary (curved arrow) and sphenoid sinus are visualized.

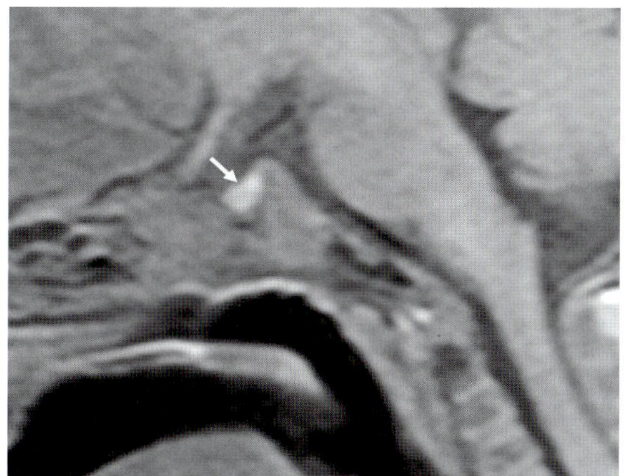

FIGURE 20.8 Normal 3-month-old male, noncontrast sagittal MR. Note the hyperintense (bright) signal of the anterior pituitary (arrow).

this was thought to be secondary to fat in the sella turcica posterior to the pituitary. Subsequently it has become clear that the high signal emanates from the posterior pituitary itself, and specifically from the phospholipid vesicles containing the neurosecretory granules [13–15]. It has been suggested that absence of high signal in the posterior pituitary reflects loss-of-function [16,17]. However, several studies have now shown that a small percentage of normal patients do not demonstrate this high signal [14,18,19]. Many, but not all, patients with diabetes insipidus lack the posterior pituitary "bright spot" [16,20]. Although the posterior pituitary may be differentiated from the anterior pituitary on MR because it displays greater signal, this is not true on contrast-enhanced MR where enhancement of the anterior pituitary reduces the contrast between the two lobes.

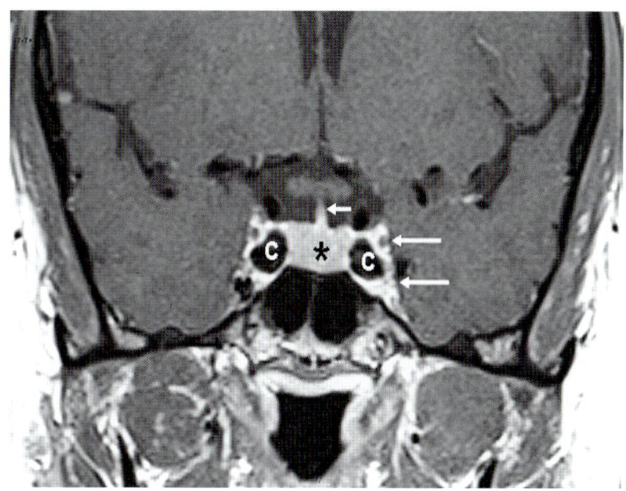

FIGURE 20.9 Normal 38-year-old woman. Coronal postcontrast MR shows homogeneously enhancing gland (*) and stalk (short arrow). Note the greater degree of contrast uptake in the cavernous sinuses, which contain the carotid arteries (C) easily depicted by their flow voids. Small hypointense dots (long arrows) are the cranial nerves within the cavernous sinuses.

Idiopathic growth hormone deficiency is often associated with a hypoplastic anterior pituitary, a thin or absent stalk and an aberrantly located posterior pituitary bright spot [21–23]. An absent or transected stalk will preclude transport of the neurosecretory granules from the hypothalamus, with development of an ectopic "bright spot" in the hypothalamus or proximal stalk (Figure 20.11). This is seen in trauma and surgical transection. A thickened stalk has been reported in idiopathic central diabetes insipidus. This is probably related to an infiltrative process including lymphocytic adenohypophysitis, Langerhans histiocytosis and tumors such as a germinoma [24].

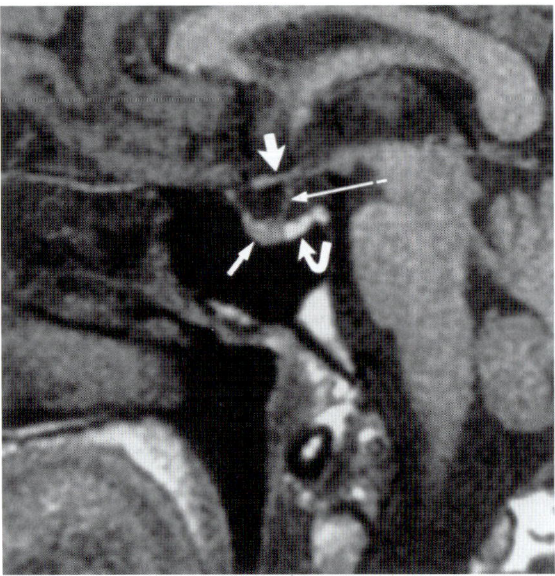

FIGURE 20.10 Normal 45-year-old man. T_1-weighted noncontrast MRI. The posterior pituitary (curved arrow) has a much higher signal (brighter) than the anterior pituitary (arrow). The superior margin of the pituitary is flat or slightly concave. The infundibular stalk (long arrow) and chiasm (broad arrow) are isointense (same intensity) to brain tissue.

Spatial resolution of MRI is not quite equivalent to CT, but definition of sellar size and shape are sufficiently clear with MRI to be diagnostic of most significant changes. Although it is true that cortical bone produces little if any signal on MRI, thus reducing fine bony detail, the significance of delineation of subtle bone changes has been markedly reduced with MRI because of its capability of directly defining pathologic changes within the tissues. Further, MRI is very effective in defining infiltration of medullary bone, exceeding CT in this respect, and this may be important in the detection of bony extension of disease processes.

TABLE 20.1 Maximum Cephalo–Caudad Dimension (mm) of "Normal" Pituitary on MRI

	Age (Year)		
	0–11	12–50	>50
Male	5	7	5
Female	5	9	5
Pregnancy	–	12	–

The above guidelines based on data from [16–23]

Nuclear medicine may play a role in pituitary evaluation. Parasellar and intrasellar masses may be detected with brain imaging radiopharmaceuticals, especially with SPECT imaging. Indium [111]-labeled octreotide may be useful in the detection of growth-hormone-secreting tumors and following their response to treatment [25].

PITUITARY SIZE AND SHAPE

Numerous studies in the literature discuss the appearance of the normal pituitary on CT and MRI (Table 20.1) [26–33]. Review of these indicates a continued evolution in assessment of normal values. Initially, gland heights of greater than 7 mm, and superior convexity of the gland, were said to be abnormal. However, the pituitary gland in females in the child-bearing years is often superiorly convex with an increased height, usually no more than 9 mm (Figure 20.12) [26,28,34]. Even in nonpregnant females, and males, superior convexity has not been verified as an absolute indicator of pituitary pathology. Both boys and girls may develop an increase in pituitary height during puberty [35]. All pituitary dimensions diminish in the elderly, and the posterior pituitary "bright spot" may be absent in as many as 29%. According to Terano

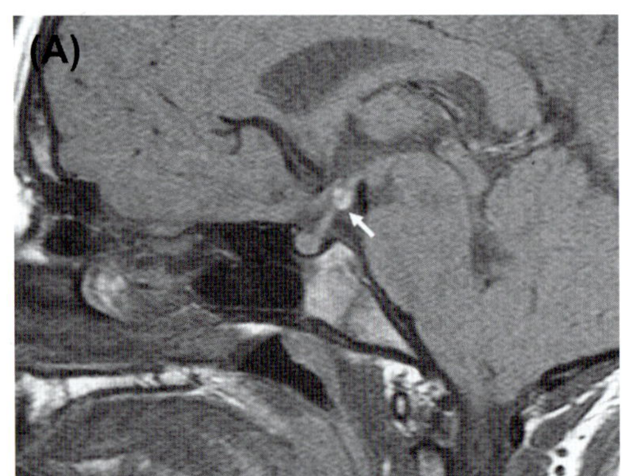

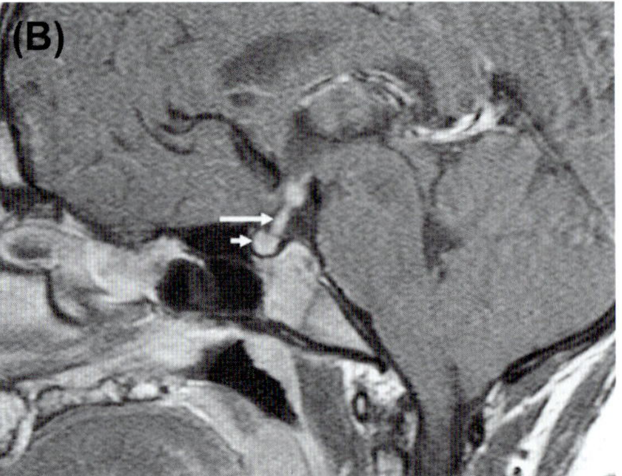

FIGURE 20.11 A 17-year-old female with hypopituitarism. Sagittal MR without (A) and with contrast (B) reveals the posterior pituitary not to be in its normal position within the sella but situated between the proximal stalk and hypothalamus (arrow). (B) Note normal enhancement of the pituitary (short arrow) and stalk (long arrow).

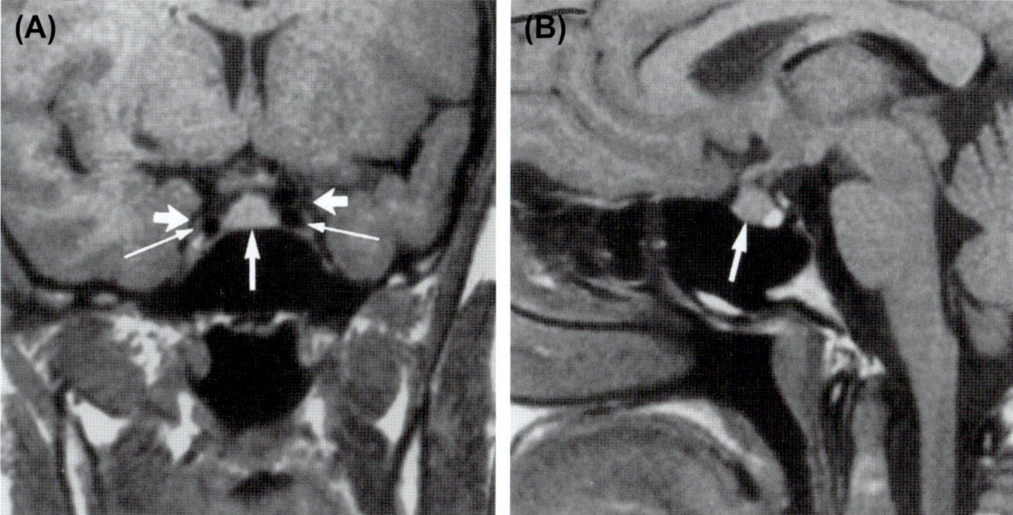

FIGURE 20.12 Normal 29-year-old woman. (A) Coronal and (B) sagittal T_1-weighted noncontrast MRI. The pituitary gland (arrow) is superiorly convex and measures 9 mm in height. However, there are no focal areas of signal abnormality. This is a common appearance in normal women of childbearing age. The cavernous sinuses are hypointense to the pituitary (short arrows), and the carotid arteries are seen as a signal void in the cavernous sinuses (long arrows).

[36] the neurosecretory granule depletion in the elderly may be secondary to persistently raised serum osmolality. Loss of glandular size with aging may result in the "empty sella."

Weiner et al. [30] reported a mean (± SD) normal gland height of 5.4 (± 0.9) mm, while Roppoll et al. [31] found a greater mean gland height for females than males (4.2 ± 1.4 mm vs. 3.6 ± 0.9 mm, respectively). The mean height was said to increase from 3.3 ± 0.4 mm, under age 11 years, 4.2 ± 1.5 mm, for ages 12 through 60 years and to decline to 3.9 ± 1.0 mm after age 60 [31,32]. Wolpert et al. [32] found females in the childbearing years to have a pituitary gland height as great as 9 mm. Swartz et al. [33] reported an average gland height of 7.1 ± 1.1 mm in women in the childbearing years; Gonzalez et al. [28] found a significant increase in pituitary dimensions in pregnant females with an increase of 2.6 mm in all three dimensions occurring by the end of pregnancy.

Pituitary enlargement may be seen in patients with intracranial hypotension. This condition may be secondary to a multitude of causes including CSF shunt procedures and spontaneous spinal CSF leaks (often associated with mesenchymal disease such as Marfan's syndrome). As a consequence of the reduced intracranial pressure pituitary hyperemia may result in a pituitary pseudomass (Figure 20.13) [37].

"Small" glands are most often normal, especially in the elderly [30,31]. They are frequently associated with intrasellar fluid, the so-called "empty sella" (Figure 20.14), which itself has no predictive value for pituitary

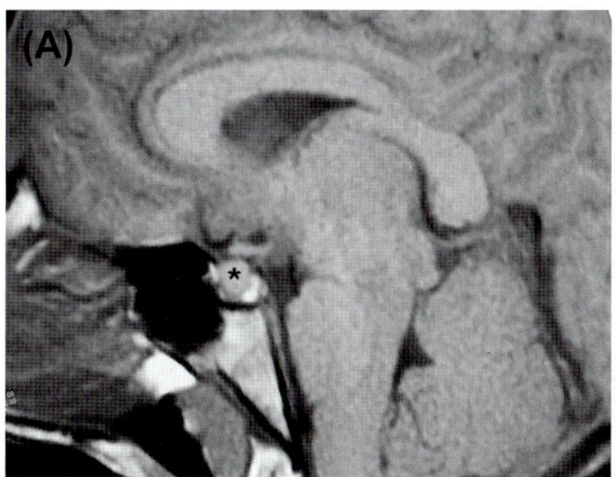

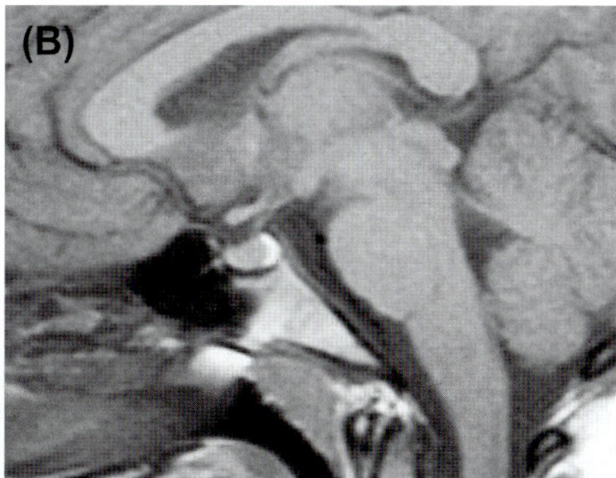

FIGURE 20.13 A 38-year-old woman with spontaneous intracranial hypotension. (A) Sagittal T_1-weighted brain MR obtained for headaches shows an enlarged and superiorly convex pituitary (*). Note the inferiorly displaced optic chiasm that is almost abutted by the gland. Sagittal T_1-weighted brain MR (B) after an epidural blood patch for CSF leak repair depicts increased CSF space between the gland and the optic chiasm. The pituitary gland is no longer superiorly convex.

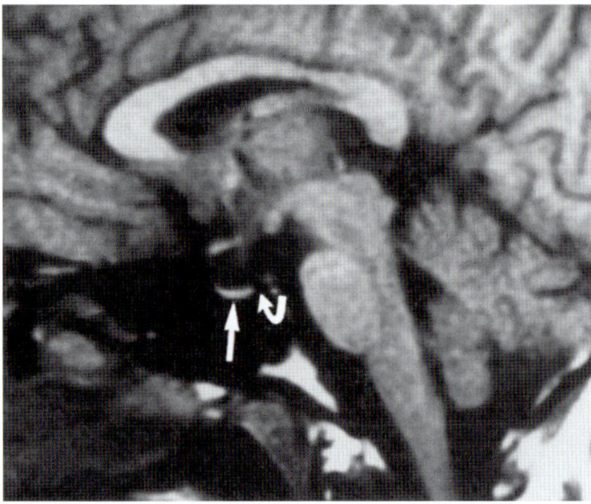

FIGURE 20.14 Midsagittal T_1-weighted noncontrast MRI of a small anterior pituitary (arrow) with no high-signal posterior pituitary visible in the posterior sella turcica (curved arrow). The patient had normal function of the anterior and posterior pituitary.

pathology (see below). Pituitary gland and infundibular hypoplasia are frequently seen in patients with pituitary dwarfism.

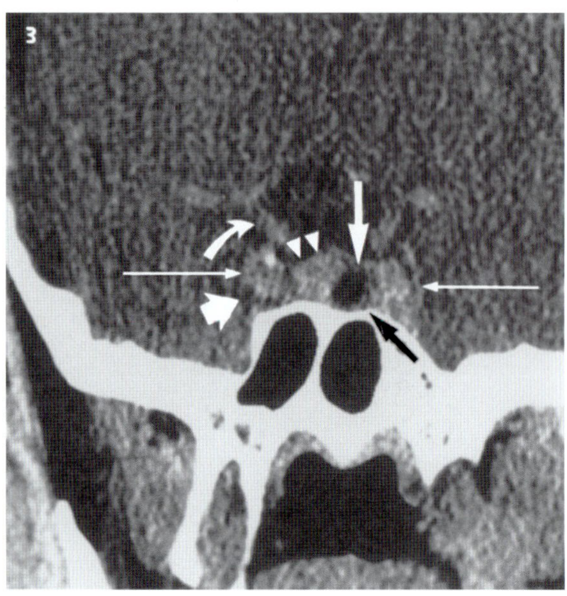

FIGURE 20.15 Contrast-enhanced direct coronal CT showing a nonenhancing microadenoma on the left (arrow). The normal pituitary enhances diffusely with the iodinated contrast (white darts). The cavernous sinuses (long arrows) and carotid arteries (curved arrows) are visualized but not as well as with MRI. Neural structures are seen as low-density (nonenhancing) areas in the cavernous sinuses (broad arrow).

MICROADENOMAS

Pituitary adenomas occur very commonly, with an incidence as high as 27% in some autopsy series. Prolactin (PRL)-containing cells are seen in up to 41% of these lesions. Therefore, the incidence of prolactinomas in the general population could be as high as 10% [38,39]. Prolactinomas have been diagnosed with an increasing frequency in recent years. Several factors may be involved, including the development of an excellent serum assay and constantly improving neuroradiologic imaging.

Prolactinomas are most often found in the posterolateral aspect of the anterior pituitary lobe. The diagnosis of a central lesion as a prolactinoma should be suspect. Lactotrophs are primarily located in the lateral aspect of the anterior lobe [40]. Growth-hormone (GH)-producing lesions may be central or lateral [40,41]. Pars media cysts are usually central, which may be their only differentiating feature from prolactinomas. These cysts occurred in 13–20% of an unselected autopsy series [42].

A number of imaging criteria have been advanced for the diagnosis of microadenomas. The most reliable, on both CT and MRI, is direct visualization of an intrapituitary lesion [43–60]. Most pituitary microadenomas are hypointense relative to the remainder of the gland on contrast-enhanced CT (Figure 20.15). A few have been reported to be hyperdense and others isodense and therefore may not be visualized unless they cause secondary findings. David et al. [58] reported that 43% of surgically proven microadenomas were isodense on noncontrast CT. Accordingly CT without contrast enhancement has a high failure rate in detection of microadenomas. In addition, technical factors, such as quantum mottle (graininess of a radiographic image attributed to the corpuscular nature of radiation [photons] and statistical variation in their distribution) and noise (spurious electrical pulses which degrade an image) [61], may result in a mottled heterogeneity of the gland on CT, thereby obscuring small hypodense lesions of 1–3 mm.

Most microadenomas detected by MRI are seen as an area of relative hypointensity on noncontrast- and contrast-enhanced T_1-weighted MRI images (Figure 20.16) but a few hyperintense lesions have been reported [51,60]. Bromocriptine therapy usually shrinks prolactinomas but may cause cellular changes and/or hemorrhage resulting in an increased signal within the gland on T_1 images (Figure 20.17) [51,62]. A case of three pituitary microadenomas has been reported [63].

Focal superior convexity of the gland without definite glandular enlargement has a greater predictive value for intraglandular pathology than does general convexity of the superior margin (Figure 20.18). However, as noted previously, superior convexity of the gland may be relatively marked in normal females of childbearing age, especially in pregnancy. Eccentric position of the

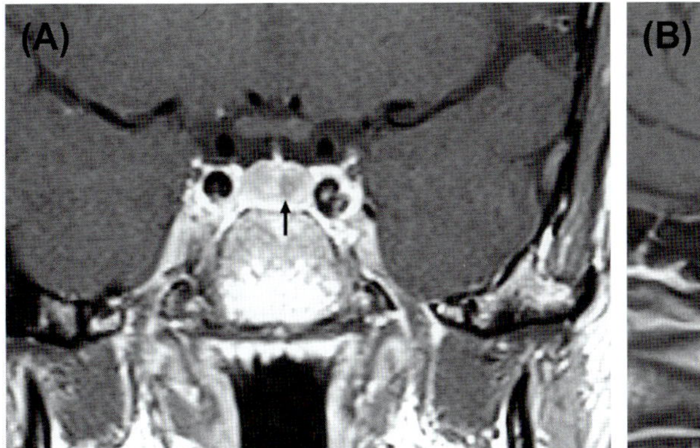

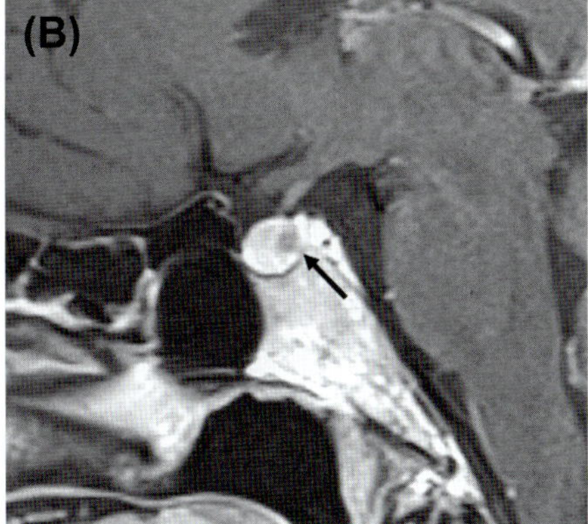

FIGURE 20.16 A 35-year-old woman with hyperprolactinemia due to microadenoma. (A) Coronal and (B) sagittal T_1-weighted contrast-enhanced MR demonstrate a hypoenhancing lesion within the pituitary gland (arrow).

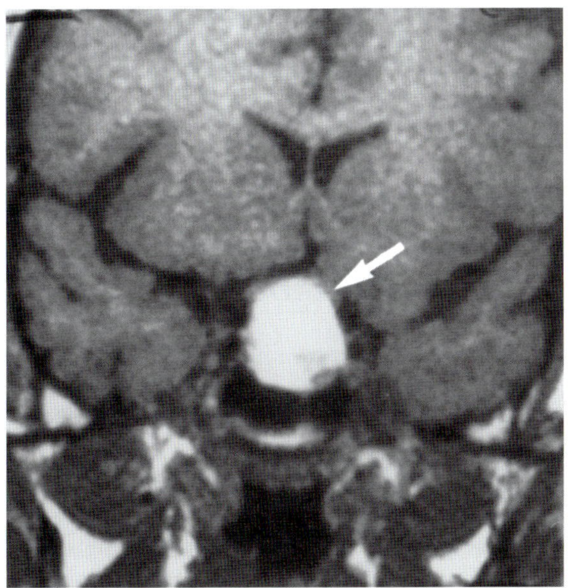

FIGURE 20.17 Effects of bromocriptine shown on a coronal T_1-weighted noncontrast MRI. A hemorrhagic pituitary mass (arrow) demonstrates high signal as a result of extracellular methemoglobin. Patient had received bromocriptine therapy to treat the mass and marked hyperprolactinemia.

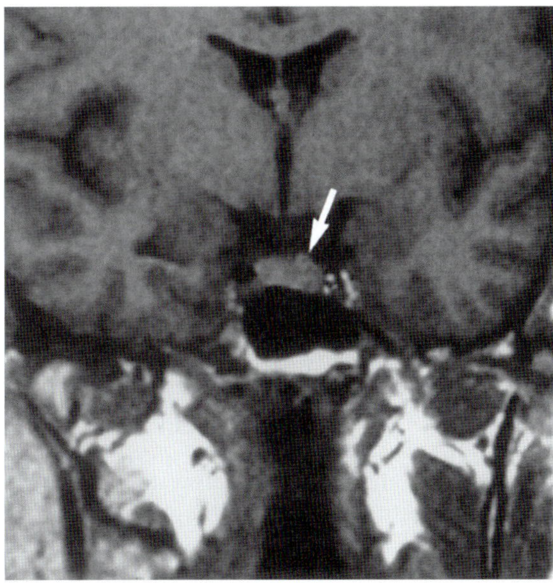

FIGURE 20.18 Coronal noncontrast T_1-weighted MRI in a patient with a left-sided isointense microadenoma suggested by focal superior convexity (arrow).

infundibulum in the transverse plane is of limited value since it is present infrequently with microadenomas [58]. However, when present and otherwise unexplained, it should increase suspicion for the presence of an intraglandular lesion. In most cases of significant infundibular displacement, it is displaced away from the lesion, but on occasion displacement may be towards the lesions. The infundibulum can be seen in virtually all T_1-weighted coronal MRI studies performed with contiguous thin sections. Since the infundibulum enhances with iodinated contrast, it is also seen in most CT studies. It may be difficult to visualize if a mass elevates or distorts it.

Enlargement of the gland to a height greater than 8 mm has also been found to be a poor criterion for microadenomas. Only five of 39 patients with proven microadenomas had gland heights greater than 8 mm [61].

Abnormality of the sellar floor and size are the least valuable indicators of glandular disease [38,47,58]. The presence of such abnormalities was frequently not correlated with the location of the lesion in the gland, and very often no such abnormalities were present in cases with proven microadenomas. The size of the sella turcica poorly correlated with pituitary size, especially when suprasellar fluid extends into the sella (partially empty sella, see below).

Gadolinium Enhancement

Gadolinium is a paramagnetic agent that can change the magnetic properties of tissues in which it collects, thereby causing enhancement of the structure on MRI (brighter image). Gadolinium enhancement has been used in an attempt to increase the conspicuity of pituitary microadenomas [41,55,58]. Greater enhancement of the normal gland relative to the lesion will result in the lesion being seen as a relatively hypointense area (Figure 20.16). The physiology of gadolinium deposition is similar to that of iodinated contrast used for CT, and therefore gadolinium enhancement with MRI can be expected to be at least as sensitive. Since contrast sensitivity of MRI is much greater than that of CT, gadolinium enhancement has the potential to add significantly to the diagnosis of intraglandular lesions. Strict attention to technical detail is required for diagnostic accuracy. Scanning must be performed within several minutes after the gadolinium is administered to allow for the greatest differential enhancement between the normal gland and the lesion. As time passes the lesion will also enhance and may become equal in intensity to the normal gland, and its conspicuity will actually decrease. Even with proper scan timing, some lesions may enhance at the same rate as the normal gland and thereby be obscured. Dynamic scanning will obviate this possibility (Figure 20.6).

In cases with suspicion of a prolactinoma, a noncontrast scan may be sufficient, even if negative, because it will exclude a mass impinging upon the chiasm or extending into the cavernous sinuses or temporal fossae. Medical therapy may then be safely instituted, based upon hormonal studies, without the necessity for absolute verification of the presence of a microadenoma. If more definite recognition of a microadenoma is needed such as with medical regimen failure or intolerance, contrast-enhanced scans are also indicated.

On the other hand, for Cushing's disease and acromegaly or gigantism, surgery is often indicated and it is highly desirable to define the exact location of the responsible lesion (Figures 20.6 and 20.18). Since excess ACTH production may occur from a pituitary tumor, or from an extrapituitary tumor ectopically secreting ACTH, treatment depends on the exact localization of the offending lesion [58]. Nonvisualization of an ACTH-producing pituitary tumor may result in an unnecessary, expensive, and, on occasion, invasive procedure to locate the lesion. It is therefore essential that the imaging of the pituitary be done with strict attention to technical detail as previously discussed. Noncontrast and gadolinium-enhanced studies with imaging immediately after the administration of the gadolinium should be performed. Dwyer et al. [51] detected a total eight of 12 pituitary Cushing's tumors on noncontrast MRI and ten of 12 only on contrast-enhanced MRI. Only after such careful evaluation of the pituitary is it appropriate to consider the MRI study negative and to proceed with additional evaluation including adrenal imaging and chest CT. Saris et al. [62] found a low sensitivity (30%) of CT in the detection of ACTH-producing tumors. Others indicated a less than 50% accuracy of CT in locating proven intrapituitary ACTH-producing tumors [64]. Dynamic imaging improves overall detectability, but due to lower resolution there is a reduced specificity [65]. Friedman et al. reported very high sensitivity and specificity in their series of mild Cushing's syndrome utilizing dynamic technique [11]. They attribute the improved specificity and sensitivity to high-field, latest-generation MR scanners. MR cannot be considered definitive in excluding pituitary sources of excess cortisol production, and if negative, venous sampling should be considered.

Fortunately most GH-producing tumors are large and easily located by CT and MRI. At presentation 75% are 1 cm or greater [66]. Careful attention to technique in imaging will improve the sensitivity for diagnosis of the few microadenomas that are found associated with excess GH production.

MACROADENOMAS

Regardless of the hormonal activity of pituitary macroadenomas, the optimal imaging technique remains the same as for microadenomas. With most macroadenomas contrast administration is desirable.

Non-contrast MRI studies of macroadenomas will demonstrate one or more of the following: (1) enlargement of the sella turcica; (2) depression or focal erosion of the sellar floor; (3) undercutting of the tuberculum; (4) erosion of the dorsum; (5) focal or diffuse superior convexity of the pituitary gland; (6) a mass extending from the sella into the suprasellar space, and/or the cavernous sinuses; (7) a focal area of decreased signal within the gland; (8) displacement of the infundibulum; (9) elevation of the chiasm; and less commonly (10), a distortion and/or displacement of the posterior pituitary bright spot (Figure 20.19) [53,55,67–70]. Whereas microadenomas are often difficult to detect, macroadenomas are easily diagnosed, but require careful delineation of the extent of the lesion. An exception is the small to moderate-sized diffuse macroadenoma and diffuse hyperplasia which may be impossible to differentiate from a normal gland in a female in the child-bearing years. Occasionally, dynamic imaging will clarify the position of the normal gland adjacent to the tumor (Figure 20.20).

Once a macroadenoma has been recognized, or gland enlargement noted, gadolinium enhancement is often of

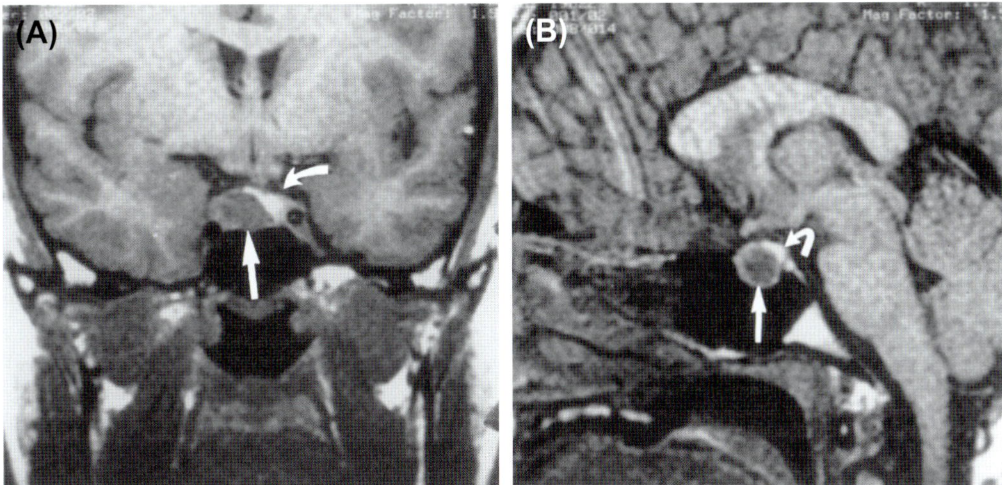

FIGURE 20.19 (A) Coronal and (B) sagittal noncontrast T_1-weighted MRI. Low-signal macroadenoma (arrow) distorts and displaces the high-signal posterior pituitary (curved arrow).

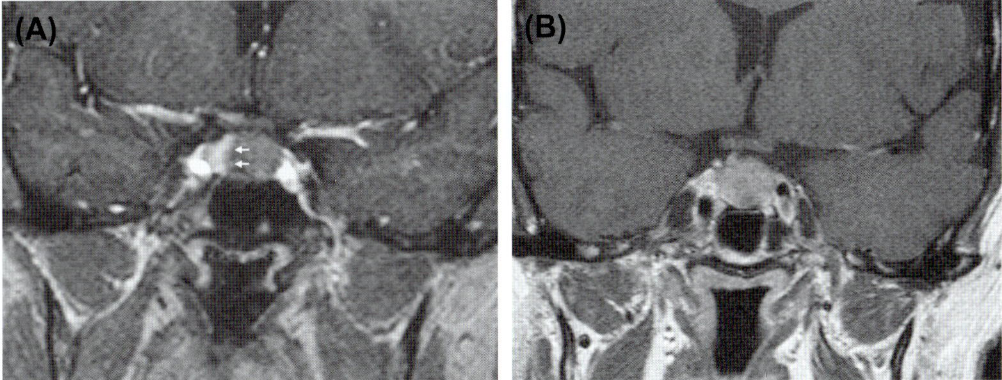

FIGURE 20.20 A 42-year-old woman with prolactinoma. Dynamic (A) and coronal conventional (B) T_1-weighted postcontrast images. Note the superior demarcation between gland and adenoma on the early phase dynamic image (arrows). This distinction is not clear on the late conventional image.

great value. It may define an otherwise isointense lesion within the gland by enhancing the normal gland to a greater extent and/or more rapidly. Gadolinium enhancement will also improve definition of the margins of large lesions extending into the suprasellar space and impressing upon the chiasm or brain parenchyma. The margins of such lesions may otherwise be indistinct on a noncontrast MRI examination (Figure 20.21).

Cavernous sinus invasion by pituitary tumors is often difficult to ascertain on CT and MRI. If lesion contrast enhancement is not as great as that of the cavernous sinus, a margin between the two may be clarified on enhanced studies (Figure 20.21) [55,67]. However, the medial dural margin of the cavernous sinuses is frequently indistinct, even in normal patients, and it is often very difficult to differentiate impingement upon the sinus from the true invasion. The most reliable criterion for sinus invasion is visualization of the lesion extending to the lateral margin of the carotid artery, and/or surrounding it. The artery is seen as a signal void on MRI, but cannot be separated from the remainder of the cavernous sinus on CT since both sinus and the vessel enhance. Even lateral bulging of the sinus could be secondary to lateral displacement of the sinus, and is not diagnostic of invasion. Recognition of sinus involvement is very important preoperatively for prognostic purposes, as the chance of total excision is greatly reduced.

Pituitary carcinomas tend to be large. The associated bony changes are often more irregular and/or infiltrative compared to the smooth enlargement and remodeling of the sellar margins seen with benign lesions. Since these rare malignancies may invade normal brain and extend through the skull base into the nasopharynx and upper neck, gadolinium enhancement is particularly valuable to define the margins of the lesion (Figure 20.22).

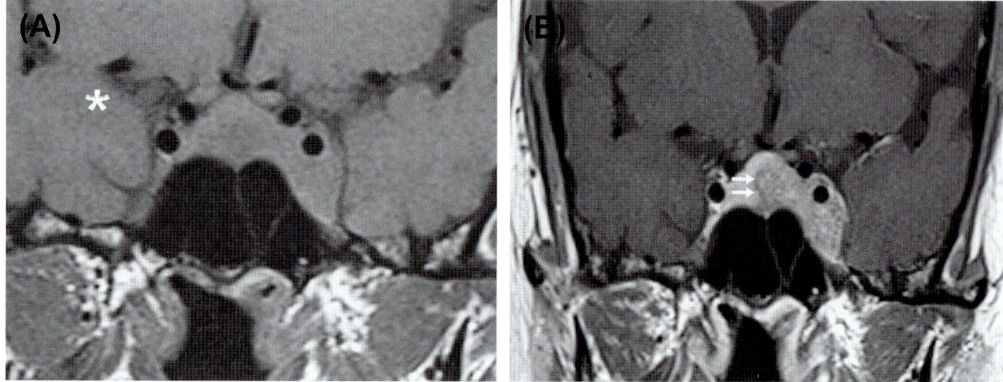

FIGURE 20.21 Left-sided macroadenoma with cavernous sinus invasion. (A) Noncontrast T_1 image shows the lesion to be isointense to the gland. (B) Postcontrast image clarifies the extent of cavernous sinus invasion (*) and the interface with adjacent gland (arrows).

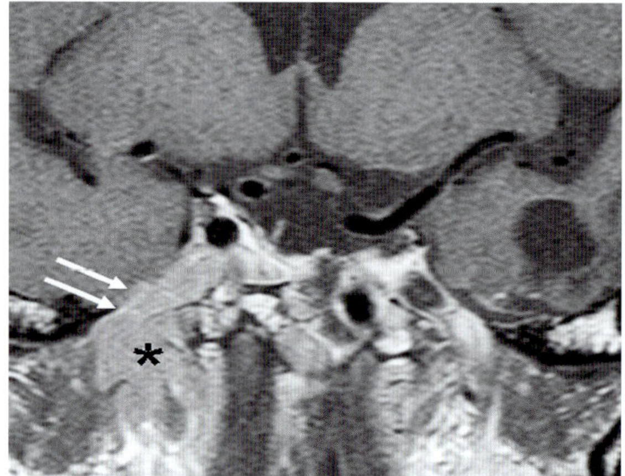

FIGURE 20.22 A 54-year-old man with pituitary carcinoma s/p pituitary surgery and radiotherapy. Note extension of cancer into the skull base and upper neck (*) through the cavernous sinus, Meckel's cave and foramen ovale (arrows).

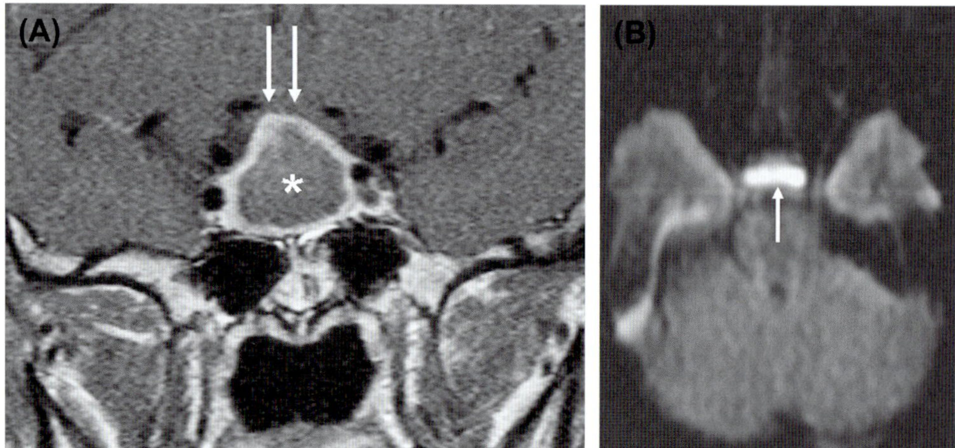

FIGURE 20.23 A 60-year-old man with pituitary abscess. (A) Coronal postcontrast T_1-weighted image shows pituitary mass (*) with suprasellar extension and chiasmatic compression (arrows), indistinguishable from a macroadenoma. (B) Axial diffusion-weighted image reveals hyperintense signal (arrow), strongly suggestive of pus contents, making the preoperative diagnosis possible.

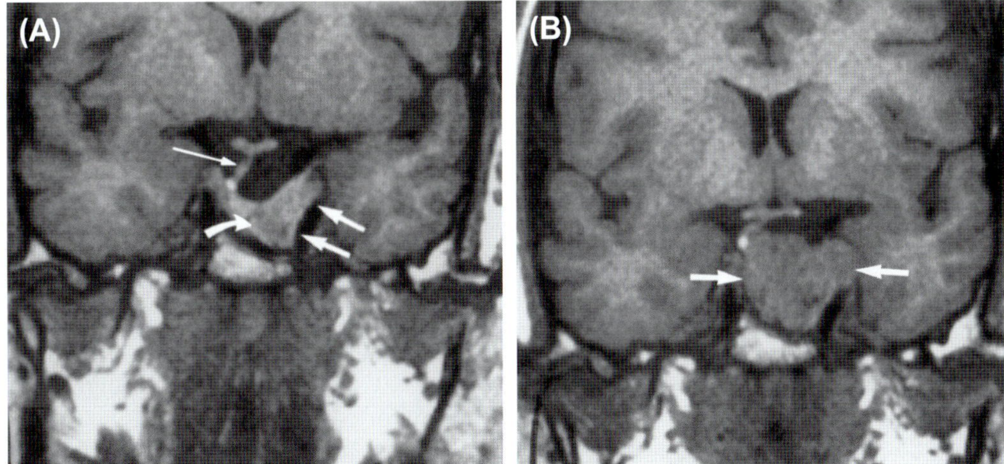

FIGURE 20.24 (A) T_1-weighted coronal noncontrast MRI of a 48-year-old woman treated with bromocriptine for hyperprolactinemia. The gland is unusual in shape (arrows), the infundibular stalk is deviated to the right (long arrow) and there is a large area of relatively decreased signal inferiorly, probably representing residual tumor (curved arrow). (B) When bromocriptine treatment was discontinued the prolactin level increased dramatically and this repeat MRI demonstrated marked tumor enlargement (arrows).

Macroadenomas, whether hormonally active or not, and whether benign or malignant, often develop cystic, necrotic and hemorrhagic areas. The former appear as low-signal regions on T_1-weighted images, and high signal on T_2-weighted images, whereas hemorrhage causes high signal on both sequences.

Pituitary hyperplasia will image as diffuse glandular enlargement. Infiltrative processes such as lymphoma, granulomatous diseases [71] and lymphocytic adenohypophysitis [72] (which is usually associated with stalk involvement and enlargement) may have a similar appearance. Clinical and hormonal information is crucial to the diagnosis and to differentiate these processes from macroadenomas. Rarely a pituitary abscess may enlarge all or part of the gland (Figure 20.23) [73].

Bromocriptine therapy for PRL-producing tumors results in an increased incidence of hemorrhage and/or other changes in the tumor that result in high signal on T_1-weighted images (Figure 20.17). Termination of bromocriptine therapy may be followed by rapid tumor enlargement (Figure 20.24). In cases of pituitary apoplexy, CT will show high density within the gland for the first 7–10 days after the hemorrhage, whereas MRI will show high intensity of the gland on T_1-weighted images obtained after the first several days. Initially, T_1-weighted images may only show an increased size of the gland or an area of relative hypointensity [74].

One of the most important considerations in evaluation of macroadenomas is the effect of the mass on the optic chiasm. In fact, a primary reason for MRI's superiority to CT for pituitary imaging is that it enables optimal evaluation of the suprasellar space and chiasm in virtually all cases, whereas with CT this is the exception rather than the rule. Elevation and deformity of the chiasm are best defined by coronal T_1-weighted images (Figure 20.25), although the sagittal plane may add additional information on some occasions.

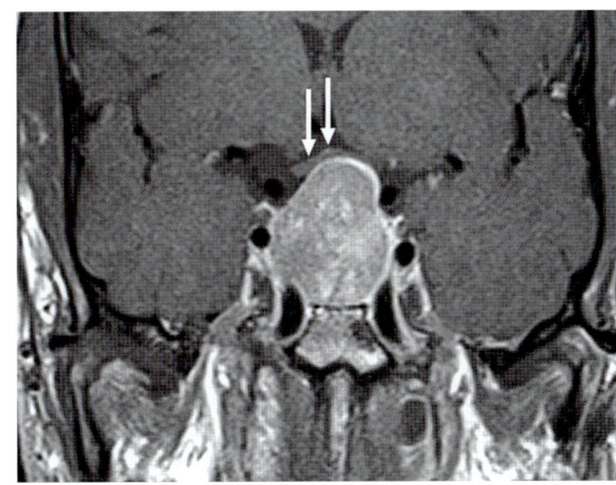

FIGURE 20.25 T_1-weighted postcontrast coronal image demonstrates large macroadenoma compressing the optic chiasm (arrows).

POSTERIOR PITUITARY

The posterior pituitary normally appears as an area of high signal on T_1-weighted images, probably reflecting the presence of neurosecretory granules (Figures 20.7 and 20.10). Specifically, it has been suggested that the phospholipid membrane of the vesicles is responsible for T_1 shortening and the attendant high signal [13–17,26,75,76]. Absence of the high signal in the posterior pituitary may be an indication of a nonfunctioning neurohypophysis, and many patients with diabetes insipidus do not show the "bright" spot of the posterior pituitary (Figure 20.26) [16,17,20,29,37,38,43,47,76].

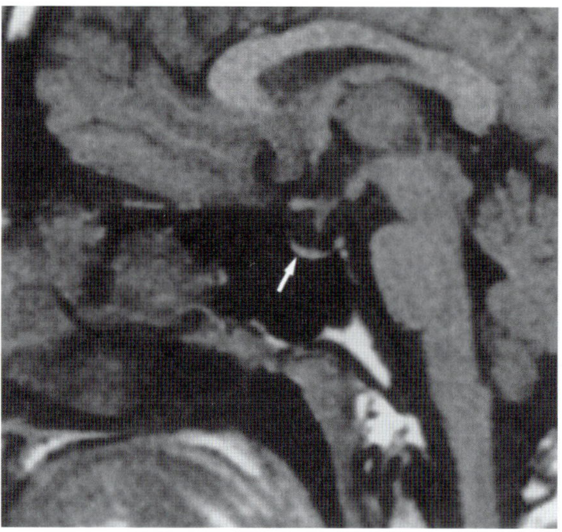

FIGURE 20.26 Sagittal T_1-weighted noncontrast MRI. A normal size "empty sella" with a thin rim of pituitary tissue inferiorly (arrow). This patient, evaluated for diabetes insipidus, does not demonstrate a posterior pituitary "bright spot."

However, a small percentage of normal patients also do not demonstrate this high-signal area.

A high-signal area in the hypothalamus or proximal infundibular stalk, thought to represent aberrant location of the pituitary, or at least of neurosecretory granules, has been reported in normal patients and in cases of presumed traumatic disruption of the pituitary stalk, hypophysectomy and pituitary tumors compressing or destroying the posterior pituitary. These patients may or may not manifest diabetes insipidus [20]. Since the high signal is related to the neurosecretory granules produced in the hypothalamus, it is not surprising that it may be seen in the stalk or in the hypothalamus if there is disruption in the normal transportation of neurosecretory products to the pituitary from the hypothalamus.

OTHER INTRASELLAR/SUPRASELLAR MASSES

Rathke's Cleft Cysts

Rathke's cleft cysts (RCC) are benign sellar cysts that arise from the invagination of Rathke's pouch, which is the precursor of anterior and intermediate lobes of the pituitary gland. They are lined with epithelium and contain serous or mucoid material. RCCs may present in the intrasellar and/or suprasellar compartments, most frequently crossing into both spaces. Purely suprasellar RCCs with a normal pituitary gland have also been reported [77].

RCC are usually a round, and sharply defined, intra- or suprasellar mass that typically lies anterior to the infundibular stalk. On CT, most are hypodense suggesting the presence of a serous fluid-filled cyst, but they may be isodense and, on a few occasions, even hyperdense with mucoid fluid. The MRI appearance is also variable, with most demonstrating hypointensity on T_1-weighted images and high signal on T_2-weighted images [78]. However, some are hyperintense on T_1-weighted images and, since they do not enhance, will appear hypointense to the enhancing gland on postcontrast T_1-weighted images (Figure 20.27). Cysts containing mucoid fluid can be hyperintense on T_1-weighted and T_2-weighted images [79], and mimic hemorrhage. In contrast to craniopharyngioma, RCCs do not calcify. Although they rarely show enhancement, RCCs occasionally have enhancing rims, which are thought to be due to normal displaced pituitary tissue [80].

Because cyst fluid of RCCs shows variable intensities on MR images, the diagnosis is often difficult when based on MR signal intensity values alone. Several authors have found a nonenhancing intracystic nodule in RCC in up to (77%) of the cases [81–83]. Detection of such intracystic nodules in lesions with signal characteristics on MR images typical of RCC, i.e., high signal

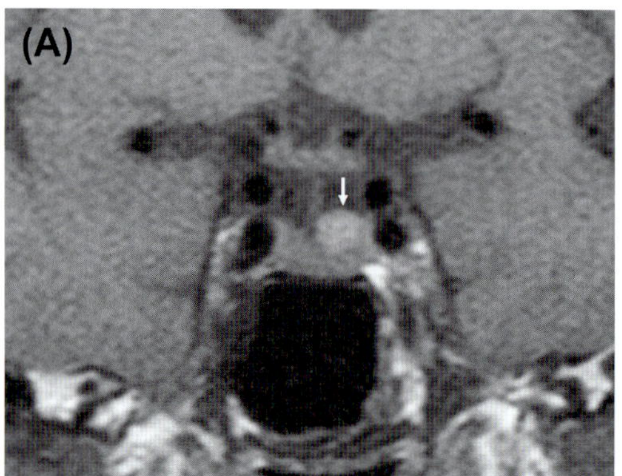

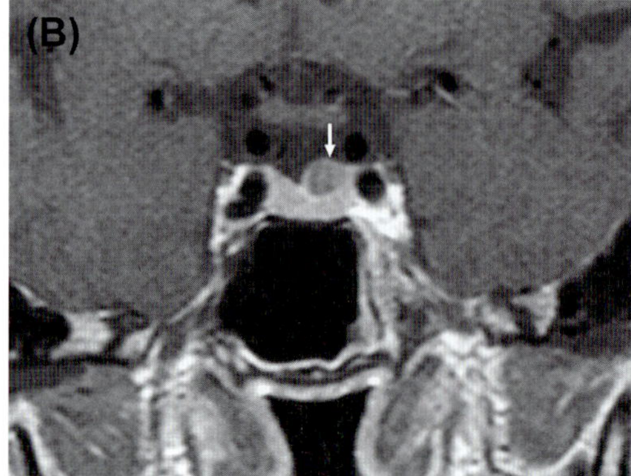

FIGURE 20.27 Sagittal (A) pre- and (B) postcontrast T_1-weighted MR of Rathke's cleft cyst Small hyperintense mass (arrow) just above the pituitary gland does not enhance with contrast on T_1-weighted postcontrast image.

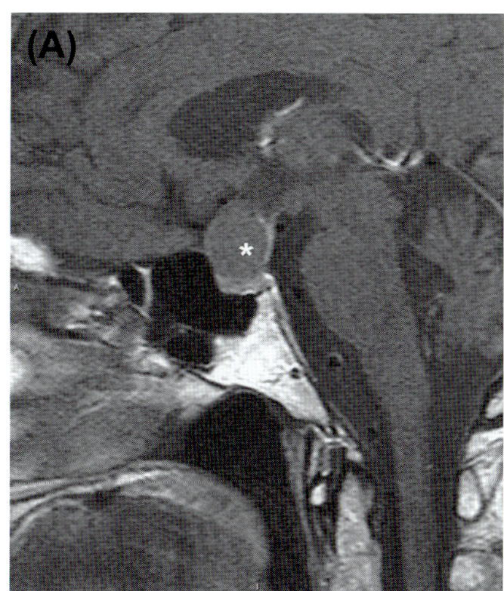

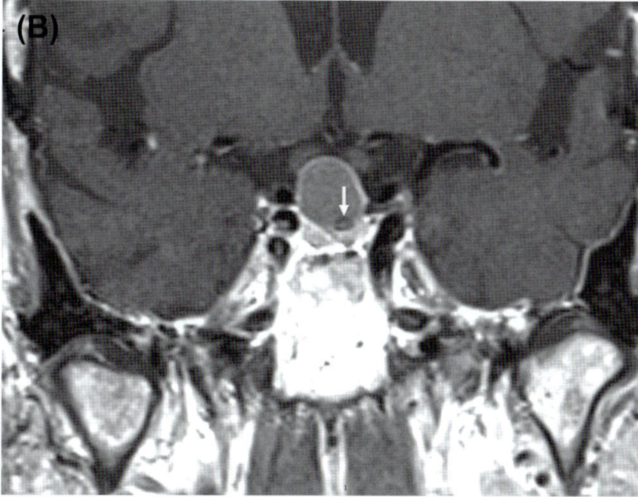

FIGURE 20.28 (A) Sagittal T_1-weighted postcontrast images demonstrate mildly hyperintense suprasellar mass (*). (B) Coronal T_1-weighted postcontrast image shows a nonenhancing intracystic nodule (arrow), typical of RCC.

intensity on T_1-weighted images and low signal intensity (nonenhancing) on T_2-weighted images, may be a diagnostic indicator of RCC (Figure 20.28). On occasion, however, they may be quite difficult to differentiate from pituitary tumors. In such cases hormonal studies may be the only differentiating feature.

Fortunately, most RCCs are asymptomatic, probably because of their relatively small size. Symptoms, when present, result from compression of optic chiasm, hypothalamus, or pituitary gland, and are indistinguishable from those caused by other sellar masses, such as craniopharyngioma or pituitary adenoma. However, cyst aspiration and partial removal of RCC generally suffices in contrast to the need for more complete resection in other sellar neoplasms.

Craniopharyngiomas

Craniopharyngiomas derive from epithelial remnants of Rathke's pouch. They may arise anywhere along the infundibular stalk from the floor of the third ventricle to the pituitary gland [18]. Although histologically benign, these tumors frequently recur after treatment. A bimodal distribution peak has been reported, with one peak at age 5–14 years and the other at age 65–74 years. Craniopharyngiomas are typically suprasellar in location but may extend into the sella. Prechiasmatic craniopharyngiomas usually result in optic atrophy and visual field defects. Retrochiasmatic craniopharyngiomas are commonly associated with signs of increased intracranial pressure (papilledema) caused by compression of the hypothalamus and protrusion into the third ventricle. Pediatric craniopharyngiomas are complex lesions containing cysts, solid components, calcification and hemorrhage. Calcification is very common, occurring in half or more of children and a lesser but significant percentage of adults (Figure 20.3). Calcification may involve the solid component or the wall of the cyst and is another differentiating feature from pituitary tumors, which infrequently calcify [84–86].

Characteristic rim and nodular calcifications are best detected on CT. On MR, these lesions have a heterogeneous appearance with a solid contrast-enhancing portion and cystic components (Figure 20.29). Cysts frequently contain high-protein, cholesterol, or blood products, which appear hyperintense on unenhanced T_1-weighted images. The solid portions and cyst wall enhance heterogeneously. Calcifications are poorly seen on MRI, whereas the CT definition of calcification is excellent, so that CT may on occasion improve the specificity of diagnosis in the case of craniopharyngiomas (Figure 20.3). However, since most craniopharyngiomas are relatively distinctive in their MRI appearance, with both cystic and solid components, lipid-like areas, and variegated signal, CT is rarely necessary. MRI with its multiplanar capability is essential for defining the tumor extension and is the most important imaging method used to plan surgical approaches.

Hamartoma

Hamartomas are rare lesions of childhood, presenting commonly with precocious puberty and gelastic seizures. They are not true neoplasms but may increase in size over time.

On both CT and MRI, hamartomas have characteristics similar to gray matter. At MR imaging they are seen as well-defined pedunculated or sessile lesions at the tuber cinereum and are isointense [23] or mildly hypointense on T_1-weighted images, and iso- to

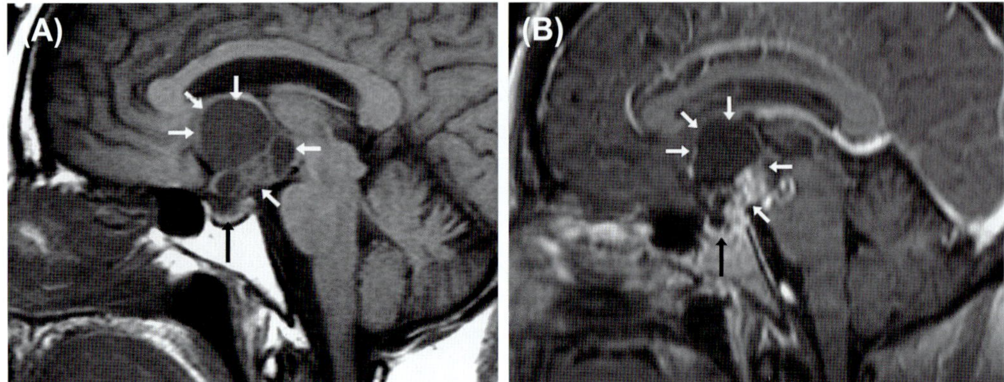

FIGURE 20.29 Craniopharyngioma. Sagittal (A) pre- and (B) postcontrast T_1-weighted MR demonstrate a multicystic suprasellar mass with enhancing solid components (arrows). Note the normal-sized and -shaped pituitary gland (black arrow).

hyperintense on T_2-weighted images, with no contrast enhancement or calcification [87]. The absence of any long-term change in the size, shape, or signal intensity of the lesion strongly supports the diagnosis of hypothalamic hamartoma [88].

Aneurysms

Intrasellar aneurysms arising from the cavernous carotid are rare. Prior to CT and MRI, the fear of such lesions or of medially positioned or tortuous carotid arteries extending into the sella turcica necessitated angiography in the preoperative evaluation for pituitary surgery. Such aneurysms may rarely cause sellar enlargement, simulating pituitary tumors. More often, and characteristically, they produce erosion along the lateral sellar margin at the carotid sulcus. CT and MRI have obviated the need for angiography in most instances because they directly demonstrate the carotid artery or the aneurysm. If an aneurysm is visualized, conventional angiography will usually be required for better definition prior to surgical or endovascular therapy. Particularly for cavernous aneurysms, endovascular therapy often may be more desirable than surgical treatment. Should there be a question as to the interpretation of CT or MRI regarding the presence of an aneurysm or tortuous vessel in the sella turcica, magnetic resonance angiography is now available and usually sufficient to clarify the diagnosis without requiring conventional angiography (Figure 20.30).

On occasion, cavernous carotid aneurysms may compress the lateral aspect of the pituitary gland sufficiently to result in elevation of the superior margin of the gland, simulating a pituitary tumor on sagittal magnetic resonance images. Such aneurysms should be easily recognizable as signal voids or mixed high and

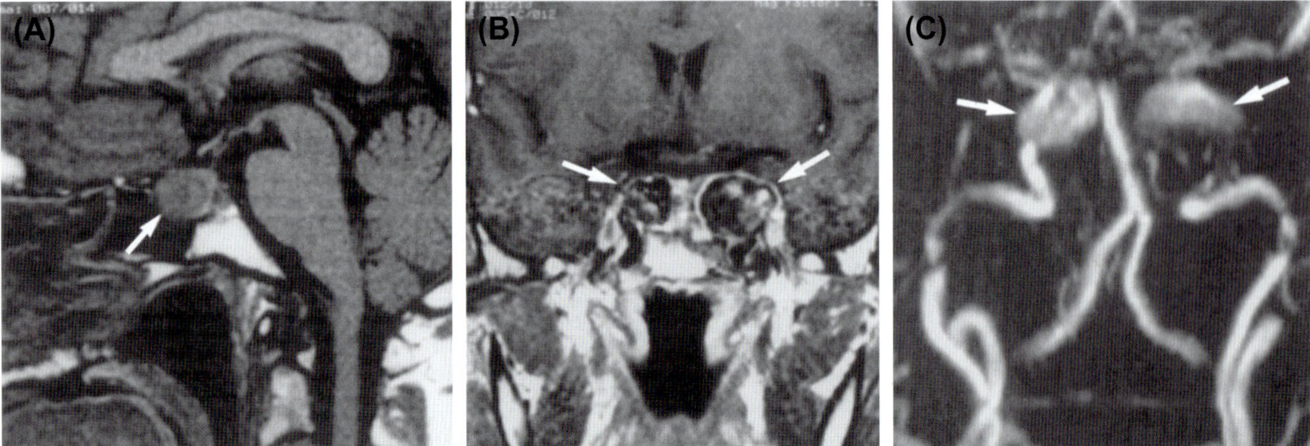

FIGURE 20.30 (A) Midline sagittal T_1-weighted noncontrast MRI suggests an enlarged pituitary (arrow) with superior convexity of the gland. (B) Coronal T_1-weighted noncontrast MRI indicates that the gland is actually compressed between two parasellar masses (arrows) which have a very variegated MRI signal. This results in the false impression of gland enlargement in the sagittal plane. (C) Magnetic resonance angiogram (MRA), coronal projection, shows these parasellar masses to be bilateral cavernous carotid aneurysms (arrows).

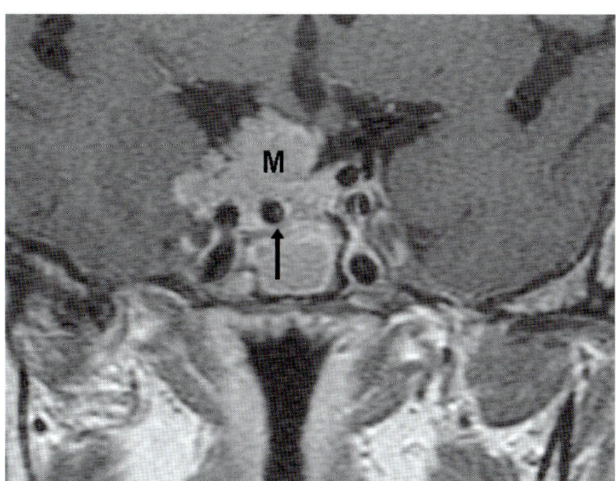

FIGURE 20.31 Pituitary meningioma. Sagittal postcontrast T_1-weighted MR image shows right-sided cavernous para- and suprasellar mass (M). Note the marked medial position of the cavernous carotid artery (arrow).

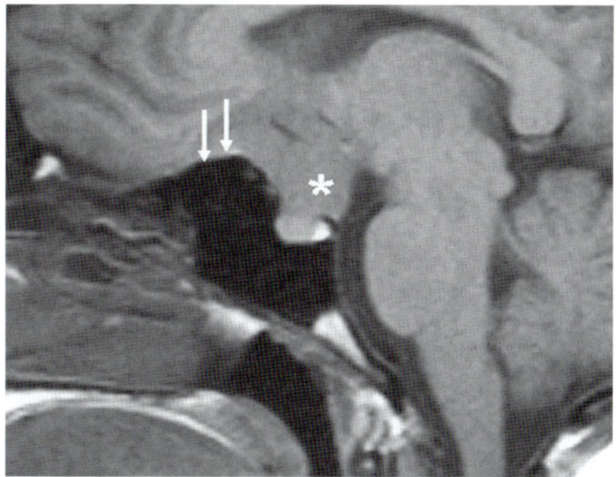

FIGURE 20.33 Meningioma. Sagittal noncontrast T_1-weighted MR depicts a suprasellar mass (*). Note the aerated expansion of the sphenoid sinus also known as pneumosinus dilatans (arrows).

low signal on MRI, or as areas of contrast enhancement deforming the normal shape of the cavernous sinus, on contrast-enhanced CT and CT angiograms.

Meningioma

Meningiomas may arise from the suprasellar (tuberculum sella, anterior clinoid process, planum sphenoidale, upper clivus, diaphragm sellae), parasellar (cavernous sinus), or intrasellar regions (diaphragm sellae) [89]. They are more common in middle age with a female preponderance. Visual loss due to involvement of the optic nerves is the most common presentation of meningiomas in this location.

On MR, meningiomas are isointense with brain parenchyma on T_1- and T_2-weighted sequences. Homogeneous, intense enhancement is seen after contrast administration. There may be a linear, enhancing dural tail extending away from the lesion. Meningiomas can be differentiated from pituitary macroadenoma by the fact that in the former the sella is usually normal in size and the pituitary gland can be identified as separate from the tumor (Figures 20.31–20.33).

CT may aid the diagnosis by revealing intratumoral calcification, hyperostosis and expansion of the sphenoid sinus (pneumosinus dilatans). Angiography shows a typical tumoral blush.

Hypothalamic–Chiasmatic Glioma

Hypothalamic and optic gliomas are childhood tumors. Males and females are approximately equally affected. At presentation, patients are usually 2–4 years of age with diminished visual acuity. Endocrine dysfunction, most commonly reduced growth hormone resulting in short stature, is present in about 20% of patients. Between 20% and 50% of patients with

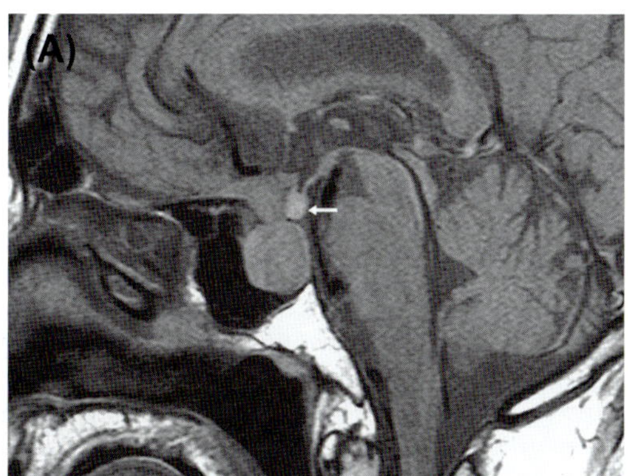

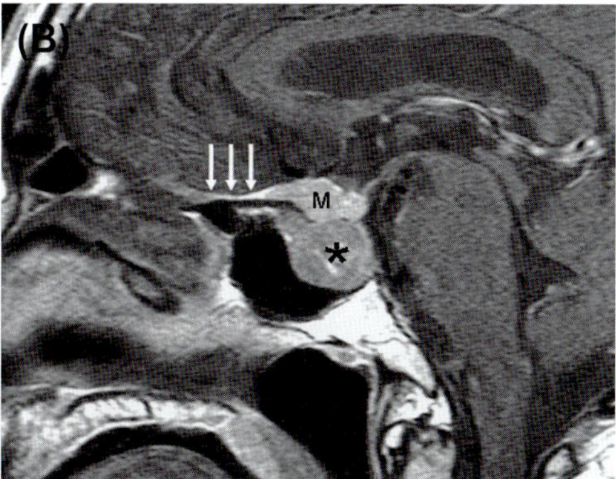

FIGURE 20.32 Tuberculum sella meningioma and pituitary adenoma. Sagittal (A) pre- and (B) postcontrast coronal T_1-weighted MR. The sella is mildly expanded due to an adenoma (*). Postcontrast images (B) best delineate a separate suprasellar mass (M) with a dural tail (arrows). Note the displaced neurohypophysis bright spot (white arrow) on precontrast image (A).

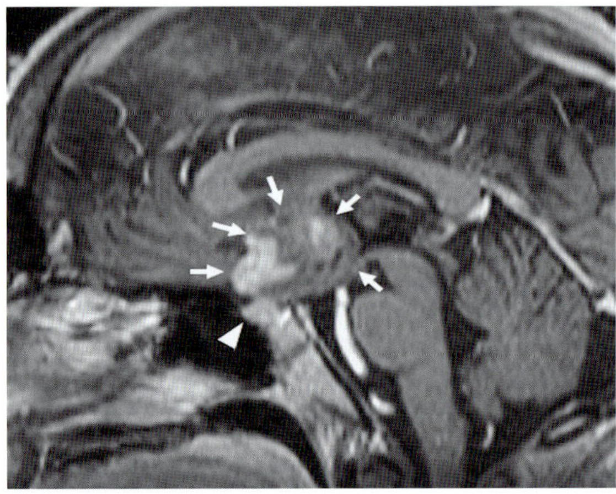

FIGURE 20.34 Hypothalamic glioma. Sagittal postcontrast T_1-weighted image demonstrates heterogeneously enhancing solid mass (arrowheads) inseparable from the optic chiasm or hypothalamus. Note the normal-sized pituitary gland (white arrow).

hypothalamic gliomas have a family history of neurofibromatosis (NF)-1 [90]. Gliomas of the optic chiasm and hypothalamus in children with NF-1 usually have a more indolent course. Tumors may grow more slowly and occasionally regress spontaneously [91]. MRI is optimal for showing the relationship of the mass to the hypothalamus, optic chiasm and infundibulum, as well as the intraorbital and intracanalicular components. Gliomas are usually iso- to slightly hypointense on T_1-weighted image and moderately hyperintense on T_2-weighted image with considerable variation. Solid or mixed enhancement is often seen following contrast medium administration although some lesions are non-enhancing (Figure 20.34). Calcification is uncommon, but can occur. Although the exact site of origin of large chiasmatic and hypothalamic gliomas cannot often be identified, the age at presentation and imaging characteristics are helpful in diagnosis.

Lymphocytic Hypophysitis

Lymphocytic hypophysitis is a rare inflammatory disorder of the pituitary gland, originally thought to occur exclusively in the adenohypophysis of young women. However, the disease is now known to be found at any age, in both sexes, and may involve neurohypophysis, as well as infundibulum. The clinical spectrum includes headaches, visual loss, hypopituitarism, diabetes insipidus, pituitary apoplexy and cranial nerve palsies [92]. In lymphocytic hypophysitis there is diffuse infiltration of the pituitary gland by inflammatory cells, predominantly lymphocytes, forming lymphoid follicles, with varying degrees of reactive fibrosis.

On MR imaging these lesions tend to mimic solid macroadenomas with prominent contrast enhancement, but not always of the entire gland. There may be thickening and enhancement of the pituitary stalk, cavernous sinus infiltration, and meningeal enhancement (Figure 20.35). The posterior pituitary bright spot may be absent due to infiltration, and this may help to differentiate this process from other conditions such as hyperplasia and physiological glandular hypertrophy of pregnancy [93,94]. When the inflammatory process is limited to the infundibulum, differentiation from other stalk lesions such as germinoma, Langerhans cell histiocytosis (LCH) and sarcoidosis may be difficult (Figure 20.36). Dynamic imaging can add to the differential diagnosis. The typical dynamic contrast enhancement pattern of hypothalamic germinomas and LCH is gradually increasing enhancement without washout, whereas hypophysitis demonstrates a sharp rise in enhancement and a steeper washout. Thus, dynamic MR imaging can help distinguish germinomas from adenohypophysitis but is not useful for differentiating them from LCH [95]. More often than not, the diagnosis is established histologically

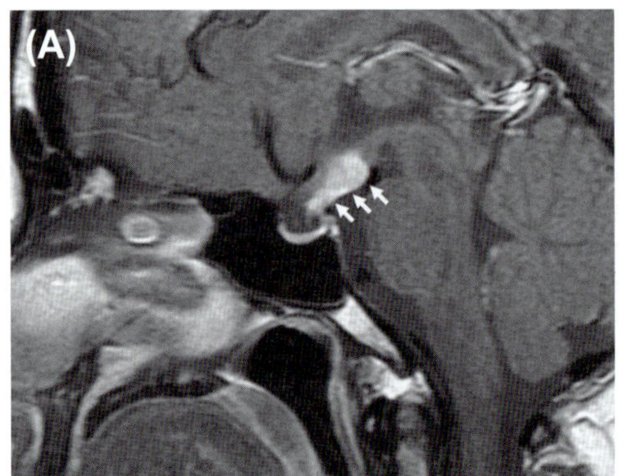

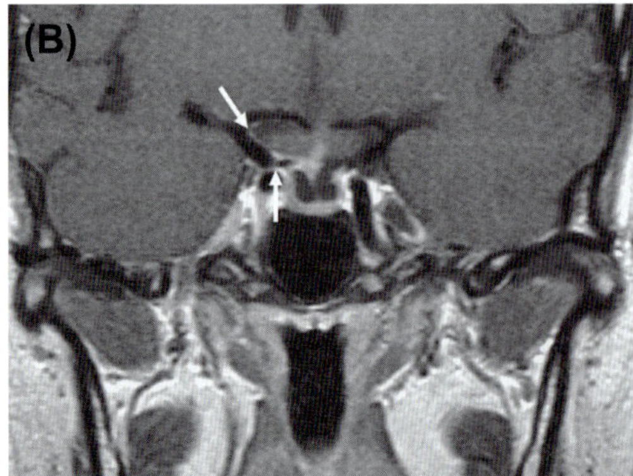

FIGURE 20.35 Hypophysitis. Sagittal (A) and coronal (B) postcontrast T_1-weighted images show a markedly thickened pituitary stalk (arrows). Note the abnormal enhancement extending to the optic chiasm (arrows).

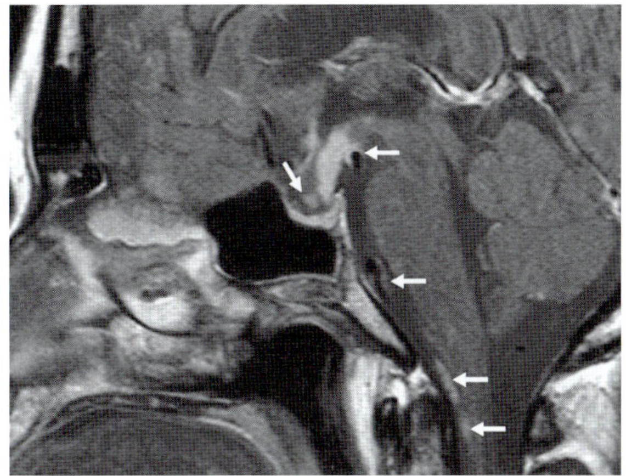

FIGURE 20.36 Sarcoidosis. Sagittal postcontrast T_1-weighted image demonstrates a very thickened infundibulum (*). Note meningeal enhancement in the suprasellar, basilar, prepontine and premedullary cisterns (arrows).

on the basis of lymphocytic infiltration of the pituitary and stalk [96].

Other

A multitude of other disease processes may occur within the pituitary or sella turcica. Abscesses are usually low density on T_1-weighted images with a thick enhancing wall [97]. Tuberculosis and Wegener's granulomatosis unusually affect the pituitary [98–100]. Primary tumors including germ cell tumors [101–103], chondrosarcoma [104], schwannoma [105,106], xanthoastrocytoma [107], pituicytoma (astrocytoma) (Figure 20.37) [108] and neuroblastoma of the pituitary/sella turcica have been reported. Metastases to the pituitary are well known, although also uncommon (Figure 20.38).

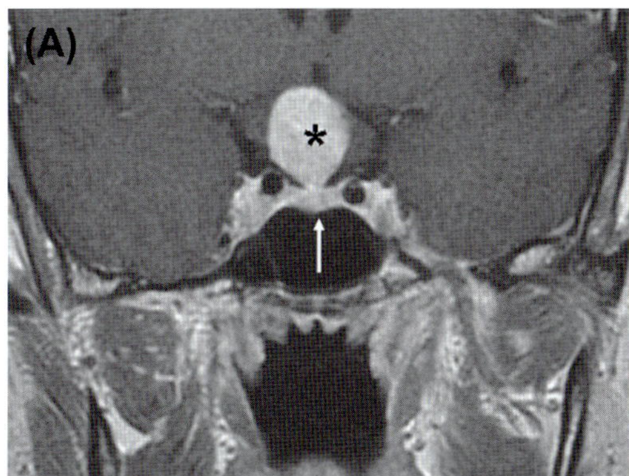

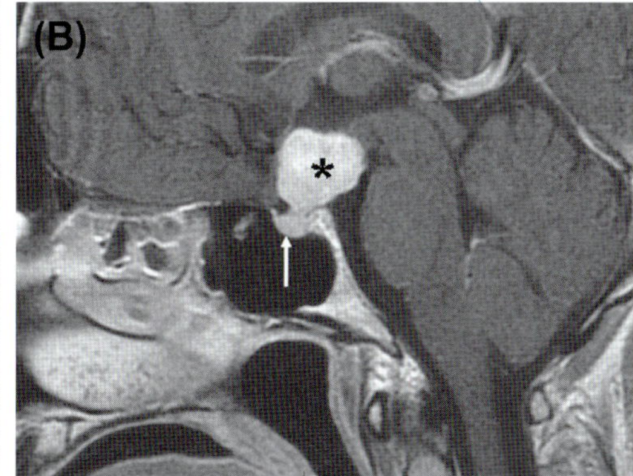

FIGURE 20.37 A 38-year-old man with pituicytoma. (A) Coronal and (B) sagittal T_1-weighted MR show a solid suprasellar mass (*) within the expected position of the stalk. The pituitary gland is normal (arrow).

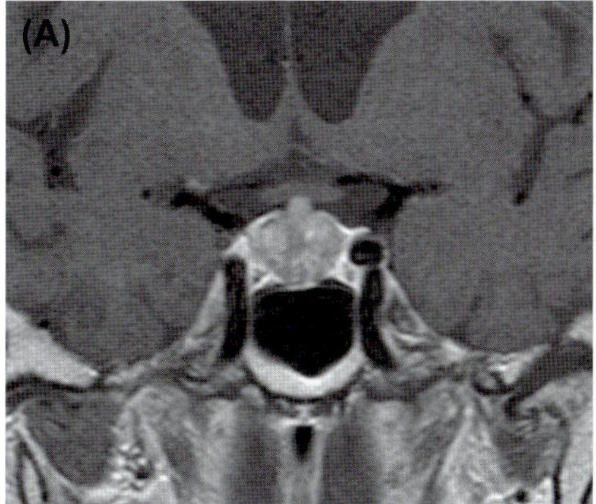

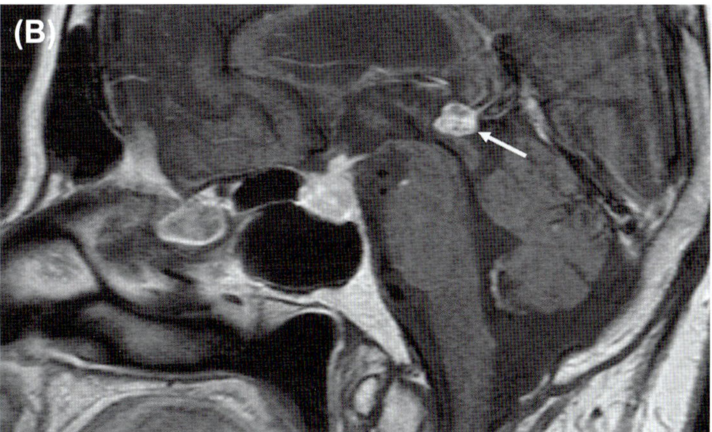

FIGURE 20.38 Pituitary metastasis. Coronal (A) and sagittal (B) T_1-weighted postcontrast images demonstrating an intrasellar mass indistinguishable from a macroadenoma. The clue to the diagnosis is the additional metastatic focus in the pineal region (arrow in B).

EMPTY SELLA

The "empty sella" refers to a sella turcica that contains CSF communicating with the suprasellar space through a normal or enlarged infundibular hiatus in the diaphragma sellae. There is almost always some pituitary tissue present, and very often the pituitary is normal in size and/or function (Figures 20.39 and 20.40).

The sella turcica may or may not be enlarged. If enlarged, it is usually symmetrically expanded, or the floor is depressed without expansion of the anterior and posterior walls. Undercutting of tuberculum and thinning of the clinoids may occur. There are no specific bony deformities that may be used to differentiate the empty sella from an expansile intrasellar mass.

In a study of 189 normal subjects by CT, it was found that there was a tendency for decreasing size of the pituitary with advancing age. Whereas in normal subjects under 29 years, especially females, the pituitary gland generally filled the sella, after age 50 years the gland was often flattened and there was increased CSF in the sella, i.e., a partially empty sella. In another study of 56 patients without a pituitary disorder, 39% had moderate or marked empty sella [109]. There are, however, a number of etiologies for the empty sella other than simply normal variation and aging, and these are classified as primary and secondary empty sella depending on the etiology.

Primary empty sella is associated with an incompetent diaphragma sellae with intrasellar extension of cisternal CSF, or a hypoplastic pituitary gland. The normal diaphragma may be a complete dural covering of the sella with only a small opening for the infundibulum. However, this opening may be wider than the infundibulum. The diaphragma may cover only a peripheral rim of the sella. In the latter two instances, which occur in approximately 40% of the population, there is a potential for downward extension of suprasellar fluid and, rarely, the suprasellar visual system (Figure 20.40). The continued pulsation of the CSF through this widened opening in the diaphragma sellae may progressively result in a partially empty sella with a depressed superior margin of the pituitary and/or an enlarged sella [110].

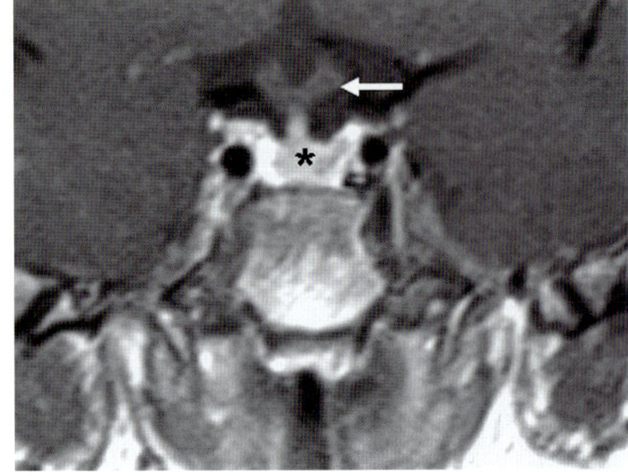

FIGURE 20.40 Secondary empty sella. Coronal T_1-weighted postcontrast image of a patient previously treated for a macroadenoma. The pituitary is normal in size (*). The optic chiasm has the distinctive "V"-shape seen in secondary empty sella (arrow).

Secondary empty sella refers to conditions in which some process has preceded and is responsible for the extension of suprasellar fluid into the sella. A multitude of etiologies have been reported to cause secondary empty sella. In these instances the sella turcica may or may not be enlarged, depending on whether the primary condition expanded the sella, e.g., macroadenoma, or the constant pulsation of the intrasellar CSF eventually resulted in an enlarged sella, e.g., pseudotumor cerebri.

Pituitary microadenomas may coexist with an empty sella. In the face of pituitary hormonal excess the finding

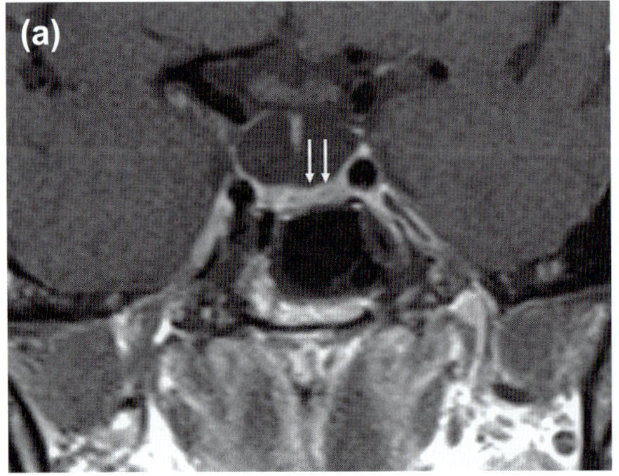

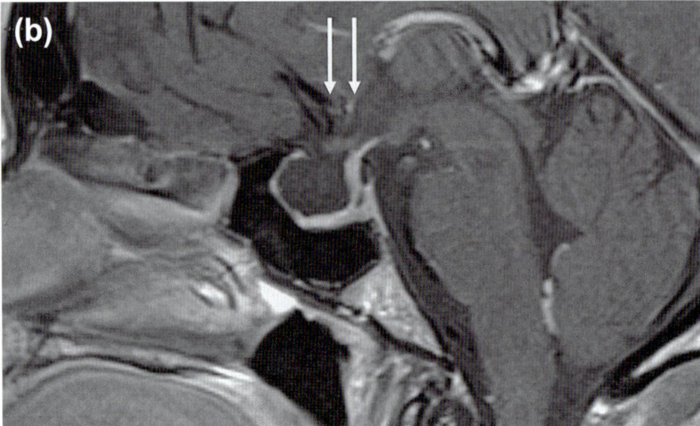

FIGURE 20.39 Primary empty sella. (A) Coronal and (B) sagittal T_1-weighted postcontrast images show expanded sella turcica, containing CSF and otherwise normal pituitary tissue (arrows). (B) Note mild displacement of the stalk posteriorly (arrow).

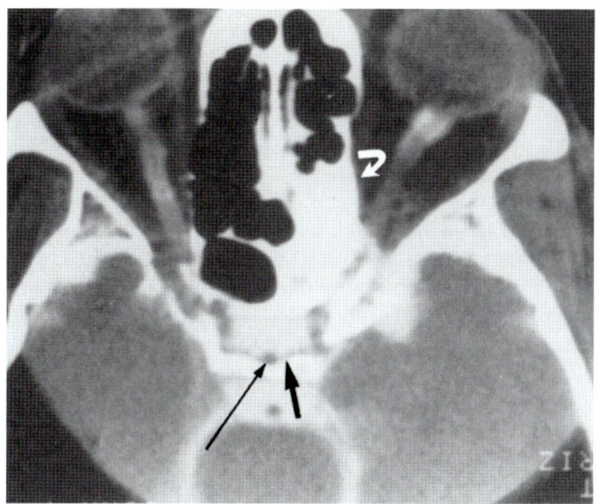

FIGURE 20.41 Axial CT through the sella turcica several minutes after lumbar instillation of intrathecal contrast agent. The empty sella (arrow) is filled with contrast-enhanced cerebrospinal fluid (CSF) and is therefore hyperdense. The infundibular stalk is visible (long arrow). The left sphenoid sinus and posterior ethmoid air cells (curved arrows) are also contrast filled, indicating that they communicate with the intracranial CSF, explaining the CSF rhinorrhea in this patient with idiopathic intracranial hypotension.

of a partially empty sella does not exclude the presence of pituitary microadenoma. A partially regressed macroadenoma may in fact be the etiology of the empty sella (Figure 20.40). In addition, hyperprolactinemia has been seen associated with an empty sella in the absence of a pituitary tumor [111].

Downward herniation of the suprasellar visual system (optic chiasm, optic nerves, optic tracts) into the sella may occur in association with primary or secondary empty sella, and is not infrequent after medical or surgical treatment of macroadenomas (Figure 20.40). Visual disturbances may or may not be present and, when present, may be progressive or static [112–114].

Imaging of the Empty Sella

MRI has made the diagnosis of empty sella quite routine. T_1-weighted images clearly define the pituitary, infundibulum and intrasellar CSF, and if there is any question of an associated mass, gadolinium enhancement will usually suffice for clarification. Furthermore, herniation of the suprasellar visual system is exquisitely defined by MRI on both coronal and sagittal T_1-weighted images that will show an empty sella when present.

Intrathecal enhanced CT is still of value in those cases of empty sella associated with CSF rhinorrhea [115–117]. This association has been extensively studied and probably does not have a single explanation. Pituitary tumor, intrasellar cyst, or increased intracranial pressure may coexist with the empty sella and be responsible for the rhinorrhea. However, there may be no associated conditions. Location of the leak is best accomplished by high-resolution, thin-section CT performed immediately after opacification of the subarachnoid cisterns by intrathecal contrast, usually administered by lumbar puncture (Figure 20.41).

References

[1] J.M. Taveras, E.H. Wood (Eds.), Diagnostic Neuroradiology, Williams and Wilkins, Baltimore, 1964.

[2] G. DiChiro, K.B. Nelson, The volume of the sella turcica, Am J Roentgenol 87 (1962) 989–1008.

[3] P. Turski, T.H. Newton, B.H. Horten, Sellar contour: Anatomic-polytomographic correlation, Am J Roentgenol 137 (1981) 213–216.

[4] G. Wortzman, N.B. Rewcastle, Tomographic abnormalities simulating pituitary microadenomas, Am J Neuroradiol 3 (1982) 505–512.

[5] W.L. Davis, J.N. Lee, B.D. King, H.R. Harnsberger, Dynamic contrast-enhanced MR imaging of the pituitary gland with fast spin-echo technique, J Magn Reson Imaging 4 (1994) 509–511.

[6] A.D. Elster, High-resolution, dynamic pituitary MR imaging: Standard of care or academic pastime? Am J Roentgenol 163 (1994) 680–682.

[7] W. Kucharczyk, J.E. Bishop, D.B. Plewes, M.A. Keller, S. George, Detection of pituitary microadenomas: Comparison of dynamic keyhole fast spin echo, unenhanced, and conventional contrast-enhanced MR imaging, Am J Roentgenol 163 (1994) 671–679.

[8] R.C. Smallridge, L.F. Czervionke, D.W. Fellows, V.J. Bernet, Corticotropin- and thyrotropin-secreting pituitary microadenomas: Detection by dynamic magnetic resonance imaging, Mayo Clin Proc 75 (2000) 521–528.

[9] T. Stadnik, D. Spruyt, A. van Binst, R. Luypaert, J. d'Haens, M. Osteaux, Pituitary microadenomas: Diagnosis with dynamic serial CT, conventional CT and T1-weighted MR imaging before and after injection of gadolinium, Eur J Radiol 18 (1994) 191–198.

[10] A. Tabarin, F. Laurent, B. Catargi, F. Olivier-Puel, R. Lescene, J. Berge, et al., Comparative evaluation of conventional and dynamic magnetic resonance imaging of the pituitary gland for the diagnosis of Cushing's disease, Clin Endocrinol (Oxf) 49 (1998) 293–300.

[11] T.C. Friedman, E. Zuckerbraun, M.L. Lee, M.S. Kabil, H. Shahinian, Dynamic pituitary MRI has high sensitivity and specificity for the diagnosis of mild cushing's syndrome and should be part of the initial workup, Horm Metab Res 39 (2007) 451–456.

[12] E. Kitamura, Y. Miki, M. Kawai, H. Itoh, S. Yura, N. Mori, et al., T_1 signal intensity and height of the anterior pituitary in neonates: Correlation with postnatal time, Am J Neuroradiol 29 (7) (2008) 1257–1260.

[13] J. Kucharczyk, W. Kucharczyk, I. Berry, et al., Histochemical characterization and functional significance of the hyperintense signal on MR images of the posterior pituitary, Am J Neuroradiol 9 (1988) 1079–1083.

[14] L.P. Mark, V.M. Haughton, The posterior pituitary bright spot; a perspective, Am J Neuroradiol 11 (1990) 701–702.

[15] W. Kucharczyk, R.E. Lenkinski, J. Kucharczyk, R.M. Henkelman, The effect of phospholipid vesicle on the NMR relaxation of water: An explanation for the MR appearance of the neurohypophysis? Am J Neuroradiol 11 (1990) 693–700.

[16] N. Colombo, I. Berry, J. Kucharczyk, et al., Posterior pituitary gland: Appearance on MR images in normal and pathologic states, Radiology 165 (1987) 481–485.

[17] I. Fujisawa, K. Nishimura, R. Asato, et al., Posterior lobe of the pituitary in diabetes insipidus: MR findings, J Comput Assist Tomogr 11 (1987) 221–225.

[18] B.S. Brooks, T.E. Gammal, J.D. Allison, W.H. Hoffman, Frequency and variation of the posterior pituitary bright signal on MR images, Am J Neuroradiol 10 (1989) 943–948.

[19] T. el Gammal, B.S. Brooks, W.H. Hoffman, MR imaging of the ectopic bright signal of posterior pituitary regeneration, Am J Neuroradiol 10 (1989) 323–328.

[20] P. Halimi, R. Sigal, D. Doyon, et al., Post-traumatic diabetes insipidus: MR demonstration of pituitary stalk rupture, J Comput Assist Tomogr 12 (1988) 135–137.

[21] J. Hamilton, D. Chitayat, S. Blaser, et al., Familial growth hormone deficiency associated with MRI abnormalities, American Journal of Medical Genetics 80 (2) (1998) 128–132.

[22] N. Kandemir, A. Cila, A. Besim, N. Yordam, Magnetic resonance imaging (MRI) findings in isolated growth hormone deficiency, Turkish Journal of Pediatrics 40 (3) (1998) 385–392.

[23] L. Kornreich, G. Horev, L. Lazar, et al., MR findings in growth hormone deficiency: Correlation with severity of hypopituitarism, Am J Neuroradiol 19 (1998) 1495–1499.

[24] J. Leger, A. Velasquez, C. Garel, et al., Thickened pituitary stalk on magnetic resonance imaging in children with central diabetes insipidus, Journal of Clinical Endocrinology and Metabolism 84 (6) (1999) 1954–1960.

[25] A. Colao, S. Lastoria, D. Ferone, et al., The pituitary uptake of (111)In-DTPA-D-Phel-octreotide in normal pituitary and in pituitary adenomas, Journal of Endocrinological Investigation 22 (3) (1999) 176–183.

[26] S.M. Wolpert, The radiology of pituitary adenomas, Endocrinology and Metabolism Clinic 16 (1987) 553–584.

[27] J.C. Chen, M. Kucharczyk, Hypothalamic—pituitary region: Magnetic resonance imaging, Clin Endocrinol Metab 3 (1989) 73–87.

[28] J.G. Gonzalez, G. Elizondo, D. Saldivar, et al., Pituitary gland growth during normal pregnancy: An in vivo study using magnetic resonance imaging, Am J Med 85 (1988) 217–220.

[29] R.G. Peyster, L.P. Adler, R.R. Viscarello, et al., CT of the normal pituitary gland, Neuroradiology 28 (1986) 161–165.

[30] S.N. Wiener, M.S. Rzeszotarski, R.T. Droege, et al., Measurement of pituitary gland height with MR imaging, Am J Neuroradiol 6 (1985) 717–722.

[31] H.M.N. Roppolo, R.E. Latchaw, J.D. Meyer, H.D. Curtin, 1. Normal pituitary gland. Macroscopic anatomy—CT correlation, Am J Neuroradiol 4 (1983) 927–935.

[32] S.M. Wolpert, M.E. Molitch, J.A. Goldman, J.B. Wood, Size, shape and appearance of the normal female pituitary gland, Am J Roentgenol 143 (1984) 377–381.

[33] J.D. Swartz, K.B. Russell, B.A. Basile, et al., High resolution computed tomographic appearance of intrasellar contents in women of childbearing years, Radiology 147 (1983) 115–117.

[34] P. Chanson, F. Daujat, J. Young, A. Bellucci, M. Kujas, D. Doyon, et al., Normal pituitary hypertrophy as a frequent cause of pituitary incidentaloma: A follow-up study, J Clin Endocrinol Metab 86 (7) (2001) 3009–3015.

[35] A. Tsunoda, O. Okuda, K. Sato, MR height of the pituitary gland as a function of age and sex: Especially physiological hypertrophy in adolescence and in climacterium, Am J Neuroradiol 18 (1997) 551–554.

[36] T. Terano, A. Seya, Y. Tamura, et al., Characteristics of the pituitary gland in elderly subjects from magnetic resonance images: Relationship to pituitary hormone secretion, Clinical Endocrinology 45 (3) (1996) 273–279.

[37] W.I. Schievink, Spontaneous spinal cerebrospinal fluid leaks, Cephalalgia 28 (12) (2008) 1345–1356.

[38] G.N. Burrow, G. Wortzman, N.B. Rewcastle, et al., Microadenomas of the pituitary and abnormal sellar tomograms in an unselected autopsy series, N Engl J Med 304 (1981) 156–158.

[39] A.D. Parent, J. Bebin, R.R. Smith, Incidental pituitary adenomas, J Neurosurg 54 (1981) 228–231.

[40] M.C. Martin, E.D. Schrlock, R.B. Jaffe, Prolactin-secreting pituitary adenomas, West J Med 139 (1983) 663–672.

[41] H. Podlas, Diagnosis of pituitary microadenomas by computed tomography, Medicamundi 26 (1981) 20–22.

[42] E.F. Chambers, P.A. Turski, D. La Masters, T.H. Newton, Region of low density in the contrast-enhanced pituitary gland: Normal and pathologic processes, Radiology 144 (1982) 109–113.

[43] P.C. Davis, J.C. Hoffman Jr., J.A. Malko, et al., Gadolinium DTPA and MR imaging of pituitary adenoma: A preliminary report, Am J Neuroradiol 8 (1987) 817–823.

[44] P.C. Davis, J.C. Hoffman Jr., G.T. Tindall, I.F. Braun, CT-surgical correlation in pituitary adenomas: Evaluation in 113 patients, Am J Neuroradiol 6 (1985) 711–716.

[45] S. Marcovitz, R. Wee, J. Chan, J. Hardy, Diagnostic accuracy of preoperative CT scanning of pituitary somatotropin adenomas, Am J Neuroradiol 9 (1988) 19–22.

[46] S. Marcovitz, R. Wee, J. Chan, J. Hardy, Diagnostic accuracy of preoperative CT scanning of pituitary prolactinomas, Am J Neuroradiol 9 (1988) 13–17.

[47] P.C. Davis, J.C. Hoffman Jr., T. Spencer, et al., MR imaging of pituitary adenoma: MR, CT, clinical and surgical correlation, Am J Neuroradiol 8 (1987) 107–112.

[48] D.A. Nichols, E.R. Laws Jr., O.W. Houser, C.F. Abboud, Comparison of magnetic resonance imaging and computed tomography in the preoperative evaluation of pituitary adenomas, Neurosurgery 22 (1988) 380–385.

[49] K.W. Pojunas, D.L. Daniels, A.L. Williams, V.M. Haughton, MR imaging of prolactin-secreting microadenomas, Am J Neuroradiol 7 (1986) 209–213.

[50] W. Kucharczyk, D.O. Davis, W.M. Kelly, et al., Pituitary adenomas: High-resolution of MR imaging at 1.5T, Radiology 161 (1986) 761–765.

[51] A.J. Dwyer, J.A. Frank, J.L. Doppman, et al., Pituitary adenomas: High-resolution MR imaging at 1.5T, Radiology 161 (1986) 761–765.

[52] M.V. Kulkarni, K.F. Lee, C.B. McArdle, et al., 1.5T MR imaging of pituitary microadenomas: Technical considerations and CT correlation, Am J Neuroradiol 9 (1988) 5–11.

[53] J.L. Doppman, J.A. Frank, A.J. Dwyer, et al., Gadolinium DTPA enhanced MR imaging of ACTH-secreting microadenomas of the pituitary gland, J Comput Assist Tomogr 12 (1988) 728–735.

[54] P. MacPherson, D.M. Hadley, E. Teasdale, G. Teasdale, Pituitary microadenomas: Does gadolinium enhance their demonstration? Am J Neuroradiol 31 (1989) 293–298.

[55] E. Steiner, H. Imhof, E. Kuosp, Gd-DTPA enhanced high resolution MR imaging of pituitary adenoma, Radiographics 9 (1989) 587–598.

[56] A.L. Stein, M.N. Levenick, O.A. Kletzky, Computed tomography versus magnetic resonance for the evaluation of suspected pituitary adenomas, Obstet Gynecol 73 (1989) 996–999.

[57] D.R. Newton, W.P. Dillon, D. Norman, et al., Gd-DTPA-enhanced MR imaging of pituitary adenomas, Am J Neuroradiol 10 (1989) 949–954.

[58] W.N. Peck, W.P. Dillon, D. Norman, et al., High-resolution MR imaging of microadenomas at 1.5T: Experience with Cushing disease, Am J Neuroradiol 9 (1988) 1085–1091.

[59] S. Marcovitz, R. Wee, J. Chan, J. Hardy, The diagnostic accuracy of pre-operative CT scanning in the evaluation of pituitary ACTH-secreting adenomas, Am J Neuroradiol 8 (1987) 641–644.
[60] P.C. Davis, J.C. Hoffman Jr., J.A. Ralko, et al., Gadolinium-DTPA and MR imaging of pituitary adenoma: A preliminary report, Am J Neuroradiol 8 (1987) 817–823.
[61] P.C. Davis, J.C. Hoffman Jr., G.T. Tindall, I.F. Braun, Prolactin-secreting pituitary microadenomas: Inaccuracy of high-resolution CT imaging, Am J Neuroradiol 5 (1984) 721–726.
[62] D.M. Yousem, J.A. Arrington, S.J. Zinreich, et al., Pituitary adenomas: Possible role of bromocriptine in intratumoral hemorrhage, Radiology 170 (1989) 239–243.
[63] S. Cannavo, L. Curto, A. Lania, et al., Unusual MRI finding of multiple adenomas in the pituitary gland: A case report and review of the literature, Magnetic Resonance Imaging 17 (4) (1999) 633–636.
[64] W.F. Chandler, P.E. Schteingart, R.V. Lyod, et al., Surgical treatment of Cushing's disease, J Neurosurg 66 (1987) 204–208.
[65] A. Tabarin, F. Laurent, B. Catargi, et al., Comparative evaluation of conventional and dynamic magnetic resonance imaging of the pituitary gland for the diagnosis of Cushing's disease, Clinical Endocrinology 49 (3) (1998) 285–286.
[66] S. Melmed, Acromegaly, New Eng J Med 355 (2006) 2558–2573.
[67] G. Scotti, C.Y. Yu, W.P. Dillon, et al., MR imaging of cavernous sinus involvement by pituitary adenomas, Am J Roentgenol 151 (1988) 799–806.
[68] S.C. Young, R.I. Grossman, H.I. Goldberg, et al., MR of vascular encasement in parasellar masses: Comparison with angiography and CT, Am J Neuroradiol 9 (1988) 35–38.
[69] B. Kaufman, B.A. Kaufman, B.M. Arafah, et al., Large pituitary gland adenomas evaluated with magnetic resonance imaging, Neurosurgery 21 (1987) 540–546.
[70] M.M.H. Teng, C. Huang, T. Chang, The pituitary mass after transsphenoidal hypophysectomy, Am J Neuroradiol 9 (1988) 23–26.
[71] M. Vasile, K. Marsot-Dupuch, M. Kujas, et al., Idiopathic granulomatous hypophysitis: Clinical and imaging features, Neuroradiology 39 (1) (1997) 7–11.
[72] J. Ahmadi, G.C. Meyers, H. Segall, et al., Lymphocytic adenohypophysitis: Contrast-enhanced MR imaging in five cases, Radiology 195 (1) (1995) 30–34.
[73] S.L. Hwang, S.L. Howng, Pituitary abscess: CT and MRI findings, Journal of Formosan Medical Association 95 (3) (1996) 267–269.
[74] S.G. Ostrov, R.M. Quencer, J.C. Hoffman, et al., Hemorrhage within pituitary adenomas: How often associated with pituitary apoplexy syndrome? Am J Neuroradiol 10 (1989) 503–510.
[75] E.R. Benshoff, B.H. Katz, Ectopia of the posterior pituitary gland as a normal variant: Assessment with MR imaging, Am J Neuroradiol 11 (1990) 709–712.
[76] F. Gudinchet, F. Burnelle, M.O. Baith, et al., MR imaging of the posterior hypophysis in children, Am J Roentgenol 153 (1989) 351–354.
[77] J.L. Voelker, R.L. Campbell, J. Muller, Clinical, radiographic, and pathological features of symptomatic Rathke's cleft tgcq [16,17,20,29,37,38,43,47,76]Basis of Disease Pathogenesis, J Neurosurg 74 (4) (1991) 535–544.
[78] Y. Nemoto, Y. Inoue, T. Fukuda, et al., MR appearances of Rathke's cleft cysts, Neuroradiology 30 (1988) 155–159.
[79] W. Kucharczyk, W.W. Peck, W.M. Kelly, et al., Rathke cleft cysts: CT, MR imaging and pathologic features, Radiology 165 (1987) 491–495.
[80] C. Christophe, J. Flamant-Durand, S. Hanquinet, C. Heinrichs, C. Raftopoulos, E. Sariban, et al., MRI in seven cases of Rathke's cleft cyst in infants and children, Pediatric Radiology 23 (1993) 79–82.
[81] W. Kucharczyk, W.W. Peck, W.M. Kelly, D. Norman, T.H. Newton, Rathke cleft cysts: CT, MR imaging, and pathologic features, Radiology 165 (1987) 491–495.
[82] W.M. Byun, O.L. Kim, D.M.R. Kim, Imaging findings of Rathke's cleft cysts: Significance of intracystic nodules, Am J Neuroradiol 21 (March 2000) 485–488.
[83] M. Sumida, T. Uozumi, K. Mukada, K. Arita, K. Kurisu, K. Eguchi, Rathke cleft cysts: Correlation of enhanced MR and surgical findings, Am J Neuroradiol 15 (1994) 525–532.
[84] M.P. Freeman, R.M. Kessler, J.H. Allen, A.C. Price, Craniopharyngioma: CT and MR imaging in nine cases, J Comput Assist Tomogr 11 (5) (1987) 810–814.
[85] R. Sorva, J.A. Jaaskinen, O. Heiskanen, Craniopharyngioma in children and adults: Correlations between radiological and clinical manifestations, Acta Neurochir 89 (1–2) (1987) 3–9.
[86] E. Pusey, K.E. Kortman, B.D. Flannigan, J. Tsuruda, W.G. Bradley, MR of craniopharyngiomas: Tumor delineation and characterization, Am J Roentgenol 149 (2) (1987) 383–388.
[87] O.B. Boyko, J.T. Curnes, W.J. Oakes, P.C. Burger, Hamartomas of the tuber cinereum: CT, MR, and pathologic findings, Am J Neuroradiol 12 (2) (1991 Mar–Apr) 309–314.
[88] J.L. Freeman, L.T. Coleman, R.M. Wellard, et al., MR imaging and spectroscopic study of epilepto-genic hypothalamic hamartomas: Analysis of 72 cases, Am J Neuroradiol 25 (3) (2004) 450–462.
[89] M. Pisaneschi, G. Kapoor, Imaging the sella and parasellar region, Neuroimag Clin N Am 15 (2005) 203–219.
[90] S. Aoki, A. Barkovich, K. Nishimura, et al., Neurofibromatosis types 1 and 2: Cranial MR findings, Radiology 172 (1989) 527–534.
[91] J.C. Allen, Initial management of children with hypothalamic and thalamic tumors and the modifying role of neurofibromatosis-1, Pediatr Neurosurg 32 (3) (2000) 154–162.
[92] Y. Nakamura, H. Okada, Y. Wada, et al., Lymphocytic hypophysitis: Its expanding features, J Endocrinol Invest 24 (2001) 262–267.
[93] C. Cheung, S. Ezzat, H.S. Smyth, S.L. Asa, The spectrum and significance of primary hypophysitis, J Clin Endocrinol Metab 86 (2001) 1048–1053.
[94] N. Sato, G. Sze, K. Endo, Hypophysitis: Endocrinologic and dynamic MR findings, Am J Neuroradiol 19 (1998) 439–444.
[95] L. Liang, Y. Korogi, T. Sugahara, et al., Dynamic MR imaging of neurohypophyseal germ cell tumors for differential diagnosis of infundibular diseases, Acta Radiol 41 (6) (2000) 562–566.
[96] J. Honegger, R. Fahlbusch, A. Bornemann, et al., Lymphocytic and granulomatous hypophysitis: Experience with nine cases, Neurosurgery 40 (1997) 713–723.
[97] L.J. Wolansky, J.D. Gallagher, R.F. Heary, G.P. Malantic, A. Dasmahapatra, P.D. Shaderowfsky, et al., MRI of pituitary abscess: Two cases and review of the literature, Neuroradiology 39 (7) (1997) 499–503.
[98] G. Stalldecker, S. Diez, A. Carabelli, R. Reynoso, R. Rey, N. Hoffman, et al., Pituitary stalk tuberculoma, Pituitary 5 (3) (2002) 155–162.
[99] F.J. Rodriguez, J.L. Atkinson, C. Giannini, Massive sellar and parasellar schwannoma, Arch Neurol 64 (8) (2007) 1198–1199.
[100] R.J. Benveniste, D. Purohit, H. Byun, Pituicytoma presenting with spontaneous hemorrhage, Pituitary 9 (1) (2006) 53–58.
[101] H. Nishioka, H. Ito, J. Haraoka, K. Akada, Immature teratoma originating from the pituitary gland: Case report, Neurosurgery 44 (3) (1999) 644–647.

[102] M.L. Policarpio-Nicolas, B.H. Le, J.W. Mandell, M.B. Lopes, Granular cell tumor of the neurohypophysis: Report of a case with intraoperative cytologic diagnosis, Diagn Cytopathol 36 (1) (2008) 58–63.

[103] L. Chimelli, M.R. Gadelha, K. Une, S. Carlos, P.J. Pereira, J.L. Santos, et al., Intra-sellar salivary gland-like pleomorphic adenoma arising within the wall of a Rathke's cleft cyst, Pituitary 3 (4) (2000) 257–261.

[104] C.A. Allan, G. Kaltsas, J. Evanson, J. Geddes, D.G. Lowe, P.N. Plowman, et al., Pituitary chondrosarcoma: An unusual cause of a sellar mass presenting as a pituitary adenoma, J Clin Endocrinol Metab 86 (1) (2001) 386–391.

[105] S.M. Whee, J.I. Lee, J.H. Kim, Intrasellar schwannoma mimicking pituitary adenoma: A case report, J Korean Med Sci 17 (1) (2002) 147–150.

[106] N.F. Maartens, D.B. Ellegala, M.L. Vance, M.B. Lopes, E.R. Laws Jr., Intrasellar schwannomas: Report of two cases, Neurosurgery 52 (5) (2003) 1200–1205.

[107] K. Arita, K. Kurisu, A. Tominaga, K. Sugiyama, M. Sumida, T. Hirose, Intrasellar pleomorphic xanthoastrocytoma: Case report, Neurosurgery 51 (4) (2002) 1079–1082.

[108] B.W. Scheithauer, B. Swearingen, E.T. Whyte, P.K. Auluck, A.O. Stemmer-Rachamimov, Ependymoma of the sella turcica: A variant of pituicytoma, Hum Pathol 40 (3) (2009) 435–440.

[109] S. Ishikawa, M. Furuse, T. Saito, K. Okada, T. Kuzuya, Empty sella in control subjects and patients with hypopituitarism, Endocrinol Jpn 35 (5) (1988) 665–674.

[110] T.H. Newton, D.G. Potts (Eds.), Radiology of the Skull and Brain, CV Mosby Company, St. Louis, 1971.

[111] H. Gharib, H.M. Frey, E.R. Laws Jr., R.V. Randall, B.W. Scheithauer, Coexistent primary empty sella syndrome and hyperprolactinemia. Report of 11 cases, Arch Intern Med 143 (7) (1983) 1383–1386.

[112] S.C. Pollock, B.S. Bromberg, Visual loss in a patient with primary empty sella. Case report, Arch Ophthalmol 105 (11) (1987) 1487–1488.

[113] E.M. Bursztyn, M.H. Lavyne, M. Aisen, Empty sella syndrome with intrasellar herniation of the optic chiasm, Am J Neuroradiol 4 (1983) 167–168.

[114] B. Kaufman, R.L. Tomsak, B.A. Kaufman, B.U. Arafah, E.M. Bellon, W.R. Selman, et al., Herniation of the suprasellar visual system and third ventricle into empty sellae: Morphologic and clinical considerations, Am J Roentgenol 152 (3) (1989) 597–608.

[115] W.F. Young Jr., L.F. Ospina, D. Wesolowski, A. Touma, The primary empty sella syndrome: Diagnosis with metrizamide cisternography, JAMA 246 (22) (1981) 2611–2612.

[116] A. Pompili, M. Iachetti, A. Riccio, S. Squillaci, Computed tomographic cisternography with iopamidol in the diagnosis of primary empty sella, Surg Neurol 24 (1) (1985) 16–22.

[117] I. Kuuliala, K. Katevuo, L. Ketonen, Metrizamide cisternography with hypocycloid and computed tomography in sellar and suprasellar lesions, Clin Radiol 32 (4) (1981) 403–407.

CHAPTER

21

Pituitary Surgery

Rudolf Fahlbusch [1], *Michael Buchfelder* [2]

[1] Endocrine Neurosurgery, International Neuroscience Institute Hannover, Germany

[2] Neurosurgical Department, University of Erlangen-Nuremberg, Germany

The goal of pituitary surgery changed tremendously during the 20th century: from 1889 onwards, pioneer pituitary surgeons searched for an approach to the sellar region and tried to decompress the optic nerves while preserving the patient's life. When mortality statistics improved, the goal was to remove as much tumor as possible in order to prevent recurrences. Low morbidity, better cosmetic results and quality of life played an important role much later. It is only in recent years that complete tumor removal and restoration of visual disturbance under preservation or even recovery of pituitary function were to become the goal to reach. A brief review of the amazing evolution of pituitary surgery, surgical anatomy, diagnostic evaluation, modern surgical techniques and the surgical results in the consecutive series of patients treated in the Neurosurgical Department of the university of Erlangen-Nürnberg are used to describe current practice and outcomes. The future of pituitary surgery is then discussed.

HISTORICAL OVERVIEW

Pituitary tumors compose approximately 15% of intracranial neoplasms. Due to their frequency, the management of these neoplasms presents a common problem in general neurosurgical practice. This is why the first surgical interventions were performed early but with great doubt that they could be successful. The first phase of pituitary tumor surgery is thus characterized by establishing approaches to the sella region. The first surgeon to operate on a pituitary tumor was Sir Victor Horsley (London) in 1889. However, he did not report this new innovative operative technique until 1906 [1]. He first used a frontal and later a temporal craniotomy to avoid vascular complications, dealing with frontal veins in a total of ten patients, with two deaths. By then, several other surgeons had developed approaches to the sella region. A right frontal osteoplastic approach was utilized by Fedor Victor Krause (Berlin), who removed a bullet located in the region of the right optic foramen in a 20-year-old patient in 1900 [2]. He quickly realized that this approach could also be used to access pituitary tumors, and operated on several cases. In 1913, Charles Frazer (Philadelphia) reported his experience with a frontal extradural approach, which was later modified to an intradural one with removal of the supraorbital ridge and parts of the orbital roof [3,4]. In 1918, George Heuer and Walter E. Dandy (Baltimore) presented 24 patients operated by a frontal intradural approach using a larger exposure of the brain than Frazer [5]. This approach was later modified by Dandy, who performed a smaller craniotomy in order to avoid extended brain trauma and to lower the risk of postoperative epidural hematoma from the large bone flap. In 1934, he mentioned in his report that "the nasal route was impractical and can never be otherwise" [6]. Even of Harvey Cushing, who established the transsphenoidal operation, we know today, that he later favored the transcranial route. A few surgeons continued to practice the transnasal approach, which later became the most frequently used surgical procedures for sellar lesions due to further technical refinements.

The first transnasal operation to remove a pituitary tumor was performed by Hermann Schloffer (Innsbruck) in Austria in 1907. The incision was performed around the left side of the nose, which was then completely dislocated and turned to the right side [7]. In the same year, Anton von Eiselsberg (Vienna) modified the approach by dislocating the nose downwards. He reported on six cases in 1910 [8,9]. An otolaryngologist, Oscar Hirsch (Vienna), developed the first approach that did not require complete dislocation of the nose in 1910 [10]. Some months later, he performed a submucous endonasal paraseptal approach, for the first time using a nasal speculum [11]. Some otolaryngologists preferred the extra-axial superior transethmoidal approach of Chiari, others

The Pituitary, Third Edition, DOI: 10.1016/B978-0-12-380926-1.10021-5

the extra-axial inferior transmaxillar approach of Denker and Hamberger. Both methods have only been used sporadically and never gained wide acceptance.

Harvey Cushing performed his first transsphenoidal approach on March 26, 1909 [12]. He refined his technique, combining methods of several other surgeons, for example the sublabial incision, the submucous paraseptal dissection towards the sphenoid sinus, the use of nasal specula and the use of an electric forehead lamp. The procedure has become known as the "Cushing's approach" to sellar lesions. Cushing later abandoned this procedure, preferring the transcranial approach, mainly because of a better normalization rate of impaired vision and a lower risk of repeat surgery [13]. This prompted neurosurgeons to also abandon the transsphenoidal approach. Sporadic reports of various modifications came from otolaryngologists like Hirsch, who in the meantime had emigrated to Boston, James from London and Hamberger from Stockholm.

The reintroduction of the so-called "Cushing's procedure" was performed by Norman Dott, the only pupil of Cushing's who continued to practice his method. Dott operated in Edinburgh on more than 100 patients with pituitary adenomas without mortality and without recurrences, due to postoperative radiotherapy. It is not clear why he never published his results. In 1956, Dott introduced Gerard Guiot to his method. It was Guiot who refined the technique, using image intensification and introducing the semisitting position [14,15].

The second phase is characterized by extended and more selective tumor removal, starting around 1965 when the introduction of the operation microscope allowed increased visualization. Jules Hardy, a fellow of Guiot, not only applied microsurgical techniques but also coined the term selective adenomectomy and proposed a classification for pituitary adenomas. He operated on several thousand patients in Canada and published extensively about all aspects of transsphenoidal surgery. Renaissance of pituitary surgery was introduced, leading to its dominant role in pituitary surgery.

The third phase is characterized by improved surgical accuracy by means of neuronavigation, intraoperative MRI and endoscopy. Endoscopy as an assisted procedure or as pure endoscopy has led to a second renaissance of transsphenoidal surgery. The direct perinasal approach became more popular. Indications were extended to craniopharyngiomas, suprasellar and cavernous sinus meningeomas, as well as other parasellar tumors which can be reached by the extended transsphenoidal approach. The extensive exposure with opening much more of the skull base than the sella floor now allowed all possible manipulations but also required extensive technical skills.

Even after the introduction of medical treatment with drugs which inhibit hormone secretion and further refinement of the techniques of radiotherapy, surgery still plays the most important role in the management of pituitary tumors.

DIAGNOSTIC EVALUATION

An overview of the interdisciplinary diagnostic procedures available is presented in Figure 21.1. Currently the most frequently used and most helpful diagnostic imaging procedure in the neuroradiological work-up of patients harboring pituitary tumors is magnetic resonance imaging (MRI) [16]. MRI not only directly depicts tumor size, extension, and characteristics such as hemorrhagic and cystic changes (T_2-weighted images), but also helps to delineate the tumor from the surrounding anatomical structures (T_1-weighted images pre- and post-gadolinium). This is important primarily in parasellar invasive tumors, where encroachment of the tumor tissue along the basal dura and localized or generalized invasion into the cavernous sinus need to be differentiated from displacement without invasion. A multinodular shape is usually considered to be very suspicious of invasive tumor growth, just as marked suprasellar extension without adequate visual compromise. The course of the major intracranial vessels may be visualized by MR angiography. Information on the exact localization of the branches of the carotid artery mostly replaces the need for conventional carotid angiography.

The value of plain skull X-rays and computerized tomography (CT) in the diagnostic evaluation of pituitary tumors has decreased. In plain skull X-rays, ballooning or even some destruction of the sella floor may be visible. However, a thin sellar floor, which is preserved in its continuity, may mimic destruction. Therefore, this finding is not conclusive of an invasive

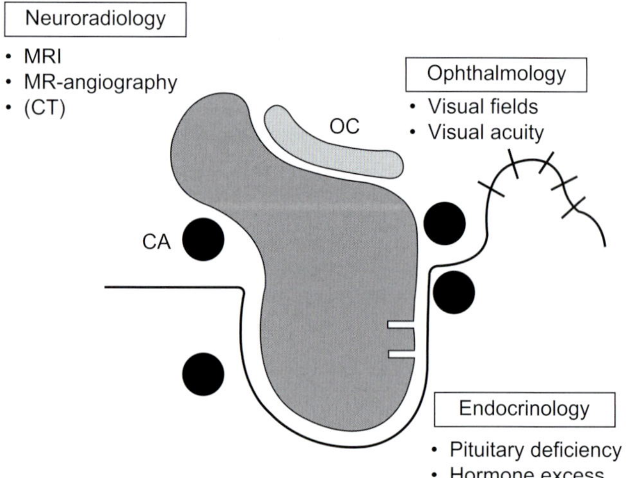

FIGURE 21.1 Interdisciplinary diagnostic evaluation of sellar tumors.

tumor. On the other hand, circumscribed penetration of the sella floor by a truly invasive tumor may not be visible in X-ray films of the sella. For planning the operative approach, a possible deviation of the osseous nasal septum, septations and also the pneumatization pattern of the sphenoid sinus are of some significance. Thin collimation CT with reconstruction of the sella may directly depict the tumor as well as the bony structures so that infiltration of the sellar floor and penetration into the sphenoid sinus may be easily detected [17].

Visual compromise develops only in tumors with a suprasellar extension of more than 10–15 mm above the plane of the diaphragma sellae. Assessment of visual fields and visual acuity is then necessary. Parasellar tumor extension sometimes leads to palsies of the cranial nerves III, IV and VI. The trigeminal nerve is rarely involved in parasellar tumors. However, many patients with infiltration or invasion of the cavernous sinus complain about periorbital pain, which in the majority of cases disappears after tumor removal. A specific situation exists in pituitary apoplexy which may either be caused by acute hemorrhage or by infarction of a pituitary adenoma. Frequently, the oculomotor nerve is involved.

Endocrine evaluation is mandatory as soon as the pituitary fossa or gland is involved in the pathological process. Anterior pituitary function and possible hormonal activity of pituitary adenomas are assessed by hormone measurements and dynamic endocrine pituitary tests, such as ACTH-, CRH- and GRH-stimulation testing, oral glucose load, insulin tolerance testing and dexamethasone suppression. In particular, the exact knowledge of the serum prolactin level is mandatory. In the case of a prolactinoma (prolactin levels > six- to tenfold elevated) medical treatment with dopamine agonists has generally to be taken into consideration as a primary therapy option. In invasive growth-hormone-producing adenomas, preoperative treatment with somatostatin analogues may be utilized to shrink the tumor within the cavernous sinus, soften its consistency, and thus allow easier surgical removal.

SURGICAL AND FUNCTIONAL ANATOMY

Understanding the anatomical relationships between the hypothalamus, the pituitary gland, the carotid artery, the optic nerve and the bony structures around them is paramount for every surgical approach to the sellar area. The hypothalamus is located behind the optic chiasm, between the optic tracts and anterior to the mammilary bodies, and can be divided into four regions: preoptic; supraoptic; tuberal; and posterior [18]. The numerous hypothalamic nuclei have connections to optic and olfactory centers and regulate body temperature, food and water intake, sleep, reproduction, the physiologic circadian rhythms and behavioral responses, by producing and releasing neurally active substances. Stimulatory and inhibitory hormones travel into the capillaries of the portal venous plexus to reach the anterior lobe of the pituitary gland. Vasopressin and oxytocin are transported to the posterior lobe by axoplasmatic flow along the hypothalamo–hypophyseal tract.

The pituitary gland or hypophysis cerebri (from the Greek υπο- (below) and φυεδθα (to grow) consists of the adeno- and the neurohypophysis. The adenohypophysis is divided into three regions: the pars distalis or anterior lobe; the pars intermedia; and the pars tuberalis, which is applied to the infundibular stem. Five distinct cell types produce different hormones: somatotrophs (growth hormone); lactotrophs (prolactin); corticotrophs (adrenocorticotropin hormone); thyrotrophs (thyroid-stimulating hormone); and gonadotrophs (luteinizing and follicle-stimulating hormone). The neurohypophysis consists of a portion of the base of the hypothalamus, the pituitary stalk and the posterior lobe of the pituitary gland, where oxytocin and vasopressin are stored. The cavernous sinus extends from the superior orbital fissure anteriorly to the petrous apex posteriorly and is conically shaped. The dura of the superior wall of the cavernous sinus forms the diaphragm sellae medially. The third, fourth, fifth and sixth cranial nerves traverse the cavernous sinus during their course. The carotid artery traverses the petrous apex region underneath the Gasserian ganglion and enters the cavernous sinus. The carotid artery exits the cavernous sinus medial to the anterior clinoid process, beneath and lateral to the optic nerves, which form the optic chiasm in their further course, that only lies some 10 mm above the diaphragm and exhibits many anatomical variations: the anterior border of the chiasma can be prefixed, just above the tuberculum, or postfixed, above the dorsum sellae. All suprasellar arteries give origin to multiple perforating branches. The thalamoperforate and the medial posterior choroid arteries are the largest of these "perforators" that arise from the posterior parts of the circle of Willis [19].

SURGICAL TECHNIQUES

The general principles of the various approaches (Figure 21.2) are similar in different centers, despite some technical variations. The most common approaches – the transsphenoidal and the transcranial pterional (frontolateral) – described herein in detail are those used in the Neurosurgical Department of the University of Erlangen-Nürnberg and at the INI –

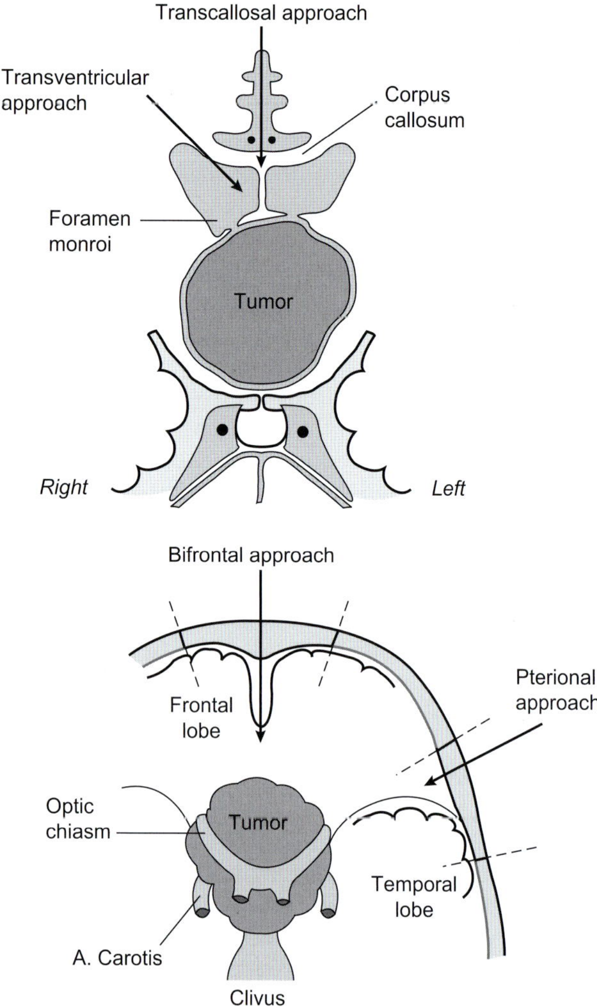

FIGURE 21.2 Different transcranial approaches to the suprasellar region.

International Neuroscience Institute of Hannover in Germany. Depending on the localization and extension of the tumors, a combination of two or three different approaches may be necessary.

TRANSSPHENOIDAL APPROACH

The original Cushing's method is used: the patient is positioned supine with the head tilted downwards about 10 degrees and the surgeon is standing behind the patient. A unilateral paraseptal approach is used. Depending on the nasal anatomy and the extent of the lesion, the mucosal incision is usually made in the vestibulum nasii along the cartilaginous nasal septum. Alternatively, a sublabial incision may be used. Under careful blunt dissection, the plane between cartilage and perichondrium is exposed. A mucosal tunnel is made without leaving this plane in order to prevent mucosal tearing. Resection of the anterior nasal spine of the maxilla gives better visualization of the tunnel. The basal cartilaginous septum is then mobilized and a Cushing-type speculum is inserted. Using the operating microscope, the tunnel is enlarged exposing the bony nasal septum, which has to be removed in order to the reach the sphenoidal sinus. We feel, however, that to date the most frequently practiced approach is the direct pernasal one. It is also used for entirely endoscopic operations. A speculum is introduced through one nasal cavity down to the anterior wall of the sphenoid sinus (optionally under fluoroscopic control) and the mucosa coagulated and incised [20].

The floor of the sphenoid sinus is then opened using a diamond drill and a larger self-retaining speculum is inserted. The sphenoid sinus is opened widely. The mucosa and all intrasphenoidal septae have to be removed, exposing the whole sella turcica from the sphenoidal plane to the clivus. In the case of incomplete pneumatization of the sphenoid sinus, the use of a drill is necessary in order to achieve such a wide exposure. The sellar floor is then opened and completely resected to the medial wall of the cavernous sinus. The basal dura is then opened and a small biopsy is taken to rule out tumor invasion histologically. The tumor is then removed using various curettes. During tumor removal, the diaphragm is usually descending into the pituitary fossa. If this does not occur spontaneously, it can usually be accomplished by an increase in intracranial pressure using positive end-expiratory pressure (PEEP) ventilation or compression of the jugular veins. In the case of a CSF leak, the surgical opening is sealed by two pieces of fascia lata fixed by fibrin glue (Figure 21.3). A lumbar drainage is then placed for CSF drainage until the third postoperative day. The mucosal incision is then closed and both nostrils are tamponaded for 24 hours [20]. Technical variations such as the use of the endoscope or the direct approach through the nasal cavity will be discussed later in this chapter.

TRANSCRANIAL PTERIONAL APPROACH

A small standard pterional craniotomy is used, but unusual extensions of large tumors may require a correspondingly designed approach, such as a bifrontal craniotomy with a subfrontal–translaminar tumor approach for tumors extending into the supra- and retrosellar region, and the transventricular approach for tumors involving the third ventricle and causing (partial) blockage of the foramen of Monro with enlarged ventricles. Following the elevation of the bone flap, the opening is expanded towards the floor of the middle fossa. The dura around the sphenoid

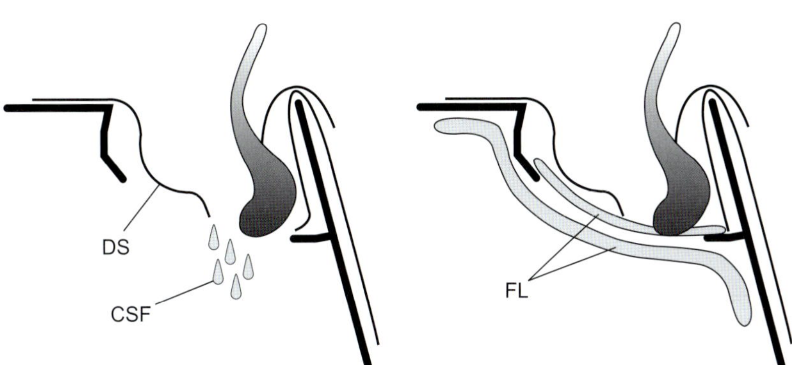

FIGURE 21.3 CSF leak during transsphenoidal surgery and repair of the sellar floor with two layers of fascia lata.

wing is separated and the spine of the wing removed by a rongeur. It is of great importance to completely flatten the posterior ridge of the greater wing in order to free the plane of vision to the suprasellar area without the need for significant retraction of the frontal lobe and to gain space for manipulations after the opening of the dura. Once the suprasellar cisterns are visible, the CSF should be drained, providing easier access by slackening of the brain. Due to the lesion, the circle of Willis and the optic apparatus are stretched. It is paramount to prevent further damage to this structure as well as to the hypothalamus. Many suprasellar tumors contact the hypothalamic area and grow adherent to it. Surgical manipulations to separate the tumor from the hypothalamus may lead to severe hypothalamic dysfunction. The tumor is usually resected piecemeal by incising the tumor capsule and performing an intracapsular evacuation of tumor tissue. The capsula is then mobilized, preserving the perforating arteries to the hypothalamic region and to the optic nerves. The stalk of the pituitary is not always easily identified; sometimes it is stretched, displaced, or even infiltrated by tumor. In some cases, complete resection of the lesion means sacrificing parts, or even complete resection of the pituitary stalk. With respect to tumors invading the cavernous sinus, the possibility of increasing the total resectable tumor mass is accompanied by a higher morbidity, particularly of optomotoric nerve dysfunction. Despite these extensive manipulations, total tumor resection and normalization of hormonal hypersecretion cannot usually be achieved by surgery alone in these cases. Authors with special anatomic experience describe extensive resection of tumors within the cavernous sinus [21]. Regarding the biological course in the case of pituitary adenomas with the availability of additional medical treatment, particularly in those tumors which secrete prolactin and growth hormone, and focused or conventional radiotherapy, the authors believe that this kind of surgery to date is rarely justified.

COMPLICATIONS

Mortality and morbidity have decreased tremendously in the microsurgical era. After transsphenoidal surgery, meningitis and CSF leak, respectively, occur in less than 1% of the cases [22]. Rebleeding is rare and must be suspected if a severe headache associated with deterioration of vision occurs postoperatively. This situation requires evacuation of the hematoma and is prevented by careful hemostasis. Ocular nerve palsies, occurring especially after transsphenoidal resection of parasellar pituitary tumors have, in our experience, been rare and transient. Deterioration of the anterior and posterior pituitary lobe may occur and may necessitate permanent replacement therapy.

FURTHER TREATMENT

Radiotherapy

Invasion, as recognized during surgery, is generally considered an indication for postoperative radiotherapy, unless only localized invasion, which could be sufficiently treated by surgery, was encountered. In the case of invasive secreting adenomas, irradiation is not mandatory of dynamic endocrine, testing postoperatively indicates a normalization of the previous excessive hormone secretion. External megavoltage radiotherapy is mostly used and a total dose ranging from 45 to 50 Gy applied in daily fractions of 1.8–2.0 Gy is recommended [23]. In cases with a distinct and small tumor remnant, focused radiation treatment with the gamma knife, the LINAC system, or the CYBER knife should be considered [24]. Severe soft tissue reactions and visual deterioration are rare, and induction of malignancies and cerebral radionecrosis are extremely rare adverse effects of radiotherapy [25]. Primary radiotherapy is used only for some patients in poor general condition and those showing signs of hypothalamic dysregulation. All other tumors should be surgically debulked before being irradiated. One goal of such decompressive operations is to create some 3–4 mm distance from the tumor surface to the visual pathway and brainstem.

Recurrences

Diagnosis of recurrent pituitary tumor depends on the surgeon's impression of complete tumor resection, normalization of hormonal hypersecretion and the absence of residual tumor in postoperative sophisticated imaging (MRI) [26]. However, even today it is not easy to differentiate between tissue suspicious of tumor recurrence and normal sellar structures, for example re-expansion of the previously compressed cavernous sinus. This fact, as well as the variable duration of follow-up intervals, explains why the percentage of recurrence reported in the literature varies considerably. Recurrence can be prevented by more radical resections, for example, surgery in two stages as well as with improved visualization: endoscopy and intraoperative resection control by MRI. Recurrence can also be prevented by postoperative radiotherapy. Histologic proof of invasion and the determination of the cell proliferation (e.g., Ki-67 or MIB1 immunohistochemistry) may also help to predict tumor recurrence [27].

Medical Treatment

In general, medical treatment supplements surgery. Defective anterior pituitary function and diabetes insipidus require compensation by adequate substitution therapy. Long-term control of tumor growth with medical treatment of pituitary tumors is well established in prolactinomas. Dopamine agonists have been shown to lower prolactin levels, to reduce the size of the adenoma, and to improve disturbed visual function in cases of visual compromise by displacement of the optic nerves or chiasm. Surgery is thus reserved for cases with intolerance to medical treatment due to side effects (e.g., orthostatic dysregulation, gastrointestinal discomfort) for nonresponders and for patients preferring operative treatment. One has to consider that in invasive prolactinomas, normoprolactinemia is very unlikely to be achieved postoperatively, so that long-term continuation of dopamine agonist treatment is necessary in almost all cases of large prolactinomas with and without surgery. Medical treatment with dopamine agonists and somatostatin analogues can be used in cases of invasive growth-hormone-producing adenomas if surgical therapy fails to restore normal growth hormone dynamics. Ketoconazole, an imidazole derivate that inhibits the synthesis of ergosterol and metyrapone, an inhibitor of the adrenocortical steroid 11-β-hydroxylation, contribute to an amelioration of clinical symptoms in cases of Cushing's disease, and both are used preoperatively in severely ill patients in order to reduce the operative risk or adjunct to external radiation.

PITUITARY TUMORS

Dealing with sellar lesions, one should distinguish between primary, metastatic and inflammatory pituitary tumors, which may mimic each other in their radiologic and clinical appearance. The relative frequency of various pituitary tumors treated in the Department of Neurosurgery of the University of Erlangen-Nürnberg in a 25 year period, from 1982–2007, is presented in Table 21.1. This statistical analysis may be used as one of the clues to the differential diagnosis of these lesions. Beginning with a comprehensive review of the surgical anatomy and continuing with the various tumor types, emphasizing the typical findings in their diagnostic endocrinological and radiological evaluation, the management of sellar and parasellar neoplasms is reviewed.

Patients with incidental tumors may remain under close observation, particularly if the tumors are small in size. However, impairment of endocrinological and ophthalmological function would add to the indications for surgical treatment. The rate of recurrence-free survival after total removal is approximately 85% after a follow-up period of 10 years (Figure 21.4).

Pituitary Adenomas

The incidence of pituitary adenomas in unselected autopsy series is almost 25%, but they account for only 15% of the intracranial tumors in neurosurgical practice [28,29]. In many cases these lesions remain undiagnosed since they do not cause clinical symptoms. Depending on their capability to produce different hormones which can be detected with routine hormone assays and histological staining methods, pituitary adenomas are classified with the most frequent being prolactinomas and null cell adenomas followed by growth-hormone-, ACTH- and TSH-producing adenomas. Some adenomas secrete more than one hormone. The most common combination is the prolactin- and growth-hormone-producing adenoma. Earlier classifications on the basis of cytoplasmatic staining affinities in acidophilic, basophilic and chromophobic adenomas are absolute due to the poor correlations with the secretory activity of the tumors [30]. In cases of hormonal hypersecretion, patients present with well-defined clinical syndromes. Other patients present with clinical symptoms of impaired pituitary function resulting from compression of the pituitary gland. In such cases, somatotrophs belong to the most vulnerable cell type causing GH deficiency, followed by gonadotrophs causing

TABLE 21.1 Classification and Incidence of Pituitary Tumors Surgically Treated in the Department of Neurosurgery of the University of Erlangen-Nürnberg from 1 December 1982–1931 December 2006 ($n = 4590$)

I. Common Tumors of the Sella Turcica	**4343**
Pituitary adenomas	3713
Nonfunctioning adenomas	1537
GH-omas	877
Prolactinomas	730
ACTH-producing adenomas	537
TSH-omas	32
Craniopharyngiomas	325
Supra- and parasellar meningiomas	199
Miscellaneous cystic lesions	106
Rathke's cleft cyst	48
Intrasellar colloid cyst	37
Arachnoid cyst	21
II. Rare Tumors of the Sella Turcica	**247**
Optico–hypothalamic gliomas	62
Metastases	41
Chordomas	37
Inflammatory lesions	35
Germinomas	24
Hypothalamic hamartomas	7
Chondromas	8
Epidermoids	7
III. Miscellaneous Pituitary Tumors	**26**
Granular cell tumor, paragangliomas, mucocele, chiasmatic cavernoma, hypothalamic lipoma, sarcoidosis	

hypogonadism, thyreotrophs causing hypothyroidism and corticotrophs causing secondary adrenocortical failure. Patients may also present with various neurologic symptoms. Tumors with marked suprasellar extension may cause impairment of visual acuity, lead to pathognomonic (bi-)temporal visual field constriction, and may even result in obstruction hydrocephalus due to compression or obstruction of the foramen of Monro. Lesions extending into the parasellar region compress the cavernous sinus and may affect the cranial nerves traversing the sinus, thus causing periorbital pain, facial hypaesthesia and diplopia. Huge invasive tumors extending into the skull base may present with obstruction of nasal airways or cerebrospinal fluid leak. In almost every type of pituitary adenoma except prolactinomas, surgery is the primary treatment of choice. Transsphenoidal surgery is the most commonly used approach. It may be applied in almost 90% of these lesions. For the remaining, a transcranial, usually pterional, approach or a combined transsphenoidal and transcranial approach is needed.

Nonfunctioning Pituitary Adenomas

Clinically nonfunctioning pituitary adenomas are also called endocrine inactive or nonsecreting adenomas, because they do not cause specific clinical syndromes of hormonal oversecretion, which can be clinically recognized or determined from tumor markers in the patient's serum. However, the majority of these tumors obviously are endocrinologically active [31]. This can be concluded from the results of cell explant culture studies and immunohistochemical examinations. However, their endocrine activity has no clinical significance until now: it neither offers a basis for efficient medical treatment (GnRH analogues, somatostatin analogues) nor provides tumor markers which would indicate complete tumor removal, tumor remnants, or recurrences [32]. In cell explant cultures, the expression of gonadotropins can most frequently be determined in older patients. Immunohistochemical examinations demonstrate gonadotropins (including α- and β-subunits) in about 80% of the tumors. Some 14% are positive for hormones other than gonadotropins, e.g., the so-called "silent" somatotroph, corticotroph and gonadotroph adenomas. Only 6% are completely negative for all pituitary hormones and thus represent pure or oncocytic null cell adenomas. Lacking clinical significance, the only difference between the two types is that in oncocytomas, there is a marked mitochondrial accumulation. Patients harboring clinically nonfunctioning pituitary adenomas present with tumors large enough to cause mass effects such as visual compromise and various degrees of hypopituitarism. In many cases the lesion is discovered incidentally when radiological evaluation is performed for an unrelated reason, such as head trauma. Patients with incidental tumors may remain under close observation, particularly if the tumors are small in size. However, impairment of endocrinological and ophthalmological function would add to the indication for surgical treatment. The rate of recurrence-free survival after total removal is approximately 85% after a follow-up period of 10 years (Figure 21.4).

Prolactinomas

Prolactinomas constitute the largest group of pituitary adenomas in autopsy series. However, their relative incidence in recent surgical series is dramatically reduced because medical treatment with dopamine

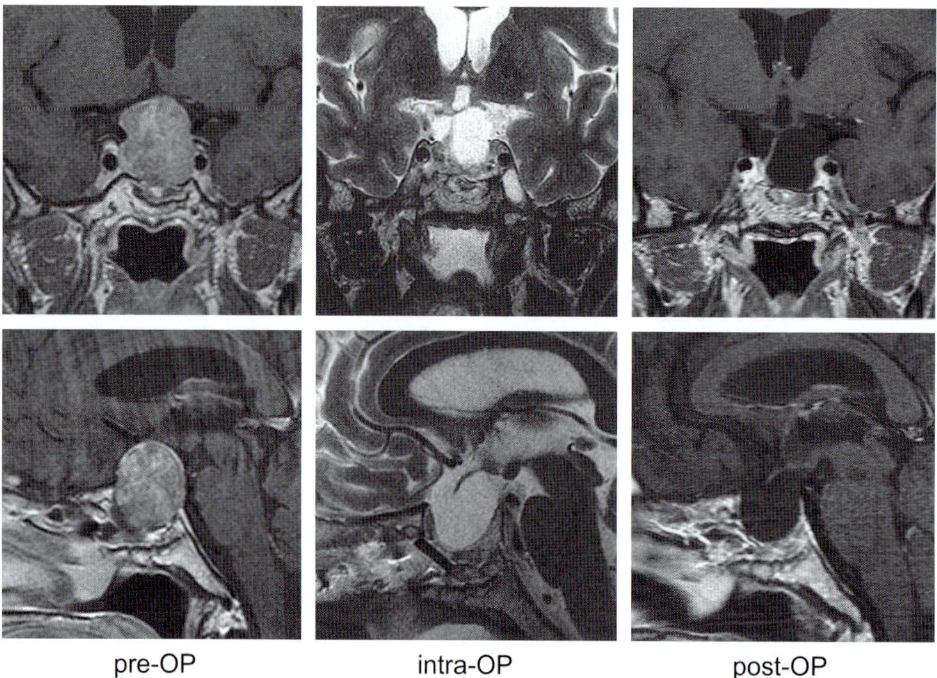

FIGURE 21.4 Pre-, peri- and intraoperative MR images of an intra- and suprasellar pituitary adenoma. Left: the large tumor is visualized preoperatively in T_1-weighted coronal and sagittal sections after contrast enhancement. Middle: after tumor resection, intraoperative images with T_2-weighted TSE sequences document a cisternal herniation, decompression of the chiasm, and preservation of the infundibulum. Right: the standard delayed postoperative T_1-weighted images after 3 months reveal a perfectly corresponding situation to the intraoperative depiction without evidence of residual tumor.

agonists is effective and safe. It leads in many cases to tumor shrinkage and normalization of prolactin levels. Patients present with the clinical symptoms of hyperprolactinemia: menstrual dysfunction and galactorrhea in women and loss of libido and potency in men. Prolactinomas may also cause various clinical symptoms due to their size, compressing surrounding structures like the pituitary gland, cavernous sinus and optic nerves. In men they tend to be diagnosed later than in woman; their tumors are larger and more frequently show an invasive growth pattern. The standard treatment is medical [33]. Disadvantages of medical therapy are side effects, like orthostatic hypotension, nausea and vomiting. In most patients the effects of dopamine agonists on prolactinomas are not tumoricidal. The therapeutic effect is only maintained as long as the drug is administered. After withdrawal of the drugs, the prolactin level is expected to rise again and the tumor frequently re-expands. Thus, in most cases, medical treatment has to be continued life-long, with a few exceptions in whom normoprolactinemia is maintained after discontinuation of dopamine agonists. The most commonly used drug was bromocriptine, but now newer-generation drugs like quinagolide and cabergoline are preferentially prescribed. Quinagolide gained considerable attention because of its extended plasma half life allowing longer application intervals [34–36]. Surgery is reserved mostly for patients with intolerance to the medication, those individually not responding to dopamine agonists (which constitute less than 10% of the cases) and those who for personal reasons reject medical treatment. A brief overview of indications of surgery in a recent series of 212 patients treated in 1990 and 2005 is presented in Table 21.2. Remission rates in large series of surgically treated prolactinomas vary between 54% and 86% [38–40]. In our consecutive series of 519 surgically treated prolactinomas, the normalization rate after transsphenoidal surgery depended on the preoperative prolactin levels, tumor size and extension (Table 21.3). The remission rate of 80% in microprolactinomas with initial prolactin levels <4000 μU/ml

TABLE 21.2 Overview of Indications for Surgical Treatment in a Recent Consecutive Series of 212 Patients Operated upon Between 1990 and 2005

Prolactinomas 1990–2005: Indications for Surgery	n = 212
Nonresponder hyperprolactinemia	27
Nonresponder tumor shrinkage	52
Cystic tumors	50
Dopamine agonists not tolerated	38
Emergency CSF fistula, diplopia, pituitary apoplexy	22
Patient's dedicated decision	23

From [37].

TABLE 21.3 Normalization of PRL Secretion in Patients with Surgically Treated Prolactinomas in Relation to the Tumor Extension and Preoperative PRL Levels after Primary Surgery

	Micro			Macro				
Tumor extension	**<4000 μU/ml**	**>4000 μU/ml**	**is**	**ps/sphe**	**S1**	**S2**	**Giant**	**Σ**
PRL <500 μU/ml	80%	49%	50%	52%	13%	17%	0%	42%

micro: <10 mm; macro: 10–40 mm; giant: >40 mm; is: intrasphenoidal; ps: parasellar; Sphe: sphenoidal; S1: suprasellar with no compression of the optic chiasm; S2: suprasellar with compression of the optic chiasm

still makes surgical treatment an interesting alternative to long-term medical treatment.

Growth-hormone-producing Pituitary Adenomas

GH-producing pituitary adenomas are the cause of almost all cases of acromegaly and gigantism. An ectopic GH-producing adenoma or a hypothalamic GHRH-producing tumor is an extreme rarity [41]. Hypersecretion of growth hormone results in enlargement of the acres (hands and feet), soft tissue swelling, hyperhidrosis, macroglossia, prognathism, retroorbital pain, carpal tunnel syndrome and metabolic disturbances. Growth hormone acts anabolically, diabetogenically and lipolytically. Acromegalic patients develop cardiac and respiratory dysfunction and have a significantly decreased life expectancy [42]. The therapy of choice is surgical treatment. Primary radiation therapy to control tumor growth and/or long-term medical treatment with octreotide is preserved for patients with severe risk factors. Octreotide and lancreotide are both somatostatin analogues, which reduce GH levels and shrink the adenomas [43,44]. The most relevant side effects are gastrointestinal discomfort, during short-term, and gallstone formation during long-term treatment. Like dopamine agonists for prolactinomas, the effect is reversible with regard to tumor extension and GH levels. Dopamine agonists may also be given to acromegalic patients but reduction of GH or IGF-1 to normal levels can be achieved in less than 20% of the cases [45]. Even in current recommendation for acromegaly, surgery plays a pivotal role. In our consecutive series of 624 GH-producing adenomas, the normalization rate after transsphenoidal surgery depended on preoperative GH levels and tumor size (Table 21.4). The most favorable remission rate was achieved in the group harboring adenomas <10 mm with an initial serum GH level of <10 ng/ml. Normalization of growth hormone secretion in patients with an initial GH level higher than 50 ng/ml is only exceptionally achieved. The remission criteria were basal GH levels <2.5 ng/ml and GH <1 ng/ml during OGTT and a normal IGF-1. Remission rates in other large published series depend on the remission criteria used and vary between 52% and 85% [47–50].

Cushing's Disease

ACTH-producing adenomas accounted for some 15% of the surgically treated pituitary adenomas in our consecutive surgical series. Cushing's disease is more common in women (8:1) [51]. The patients present with typical clinical symptoms due to hypercortisolism: weight gain, centripetal obesity with moon face and buffalo hump, acne, purple striae, ecchymoses, hirsutism, menstrual disturbances, loss of libido, osteoporosis with pathologic fractures, glucose intolerance and arterial hypertension [52]. In about 80% of patients the endogenous Cushing's syndrome is ACTH-dependent (pituitary adenomas 85%, ectopic ACTH syndrome 15%, ectopic CRH-syndrome <1%). ACTH-independent Cushing's syndrome caused by adrenal adenomas or carcinomas is present in 20% of cases [53]. Therefore, sophisticated endocrinological testing is necessary to diagnose the condition and to identify the cause. Circadian rhythm studies of serum and urine cortisol and the low-dose dexamethasone suppression test confirm the diagnosis of Cushing's syndrome. High-dose dexamethasone and ACTH-stimulation after administration of CRH lead to the diagnosis of pituitary-dependent Cushing's syndrome (Cushing's disease). In the vast majority of cases, the cause is a pituitary microadenoma. If thin collimation MRI fails to demonstrate the lesion (<2–3 mm), then bilateral blood sampling from the inferior petrosal sinuses should be performed. A gradient between central and peripheral ACTH levels confirms the diagnosis. A gradient between right and left petrosal sinus helps to identify the site of the lesion intraoperatively and offers the

TABLE 21.4 Normalization of GH Secretion in Patients with Acromegaly in Relation to the Tumor Extension and Preoperative GH Levels after Primary Surgery

	Micro		Macro				
Tumor extension		**is**	**ps/sphe**	**S1**	**S2**	**Giant**	**Σ**
GH (OGT) <1 ng/ml IGF-1 n	75%	74%	42%	45%	33%	10%	57%
Preoperative GH level ng/ml	<10	10–50	50–125			>125	Σ
GH (OGTT) <2 g/ml	90%	74%	25%			0%	57%

From [48].

TABLE 21.5 Normalization of ACTH Secretion in Patients with Cushing's Disease after Primary Surgery

Primary Surgery for Cushing's Disease n = 347	%
Selective adenomectomy (295/347)	85
No tumor found 15% (52/347)	
Partial hypophysectomy (n = 31)	
Remission (217/295)	74
Persistence (78/295)	27
Remission (10/31)	30
Persistence (21/31)	68

option of a hemihypophysectomy if no adenoma is identified. In most large series, a remission of hypercortisolism can be induced in between 70% and 86% of patients [53–58]. The summary of the results of our series of 382 surgically treated patients is demonstrated in Table 21.5. Because of the severity of the disease, patients are almost always in reduced general condition and need specific expert peri- and postoperative care. After endocrinological remission, the high recurrence rate of up to 25% in 5 years makes long-term postoperative endocrinological follow-up necessary [58]. In the case of persistence or recurrence of the disease the treatment options include second-look surgery, bilateral adrenalectomy, medical treatment and radiotherapy [59].

Rare Pituitary Adenomas

NELSON'S SYNDROME

First reported by Nelson, the syndrome was originally characterized by the classic triad of cutaneous hyperpigmentation, considerable elevated ACTH levels and an enlarged sella turcica months or years after Cushing's disease was treated by bilateral adrenalectomy [60]. The association of increasing hyperpigmentation in patients with an enlarging ACTH-producing adenoma could be better monitored when direct imaging became available. These tumors are usually invasive macroadenomas and the patients develop extremely high ACTH levels. In our series the incidence of this syndrome was 1.3%. The patients should eventually be treated surgically. Normalization of ACTH levels is hardly ever achieved, since the postadrenalectomy condition persists. Radiation therapy should be routinely utilized postoperatively in these tumors, since ACTH levels remain elevated and in respect of the aggressive biologic behavior of these lesions [61].

TSH-PRODUCING ADENOMAS

The first case with TSH secretion proven by radioimmunoassay was reported in 1970 [62]. Since then only a few hundred patients with TSH-producing adenomas have been reported in the medical literature; 22 such patients underwent surgery in our department and remission was achieved in 14 of them. The patients usually present with signs and symptoms of hyperthyroidism in the presence of elevated TSH levels. Many patients have a history of surgically treated goiter. The pituitary tumors are frequently invasive macroadenomas and respond well to octreotide, which has been used successfully before surgery to suppress TSH, normalize the peripheral thyroid hormones, and shrink the tumor [63]. In the case of residual tumor and persistently elevated TSH levels medical treatment with octreotide and radiation therapy are utilized. Previous therapies sometimes make the clinical problems very complex.

GONADOTROPIN-PRODUCING ADENOMAS

These are uncommon and mostly remain undetected because of the lack of specific symptoms. LH and FSH levels, respectively, are clearly elevated in the serum. These lesions have to be differentiated from nonfunctioning pituitary adenomas with only immunohistochemical evidence of FSH and LH ("silent" gonadotroph pituitary adenomas). Patients usually present with visual compromise. Gonadotropin- and TSH-producing adenomas may additionally produce the α- and ß-subunits, which does not imply therapeutical significance [64].

Craniopharyngiomas

Craniopharyngiomas arise from remnants of Rathke's pouch and account for 3% of all intracranial tumors. They can be differentiated into adamantinomatous and papillary craniopharyngiomas. The adamantinomatous type is more frequent and usually presents as a cystic, partially calcified lesion containing cholesterol crystals. Only 10% of the craniopharyngiomas are of the papillary type [65]. They occur only in adults and frequently involve the third ventricle. Both types develop in the intra- and suprasellar region, thus causing visual compromise and endocrine deficiencies (Figure 21.5). They may cause hydrocephalus by obstruction of the cerebrospinal fluid circulation in cases in which the third ventricle is involved. They may extend into the hypothalamic area and may cause vegetative dysregulation as well as endocrine hypothalamic syndromes, like Fröhlich syndrome (hypothalamic–hypogonadal adiposity). As much as one-half of the newly diagnosed craniopharyngiomas are predominantly cystic. In about 60% of the tumors, different degrees of calcification are encountered. The patients' age distribution shows peak incidences between 15 and 20 years and between 50 and 55 years [66]. Approximately 40% of the patients are children aged less than 16 years at the time of surgery. The vast majority of patients harboring such a lesion present

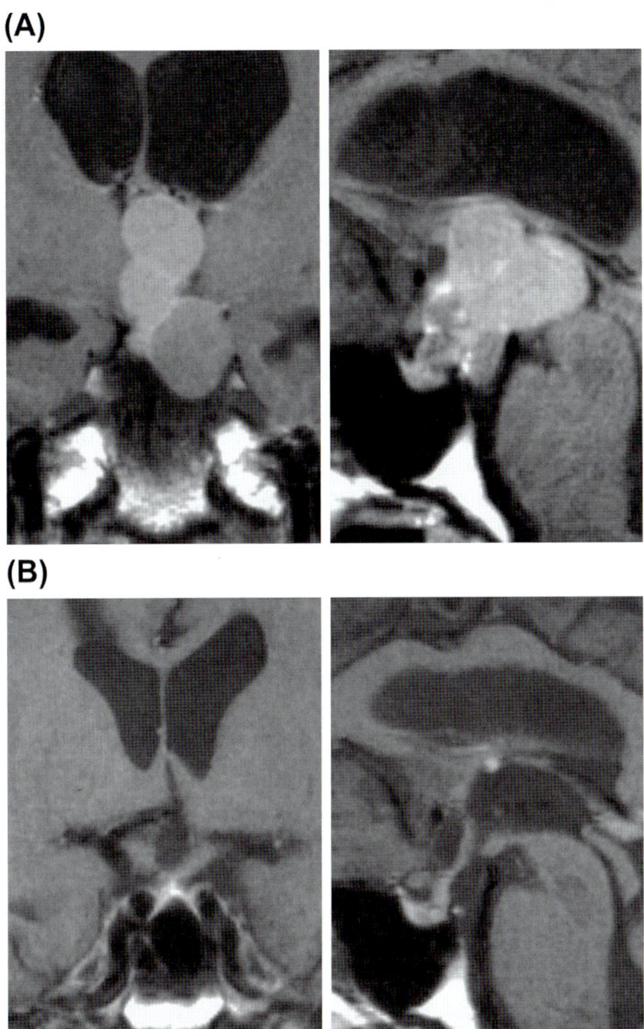

FIGURE 21.5 Giant supra- and retrosellar craniopharyngioma before (A) and after (B) total removal via a right frontolateral approach with preservation of pituitary stalk (perioperative temporary drainage of the enlarged lateral ventricles).

with impairment of anterior pituitary function, hypogonadism being the most frequent deficiency, followed by failure of the corticotrope and thyrotrope axis. Many patients present with diabetes insipidus [67]. Surgical treatment still remains a technical challenge and a subject of controversy. In many early reports, radical surgery led to an unacceptably high mortality and morbidity because of the involvement of both the hypothalamus and the pituitary gland. For this reason, other authors favored the therapeutic concept of conservative incomplete surgery followed by radiotherapy [68,69]. Concerning the many improvements which have been made in recent years, the goal of therapy should be selective removal of the tumor with preservation of the hypothalamus, midbrain, perforating vessels of the circle of Willis, optic pathways, pituitary stalk and pituitary gland. Depending on the tumor location, all available surgical approaches to the sellar region may be used. In many instances, combined approaches are necessary. The cases (up to 40%) in which the transsphenoidal approach is suitable have the advantage of a favorably low morbidity and mortality. The rate of recurrence-free survival after total removal of the tumors may attain 80% after a follow-up interval of 10 years.

Supra- and Parasellar Meningiomas

Meningiomas originate from arachnoidal cap cells and are surgically classified by their site of origin. They account for about 15% of all intracranial tumors. Some 10% of meningiomas involve sellar and parasellar structures [70]. The tuberculum sellae meningioma is the classic suprasellar meningioma, causing slowly progressive loss of vision and headache. These tumors may invade the bony skull base, causing hyperostosis of the sphenoidal plane, may extend into the optic canal and displace the carotid and the anterior cerebral arteries and the pituitary stalk. They thus cause hyperprolactinemia, which is the only endocrine disturbance that usually can be detected. Meningiomas of the cavernous sinus usually cause the so-called cavernous sinus syndrome: diplopia and proptosis due to palsy of the sixth and third, and periorbital pain and numbness due to compression of the fifth cranial nerves [71]. Patients with optic sheath meningiomas present with progressive and painless loss of vision but orbital pain, exophthalmus and ophthalmoplegia may also occur. Meningiomas of the clinoid process, however, expand into the suprasellar cistern, the optic canal and invade the cavernous sinus. Diaphragma sellae and intrasellar meningiomas are rarely found. Various histology types including the rare hemangiopericytoma and malignant meningioma can be found. Surgery is the treatment of choice in sellar and parasellar meningiomas. Depending on several factors, like the site of origin, extension, consistency, vascularization, but also dura, bone and soft tissue infiltration, several meningiomas can be totally removed; others cannot, at least not without unacceptable morbidity. The best results are obtained in suprasellar meningiomas, in which the tumor can be completely resected under preservation of the optic and oculomotor nerves. Treatment of meningiomas of the cavernous sinus is handled controversially among neurosurgeons, complete removal may lead to significant new neurological deficits and ischemia. The authors thus frequently prefer to perform a "slice technique," transsphenoidal decompression of the cavernous sinus and the pituitary gland in tumors with intra- and parasellar extensions [72,73]. In cases with progressive neurological deficit, transcranial decompression by resection of the lateral portions of the cavernous sinus meningioma is performed, followed by radiotherapy. Medical treatment with hydroxyurea for tumor shrinkage may be useful, especially in combination with radiotherapy [74].

Miscellaneous Cystic Lesions

Rathke's Cleft Cysts

These are found in up to 20% of the specimens as any intrasellar lesions in large autopsy series, but it is unusual for them to enlarge and become symptomatic due to compression of the pituitary gland, the optic system and the hypothalamus [75]. Rathke's cleft cysts are lined by epithelial cells that consist of a single layer of cuboid and columnar epithelium on a basal membrane. In their radiologic appearance they may mimic craniopharyngiomas. Surgical treatment is suggested, when they become symptomatic. Depending on their location some 90% of these lesions can be removed by the transsphenoidal approach. Only exceptionally a recurrence occurs [76].

Intra- and Suprasellar Colloid Cysts

Also termed pars intermedia cysts, they consist of a circumscribed collection of colloid material within the pituitary gland that lacks a cyst wall [77]. Some of these patients harbor a concomitant pituitary adenoma. The most frequent presenting symptoms are oligomenorrhea, galactorrhea and headache, but panhypopituitarism may also accur. Postoperatively, a normalization of pituitary function is observed in more than 80% of patients. Again, transsphenoidal surgery is indicated when the lesion becomes symptomatic.

Arachnoid Cysts

These only sporadically involve the sellar region. Then, they are usually located in the suprasellar area. These patients present with headache, visual disturbances and hypopituitarism. Frequently the radiological diagnosis is difficult, because in the MRI they appear as lesions with a signal identical to CSF. Empty sella therefore is the most important differential diagnosis. In such a case, metrizamide cisternography provides a reliable preoperative diagnosis. Transsphenoidal or transcranial approaches are used in symptomatic arachnoid cysts for drainage, partial removal of the cyst wall and fenestration to the suprasellar cisterns [78].

Rare Pituitary Tumors

Optico–Hypothalamic Gliomas

Optico–hypothalamic gliomas are mostly pilocytic astrocytomas arising from the optic nerves, the chiasm, the walls of the third ventricle or the tuber cinereum. The patients present with visual disturbances (loss of vision, papilledema, optic atrophy, visual field defects). Frequently, hypothalamo–pituitary function remains unaffected despite the considerable size of the lesion. However, various endocrine disturbances including hypopituitarism, diabetes insipidus or even Russell syndrome (hypothalamic cachexia) and precocious puberty may occur. In some cases hydrocephalus is present due to obstruction of the foramen of Monro. Neurofibromatosis type 1 is not uncommon among patients harboring optico–hypothalamic gliomas [79,80]. The treatment is handled controversially and depends on the location and clinical symptoms. Treatment options include total surgical removal (intraorbital gliomas), removal of exophytic tumor parts (chiasmatic gliomas), chemotherapy (usually vincristine and carboplastine), or radiation therapy, which is reserved for older patients. In cases without progressive neurologic deficit, observation is recommended since many tumors do not enlarge during a long-term follow-up interval.

Metastatic Tumors

Symptomatic metastatic tumors to the sella area are rare lesions, but in autopsy series of patients with various types of cancer the incidence is reported to be as high as 27% [81]. The most common cancers that metastasize to the pituitary region are lung, prostate and stomach cancer in men; and breast, lung and stomach cancer in women [82]. Sellar metastases are usually invasive tumors involving osseous structures as well as the pituitary gland. Patients present with diabetes insipidus and ophthalmological symptoms. Surgery is indicated to decompress surrounding tissue followed by radiotherapy. Involvement of the sellar region in metastasis of hematopoietic neoplasms is rarely observed [83]. However, lymphomas, which involve the hypothalamic area, and plasmocytomas both occur and are associated with poor prognosis whatever treatment is chosen [84].

Chordomas

Chordomas are histologically benign tumors that are derived from notochondral remnants and almost always involve the clival area. Their biologic character is extremely aggressive, which is expressed by bone destruction, infiltration of the cavernous sinus and basal dura, and extension into all cranial fossae [85]. Depending on the location of the chordomas, patients may present with visual compromise, pituitary deficiencies and ophthalmoplegia. Because of the invasive growth pattern total removal is not possible without high mortality and morbidity. Even after radiotherapy, the recurrence rate in our series is found to be 80% in 5 years. The survival rate after a follow-up period of 10 years is lower than 30%, but in individual patients no tumor progression is observed even after 15 years.

Inflammatory Lesions

HYPOPHYSITIS

Lymphocytic hypophysitis is histologically characterized by infiltration of the pituitary gland by lymphocytes and plasma cells, and by fibrosis. An autoimmune background and a relation to pregnancy have been suggested [86,87]. The granulomatous hypophysitis is characterized by granulomas with histiocytes and multinucleated giant cells but also shows a collection of lymphocytes. The most frequent presenting syndrome is headache occurring in a fluctuating course due to recurrent aseptic meningitis, followed by diabetes insipidus, menstrual irregularities and visual compromise. Radiologically a dumbbell-shaped lesion with a tongue-like supra- and retrosellar extension in the MRI is a characteristic finding that is seen in more than 60% of cases (Figure 21.6). After surgical treatment, recurrence occurs in some 10% of patients [88,89]. Repeat surgery, medical treatment with corticosteroids and radiation therapy are additional treatment options.

PITUITARY ABSCESS

Pituitary abscesses may be a rare manifestation of an acute bacterial infection that develops per continuitatem in cases with perisellar infections like sinusitis and mastoiditis. However, this entity is not clearly defined and thus significant confusion exists. A pre-existing tumor seems to be evident in many cases. The diagnosis is made intraoperatively and histologically because the pituitary abscess mimics nonfunctional pituitary tumors in radiological and endocrinological evaluations [90]. After surgical removal the patient should receive antibiotics. *Staphylococcus aureus* is the most relevant microorganism and can be isolated from bacterial cultures, but in many cases these cultures remain sterile.

Hypothalamic Hamartomas

Hamartomas are neuronal lesions consisting of neurons within a stroma of axons and astroglial elements. In the few known cases the lesions led to precocious puberty in young males as a result of hypothalamic compression [91]. They may also cause epilepsy with gelastic and complex partial seizures. In some cases gonadotropin-releasing hormone could be detected immunohistochemically. Rarely, growth-hormone-releasing hormones are secreted, causing acromegaly either from pituitary hyperplasia or to pituitary adenoma [92]. Effective medical treatment with gonadotropin-releasing hormone analogues for precocious puberty and anticonvulsants for gelastic seizures mean that surgery is no longer the preferred initial management for these lesions [93,94].

Germ Cell Tumors

Germ cell tumors develop in the midline and affect the pineal, the suprasellar, or both, regions simultaneously [95]. Seventy percent of the lesions are germinomas. The 30% nongerminomatous lesions include teratomas, embryonal carcinomas, endodermal sinus tumors and choriocarcinomas. Germinomas show an invasive growth pattern and infiltrate the surrounding tissue causing typical clinical symptoms like visual disturbances, diabetes insipidus, hypopituitarism and hydrocephalus [96]. Occasionally biochemical tumor markers like α-fetoprotein, human chorionic gonadotropine and placental alkaline phosphatase may be detected in both serum and CSF [97]. In these patients,

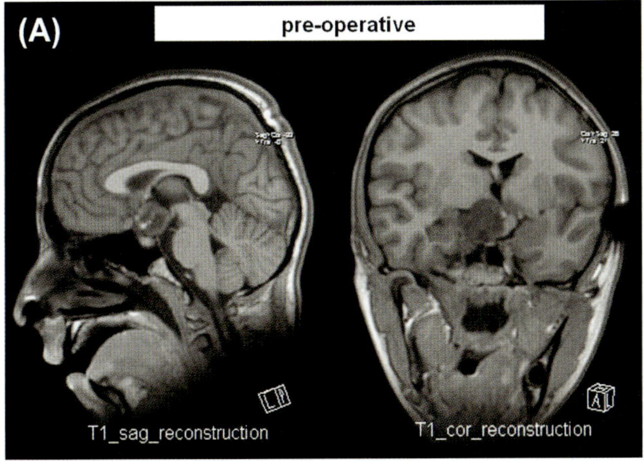

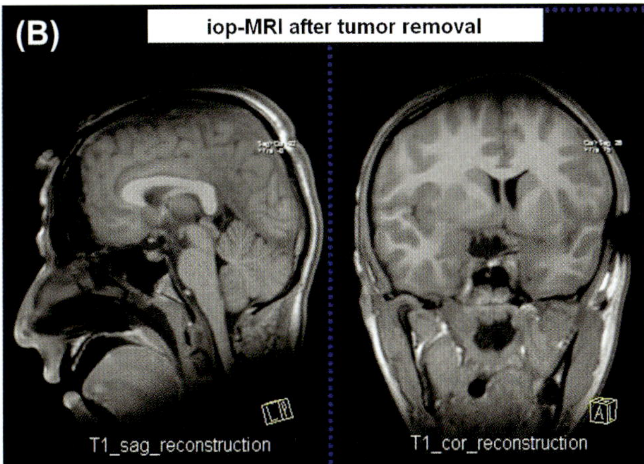

FIGURE 21.6 Left suprasellar craniopharygoima with displacement of optic chiasma and pituitary stalk to the left side and N6 paresis, (A) before, (B) after total removal via a right pterional approach with preservation of pituitary stalk and pituitary as well as optomotoric functions.

a biopsy is usually necessary to confirm the diagnosis. These lesions are extremely radiosensitive. Long-term control of tumor growth is achieved with primary radiation therapy. After a few fractions, the MRI should confirm tumor shrinkage. Radiotherapy of the neuroaxis should be performed due to the possibility of metastatic dissemination CSF pathways. Nongerminomatous germ cell tumors are rare lesions with high malignancy. Dermoid cysts are entire via the distinct noninfiltrative lesions containing hair, bone, or even teeth.

Epidermoid Cysts

Epidermoid cysts are uncommon lesions of the sellar area [98]. They grow slowly and become manifest in the fourth and fifth decades of life causing visual compromise, hypopituitarism and episodes of aseptic meningitis due to leakage of the cyst content into the CSF. The treatment is surgical. Recurrence in case of incomplete removal is probable, thus necessitating repeat surgery.

EVOLVING TECHNOLOGIES

Just like in other surgical specialities, a variety of novel technical developments were introduced for surgery of the pituitary gland and its tumours. One unequivocal major progress is the use of the endoscope. Endoscope-assisted microsurgery means that an endoscope is used within the classical microsurgical operation, when the surgeon feels that the additional assets of the endoscope could be helpful. The visual field is no more restricted by the straight beam of light within the nasal tunnel maintained open by the speculum. Introduction of an endoscope into the sphenoid sinus allows a more panoramic visualization of the anatomy, an excellent orientation, and additional control of the radicality of tumor resection. The visual field of the surgeon is thus considerably extended [26]. Alternatively, fully endoscopic procedures no longer require septal dissections and the use of a speculum [99]. A direct perinasal route is chosen and a sphenoidotomy performed. Rather than an operating microscope a monitor is used. To date, few data are available on the hormonal and imaging outcomes which allow a comparison of remission and complication rates, respectively, of open microsurgical procedures and entirely endoscopic operations [100]. One disadvantage of the endoscopic technique is the learning curve with a technically somewhat different procedure during which the surgeon controls his instruments from a screen rather than from the lenses of the operating microscope. Thus, the operating time is frequently extended. The three-dimensional view, which the operating microscope allows, is lost and the color information is inferior to that obtained with sophisticated microscopic equipment. With "extended" nasal approaches, lesions become accessible transsphenoidally which have previously been considered contraindications for nasal approaches [102]. However, to date still most of the data available on safety and efficacy of pituitary operations come from microsurgical operations.

Neuronavigation is to date widely used in the entire field of microneurosurgery and may be used during pituitary operations. The three-dimensional data set provided by preoperative imaging is related to the patient's head in the operation room. Critical structures such as the tumor shape or the brain-supplying major arteries can be localized with a "pointer" or segmented and superimposed onto the surgical field [26,103]. Thus, additional anatomical orientation is gained. Image-guided surgery can be used in each and every case, but is associated with increased costs and might not be always needed. It is certainly particularly helpful in anatomical variants and reoperations. Neuronavigation to date is highly reliable and substitutes for the traditional fluoroscopic control [104].

The microdoppler system, which is widely used in neurovascular microsurgery, can also be considered a useful technical tool for pituitary operations. It allows localization of the carotid artery within the cavernous sinus or within parasellar tumor. Thus, the likelihood of an arterial lesion is further minimized [105].

Intraoperative magnetic resonance imaging is receiving increasing recognition. Dedicated MR scanners were developed for intraoperative imaging and diagnostic scanners systems were modified for intraoperative use in pituitary surgery [106,107]. While in an ideal case of an intra- and suprasellar adenoma, the elevated arachnoid descends into the sella in only one smooth arachnoidal plane, a complex situation may occur in which residual tumor cannot be directly visualized. There might be tumor hidden below any one of the arachnoidal pouches or in the lateral, anterior, or posterior portions of the sella. Both low- and high-field MR systems are able to detect such residual tumor intraoperatively and thus allow improvement of the radicality of tumor excision, particularly in large tumors [107,108]. Only high-field systems can also depict the parasellar structures with sufficient image quality and thus allow a decision about total removal of intra- and parasellar lesions. In a modern high-field system intraoperative images can be obtained that correspond perfectly to the delayed postoperative scans which constitute the standard of postoperative imaging [108,109]. The relatively high costs of the devices and the necessity of at least partially rebuilding the operating room to make it suitable for the MR are clearly disadvantages of this technology. In several reports, it has been convincingly demonstrated, that even in experienced hands, the rate of total tumor resections could be increased by about one-third [109]. However, even with all the technical refinements in the surgery of pituitary adenomas, the factors defined by the tumor growth characteristics and location and the individual experience and technical skills of the surgeon are still the main determinants of the surgical outcome for an individual patient. Centers with a high case load and experienced neurosurgeons have less complications and achieve a more efficient outcome in terms of both the extent of tumor resection as visualized by imaging and normalization of hormonal oversecretion [110,111].

References

[1] V. Horsley, On operative technique of operations on the central nervous system, Br Med J 2 (1906) 411–423.

[2] O.G.T. Kiliani, Some remarks on tumors of the chiasm, with a proposal on how to reach the same by operation, Ann Surg 40 (1904) 35–43.

[3] C.H. Frazier, Choice of method in operations upon the pituitary body, Surg Gynecol Obstet 29 (1919) 9–16.

[4] C.H. Frazier, Lesions of the hypophysis from the viewpoint of a surgeon, Surg Gynecol Obstet 17 (1913) 724–736.

[5] W.E. Dandy, A new hypophysis operation, Bull Johns Hopkins Hosp 29 (1918) 151–155.

[6] W.E. Dandy, The brain, in: D. Lewis (Ed.), Practise of Surgery, WF Prior, Hagerstown, MD, 1934, pp. 556–605.

[7] H. Schloffer, Erfolgreiche Operation eines Hypophysentumors auf nasalem Wege, Wien Klin Wochensch 20 (1907) 621–624.

[8] A.H. von Eiselsberg, Über den Endausgang und Obduktion meines ersten operativen Falles von Hypophyentumor, Beitr Pathol Anat 71 (1922) 619–624.

[9] A.H. von Eiselsberg, My experience about operation upon the hypophysis, Ann Surg 52 (1910) 1–14.

[10] O. Hirsch, Endonasal method of removal of hypophyseal tumors: With report of two cases, JAMA 55 (1910) 772–774.

[11] O. Hirsch, Über Methoden der Behandlung von Hypophysistumoren auf endonasalem Wege, Arch Laryngol Rhinol 24 (1911) 129–177.

[12] H. Cushing, Partial hypophysectomy for acromegaly: With remarks on the functions of the hypophysis, Ann Surg 50 (1909) 1002–1017.

[13] H. Cushing, Intracranial tumours. Notes upon a series of two thousand verified cases with surgical-mortality percentages pertaining thereto, Ch.C. Thomas, Springfield, 1932, pp. 69–79.

[14] G. Guiot, G. Arfel, S. Brion, et al., Adenomes hypophysarires, Masson, Paris, 1958, pp. 1–276.

[15] G. Guiot, Considerations on the surgical treatment of pituitary adenomas, in: R. Fahlbusch, K. von Werder (Eds.), Treatment of pituitary adenomas, Thieme, Stuttgart, 1978, pp. 202–218.

[16] E. Knosp, E. Steiner, K. Kitz, C. Matula, Pituitary adenomas with invasion of the cavernous sinus space: A magnetic resonance imaging classification compared with surgical findings, Neurosurgery 33 (1993) 610–617.

[17] M. Buchfelder, R. Fahlbusch, P. Nomikos, et al., Recent Advances in CT and MRI in the diagnosis and follow-up of hypothalamo–pituitary disease, in: K. von Werder, R. Fahlbusch (Eds.), Pituitary adenomas, Excerpta Media Elsevier, Amsterdam, 1996, pp. 132–145.

[18] A.L. Rhoton, D.G. Hardy, S.M. Chambers, Microsurgery anatomy and dissection of the sphenoid bone, cavernous sinus and sellar region, Surg Neurol 12 (1979) 63–104.

[19] A.L. Rhoton, F.S. Harris, W.H. Rehn, Microsurgical anatomy of the sellar region and cavernous sinus, Clin Neurosurg 24 (1977) 54–85.

[20] M. Buchfelder, R. Fahlbusch, The "classic" transsphenoidal approach for resection of pituitary tumors, Operat Techn Neurosurg 5 (2002) 210–217.

[21] V.V. Dolenc, Transcranial epidural approach to pituitary tumors extending beyond the sella, Neurosurgery 41 (1997) 542–550.

[22] R. Fahlbusch, M. Buchfelder, Surgical complications, in: A.M. Landolt, M.L. Vance, P.L. Reilly (Eds.), Pituitary adenoma, Churchill Livingstone, New York, 1996, pp. 395–408.

[23] R.W. Tsang, J.D. Brierley, T. Panzarella, et al., Role of radiation therapy in clinical hormonally-active pituitary adenomas, Radiother Oncol 41 (1996) 45–53.

[24] B.E. Pollock, D. Kondzialka, L.D. Lundsford, J.C. Flickinger, Stereotactic radiosurgery for pituitary adenomas: Imaging, visual and endocrine results, Acta Neurochir 62 (Suppl) (1994) 33–38.

[25] J.C. Flickinger, P.B. Nelson, F.H. Taylor, A. Robinson, Incidence of cerebral infarction after radiotherapy for pituitary adenoma, Cancer 63 (1989) 2404–2408.

[26] R. Fahlbusch, T. Heigl, W.J. Huk, et al., The role of endoscopy and intraoperative MRI in transsphenoidal pituitary surgery, in: K. von Werder, R. Fahlbusch (Eds.), Pituitary adenomas, Excerpta Medica Elsevier, Amsterdam, 1996, pp. 237–244.

[27] M. Buchfelder, R. Fahlbusch, E.F. Adams, et al., Proliferation parameters for pituitary adenomas, Acta Neurochir 65 (Suppl) (1996) 18–21.

[28] G.N. Burrow, G. Wortzman, N.B. Rewcastle, et al., Microadenomas of the pituitary and abnormal sellar tomograms in an unselected autopsy series, N Engl J Med 304 (1981) 156–158.

[29] S.L. Asa, Tumors of the pituitary gland. *Atlas of tumor pathology*. Fascicle 22, third series ed., Armed Forces Institute of Pathology, Washington DC, 1989.

[30] K. Thapar, K. Kovacs, E.R. Laws, Jr., P.J. Müller, Pituitary adenomas: Current concepts in classification, histopathology and molecular biology, The Endocrinologist 3 (1993) 39–57.

[31] T. Sano, S. Yamada, Histologic and immunohistochemical study of clinically non-functioning pituitary adenomas: Special reference to gonadotropin-positive adenomas, Pathol Int 44 (1994) 697–703.

[32] P. Colombo, B. Ambrosi, K. Saccomanno, et al., Effects of long-term treatment with the gonadotropin-releasing hormone analog nafarelin in patients with non-functioning pituitary adenomas, Eur J Endocrinol 130 (1994) 339–345.

[33] F.F. Casanueva, M.E. Molitch, J.A. Schlechte, et al., Guidelines of the Pituitary Society for the diagnosis and management of prolactinomas, Clin Endocrinol (Oxf) 65 (2006) 265–273.

[34] G.W. Bodner, S.L. Atkin, M.W. Savage, et al., Effects of quinagolide (CV 205-502), a selective D2-agonist, on vascular reactivity in patients with a prolactin-secreting adenoma, Clin Endocrinol (Oxf) 43 (1995) 49–53.

[35] J. Webster, Cabergoline and quinagolide therapy for prolactinomas, Clin Endocrinol (Oxf) 53 (2000) 549–550.

[36] E. Ciccarelli, F. Camanni, Diagnosis and drug therapy of prolactinoma, Drugs 51 (1996) 954–965.

[37] J. Kreutzer, R. Buslei, H. Wallaschowski, et al., Operative treatment of prolactinomas: Indications and results in a current consecutive series of 212 patients, Eur J Endocrinol 158 (2008) 11–18.

[38] R. Fahlbusch, M. Buchfelder, Present status of neurosurgery in the treatment of prolactinomas, Neurosurg Rev 8 (1985) 195–205.

[39] G. Charpentier, T. de Plunkert, P. Jedynak, et al., Surgical treatment of prolactinomas. Short- and long-term results, prognostic factors, Horm Res 22 (1985) 222–227.

[40] B. Guidetti, B. Fraioli, G.P. Cantore, Results of surgical management of 319 pituitary adenomas, Acta Neurochir (Wien) 85 (1987) 117–124.

[41] T. Sano, S.L. Asa, K. Kovacs, Growth hormone-releasing hormone producing tumors: Clinical, biochemical and morphological manifestations, Endocr Rev 9 (1988) 357–373.

[42] A.D. Wright, D.M. Hill, C. Lowy, T.R. Fraser, Mortality in acromegaly, Q J Med 39 (1970) 1–16.

[43] O. Plewe, J. Beyer, U. Krause, et al., Long-acting and selective suppression of growth hormone secretion by somatostatin analogue SMS 201-995 in acromegaly, Lancet 2 (1984) 782–784.

[44] I. Morange, F. De Boisvilliers, P. Chanson, et al., Slow release lanreotide treatment in acromegalic patients previously normalized by octreotide, J Clin Endocrinol Metab 79 (1994) 145–151.

[45] A.L. Barkan, Acromegaly. Diagnosis and therapy, Endocrinol Metab Clin North Am 18 (1989) 277–310.

[46] S. Melmed, A. Colao, A. Barkan, M. Molitch, et al., Acromegaly Consensus Group: Guidelines for acromegaly management: An update, J Clin Endocrinol Metab 94 (2009) 1509–1517.

[47] A. Giustina, A. Barkan, F.F. Casanueva, et al., Criteria for cure of acromegaly: A consensus statement, J Clin Endocrinol Metab 85 (2000) 526–529.

[48] P. Nomikos, M. Buchfelder, R. Fahlbusch, The outcome of surgery in 668 patients with acromegaly using current criteria of biochemical cure, Eur J Endocrinol 152 (2005) 379–387.

[49] D.H. Davis, E.R. Laws, Jr., D.M. Ilstrup, et al., Results of surgical treatment for growth hormone-secreting pituitary adenomas, J Neurosurg 79 (1993) 70–75.

[50] P.R. Bates, M.N. Carson, P.J. Trainer, J.A. Wass, UK National Acromegaly Register Study Group (UKAR-2): Wide variation in surgical outcomes for acromegaly in the UK, Clin Endocrinol (Oxf) 68 (2008) 136–142.

[51] D.C. Aron, J.W. Findling, J.B. Tyrrell, Cushing's disease, Endocrinol Metab Clin North Am 16 (1987) 705–730.

[52] D.N. Orth, Cushing's syndrome, N Engl J Med 332 (1995) 791–803.

[53] B.M. Biller, A.B. Grossman, P.M. Stewart, et al., Treatment of adrenocorticotropin-dependent Cushing's syndrome: A consensus statement, J Clin Endocrinol Metab 93 (2008) 2454–2462.

[54] R. Fahlbusch, M. Buchfelder, O.A. Müller, Transsphenoidal surgery for Cushing's disease, J Royal Soc Med 79 (1986) 262–269.

[55] W.F. Chandler, D.E. Schteingart, R.V. Lloyd, et al., Surgical treatment of Cushing's disease, J Neurosurg 66 (1987) 204–212.

[56] T.J. Mampalam, J.B. Tyrrell, C.B. Wilson, Transsphenoidal microsurgery for Cushing's disease. A report of 216 cases, Ann Intern Med 109 (1988) 487–493.

[57] B. Guilhaume, X. Bertagna, M. Thomsen, et al., Transsphenoidal pituitary surgery for the treatment of Cushing's disease: Results in 64 patients and long-term follow-up studies, J Clin Endocrinol Metab 66 (1988) 1056–1064.

[58] C.G. Patel, D.M. Prevedello, S.P. Lad, et al., Late recurrences of Cushing's disease after initial successful transsphenoidal surgery, J Clin Endocrinol Metab 93 (2008) 358–362.

[59] B.M. Hofmann, M. Hlavac, J. Kreutzer, Surgical treatment of recurrent Cushing's disease, Neurosurgery 58 (2006) 1108–1118.

[60] D.H. Nelson, J.W. Meakin, J.B. Dealy, et al., ACTH producing tumor of the pituitary gland, Ann Intern Med 52 (1958) 560–569.

[61] M. Buchfelder, R. Fahlbusch, P. Thierauf, O.A. Müller, Observations on the pathophysiology of Nelson's syndrome: A report of three cases, Neurosurgery 27 (1990) 961–968.

[62] P. Beck-Peccoz, L. Persani, TSH-induced hyperthyroidism caused by a pituitary tumor, Nat Clin Pract Endocrinol Metab 2 (2006) 524–528.

[63] R.J. Comi, N. Gesundheit, L. Murray, et al., Response of thyrotropin-secreting pituitary adenomas to a long-acting somatostatin analogue, N Engl J Med 319 (1987) 12–17.

[64] M.E. Molitch, Gonadotroph-cell pituitary adenomas (editorial; comment), N Engl J Med 324 (1991) 626–627.

[65] K. Thapar, K. Kovacs, B.W. Scheithauer, et al., Classification and pathology of sellar and parasellar tumors, in: G.T. Tindall, P. Cooper, D.L. Barrow (Eds.), The practice of neurosurgery, Williams & Willkins, Baltimore, 1996, pp. 1021–1070.

[66] R. Fahlbusch, J. Honegger, W. Paulus, et al., Surgical treatment of craniopharyngiomas: Experience with 168 patients, J Neurosurg 90 (1999) 237–250.

[67] J. Honegger, M. Buchfelder, R. Fahlbusch, Surgical treatment of craniopharyngiomas: Endocrinological results, J Neurosurg 90 (1999) 251–257.

[68] E.G. Fischer, K. Welch, J. Shillito, et al., Craniopharyngiomas in children. Long-term effects of conservative surgical procedures combined with radiation therapy, J Neurosurg 73 (1990) 534–540.

[69] A.J. Raimondi, Craniopharyngioma: Complications and treatment failures weaken case for aggressive surgery, Crit Rev Neurosurg 3 (1993) 7–24.

[70] H. Cushing, L. Eisenhardt, Meningiomas. Their classifications, regional behaviour, life history and surgical end results, Charles C. Thomas, Springfield IL, 1938, pp. 298–319.

[71] L.N. Sekhar, C.N. Sen, H.D. Jho, I.P. Janecka, Surgical treatment of intracavernous neoplasms: A four-year experience, Neurosurgery 24 (1989) 18–30.

[72] J. Honegger, R. Fahlbusch, M. Buchfelder, et al., The role of transsphenoidal microsurgery in the management of sellar and parasellar meningioma, Surg Neurol 39 (1993) 18–24.

[73] H. Akutsu, J. Kreutzer, R. Fahlbusch, M. Buchfelder, Transsphenoidal decompression of the sellar floor for cavernous sinus meningiomas: Experience with 21 patients, Neurosurgery 65 (2009) 54–62.

[74] U.M. Schrell, M.G. Rittig, M. Anders, et al., Hydroxyurea for treatment of unresectable and recurrent meningiomas. I. Inhibition of primary human meningioma cells in culture and in meningioma transplants by induction of the apoptotic pathway, J Neurosurg 86 (1997) 845–852.

[75] B. McGrath, Cysts of sellar and pharyngeal hypophyses, Pathology 3 (1971) 123–131.

[76] J.L. Voelker, R.L. Campbell, J. Muller, Clinical, radiographic and pathological features of symptomatic Rathke's cleft cysts, J Neurosurg 74 (1991) 535–544.

[77] P. Nomikos, M. Buchfelder, R. Fahlbusch, Intra- and suprasellar colloid cysts, Pituitary 2 (1999) 123–125.

[78] D.S. Baskin, C.B. Wilson, Transsphenoidal treatment of nonneoplastic intrasellar cysts. A report of 38 cases, J Neurosurg 60 (1984) 8–13.

[79] J. Jafar, R. Crowell, Parasellar and optic nerve lesions: The neurosurgeon's perspective, Radiol Clin North Am 25 (1987) 877–885.

[80] J. Rutka, H. Hoffman, J. Drake, Suprasellar and sellar tumors in childhood and adolescence, Neurosurg Clin N Am 3 (1992) 103–115.

[81] U. Roessmann, B. Kaufman, R.T. Friede, Metastatic lesions in the sella turcica and pituitary gland, Cancer 25 (1970) 478–480.

[82] R.J. Teears, E.M. Silverman, Clinicopathologic review of 88 cases of carcinoma metastatic to the pituitary gland, Cancer 36 (1975) 216–220.
[83] B. Maiuri, Primary cerebral lymphoma presenting as steroid-responsive chiasmal syndrome, Br J Neurosurg 1 (1987) 499–502.
[84] A.-N.N. Dhanani, J.M. Bilbao, K. Kovacs, Multiple myeloma presenting as a sellar plasmocytoma and mimicking a pituitary tumor: Report of a case and review of the literature, Endocr Pathol 1 (1990) 245–248.
[85] L.F. Wold, E.R. Laws, Jr., Cranial chordomas in children and young adults, J Neurosurg 59 (1983) 1043–1047.
[86] F. Cosman, K.D. Post, D.A. Holub, S.L. Wardlaw, Lymphocytic hypophysitis. Report of 3 new cases and review of the literature, Medicine Baltimore 68 (1989) 240–256.
[87] S.L. Asa, J.M. Bilbao, K. Kovacs, et al., Lymphocyic hypophysitis of pregnancy resulting in hypopituitarism, Ann Intern Med 95 (1981) 166–171.
[88] J. Honegger, R. Fahlbusch, A. Bornemann, et al., Lymphocytic and granulomatous hypophysitis, experience with nine cases, Neurosurgery 40 (1997) 713–722.
[89] A. Gutenberg, V. Hans, M.J. Puchner, et al., Primary hypophysitis: Clinical–pathological correlations, Eur J Endocrinol 155 (2006) 101–107.
[90] S.A. Berger, S.C. Edberg, G. David, Infectious disease in the sella turcica, Rev Infect Dis 8 (1986) 747–755.
[91] A.L. Albright, P.A. Lee, Neurosurgical treatment of hypothalamic hamartoma causing precocious puberty, J Neurosurg 78 (1993) 77–82.
[92] S.L. Asa, B.W. Scheithauer, J.M. Bilbao, et al., A case for hypothalamic acromegaly: A clinico-pathological study of six patients with hypothalamic gangliocytomas producing growth hormone-releasing factor, J Clin Endocrinol Metab 58 (1984) 796–803.
[93] N. Georgakoulias, C. Vize, A. Jenkins, B. Singounas, Hypothalamic hamartomas causing gelastic epilepsy: Two cases and a review of the literature, Seizure 7 (1998) 167–171.
[94] L. Stewart, P. Steinbok, J. Daaboul, Role of surgical resection in the treatment of hypothalamic hamartomas causing precocious puberty. Report of six cases, J Neurosurg 88 (1998) 340–345.
[95] M.T. Jennings, R. Gelman, F. Hochberg, Intracranial germ-cell tumors: Natural history and pathogenesis, J Neurosurg 63 (1985) 155–167.
[96] M. Buchfelder, R. Fahlbusch, M. Walther, K. Mann, Endocrine disturbances in suprasellar germinomas, Acta Endocrinol (Copenh) 120 (1989) 337–342.
[97] J.E. Baumgartner, M.S. Edwards, Pineal tumors, Neurosurg Clin N Am 3 (1992) 853–862.
[98] J.E. Boggan, R.L. Davis, G. Zorman, C.B. Wilson, Intrasellar epidermoid cyst. Case report, J Neurosurg 58 (1983) 411–415.
[99] H.D. Jho, R.L. Carrau, Endoscopic endonasal transsphenoidal surgery, J Neurosurg 87 (1997) 44–51.
[100] A. Rudnik, B. Kos-Kudla, D. Larysz, et al., Endoscopic transsphenoidal treatment of hormonally active pituitary adenomas, Neuro Endocrinol Lett 28 (2007) 438–444.
[101] G. Zada, D.F. Kelly, P. Cohan, et al., Endonasal transspenoidal approach for pituitary adenomas and other sellar lesions: An assessment of efficacy, safety and patient impressions, J Neurosurg 98 (2003) 350–358.
[102] L.M. Cavallo, D.M. Prevedello, D. Solari, et al., Extended endoscopic endonasal transsphenoidal approach for residual or recurrent craniopharyngiomas, J Neurosurg 111 (2009) 578–589.
[103] W.J. Elias, J.B. Chadduck, T.D. Alden, E.R. Laws, Jr., Frameless stereotaxy for transsphenoidal surgery, Neurosurgery 45 (1999) 271–275.
[104] Y. Carvi, M.N. Nievas, H.G. Höllerhage, Reliability of neuronavigation-assisted trans-sphenoidal tumor resection, Neurol Res 29 (2007) 557–562.
[105] T. Yamasaki, K. Moritake, J. Hatta, H. Nagai, Intraoperative monitoring with pulse Doppler ultrasonography in transsphenoidal surgery: Technique application, Neurosurgery 38 (1996) 95–97.
[106] R.J. Bohinski, R.E. Warnick, M.F. Gaskill-Shipley, et al., Intraoperative magnetic resonance imaging to determine the extent of resection of pituitary macroadenomas during transsphenoidal microsurgery, Neurosurgery 49 (2001) 1133–1143.
[107] R. Fahlbusch, O. Ganslandt, M. Buchfelder, et al., Intraoperative magnetic resonance imaging during transsphenoidal surgery, J Neurosurg 95 (2001) 381–390.
[108] C. Nimsky, O. Ganslandt, R. Fahlbusch, Comparing 0.2 tesla with 1.5 tesla intraoperative magnetic resonance imaging analysis of setup, workflow and efficiency, Acad Radiol 12 (2005) 1065–1079.
[109] C. Nimsky, B. von Keller, O. Ganslandt, R. Fahlbusch, Intraoperative high-field magnetic resonance imaging in transsphenoidal surgery of hormonally inactive pituitary macroadenomas, Neurosurgery 59 (2006) 105–114.
[110] F.G. Barker 2nd, A. Klibanski, B. Swearingen, Transsphenoidal surgery for pituitary tumors in the United States, 1996–2000: Mortality, morbidity and the effects of hospital and surgeon volume, J Clin Endocrinol Metab 88 (2003) 4709–4719.
[111] P. Mortini, M. Losa, R. Barzaghi, et al., Results of transsphenoidal surgery in a large series of patients with pituitary adenoma, Neurosurgery 56 (2005) 1222–1233.

Index